T0373111

BLACKWELL'S FIVE-MINUTE VETERINARY CONSULT: LABORATORY TESTS AND DIAGNOSTIC PROCEDURES: CANINE & FELINE

BLACKWELL'S FIVE-MINUTE VETERINARY CONSULT: LABORATORY TESTS AND DIAGNOSTIC PROCEDURES: CANINE & FELINE

Shelly L. Vaden
Joyce S. Knoll
Francis W.K. Smith, Jr.
Larry P. Tilley

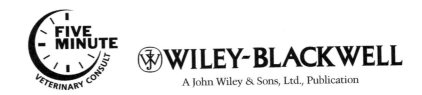

WILEY-BLACKWELL

A John Wiley & Sons, Ltd., Publication

Edition first published 2009
© 2009 Wiley-Blackwell

Blackwell Publishing was acquired by John Wiley & Sons in February 2007. Blackwell's publishing program has been merged with Wiley's global Scientific, Technical, and Medical business to form Wiley-Blackwell.

Editorial Office
2121 State Avenue, Ames, Iowa 50014-8300, USA

For details of our global editorial offices, for customer services, and for information about how to apply for permission to reuse the copyright material in this book, please see our website at www.wiley.com/wiley-blackwell.

Authorization to photocopy items for internal or personal use, or the internal or personal use of specific clients, is granted by Blackwell Publishing, provided that the base fee is paid directly to the Copyright Clearance Center, 222 Rosewood Drive, Danvers, MA 01923. For those organizations that have been granted a photocopy license by CCC, a separate system of payments has been arranged. The fee codes for users of the Transactional Reporting Service are ISBN-13: 978-0-8138-1748-4/2009.

Designations used by companies to distinguish their products are often claimed as trademarks. All brand names and product names used in this book are trade names, service marks, trademarks or registered trademarks of their respective owners. The publisher is not associated with any product or vendor mentioned in this book. This publication is designed to provide accurate and authoritative information in regard to the subject matter covered. It is sold on the understanding that the publisher is not engaged in rendering professional services. If professional advice or other expert assistance is required, the services of a competent professional should be sought.

Library of Congress Cataloging-in-Publication Data

Blackwell's five-minute veterinary consult. Lab tests and diagnostic procedures / Shelly Vaden . . . [et al.].
  p. ; cm.
  Includes bibliographical references and index.
  ISBN-13: 978-0-8138-1748-4 (alk. paper)
  ISBN-10: 0-8138-1748-X (alk. paper)
  1. Veterinary clinical pathology–Laboratory manuals. I. Vaden, Shelly L. II. Title: Five-minute veterinary consult. Lab tests and diagnostic procedures.
III. Title: Lab tests and diagnostic procedures.
  [DNLM: 1. Laboratory Techniques and Procedures–Veterinary–Handbooks. 2. Animal Diseases–Diagnosis–Handbooks. SF 772.6 B632 2008]
  SF772.6.B53 2008
  636.089′6075–dc22

A catalog record for this book is available from the U.S. Library of Congress.

Set in 9/10 pt Adobe Garamond by Aptara® Inc., New Delhi, India
Printed in Singapore by Fabulous Printers Pte Ltd

Disclaimer

The contents of this work are intended to further general scientific research, understanding, and discussion only and are not intended and should not be relied upon as recommending or promoting a specific method, diagnosis, or treatment by practitioners for any particular patient. The publisher and the author make no representations or warranties with respect to the accuracy or completeness of the contents of this work and specifically disclaim all warranties, including without limitation any implied warranties of fitness for a particular purpose. In view of ongoing research, equipment modifications, changes in governmental regulations, and the constant flow of information relating to the use of medicines, equipment, and devices, the reader is urged to review and evaluate the information provided in the package insert or instructions for each medicine, equipment, or device for, among other things, any changes in the instructions or indication of usage and for added warnings and precautions. Readers should consult with a specialist where appropriate. The fact that an organization or Website is referred to in this work as a citation and/or a potential source of further information does not mean that the author or the publisher endorses the information the organization or Website may provide or recommendations it may make. Further, readers should be aware that Internet Websites listed in this work may have changed or disappeared between when this work was written and when it is read. No warranty may be created or extended by any promotional statements for this work. Neither the publisher nor the author shall be liable for any damages arising herefrom.

Printed and bound by CPI Group (UK) Ltd, Croydon, CR0 4YY

C9780813817484_201123

CONTENTS

TOPIC	

TOPIC	

TOPIC	

TOPIC	

CONTENTS *by Subject*

TOPIC	

TOPIC	

TOPIC	

DIAGNOSTIC PROCEDURES

TOPIC	

TOPIC	

PREFACE

Blackwell's Five-Minute Veterinary Consult: Laboratory Tests and Diagnostic Procedures: Canine & Feline is designed to provide busy veterinary practitioners and students with a complete and quick reference to diagnostic procedures and laboratory tests that are used daily in the diagnosis and management of medical problems of dogs and cats. Our goal in creating this textbook is also to provide up-to-date information in an easy-to-use format. Prior to the publication of this book, this information could be found scattered throughout a variety of clinical resources. We are unaware of another comprehensive book that brings all of these diagnostic procedures and laboratory tests under one cover. The laboratory tests section of the book enables rapid access to clinically relevant laboratory tests, with comprehensive information on test preparation, performance, factors that affect each test, and a brief guide to test interpretation. This information can be used to optimize results, while avoiding repeat testing necessitated by problems in sample handling or patient preparation. The diagnostic procedures section is intended to provide clinically relevant information that will enable practitioners to determine quickly whether a procedure is indicated in a particular case. In many chapters, enough information is included to enable veterinary practitioners or technicians to perform a procedure in house. Other chapters provide practicing veterinarians with sufficient information to understand a procedure and prepare clients and patients for a possible referral.

The book is intended to serve as a companion to *Blackwell's Five-Minute Veterinary Consult: Canine and Feline*, 4th Edition. The uniqueness and value of *Blackwell's Five-Minute Veterinary Consult* approach as a quick reference are based on the consistency of presentation, the breadth of coverage, the contribution of large numbers of experts, and the timely preparation of the topics. The format of every topic is identical, making it easy to find information. An extensive list of topic headings ensures complete coverage of each topic.

This book contains information about more than 250 diagnostic procedures and laboratory tests. As the title implies, one objective of this book is to make information available quickly. To this end, we have organized topics alphabetically. Most topics can be found without using the index. General information concerning appropriate test collection and principles that can be applied to major procedures such as ultrasonography, radiography, and endoscopy can be found in the front section of the book. Appendices at the end of the book contain tables of laboratory normal values, therapeutic drug concentrations, and a list of diagnostic laboratories.

Each topic is presented in a standardized fashion that enables rapid and easy localization of specific information. All chapters provide information about related physiology, indications, contraindications, potential complications, and client education related to the subject. The laboratory test chapters include sections that are uniquely applicable to a laboratory test: the type of specimen required; information about sample collection, handling, storage, and stability; the protocol for running the test; and important test limitations, as well as a table that lists causes of test abnormalities. Information specific to diagnostic procedures is included in those chapters: patient preparation, detailed description of the technique, sample handling, and appropriate aftercare. All chapters include sections that provide guidance during interpretation of the test or procedural results, including normal findings or range, abnormal findings, critical values that would prompt immediate intervention, and lists of drugs or other factors that may interfere with results, performance, or interpretation of the test or procedure. Each chapter also contains a clinical perspective section that provides clinical wisdom about the use and interpretation of the test or procedure. The chapters end with information about ancillary tests, related topics, and suggested reading and Internet resources. To this end, the chapters should provide practitioners with enough information to understand and apply a laboratory test or diagnostic procedure to the daily practice of veterinary medicine.

We are delighted and privileged to have had the assistance of numerous experts in veterinary medicine from around the world. More than 125 veterinary specialists contributed to this text, allowing each chapter to be written by an expert on the subject. In addition to providing outstanding information, this large pool of experts enabled us to publish this major text in a timely manner. Each chapter was written by an expert in the field, which allows for insight into each subject that only experience can provide.

This first edition constitutes an important, up-to-date medical reference source for your practice and clinical education. We strived to make it complete, yet practical and easy to use. Our dreams are realized if this text helps you to quickly locate and use the momentarily important information that is essential to the practice of high-quality veterinary medicine. We would appreciate your input so that we can make future editions even more useful. If you would like to see any changes in content or format, additions, or deletions, please let us know. Send comments to the following:

Wiley-Blackwell
2121 State Avenue
Ames, IA 50014

Editors
Shelly L. Vaden
Joyce S. Knoll
Francis W.K. Smith, Jr.
Larry P. Tilley

ACKNOWLEDGEMENTS

The completion of this textbook provides a welcome opportunity to recognize in writing the many individuals who have helped along the way. The editors gratefully acknowledge the contributors who, by their expertise, have so unmistakably enhanced the quality of this textbook. In addition, we would like to thank Beth Mellor, the medical illustrator who provided line drawings for several of the laboratory test chapters, including those on erythrocyte morphology and urine sediment.

We would also like to acknowledge and thank our families and colleagues for their support of this project and the sacrifices they made to allow us the time to complete the book.

In addition to thanking veterinarians who have referred patients to us, we would like to express our gratitude to each of the veterinary students, interns, and residents whom we have had the privilege of teaching. Their curiosity and intellectual stimulation have enabled us to grow and have prompted us to undertake the task of writing this book.

We would also like to acknowledge all of the small-animal patients and the pet owners that have allowed us to gain the knowledge and expertise necessary to practice high-quality medicine and amass a resource such as this textbook.

Finally, a special thank you goes to Antonia Seymour, Nancy Simmerman, Erin Gardner, and all the rest of the staff at Wiley-Blackwell and everyone in the production and editing departments. The marketing and sales departments also must be acknowledged for generating such an interest in this book. We are grateful to the copy editor, John Flukas, whose eye for detail enhanced the final product. They are all meticulous workers and kind people who have made the final stages of preparing this book both inspiring and fun. An important life goal of ours has been fulfilled: to provide expertise in veterinary medicine worldwide and to teach the principles contained in this textbook to veterinarians and students everywhere.

Editors
Shelly L. Vaden
Joyce S. Knoll
Francis W.K. Smith, Jr.
Larry P. Tilley

CONTRIBUTORS LIST

KARIN ALLENSPACH, DrMedVet, PhD
Diplomate, ECVIM
Lecturer in Internal Medicine
Department of Veterinary Clinical Sciences
Royal Veterinary College
University of London
North Mymms, England, UK

JANICE M. ANDREWS, DVM, PhD
Diplomate, ACVP (Clinical Pathology)
Laboratory Director
North Carolina Laboratory
Antech Diagnostics
Cary, NC, USA

ANNE BAHR, DVM, MS
Diplomate, ACVR
Assistant Professor; Chief of Radiology
Department of Large Animal Clinical Sciences
Texas A&M University
College Station, TX, USA

NATHAN L. BAILIFF, DVM
Diplomate, ACVIM
VCA Sacramento Veterinary Referral Center
Sacramento, CA, USA

PERRY JAMES BAIN, DVM, PhD
Diplomate, ACVP (Clinical Pathology)
Assistant Professor
Department of Biomedical Sciences
Cummings School of Veterinary Medicine
Tufts University
North Grafton, MA, USA

VANESSA R.D. BARRS, BVSc, MVCS
FACVSc (Feline Medicine)
Senior Lecturer in Small Animal Medicine
Faculty of Veterinary Science
Valentine Charlton Cat Centre
University of Sydney
Sydney, Australia

A. BRADY BEALE, VMD
Diplomate, ACVO
Hope Center for Advanced Veterinary Medicine
Vienna, VA, USA

JEROLD S. BELL, DVM
Clinical Associate Professor
Department of Clinical Sciences
Cummings School of Veterinary Medicine
Tufts University
North Grafton, MA, USA
and
Freshwater Veterinary Hospital
Enfold, CT, USA

NORA BERGHOFF, DrMedVet
Graduate Assistant
Gastrointestinal Laboratory
Department of Small Animal Clinical Sciences
Texas A&M University
College Station, TX, USA

CLIFFORD R. BERRY, DVM
Diplomate, ACVR
Central Florida Veterinary Radiology, PA
Winter Park, FL, USA

ADAM J. BIRKENHEUER, DVM, PhD
Diplomate, ACVIM
Assistant Professor
Department of Clinical Sciences
College of Veterinary Medicine
North Carolina State University
Raleigh, NC, USA

KARYN BISCHOFF, DVM, MS
Assistant Professor
Department of Population Medicine and Diagnostic Sciences
Cornell University
Ithaca, NY, USA

SALLY A. BISSETT, BVSc, MVSc
Diplomate, ACVIM
Assistant Professor
Department of Clinical Sciences
North Carolina State University
Raleigh, NC, USA

MARIE-CLAUDE BLAIS, DMV
Diplomate, ACVIM
Professeure adjointe
Département de sciences cliniques
Université de Montreal
Québec, Canada

ADRIAN BOSWOOD, MA, VetMB, DVC, FHEA, MRCVS
Diplomate, ECVIM (Cardiology)
RCVS Specialist in Veterinary Cardiology
Senior Lecturer in Internal Medicine and Cardiology
Royal Veterinary College
University of London
London, England, UK

JENNIFER L. BRAZZELL, DVM
Diplomate, ACVP (Clinical Pathology)
Research Assistant
Department of Veterinary Population Medicine
University of Minnesota
St. Paul, MN, USA

BARBARA P. BREWER, BA, BS, CVT, VTS (Cardiology)
Cardiology Technician
Department of Cardiology
Cummings School of Veterinary Medicine
Tufts University
North Grafton, MA, USA

MARJORY B. BROOKS, DVM
Diplomate, ACVIM
Associate Director
Department of Population Medicine and Diagnostic Science
Animal Health Diagnostic Center
Cornell University
Ithaca, NY, USA

DONALD J. BROWN, DVM, PhD
Diplomate, ACVIM (Cardiology)
Assistant Professor
Department of Clinical Sciences
Cummings School of Veterinary Medicine
Tufts University
North Grafton, MA, USA

SCOTT A. BROWN, VMD, PhD
Diplomate, ACVIM
Josiah Meigs Distinguished Professor
Department of Small Animal Medicine and Surgery
College of Veterinary Medicine
University of Georgia
Athens, GA, USA

COLIN F. BURROWS, BVetMed, PhD, MRCVS
Diplomate, ACVIM
Professor and Chair; Chief of Staff
Department of Small Animal Clinical Sciences
College of Veterinary Medicine
Small Animal Hospital
Veterinary Medical Center
University of Florida
Gainesville, FL, USA

ANTHONY P. CARR, DMV
Diplomate, ACVIM (Small Animal Internal Medicine)
Associate Professor
Department of Small Animal Clinical Sciences
Western College of Veterinary Medicine
Saskatoon, SK, Canada

SHARON A. CENTER, DVM
Diplomate, ACVIM (Small Animal Internal Medicine)
Professor of Medicine
Department of Clinical Sciences
College of Veterinary Medicine
Cornell University
Ithaca, NY, USA

JOSE JOAQUIN CERON, DVM, PhD
Diplomate, ECVCP
Associate Professor
Department of Animal Medicine and Surgery
Murcia Veterinary School
University of Murcia
Murcia, Spain

DANIEL L. CHAN, DVM, MRCVS
Diplomate, ACVECC; Diplomate, ACVN
Lecturer
Department of Clinical Sciences
Queen Mother Hospital
Royal Veterinary College
University of London
North Mymms, England, UK

SETH E. CHAPMAN, DVM
Clinical Pathology Resident
Department of Veterinary Pathobiology
Veterinary Teaching Hospital
Texas A&M University
College Station, TX, USA

ALISON B. CLODE, DVM
Diplomate, ACVO
Assistant Professor
Department of Ophthalmology
College of Veterinary Medicine
North Carolina State University
Raleigh, NC, USA

MICHAEL G. CONZEMIUS, DVM, PhD
Diplomate, ACVS
Associate Professor
Department of Veterinary Clinical Sciences
College of Veterinary Medicine
Iowa State University
Ames, IA, USA

STEPHANIE C. CORN, DVM
Diplomate, ACVP (Clinical Pathology)
Clinical Pathologist
IDEXX Laboratories
Worthington, OH, USA

DEBORAH GROPPE DAVIS, DVM
Diplomate, ACVP (Clinical Pathology)
Clinical Pathologist
IDEXX Laboratories
North Grafton, MA, USA

RYAN M. DICKINSON, DVM
Diplomate, ACVP (Clinical Pathology)
Prairie Diagnostic Services
and
Adjunct Professor
Western College of Veterinary Medicine
Saskatoon, SK, Canada

WM TOD DROST, DVM
Diplomate, ACVR
Associate Professor in Radiology
Department of Veterinary Clinical Sciences
Ohio State University
Columbus, OH, USA

CHARLOTTE DYE, BVMAS, PhD,
CestSAM, MRCVS
Clinical Associate in Small Animal Medicine
Department of Clinical Veterinary Science
University of Bristol
Bristol, England, UK

JANICE A. DYE, DVM, MS, PhD
Diplomate, ACVIM (Small Animal
Internal Medicine)
Pulmonary Toxicology Branch
US Environmental Protection Agency
Research Triangle Park, NC, USA

JAMES ROGER EASLEY, DVM, MS
Diplomate, ACVP (Clinical Pathology)
Adjunct Professor
Department of Physiological Sciences
College of Veterinary Medicine
University of Florida
Gainesville, FL, USA

PETER DAVID ECKERSALL, BSc, MBA, PhD, MRCPath
Professor of Veterinary Biochemistry
Department of Animal Production and Public Health
Faculty of Veterinary Medicine
University of Glasgow
Glasgow, Scotland, UK

PATTY J. EWING, DVM
Diplomate, ACVP (Anatomic and Clinical Pathology)
Department of Pathology
Angell Animal Medical Center
Boston, MA, USA

DANIEL A. FEENEY, DVM, MS
Diplomate, ACVR
Professor of Medical Imaging
Department of Veterinary Clinical Sciences
College of Veterinary Medicine
University of Minnesota
St. Paul, MN, USA

THERESA W. FOSSUM, DVM, MS, PhD
Diplomate, ACVS
Tom and Joan Read Chair in Veterinary Surgery;
Professor of Surgery
Department of Small Animal Clinical Sciences
College of Veterinary Medicine and Biomedical Sciences
Texas A&M University
College Station, TX, USA

KRISTEN RAE FRIEDRICHS, DVM
Diplomate, ACVP (Clinical Pathology)
Clinical Assistant Professor
Department of Pathobiological Sciences
School of Veterinary Medicine
University of Wisconsin
Madison, WI, USA

LORRIE GASCHEN, DVM, PhD, Diplomate, ECVDI
Associate Professor
Department of Veterinary Clinical Sciences
Division of Radiology
School of Veterinary Medicine
Louisiana State University
Baton Rouge, LA, USA

CARLOS M. GRADIL, DVM, MS, PhD
Diplomate, ACT
Assistant Professor Department of
Veterinary and Animal Sciences
University of Massachusetts
Amherst, MA, USA

REBEKAH GRAY GUNN-CHRISTIE, DVM
Diplomate, ACVP (Clinical Pathology)
Antech Diagnostics
Cary, NC, USA

ELIZABETH M. HARDIE, DVM, PhD
Diplomate, ACVS
Professor
Department of Clinical Sciences
Veterinary Teaching Hospital
North Carolina State University
Raleigh, NC, USA

KARYN HARRELL, DVM
Diplomate, ACVIM
Clinical Assistant Professor of
Internal Medicine
Department of Clinical Sciences
College of Veterinary Medicine
North Carolina State University
Raleigh, NC, USA

ANDREA HARVEY, BVSc, DSAM (Feline)
Diplomate, ECVIM-CA, MRCVS
FAB Clinical Associate in Feline Medicine
Department of Clinical Veterinary Science
Division of Companion Animals
University of Bristol
Bristol, England, UK

JOHN W. HARVEY, DVM, PhD
Diplomate, ACVP (Clinical Pathology)
Professor and Chair
Department of Physiological Sciences
College of Veterinary Medicine
and
Chief, Clinical Pathology Service
UF Veterinary Medical Center
University of Florida
Gainesville, FL, USA

ELEANOR C. HAWKINS, DVM
Diplomate, ACVIM (Small Animal
Internal Medicine)
Professor
Department of Clinical Sciences
College of Veterinary Medicine
North Carolina State University
Raleigh, NC, USA

ROSEMARY A. HENIK, DVM, MS
Diplomate, ACVIM
Clinical Associate Professor
Department of Medical Sciences
Veterinary Medical Teaching Hospital
University of Wisconsin–Madison
Madison, WI, USA

GEORGE A. HENRY, DVM
Diplomate, ACVR
Associate Professor of Radiology
Department of Small Animal Clinical Sciences
University of Tennessee
Knoxville, TN, USA

LEE V. HEROLD, DVM
Diplomate, ACVECC
Dove Lewis Emergency Animal Hospital
Portland, OR, USA

MARK E. HITT, DVM, MS
Diplomate, ACVIM (Small Animal
Internal Medicine)
Head of Medicine
Atlantic Veterinary Internal Medicine, LLC
Annapolis, MD, USA

HILARY A. JACKSON, BVM&S, DVD
Diplomate, ACVD, MRCVS
Honorary Teacher
Faculty of Veterinary Medicine
Dermatology Referral Services
University of Glasgow
Glasgow, Scotland, UK

CHERI A. JOHNSON, DVM, MS
Diplomate, ACVIM
Professor; Chief of Staff
Department of Small Animal Clinical Sciences
College of Veterinary Medicine
Michigan State University
East Lansing, MI, USA

LYNELLE R. JOHNSON, DVM, PhD
Diplomate, ACVIM (Small Animal Internal Medicine)
Assistant Professor
Department of Medicine and Epidemiology
University of California–Davis
Davis, CA, USA

JOYCE S. KNOLL, VMD, PhD
Diplomate, ACVP (Clinical Pathology)
Associate Professor; Clinical Pathology Section Head
Department of Biomedical Sciences
Cummings School of Veterinary Medicine
Tufts University
North Grafton, MA, USA

MICHAEL STEPHEN LAGUTCHIK, DVM, MS
Diplomate, ACVECC
Lieutenant Colonel
Department of Defense Veterinary Service Activity
Lackland Air Force Base, TX, USA

ALLISON LAMB, BA
Research Associate
College of Veterinary Medicine
Ohio State University
Columbus, OH, USA

INDIA F. LANE, DVM, MS
Diplomate, ACVIM (Small Animal Internal Medicine)
Associate Professor; Internist and
Director of Medical Services
Department of Small Animal Clinical Sciences
College of Veterinary Medicine
W.W. Armistead Veterinary Teaching Hospital
University of Tennessee
Knoxville, TN, USA

ROBIN LAZARO, RVT, VTS (ECC)
Veterinary Teaching Hospital
College of Veterinary
North Carolina State University
Raleigh, NC, USA

ANDREW K.J. LINKLATER, DVM
Clinical Instructor
Animal Emergency Center
Milwaukee, WI, USA

MARLA K. LICHTENBERGER, DVM
Diplomate, ACVECC
Emergency and Critical Care Specialist
Milwaukee Emergency Center for Animals and Specialty Services
Milwaukee, WI, USA

SOFIJA ROCKOV LILES, DVM
Radiology Resident
Department of Biomedical Sciences
College of Veterinary Medicine
North Carolina State University
Raleigh, NC, USA

HEIDI B. LOBPRISE, DVM
Diplomate, AVDC
Senior Veterinary Specialist
Veterinary Specialty Team
Pfizer Animal Health
McKinney, TX, USA

MICHAEL LOGAN, DVM
Diplomate, ACVP (Clinical Pathology)
Graduate Student
Department of Veterinary Pathobiology
School of Veterinary Medicine
Purdue University
West Lafayette, IN, USA

JODY P. LULICH, DVM, PhD
Diplomate, ACVIM
Professor
Department of Clinical Sciences
College of Veterinary Medicine
University of Minnesota
St. Paul, MN, USA

ORLA M. MAHONY, MVB, MRCVS
Diplomate, ACVIM; Diplomate, ECVIM
Clinical Assistant Professor
Department of Small Animal Clinical Sciences
Cummings School of Veterinary Medicine
Tufts University
North Grafton, MA, USA

KATHRYN M. MEURS, DVM, PhD
Diplomate, ACVIM (Cardiology)
Professor and Ott Chair of Small Animal Medicine and Research
Department of Veterinary Clinical Sciences
College of Veterinary Medicine
Washington State University
Pullman, WA, USA

TAMMY MILLER MICHAU, DVM, MS, MSpVM
Diplomate, ACVO
Assistant Professor
Department of Clinical Sciences
College of Veterinary Medicine
North Carolina State University
Raleigh, NC, USA

JAN A. MOL, PhD
Associate Professor
Department of Clinical Sciences of Companion Animals
Faculty of Veterinary Medicine
Utrecht University
Utrecht, The Netherlands

LISA MOSES, VMD
Diplomate, ACVIM
Staff Veterinarian
Angell Animal Medical Center
Jamaica Plain, MA, USA

KAREN R. MUÑANA, DVM, MS
Diplomate, ACVIM (Neurology)
Associate Professor
Department of Clinical Sciences
College of Veterinary Medicine
North Carolina State University
Raleigh, NC, USA

MARY B. NABITY, DVM
Diplomate, ACVP (Clinical Pathology)
Postdoctoral Research Associate
Department of Veterinary Pathobiology
College of Veterinary Medicine
Texas A&M University
College Station, TX, USA

JACQUELINE M. NORRIS, BVSC, MVST, PhD
Senior Lecturer in Veterinary Microbiology
Faculty of Veterinary Sciences
University of Sydney
Sydney, Australia

NATASHA JANE OLBY, VET MB, PhD
Diplomate, ACVIM (Neurology)
Associate Professor
Department of Clinical Sciences
College of Veterinary Medicine
North Carolina State University
Raleigh, NC, USA

CARL A. OSBORNE, DVM, PhD
Diplomate, ACVIM
Professor
Veterinary Clinical Sciences Department
College of Veterinary Medicine
University of Minnesota
St. Paul, MN, USA

JED OVERMANN, DVM
Diplomate, ACVP (Clinical Pathology)
Instructor, Clinical Pathology
Veterinary Clinical Sciences Department
College of Veterinary Medicine
University of Minnesota
St. Paul, MN, USA

JERRY M. OWENS, DVM
Diplomate, ACVR
Staff Radiologist
Veterinary Radiology Services
San Rafael, CA, USA

MARK A. OYAMA, DVM
Diplomate, ACVIM (Cardiology)
Associate Professor
Department of Clinical Studies
School of Veterinary Medicine
University of Pennsylvania
Philadelphia, PA, USA

PHILIP PADRID, DVM
Associate Professor of Molecular Medicine (Adjunct)
University of Chicago
and
Associate Professor of Small Animal Medicine (Adjunct)
Ohio State University School of Veterinary Medicine
Columbus, OH, USA
and
Family Pet Animal Hospital
Chicago, IL, USA

MARK PAPICH, DVM, MS
Diplomate, ACVCP
Professor
Department of Molecular Biomedical Sciences
College of Veterinary Medicine
North Carolina State University
Raleigh, NC, USA

CECILIA PARRULA
Resident
Department of Veterinary Biosciences
College of Veterinary Medicine
Ohio State University
Columbus, OH, USA

PATRICIA A. PAYNE, DVM, PhD
Assistant Professor
Department of Diagnostic Medicine/Pathobiology
College of Veterinary Medicine
Kansas State University
Manhattan, KS, USA

ANTHONY PEASE, DVM, MS
Diplomate, ACVR
Assistant Professor in Diagnostic Imaging
Department of Molecular Biomedical Sciences
College of Veterinary Medicine
North Carolina State University
Raleigh, NC, USA

BARRAK M. PRESSLER, DVM, PhD
Diplomate, ACVIM
Assistant Professor
Department of Veterinary Clinical Sciences
School of Veterinary Medicine
Purdue University
West Lafayette, IN, USA

M. JUDITH RADIN, DVM, PhD
Diplomate, ACVP (Clinical Pathology)
Professor
Department of Veterinary Biosciences
Ohio State University
Columbus, OH, USA

PAUL M. RIST, DVM
Diplomate, ACVR
Assistant Professor
Department of Clinical Sciences
College of Veterinary Medicine
Oregon State University
Corvallis, OR, USA

IAN DOUGLAS ROBERTSON, BVSc
Diplomate, ACVR
Assistant Professor
Department of Molecular Biomedical Sciences
North Carolina State University
Raleigh, NC, USA

DUANE A. ROBINSON, DVM
Research Fellow/Clinician
Department of Veterinary Sciences
College of Veterinary Medicine
Iowa State University
Ames, IA, USA

SIMON C. ROE, BVSC, PhD
Diplomate, ACVS
Department of Clinical Science
North Carolina State University
Raleigh, NC, USA

ELIZABETH ROZANSKI, DVM
Diplomate, ACVIM (Internal Medicine); Diplomate, ACVECC
Assistant Professor
Department of Clinical Sciences
Cummings School of Veterinary Medicine
Tufts University
North Grafton, MA, USA

JOHN E. RUSH, DVM, MS
Diplomate, ACVIM (Cardiology); Diplomate, ACVECC
Associate Chair
Department of Clinical Sciences
Cummings School of Veterinary Medicine
Tufts University
North Grafton, MA, USA

KAREN ELIZABETH RUSSELL, DVM, PhD
Diplomate, ACVP (Clinical Pathology)
Assistant Professor
Department of Pathobiology
College of Veterinary Medicine
Texas A&M University
College Station, TX, USA

SHERRY LYNN SANDERSON, DVM, PhD
Diplomate, ACVIM; Diplomate, ACVN
Associate Professor
Department of Physiology and Pharmacology
College of Veterinary Medicine
University of Georgia
Athens, GA, USA

H. MARK SAUNDERS, VMD, MS
Diplomate, ACVR
Lynks Group—Veterinary Imaging
Shelburne, VT, USA

KARINE SAVARY-BATAILLE, DVM
Diplomate, ACVIM (Internal Medicine); Diplomate, ECVIM-CA
Department of Medicine and Clinical Biology of Small Animals
Ghent University
Merelbeke, Belgium

DEANNA M.W. SCHAEFER, DVM, MT (ASCP)
Diplomate, ACVP (Clinical Pathology)
Lecturer
Department of Population Medicine and Diagnostic Sciences
Cornell University
Ithaca, NY, USA

KIELYN SCOTT, DVM
Resident, Emergency and Critical Care
Department of Clinical Science
North Carolina State University
Raleigh, NC, USA

PETER V. SCRIVANI, DVM
Diplomate, ACVR
Assistant Professor of Imaging
Department of Clinical Sciences
College of Veterinary Medicine
Cornell University
Ithaca, NY, USA

LESLIE C. SHARKEY, DVM, PhD
Diplomate, ACVP (Clinical Pathology)
Associate Professor
Department of Veterinary Population Medicine
University of Minnesota
St. Paul, MN, USA

G. DIANE SHELTON, DVM, PhD
Diplomate, ACVIM
Professor
Department of Pathology
University of California–San Diego
La Jolla, CA, USA

ROB SIMONI, DVM
Clinical Pathology Resident
Department of Biomedical Sciences
Cummings School of Veterinary Medicine
Tufts University, Large Animal Hospital
North Grafton, MA, USA

DAVID SISSON, DVM
Diplomate, ACVIM (Cardiology)
Professor of Cardiovascular Medicine; Director, Small Animal Hospital
Department of Clinical Sciences
College of Veterinary Medicine
Oregon State University
Corvallis, OR, USA

FRANCIS W.K. SMITH JR., DVM
Diplomate, ACVIM (Cardiology and Small Animal Internal Medicine)
Vice President, VetMed Consultants
Lexington, MA, USA
and
Clinical Assistant Professor
Cummings School of Veterinary Medicine
Tufts University
North Grafton, MA, USA

KATHY ANN SPAULDING, DVM
Diplomate, ACVR
Professor of Radiology
Department of Molecular Biomedical Sciences
North Carolina State University
Raleigh, NC, USA

JENNIFER D. STEINBERG, DVM
Diplomate, ACVP (Clinical Pathology)
IDEXX Laboratories
Glen Burnie, MD, USA

JÖRG M. STEINER, Med Vet, Dr Med Vet, PhD
Diplomate, ACVIM (Small Animal Internal Medicine); Diplomate,
ECVIM-CA
Associate Professor; Director, Gastrointestinal Laboratory
Department of Small Animal Clinical Sciences
Texas A&M University
College Station, TX, USA

CHERYL MACCABE STOCKMAN, MT (ASCP), BS
Supervisor Clinical Pathology Laboratory
Department of Biomedical Sciences
Cummings School of Veterinary Medicine
Tufts University
North Grafton, MA, USA

TRACY STOKOL, BVSc, PhD
Diplomate, ACVP (Clinical Pathology)
Assistant Professor
Department of Population
Medicine and Diagnostic Sciences
College of Veterinary Medicine
Cornell University
Ithaca, NY, USA

JAN S. SUCHODOLSKI, DVM, PhD
Research Assistant Professor; Associate Director
Gastrointestinal Laboratory
Department of Small Animal Clinical Sciences
Texas A&M University
College Station, TX, USA

STACEY A. SULLIVAN, DVM
Diplomate, ACVIM (Neurology)
Animal Specialty Group
Los Angeles, CA, USA

SÉVERINE TASKER, BSc, BVSc, PhD
Diplomate, ACVIM (Small Animal Internal Medicine);
Diplomate, ECVIM, MRCVS
Lecturer in Small Animal Medicine
Department of Clinical Veterinary Science
University of Bristol
Bristol, England, UK

KATHY C. TATER, DVM
Diplomate, ACVD
Staff Dermatologist
Angell Animal Medical Center
Boston, MA, USA

LARRY PATRICK TILLEY, DVM
Diplomate, ACVIM (Small Animal Internal Medicine)
President
VetMed Consultants
Consultant, New Mexico
Veterinary Specialty Referral Center
Santa Fe, NM, USA

REID TYSON, DVM
Diplomate, ACVR
Assistant Professor
Department of Clinical Sciences
College of Veterinary Medicine
Oregon State University
Corvallis, OR, USA

LISA K. ULRICH, CVT
Principle Veterinary Technician
Minnesota Urolith Center
Department of Veterinary Clinical Sciences
College of Veterinary Medicine
University of Minnesota
St. Paul, MN, USA

SHELLY L. VADEN, DVM, PhD
Diplomate, ACVIM (Small Animal Internal Medicine)
Professor, Internal Medicine
Department of Clinical Sciences
College of Veterinary Medicine
North Carolina State University
Raleigh, NC, USA

MARIA A. VANDIS, DVM
Clinical Pathology Resident
Department of Pathology
Cummings School of Veterinary Medicine
Tufts University
North Grafton, MA, USA

HEATHER L. WAMSLEY, DVM
Diplomate, ACVP (Clinical Pathology)
Clinical Instructor of Veterinary Clinical Pathology
Department of Physiological Sciences
Veterinary Medical Center
University of Florida
Gainesville, FL, USA

MAXEY LEE WELLMAN, DVM, PhD
Diplomate, ACVP (Clinical Pathology)
Associate Professor
Department of Veterinary Biosciences
Ohio State University
Columbus, OH, USA

TERRI ANN WHEELER, MA, DVM
Area Veterinarian, New England
Pfizer Animal Health
Northbridge, MA, USA

ANGELA L. WILCOX, BVSc
Assistant Lecturer
Department of Veterinary Pathobiology
Veterinary Teaching Hospital
Texas A&M University
College Station, TX, USA

MICHAEL D. WILLARD, DVM
Diplomate, ACVIM (Small Animal Internal Medicine)
Professor
Department of Small Animal Medicine and Surgery
Texas Veterinary Medical Center
Texas A&M University
College Station, TX, USA

DIANE COLETTE WILLIAMS, PhD
Staff Research Associate III
Department of Electrophysiology Laboratory/
Neuromuscular Diseases
Veterinary Medical Teaching Hospital
University of California–Davis
Davis, CA, USA

LAUREL E. WILLIAMS, DVM
Diplomate, ACVIM (Oncology)
Associate Professor
Department of Clinical Sciences
College of Veterinary Medicine
North Carolina State University
Raleigh, NC, USA

MICHAEL W. WOOD, DVM
Diplomate, ACVIM (Small Animal Internal Medicine)
Clinical Investigator
Department of Clinical Sciences
College of Veterinary Medicine
North Carolina State University
Raleigh, NC, USA

DENISE WUNN, DVM, MS
Diplomate, ACVP (Clinical Pathology)
Head of Clinical Pathology, Eastern Region
IDEXX Laboratories
North Grafton, MA, USA

BRENDA MICHIYO YAMAMOTO, DVM
Research Associate; Clinical Pathology Resident
Department of Veterinary Biosciences
Ohio State University
Columbus, OH, USA

PANAGIOTIS G. XENOULIS, DVM, DrMedVet
Research Assistant
Gastrointestinal Laboratory
Department of Small Animal Clinical Sciences
College of Veterinary Medicine and Biomedical Sciences
Texas A&M University
College Station, TX, USA

KAREN L. ZAKS, DVM
Diplomate, ACVP (Clinical Pathology)
Veterinary Specialists of Northern Colorado
Antech Diagnostics
Loveland, CO, USA

STANDARD ABBREVIATIONS

ALT: alanine aminotransferase
ANOVA: analysis of variance
AST: aspartate aminotransferase
ATP: adenosine triphosphate
BUN: blood urea nitrogen
CBC: complete blood count
DNA: deoxyribonucleic acid
ECG: electrocardiogram, electrocardiograph, electrocardiographic
EDTA: ethylenediaminetetraacetic acid
ELISA: enzyme-linked immunosorbent assay
FeLV: feline leukemia virus
FIP: feline infectious peritonitis
FIV: feline immunodeficiency virus
g: force of gravity
GGT: γ-glutamyltransferase
GI: gastrointestinal
H&E: hematoxylin-eosin
Hct: hematocrit
IFA: indirect fluorescent antibody [test]
Ig: immunoglobulin
IgA: immunoglobulin A

IgE: immunoglobulin E
IgG: immunoglobulin G
IgM: immunoglobulin M
IM: intramuscular, intramuscularly
IV: intravenous, intravenously
MCH: mean cell hemoglobin
MCHC: mean cell hemoglobin concentration
MCV: mean cell volume
MW: molecular weight
N/A: not applicable
NADH: reduced form of nicotinamide-adenine dinucleotide
NADPH: nicotinamide-adenine dinucleotide phosphate
NSAIDs: nonsteroidal anti-inflammatory drugs
PCR: polymerase chain reaction
PCV: packed cell volume
RBC: red blood cell
RNA: ribonucleic acid
RPM: revolutions per minute
SC: subcutaneous, subcutaneously
SD: standard deviation
WBC: white blood cell

GETTING THE MOST OUT OF YOUR DIAGNOSTIC LABORATORY

In this day and age, with the proliferation of in-house equipment, practitioners can choose between performing routine laboratory tests in their practice or sending these samples to a commercial laboratory. Often, using a reference laboratory, with trained personnel and a strictly enforced quality assurance program, will enhance the quality of patient care that the facility can provide. In most areas, practitioners have a choice of several different commercial veterinary diagnostic laboratories that provide extensive testing menus, often including tests not available in the ordinary in-house laboratory. When selecting a laboratory, it is important to consider the turnaround time for routine assays such as CBCs, chemistry profiles, and urinalysis. Will results be available in a reasonable time frame? Larger laboratories can often provide these results by the next morning, with longer turnaround times for cultures, biopsies, and relatively uncommon tests. Is a courier pickup available and, if so, are the pickup times appropriate for your hours of operation? If there is only 1 pickup, the end of the business day is generally preferred because any samples collected after the pickup will wait until the next day for transport to the lab. Sample integrity is best if analysis is performed as close to the collection time as possible. If there is no courier pickup, will the lab offer a discounted cost for express shipment?

Unlike human diagnostic laboratories, veterinary diagnostic laboratories have no regulatory oversight, and it may be up to the clinician to investigate and compare the services provided, through phone calls to laboratory management or discussions with local colleagues. Without proper investigation and true comparison of the different laboratory services being offered, the price of the laboratory testing often becomes the unfortunate deciding factor. The appealing discounts, incentives, special offers, and placement of laboratory equipment help some commercial laboratories remain competitive. However, these incentives do not necessarily speak to the quality of the laboratory's service or the accuracy of their testing methods and results, the true reason to use an external laboratory service.

The following things are important considerations when assessing laboratory reliability:

1. What are the credentials of the staff performing the actual testing and interpreting the results? Board-certified pathologists and licensed medical technology staff (MT or MLT degrees) are usually the most qualified laboratory personnel.

2. What type of personnel training does the laboratory provide? Since medical technology programs are based on human samples, even these highly qualified individuals may require additional training before they will be proficient in all facets of veterinary testing.

3. Does the CBC include an automatic microscopic smear review? Heavy reliance on instrumentation, without a microscopic double check, can be labor (and cost) saving, but important abnormalities such as platelet clumps, microfilariae, hemoparasites, cellular inclusions (e.g., *Ehrlichia* or *Anaplasma*, Heinz bodies), and low numbers of abnormal cells (e.g., bands, blasts, mast cells) may go undetected. If a microscopic exam is not part of the routine package, consider requesting this service for an additional fee or screen blood smears yourself.

4. Is the laboratory using technology appropriate for veterinary specimens? This is a particularly important question when a human diagnostic laboratory is used. Most clinical chemistry assays will work regardless of the species, but hematology, endocrinology, and serology assays require specific assays validated for veterinary species.

5. How does the laboratory determine reference intervals? Reference intervals should be obtained by each lab, with its own instrumentation and reagent system, optimally using clinically normal patients that are not on medication or have no inherent disease. Ideally, these ranges are generated using >100 *healthy* individuals of each species, including a mix of different breeds and ages. This can be a challenge for any laboratory, and when healthy animals are not available, laboratories may resort to statistical manipulation of large data sets that include a mix of healthy and sick individuals. Since laboratory data can vary depending on the specific instrument and reagents used, reference values obtained from literature need careful consideration with respect to usefulness, although it may be necessary to resort to literature values when dealing with rare and/or exotic species.

6. Does the laboratory participate in proficiency surveys? These programs involve quarterly testing of unknown specimens, with results compared against those from other laboratories using the same methodology. Although it is a requirement for human laboratories to have acceptable performance in these surveys, veterinary labs have no such requirement. Voluntary participation in proficiency surveys often suggests a commitment to quality testing. Both human [e.g., College of American Pathologists (CAP)] and veterinary [e.g., Veterinary Laboratory Association (VLA)] proficiency programs are available, and each has potential merits of use in a veterinary laboratory.

It is important to maintain an open dialogue with your diagnostic laboratory, and ease of communication with customer service representatives should be an important consideration when choosing a lab. Keep in mind that a laboratory cannot fix a problem if it doesn't know the problem exists, so the laboratory manager or pathologist should be notified if results don't match clinical signs and/or biologic behavior of the lesion or if there is an unexpected level of day-to-day variation in results from a given patient. A good lab should be willing to rerun a sample if results are questionable. Do not be shy about requesting that the pathologist review a sample. Suspected problems with reference intervals should also be brought to the attention of lab management, but remember that the lab may need the assistance of clinicians to obtain sufficient samples from healthy animals.

Finally, optimal laboratory service requires some cooperation on the part of the veterinarian and his or her practice. To ensure timely results, the practice needs to have samples ready for the courier at the designated pickup time. Lab couriers are usually placed on a very tight schedule, and each delay along the way prevents timely delivery of samples to the lab for analysis. Incomplete paperwork, inappropriate labeling of the specimen type, or incorrect labeling of the specimen with owner and pet information are all instances in which laboratory data can be delayed or compromised. Missing or inappropriate information may trigger a phone call to the practice for clarification, which incurs a delay in testing. In addition to owner and animal identification, at minimum paperwork should indicate species, age, gender, and breed. For samples requiring interpretation (e.g., cytology and biopsy samples), details about the physical location, description, and duration of the lesion, as well as clinical information about response to treatment or tentative differential diagnoses, can also be helpful. Although the absence of this information does not alter what is on the slide, the interpretation can be greatly affected and, in general, the more information you provide, the more accurate the resulting differentials will be. For example, some diseases are more likely to occur in a dog than in a cat, or in a geriatric patient rather than in a young one.

Lastly, be sure to provide the appropriate sample for the required testing. The usefulness of laboratory data depends not only on the laboratory analysis of the specimen, but also the validity of the specimen. Is the owner information on the label accurate or will the lab be inadvertently reporting results from another patient? Was the proper anticoagulant used? Is the sample too old to provide valid results? Simply stated, bad laboratory data is dangerous. Interpretation of invalid data is impossible, misleading, and could be deadly. Therefore, strict attention needs to be maintained during the collection, storage, and appropriate shipment of the laboratory specimens in order to provide accurate, reliable information. If there is uncertainty about the correct sample or optimal handling of a specimen, check with the lab prior to obtaining the specimen. Quality lab results begin with quality patient specimens.

AUTHOR NAMES
Cheryl Stockman and Joyce S. Knoll

GENERAL PRINCIPLES FOR PERFORMING BLOOD TESTS

Blood is the most common sample used for analytical testing, and as it flows through out the body, it is affected by many medical conditions. Collection of blood provides a relatively noninvasive way to assess RBCs and WBCs, as well as enzymes, lipids, clotting factors, hormones, and antibody levels.

PREPARATION FOR SAMPLE COLLECTION

Prior to the actual phlebotomy, the appropriate supplies should be collected, including tubes appropriate for the ordered tests, skin disinfectant, and laboratory requisition forms. For uncommon tests, research may need to be done beforehand to determine the correct blood tubes and sample-handling requirements. Many reference laboratories provide a manual with collection and storage guidelines, but if information on a particular test is not available, contact a laboratory customer service representative for specific instructions. Do not assume that the sample requirements and handling are similar from lab to lab. Two different laboratories may offer the same test, but use different methodologies with different specimen requirements. It cannot be overstated that only submission of the correct specimen the first time can ensure accurate results and prevent the frustration and delay of having to perform a second patient venipuncture.

Although it may seem obvious, it is important to draw blood from the correct patient, and it is recommended that the hospital's standard operating procedure include some system for confirming patient identity (e.g., neck band, or simply double check with owner before returning the animal to the room). To further aid in patient identification, the use of a unique patient and owner identification number associated with that patient is also recommended. Many of the available practice management or medical record systems offer this service. This medical record number should be linked to patient identification on every level of patient transaction. There is bound to be a time when more than one "Max" or Smith is having blood tests performed.

Depending on the test, special procedures may need to be followed either before or after sample collection that may require advanced planning. For example, blood cultures require very particular phlebotomy cleansing procedures to lessen the risk of sample contamination with cutaneous flora. Patient fasting is recommended or required for a number of tests. Some tests require that samples be quickly separated from RBCs or immediately placed on ice and/or frozen, whereas other tests are adversely affected by contact with glass or the rubber tube caps. Many drug-testing procedures should not be performed on serum obtained from serum-separator gel tubes, because the gel has been shown to interfere with accurate drug recovery. The list of specific testing requirements is lengthy and specific, but these few examples reinforce the need for understanding of each test procedure prior to phlebotomy.

COLLECTION TUBES

Details regarding the actual technique of phlebotomy can be found in the "Blood Sample Collection" chapter. However, it is critical that the right tubes are selected for the blood samples needed in the test. Anticoagulated blood is needed for any test that involves cell counts or isolated WBCs or their DNA. Plasma comes from those tubes, too, and is the required sample for some tests (e.g., tests evaluating clotting proteins, which will be consumed in the clotting reaction). Serum comes from whole blood that has been allowed to clot.

Listed in Table 1 are the most commonly used blood-collection tubes, along with their most common uses and special notes. This list of collection tubes does not include the specialty tubes for less commonly performed testing. When a sample must be collected into several different types of collection tubes, follow the universal

guidelines regarding the order in which tubes should be filled. As the collection syringe is pushed into each successive tube, the potential exists for anticoagulant carryover into the next tube. To minimize this risk, tubes should be filled in the following order:

1. Blood culture tubes: Sterility must be maintained during sample collection.
2. Anticoagulant-free tubes [plain red-top tube and serum-separator tubes (SSTs)]: Carryover of anticoagulant, especially EDTA, risks chelation and a falsely decreased recovery of serum calcium and magnesium. The potassium in the EDTA anticoagulant falsely elevates the reported potassium value.
3. Coagulation tubes (sodium citrate): These are filled after tubes without anticoagulant to lessen sample contamination with tissue thromboplastin that may be released during the trauma of the venipuncture and falsely elevate clotting times.
4. Heparin
5. EDTA tubes
6. Oxalate-fluoride tubes

An alternate way to avoid contamination from a common dispensing needle is to fill the EDTA tube and then replace the drawing needle with a fresh one for filling any remaining tubes. Filling blood tubes with a needle and a syringe needs to be done with care. If the phlebotomist opts to fill the tubes by piercing the blood-tube cap with the needle, the vacuum in the tube should be allowed to take the correct amount of blood from the syringe without depressing the syringe plunger. Overfilling and therefore overwhelming the anticoagulant may cause subsequent, unwanted clotting of the blood sample. Also, the extra pressure exerted on the blood specimen as it is forced back through the needle may cause hemolysis of the specimen, which is undesirable for most test procedures.

Underfilling tubes containing anticoagulants can also result in a number of sample artifacts. Excess EDTA (tube < one-quarter full) can cause RBC distortion, altered RBC indices (MCV and MCHC) and can elevate protein measurements as determined by refractometer. The excess amount of anticoagulant in an underfilled citrate tube can dilute out coagulation factors, falsely prolonging clotting times.

SAMPLE HANDLING AND STORAGE

It is vital that any unique handling requirements are followed before shipping a sample to the reference laboratory for testing. If the test calls for serum or plasma, the sample should be centrifuged for 10–15 min at about 1,300–1,800 g. Centrifuge RPM differ depending on the size of the centrifuge rotor (rotor arm length). Some artifacts can be seen with a delay in centrifugation, because blood cells will metabolize analytes, such as glucose and certain hormones, artificially decreasing their levels in the sample. Depending on the test, serum in plain red-top tubes and some plasma samples (e.g., EDTA, citrate, or heparin anticoagulant) may need to be transferred into a clean anticoagulant-free tube away from the RBCs. Use polypropylene tubes for serum that cannot be kept in glass tubes. When using an SST, first gently invert the filled tube several times to mix blood with clot activator. Allow samples in SST and plain red-top tubes to clot for 20–30 min, preferably while vertical, prior to centrifugation. If a sample is centrifuged prior to complete clot formation and retraction, serum can become trapped in a gelatinous fibrin clot. Although serum can still be released by compressing the clot, the yield of serum will be inevitably decreased. Successful centrifugation of an SST will result in a gel barrier separating serum from the clot. In general, serum in these tubes does not need to be transferred into a transport tube unless the serum is to be stored frozen. If necessary, samples can be protected from light by wrapping the specimen in aluminum foil. If the sample

Table 1 Common blood-collection tubes

Type	Cap color	Sample type	Common use	Notes
SST	Red/black marble	Serum	Chemistry profiles Serologic testing	Not appropriate for therapeutic drug testing, because of gel interference with drug recovery.
Plain	Red	Serum	Chemistry profiles Serologic testing Therapeutic drug testing Fluid analysis	Serum usually needs to be separated from RBCs to prevent contamination with RBC breakdown products. Serum should be transferred to a clean red-top tube after centrifugation.
EDTA	Lavender	Plasma or whole blood	Hematology tests; e.g., CBC, platelet count, reticulocyte count PCR testing Coombs' testing Blood typing and crossmatching Fluid analysis	EDTA is *not* the preferred specimen for certain avian or reptile species such as crows, tortoises, or turtles. PCR specimens should not be allowed any contact with formalin or its fumes.
Sodium citrate	Light blue	Plasma or whole blood	Coagulation tests; e.g., PT, PTT, D-dimer, fibrinogen, FDP	For accurate results, a strict 1:9 ratio of blood to anticoagulant is required. Underfilling tubes causes a dilution effect and falsely extended coagulation times. Overfilling can overdilute the anticoagulant and allow premature clot formation, which consumes clotting factors and can also result in a prolonged coagulation time.
Lithium heparin	Green	Plasma or whole blood	Chemistry profiles on plasma CBCs on whole blood	Sodium heparin tubes have the same cap and their use should be avoided for electrolyte determinations. Sample of choice for certain avian or reptile species.
Blood culture bottles	Various cap colors; bottles contain supportive culture media	Whole blood in culture media	Blood cultures Synovial fluid culture	Stringent cleansing procedures are required prior to phlebotomy for blood cultures. Draw tube/bottles in pairs for aerobic and anaerobic testing. Larger volumes of blood are more likely to detect bloodborne infections. Blood culture tubes or bottles should not be refrigerated.
Sodium fluoride oxalate	Gray	Plasma	Glucose tolerance test	Sodium fluoride prevents glucose metabolism by RBCs (glycolysis).

FDP, fibrin degradation product; PT, prothrombin time; PTT, partial thromboplastin time; and SST, serum-separator tube.

is to be frozen, avoid repeated freeze-thaw cycles, which could cause sample degradation. Optimally, specimens should be stored in a freezer that does not self-defrost.

SENDING SPECIMENS WITH THE LAB COURIER

It is important to be sure that blood samples to be picked up by a courier are packaged correctly for their trip. Each specimen needs to be maintained at the correct temperature for the entire trip. Although the courier should have a cooler, specimens may be exposed to a long period of storage in a cooler that is opened and closed many times before reaching the laboratory. Frozen samples may need to be sandwiched between ice packs or, with advanced notice, arrangements can be made for the courier to bring dry ice. Alternatively, whole blood for cell counts should not be placed directly against an ice pack, because

cells will lyse if the sample freezes. Keep prepared blood smears out of the ice bag and never place the slides with blood tubes in the refrigerator. If condensation forms on the slides when they are removed from the refrigerator or moved off of an ice pack, the water droplets can destroy cells on the premade slides. Finally, if samples are left outside for the courier to pick up after the practice has closed, be aware of any extreme weather conditions (e.g., a heat wave or a cold snap) that might compromise the condition of samples. If questions arise about the best way to prepare specimens for the courier trip, consult with the customer service representative at the reference lab for specific details.

AUTHOR NAMES

Cheryl Stockman and Joyce S. Knoll

General Principles for Performing Fecal Tests

Although somewhat unpleasant to handle, fecal testing is a valuable tool for assessing the function and integrity of the bowel and is a routine part of the workup in patients with signs of GI disease. Several different types of tests can be performed on feces. Depending on the assay technique chosen, examination of stool may provide a relatively noninvasive method of screening for evidence of intestinal bleeding, infection (viral, bacterial, protozoal, or parasitic), inflammation, or malabsorption. Like other tests, the validity of fecal tests can depend on how the sample has been collected and handled. Microscopic techniques rely heavily on the observational skills and knowledge of the person performing the analysis.

SAMPLE COLLECTION

When possible, a fresh sample should be collected at the time of examination. This minimizes problems associated with sample age and eliminates questions about where the sample came from and how it was stored. However, this may be impractical for techniques such as fecal flotation or sedimentation, which require large sample volumes (2–10 g, equivalent to 0.5–2.5 teaspoons). For these assays, smaller samples may result in false-negative results, especially if an animal has a light infection or if ova are unevenly distributed throughout the feces. Typically, large samples are obtained by collecting voided feces. It is important that the patient defecates in a clean area and that the sample is immediately collected and placed in a clean, airtight container (e.g., screw-top jar, ziplock bag) and stored appropriately.

Smaller samples, for assays such as an occult blood test or a direct fecal smear, can be collected directly from the rectum by using a slightly moistened cotton-tipped applicator, a fecal loop, or gloved fingertip during digital rectal examination. Rectal lavage with saline is another option. With this procedure, 6–12 mL of saline is infused into the rectum or colon by using a lubricated 8F red rubber catheter. Saline is infused and aspirated several times to obtain a mudlike sample containing a mixture of mucus from the mucosal surface and lesser amounts of fecal material. This material can be used for direct smears or stored in a sterile red-top tube. This is a particularly good type of sample for identifying motile protozoa (e.g., *Giardia* trophozoites) and bacteria, but is less reliable for fecal floatation, because parasite eggs and cysts are more prevalent in fecal material and are less numerous in flush samples.

Specimen containers must be properly labeled. When a specimen cup or jar is used, labels should be placed on the side of the container and not on the lid because, when the lid is removed, the specimen is unlabeled.

SAMPLE STORAGE

Ideally, analysis should be performed as soon as possible after collection, because feces undergo a variety of changes as soon as the stool is passed. Cells and fragile organisms such as *Giardia* trophozoites and trichomonads deteriorate rapidly and become difficult to identify. Nematode eggs continue to develop over time and may be more difficult to recognize. Hookworm eggs hatch within 1 day in a warm environment, whereas *Toxascaris* eggs embryonate within a few days. In addition, bacterial flora continue to grow, potentially leading to overgrowth of a particular type of bacteria or yeast. Some bacterial species will sporulate.

Immediate analysis is more important for some assays than others. For wet preparations used in looking for motile protozoa, accurate results require feces to be absolutely fresh (<5 min old), but appropriate storage methods are available for many other types of fecal tests. Cytologic smears may be fixed in ethanol or stained (e.g., with Romanovsky stain or acid-fast stain). Special transport media are available for fecal cultures. Freezing will preserve feces for antigen-detection methods. Eggs and oocytes are resistant to degradation, and refrigeration will slow down embryonation, adequately stabilizing feces up to 1 day for flotation or sedimentation procedures. A variety of fixatives are also available to preserve feces for longer periods prior to flotation and/or sedimentation. Historically, formalin and mercuric chloride–based low-viscosity polyvinyl alcohol fixatives have been most widely used by parasitology laboratories for preservation of helminth eggs, protozoan cysts, and trophozoites in fecal specimens. However, in response to concerns about formalin toxicity and the difficulty in disposing of mercuric chloride solutions safely, several alternative preservatives are now available (e.g., Ecofix, from Meridian; Parasafe, from Scientific Device Laboratories; Proto-fix, from Alpha Tec Systems).

SAMPLE HANDLING

Although some may joke about veterinarians being "the ones willing to pick up dog poop with their bare hands," this is generally not advised, and all samples should be treated as though infectious. Although many of the organisms in feces are harmless, some can cause disease, especially in an immunocompromised person. Examples of possible pathogens include *Salmonella*, some strains of *Escherichia coli*, and *Cryptosporidia*. *Strongyloides* sp. is zoonotic to humans, and infective worms can burrow through skin and migrate through the body, potentially causing a lifelong infection. Therefore, it is recommended that gloves always be worn when handling feces and hands washed afterward. Owners who are asked to collect fecal samples should also be advised to use these universal precautions.

AUTHOR NAME
Joyce S. Knoll

GENERAL PRINCIPLES FOR PERFORMING URINE TESTS

Urine is obtained easily and can provide clinicians with a wealth of information. Urinalysis is an essential part of a routine workup and aids in diagnosing urinary tract inflammation, renal tubular dysfunction, and glomerular disease. In addition, since urine is derived through filtration of blood, urine can often provide valuable information about metabolic derangements or disorders of other organ systems, aiding in diagnosis of such conditions as liver disease, muscle disease, endocrine disease, and hemolysis. Evaluation of urine can be advantageous because urine contains compounds (e.g., cortisol, bile acids) filtered from the blood over several hours. This may provide a better reflection of homeostasis and disease than a does single random blood sample. In addition, renal clearance may affect blood levels of some compounds. Rapidly cleared molecules, such as Bence-Jones protein, may be found in urine but be undetectable in a serum sample. Finally, comparison of the concentration of an analyte, such as creatinine or sodium, in concurrent urine and serum samples may provide significantly more information about renal clearance than that provided by a serum sample alone. By itself, urine analysis rarely provides a specific diagnosis, but must instead be interpreted in conjunction with physical exam findings, CBC data, serum chemistry test results, and imaging techniques such as ultrasonography or contrast radiographs.

Like other tests, urine tests must be performed properly and controlled carefully. Use of incorrect techniques or outdated reagents can produce misleading results, and how the sample is collected can significantly affect results. The value of urinalysis is directly proportional to the quality of the sample and observational skills of the person performing the analysis.

COLLECTION TIMING

Timing of sample collection may depend on the test ordered. In general, 24-h urine collection is more accurate than collection of a random sample. This technique corrects for variations in analyte excretion at different times of day, and, since a 24-h sample tends to contain greater concentrations of an analyte, there is less chance of a false negative. However, this method is extremely cumbersome and thus impractical for most veterinary patients.

A sample collected first thing in the morning will be most closely reflective of a 24-h sample because the bladder will have accumulated urine over the previous 6–8 h. Also, because this urine was produced during an overnight fast, it is usually concentrated, and testing is more likely to detect positive findings that might be missed in a dilute sample. However, morning samples, which are usually collected by owners, are typically voided and therefore may not be ideal when looking for evidence of a urinary tract infection. Furthermore, morning collection often requires assistance by the owner, who must be given instructions and a proper collection container at least 1 day before the sample is collected. Depending on the test, the additional delay in sample analysis as a result of sample collection at home may also affect the accuracy of results.

For ease and convenience, routine urine screening is most often performed on a random specimen.

COLLECTION METHODS

VOIDED URINE

Collection of voided urine is safe, simple, and can be performed by owners, assuming they have cooperative pets. The first portion of the urine stream should be excluded from the sample because that portion is often contaminated by contact with the genital tract, skin, and hair. Inherent in the voided sample is the increased number of epithelial cells and sometimes WBCs picked up by urine as it travels through the lower urogenital tract. The vagina, prostate, and lower portion of the urethra are lined with squamous cells, which readily shed into a voided urine sample. The prepuce and vagina normally contain low levels of bacteria that can be picked up in a voided sample. Voided samples are therefore not optimal for culturing, although bacteria in a voided sample can still be suggestive of infection if present in large enough numbers. Although small numbers of bacteria and WBCs can be normal in a voided sample, more severe abnormalities can be caused by disease occurring at any portion of the urogenital tract, including the prostate, distal urethra, vagina, or prepuce. Localization of the problem to the bladder or kidney is therefore more difficult. A voided sample from a bitch in heat may contain increased numbers of RBCs. Voided samples can also sometimes include materials from the environment, such as pollen and plant fibers.

Samples collected from the top of an exam table may contain residual disinfectants that affect chemical tests. For example, hydrogen peroxide–based cleaning solutions can cause a false-positive heme/blood reaction. Some types of detergent can interfere with the glucose reaction. Samples from a litterbox can be contaminated with dust, bacteria, or other debris. When a patient is uncooperative or unable to urinate, samples can sometimes be collected by manual compression of the bladder, if it is distended. Although this method can be convenient for obtaining a sample, there are some drawbacks. Just as with a typical voided sample, these samples are often contaminated with materials from the genital tract. In addition, excessive compression can cause bladder trauma, increasing the numbers of RBCs in the sample. If a patient has a urinary tract infection, the high pressures that develop may force infected urine into the kidneys or prostate, spreading the infection.

CATHETERIZED SAMPLE

Catheterized specimens routinely contain an increased number of epithelial cells and can also be contaminated with bacteria and WBCs from the lower urogenital tract. Epithelial cells can include squamous cells from the lower urinary tract or transitional cells from the upper urethra and/or bladder. Because of the potential for sample contamination, these cells are not optimal for culturing. The quality of the sample can be improved by discarding the first few milliliters of urine, which are most likely to include genital tract contaminants. In addition to the risks of sample contamination, there is some risk to patients that the catheter either will traumatize the bladder, causing hemorrhage into the sample, or might introduce normal bacteria from the genital tract, inducing a urinary tract infection.

In patients with an indwelling catheter, urine should be aspirated from the catheter at a point distal to the sleeve leading to the balloon. Catheters often have a rubber access port for this purpose. It may be necessary to first clamp off the distal end of the catheter for 15–30 min, allowing urine to fill the tubing. The clamp should be removed after withdrawing the sample. Urine in the plastic reservoir bag should never be used for a urine test.

CYSTOCENTESIS

Percutaneous aspiration of the bladder (i.e., cystocentesis) is the most accurate representative of bladder contents so long as incidental capillary blood does not become part of the aspirated urine sample. Transitional cells can be included in the sample if the needle scratches the bladder wall or aspirates cells from the mucosal surface. It is important to stop aspiration prior to withdrawing the needle so that epithelial cells and capillary blood are not aspirated as the needle is pulled back through the bladder wall. This is the sample of choice for culturing and can be useful in localizing any visible inflammation to the kidney and/or bladder, as opposed to inflammation originating in the genital tract. RBCs are more difficult to interpret: Are they present because of hemorrhage into the urinary tract or was a blood vessel accidentally nicked during passage of the needle through the body wall? Occasionally, a cystocentesis specimen can be contaminated with fecal material from a misguided needle that enters the intestine prior to tapping the bladder. This might occur during a "blind stick," but is unlikely if the sample is ultrasound guided or if the bladder is immobilized during the procedure.

CHOICE OF COLLECTION CONTAINER

Results can be affected by the choice of collection container. Ideally, a rigid, opaque plastic container should be used, preferably with a screw-top lid to minimize the risk of leakage during transportation. Unless otherwise instructed, owners might choose collection containers that have been recycled from the kitchen and have not been properly washed. Residual food may affect results by introducing glucose into the collected urine specimen or by altering pH (e.g., pickled samples). Residual detergents used to clean the container may interfere with chemical tests. Although clear containers are adequate for most purposes, opaque containers are preferred, especially if analysis cannot be performed within 30–60 min, because they minimize photochemical breakdown of components, such as bilirubin, in the urine. Urine for culturing should be collected into a sterilized container (syringe or cup with a tight-fitting lid). Samples collected into an absorbent sponge are acceptable for chemical analysis, but the sediment analysis is less accurate because elements such as cells, casts, or crystals might become trapped within the sponge. Containers designed specifically for urine collection are available commercially and their use avoids many of these problems. Although these containers are disposable, they can be sterilized with ethylene oxide gas. Samples collected by catheterization or cystocentesis may be transported in a collection syringe, although, for safety reasons, any needles should be removed and the syringe

end capped or sealed with Parafilm prior to shipping. Alternatively, these samples can be transferred into a sterile tube (e.g., a red-top tube lacking anticoagulant).

Specimen containers must be properly labeled. When a cup or bottle is used, labels should be placed on the side of the container and not on the lid because, when the lid is removed, the specimen is unlabeled.

SAMPLE STORAGE AND TRANSPORT

Sample stability varies depending on the test. Ideally, urine for routine urinalysis should be analyzed within 2 h of collection to avoid alterations as a result of oxidation, precipitation of minerals (crystal formation), photolytic reactions, and/or the effects of bacterial metabolism. Urine left at room temperature loses carbon dioxide into the environment, increasing the pH. Crystals can increase or decrease over time, depending on the concentration of minerals and crystal solubility in alkaline urine. In addition, alkaline urine can result in false-positive dipstick results (especially protein determination) and lysis of RBCs, casts, and WBCs. Over time, any bacteria contaminating the sample may overgrow, especially if urine is not refrigerated. Depending on the type of bacteria present, they could metabolize glucose or ketones, changing the concentration of these substances in the urine.

Refrigeration is recommended to preserve sample integrity if processing must be delayed by >2 h. Preservatives are available, but these generally adversely affect chemical assays, and no single preservative suits all testing requirements. Freezing can preserve chemical components (e.g., catecholamines) in urine, but will cause cellular disruption.

AUTHOR NAME
Joyce S. Knoll

GENERAL PRINCIPLES OF ENDOSCOPY

INDICATIONS FOR ENDOSCOPY

Diagnostic endoscopy consists of using an instrument to visualize parts of the body that otherwise cannot be visualized without surgery. Endoscopy can also be used to perform certain procedures (e.g., biopsy tissue, obtain cells for cytology or culture, or remove a foreign object) that would normally require surgery. There are various types of endoscopy, each named after the part(s) of the body being examined (e.g., *gastroscopy* is endoscopy of the stomach, and *arthroscopy* is endoscopy of joints). Interventional endoscopy consists of using an endoscope to correct a problem or remove tissue so that more invasive, routine surgery can be avoided. Interventional endoscopy of the abdomen (*laparoscopy*) and chest (*thoracoscopy*) is sometimes called *minimally invasive surgery*. The major indications for endoscopy in dogs and cats are listed in Table 1.

A good endoscopist is not necessarily someone who tries to make endoscopy do everything. Rather, a good endoscopist knows when endoscopy can accomplish what is needed, as well as when endoscopy is not in the patient's best interests. Assuming that endoscopy is appropriate for a particular patient (i.e., it is expected that endoscopy can be used to diagnose 1 or more of the important differentials or accomplish what would otherwise require surgery), a few important questions should be asked before performing the procedure. Here are 3 important considerations before any endoscopic procedure:

1. Do you have equipment that will enable you to perform the procedure successfully and safely?
2. Is the patient likely to bleed excessively during or after the procedure?
3. Is the patient an acceptable anesthetic risk?

Additional questions and considerations are specific for each type of endoscopy. For example, 2 important considerations for gastro-duodenoscopy and colonoileoscopy are (1) whether a lesion is beyond reach of the endoscope, and (2) whether a less invasive procedure (e.g., transabdominal fine-needle aspiration) could be used to determine the diagnosis. Imaging, especially ultrasonography, is usually the best way to answer these questions for gastroduodenoscopy and colonoileoscopy. For colonoscopy, knowing what kind of lesion is suspected is particularly important. If the clinician is concerned about a dense, submucosal lesion near the rectum (e.g., a scirrhous carcinoma or pythiosis) or about determining whether a proliferative growth near the rectum is malignant or a benign polyp, flexible endoscopic forceps are often inadequate; yet rigid biopsy forceps increase the chance of making an accurate diagnosis. For bronchoscopy, a major question is whether performing a bronchoalveolar lavage will cause or worsen dyspnea.

INSTRUMENTATION

There are 2 main types of endoscopes: flexible and rigid. Esophagoscopy, gastroduodenoscopy, colonoileoscopy, bronchoscopy, and examination of the choana are performed primarily with flexible endoscopes. Proctoscopy, pharyngoscopy, laryngoscopy, laparoscopy, thoracoscopy, and arthroscopy are performed primarily with rigid endoscopes. Rhinoscopy, colonoscopy, cystoscopy, and vaginoscopy are performed routinely with either type.

An endoscope basically consists of something through which a clinician can look into a cavity. One can look through a hollow metal or plastic tube (e.g., a rigid colonoscope), through a solid metal or plastic tube that has lenses or a fiberoptic bundle running through it (e.g., a rigid laparoscope or a flexible fiberoptic gastroscope, respectively), or by means of a small liquid crystal display (LCD) camera placed at the end of a solid tube (e.g., a flexible videogastroscope). There must also be a light source that illuminates the cavity being examined through this same tube. Flexible scopes generally have 1 or more channels that are used to insufflate air, wash off the viewing lens, wash debris off the mucosa, aspirate debris, or insert a device (e.g.,

a biopsy forceps, a foreign body retrieval device, a cautery device, or a tube for instilling and recovering fluid). The tip of a flexible scope can generally be directed in either 1 plane (i.e., 2-way deflection) or 2 planes (i.e., 4-way deflection) by knobs on the handle. In general, the largest-diameter endoscope that can safely be used often provides the best visualization and enables better biopsies or more successful foreign body retrieval. However, larger-diameter scopes can be harder to pass into the desired area (e.g., through the pylorus into the duodenum or between nasal turbinates) or may limit maneuverability once in place. Cameras placed over the eyepiece of the scope or in the tip of the scope enable the image to be displayed on a monitor so that more people can observe and possibly assist the procedure. Hard-copy photographs, video, and computer images can be taken during the endoscopic examination. There are numerous types of biopsy forceps, foreign body retrieval devices, cautery devices, forceps, stapling devices, and the like, so that a multitude of procedures can be performed.

Flexible endoscopes that will be used in the GI tract minimally need to be able to insufflate air to inflate the viscus; wash off the viewing lens; aspirate fluid, debris, and air; and enable the use of various biopsy forceps or foreign body retrieval devices; as well as have 4-way deflection of the tip. Flexible bronchoscopes minimally need to have 2-way deflection and a channel that will enable aspiration of air or fluid, as well as the use of various forceps, tubes, brushes, and retrieval devices. Rigid colonoscopes need to be able to be closed off so that air can be insufflated during visualization of the colonic lumen. Laparoscopy, thoracoscopy, arthroscopy, and cystoscopy each have very specialized needs, which will be considered under their respective sections.

Because of the wide range of patients seen by veterinarians, sometimes one must adapt scopes for uses for which they were not originally intended. For example, when attempting to remove gastric foreign bodies from very small patients (e.g., a ferret or small bird), one must often use a bronchoscope despite it not having all the features expected in gastroscopes. Likewise, sometimes it becomes necessary to use small-diameter gastroscopes when performing bronchoscopy in long-bodied, large-breed dogs (e.g., Great Danes).

PROCEDURAL CARE OF PATIENT AND ENDOSCOPE

BEFORE THE PROCEDURE

Sterilization or disinfection of endoscopes is important in veterinary medicine, but fortunately it usually is not as critical as in human medicine, where there is the concern about human immunodeficiency virus (HIV) and a plethora of transmissible agents. *Sterilization* refers to the complete elimination and destruction of all living organisms, including viral particles and bacterial spores. *Disinfection* refers to eliminating or reducing numbers of potentially pathogenic organisms. If something has been sterilized, it has also been disinfected. However, something that has been disinfected is usually not sterilized. One can refer to *low-level* or *high-level* disinfection, which are degrees to which organisms have been reduced in number. Flexible scopes in particular are relatively delicate instruments, and improper cleaning, disinfection, and sterilization will damage or destroy the equipment. It is critically important that the manufacturers' recommendations be consulted regarding cleaning, disinfecting, and sterilizing all scopes. To prevent debris from drying in place and forming biofilms, proper cleaning should occur quickly after the procedure. Thorough drying is important because it is almost impossible to sterilize or adequately disinfect equipment that has retained moisture.

The degree of sterilization or disinfection required for an endoscope depends on the procedures that have been or will be performed, as well as on the potential disease(s) of the prior patients. Instruments (i.e., laparoscopes, thoracoscopes, cystoscopes, and arthroscopes) to be inserted into sterile body cavities must be sterilized. Instruments

Table 1   Principal indications for different types of endoscopy in veterinary medicine

Laryngoscopy or pharyngoscopy	Diagnose mass, laryngeal paralysis, or elongated soft palate
	Diagnose and remove a laryngeal or pharyngeal foreign body
Esophagoscopy	Diagnose esophagitis, esophageal mass, hiatal hernia, or *Spirocerca*
	Diagnose and remove a foreign body
	Diagnose and dilate an esophageal stricture
Gastroscopy or gastroduodenoscopy	Biopsy mucosa when looking for infiltrative upper GI disease
	Look for and biopsy an ulcer, erosion, or mass
	Diagnose lymphangiectasia (visual or biopsy)
	Diagnose and remove a foreign body
	Place a gastrostomy feeding tube
Proctoscopy	Biopsy proliferative lesions
	Biopsy mucosa when looking for infiltrative lower colonic disease
Colonoileoscopy	Biopsy mucosa when looking for infiltrative disease
	Look for intussusception
Bronchoscopy	Diagnose tracheal or bronchial collapse missed by imaging
	Obtain samples for cytology and culture when looking for inflammatory or neoplastic disease of the airways or pulmonary parenchyma
	Diagnose and remove a foreign body
Rhinoscopy	Biopsy mucosa when looking for inflammatory or neoplastic disease
	Look for turbinate destruction and fungal plaques
	Look for masses
	Look for a cause of epistaxis
	Diagnose and remove a foreign body
	Examine the choana for masses, mites, or foreign objects
Laparoscopy	Biopsy the liver (most common), pancreas, kidney, small intestine, or mass
	Perform gastropexy
	Place a jejunostomy feeding tube
Thoracoscopy	Biopsy lung, lymph nodes, pericardial sac, or masses
	Find all pulmonary bullae prior to thoracotomy
	Perform partial pericardectomy or partial lung lobectomy
	Aid in placing a chest tube
Cystoscopy	Look for ectopic ureters
	Biopsy a mass, primarily when looking for transitional cell carcinoma
	Remove small cystoliths
Vaginoscopy	Diagnose and biopsy tumors
Arthroscopy	Diagnose and treat osteochondritis dissecans, ligament tears, or meniscus abnormalities
Otoscopy	Examine the tympanic membrane and horizontal ear canal for evidence of disease
	Diagnose and remove foreign bodies

to be inserted into body cavities that are already contaminated do not necessarily require sterilization unless the scope was previously used in a patient with an infectious agent that mandates such action (e.g., parvovirus or herpes B virus). Sterilization is never wrong, but disinfection is typically performed when it is adequate for the procedure because disinfection is quicker, simpler, and less expensive. If the scope will be placed into a body cavity in which transmitting an infection is more of a concern (e.g., bronchoscopy), then high-level disinfection is recommended. High-level disinfection may consist of exposing the scope to a glutaraldehyde solution followed by sterile water. If the scope will be placed into a body cavity in which transmitting an infection is of minimal concern (e.g., gastroduodenoscopy or colonoscopy), then low-level disinfection (e.g., adequate cleaning followed by alcohol and drying) is more typical. Regardless of what level of disinfection or sterilization is performed, it is important that no chemical residues that may injure the patient remain in or on the endoscope.

Assuming the patient is not suspected of having a coagulopathy, excessive hemorrhage is seldom a concern except when performing rhinoscopy for epistaxis or performing laparoscopy or thoracoscopy for any reason. In most cases, a platelet count and a patient history that do not support a coagulopathy are sufficient. In patients to undergo rhinoscopy for epistaxis or a laparoscopy or thoracoscopy, determi-

nation of a mucosal bleeding time is advisable in addition to the platelet count. Laboratory tests of clotting [i.e., PT, PTT, and PIVKA (*protein induced by vitamin K absence*)] generally do not correlate well with potential for bleeding during or after endoscopy and are seldom necessary for endoscopists (except to diagnose the cause of the bleeding). If severe clinical bleeding is a concern and endoscopy is still warranted, then blood products for transfusion, or electrocautery, or both, as well as surgical instruments, should be readily available.

DURING THE PROCEDURE

At least 2 people should be involved in almost every endoscopy. One person should be dedicated to maintaining anesthesia and monitoring the patient's vital signs while another performs the endoscopy. What constitutes adequate anesthetic monitoring of the patient depends on many factors and is not addressed here. However, clinicians should be prepared for resuscitative measures. Having 1 or more other people who can assist (e.g., to work biopsy forceps and other devices, to retrieve biopsy samples, and to obtain needed equipment) is clearly advantageous. In particular, when air is being insufflated into a body cavity, it is very desirable to have a third person who can watch to ensure that excessive insufflation does not compromise the patient (e.g., iatrogenic gastric dilatation).

AFTER THE PROCEDURE

The patient should be recovered from anesthesia and watched for anesthetic, as well as endoscopic, complications (see the next section). This will vary with the procedure and the patient. As part of the endoscopic procedure, owners should be counseled as to what is expected (i.e., is unimportant) and what is unexpected (i.e., warrants communication with the veterinarian) during the 8–24 h following endoscopy.

POTENTIAL COMPLICATIONS

Each type of endoscopy has its own set of potential complications. However, some complications are concerns with almost any endoscopic procedure.

• Anesthetic death is the most devastating complication. It can occur anytime, but patients with severe hypoalbuminemia (i.e., serum albumin, <1.3 g/dL), severe cardiac disease or failure (especially patients with severe arrhythmias), severe respiratory dysfunction, or severe organ dysfunction (especially renal failure and hepatic failure) seem to be at greatest risk.

• Perforation is potentially fatal, but quick action can often avert mortality. Endoscopy is best accomplished by skill and finesse as opposed to brute force, and perforation seems rare among experienced endoscopists. However, sometimes perforation occurs due to diseased tissue that cannot tolerate what would normally be a reasonable amount of pressure. If there is any concern about the possibility of perforation (e.g., removal of an esophageal foreign body that caused substantial ulceration, biopsy of the center of a deep ulcer, or removal of a linear foreign object), looking for free thoracic or abdominal gas via radiography is a reasonable way to evaluate for perforation when air was insufflated as part of the endoscopic procedure.

• Persistent bleeding from a biopsy site is uncommon unless an artery or major vein has been torn or there is a coagulopathy. It must be remembered that the PCV will not change substantially in acute hemorrhage; rather, one must monitor mucous membrane color, pulse quality, heart rate, and possibly blood pressure to detect excessive postprocedural hemorrhage.

• Infection following endoscopy is primarily a concern when laparoscopy, thoracoscopy, arthroscopy, or cystoscopy has been performed. Nonetheless, routine antibiotic administration is not warranted during or after these procedures unless there was a known risk factor (e.g., a break in sterile technique). Some procedures and situations in people are recognized to cause bacteremia or put patients at increased risk for postprocedural infections (e.g., dilating esophageal strictures or patients with prosthetic joints or heart valves). Antibiotics can reasonably be used in these same situations in veterinary medicine, as well as when circumstances and common sense dictate them (e.g., cystoscopy of a patient with an ongoing urinary tract infection). However, antibiotics are generally rarely required with veterinary endoscopic procedures.

• Anesthesia-associated gastroesophageal reflux and subsequent esophagitis or stricture is a very rare, but potentially devastating, complication of any anesthetic procedure. It is easy to detect after gastroduodenoscopy as the scope is withdrawn from the stomach.

Table 2 Basic information for an endoscopy report

1. Patient information (e.g., case number) and the date of the examination
2. Equipment information (i.e., which scope and which retrieval device were used)
3. Gross endoscopic appearance of organs examined
   a. Which organs were examined?
   b. How much of the organ could be visualized and its gross appearance
   c. Presence of foreign objects
   d. Presence of debris (e.g., food, fluid, feces, grass, or barium) obscuring visualization
4. How successful was the procedure?
   a. What was biopsied?
   b. What foreign objects were removed?
5. Complications or problems that occurred
   a. Procedure stopped because of anesthetic complications
   b. Endoscope could not be passed to a desired point.
   c. Excessive bleeding was caused by biopsy or foreign object removal or by perforation.
6. Endoscopist's signature

Otherwise, having a patient that becomes anorexic and starts regurgitating hours to days following anesthesia warrants consideration of this complication.

REPORTING RESULTS

An endoscopy report is an integral part of the medical record and is critically important for documenting what was performed and how it was performed. This information is necessary for making diagnostic and therapeutic recommendations (especially days or weeks after a patient has been discharged and the clients or referring veterinarian are asking for advice), as well as for evaluating patients accurately at recheck (especially when endoscopy is repeated). Issues of quality assurance and medicolegal documentation historically have not been driving factors in veterinary endoscopy, but this may change with time. The absolute minimal for an endoscopy report should probably include the items in Table 2.

Photographic documentation is desirable for the endoscopy record, but currently is not considered the standard of practice for veterinary medicine. Likewise, additional information (e.g., history, indication for endoscopy, anesthetic drugs used, people assisting in endoscopy, and recommendations by the endoscopist) may be added and will enhance the endoscopy record. However, since most of this information is available elsewhere in the medical record, it is not absolutely required for the endoscopy report.

AUTHOR NAME
Michael Willard

GENERAL PRINCIPLES OF RADIOGRAPHY

INDICATIONS FOR PERFORMING RADIOGRAPHIC PROCEDURES

Radiology (the art of radiographic interpretation) is an integral part of companion animal practice. Generating high-quality diagnostic radiographs (radiography) is the first step in maximizing the diagnostic potential of this modality. A thorough understanding of the principles of radiography and radiographic interpretation is the first step in the interpretation process. Although radiology is not the gold standard when evaluating many disorders, it is often the first imaging modality used in the diagnostic workup. Indications for radiographic procedures include the following:

- Cardiorespiratory compromise
- Tumor staging
- Assessment of the skull and extracranial structures
- Abdominal pain
- Abdominal mass(es)
- GI dysfunction
- Urogenital dysfunction
- Musculoskeletal disorders
- Spinal disorders
- Screening of juvenile orthopedic disorders

Many practices invest in physical resources, but fail to invest sufficient time and resources into technician training and clinician continuing education. A well-functioning radiography suite that consistently produces good-quality images is a commonly undervalued resource in veterinary medicine.

PRINCIPLES OF RADIOLOGY

All other factors being equal, the most important parameters that determine radiographic quality are selection of kVp, mAs, film and screen type, and use of a grid. *K*ilo*v*oltage *p*eak (kVp) primarily controls photon energy. The penetrating power of the beam increases as the kVp increases. This results in a relative increase in the number of shades of gray and a radiograph with more latitude. The other important parameter is *mAs*: *mA* means *milli*ampere and relates to the number of photons generated per unit time. The *s* designates the exposure time (seconds). Together it (mA multiplied by s) primarily controls film blackness (essentially the number of photons hitting the film), although increasing kVp does also increase film blackness (more photons generated at the anode and more photons penetrate the patient because of increased photon energy).

The selection of *film type* is important. The film and screen together have a designated system speed relative to an industry standard. High-detail systems require more exposure and usually have a speed designation of less than 100. Faster systems require less exposure, but there is a relative loss of detail (spatial resolution). There is a trade-off between detail and exposure. Higher exposures mean increased exposure time, an increased chance of motion artifact and, potentially, increased personnel exposure. In addition to system speed, film type can significantly affect the latitude of the resulting radiograph. Film designed for human chest imaging has more latitude than general-purpose orthopedic film. While such latitude radiographs are not as dramatic to look at and appear dull, there is inherently more information relative to a high-contrast radiograph made using general-purpose or orthopedic or mammography film.

Scatter (photons causing unwanted film exposure) is best controlled by the use of a *grid*. A grid, placed between the patient and film, should be used when patient thickness exceeds 10 cm. (A grid may not be necessary with some digital systems.) This device, usually comprising fine interleaves of lead and nonradiopaque material, removes a significant proportion of scatter radiation from the primary beam before the scatter hits the receiver device [film/screen cassette, computed radiography (CR) cassette, or direct digital radiography image plate]. Unfortunately, a grid also attenuates the primary beam, necessitating

an adjustment in mAs—usually in the order of a 3- or 4-fold increase. However, the improved contrast and detail afforded by a grid usually outweighs the resulting exposure penalty.

Collimation of the beam inside the film border potentially reduces personnel exposure. Collimation inside patient anatomy reduces scatter and increases image detail and contrast.

The technique used for making radiographs will vary with the region of interest. Thoracic radiographs should be made with a high kVp, at the maximum mA the machine can produce. This results in as short an exposure time as possible. The thorax has high inherent subject contrast, and a high-kVp low-mAs technique is well suited to thoracic imaging. The exposure should be made during peak inspiration to ensure maximal lung aeration. This affords the best opportunity to see most pulmonary pathology. Abdominal radiographs should be made during peak expiration. The patient is still for a longer period between breaths, which is important because abdominal radiographs typically require a larger mAs (therefore longer exposure time) when compared to thoracic radiographs. This is because the abdomen comprises more soft tissue than the thorax, and a lower kVp is often used to accentuate image contrast.

A *radiographic technique chart* should be maintained and used to calculate the optimum machine settings. Variable kVp techniques are most commonly employed in animals because they enable more exposure variation. Once an optimal radiograph of any given region has been generated with an appropriate kVp and mAs, a general technique chart can be generated by using the following relationship between kVp and patient thickness (cm).

Up to 80 kVp	+/−	2 kVp/cm thickness
80−100 kVp	+/−	3 Vp/cm thickness
100+kVp	+/−	4 kVp/cm thickness

To maintain the same film blackness and for changes in techniques, the following rules can be applied:
- If you decrease mAs by 50%, increase kVp by 20%.
- If you double the mAs, decrease kVp by 16%.
- If a radiograph is useful, but either too dark or too light, use the 10% rule:
  - If too dark, decrease kVp by 10%.
  - If too light, increase the kVp by 10%.

RADIOGRAPHIC EQUIPMENT

Poor darkroom technique, aged cassettes and screens, and low-output radiographic machines are the 3 major limiting factors to improving radiographic quality, with respect to equipment. A well-maintained automatic processor, appropriate film handling, and a modern film/screen system will eliminate many variables that adversely affect image quality.

Generally, less expensive machines create a smaller current at the filament (less mA) which results in a lower X-ray photon output per unit time. This necessitates a longer exposure time for a given patient thickness or body part. With respect to the thorax and abdomen, this increases the likelihood of motion artifact (radiographic blur). This can be negated, at least in part, by using a modern rare earth film/screen system (medium or high speed) and optimizing darkroom technique. Radiographic machines should be checked for output consistency annually by a licensed inspector.

The use of digital imaging is growing rapidly. Many digital imaging products are available to practicing veterinarians, and the cost of this technology is stabilizing. Investment in good-quality digital imaging equipment can reap significant and consistent improvements in image quality and increased throughput. However, investment in inferior products and vendors that use non–industry-standard image file formats should be avoided. *D*iagnostic *I*mage and *Co*mmunications in *M*edicine (DICOM) is the image file format endorsed by the

American College of Radiology (ACR) and the American College of Veterinary Radiology (ACVR), and, for many reasons, is the only file format that should be considered.

The DICOM standard allows for the identification, storage, viewing, and dissemination of medical images across local area networks and the Internet in a highly efficient and simplistic manner. Images generated from all radiographic modalities and any vendor conforming to the DICOM standard can be managed similarly.

There are 2 broad categories of primary acquisition digital equipment. *Computed radiography* uses a photosensitive phosphor plate within a cassette. Once exposed, the cassette is placed into a reader and an image generated in about a minute, depending on the system. *Direct digital radiography* comprises an imaging plate connected by a cable to a processing computer. The plate, similar in size to a large cassette, replaces the self-centering cassette tray under the table. Images are usually generated within 3–5 s, and the plate can usually be reexposed within approximately 15 s. Another popular direct digital configuration is the *c*harged *c*ouple *d*evice), whereby a digital camera and lens system records (photographs) an image-intensifying screen as it fluoresces during exposure. There are significant differences in image quality and performance of veterinary digital imaging systems, particularly the lower-end CCD systems, so an extensive investigation of the options available before purchase is highly recommended. (An invaluable resource is http://www.animalinsides.com.)

Digital imaging systems provide many advantages over traditional film/screen systems. From an image-quality perspective, digital systems have a wide tolerance to exposure error. Nondiagnostic images caused by exposure errors are all but eliminated, particularly with the digital plate technology. In addition to exposure tolerance, digital systems have much more dynamic range (image latitude) when compared to traditional film/screen systems. The ability to manipulate the image electronically enables the image to be normalized, whereby regions that are seemingly overexposed or too dark are made lighter and vice versa. This is done automatically according to preset parameters, and, in well-configured systems, most every image should appear perfectly exposed. In any practice, but particularly in practices struggling to maintain satisfactory image quality, this is a tremendous advantage.

There are many other advantages of digital systems, not the least of which is easy image storage, dissemination, and viewing. The ability to *soft-copy review* (view on a computer monitor) anywhere in the clinic (and beyond) within seconds of image generation makes obtaining a second opinion from a boarded radiologist much easier than possible previously, and this is considered a significant advantage of digital technology. Many teleradiology interpretation services are available, some provided by vendors of imaging equipment and some independently by diplomates of the ACVR. It is expected that the use of such services will dramatically increase in the next decade as more veterinary clinics go online with digital imaging equipment and broadband Internet connections.

In addition to enhanced image quality, veterinarians report significant improvements in patient throughput with DR. Because the CR cassette must be run through a reader, which takes approximately 1 min, only modest improvements in throughput with CR are seen.

RADIOGRAPHIC INTERPRETATION

An understanding of normal anatomy is essential before an accurate radiographic interpretation is possible. Many readily available textbooks include images of normal radiographic anatomy. Consideration should be given to maintaining a bone bank or assembled skeleton to assist in radiographic anatomy. A library of normal images can be an invaluable resource. When pathology is unilateral, radiographs of the contralateral limb may act as normal controls. Conversely, radiographs of normal littermates may be useful when reference texts are not available.

The viewing environment is particularly important. Analog radiographs should be viewed on good-quality viewing boxes in a quiet room with control of ambient lighting. Digital images should be viewed on well-calibrated monitors of adequate size, brightness, and pixel density.

Radiographs should not be interpreted hastily. Sufficient time and attention should be dedicated to the exam. Images should be assessed for radiographic quality before interpretation. The initial radiographic evaluation should address such issues as these:
- Are there sufficient views?
- Is patient positioning adequate?
- Are the images adequately identified?
- Are there any artifacts? Is there sufficient contrast and detail?
- Is there sufficient film blackness?

A systematic approach to radiographic evaluation is paramount in order to prevent important abnormalities from being overlooked.

Radiographic interpretation is a skill that requires much time to master. Numerous textbooks are available that detail the radiographic manifestations of the common disorders of cats and dogs. These texts should be kept readily available to interpreting clinicians. Continuing education courses on all aspects of radiographic interpretation should be pursued.

RISKS OF RADIATION EXPOSURE

The practice should comply with local regulations with respect to radiation safety. Protective gloves and aprons should be worn at all times by all personnel involved in the physical restraint of patients. Some states do not allow personnel in the room during radiography. Good radiographic practices should be employed so as to minimize potential personnel exposure, and under no circumstances should personnel be exposed to the primary beam. Radiation dosimeters should be used, and the personnel dose monitored regularly.

CONTRAINDICATIONS

There are no specific contraindications to radiography. Unnecessary irradiation of pregnant bitches, particularly in the first trimester, should be avoided. Although there are no comprehensive veterinary studies documenting the risk of clinical imaging to pregnancy, common sense suggests that the use of unnecessary irradiation should be avoided.

INTERFERING FACTORS

DRUGS
- Many drugs or compounds used in the management of GI disorders are radiopaque and therefore apparent on survey radiographs. This may lead to confusion during radiographic interpretation.
- Drugs used to modify GI motility and drugs used for chemical restraint can alter gastric and intestinal gas patterns and may lead to a false diagnosis of GI disease.

CONDITIONS
Anesthesia and sedation of noncompliant patients for thoracic radiographs may result in transient pulmonary atelectasis related to anesthesia. This may not be clinically important but difficult to differentiate from real pathology. This is exacerbated if the patient is maintained in lateral recumbency for prolonged periods before radiography.

PROCEDURE TECHNIQUES OR HANDLING
Problems can arise from the use of improper technique or improper patient positioning. A thorough understanding of the physics of radiography will enable clinicians to better troubleshoot these problems.

INFLUENCE OF SIGNALMENT ON PERFORMING AND INTERPRETING THE PROCEDURE

SPECIES
High-detail systems are needed to critically evaluate the fine trabecular detail in small bones, as well as the subtle pulmonary architecture in cats.

BREED

Large dogs are more difficult to image than small dogs. The region of interest may not fit on 1 cassette. A higher exposure is required because the body part being imaged is often thicker (e.g., spine, thorax, abdomen, pelvis). If a slow imaging system is used or the radiographic machine is low in mA output, there may be motion artifact.

AGE

One must be aware of the changes in skeletal maturation with age in order to interpret radiographs accurately. Young and thin patients have less abdominal fat, resulting in less image contrast, sometimes compromising radiographic interpretation.

GENDER

When evaluating the male lower urinary tract, images of the entire perineum and os penis are required.

PROCEDURE AND PATIENT CARE

Specific procedures are detailed in the individual chapters.

BEFORE

• The client should be informed of the procedure and any specific fasting requirements.
• Many radiographic exams necessitate the administration of chemical or physical restraint. Clients should be made aware of the risks of sedation in patients with cardiopulmonary compromise.
• No specific patient preparation is required for survey radiographs. Collars, harnesses, etc., should be removed prior to imaging.
• Where practical, bandage material should be removed.
• Ideally, food should be withheld for 12 h before patients undergo elective abdominal radiography.
• For elective contrast studies involving the abdomen, food should be withheld for 12 h and a cleansing enema may be required.
• Survey radiographs should always be made before any contrast medium is administered. This gives an opportunity to optimize radiographic technique, ensure optimal patient preparation, and act as a baseline for later comparison.
• Anesthesia or heavy sedation is required when optimal positioning is critical and when the patient is in pain. This is particularly important when imaging the skull and spine.

DURING

• To minimize the effects of recumbency-related pulmonary atelectasis, nonambulatory or moribund patients undergoing thoracic radiographs should be maintained in sternal recumbency for several minutes before radiography.
• Generally, a minimum of 2 orthogonal views are required to assess a given region. The few exceptions to this rule include examinations made in the screening of orthopedic disorders (e.g., hip extended view for evaluation of canine hip dysplasia, flexed lateral view in the assessment of elbow dysplasia). Acquiring sufficient radiographic projections is an often-overlooked aspect of the radiographic evaluation.
• Accurate patient positioning is extremely important in the generation of good-quality radiographs. Poorly positioned radiographs, and radiographs with poor contrast and detail, increase the chances of important radiographic anomalies being overlooked or incorrect assessments. This can lead to inappropriate patient management.
• Routine monitoring is required for sedated and anesthetized patients.
• Patients receiving IV radiographic contrast media should be monitored for evidence of an adverse reaction.

AFTER

• Patients receiving IV contrast media are at some risk, albeit minimal, of an adverse reaction to iodine and should be monitored for such complications. Nausea and vomiting are the most common mild reactions. Anaphylaxis and contrast medium–induced renal failure are uncommon but potentially severe adverse reactions.
• Patients receiving oral barium products should be monitored for potential barium inhalation. This is most important in patients with esophageal dysfunction or proximal upper GI obstruction.

POTENTIAL COMPLICATIONS

Few complications are associated with radiography. Physical and chemical restraint, combined with forced positioning of patients with cardiorespiratory compromise, can result in decompensation. Forced positioning of patients with unstable fractures (appendicular or spinal) can exacerbate soft tissue injuries.

REPORTING OF RESULTS

Radiographic images are part of the legal medical record and must be permanently identified and archived. Archiving should comply with local regulations. A significant advantage of digital imaging using the DICOM standard is that studies are permanently identified electronically. Furthermore, patient data can be edited only by specific header editing software, which is usually accessible only to system administrators. If images are acquired and stored in digital format, consideration must be given to ensuring that adequate archiving resources and system redundancy are available. Archive servers should use a *r*edundant *a*rray of *i*ndependent *d*isks (RAID) configuration to minimize the chances of data loss associated with hard-drive failure. Adequate planning with respect to disaster recovery is mandatory and should include some type of off-site repository.

AUTHOR NAME

Ian D. Robertson

GENERAL PRINCIPLES OF ULTRASONOGRAPHY

INDICATIONS FOR PERFORMING ULTRASONOGRAPHY

Ultrasonography is frequently performed in veterinary medicine as a complementary diagnostic procedure to radiography for a large number of diseases. Ultrasound may be the sole modality used, however, for the detection of small amounts of free pleural or peritoneal fluid, early pregnancy detection, and determination of fetal viability, as well as for diagnosis of pyometra. Both radiography and ultrasound provide information as to the size, shape, and location of organs. Ultrasound, however, is superior to radiography for the examination of the internal structure of organs and differentiation of fluid-filled versus solid space-occupying lesions.

Frequent indications for performing abdominal ultrasound include the following:

- Hepatic disease
- Icterus
- Pancreatitis
- Detection of portosystemic shunts
- Determination of the origin of abdominal masses
- Chronic vomiting and diarrhea
- Renal failure
- Urinary tract obstruction
- Detection of pyometra
- Prostatomegaly
- Hyperadrenocorticism
- Cancer staging
- Ultrasound-guided tissue sampling
- Detection of small amounts of free fluid

The ultrasound examination of the thorax is not only limited to echocardiography. The lung surface, as well as its inner architecture, can be examined with ultrasound under certain conditions. Furthermore, cranial mediastinal masses can also be detected.

Although well established in equine sports medicine, ultrasound is used with increasing frequency in small-animal orthopedics for the diagnosis of many musculoskeletal diseases. The diagnosis of ligamentous or tendinous trauma of both the front and hind limbs is greatly aided with ultrasound.

Ocular ultrasound has become an integral part of the ophthalmic examination for the detection of retinal detachment, retrobulbar disease, and other intraocular manifestations.

Ultrasound-guided tissue sampling is often used in either fine-needle aspirations or Tru-cut biopsies of many organs and structures. The liver and kidneys are the organs most frequently biopsied. Fine-needle aspirations for cytology can be carried out on most organs and structures, provided that overlying organs or vessels do not obstruct the region of interest.

PHYSICAL PRINCIPLES OF ULTRASONOGRAPHY

Mechanical waves produced from the expansion and contraction of piezoelectric crystals in the ultrasound transducer, or *probe*, are transmitted into the body and then are reflected by internal structures. A mechanical wave from the sound beam reflection, or *echo*, is transmitted back to the ultrasound probe and converted into an electrical signal due to the piezoelectric effect. The received signal contains beam intensity, depth, and frequency information that enables the images of the internal organs to be formed. The intensity or amplitude of the returning echo determines the shade of gray from white to black to be assigned to various structures. Changes in acoustic impedance of the beam as it passes through different structures and organs determine how much of the sound beam is reflected back to the transducer.

Highly reflecting structures such as air or bone are hyperechoic or white. Fluid such as urine or bile will allow almost complete transmission of the beam and will therefore appear black. The varying impedance of different parenchymal structures such as the liver, spleen, and kidney results in the differences in the shades of gray assigned to them.

The ultrasound beam is produced as a mechanical wave with a frequency, speed, and wavelength. The velocity of a sound beam traveling through the body is given as a constant of 1540 m/s and is the speed used in all ultrasound machines for calculations.

The *frequency* refers to the number of cycles per second and is expressed in hertz (Hz) or megahertz (MHz). Today, probe frequencies generally range between 2 and 17. Very high frequency probes from 20 to 100 MHz are available for specialized purposed. High-frequency probes have a short wavelength (expressed in millimeters) and low-frequency probes have a longer wavelength: the shorter the wavelength, the higher the resolution and lower the depth penetration. An example of this principle is the requirement of low-frequency transducers for examining the liver of larger dogs. A compromise exists between obtaining high resolution and good depth penetration. Therefore, ultrasound machines must generally be equipped with multiple probes for examining different regions of the body and different sized patients.

Electronic ultrasound probes are the type of transducer most commonly used today. They are available in a variety of formats, shapes, and sizes. Sector probes have a pie-shaped scan field with a narrow near field and wide far field. These are ideal for imaging deep structures or between the ribs, such as for echocardiography. Linear array transducers produce a rectangular scan field with excellent near field imaging for examination of superficial structures. These probes are ideal for examination of musculoskeletal structures, as well as superficial abdominal organs such as the spleen and intestines or urinary bladder wall. The probes have a rectangular surface, which does not allow all parts of the abdomen to be examined, especially the liver, because of the body conformation of the cranial abdomen. Convex probes are curved linear arrays with a small curved probe tip that are ideal for imaging the entire abdomen of cats and dogs.

PATIENT PREPARATION AND CARE

Hair traps air and prevents good coupling between the skin and probe and transmission of the ultrasound beam. Therefore, the hair over the region to be examined must be clipped. Wiping the skin with alcohol (not greater than 70%) will improve beam transmission with or without coupling gel. Animals with thin or sparse hair may be examined by applying only alcohol. Clients should be made aware, however, that their animals will require clipping in most cases.

Patients should be fasted for 12 h prior to the examination. Water may be given, however, up to a few hours in advance except in special situations, such as gastric distention or delayed outflow. A moderately full bladder is necessary for complete examination of the urinary tract. However, an extremely full bladder will impede examination of both the bladder and the remainder of the abdomen.

TECHINIQUE

Ultrasound is highly user dependent and, compared to radiography, ultrasonography requires greater user experience for both performing the procedure and for recognizing and interpreting findings. Good knowledge of cross-sectional anatomy is required because the images are obtained in thin slices through the body. Furthermore, excellent hand-eye coordination and dexterity with the ultrasound probe are advantageous. Image quality depends on multiple factors such as quality of the machine and probes, probe selection for the body part, and proper adjustment of the machine settings, as well as experience of the sonographer.

Patients are generally examined without being sedated and are positioned in either dorsal or right lateral recumbency. Alternate positions may be required to examine certain regions of the abdomen, depending on the circumstances and the patient's body conformation.

Ultrasound images can be displayed in a number of real-time modes. These are the most common:

TWO-DIMENSIONAL GRAY SCALE

Multiple dots along multiple parallel image lines correspond to the intensity of the returning echoes, which are assigned various shades of gray. The strongest echoes are depicted as white and the weakest as black. The depth of each dot in each image line is determined by the amount of time the echo from each point takes to return to the transducer. The multiple scan lines make up the slice of tissue seen on the monitor.

M-MODE

The transducer is held stationary, and 1 image line is displayed over time in a gray-scale format. The resulting image is displayed on a y- and x-axis and moves along the x-axis over time. The y-axis represents depth. This mode is frequently used in echocardiography to examine movement of the heart valves and ventricular walls.

DOPPLER ULTRASOUND

The RBCs within the vessels reflect the ultrasound beam. Because the blood cells are moving and the transducer is fixed in position, the frequency of the returning echo is shifted from that of the source. This Doppler shift is recorded by the machine and is negative if the blood is flowing away from the transducer and positive if toward it. Therefore, the presence, direction, and velocity of moving blood can be determined. The blood flow can be displayed as a spectral format or as a color map. In the spectral format, the arterial and venous waveforms can be observed on an x- and y-axis over time for quantitative and semiquantitative analysis. Color Doppler maps the frequency shifts as red and blue over the two-dimensional gray-scale image, allowing appreciation of the anatomy and regions of blood flow simultaneously.

INTERFERING FACTORS

AIR

Subcutaneous air or skin wounds and defects may impede good transducer coupling and beam transmission. However, these are encountered infrequently.

Gas-filled GI tract can be a major barrier to a complete examination of the abdomen. Intestinal segments filled or dilated with gas will prevent many organs from being visualized. Furthermore, the mesentery and small lymph nodes may not be visualized. Excitement, aerophagia, or gastroenteritis may lead to such situations.

BARIUM

This should not be administered prior to ultrasonography because barium will prevent beam transmission, making some regions of the abdomen and GI tract not visible.

HAIR

This is a major barrier to transmission of the ultrasound beam. Even small amounts of hair left after clipping may cause interference. Wetting with alcohol (<70%) will help improve coupling.

OBESITY

A large amount of subcutaneous and intra-abdominal fat may greatly reduce image quality. Low-frequency transducers are required, and image resolution is low. In some obese patients, intracavitary ultrasound examination using endoscopic probes is required. Otherwise, computed tomography is a good alternative for abdominal and thoracic imaging in obese patients.

PAIN

Patients with acute abdomen are difficult to examine with ultrasound because of constant abdominal pressing as a reaction to pain or discomfort. Examining some patients may be impossible under these circumstances. Premedication with analgesics is often indicated to enable the examination to be performed.

PANTING OR PATIENT MOTION

Heavy breathing, panting, and movement in uncooperative patients make the examination frustrating and oftentimes short and incomplete. Sedation may be required if panting or fractious behavior cannot be controlled.

ARTIFACTS

The ultrasound examination produces more artifacts than conventional radiography, so it is important to recognize common artifacts to interpret images properly. Artifacts may cause misrepresentation of normal structures. However, some artifacts can also be helpful, aiding the sonographer in recognition of certain structures or abnormalities. These artifacts are commonly encountered:

REVERBERATION

When the sound beam encounters highly reflective structures, the echoes are reflected back and forth between the transducer and the reflective areas. This is commonly seen with gas-filled structures and results in regularly occurring hyperechoic regions distal to the origin of the artifact. Structures distal to gas-filled intestines are, therefore, difficult to assess.

MIRROR IMAGE

The liver is often seen on the monitor as a mirror image of itself on the opposite side of the diaphragm. This occurs because the diaphragm is a highly reflective surface, which causes the ultrasound beam to be bounced back and forth between it and the liver. These echoes take longer to travel back to the transducer and are therefore positioned deeper on the image than they actually are.

ACOUSTIC ENHANCEMENT

An ultrasound beam that passes though a fluid-filled structure is not attenuated to the same degree as one that passes through solid structures. Therefore, the intensity of the signal distal to the gallbladder, for example, is greater and that region in the liver will appear hyperechoic compared to the neighboring parenchyma.

SHADOWING

Decreased echogenicity occurs distal to objects that are highly reflective such that the beam is either completely reflected or absorbed, resulting in a loss in the signal of the returning echo. This can occur distal to mineralized structures in the soft tissues or uroliths or in gas or solid foreign material (wood, plastic, synthetics).

SLICE-THICKNESS ARTIFACT

Since the thickness of the ultrasound beam creates the image slice, different parts of the same object are recorded as being from the same section. In the urinary bladder, this may appear as hyperechoic sediment within the lumen, although the echoes are actually originating from the urinary bladder wall.

POTENTIAL COMPLICATIONS

Complications from performing routine ultrasound examinations in the diagnostic frequency ranges do not occur. Unstable patients, especially those with pain or respiratory difficulty, may not be able to withstand a lengthy examination. Furthermore, examining such patients in conventional positions may not be possible. Patients with dyspnea may need to be in sternal recumbency for examination of the thorax.

Interventional procedures may cause minor bleeding. Prior to biopsy procedures, the coagulation status of the patients should be verified.

DOCUMENTATION

The ultrasound examination requires documentation for purposes of record keeping and reporting. Unlike the radiograph, which can be archived and reevaluated by another individual years later, the ultrasound examination is more difficult to preserve in its entirety. A written summary of the findings and diagnoses should be archived either electronically or as hard copies in the patient records. Electronic archiving in a Picture Archiving Communications System (PACS) is becoming more common in veterinary practice since the advent of digital imaging technology. Modern ultrasound equipment generally enables images and video clips to be stored as Diagnostic Image and Communications in Medicine (DICOM) files for storage in a PACS. Backup of the information on these storage devices is necessary.

Images can also be printed out and stored in the patient records. Static ultrasound images are difficult to interpret because they represent only a small part of the entire exam. Video documentation is preferable for reviewing the full examination at a later date. Video libraries, however, require good organization and space to maintain them and retrieve studies easily. Electronic storage of multiple image frames as a clip is preferable because it takes up less space than a video library.

SAFETY

Abdominal and thoracic diagnostic ultrasound procedures with commercially available equipment and diagnostic frequency ranges have not been associated with health-related problems. The procedures are safe and noninvasive.

AUTHOR NAME

Lorrie Gaschen

ABDOMINAL RADIOGRAPHY

BASICS

TYPE OF PROCEDURE
Radiographic

PROCEDURE EXPLANATION AND RELATED PHYSIOLOGY
The procedure consists of 2 orthogonal projections of the abdomen, right or left lateral and ventrodorsal (VD) projections. These projections include the structures from the cranial-most aspect of the diaphragm to the pelvic inlet. Radiographic techniques are based on patient thickness. The patient's hind legs are gently pulled caudally to avoid their superimposition on the caudal abdomen and to spread out the abdominal contents. Abdominal radiographs are made at full respiratory expiration.

INDICATIONS
• To confirm or differentiate cause of clinical signs referable to abdominal organs. Vomiting and diarrhea are most common.
• To determine origin of palpable abdominal mass.
• To determine the extent of abdominal disease, including metastasis evaluation.

CONTRAINDICATIONS
None

POTENTIAL COMPLICATIONS
None

CLIENT EDUCATION
• Ideally, food is withheld from the patients for 12–24 h, and an enema is administered before the radiographs are made.
• Sedation may be required.

BODY SYSTEMS ASSESSED
• Cardiovascular
• Endocrine and metabolic
• Gastrointestinal
• Hemic, lymphatic, and immune
• Hepatobiliary
• Renal and urologic
• Reproductive

PROCEDURE

PATIENT PREPARATION
Preprocedure Medication or Preparation
• Food is withheld from the patient for 12–24 h before imaging.
• An enema is ideally administered 1–2 h before the radiographs are made.
• *Note*: Withholding food and administering enemas are not always practical.

Anesthesia or Sedation
As needed. Some sedatives will affect GI motility (see Hall & Watrous 2000).

Patient Positioning
• Lateral projections: left or right lateral recumbency. The hind legs are gently extended caudally to minimize superimposition on the caudal abdomen.
• VD projection: dorsal recumbency. The hind legs are gently extended caudally to minimize superimposition on the caudal abdomen.

Patient Monitoring
N/A

Equipment or Supplies
• X-ray machine
• X-ray cassette loaded with film or digital x-ray detector
• Grid—for animals that are >10 cm thick
• Patient restraint devices—tape and sand bags—help minimize radiation exposure to personnel.

TECHNIQUE
• This consists of 2 orthogonal projections of the abdomen, right or left lateral and VD projections. These projections include the structures from the cranial-most aspect of the diaphragm to the pelvic inlet. Radiographic techniques are based on patient thickness. The patient's hind legs are gently pulled caudally to avoid their superimposition on the caudal abdomen and to spread out the abdominal contents. Abdominal radiographs are produced at full respiratory expiration.

SAMPLE HANDLING
N/A

APPROPRIATE AFTERCARE
Postprocedure Patient Monitoring
None

Nursing Care
None

Dietary Modification
None

Medication Requirements
None

Restrictions on Activity
None

Anticipated Recovery Time
Recovery is immediate or determined by the sedative used.

INTERPRETATION

NORMAL FINDINGS OR RANGE
• Use a systematic technique for interpreting abdominal radiographs. Some organs are seen routinely. Others are not seen routinely and should be considered every time an abdominal radiograph is interpreted.

- Abdominal organs normally seen: liver, stomach, spleen, kidneys, urinary bladder, prostate, and intestines.
- Abdominal organs not normally seen: ureters, urethra, ovaries, pancreas, and lymph nodes.

ABNORMAL VALUES
Peritoneal Cavity
- Normal appearance: Margins of abdominal organs are discernible. Many structures overlie each other, partially obscuring organ margins.
- Radiographic abnormality: decreased serosal margin detail. The abdomen has homogeneous, soft tissue opacity. Abdominal organs are not discernible from one another. They may be diffuse or focal.
  - Causes
    - Normal condition: young animal
    - Abnormal conditions: peritoneal effusion, lack of intra-abdominal fat, emaciation
  - Plan
    - Abdominal ultrasound, abdominocentesis (if peritoneal effusion present)
- Radiographic abnormality: increased serosal margin detail (pneumoperitoneum). Gas in the peritoneal cavity enhances visualization of abdominal organs.
  - Causes
    - Postoperatively, gas remains in peritoneal cavity for 3–5 days. Gas may persist for 2 weeks.
    - Ruptured GI tract: usually a surgical emergency
    - Penetrating abdominal wall wound
  - Plan
    - Horizontal beam radiography to confirm pneumoperitoneum

Abdominal Masses
- Normal appearance: no abdominal masses
- Radiographic abnormality: Masses are usually soft tissue opaque and cause displacement of adjacent organs, especially intestinal displacement. One can divide the abdomen into regions and determine the potential origin of an abdominal mass by what should normally be present in that region. The regions are cranial, middle, caudal, dorsal, ventral, left, and right.
  - Causes
    - Neoplasia, hyperplasia, abscess, hematoma
  - Plan
    - Abdominal ultrasound, contrast procedures (upper GI, excretory urogram, cystogram, etc.), FNA, or biopsy

Organs Normally Seen on Abdominal Radiographs
Liver
- Normal appearance: homogeneous soft tissue opacity caudal to the diaphragm and cranial to the stomach. Liver size is usually determined by the position of the stomach. On the lateral projection, the stomach should be parallel to the intercostal spaces.
- Radiographic abnormality: Hepatomegaly causes caudal displacement of gastric axis. The pylorus is displaced caudodorsally on lateral projections, and the stomach is displaces caudally on VD projections. Involvement may be diffuse or focal.

- Causes
  - Diffuse: fat or glycogen infiltration, neoplasia (primary or metastatic), hepatic congestion (right heart failure), hepatitis
  - Focal: neoplasia (primary or metastatic), cysts, abscess, nodular hyperplasia
- Plan
  - Abdominal ultrasound, FNA, or biopsy
- Radiographic abnormality: Microhepatica causes cranial displacement of gastric axis and allows cranial displacement of stomach on VD projection. The liver is typically 1 intercostal space wide.
  - Causes
    - Portosystemic shunt
    - Cirrhosis
  - Plan
    - Transsplenic nuclear portography, positive-contrast portography

Stomach
- Normal appearance: The stomach has various appearances based on its contents. The stomach usually contains gas and fluid (soft tissue) and may contain mineral. The stomach size is varied based on the amount of material within its lumen. The stomach can distend quite remarkably, so it is often warranted to reradiograph the animal several hours later to gauge the degree of gastric emptying and determine whether the gastric enlargement was due to pathology or physiology.
- Radiographic abnormality: gastric dilation—gas, fluid, ingesta, or a combination. The pylorus remains in the right cranioventral aspect of the abdomen. The enlarged stomach causes caudal displacement of abdominal organs, except the liver.
  - Causes
    - A recent meal will cause gastric distention that resolves with time.
    - Aerophagia
- Radiographic abnormality: GDV. The pylorus is rotated into the left craniodorsal aspect of the abdomen. The stomach is usually compartmentalized. The spleen is often malpositioned, too. The enlarged stomach causes caudal displacement of abdominal organs, except the liver.
- Radiographic abnormality: gastric outflow obstruction—fluid or ingesta or both. The stomach size is based on degree of outflow obstruction. The diagnosis is made using serial abdominal radiographs while withholding food from the animal. Alternatively, an upper GI exam is performed.
  - Causes
    - Hypertrophic pyloric stenosis, pylorospasm, pyloric inflammation or fibrosis, neoplasia
  - Plan
    - Positive-contrast gastrogram, gastric ultrasound, endoscopy
- Radiographic abnormality: gastric foreign body—various opacities. Metallic and mineral foreign bodies are easiest to detect. Soft tissue foreign bodies silhouette with gastric fluid.

- Plan
  - A positive- or a negative-contrast gastrogram is useful for evaluation of a nonmetal gastric foreign body.
- Radiographic abnormality: gastric wall abnormalities. Survey abdominal radiographs are not useful for evaluation of the gastric wall. Gastric fluid and the stomach wall silhouette make determination of gastric wall thickness very inaccurate.
  - Causes
    - Neoplasia, inflammation, fibrosis
  - Plan
    - Positive contrast gastrogram, gastric ultrasonography

Spleen
- Normal appearance: homogeneous soft tissue opacity. The head of the spleen is in the left dorsal abdomen, slightly caudolateral to the stomach. The body and tail of the spleen are fairly mobile and may be located anywhere between the stomach and urinary bladder.
- Radiographic abnormality: generalized splenomegaly. The spleen retains its normal shape while increasing its size.
  - Causes
    - Physiologic, drugs, neoplasia, congestion, hemolytic anemia, infections
- Radiographic abnormality: focal enlargement—creates a soft tissue abdominal mass effect. The mass may be anywhere in the abdomen between the liver and urinary bladder.
  - Causes
    - Hematoma, hyperplasia, neoplasia, abscess (often contains gas)
  - Plan
  - Splenic ultrasonography with or without FNA

Kidneys
- Normal appearance: bean-shaped, homogeneous soft tissue opacities in the right and left middorsal abdomen, respectively. The kidneys are in the retroperitoneal space.
- Radiographic sign: normal size and shape
  - Causes
    - Normal
    - Possible diseases: amyloidosis, glomerulonephritis, acute pyelonephritis, familial renal disease
- Radiographic abnormality: normal size, irregular shape
  - Causes
    - Focal: infarct, abscess
    - Diffuse: chronic pyelonephritis, polycystic kidney disease, tubulointerstitial disease, or glomerular disease
- Radiographic abnormality: small, regular shape
  - Causes
    - Hypoplasia, glomerulonephritis, amyloidosis, familial renal disease
- Radiographic abnormality: small, irregular shape
  - Causes
    - End-stage renal disease, renal dysplasia
- Radiographic abnormality: large, regular shape
  - Causes

- Compensatory hypertrophy, lymphoma, hydronephrosis, *Dioctophyma renale* (giant kidney worm), amyloidosis, glomerulonephritis, perirenal pseudocyst, solitary cyst
- Radiographic abnormality: large, irregular shape
  - Causes
    - Focal: primary tumor, metastatic tumor, hematoma
    - Diffuse: polycystic kidney disease, FIP, lymphoma
- Radiographic abnormality: renal mineralization
  - Causes
    - Nephrocalcinosis: diffuse mineralization of the renal parenchyma
    - Hyperadrenocorticism, hyperparathyroidism, hypercalcemia, ethylene glycol toxicity, renal tubular defects, hypervitaminosis D, chronic renal failure
    - Renal calculi: found in the renal pelvis
    - Diverticular mineralization: linear mineralization in the middle to peripheral aspect of the kidney
  - Plan
    - Renal ultrasonography, excretory urography, FNA, biopsy

Urinary Bladder
- Normal appearance: teardrop-shaped soft tissue opacity in caudoventral abdomen
- Radiographic abnormality: urinary bladder not seen
  - Causes
    - Normal empty bladder, displaced (hernia), hypoplastic (usually associated with ectopic ureters)
    - Peritoneal effusion
    - Emaciation
    - Ruptured urinary bladder
- Radiographic abnormality: abnormal shape
  - Causes
    - Impingement from abdominal mass
    - Urachal diverticulum
- Radiographic abnormality: enlarged urinary bladder
  - Causes
    - Need to urinate
    - Bladder neck obstruction (calculus, neoplasia, functional)
    - Neurogenic atony
- Radiographic abnormality: increased opacity
  - Cause
    - Calculi
- Radiographic abnormality: decreased opacity
  - Causes
    - Luminal gas: iatrogenic (cystocentesis, catheterization)
    - Mural gas: emphysematous cystitis (gas-producing bacteria secondary to diabetes mellitus)
- Radiographic abnormality: urinary bladder wall abnormalities. Survey abdominal radiographs are not useful for evaluation of the urinary bladder wall. The urine and the urinary bladder wall silhouette making determination of urinary bladder wall thickness very inaccurate.

- Plan
  - Urinary bladder sonography, cystography (positive, negative, double contrast)

Prostate Gland
- Normal appearance: round, soft tissue opacity ventral to the colon and cranial to or within the pelvic canal
- Radiographic abnormality: soft tissue enlargement that causes cranial displacement of the urinary bladder and dorsal displacement or compression of the colon
  - Causes
    - Benign prostatic hyperplasia, prostatitis, neoplasia, prostatic cyst
- Radiographic abnormality: small prostate
  - Cause
    - Secondary to castration
- Radiographic abnormality: mineralization
  - Causes
    - Neoplasia, calculus in prostatic urethra, chronic prostatitis

Small Intestine
- Normal appearance: tubular soft tissue opacity with various amounts of gas or mineral or both. The diameter of the small intestines varies with peristalsis.
- *Important*: Intestinal wall thickness cannot be determined by using survey radiographs. The intestinal fluid silhouettes with the intestinal wall. To determine wall thickness, perform an upper GI or intestinal ultrasonography.
- Radiographic abnormality: diameter of intestine excessively increased
  - Dogs: Normal intestinal diameter should not exceed the height of the central aspect of a lumbar vertebral body or should not be >50% larger than adjacent bowel.
  - Cats: Normal intestinal diameter should not exceed twice the height of the central aspect L4 vertebral body or 12 mm.
  - Degree of dilation depends on the cause of ileus, lesion location, and lesion extent.
  - *Remember*: Intestines are dynamic. Repeat radiographs of the animal made 2–12 h later will help evaluate the importance of intestinal size. Segments remaining enlarged on subsequent films have a higher likelihood of being truly obstructed.
  - Causes of intestinal obstruction (ileus)
    - Mechanical (obstructive, dynamic): intraluminal (foreign bodies, enteroliths, parasites), mural (neoplasia, granulomas, stricture), extramural (compression by mass, hernia entrapment), volvulus, intussusception
    - Paralytic (functional, adynamic): peritonitis, severe viral enteritis (parvovirus), bowel infarction, postoperative
    - Linear foreign body: intestines will plicate or pleat on a foreign body; abnormal pockets of gas within the intestines. Intestines are bunched with multiple, sharp, hairpin turns.

- Plan
  - Upper GI (use iodinated contrast medium if intestinal perforation suspected), intestinal ultrasonography, endoscopy

Large Intestine
- Normal appearance: tubular, soft tissue opacity with various amounts of gas, mineral, or both
- *Important*: Intestinal wall thickness cannot be determined by using survey radiographs. The intestinal fluid silhouettes with the intestinal wall. To determine wall thickness, perform a barium enema or intestinal ultrasonography.
- Radiographic abnormality: abnormal dilation of the colon. Normally, the colon should not be greater than length of L7 or 3 times the width of small intestine. Fecal material usually is mineral opaque because of inspissation.
  - Causes
    - Chronic constipation or obstipation, pelvic canal narrowing (stricture, neoplasia, pelvic fractures), neurologic disease, idiopathic.

Organs Not Normally Seen on Abdominal Radiographs
Pancreas
- Radiographic abnormalities: increased soft tissue opacity (focal peritoneal effusion) in the right cranial abdomen; displacement of the duodenum to right and the stomach antrum to left; persistent, mild gas dilation of the proximal duodenum
  - Cause
    - Pancreatitis
- Radiographic abnormality: A soft tissue mass effect in right cranial abdomen displaces the duodenum to right and the stomach to left.
  - Cause
    - Neoplasia
  - Plan
    - Pancreatic sonography, CT

Adrenal Glands
- Radiographic abnormality: increased mineral craniomedial to a kidney
  - Cause
    - Mineralization
- Radiographic abnormality: a soft tissue mass craniomedial to a kidney
  - Cause
    - Neoplasia, adenoma, hypertrophy as found with hyperadrenocortism
  - Plan
    - Adrenal gland sonography, CT

Ureters
- Radiographic abnormality: focal mineral opacity in the caudodorsal abdomen between the kidneys and the neck of the urinary bladder

ABDOMINAL RADIOGRAPHY

- Cause
  - Ureteral calculus
- Radiographic abnormality: a tortuous, tubular soft tissue opacity in caudodorsal abdomen
  - Cause
    - Ureteral obstruction (calculus, neoplasia, urinary bladder abnormality, iatrogenic after surgery)
  - Plan
    - Urinary sonography, excretory urogram, CT

Urethra
- Normal appearance: silhouettes with the surrounding soft tissues. To evaluate the entire urethra, include the perineal region. For male dogs, pull their hind limbs cranially on a supplemental lateral projection that includes the perineal region.
- Radiographic abnormality: focal mineral opacity
  - Cause
    - Calculi, frequently lodged at the base of os penis

Uterus
- Radiographic abnormality: a tubular soft tissue mass between the urinary bladder and the colon
  - Causes
    - Pyometra, early pregnancy
- Radiographic abnormality: a tubular soft tissue mass in the caudal abdomen with mineralization (fetuses)
  - Cause
    - Pregnancy
- Radiographic abnormalities: gas within the uterus or any part of the fetus, overlapping the fetal skull bones, lysis of the fetal skeleton, abnormal fetal spine angulation
  - Cause
    - Fetal death
  - Plan
    - Uterine ultrasonography

Lymph Nodes
- Radiographic abnormality: soft tissue mass effect, displacing adjacent organs in the following locations. Mesenteric lymph nodes are in central abdomen. Sublumbar lymph nodes are ventral to L6-sacrum and dorsal to colon.
  - Causes
    - Neoplasia (lymphoma), reactivity
  - Plan
    - Abdominal sonography, CT

CRITICAL VALUES
- Pneumoperitoneum in an animal that has not had recent surgery
- GDV
- GI obstruction

INTERFERING FACTORS
Drugs That May Alter Results of the Procedure
GI modulating drugs (Hall & Watrous 2000)

Conditions That May Interfere with Performing the Procedure
None

Procedure Techniques or Handling That May Alter Results
- None

Influence of Signalment on Performing and Interpreting the Procedure

Species
None

Breed
None

Age
None

Gender
None

Pregnancy
None

CLINICAL PERSPECTIVE
Abdominal ultrasound is not a substitute for abdominal radiography and vice versa. By the use of abdominal radiographs, the spatial relationship of the abdominal organs is maintained. For intestinal obstruction, the size of the intestines is evaluated better by using radiographs because one can compare various segments of bowel to one another. Using ultrasound, it is not possible to visualize the entire abdomen on 1 image. The strengths of abdominal ultrasound are the characterization of organ internal architecture and evaluation of abdominal structures not normally seen on radiographs (e.g., adrenal glands). Abdominal CT is an emerging imaging modality for veterinary medicine. By using CT, the spatial relationship of the abdominal organs can be understood and information gained about the internal architecture of these organs.

MISCELLANEOUS

ANCILLARY TESTS
The tests used depend on the abnormality. Plans are provided in the foregoing text.

SYNONYMS
None

SEE ALSO
Blackwell's Five-Minute Veterinary Consult: Canine and Feline Topics
Many

Related Topics in This Book
- General Principles of Radiography
- Abdominal Ultrasonography
- Abdominocentesis and Fluid Analysis
- Adrenal Ultrasonography
- Barium-Impregnated Polyethylene Spheres (BIPS)
- Computed Tomography
- Cystourethrography (male, female, canine, feline)
- Excretory Urography
- Gastrointestinal Ultrasonography
- Horizontal Beam Radiography
- Liver and Gallbladder Ultrasonography (including portohepatic shunts)
- Lower Gastrointestinal Radiographic Contrast Studies (includes air and barium)
- Lower Urinary Tract Ultrasonography (bladder, prostate, urethra)
- Pancreatic Ultrasonography
- Renal Ultrasonography (including comments on ureters)
- Splenic Ultrasonography
- Ultrasound-Guided Mass or Organ Aspiration
- Upper Gastrointestinal Radiographic Contrast Studies (including pneumogastrogram)
- Uterine Ultrasonography
- Vaginography

ABBREVIATIONS
- CT = computed tomography
- FNA = fine-needle aspiration
- GDV = gastric dilatation and volvulus syndrome
- VD = ventrodorsal

Suggested Reading
Burk RL, Ackerman N, eds. *Small Animal Radiology and Ultrasonography: A Diagnostic Atlas and Text,* 2nd ed. Philadelphia: WB Saunders, 1996.
Hall SA, Watrous BA. Effect of pharmaceuticals on radiographic appearance of selected examinations of the abdomen and thorax. *Vet Clin North Am Small Anim Pract* 2000; 30: 349–378.
O'Brien TR. *Radiographic Diagnosis of Abdominal Disorders in the Dog and Cat.* Philadelphia: WB Saunders, 1978.
Owens JM, Biery DN. *Radiographic Interpretation for the Small Animal Clinician,* 2nd ed. Baltimore: Williams & Wilkins, 1999.
Thrall DE, ed. *Textbook of Veterinary Diagnostic Radiology, 5th ed.* Philadelphia: WB Saunders, 2007.

INTERNET RESOURCES
None

AUTHOR NAME
Wm Tod Drost

ABDOMINAL ULTRASONOGRAPHY

 BASICS

TYPE OF PROCEDURE
Ultrasonographic

PROCEDURE EXPLANATION AND RELATED PHYSIOLOGY
Abdominal ultrasound is an extremely useful diagnostic tool because it enables noninvasive evaluation of the internal structure of the abdominal organs and ultimately provides a means to obtain etiologic information through percutaneous aspiration. In many instances, ultrasound examination has virtually replaced the need for special radiographic procedures such as negative-contrast peritoneography, excretory urography, and GI contrast studies.

INDICATIONS
- Suspected abnormalities involving the abdominal structures based on physical examination, clinical pathologic examination, or abdominal survey radiography. For example,
  - Hepatomegaly, hepatic mass, or increased liver enzyme activity or bilirubin concentration
  - Splenomegaly or splenic mass
  - Renomegaly, small kidneys, renal masses, proteinuria, or renal insufficiency or failure
  - Stranguria, pollakiuria, or urinary incontinence
  - Vomiting, diarrhea, or both
  - Ascites
- Evaluation for primary or metastatic neoplasia

CONTRAINDICATIONS
None

POTENTIAL COMPLICATIONS
None

CLIENT EDUCATION
- This is a noninvasive study and is tolerated well by most animals.
- Withholding food is helpful to improve the quality of the study.
- The hair must be clipped in the area to be imaged in order to obtain a diagnostic examination.

BODY SYSTEMS ASSESSED
- Endocrine and metabolic
- Gastrointestinal
- Hemic, lymphatic, and immune
- Hepatobiliary
- Renal and urologic
- Reproductive

 PROCEDURE

PATIENT PREPARATION
Preprocedure Medication or Preparation
- Withhold food for 12 h prior to examination to improve quality of the study.
- Removal of hair over the ventral abdomen, if scanning in ventrodorsal recumbency, or toward the spine, if scanning from a lateral aspect, is necessary in order to visualize all structures (kidneys, adrenal glands, etc.).

Anesthesia or Sedation
Most examinations may be performed without the animal being under any sedation or general anesthesia. However, these may be required for animals that are anxious or in pain. Sedate or place an animal under general anesthesia as needed to control its motion.

Patient Positioning
Animals may be scanned in ventrodorsal or lateral recumbency.

Patient Monitoring
None

Equipment or Supplies
- Ultrasound machine
- Initial scanning is usually performed using the highest-frequency transducer possible. A sector/vector transducer is useful because it enables a broad view of the organs being imaged. Also, sector/vector transducers usually have a relatively small footprint, which makes it easier to maintain good contact (see Figure 1). The following can be used as a general guideline:
  - 7–10 MHz (or higher)—cats and small dogs
  - 5 MHz—medium-sized dogs [30–100 lb (13.5–45.5 kg)]
  - 3 MHz—large or giant dogs
- An appropriate transducer for patient imaging
- A linear format best for near-field imaging
- A sector/vector format best for overall imaging
- High frequency (>7.5 MHz) best for resolution
- Low frequency (<7.5 MHz) best for penetration
- Clippers to remove hair
- Acoustic coupling gel

TECHNIQUE
Each of the major organs should be as completely evaluated as possible. This includes imaging all organs in 2 planes. The sagittal plane splits the view of the animal into 2 parts running along or parallel to the spine. All sagittal or parasagittal images should be oriented so that the cranial portion of the patient's body is toward the left side of the image. The transverse plane is 90° to the sagittal plane. Transverse images should be oriented with the left side of the animal to the right side of the screen. If these orientations are maintained, the primary transducer movement will be rotating the transducer 90° from a sagittal plane (counterclockwise) and back clockwise from a transverse plane. Also, if the transducer is moved from the ventral aspect of the abdomen laterally toward the dorsum, the dorsal planes will be properly oriented (see Figures 2 and 3). (Select images of these organs may be found in their respective chapters.)

Liver
The liver can be found by placing the transducer immediately caudal to the xiphoid and pointing the probe cranially. Significant pressure may be required in order to visualize the liver particularly in larger patients. The probe is pointed or fanned or moved slightly across the abdominal surface in order to visualize the entire liver. In patients with a deep-chested conformation or a small liver, an intercostal approach may be necessary (place the probe between the ribs toward the ventral aspect).

Spleen
The size may vary significantly especially in dogs. The head of the spleen is always found just caudolateral to the stomach. The tail may be located along the left body wall or may move around the ventral abdomen.

Kidneys
In dogs, the left kidney is located in the middorsal abdomen and is often found medial to the spleen. The right kidney is found in the fossa of the caudate liver lobe, and 1 technique for visualization is to follow the costal arch along the right side until kidney is identified. The right kidney is usually located deeper than the left kidney. In cats, the kidneys often have long pedicles and are mobile. Excessive transducer pressure may push the kidneys and make them difficult to identify. Minimal pressure is typically required when imaging cats.

Urinary Bladder
The urinary bladder is found ventral to the colon (and uterus in females). Its size is variable. Transducer pressure should be light to avoid completely compressing the bladder if it is small. Typically, the midcaudal abdomen is searched for until a fluid filled structure is found.

Prostate
The prostate is best identified by first finding the neck of the urinary bladder. Once midline is identified, the transducer is then pointed caudally into the pelvic inlet. If the prostate is abdominal or in the cranial pelvic inlet, it should be identified in this manner.

Uterus
The uterus, which is found by first identifying the urinary bladder, is typically found dorsal or dorsolateral to the bladder. It is easiest to find

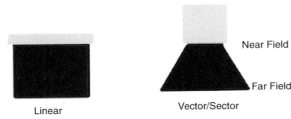

Near Field

Far Field

Linear   Vector/Sector

Figure 1

This diagram depicts the general image shape that is formed by the linear vs sector/vector format. Notice that the image is wider in the far field for the vector/sector format. This allows for a more overall view of these deeper structures and is usually used for initial imaging of the patient. The linear format is better for evaluation of more specific areas.

initially in a transverse plane and will appear as a circular structure adjacent to the urinary bladder.

Pancreas
The right limb of the pancreas is typically found by identifying the descending duodenum in the right cranial abdomen. The duodenum is the most lateral loop of small intestine and typically is seen ventral to the right kidney. The pancreas will be adjacent to the duodenum. Visualization of the body and the left limb of the pancreas may be variable particularly with large amounts of gastric gas.

Adrenal Glands
The left adrenal gland is found by first identifying the cranial pole of the left kidney in a sagittal plane. The transducer is then fanned medially until the aorta is identified. The left adrenal gland will be seen adjacent to the aorta just cranial to the left renal artery. A slight clockwise rotation of the transducer usually produces an elongated view of the adrenal gland. To identify the right adrenal gland, the cranial pole of the right kidney is first located in a sagittal plane. The probe is then fanned medially until the caudal vena cava is identified. The ultrasound beam is then fanned slightly laterally to identify the right adrenal gland.

SAMPLE HANDLING
N/A

APPROPRIATE AFTERCARE
Postprocedure Patient Monitoring
N/A

Nursing Care
N/A

Dietary Modification
N/A

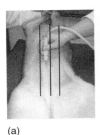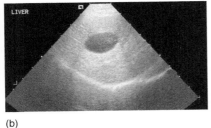

(a)   (b)

Figure 2

A: Orientation of the ultrasound probe in a sagittal and parasagittal planes is indicated by the *black lines*. The probe must be oriented so that the patient's head is projected to the left of the image and the patient's tail is oriented to the right of the screen. **B:** This parasagittal image of the liver shows the normal orientation.

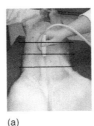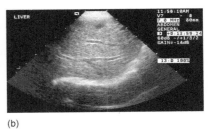

(a)   (b)

Figure 3

A: Orientation of the ultrasound probe in a transverse plane is indicated by the *black lines*. The probe must be oriented so that the patient's right side is projected to the left of the image and the left side of the patient is on the right side of the image. **B:** This is a transverse view of the left liver. The patient's left side is projected on the right side of the image and the right side is toward the left.

Medication Requirements
N/A

Restrictions on Activity
None

Anticipated Recovery Time
None

INTERPRETATION

NORMAL FINDINGS OR RANGE
• In general, sonographic interrogation can be used to evaluate the echotexture of a structure, as well as the margination and internal derangement of normal architecture. In the abdomen, the relative echogenicity of organs is a mainstay in evaluation. The common terminology would include (1) hyperechoic—bright strong echos, (2) hypoechoic—weak, dark echos, (3) isoechoic—structures of the same echogenicity (does not necessarily convey brightness or darkness), and (4) heterochoic—a combination of hyper- and hypoechogenicities. The spleen is the most echogenic organ, whereas the liver and renal cortex are of approximately the same echogenicity and are hypoechoic compared to the spleen.
• All organs should be evaluated in their entirety in 2 planes: sagittal and transverse. Additional imaging planes may be used as necessary. They should be assessed for size, margination, and changes in internal architecture.

Liver
The liver is bounded by the diaphragm cranially and the stomach caudally. The right kidney is adjacent to the caudate liver lobe. The falciform fat is typically found ventrally. Sonographically, the liver has a coarse uniform echotexture. The prominent vascular structures that are visualized are the portal veins (denoted by hyperechoic walls) and the hepatic veins (isoechoic walls). In normal dogs and cats, hepatic arteries and bile ducts are not visualized. The gallbladder is typically teardrop shaped and thin walled.

Spleen
Sonographically, the spleen has a uniform echotexture and is the most echogenic organ in the abdomen. Splenic veins can be easily seen entering the hilus. The capsular margin is normally smooth, with gradation of thickness from the extremities to the center.

Kidneys
The cortex and medulla can be seen distinctly. The cortex has a fine, homogeneous echotexture, which is approximately isoechoic to the liver. The medulla is anechoic to hypoechoic. The pelvis is usually filled with fat, with no dilation. There is no reliable method to evaluate kidney size

sonographically. In cats, a general rule is that the sagittal length should be approximately 4 cm.

Urinary Bladder
The wall is normally thin (<2–3 mm) and should have anechoic contents. In cats, the urine may contain some echoes, which may be clinically insignificant.

GI Tract
Visualization of the structures depends on the luminal contents and the amount of gas present. The duodenum is typically the most lateral loop of small intestine in the right cranial quadrant. The small intestine typically shows a laminar arrangement of the layers. The luminal or mucosal surface is hyperechoic. The next layer is the mucosa, which is hypoechoic. The next layer is the submucosa, which is hyperechoic. The muscularis is hypoechoic, and the outer layer is the serosa, which is hyperechoic. The typical, normal thickness of the stomach is 3–5 mm. The intestines are 2–3 mm thick (except the duodenum, which can be 1–2 mm thicker).

Prostate
The normal prostate is bilobed with a relatively uniform echotexture with the exception of the muscular fibers around the urethra as it traverses the prostate. Size is variable, depending on the reproductive status of the animal. Castrated dogs typically have a very small prostate, which may not be visible abdominally.

Uterus
The normal uterus will be completely collapsed. Fluid or material in the lumen may be pathologic or may be visualized, depending on the reproductive status of the patient.

Pancreas
In normal animals, the echogenicity of the pancreas may be similar to that of the surrounding fat. Visualization of the pancreaticoduodenal vessels can help in identification.

Adrenal Glands
The left gland is peanut shaped and has a cortex and a medulla. The right gland is arrow shaped.

ABNORMAL VALUES
Abnormalities can be reviewed in the individual chapters.

CRITICAL VALUES
None

INTERFERING FACTORS
Drugs That May Alter Results of the Procedure
Anesthesia and or sedation may alter GI motility. In addition, splenic size may vary, depending on the pharmaceuticals used.

Conditions That May Interfere with Performing the Procedure
• Free peritoneal gas
• Severe gas dilation of the GI tract
• Patient noncompliance (panting, dyspnea, struggling, resisting restraint)

Procedure Techniques or Handling That May Alter Results
None

Influence of Signalment on Performing and Interpreting the Procedure
Species
Larger dogs will require the use of lower-frequency transducers, which may impact the resolution and thus quality of the images. Better image quality is typically produced in smaller dogs and cats because of their small size and the capability of higher-frequency transducers with superior resolution being used.

Breed
None

Age
None

Gender
None

Pregnancy
Near-term pregnancy, particularly with large litter numbers, may preclude complete evaluation of the abdomen

CLINICAL PERSPECTIVE
• The significance of abdominal sonographic findings should be interpreted in conjunction with other diagnostic tests such as abdominal radiographs or laboratory data.
• Complete evaluation of all organs (as is possible) is recommended, even if clinical signs are referable to only 1 area, to decrease the chance of missing a clinically silent but significant finding.
• Negative findings on sonographic examination do not exclude the possibility of disease. Remember that ultrasound examination is operator dependent, but, more importantly, it is not specific, and additional tests or procedures are usually required for a final diagnosis.

MISCELLANEOUS

ANCILLARY TESTS
Ultrasound examination may be used to guide obtaining aspirates or biopsy samples of potential lesions.

SYNONYMS
Abdominal sonography

SEE ALSO
Blackwell's Five-Minute Veterinary Consult: Canine and Feline Topics
Many

Related Topics in This Book
• General Principles of Ultrasonography
• Adrenal Ultrasonography
• Gastrointestinal Ultrasonography
• Liver and Gallbladder Ultrasonography
• Pancreatic Ultrasonography
• Renal Ultrasonography
• Splenic Ultrasonography
• Ultrasound-Guided Mass or Organ Aspiration

ABBREVIATIONS
None

Suggested Reading
Mattoon JS, Auld DM, Nyland TG. Abdominal ultrasound scanning techniques. In: Nyland TG, Mattoon JS, eds. *Small Animal Diagnostic Ultrasound*, 2nd ed. Philadelphia: WB Saunders, 2002: 49–81.

INTERNET RESOURCES
None

AUTHOR NAME
Anne Bahr

BASICS

TYPE OF PROCEDURE
Diagnostic sample collection

PROCEDURE EXPLANATION AND RELATED PHYSIOLOGY
• Acute or chronic abdominal fluid accumulation complicates numerous intra-abdominal or extra-abdominal disease processes and traumas.
• To achieve a definitive diagnosis, abdominal fluid characterization is necessary to elucidate the primary disease process or pathophysiologic mechanism responsible for fluid accumulation.
• In the case of acute abdomen, abdominal fluid characterization will influence the therapeutic approach, such as the decision to perform emergency exploratory celiotomy.
• Abdominocentesis is the percutaneous removal of intra-abdominal fluid, most often for diagnostics purposes, although in some cases it is therapeutic.
• Blind abdominocentesis is easily performed when a large amount of fluid is present, and ultrasound-guided abdominocentesis is useful when the fluid volume is limited.
• Diagnostic peritoneal lavage (DPL) is most often used in acute settings, if 4-quadrant abdominocentesis has failed to yield any fluid or if undiagnosed intra-abdominal disease is suspected.
• Therapeutic abdominocentesis (e.g., to remove a large volume of ascites) can improve an animal's quality of life when used in addition to medical management.

INDICATIONS
• Intra-abdominal fluid accumulation detected upon physical examination (abdominal distention, positive fluid wave, slippery sensation) or diagnostic imaging (abdominal radiography or ultrasound)
• Blunt or penetrating abdominal trauma (e.g., dog bite, gunshot wound, car accident)
• Suspicion of ruptured bowel, peritonitis, or postoperative GI dehiscence
• Acute abdomen
• Persistent acute abdominal pain or shock without apparent cause
• DPL is indicated when it is suspected that intra-abdominal disease has remained undiagnosed (e.g., a limited amount of intra-abdominal fluid has led to false-negative 4-quadrant abdominocentesis).
• Therapeutic abdominocentesis is indicated when respiratory distress and patient discomfort result from large fluid volume, despite appropriate medical therapy.

CONTRAINDICATIONS
• There are few contraindications for abdominocentesis and DPL.
• The procedures should be performed with caution or are contraindicated if any of the following are present:
  • Dilated bowel loops, generalized ileus
  • Organomegaly
  • An enlarged uterus because of pregnancy or pyometra

• An uncharacterized large intra-abdominal mass is a contraindication for blind abdominocentesis.
• Avoid the use of DPL if diaphragmatic hernia, advanced coagulopathy or body wall adhesion is suspected.
• Avoid removing a large fluid volume quickly, especially without previous sodium restriction.

POTENTIAL COMPLICATIONS
• Laceration of abdominal organ (spleen, liver, tumor, vessels) with subsequent hemorrhage
• Perforation of a hollow viscus (bowel, bladder) and iatrogenic peritonitis (the bowel loops usually move away from the needle during puncture)
• Spreading of infection from a localized lesion (e.g., abscess, pyometra)
• Tearing of the catheter in the abdomen during removal, when using a fenestrated over-the-needle catheter

For DPL
• An increased risk of previously mentioned complications when compared with abdominocentesis
• Patient discomfort
• SC hematoma formation
• SC leakage of lavage fluid
• Serious complications of therapeutic abdominocentesis, such as hypovolemia and renal failure reported in some people after rapid removal of large volumes of abdominal fluid, have not been described in dogs with chronic hepatic failure. However, most clinicians avoid removing large volumes from animals that have a serum albumin of ≤2 g/dL.

CLIENT EDUCATION
• Abdominocentesis is a minimally invasive diagnostic procedure that is easy to perform and is associated with minimal risk and discomfort for the animal.
• Abdominocentesis is usually performed in awake patients, but sedation might be required if an animal is fractious or in pain.

BODY SYSTEMS ASSESSED
• Hepatobiliary
• Renal and urologic

PROCEDURE

PATIENT PREPARATION
Preprocedure Medication or Preparation
• The urinary bladder should be palpated and emptied if distended (void, manual expression, or urethral catheterization) prior to abdominocentesis or DPL.
• To avoid puncture, the size and position of the spleen should be noted via palpation.

ABDOMINOCENTESIS AND FLUID ANALYSIS

Anesthesia or Sedation
To prevent any unwanted motion that could increase the risk of organ puncture, sedation might be required if an animal is fractious or in pain. This needs to be tailored to the patient's general and cardiovascular condition (e.g., shock) and to the procedure (sedation may be needed for DPL).

Patient Positioning
The patient is positioned in left lateral recumbency (to prevent splenic puncture) or can remain standing to improve gravity-dependent fluid retrieval. However, any position that is comfortable for the animal and allows pooling of fluid is satisfactory.

Patient Monitoring
Patient monitoring (e.g., blood pressure and central venous pressure (CVP) measurement) needs to be tailored to an animal's general and cardiovascular condition.

Equipment or Supplies
- Clippers
- Surgical skin-preparation supplies [e.g., povidone-iodine (Betadine) scrub and solution, isopropyl alcohol]
- Sterile gloves
- Number 11 scalpel blade
- Appropriately sized syringe (3, 6, or 12 mL)
- Glass slides
- EDTA and serum tubes and Port-A-Cul vials

For Abdominocentesis
- Hypodermic 18-, 20-, to 22-gauge, 1- to 1 $1/2$-inch (25.4–38.1 mm) needle or alternatively an over-the-needle IV catheter in which side holes have been added with a scalpel blade. Use of a fenestrated catheter instead of needle might lower the incidence of certain complications. The added side holes should be small and smooth to prevent kinking and tearing of the catheter within the abdomen.
- Optional: an extension set mounted on the syringe.
- For therapeutic abdominocentesis, a 3-way stopcock and a 60-mL syringe.

For DPL
- A commercially available dialysis catheter [peritoneal lavage catheter (Global Veterinary Products, Waukesha, WI) and Argyle Turkel Safety Thoracocentesis System (Sherwood Davis and Geck, St. Louis, MO)] or alternatively a 20- to 14-gauge, over-the-needle, 1 $1/2$- to 2-inch (38.1–50.8 mm) IV catheter, fenestrated as described previously.
- A bag of warmed sterile isotonic saline solution with an IV perfusion set.
- A 12-mL syringe.
- A 3-way stopcock attached to an extension set (optional).

TECHNIQUE

Simple Needle Abdominocentesis
- The abdominocentesis site is just caudal to the umbilicus, on the ventral midline or slightly lateral to the right (2–3 cm in mid-sized dogs), unless the animal is standing, in which case the site would be at the most dependent part the abdomen.
- Hair is clipped on a 10×10-cm^2 area, and the skin is prepared aseptically.
- The needle, which is inserted through the skin and abdominal wall, may or may not be attached to the syringe.
  - If it is not attached to the syringe, collect the fluid into a sterile tube as it drips from the needle's hub.
  - If it is attached to the syringe, apply gentle suction with the syringe, and avoid vigorous suction to prevent a false-negative result (i.e., dry tap).
- Fluid is collected aseptically and submitted for relevant analysis. Usually a 10-mL sample is necessary for complete analysis.
- For therapeutic abdominocentesis, the extension set and 3-way stopcock are mounted on the catheter. Fluid is aspirated gently with the syringe and discarded subjectively until the abdomen feels less tense and the animal appears more comfortable.
- When using an over-the-needle catheter with added side holes, take care to remove the catheter completely by gently rotating it or dissecting it from the subcutaneous tissue.

Four-Quadrant Abdominocentesis
- The ventral surface of the abdomen is divided into 4 quadrants by an imaginary line that bisects the linea alba through the umbilicus.
- A small area (4–6 cm^2) of hair is shaved in each quadrant and the skin prepared aseptically.
- Each site is punctured and aspirated gently with a syringe.
- Repeat until fluid is retrieved or all 4 sites have been aspirated.
- In case of a negative tap, abdominal ultrasound, DPL, or both should be considered.

Ultrasound-Guided Abdominocentesis
- Ultrasonography is used to locate small volume or localized effusion.
- The hair is clipped on a 10×10-cm^2 area, and the skin is prepared aseptically.
- The needle mounted on a syringe is inserted under ultrasound guidance into the pocket of fluid and fluid is gently aspirated.
- Aspiration is stopped when sufficient fluid volume is collected.

Diagnostic Peritoneal Lavage (Closed Technique)
- Make any necessary abdominal radiographs or ultrasound before the procedure because DPL will alter the results.
- The site for DPL is 1–3 cm caudal to the umbilicus, on the midline or just right off the midline. Avoid using scarred areas from previous surgeries.

- The hair is clipped, and the skin is prepared aseptically.
- Infiltrate the skin and abdominal wall with enough local anesthetic (e.g., 2% lidocaine) to make a small bleb.
- At the catheter entry site, make a 0.5- to 1-cm stab incision through the skin with a number 11 scalpel blade.
- Thrust the catheter with stylet into the abdomen through the stab incision and abdominal wall.
- Remove the stylet and slide the catheter dorsocaudally into the abdomen.
- Once the catheter is in the abdomen, attach a syringe and aspirate gently. If fluid is retrieved, there is no need to pursue with lavage.
- In the absence of fluid, infuse 20–22 mL of warmed sterile isotonic saline solution per kilogram of body weight through the catheter via an IV infusion set with rapid gravity flow or by applying moderate pressure to the bag for 1–2 min.
- After completing the infusion, roll the animal gently from side to side to disperse the fluid and ballot the abdomen for 1–2 min, taking care not to dislodge the catheter.
- Lower the fluid bag to the floor and allow the fluid to drain into the bag or aspirate the catheter slowly with a syringe to remove a fluid sample. Most often, only a small portion of the instilled fluid is retrieved; the remaining fluid will be reabsorbed by the peritoneum.
- Lavage fluid is collected aseptically and submitted for relevant analysis.
- The catheter can remain in place temporarily for serial fluid evaluation (e.g., ongoing hemorrhage), if needed.
- Withdraw the catheter when sampling is complete, and suture the skin incision, if needed.

SAMPLE HANDLING
- Abdominal or lavage fluid is inspected macroscopically for clarity and color.
- Specific gravity is determined and total solids are quantified via refractometry.
- PCV is measured in hemorrhagic fluids by using a microhematocrit tube.
- Some fluid is processed for direct microscopic cytologic evaluation by smearing a small drop of fluid across a slide, allowing the smear to air-dry, and applying Romanovsky-type stain (Diff-Quick, Hema III, Giemsa, or Wright stain). For very cellular fluids (>50,000 cells/μL), cytologic evaluation of a direct smear is likely to be adequate.
- Abdominal fluid is split into aliquots and placed into the following:
  - An EDTA tube for cytologic evaluation, including RBCs and nucleated cell counts and differential, after concentration technique (if 2,000–50,000 cells/μL) or cytospin (if<2,000 cells/μL).

- A clot tube for biochemical analysis, depending on differential diagnoses. Analyses are performed simultaneously on fluid supernatant and blood. These should be evaluated for the given differential diagnoses:
  - Uroabdomen: creatinine, potassium
  - Bile peritonitis: bilirubin
  - Pancreatitis: lipase, amylase
  - Chyloabdomen: triglycerides, cholesterol
  - Septic peritonitis: glucose, lactate
  - FIP: protein electrophoresis
- A Port-A-Cul tube or a clot tub for aerobic and anaerobic bacterial culture, depending on clinical suspicion and fluid characteristics. Avoid the use of an EDTA tube because EDTA is bacteriostatic.

APPROPRIATE AFTERCARE
Postprocedure Patient Monitoring
Usually none for diagnostic abdominocentesis, but needs to be tailored to the patient's general and cardiovascular condition (e.g., shock)

Nursing Care
None

Dietary Modification
None

Medication Requirements
Adequate analgesia might be required following DLP.

Restrictions on Activity
Keep the patient cage rested, depending on the animal.

Anticipated Recovery Time
Recovery should be immediate.

INTERPRETATION
NORMAL FINDINGS OR RANGE
- Absence of free intra-abdominal fluid
- In normal dogs, the lavage fluid WBC count is <500–1,000 cells/μL.
- The postsurgery lavage fluid WBC count can be up to 10,000 cells/μL in dogs. Cytologic characteristics are more meaningful than cell count in differentiating septic vs nonseptic peritonitis.

ABNORMAL VALUES
- The presence of free intra-abdominal fluid
- Lavage fluid with >1,000 WBCs/μL or that is grossly abnormal (e.g., hemorrhagic, greenish, cloudy, purulent)

ABDOMINOCENTESIS AND FLUID ANALYSIS

- Depending on macroscopic appearance, specific gravity, protein content, cellularity, and cytologic findings, abdominal effusion is classified as pure transudate, modified transudate, and exudate (septic and nonseptic). Its etiology can sometimes be determined.

Additional Results for Specific Conditions
- Chyloabdomen: The concentration of abdominal fluid triglycerides is higher than the serum triglyceride concentration, and the fluid often contains a triglyceride concentration of >100 mg/dL.
- FIP: An abdominal fluid albumin/globulin ratio of <0.8 is highly suggestive of FIP.
- Hemoabdomen: The PCV of abdominal fluid is greater than the PCV of peripheral blood after a patient's peripheral volume has been restored. For DPL, the lavage fluid PCV is >2%–5% or if newsprint cannot be read through the lavage fluid and the volume of blood present in the abdomen is >2 mL/kg.
- Uroabdomen: The abdominal fluid creatinine concentration is higher than serum creatinine concentration (usually 2-fold greater in dogs). A similar result is obtained with potassium. In cats, the serum to abdominal fluid creatinine ratio and the serum to potassium ratio might be small. Comparatively, there is little to no difference between fluid and blood urea nitrogen.
- Bile peritonitis: The fluid bilirubin concentration is higher than that of serum, and extra- or intracellular bile pigment is usually found via cytologic examination.
- Pancreatitis: Higher fluid amylase and lipase concentrations than that of serum are suggestive of pancreatitis.
- Peritonitis: >1,000 WBCs/μL in lavage fluid
- Septic peritonitis: Cytologic findings include food fibers, degenerate neutrophils, and intracellular bacteria. The fluid lactate concentration is higher in septic vs nonseptic effusion. In dogs, a fluid lactate concentration of >2.5 mmol/L has a 100% sensitivity and a 91% specificity for diagnosing septic effusion. Also in dogs, a blood-to-fluid lactate difference of >2 mmol/L is 100% sensitive and specific for a diagnosis of septic effusion. Fluid lactate concentration is probably less reliable in cats. A blood-to-fluid glucose difference of >20 mg/dL is 100% sensitive and 100% specific for the diagnosis of septic peritoneal effusion in dogs and 86% sensitive and 100% specific for a diagnosis of septic peritonitis in cats.
- Eosinophilic effusion: >10% eosinophils in abdominal fluid, regardless of the protein content or cell count
- Aberrant cestodiasis infection: the presence of *Mesocestoides* spp. (motile cestodes seen with unaided eye or with microscopic examination) or calcareous corpuscles in abdominal fluid

CRITICAL VALUES
- After adequate cardiovascular resuscitation, the following conditions need immediate attention and might require exploratory celiotomy.
- Traumatic hemoabdomen
- Bacterial peritonitis
- Uroabdomen
- Bile peritonitis

INTERFERING FACTORS
Drugs That May Alter Results of the Procedure
Avoid sedative agents that can induce splenomegaly.

Conditions That May Interfere with Performing the Procedure
- If there is abdominal distention, differentiation between organomegaly, intra-abdominal fat accumulation (can appear to ripple on abdominal ballottement), and fluid accumulation should be made before abdominocentesis is performed.
- Previous surgeries may interfere with DPL.
- Differential diagnosis for false-negative abdominocentesis or DPL.
- Fluid quantity and technique used: Needle abdominocentesis detects an abdominal fluid volume of >5.2–6.6 mL/kg of body weight; a dialysis catheter, >1.0–4.4 mL/kg; and a catheter and lavage combination, 0.8 mL/kg.
- Flocculent fluid
- Fluid localized in a difficult access space (e.g., retroperitoneally).
- An early disease process that is <3–6h after injury. Repeating DPL 1–2h later might help in patients with an initial negative DPL and persistent abdominal pain.

Procedure Techniques or Handling That May Alter Results
- False-negative abdominocentesis or DPL can be caused by too vigorous suction being applied to the syringe, resulting in needle blockage by omentum or viscera.
- Differential diagnosis for false-positive DPL
- Hemoabdomen vs hemorrhage from traumatic sampling: In the absence of coagulopathy, blood from traumatic sampling will usually clot when exposed to an artificial surface, whereas effusion will not. Platelets are usually present in iatrogenic sample.
- Bacterial peritonitis vs bowel-loop puncture: Toxic degenerate neutrophils and intracellular bacteria are signs of bacterial peritonitis and are not present in bowel-loop puncture (usually bacteria and debris are present).

ABDOMINOCENTESIS AND FLUID ANALYSIS

Influence of Signalment on Performing and Interpreting the Procedure

Species
None

Breed
None

Age
None

Gender
None

Pregnancy
Relative contraindication because of an enlarged uterus

Clinical Perspective
- The principal disadvantage of abdominocentesis is its poor sensitivity (a low diagnostic accuracy rate of 47.3%) because of frequent false-negative results.
- The use of a fenestrated catheter versus a needle increases the likelihood of fluid retrieval (47.3% and 82.9%, respectively).
- Diagnostic accuracy is doubled by the use of DLP versus simple needle paracentesis (47.3% and 94.6%, respectively), although its interpretation might be more difficult because of dilution of the sample. The sensitivity of DLP provides clinicians with a >90% assurance of making the correct decision regarding surgical exploration in the animal with acute abdomen.

MISCELLANEOUS

ANCILLARY TESTS
- CBC, complete chemistry, and urinalysis to reach a definitive diagnosis and provide a patient's accurate hematologic and metabolic status.
- Abdominal ultrasonography to assess an organ's integrity and identify small fluid volume.
- Any additional testing that is deemed necessary upon history, physical examination, and fluid characteristics to determine the primary etiology of abdominal effusion (nonexhaustive list):
  - Chest radiography, echocardiogram, ECG, and heartworm test, if heart failure is suspected.
  - Chest radiography, if neoplasia is suspected.

- Contrast excretory urography or cystourethrogram to localize the site of rupture if uroabdomen is suspected.
- Tests of preprandial and postprandial serum bile acids if liver failure associated with portal hypertension is suspected.
- Biopsies, FIP serology, PCR testing, or a combination of these tests if FIP is suspected.

SYNONYMS
- Abdominal tap
- Abdominoparacentesis
- Coeliocentesis
- Intraperitoneal fluid aspiration
- Peritoneocentesis

SEE ALSO
Blackwell's Five-Minute Veterinary Consult: Canine and Feline
Topics
Ascites
Related Topics in This Book
Fluid Analysis

ABBREVIATIONS
DPL = diagnostic peritoneal lavage

Suggested Reading
Bjorling DE, Latimer KS, Rawlings CA, *et al.* Diagnostic peritoneal lavage before and after abdominal surgery in dogs. *Am J Vet Res* 1983; 44: 816–820.
Bonczynski JJ, Ludwig LL, Barton LJ, *et al.* Comparison of peritoneal fluid and peripheral blood pH, bicarbonate, glucose, and lactate concentration as a diagnostic tool for septic peritonitis in dogs and cats. *Vet Surg* 2003; 32: 161–166.
Connally HE. Cytology and fluid analysis of the acute abdomen. *Clin Tech Small Anim Pract* 2003; 18: 39–44.
Crowe DT. Diagnostic abdominal paracentesis techniques: Clinical evaluation in 129 dogs and cats. *J Am Anim Hosp Assoc* 1984; 20: 223–230.
Dye T. The acute abdomen: A surgeon's approach to diagnosis and treatment. *Clin Tech Small Anim Pract* 2003; 18: 53–65.
Levin GM, Bonczynski JJ, Ludwig LL, *et al.* Lactate as a diagnostic test for septic peritoneal effusions in dogs and cats. *J Am Anim Hosp Assoc* 2004; 40: 364371.

INTERNET RESOURCES
None

AUTHOR NAME
Karine Savary-Bataille

ACETYLCHOLINE RECEPTOR ANTIBODY

BASICS

TYPE OF SPECIMEN
Blood

TEST EXPLANATION AND RELATED PHYSIOLOGY
The acetylcholine receptor (AChR) antibody test by immunoprecipitation radioimmunoassay is the gold standard for the diagnosis of acquired, immune-mediated myasthenia gravis (MG). The nicotinic AChR plays a central role in neuromuscular transmission, and any disruption of structure or function can interfere with the overall control of muscle contraction and cause muscle weakness. Pathogenic autoantibodies bind muscle AChRs and destroy these receptors by various mechanisms, including cross-linking, complement activation, and increased internalization.

INDICATIONS
- Regurgitation from esophageal dilatation
- Generalized weakness
- Exercise intolerance
- Dysphagia
- Voice change
- Inability to blink
- Cranial mediastinal mass

CONTRAINDICATION
Chronic muscle atrophy

POTENTIAL COMPLICATIONS
None

CLIENT EDUCATION
- 12-h fast
- A negative AChR antibody titer does not completely rule out a diagnosis of acquired MG.

BODY SYSTEMS ASSESSED
- Gastrointestinal
- Neuromuscular
- Respiratory

SAMPLE

COLLECTION
1–2 mL of venous blood

HANDLING
- Red-top tube or serum-separator tube
- Separate serum from cells.

STORAGE
Refrigerate or freeze.

STABILITY
- 3–5 days at room temperature
- 1–2 weeks at 2°–8°C (refrigerated)
- Years at −20°C (frozen)

PROTOCOL
None

INTERPRETATION

NORMAL FINDINGS OR RANGE
- Dogs: <0.6 nmol/L
- Cats: <0.3 nmol/L

These values were valid for the Comparative Neuromuscular Laboratory, University of California–San Diego. Values may vary, depending on the laboratory and the assay.

ABNORMAL VALUES
Values above the reference range

CRITICAL VALUES
None

INTERFERING FACTORS
Drugs That May Alter Results or Interpretation
Drugs That Interfere with Test Methodology
None

Drugs That Alter Physiology
Corticosteroid therapy at immunosuppressive dosages for longer than 7–10 days will lower autoantibody levels. Effects of other immunosuppressive agents have not been evaluated but likely also lower antibody concentrations.

Disorders That May Alter Results
Severe hemolysis or lipemia

Collection Techniques or Handling That May Alter Results
- Failure to separate serum from cells may cause severe hemolysis.
- Serum held at room temperature for longer than advised

Influence of Signalment
Species
None

Breed
- All breeds of dogs and cats may be affected.
- Dog breeds predisposed to acquiring MG include German shepherds, golden retrievers, Akitas, the terrier group, Scottish terriers, German shorthaired pointers, and Chihuahuas.
- An increased incidence of MG has been reported in Abyssinians and Somalis cats.

Age
- Dogs or cats <3 months of age are unlikely to have acquired MG.
- A bimodal age of onset in acquired MG has been described with young dogs (4 months to 4 years) and older dogs (9–13 years) affected.

Gender
Both genders may be affected, with a slight female predominance.

Pregnancy
Pregnancy may unmask subclinical MG.

LIMITATIONS OF THE TEST
- Corticosteroid therapy may lower antibody titers.
- A negative AChR antibody titer does not eliminate a diagnosis of MG. Response to edrophonium chloride challenge, and electrodiagnostic testing, may help confirm the diagnosis.

Sensitivity, Specificity, and Positive and Negative Predictive Values
- 98% sensitivity in generalized MG
- Unknown for focal MG but likely 70%–80%
- A positive AChR antibody titer is diagnostic of acquired MG.
- False-positive results are very rare.

Valid If Run in a Human Lab?
No. Although there is some cross-reactivity between species, the test is relatively species specific. High positive antibody titers may be detected, but lower antibody titers may be missed.

Causes of Abnormal Findings

High values	Low values
Acquired MG	Seronegative MG
Rarely in other muscular diseases	Corticosteroids

ACETYLCHOLINE RECEPTOR ANTIBODY

CLINICAL PERSPECTIVE
• Any antibody titer of >0.6 nmol/L for dogs or >0.3 nmol/L for cats is a positive titer, diagnostic of MG, and requires treatment.
• A diagnosis of seronegative MG should not be made until there are 2 negative AChR antibody titers collected 3–4 weeks apart.
• Because of the large size of the AChR and the variability in pathogenic potential of antibodies against different sites, there is no correlation between severity of MG and the antibody titer.
• In the absence of corticosteroid therapy, there is a good correlation in an individual animal between antibody titer and course of the disease.
• Vaccination during active disease can exacerbate MG and increase the antibody titer. It is not yet known whether vaccination can precipitate the disease.
• Intact females should be spayed as soon as clinically feasible because heat cycles can exacerbate MG and increase antibody titers.

MISCELLANEOUS

ANCILLARY TESTS
• Thoracic radiographs as a cranial mediastinal mass may be associated with paraneoplastic MG.
• Evaluation of thyroid status as hypothyroidism may occur concurrently in patients with MG.
• If clinically indicated, search for other autoimmune diseases, such as autoimmune hemolytic anemia, thrombocytopenia, and inflammatory bowel disease, that can occur concurrently with MG.
• Serum creatine kinase concentration as inflammatory myopathy can occur along with paraneoplastic MG associated with thymoma.

SYNONYMS
AChR Ab

SEE ALSO
Blackwell's Five-Minute Veterinary Consult: Canine and Feline Topics
• Dysphagia
• Megaesophagus
• Myasthenia Gravis
• Pneumonia, Aspiration

Related Topics in This Book
• Masticatory Muscle Myositis (2M Antibody Assay)
• Thyroglobulin Autoantibody

ABBREVIATIONS
• AChR = acetylcholine receptor
• MG = myasthenia gravis

Suggested Reading
Lipsitz D, Berry JL, Shelton GD. Inherited predisposition to myasthenia gravis in Newfoundlands. *J Am Vet Med Assoc* 1999; 215: 956–958.
Shelton GD. Myasthenia gravis and disorders of neuromuscular transmission. *Vet Clin North Am* 2002; 32: 189–206.
Shelton GD, Ho M, Kass PH. Risk factors for acquired myasthenia gravis in cats: 105 cases (1986–1998). *J Am Vet Med Assoc* 2000; 216: 55–57.
Shelton GD, Lindstrom JM. Spontaneous remission in canine myasthenia gravis: Implications for assessing human MG therapies. *Neurology* 2001; 57: 2139–2141.
Shelton GD, Schule A, Kass PH. Risk factors for acquired myasthenia gravis in dogs: 1,154 cases (1991–1995). *J Am Vet Med Assoc* 1997; 211: 1428–1431.

INTERNET RESOURCES
University of California–San Diego, Department of Pathology, School of Medicine, Comparative Neuromuscular Laboratory: Companion animal diagnostics, http://medicine.ucsd.edu/vet_neuromuscular.

AUTHOR NAME
G. Diane Shelton

ACETYLCHOLINESTERASE

BASICS

TYPE OF SPECIMEN
Blood
Tissue

TEST EXPLANATION AND RELATED PHYSIOLOGY
Certain toxic compounds, particularly organophosphorus insecticide (OP) and carbamate insecticides, act as cholinesterase inhibitors (ChEIs) by competitive inhibition at the active site of acetylcholinesterase (AChE). AChE, or true ChE, catabolizes the neurotransmitter acetylcholine at the synapses and neuromuscular junction. Inhibition of AChE therefore leads to overstimulation of the cholinergic nervous system. Salivation, lacrimation, urination, and defecation (SLUD), muscle tremors, and dyspnea are the predominant clinical signs in most cases. Clinical signs often progress rapidly and usually require treatment before a conclusive diagnosis can be made.

    AChEs are found in the nervous tissue and in red blood cells. Pseudocholinesterases (pChEs) are found in plasma or serum and are more sensitive to inhibition. Decreased AChE activity correlates more strongly with clinical signs than does decreased pChE activity, but pChE activity is a sensitive indicator of exposure to a ChEI.

    Other ChEIs include the drug physostigmine and the cyanobacterial (blue-green algal) toxin anatoxin-a(s), produced by *Anabaena flos-aquae*. Unlike the compounds just listed, anatoxin-a(s) does not cross the blood-brain barrier under normal circumstances.

    Techniques used to determine ChE activity vary among laboratories. Generally, a substrate for ChE is added to a sample, and the hydrolysis of this substrate is measured based on a change in the mixture's pH or a color-change reaction. The Ellman method, which measures a change in color with a spectrophotometer, is commonly used.

INDICATIONS
- SLUD
- Exposure to an OP or carbamate insecticide

CONTRAINDICATIONS
None

POTENTIAL COMPLICATIONS
None

CLIENT EDUCATION
- OP and carbamate poisonings may cause severe clinical signs, and treatment may be required before confirmation of the diagnosis.
- False negatives are possible with this test.

BODY SYSTEMS ASSESSED
- Behavioral
- Gastrointestinal
- Musculoskeletal
- Nervous
- Neuromuscular
- Respiratory

SAMPLE

COLLECTION
- 1 mL of whole blood in heparin or EDTA for AChE activity
- 1/2 brain for AChE activity
- 1 mL serum of heparinized plasma for pChE activity

HANDLING
- Submit whole blood, serum, or plasma on ice.
- Submit brain frozen.

STORAGE
Store frozen.

STABILITY
- Samples should be analyzed as soon as possible.
- Carbamate insecticides bind reversibly to ChE and will be hydrolyzed over time. Hence, ChE activity may increase in samples stored for a prolonged period.
- OP binding, on the other hand, is usually irreversible. Changes in ChE activity are more likely to be maintained during storage.
- A study of stored blood from horses exposed to an OP found loss of activity after:
  - 1 day at room temperature
  - 1 week at 2°–0°C (refrigerated)

PROTOCOL
None

INTERPRETATION

NORMAL FINDINGS OR RANGE
Reference ranges for normal ChE activity vary between laboratories and depend on analytical technique.

ABNORMAL VALUES
Blood ChE <50% of control values is suspicious for ChEI exposure.

CRITICAL VALUES
Blood ChE <25% of control may be associated with severe toxicosis.

INTERFERING FACTORS
Drugs That May Alter Results or Interpretation
Drugs That Interfere with Test Methodology
None

Drugs That Alter Physiology
Physostigmine and related drugs inhibit ChE.

Disorders That May Alter Results
None

Collection Techniques or Handling That May Alter Results
- Blood samples collected in citrate may produce lower ChE values.
- Prolonged storage may decrease ChE values, particularly if a carbamate insecticide is involved.

Influence of Signalment
Species
None

Breed
None

Age
None

Gender
None

Pregnancy
None

LIMITATIONS OF THE TEST
False-negative results are common, particularly after carbamate exposure. Carbamates may have dissociated or been hydrolyzed from the active site of the ChE during sample transport or testing.

Sensitivity, Specificity, and Positive and Negative Predictive Values
N/A

Valid If Run in a Human Lab?
Yes—but conversion factors may be different for canine versus human samples. A control sample from an unaffected individual of the same species should be submitted with the sample.

Causes of Abnormal Findings

High values	Low values
None	OPs
	Carbamate insecticides
	Physostigmine and related drugs
	Anabaena flos-aquae (blue-green algae) anatoxin-a(s)

CLINICAL PERSPECTIVE
- OP and carbamate insecticides inhibit ChE activity.
- AChE activity can be tested on blood or brain, and decreased activity is likely to correspond with the severity of the clinical signs.
- pChE is tested on serum or plasma and is more sensitive to inhibition, and thus is a more sensitive indicator of exposure.
- False-negative ChE activity assays are common.

MISCELLANEOUS
ANCILLARY TESTS
- Atropine test dose
  - Resolution of clinical signs and normal atropinization with a preanesthetic dose of atropine is inconsistent with OP or carbamate exposure.
  - Animals exposed to ChE inhibitors respond only to high doses of atropine.
- Gas chromatography/mass spectroscopy insecticide screen on stomach content or tissue

SYNONYMS
- AChE
- Cholinesterase
- Pseudocholinesterase

SEE ALSO
Blackwell's Five-Minute Veterinary Consult: Canine and Feline Topics
Organophosphate and Carbamate Toxicity
Related Topics in This Book
None

ABBREVIATIONS
- AChE = acetylcholinesterase
- ChE = cholinesterase
- ChEI = cholinesterase inhibitor
- OP = organophosphorus insecticide
- pChE = pseudocholinesterase
- SLUD = salivation, lacrimation, urination, and defecation

Suggested Reading
Blodgett DJ. Organophosphate and carbamate insecticides. In: Peterson ME, Talcott PA, eds. *Small Animal Toxicology*, 2nd ed. Philadelphia: WB Saunders, 2005: 941–955.
Meerdink GL. Anticholinesterase insecticides. In: Plumlee KH, ed. *Clinical Veterinary Toxicology*, 1st ed. St Louis: CV Mosby, 2003: 178–180.
Plumlee KH, Richardson AR, Gardner IA, Galey FD. Effect of time and storage temperature on cholinesterase activity in blood from normal and organophosphorus insecticide–treated horses. *J Vet Diagn Invest* 1994; **6**: 247–249.
Tecles F, Gutierrez PC, Martinez SS, Ceron JJ. Effects of different variables on whole blood cholinesterase analysis in dogs. J Vet Diagn Invest 2002; **14**: 132–139.

INTERNET RESOURCES
Braund KG. Neurotoxic disorders. In: Braunder KG, ed. Clinical Neurology in Small Animals: Localization, Diagnosis and Treatment. Ithaca, NY: International Veterinary Information Service (IVIS), 2003, http://www.ivis.org/advances/Vite/braund22/ivis.pdf.
Carbamate insecticides. In: Merck Veterinary Manual, 9th ed. Whitehouse Station, NJ: Merck, 2008, http://www.merckvetmanual.com/mvm/index.jsp?cfile = htm/bc/211602.htm.
Organophosphates: Overview. In: Merck Veterinary Manual, 9th ed. Whitehouse Station, NJ: Merck, 2008, http://www.merckvetmanual.com/mvm/index.jsp?cfile = htm/bc/211605.htm&word = cholinesterase%2cinhibitors.

AUTHOR NAME
Karyn Bischoff

BASICS

TYPE OF SPECIMEN
Blood

TEST EXPLANATION AND RELATED PHYSIOLOGY
Adrenal cortisol secretion is stimulated by ACTH release from the anterior pituitary gland. Cortisol then inhibits further release of ACTH (negative-feedback inhibition). Hyperadrenocorticism (HAC) is a clinical disorder resulting from excessive glucocorticoids. Naturally occurring HAC is a result of either an ACTH-secreting pituitary adenoma (PDH), causing bilateral adrenal hypertrophy, or a functional adrenal cortical tumor. PDH is the most common form of HAC in both dogs and cats. Iatrogenic HAC occurs secondary to administration of excessive corticosteroids and is seen almost exclusively in dogs. Screening tests, such as the ACTH stimulation test and LDDST, are performed initially to confirm a diagnosis of HAC and are followed by differentiating tests to determine the cause. Differentiating tests include measuring endogenous ACTH, the HDDST, and adrenal ultrasonography. Endogenous ACTH is increased or high-normal in PDH, owing to uninhibited production by the pituitary tumor, and low in adrenal tumors, because of negative-feedback inhibition.

The endogenous ACTH test can also differentiate between primary and secondary hypoadrenocorticism. Primary hypoadrenocorticism results from idiopathic destruction of the adrenal cortex, leading to absence of aldosterone and glucocorticoids and to increased ACTH owing to loss of negative inhibition. The rare, secondary form results from a pituitary lesion; the absence of pituitary ACTH leads to atrophy only of the cortisol-secreting layers of the adrenal cortex.

Endogenous ACTH is measured by immunoassay. ACTH assays developed for humans have been validated for the veterinary market.

INDICATIONS
• Differentiation between PDH and HAC caused by an adrenal tumor
• Differentiation between primary and secondary hypoadrenocorticism

CONTRAINDICATIONS
Cannot be used as a preliminary screening test for HAC

POTENTIAL COMPLICATIONS
None

CLIENT EDUCATION
Collecting sample between 8 and 9 a.m. after overnight hospitalization should minimize effects of transportation stress and daily fluctuation.

BODY SYSTEMS ASSESSED
Endocrine or metabolic

SAMPLE

COLLECTION
2.0 mL of venous blood

HANDLING
• Collect into a prechilled, silicone-coated EDTA tube. Keep blood chilled throughout handling.
• Invert the tube several times, centrifuge within 5 min, and transfer the plasma to a plastic tube.
• Freeze the plasma.
• Ship overnight on ice packs or dry ice. The sample must arrive with a temperature of <16°C.
• EDTA tubes containing aprotinin, an enzyme inhibitor, may improve stability; however, aprotinin may interfere with certain analytical methods.

STORAGE
Freeze

STABILITY
• <1 day in a refrigerator (4°C) without aprotinin
• ≤4 days at 4°C with aprotinin
• ≤1 month in a freezer (−20°C)

PROTOCOL
Collect blood between 8 and 9 a.m. after overnight hopitalization and fast

INTERPRETATION

NORMAL FINDINGS OR RANGE
• Dogs: 10–80 pg/mL (2.2–17.8 pmol/L)
• Cats: 10–60 pg/mL (2.2–13.3 pmol/L)
• Reference intervals may vary, depending on the laboratory and the assay.

ABNORMAL VALUES
HAC
• PDH: >45 pg/mL (>10 pmol/L)
• Adrenal tumor: <10 pg/mL (<2.2 pmol/L)
• A result of 10–45 pg/mL is inconclusive; repeat or perform another differentiating test.

Hypoadrenocorticism
• Primary: >45 pg/mL (>10 pmol/L), usually >450 pg/mL
• Secondary: <10 pg/mL (<22.2 pmol/L)

CRITICAL VALUES
None

INTERFERING FACTORS
Drugs That May Alter Results or Interpretation
Drugs That Interfere with Test Methodology
Exogenous ACTH—wait at least 1 day after the ACTH stimulation test.

Drugs That Alter Physiology
• Prolonged and/or high-dose glucocorticoid administration interferes with the hypothalamic-pituitary-adrenal axis. Withhold all formulations of glucocorticoids for 2–4 weeks prior to testing.
• Progestins

Disorders That May Alter Results
Lipemia

Collection Techniques or Handling That May Alter Results
- Delayed separation, use of nonsiliconized glass tubes, and warming of the specimen
- Aprotinin interferes with some assay methods (chemiluminescent).

Influence of Signalment

Species
Adrenal disease is common is dogs and rare in cats.

Breed
None

Age
None

Gender
None

Pregnancy
The hypothalamic-pituitary-adrenal axis is altered during pregnancy. Delay adrenal function testing.

LIMITATIONS OF THE TEST
- Endogenous ACTH is very labile, making appropriate sample handling crucial.
- Results are occasionally inconclusive.

Sensitivity, Specificity, and Positive and Negative Predictive Values in Dogs
- PDH is >45 pg/mL in about 85%–90% of dogs; 35%–40% have ACTH above reference limits.
- Adrenal tumors: 58% have undetectable ACTH.

Valid If Run in a Human Lab?
Yes, if the assay is validated in animals.

Causes of Abnormal Findings

High values	Low values
PDH	Adrenal tumor
Primary hypoadrenocorticism	Iatrogenic HAC
Exogenous ACTH (ACTH stimulation test)	Secondary hypoadrenocorticism

CLINICAL PERSPECTIVE
- Since many dogs with PDH have high-normal ACTH levels, endogenous ACTH cannot be used to diagnose HAC.
  - Once HAC is diagnosed, patients with high-normal to elevated ACTH have PDH, whereas those with low ACTH most likely have an adrenal tumor.
- Special handling requirements can limit the feasibility of this assay.

MISCELLANEOUS

ANCILLARY TESTS
- LDDST
- ACTH stimulation test
- Ultrasonographic examination of the adrenal glands
  - Bilateral adrenal hypertrophy detected in PDH
  - Adrenal tumor appears as 1 enlarged adrenal gland and 1 atrophied gland.

SYNONYMS
- Endogenous ACTH
- Plasma ACTH

SEE ALSO

Blackwell's Five-Minute Veterinary Consult: Canine and Feline Topics
- Hyperadrenocorticism (Cushing's Disease)—Cats
- Hyperadrenocorticism (Cushing's Disease)—Dogs
- Hypoadrenocorticism (Addison's Disease)

Related Topics in This Book
- ACTH Stimulation Test
- Adrenal Ultrasonography
- High-Dose Dexamethasone Suppression Test
- Low-Dose Dexamethasone Suppression Test
- Cortisol/Creatinine Ratio

ABBREVIATIONS
- ACTH = adrenocorticotropic hormone
- HAC = hyperadrenocorticism
- HDDST = high-dosage dexamethasone suppression test
- LDDST = low-dose dexamethasone suppression test
- PDH = pituitary-dependent hyperadrenocorticism

Suggested Reading
Feldman EC, Nelson RW. *Canine and Feline Endocrinology and Reproduction*, 3rd ed. St Louis: Saunders Elsevier, 2004.

INTERNET RESOURCES
Antech Diagnostics Newsletter, June 1997: Canine hyperadrenocorticism (Cushing's syndrome), http://www. antechdiagnostics. com/clients/antechNews/1997/6–97.htm.
Michigan State University, Diagnostic Center for Population and Animal Health, http://www.animalhealth.msu.edu.

AUTHOR NAME
Kristen R. Friedrichs

ACTH STIMULATION TEST

BASICS

TYPE OF SPECIMEN
Blood

TEST EXPLANATION AND RELATED PHYSIOLOGY
Cortisol is the major glucocorticoid secreted by the adrenal cortex. This test determines the ability of the adrenal gland to secrete endogenous cortisol in response to exogenous ACTH. Additionally, this test can be used to evaluate the ability of the adrenal glands to produce other steroid hormones.

INDICATIONS
- Screening test for hyperadrenocorticism (Cushing's disease)
- Monitoring therapy for hyperadrenocorticism
- Confirmation test for iatrogenic hyperadrenocorticism
- Confirmation test for hypoadrenocorticism (Addison's disease)
- Screening test for atypical hyperadrenocorticism or alopecia X

CONTRAINDICATIONS
None

POTENTIAL COMPLICATIONS
None

CLIENT EDUCATION
- Basal levels of cortisol provide limited information regarding adrenocortical function.
- A normal response to ACTH may necessitate an LDDST to rule out spontaneous hyperadrenocorticism.

BODY SYSTEMS ASSESSED
Endocrine or metabolic

SAMPLE

COLLECTION
0.5–1.0 mL of venous blood

HANDLING
- Collected into EDTA or a red-top tube; check with the lab about preference.
- Centrifuge within 1h and separate serum or plasma from RBCs.
- Cortisol: Refrigerate and ship overnight.
- Other steroid hormones: Freeze and ship in an insulated container with ice packs.

STORAGE
- Cortisol: Refrigerate or freeze.
- Other steroids: Freeze.

STABILITY
- Cortisol
  - Refrigerated (4°C): 5 days
  - Frozen: >5 days
- Other steroids: N/A

PROTOCOL
Dogs
1. Collect a baseline sample.
2. Administer ACTH IM.
   - Administer ACTH gel at 2.2 IU/kg.
   - Administer synthetic ACTH (Cortrosyn) at 0.25 mg/dog.
3. Collect the sample 1h (Cortrosyn) or 2h (gel) after ACTH administration.
4. Submit both samples for measurement of cortisol.

5. For alopecia-X or atypical hyperadrenocorticism, follow this protocol, but submit both samples for measurement of estradiol, androstendione, 17-hydroxyprogesterone, progesterone, and aldosterone.

Cats
1. Collect a baseline sample.
2. Administer synthetic ACTH (Cortrosyn) at 0.125 mg/cat IM.
3. Collect samples at 30 min and 1h after ACTH administration.
4. Submit both samples for measurement of cortisol.

INTERPRETATION

NORMAL FINDINGS OR RANGE
- Typical basal cortisol levels: 0.6–6.0 μg/dL
- Post-ACTH cortisol levels
  - Dogs: 5.5–20.0 μg/dL
  - Cats: 4.5–15.0 μg/dL
  - Levels may vary, depending on laboratory and assay.
  - Following treatment of hyperadrenocorticism: the post ACTH cortisol level should be in the basal cortisol range (1–5 μg/dL)
- Other steroid levels are laboratory dependent.

ABNORMAL VALUES
- Hypoadrenocorticism: post-ACTH cortisol < 1.0 μg/dL
- Hyperadrenocorticism
  - Dogs: post-ACTH cortisol, >20.0 μg/dL
  - Cat: post-ACTH cortisol, >15.0 μg/dL
  - Iatrogenic Cushing's disease: post-ACTH cortisol; little or no response to ACTH, usually 1–5 μg/dL
- Following treatment of hyperadrenocorticism: basal cortisol and post-ACTH cortisol above the basal cortisol range

CRITICAL VALUES
None

INTERFERING FACTORS
Drugs That May Alter Results or Interpretation
Drugs That Interfere with Test Methodology
Prednisone or prednisolone (or structurally related steroids) cross-reacts in the cortisol assay and falsely elevates results; dexamethasone does not interfere.

Drugs That Alter Physiology
Anticonvulsant therapy

Disorders That May Alter Results
- Excessive lipemia or hemolysis
- Stress and nonadrenal illness

Collection Techniques or Handling That May Alter Results
Storage of serum in a serum-separator tube or delayed separation of serum

Influence of Signalment
Species
None

Breed
None

Age
None

Gender
None

Pregnancy
None

LIMITATIONS OF THE TEST
- This test often fails to diagnose adrenal tumors and can miss early PDH.
- The test will not differentiate PDH vs. AT.

Sensitivity, Specificity, and Positive and Negative Predictive Values
Hyperadrenocorticism: Dogs
- Overall sensitivity approximately 80%
- AT sensitivity approximately 60%
- PDH sensitivity approximately 85%
- Specificity approximately 85%

Hyperadrenocorticism: Cats
- Overall sensitivity approximately 81%
- Specificity unknown

Valid If Run in a Human Lab?
Yes—if cortisol assay is validated for dogs and cats.

Causes of Abnormal Findings

High values	Low values
Hyperadrenocorticism	Hypoadrenocorticism
Chronic stress	Iatrogenic hyperadrenocorticism
Nonadrenal illness	Improper handling and/or storage
Prednisone, prednisolone, or related steroids	Improper handling or administration of ACTH
Improper handling and/or storage	

CLINICAL PERSPECTIVE
- This is the test of choice for diagnosis of hypoadrenocorticism
- With hyperadrenocorticism, interpret in context with history and clinical signs since false positives occur in animals with nonadrenal illness.
- Discontinue prednisone or structurally related steroids 2 days prior to performing test.
- Pre- and post-ACTH levels of 17-hydroxyprogesterone and other steroids may aid in the diagnosis of hyperadrenocorticism missed by other tests.

 MISCELLANEOUS

ANCILLARY TESTS
- CBC and chemistry profile for supportive evidence of hyperadrenocorticism

- LDDST may be needed to confirm hyperadrenocorticism.
- Endogenous ACTH to distinguish primary vs. secondary hypoadrenocorticism
- Endogenous ACTH or HDDST to differentiate PDH vs. AT
- Adrenal ultrasound

SYNONYMS
ACTH Stim

SEE ALSO
Blackwell's Five-Minute Veterinary Consult: Canine and Feline Topics
- Growth Hormone–Responsive Dermatoses
- Hyperadrenocorticism (Cushing's Disease)—Cats
- Hyperadrenocorticism (Cushing's Disease)—Dogs
- Hypoadrenocorticism (Addison's Disease)
- Sex Hormone–Responsive Dermatoses

Related Topics in This Book
- ACTH Assay
- Adrenal Ultrasonography
- Cortisol
- Low-Dose Dexamethasone Suppression Test
- High-Dose Dexamethasone Suppression Test

ABBREVIATIONS
- ACTH = adrenocorticotropic hormone
- AT = adrenal tumor
- HDDT = high-dose dexamethasone suppression test
- LDDT = low-dose dexamethasone suppression test
- PDH = pituitary-dependent hyperadrenocorticism

Suggested Reading

Benitah N, Feldman EC, Kass PH, Nelson RW. Evaluation of serum 17-hydroxyprogesterone concentration after administration of ACTH in dogs with hyperadrenocorticism. *J Am Vet Med Assoc* 2005; 227: 1095–1101.

Feldman EC, Nelson RW. Canine hyperadrenocorticism (Cushing's syndrome). In: Feldman EC, Nelson RW, eds. *Canine and Feline Endocrinology and Reproduction*, 3rd ed. St Louis: Saunders Elsevier, 2004: 252–357.

Feldman EC, Nelson RW. Hyperadrenocorticism in cats (Cushing's syndrome). In: Feldman EC, Nelson RW, eds. *Canine and Feline Endocrinology and Reproduction*, 3rd ed. St Louis: Saunders Elsevier, 2004: 358–393.

INTERNET RESOURCES
Kintzer P. Beware of false positives, negatives in canine hyperadrenocorticism testing. DVM Newsmagazine, 2003, http://www.dvm-newsmagazine.com/dvm/article/articleDetail.jsp?id = 70245.

AUTHOR NAME
Janice M. Andrews

ACTIVATED CLOTTING TIME

BASICS

TYPE OF PROCEDURE
Function test

PROCEDURE EXPLANATION AND RELATED PHYSIOLOGY
Patients with bleeding disorders are often evaluated for life-threatening emergencies. A quick and organized assessment of hemostasis in these patients is crucial for their survival. The activated clotting time (ACT) is an easy, benchtop test requiring minimal equipment that enables rapid, in-house evaluation of the intrinsic and common pathways. It is less sensitive than the activated partial thromboplastin time (aPTT), but both tests assess all factors except for factor VII. The ACT is a function test that measures the amount of time it takes for whole blood to form a clot when it comes into contact with a surface activator at 37°C. Although the ACT is not prolonged until severe factor deficiencies are present, it is an excellent screening test for both inherited and acquired coagulation disorders. When the ACT has been determined, a preliminary diagnosis often can be obtained, and appropriate treatment can be instituted rapidly. Once the patient is stabilized, steps can then be taken to further characterize the specific disease process or factor deficiency with more sensitive tests.

INDICATIONS
- A screening test for evaluation of suspected coagulopathies
- Bleeding into body cavities, joints, or subcutaneous tissue
- Prolonged bleeding after venipuncture, trauma, or surgery
- A history of anticoagulant ingestion [determination of prothrombin time (PT) is preferred if available]
- Presurgical evaluation
- Evaluation of potential coagulopathy in liver disease, neoplasia, or suspected DIC

CONTRAINDICATIONS
None

POTENTIAL COMPLICATIONS
Prolonged bleeding from the venipuncture site

CLIENT EDUCATION
None

BODY SYSTEMS ASSESSED
Hemic, lymphatic, and immune

PROCEDURE

PATIENT PREPARATION
Preprocedure Medication or Preparation
Standard blood sample collection technique

Anesthesia or Sedation
Usually none

Patient Positioning
Standard blood sample collection technique

Patient Monitoring
None

Equipment or Supplies
- A needle and syringe or a Vacutainer system (Becton Dickinson)
- Clotting-time Vacutainer tubes, which contain diatomaceous earth as a contact activator
- A 37°C heating block or a water bath
- A watch with a second hand

TECHNIQUE
- Preheat specialized tubes in a heating block or water bath set at 37°C.
- Collect blood via atraumatic venipuncture.
- Add 2 mL of whole blood to the sample tube and begin timing.
- Invert the tube 3–5 times to mix and then place back in the heating source.
- Remove the tube from heating block at 60 s (45 s for cats) and invert once to check for clot formation. Repeat every 10 s thereafter until clot formation is seen. Record the elapsed time.
- If a clot has not formed, continue timing up to 3 min for dogs and 4 min for cats.

SAMPLE HANDLING
See Technique, the preceding section.

APPROPRIATE AFTERCARE
Postprocedure Patient Monitoring
Monitor for prolonged bleeding.

Nursing Care
Apply a pressure wrap to the venipuncture site.

Dietary Modification
None

Medication Requirements
None

Restrictions on Activity
If the ACT is prolonged, the animal should remain quiet for 30–60 min after the procedure.

Anticipated Recovery Time
N/A

INTERPRETATION

NORMAL FINDINGS OR RANGE
- Dogs: 60–90s
- Cats: 45–160s

ABNORMAL VALUES
- Values above the normal range are considered to be suspicious for coagulation abnormalities.
- Values below normal range are difficult to interpret.

CRITICAL VALUES
Animals with values $1\frac{1}{2}$ times normal are more likely to have spontaneous or prolonged bleeding than are those with lower values.

INTERFERING FACTORS
Drugs That May Alter Results of the Procedure
Heparin or other anticoagulants

Conditions That May Interfere with Performing the Procedure
Platelet phospholipids are a necessary component of the reaction. Platelet counts of <10,000 may delay clot formation by 10–20s.

Procedure Techniques or Handling That May Alter Results
- Inadequate warming of the tube will prolong the ACT.
- Multiple venipuncture attempts or difficulty in drawing blood will activate the hemostatic system and can lead to inaccurate results. Blood collection should be done cleanly and quickly.

Influence of Signalment on Performing and Interpreting the Procedure
Species
- Normal values differ for cats and dogs.
- Some cats have a factor XII deficiency, which results in a prolonged ACT but does not result in clinical signs.

Breed
None

Age
None

Gender
None

Pregnancy
None

CLINICAL PERSPECTIVE

- Animals with bleeding disorders are fairly common in all practices. As these patients are often critical, it is essential to have an easily accessible method to assess these patients quickly.
- The ACT is a quick and easy screening test that is very good at picking up severe factor deficiencies but is insensitive. If a coagulopathy is still suspected in a patient with a normal ACT, more sensitive tests for factor analysis should be considered.
- The ACT is also nonspecific. If the ACT is prolonged, additional factor analyses can be performed to determine more accurately which factor(s) is affected.
- Some clinicians use body heat (e.g., from hands or armpits) to warm the tubes; however, inappropriate temperatures may affect the validity of results.

MISCELLANEOUS

ANCILLARY TESTS

- aPTT tests for similar factor deficiencies and is more sensitive.
- PT will test for factor VII.
- Specific factor analysis may be needed for exact diagnosis.
- Fibrin degradation products and D-dimer (canine) can further delineate the coagulopathy.

SYNONYMS

Activated coagulation time (ACT)

SEE ALSO

Blackwell's Five-Minute Veterinary Consult: Canine and Feline Topics

- Anticoagulant Rodenticide Poisoning
- Coagulation Factor Deficiency
- Coagulopathy of Liver Disease
- Hemothorax

Related Topics in This Book

- Anticoagulant Screen
- Blood Sample Collection
- Coagulation Factors
- D-Dimer
- Fibrin Degradation Products
- Partial Thromboplastin Time, Activated
- PIVKA (protein induced by vitamin K absence or antagonism) Test
- Platelet Count and Volume
- Platelet Function Tests
- Prothrombin Time

ABBREVIATIONS

- ACT = activated clotting time
- aPTT = activated partial thromboplastin time
- PT = prothrombin time

Suggested Reading
Couto CG. Disorders of hemostasis. In: Nelson RW, Couto CG, eds. *Small Animal Internal Medicine*. St Louis: CV Mosby, 2003: 1185–1199.
Fogh JM, Fogh IT. Inherited coagulation disorders. *Vet Clin North Am Small Anim* 1988; 18: 231–243.
Stockham SL, Scott MA. In: *Fundamentals of Veterinary Clinical Pathology*. Ames: Iowa State Press, 2002: 188–193.
Tvedten H, Willard MD. Hemostatic abnormalities. In: *Small Animal Clinical Diagnosis by Laboratory Methods*. Philadelphia: WB Saunders, 2004: 92–112.

INTERNET RESOURCES

Cornell University, College of Medicine: Hemostasis, http://www.diaglab.vet.cornell.edu/clinpath/modules/coags/coag.htm.

AUTHOR NAME

Karyn Harrell

ACUTE PHASE PROTEINS

BASICS

TYPE OF SPECIMEN
Blood

TEST EXPLANATION AND RELATED PHYSIOLOGY
Following infection, inflammation or trauma, release of proinflammatory cytokines such as interleukin 1, interleukin 6, and tumor necrosis factor α stimulate hepatocytes to increase synthesis and secretion of a number of acute phase proteins (APPs). Moderate APPs, including haptoglobin (Hp), α_1-acid glycoprotein (AGP), and fibrinogen, are present in the blood of healthy animals, but may increase 2- to 10-fold in concentration after stimulation. Major APPs, including C-reactive protein (CRP) and serum amyloid A (SAA), usually are virtually undetectable in the blood of healthy animals, but the concentration can increase 10- to 1,000-fold on stimulation. Major APPs have an early and high rise in concentration and a very rapid decline, whereas moderate APPs need more time to increase and return to normal values. APPs have different profiles between species.

INDICATIONS
• Detection of clinical or subclinical inflammation due to any cause, for example,
  • Infectious disease
  • Autoimmune disease
  • Neoplastic disease
  • Endocrine disease
  • GI disease
• Treatment monitoring of any inflammatory process

CONTRAINDICATIONS
None

POTENTIAL COMPLICATIONS
None

CLIENT EDUCATION
None

BODY SYSTEMS ASSESSED
Hemic, lymphatic, and immune

SAMPLE

COLLECTION
1–2 mL of venous blood

HANDLING
• Plain red-top tube or serum-separator tube for most APPs
• EDTA, heparin, or citrate for fibrinogen; plasma required
• Best if the sample is analyzed within 2 days
• Avoid hemolysis, especially if using immunoturbidimetric methods.

STORAGE
Refrigerate or freeze.

STABILITY
• Refrigerated (2°– 8°C): several days
• Frozen (−20°C): Serum and/or plasma stable for long periods

PROTOCOL
None

INTERPRETATION

NORMAL FINDINGS AND REFERENCE RANGE
Reference intervals may vary depending on the laboratory and assay.
Dogs
• CRP: <10 mg/L
• SAA: <3 mg/L
• Hp: <3 g/L
• α_1-Acid glycoprotein: <1.5 g/L
• Fibrinogen: 120–300 mg/dL (1.2–3.0 g/L)
Cats
• SAA: <10 mg/L
• Hp: <2 g/L
• α_1-Acid glycoprotein: <1.5 g/L
• Fibrinogen: 100–400 mg/dL (1–4 g/L)

ABNORMAL VALUES
Values above reference ranges indicate inflammatory conditions. High-fold increases can indicate severe infective and/or inflammatory conditions, whereas increases of low magnitude can be associated with subclinical or mild inflammatory conditions.

INTERFERING FACTORS
Drugs That May Alter Results or Interpretation
Drugs That Interfere with Test Methodology
None

Drugs That Alter Physiology
• Corticosteroids induce the production of Hp and can inhibit CRP synthesis in dogs (effect in cats unknown).
• Phenobarbital increases canine AGP.
• Anthelmintics increase canine Hp.

Disorders That May Alter Results
• Cushing's syndrome leads to elevation of Hp in dogs, and CRP response to an inflammatory condition is of lower magnitude in dogs with Cushing's disease or after glucocorticoid administration.
• Liver failure can reduce the APP response.
• Hemolysis can reduce Hp values.

Collection Techniques or Handling That May Alter Results
Hemolysis

Influence of Signalment
Species
• In dogs, CRP and SAA are major, and Hp, fibrinogen, and AGP are moderate, APPs.
• In cats, CRP is not an APP, whereas SAA and AGP are major, and Hp and fibrinogen are moderate, APPs.

Breed
Greyhounds have lower Hp concentrations than other dog breeds. Yorkshire terriers and dachshunds have lower AGP concentrations than other dog breeds.

Age
None

Gender
None

Pregnancy
In pregnant bitches, an acute phase response occurs around 3 weeks after fertilization, and the serum concentrations of CRP and Hp increase. This has been used as a test for pregnancy.

LIMITATIONS OF THE TEST
Sensitivity, Specificity, and Positive and Negative Predictive Values
- High sensitivity (higher than WBC and differential counts) to detect any inflammatory process
  - For example, CRP had sensitivities of 93% and 82% in symptomatic and asymptomatic dogs naturally infected with *Leishmania infantum.*
- Low specificity to detect the cause of the inflammation

Valid If Run in a Human Lab?
The APP tests are not valid if run in a human laboratory unless each assay is validated for the species being tested. The proteins have variable cross-reactivities to antisera to the human proteins, different reaction profiles, and different reference ranges. Use of species-specific antibodies, standards, and controls is highly recommended.

CLINICAL PERSPECTIVE
- APP tests are not specific for one disease.
- The tests detect the presence of an inflammatory and/or infectious disease or subclinical disease.
- For monitoring treatment, decreasing concentrations suggest patient recovery, whereas rising concentrations suggest continued disease or relapse.

MISCELLANEOUS
ANCILLARY TESTS
None

SYNONYMS
- α_1-Acid glycoprotein
- C-reactive protein
- Fibrinogen
- Haptoglobin
- Serum amyloid A

SEE ALSO
Blackwell's Five-Minute Veterinary Consult: Canine and Feline Topics
- Chapters relating to inflammation, infection, and neoplasia

- Hyperadrenocorticism (Cushing's Disease)—Cats
- Hyperadrenocorticism (Cushing's Disease)—Dogs

Related Topics in This Book
- White Blood Cells and Differential
- White Blood Cells: Lymphocytes
- White Blood Cells: Monocytes
- White Blood Cells: Neutrophils

ABBREVIATIONS
- AGP = α_1-acid glycoprotein
- APP = acute phase protein
- CRP = C-reactive protein
- Hp = haptoglobin
- SAA = serum amyloid A

Suggested Reading
Caldin M, Tasca S, Carli E, *et al.* Acute phase proteins in dogs with hyperadrenocorticism: A particular profile? [Abstract]. *Vet Clin Pathol* 2006; 35: 477.
Ceron JJ, Eckersall PD, Martinez-Subiela S. Acute phase proteins in dogs and cats: Current knowledge and future perspectives. *Vet Clin Pathol* 2005; 34: 85–99.
Duthie S, Eckersall PD, Addie DD, *et al.* Value of alpha 1-acid glycoprotein in the diagnosis of feline infectious peritonitis. *Vet Rec* 1997; 141: 299–303.
Eckersall PD. The time is right for acute phase protein assays. *Vet J* 2004; 168: 3–5.
Jergens AE, Schreiner CA, Frank DE, *et al.* A scoring index for disease activity in canine inflammatory bowel disease. J *Vet Intern Med* 2003; 17: 291–297.

INTERNET RESOURCES
University of Glasgow, Faculty of Veterinary Medicine, Acute Phase Protein Laboratory within the Veterinary Genes and Proteins Group: Acute phase proteins, http://www.gla.ac.uk/vet/acutephaseproteins.

AUTHOR NAMES
Peter David Eckersall and Jose Joaquin Ceron

BASICS

TYPE OF PROCEDURE
Ultrasonographic

PROCEDURE EXPLANATION AND RELATED PHYSIOLOGY
Each adrenal gland is imaged with a high-resolution transducer. The normal adrenal glands are included in imaging in the abdominal ultrasound examination. The appearance of each gland may be determined and, from the size and shape and echogenicity, a specific diagnosis may be made. This is the best modality to image the adrenal glands. Other modalities, including computed tomography and magnetic resonance imaging, may also be used to image the glands. Ultrasound is often used to determine whether hyperadrenocorticism is caused by an adrenal tumor or adenoma or is pituitary dependent. The size, shape, and echogenicity of the adrenal gland are used to assist in the diagnosis. Ultrasound may also be used to confirm small adrenal glands. Small adrenal glands may be indicative of hypoadrenocorticism, exogenous steroids, or related to drug therapy.

INDICATIONS
Clinical signs supportive of the following:
- Hyperadrenocorticism
- Hyperaldosteronism
- A pheochromocytoma
- Hypoadrenocorticism

CONTRAINDICATIONS
If the patient is severely thrombocytopenic, bruising may occur due to transducer pressure on the skin. This is rarely a contraindication to using the procedure.

POTENTIAL COMPLICATIONS
Bruising of the subcutaneous tissue on patients that have a bleeding abnormality

CLIENT EDUCATION
- The study requires clipping of the abdominal hair in most patients.
- The patient may need chemical restraint if unruly, in pain, or uncooperative.
- Fine-needle aspirates may be needed if hepatomegaly or lymphadenopathy is also detected.
- Further imaging of the brain (computed tomography or magnetic resonance imaging) may be needed to evaluate the pituitary gland.

BODY SYSTEMS ASSESSED
Endocrine and metabolic

PROCEDURE

PATIENT PREPARATION

Preprocedure Medication or Preparation
The hair is clipped over the entire abdomen in sufficient quantity to image the entire abdomen.

Anesthesia or Sedation
Sedation may be required if fine-needle aspirates of the liver or lymph nodes are obtained. The adrenal glands usually are not aspirated.

Patient Positioning
Depending on the sonologist, the patient may be imaged in lateral or dorsal recumbency. An assistant holds the patient in position during the procedure.

Patient Monitoring
If aspirates are performed, the patient should be monitored for excessive bleeding.

Equipment or Supplies
- An ultrasound unit with transducers that are of sufficient resolution to image the adrenal glands is required. This is usually 7 MHz or higher, depending on the size and conformation of the patient.
- Ultrasound gel is needed for acoustic coupling.
- Clippers
- Alcohol for skin cleansing

TECHNIQUE
- The hair is clipped with a surgical blade at the level of the diaphragm from the epaxial muscles to the pelvic limbs.
- The animal is placed in right lateral recumbency.
- The skin is cleaned with alcohol.
- Ample ultrasound gel is applied.
- The transducer with the highest resolution is chosen (7–13 MHz).
- The gland should be imaged throughout its length and measurements obtained on the gland's width and length.
- The image is oriented such that the left side of the image should represent the cranial or dorsal aspect of the gland.
- Right or left indicator markers are recorded on the image.
- The patient is placed in right lateral recumbency. The left adrenal gland is located by scanning in the dorsal caudal quadrant of the abdomen. The aorta and caudal vena cava are identified as tubular parallel vascular structures coursing in a cranial to caudal direction. From the left side, the aorta is in the near field. The aorta is traced cranially to the level of the left renal artery. This small vessel will branch off the aorta and then course cranially and laterally. There is often a bend or hook

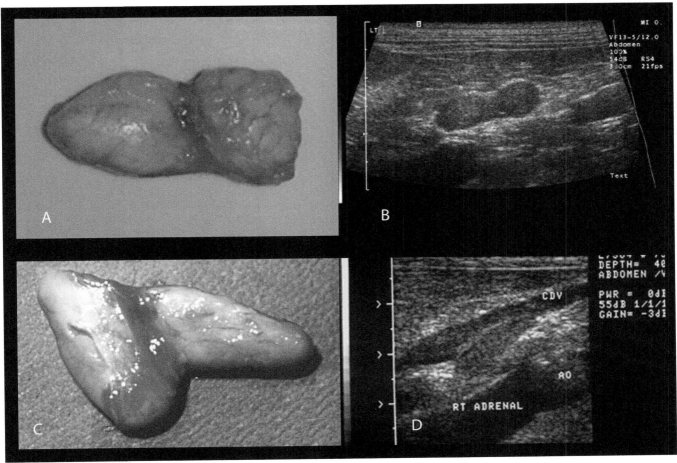

Figure 1

A: The left adrenal gland has a dumbbell or bean shape with an indentation in the center where the phrenicoabdominal vein crosses the gland. **B**: An ultrasound image of the left adrenal gland demonstrates the bilobed appearance of the gland, which is hypoechoic relative to the surrounding fat. **C**: The right adrenal gland has a bent-arrow or a backward-L shape. The longest segment is adjacent to the caudal vena cava. The indentation over the central part of the gland is from the phrenicoabdominal vein crossing the gland. **D**: The right adrenal gland lies adjacent to the caudal vena cava. A tumor affecting the adrenal gland has a short distance to track to the caudal vena cava.

in the left renal artery after it arises from the aorta and before it connects to the kidney. The corresponding vein may be slightly larger and parallels the artery. Located just cranial to these vessels is the left adrenal gland. Once the renal artery is located, sliding the probe to the area just cranial to the renal vessel and then rotating the transducer often in a clockwise direction is helpful in locating the adrenal gland. The gland is bilobed (Figure 1A and B). Once the gland is identified, optimization of the gland is attempted by imaging the gland in its longitudinal axis. The gland's length and width are measured. A transverse image of the gland will enable a height measurement. The surrounding tissue vessels and organs are evaluated especially if the gland is abnormal in echogenicity, shape, or size.

• The right adrenal gland is evaluated by placing the patient in left lateral recumbency. The caudal vena cava and aorta are identified: The caudal vena cava will be in the near field, and the aorta will be in the far field. The vessels are traced cranially to where the right renal artery branches off the aorta, crosses the caudal vena cava, and courses through the near field to the right kidney. At this point, the aorta and caudal vena cava diverge, with the aorta coursing deeper. As the aorta is traced cranially, the celiac and the cranial mesenteric arteries will be identified arising from the aorta. The transducer is then moved cranially and angled slightly away from the table and toward the image of the caudal vena cava. The right adrenal gland will be in close apposition to the caudal vena cava and cranial to the celiac artery.

ADRENAL ULTRASONOGRAPHY

The gland has reverse-L shape, with the longest segment adjacent to the caudal vena cava (Figure 1C and D). The caudal pole, or any mass that may be present, is measured. The left gland may also be imaged from the right side by sliding the transducer caudal to the celiac and cranial mesenteric arteries and aiming the transducer more ventrally.

SAMPLE HANDLING
N/A

APPROPRIATE AFTERCARE
Postprocedure Patient Monitoring
If aspirates are obtained, then the patient may be monitored for postaspiration bleeding.

Nursing Care
None

Dietary Modification
None

Medication Requirements
None

Restrictions on Activity
None

Anticipated Recovery Time
Immediate

 INTERPRETATION

NORMAL FINDINGS OR RANGE
• The adrenal gland size varies with weight.
• The normal range for adrenal gland thickness is 3.0–5.2 mm for the left gland in small dogs and up to 7.4 in larger dogs, and 3.1–6.0 mm for the right gland in small dogs and 7.4 for dogs that weigh >50 lb (>22.7 kg).
• The glands should be mildly hypoechoic relative to the surrounding tissue. They should be of uniform echogenicity. The margins should be smooth.
• One adrenal gland should be interpreted in light of the opposite gland's appearance.

ABNORMAL VALUES
• A change in size either focally or generally (focally enlarged or uniformly enlarged and >7.5 mm for most mid-sized dogs)
• A small gland usually <3 mm thick
• A change in echogenicity—especially areas of mineralization
• A change in shape indicating that a mass may be present

CRITICAL VALUES
Vascular invasion of the mass especially into the caudal vena cava

INTERFERING FACTORS
Drugs That May Alter Results of the Procedure
• Corticosteroids
• Lysodren

Conditions That May Interfere with Performing the Procedure
• A very critically ill patient
• An inability to apply any pressure to the abdominal cavity
• An intractable patient
• Panting
• Excessive intestinal or intra-abdominal gas may prevent identification of the glands.
• A very tense abdomen or a painful abdomen such as with pancreatitis
• Another mass, such as a splenic hemangiosarcoma, that may rupture if pressure is applied while searching for the adrenal gland

Procedure Techniques or Handling That May Alter Results
• Mistaking a periaortic or perirenal lymph node for the glands will alter the results.
• Repeated measurements of the width and height may yield different results. The gland has three specific different measurements: length, width, and height. The width and height are often slightly different in size. One report suggests that height is more specific than width. It is not always possible to be sure that the measurement procured is height vs width. This may result in minor changes in the exact measurement recorded.
• Failure to ensure that the true length of the gland is measured

Influence of Signalment on Performing and Interpreting the Procedure
Species
Dogs, cats, and ferrets each have species-specific documented measurements.

Breed
Specific breeds have a predilection for hyperadrenocorticism or hypoadrenocorticism (especially small-breed dogs).

Age
• The adrenal glands are often easier to see in young patients with a compliant abdomen.
• Older patients often have more degenerative changes.
• The glands of older cats may have mineralization.

Pregnancy
Adequate imaging of the adrenal gland may be more difficult later in gestation, and the larger and more fetuses present.

CLINICAL PERSPECTIVE
• The adrenals are included in the routine abdominal ultrasound study. Changes in the size and shape of the gland are the most

common abnormalities detected. Hyperechoic nodules that are within a lobe or that mildly increase the size of the gland will often represent benign nodules from adenomas. If the nodule is >2 cm, then it is more often a malignant tumor. However, a malignant tumor can be <2 cm. The types of tumors that create a mass include a pheochromocytoma, cortisol-secreting carcinoma, aldosterone-secreting tumor, or metastasis.

• A pituitary-dependent or adrenal-based cause for the suspected hyperadrenocorticism is a common reason for the examination. Comparing the size of one gland to the other may also assist in determining the primary location of the disease. The contralateral gland may be smaller or normal in a patient with a cortisol-secreting tumor in one adrenal gland. If both glands are uniformly enlarged, then they may be responding to a pituitary-dependent hyperadrenocortical process. If there is a mass in one gland and the opposite gland is uniformly enlarged, then the possibility of a pheochromocytoma and pituitary-dependent hyperadrenocorticism should be considered. Tumors may be unilateral or bilateral. Mineralization that has an eggshell appearance is more often seen with a benign process, whereas amorphous mineralization is more frequently seen with a neoplastic process. Older cats may have foci of mineral present as result of a degenerative process.

• The appearance of the glands should be interpreted in light of the laboratory and clinical findings. When each gland is uniformly enlarged, then pituitary-dependent hyperadrenocorticism is most likely. If one gland is enlarged and has lost its normal shape, this is most consistent with an adrenal mass. Adenomas are often hyperechoic and may lead to a minor change in the size of the lobe where it is located. Masses may be a primary adrenal tumor such as a pheochromocytoma, or a cortisol-secreting tumor or a metastatic lesion. The pheochromocytoma and the carcinomas may invade local vessels and may partially or completely occlude the caudal vena cava. Surrounding organs to evaluate include the kidneys for potential invasion and the regional lymph nodes for metastasis. With hyperadrenocorticism, the liver is often hyperechoic and enlarged and contains hypoechoic subtle nodules consistent with steroid hepatopathy and focal hyperplasia. There may be evidence of one or more thrombi in the portal or splenic veins.

• Adrenal size may be normal, and yet the clinical picture and the laboratory values support hyperadrenocorticism. Conversely, the glands may be mildly enlarged and not be associated with hyperadrenocorticism. The appearance of the glands needs to be evaluated in light of the other ultrasound findings, the clinical picture, and the laboratory values. Aspirating the liver may be beneficial in diagnosing steroid hepatopathy. An adrenal tumor is not typically aspirated with ultrasound guidance.

ANCILLARY TESTS

• Liver enzyme tests
• Adrenocorticotropic hormone (ACTH) assay
• ACTH stimulation test
• Dexamethasone suppression testing
• Urine cortisol/creatinine ratio
• Magnetic resonance imaging or computed tomography of the brain
• Abdominal or thoracic radiographs

SYNONYMS

Adrenal sonography

SEE ALSO

Blackwell's Five-Minute Veterinary Consult: Canine and Feline Topics

• Hyperadrenocorticism (Cushing's Disease)—Cats
• Hyperadrenocorticism (Cushing's Disease)—Dogs
• Hypoadrenocorticism (Addison's Disease)
• Pheochromocytoma

Related Topics in This Book

• General Principles of Ultrasonography
• ACTH Assay
• ACTH Stimulation Test
• Alanine Aminotransferase
• Alkaline Phosphatase
• Computed Tomography
• Cortisol
• Cortisol/Creatinine Ratio
• High-Dose Dexamethasone Suppression Test
• Low-Dose Dexamethasone Suppression Test
• Magnetic Resonance Imaging

ABBREVIATIONS

ACTH = adrenocorticotropic hormone

Suggested Reading
Nyland TG, Mattoon JS, eds. *Small Animal Diagnostic Ultrasound.* Philadelphia: WB Saunders, 2002.

INTERNET RESOURCES

None

AUTHOR NAME

Kathy Spaulding

ALANINE AMINOTRANSFERASE

BASICS

TYPE OF SPECIMEN
Blood

TEST EXPLANATION AND RELATED PHYSIOLOGY
ALT is an enzyme located in the cytosol of many cell types, with a relatively high concentration in liver and lesser quantities in the kidneys, heart, skeletal muscle, and RBCs. As a result, ALT is a more specific indicator of liver damage than is AST. ALT may be released from cells with either sublethal cell injury (leakage) or necrosis or through enzyme induction (increased synthesis). Cholestasis and biliary tract obstruction can increase ALT by means of toxic effects of bile salts on hepatocytes. Serum ALT levels are not generally regarded as significant unless they are 2–3 times normal.

ALT has a serum half-life of approximately 5 days (dogs). Enzyme levels should increase by 12 h after hepatocellular damage and peak within 1–2 days, returning to normal in 1–3 weeks if hepatic insult resolves.

ALT will increase in dogs with severe muscle injury, and this may also occur in cats, but is not well documented (perhaps because of the cat lower muscle mass). Intravascular hemolysis can also increase ALT, especially in cats. ALT in renal epithelium can leak into urine, but does not affect serum levels.

INDICATIONS
Suspected hepatic disease

CONTRAINDICATIONS
None

POTENTIAL COMPLICATIONS
None

CLIENT EDUCATION
None

BODY SYSTEMS ASSESSED
- Hepatobiliary
- Musculoskeletal

SAMPLE

COLLECTION
0.5–2.0 mL of venous blood

HANDLING
- A plain red-top tube or serum-separator tube
- EDTA, sodium heparin, or lithium heparin are acceptable anticoagulants.
- Separate refrigerated serum or plasma from cells within 2 days.

STORAGE
Refrigerate or freeze serum or plasma for long-term storage.

STABILITY
- Room temperature: 1 day
- Refrigerated (2°–8°C): 1 week
- Frozen (−20°C): >1 week

PROTOCOL
None

INTERPRETATION

NORMAL FINDINGS OR RANGE
- Dogs: 18–86 IU/L
- Cats: 29–145 IU/L
- Reference intervals may vary, depending on the laboratory and assay.

ABNORMAL VALUES
Values above the reference interval

CRITICAL VALUES
None

INTERFERING FACTORS
Drugs That May Alter Results or Interpretation
Drugs That Interfere With Test Methodology
- Metronidazole may artifactually depress AST activity as determined by reduced NADH-coupled analytical methods. Interference is from similarity in absorbance peaks of NADH (340 nm) and metronidazole (322 nm).
- AST activity can be decreased by drugs (e.g., cephalosporin, cyclosporine, isoniazide) that impair activation of vitamin B_6 to pyridoxal 5′-phosphate (P5P). This effect can be avoided if P5P is added as an assay cofactor.

Drugs That Alter Physiology
- Corticosteroids may increase ALT by possible induction or cell injury (steroid hepatopathy).
- Phenobarbitol treatment may increase ALT by induction or cell injury.
- ALT activity can be increased by a variety of hepatotoxic drugs (e.g., erythromycin, rifampin, sulfonamides, acetaminophen, caparsolate).

Disorders That May Alter Results
- Hemolysis can cause a mild increase in ALT activity.
- Lipemia can cause an artifactual increase in ALT activity.
- Low vitamin B_6 levels may decrease ALT activity, as this is an essential cofactor for the enzyme (rare—occurs idiopathically and in humans undergoing hemodialysis).

Collection Techniques or Handling That May Alter Results
Hemolysis or severe lipemia

Influence of Signalment
Species
None

Breed
None

Age
None

Gender
None

Pregnancy
None

LIMITATIONS OF THE TEST
It is relatively specific and sensitive for liver damage, but ALT activity may be normal or only slightly increased with significant chronic disease associated with decreased hepatic mass.

Sensitivity, Specificity, and Positive and Negative Predictive Values
N/A

ALANINE AMINOTRANSFERASE

Valid If Run in a Human Lab?
Yes.

Causes of Abnormal Findings

High values	Low values
Hepatocellular injury or leakage	Hepatic atrophy (as in chronic congenital portosystemic shunts)
Inflammation (hepatitis)	Decreased P5P levels (if not added to assay)
Toxin or drug reactions	
Hepatic or biliary neoplasia	
Corticosteroid hepatopathy	
Hepatic lipidosis	
Hypoxia (anemia, cardiovascular disease)	
Pancreatitis	
Trauma	
Liver flukes	
Cirrhosis	
Copper storage disease	
Drug treatment (phenobarbitol, glucocorticoids)	
Muscle injury or necrosis (severe)	
Trauma	
Overexertion	
Myositis	

CLINICAL PERSPECTIVE
• ALT is fairly specific for hepatocellular injury in dogs and cats.
• Severe muscle injury elevates AST and creatine kinase also, but the ALT increase is less than the AST increase.
• Increased ALT levels in liver disease are proportional to the number of necrotic or damaged cells. Low-level, chronic liver disease may eventually result in hepatic failure with little to no increase in "leakage" enzymes.

MISCELLANEOUS

ANCILLARY TESTS
• AST may be measured concurrently to help confirm hepatocellular injury.
• Assaying creatine kinase levels may be useful to rule in or rule out muscle necrosis as a possible cause for an increased ALT level.

• Assay alkaline phosphatase or GGT level to detect any cholestatic component of liver disease.
• Assay serum bile acids or plasma ammonia levels to assess hepatic function.

SYNONYMS
• ALT
• Serum glutamic pyruvic transaminase (SGPT)

SEE ALSO
Blackwell's Five-Minute Veterinary Consult: Canine and Feline Topics
• Chapters on hepatic diseases
• Myocardial Infarction
• Myocarditis
• Myopathy, Focal Inflammatory—Masticatory Muscle Myositis and Extraocular Myositis
• Myopathy, Generalized Inflammatory—Polymyositis and Dermatomyositis

Related Topics in This Book
• Ammonia
• Aspartate Aminotransferase
• Bile Acids
• Bilirubin
• Creatine Kinase

ABBREVIATIONS
P5P = pyridoxal 5'-phosphate

Suggested Reading
Bain PJ. Liver. In: Latimer KS, ed. *Duncan and Prasse's Veterinary Laboratory Medicine: Clinical Pathology*, 4th ed. Ames: Iowa State Press, 2003: 193–214.
Center SA. Diagnostic procedures for evaluation of hepatic disease. In: Guilford WG, Center SA, Strombeck DR, *et al.*, eds. *Strombeck's Small Animal Gastroenterology*. Philadelphia: WB Saunders, 1996: 130–188.
Swenson CL, Graves ST. Absence of liver specificity for canine alanine aminotransferase (ALT). *Vet Clin Pathol* 1997; **26**: 26–28.
Willard MD, Twedt DC. Gastrointestinal, pancreatic, and hepatic disorders. In: Willard MD, Tvedten H, eds. *Small animal Clinical Diagnosis by Laboratory Methods*, 4th ed. St Louis: Saunders Elsevier, 2004: 208–246.

INTERNET RESOURCES
Tams TR. Liver disease: Diagnostic evaluation [Abstract]. In: 2001 Atlantic Coast Veterinary Conference, http://www.vin.com/VINDBPub/SearchPB/Proceedings/PR05000/PR00429.htm.

AUTHOR NAME
Perry J. Bain

ALBUMIN

BASICS

TYPE OF SPECIMEN
Blood

TEST EXPLANATION AND RELATED PHYSIOLOGY
Albumin is a small, water-soluble globular protein that accounts for approximately 75%–80% of the oncotic pressure of plasma. Manufactured in the liver, this negatively charged molecule is an important carrier protein for free fatty acids, Ca^{2+}, Mg^{2+}, bile acids, unconjugated bilirubin, thyroxine, and certain drugs. Albumin is catabolized in most tissues, and its half-life varies depending on the species. There appears to be a direct correlation between albumin turnover rate and body size; that is, larger animals have a slower replacement time and therefore are more susceptible to hypoalbuminemic edema than are smaller animals.

Most automated chemistry analyzers measure albumin spectrophotometrically. The BCG method is employed most commonly and involves preferential binding of BCG to albumin and detection of a subsequent color change. The quantity of albumin-bound dye is proportional to the concentration of albumin in the sample. Albumin concentration can also be evaluated with serum protein electrophoresis. Albumin migrates the farthest through cellulose acetate or agarose gel because of the combination of its relatively small size and anionic charge (see the "Protein Electrophoresis" chapter for more information on this method).

As a negative acute phase protein, albumin can decrease with inflammatory diseases.

INDICATIONS
- To assess hydration status
- To evaluate patients with anemia, cavity effusions, liver disease, renal disease, weight loss, and/or edema

CONTRAINDICATIONS
None

POTENTIAL COMPLICATIONS
None

CLIENT EDUCATION
None

BODY SYSTEMS ASSESSED
- Gastrointestinal
- Hepatobiliary
- Renal or urologic

SAMPLE

COLLECTION
0.5–2.0 mL of venous blood

HANDLING
- Plain red-top tube or serum-separator tube
- Sodium heparin, or lithium heparin anticoagulant also acceptable

STORAGE
- Store at room temperature for short-term use.
- Refrigerate for up to 1 month.
- Freeze for the long term.

STABILITY
- Room temperature: 1 week
- Refrigerated (2°–8°C): 1 month
- Frozen (−18°C): >1 month

PROTOCOL
None

INTERPRETATION

NORMAL FINDINGS OR RANGE
- Dogs: 2.8–4.0 g/dL (28–40 g/L)
- Cats: 2.4–3.9 g/dL (24–39 g/L)
- Reference intervals may vary, depending on the laboratory and assay.

ABNORMAL VALUES
Values above or below reference interval

CRITICAL VALUES
None

INTERFERING FACTORS
Drugs That May Alter Results or Interpretation
Drugs That Interfere with Test Methodology
Acetylsalicylic acid at higher than therapeutic doses—decreased levels

Drugs That Alter Physiology
- High-dose glucocorticoids can cause a slight increase.
- Testosterone, estrogen, or growth hormone may cause mild increases.

Disorders That May Alter Results
- Hemolysis or hemoglobinemia can cause false increases.
- Marked lipemia or hypertriglyceridemia can cause false decreases.
- With severe hypoalbuminemia (i.e., <1 g/dL), BCG may bind to globulins, causing a falsely elevated albumin concentration.

Collection Techniques or Handling That May Alter Results
- Marked hemolysis can cause false increases.
- Failure to fast a patient may result in lipemia.

Influence of Signalment
Species
None

Breed
None

Age
- Puppies, kittens, calves, and foals may have lower albumin concentrations than adult animals.
- In adult animals, a slight decrease in albumin occurs with advancing age.

Gender
None

Pregnancy
Decreases occur with pregnancy and lactation.

LIMITATIONS OF THE TEST
Sensitivity, Specificity, and Positive and Negative Predictive Values
Not available

Valid If Run in a Human Lab?
Yes, if the lab uses the BCG method. The bromcresol purple method commonly used in human laboratories may give falsely low levels in

some domestic species (e.g., dogs) because BCG does not reliably bind with all mammalian albumin molecules.

Causes of Abnormal Findings

High values	Low values
Hemoconcentration due to dehydration	Decreased production
	Hepatic insufficiency or failure
	Intestinal malabsorption
	Exocrine pancreatic insufficiency
	Inflammation
	Increased loss
	Blood loss
	Protein-losing nephropathy
	Glomerulonephritis (immune mediated or congenital)
	Amyloidosis
	Protein-losing enteropathy
	Small intestinal mucosal disease (inflammation, neoplasia)
	Lymphangiectasia
	Intestinal hemorrhage (intestinal parasites)
	Protein-losing dermatopathy: burns, generalized exudative skin disease
	Vasculitis
	Hemodilution
	Excessive IV fluid administration
	SIADH
	Edematous disorders: congestive heart failure

CLINICAL PERSPECTIVE

- Albumin accounts for the majority of plasma oncotic pressure.
- Hypoalbuminemia is often accompanied by hypoglobulinemia, with some exceptions:
  - Antigenic stimulation can increase immunoglobulin production, masking globulin losses.
  - Globulin levels are usually normal with renal disease because globulins are too large to pass through the glomerulus even when damaged.
  - Although most serum globulins are synthesized in the liver, because of concurrent systemic immunoglobulin synthesis, animals with hepatobiliary disease often have normal or even increased globulin concentrations.
- With liver disease, hypoalbuminemia is not seen until >70% of hepatobiliary function has been compromised.

MISCELLANEOUS

ANCILLARY TESTS
- Liver enyzmes and bile acids
- Total protein and globulins
- Urinalysis
- Urine protein/creatinine ratio

SYNONYMS
None

SEE ALSO

Blackwell's Five-Minute Veterinary Consult: Canine and Feline Topics
- Specific chapters on hepatic disease
- Glomerulonephritis
- Hypoalbuminemia
- Protein-Losing Enteropathy
- Proteinuria

Related Topics in This Book
- Globulins
- Protein Electrophoresis
- Total Protein
- Urine Protein

ABBREVIATIONS
- BCG = bromcresol green
- SIADH = syndrome of inappropriate antidiuretic hormone secretion

Suggested Reading

Evans EW, Duncan JR. Proteins, lipids and carbohydrates. In: Latimer KS, Mahaffey EA, Prasse KW, eds. *Duncan and Prasse's Veterinary Laboratory Medicine Clinical Pathology,* 4th ed. Ames: Iowa State Press, 2003: 162–192.

Lassen ED. Laboratory evaluation of plasma and serum proteins. In: Thrall MA, ed. *Veterinary Hematology and Clinical Chemistry*. Philadelphia: Lippincott Williams & Wilkins, 2004: 401–412.

Werner LL, Turnwald GH, Willard MD. Immunologic and plasma protein disorders. In: Willard MD, Tvedten H, eds. *Small Animal Clinical Diagnosis by Laboratory Methods,* 4th ed. St Louis: Saunders Elsevier, 2004: 290–305.

INTERNET RESOURCES
None

AUTHOR NAME
Jennifer Steinberg

ALKALINE PHOSPHATASE

BASICS

TYPE OF SPECIMEN
Blood

TEST EXPLANATION AND RELATED PHYSIOLOGY
Alkaline phosphatase is an enzyme present in many cells. Its biologic function in the cell is unknown, but it is a membrane-bound enzyme and its production and release into serum can be induced by cholestasis, drug treatment, corticosteroids, etc. Because it is a membrane-bound enzyme, increased serum enzyme activity should not occur with cell injury or necrosis, unless cholestasis (or other induction) also occurs. Variable forms of ALP (isoenzymes) are produced in different tissues and with different inducing agents. The most common isoenzymes found in serum of dogs and cats are the liver isoenzyme (increased in cholestasis, etc.), the bone isoenzyme (increased with bone remodeling), and, in dogs only, a corticosteroid-induced isoenzyme (produced in the liver). Although total serum ALP is typically measured in serum, increases in specific ALP isoenzymes can be differentiated by electrophoresis or by selective isoenzyme-inhibition tests.

INDICATIONS
- Suspected hepatic or biliary disease
- Suspected Cushing's syndrome

CONTRAINDICATIONS
None

POTENTIAL COMPLICATIONS
None

CLIENT EDUCATION
None

BODY SYSTEMS ASSESSED
- Hepatobiliary
- Musculoskeletal
- Endocrine or metabolic

SAMPLE

COLLECTION
0.5–2 mL of venous blood

HANDLING
Collect into a plain red-top tube or serum-separator tube.

STORAGE
Refrigerate for short-term storage, and freeze for long-term storage.

STABILITY
- Room temperature or refrigerated: 1 week
- Frozen (−20°C): 2 months

PROTOCOL
None

INTERPRETATION

NORMAL FINDINGS OR RANGE
- Dogs: 12–121 IU/L
- Cats: 10–72 IU/L
- Reference intervals may vary, depending on the laboratory and assay.

ABNORMAL VALUES
Values above the reference interval

CRITICAL VALUES
None

INTERFERING FACTORS
Drugs That May Alter Results or Interpretation
Drugs That Interfere with Test Methodology
None

Drugs That Alter Physiology
- In dogs, any corticosteroid treatment (even topical or ophthalmic treatments) increases ALP levels. Effects may persist for weeks after discontinuation of the drug, particularly with "depo"-type formulations.
- Anticonvulsants and barbiturates (phenobarbital, phenytoin, primidone) may also cause ALP increases.

Disorders That May Alter Results
None

Collection Techniques or Handling That May Alter Results
None

Influence of Signalment
Species
- ALP is relatively insensitive for cholestasis in cats.
- Dogs are unique in producing a corticosteroid isoenzyme of ALP (CALP) in response to corticosteroid treatment or increased endogenous corticosteroids.

Breed
Some families of Siberian huskies and Scottish terriers have ALP levels 1.5- to 17-fold normal and no evidence of hepatic abnormalities or increased cortisol concentration.

Age
- Young, rapidly growing animals (<12–15 months) commonly have increased serum ALP levels (bone isoenzyme).
- Geriatric dogs often have elevated ALP because of hepatic nodular hyperplasia.

Gender
None

Pregnancy
Pregnant, nursing animals may have increased ALP (bone remodeling, etc.).

LIMITATIONS OF THE TEST

Sensitivity, Specificity, and Positive and Negative Predictive Values

- For cholestatic disease in dogs:
  - Sensitivity, 96%
  - Positive predictive value, 61%
  - Negative predictive value, 94%
- Relatively insensitive for cholestasis in the cat.

Valid If Run in a Human Lab?
Yes.

Causes of Abnormal Findings

High values	Low values
Liver ALP	No significance
Corticosteroid treatment or increased endogenous corticosteroids (early)	
Corticosteroid hepatopathy (cholestasis)	
Hepatic nodular hyperplasia	
Hepatic lipidosis	
Cirrhosis	
Hepatitis or cholangiohepatitis	
Gallstones	
Cholecystitis	
Hepatic or biliary neoplasia	
Pancreatitis	
Anticonvulsant therapy	
Hyperthyroidism	
Copper storage disease	
Bone ALP	
Young, growing animals	
Fracture repair	
Bone neoplasia	
Metabolic bone disease (resorption)	
Hyperthyroidism	
Pregnancy	
Familial hyperphosphatemia (Siberian huskies, Scottish terriers)	
Corticosteroid ALP (canine only)	
Hyperadrenocorticism	
Glucocorticoid therapy	

Severe non-adrenal disease (stress of
    disease causes increased
    cortisol secretion)	

CLINICAL PERSPECTIVE

- Bone ALP increases tend to be mild (up to 2- to 3-fold normal).
- Large increases in ALP (10-fold or greater) are typically caused either by hepatic or cholestatic disease or by corticosteroid induction.
- Massive ALP increases (up to 100-fold normal) may be seen with corticosteroid treatment or Cushing's disease in dogs. Increased endogenous corticosteroids caused by stress of disease may cause smaller increases (<3-fold normal).
- Corticosteroids in dogs cause an initial increase in the liver isoenzyme. The corticosteroid isoenzyme becomes the predominant form over 2–3 weeks.

- Even mild increases in ALP should be considered significant in cats.
- Cats with hepatic lipidosis often exhibit an increased ALP level with a normal or mildly increased GGT level.

 MISCELLANEOUS

ANCILLARY TESTS

- Levamisole-inhibition test and heat-inactivation test to measure CALP: Levamisole and heat both selectively inhibit noncorticosteroid isoenzymes of ALP.
- Isoenzyme electrophoresis to quantify various ALP enzymes
- GGT and/or bilirubin levels to confirm a cholestasis
- ALT and AST to detect hepatocellular injury
- Urine cortisol/creatinine ratio to screen for hyperadrenocorticism

SYNONYMS

- Alk Phos
- ALP
- AP
- Serum alkaline phosphatase (SAP)

SEE ALSO

Blackwell's Five-Minute Veterinary Consult: Canine and Feline Topics
- Specific chapters on hepatic and biliary diseases
- Hyperadrenocorticism (Cushing's Disease)—Dogs

Related Topics in This Book
- Alanine Aminotransferase
- Bilirubin
- Cortisol/Creatinine Ratio
- Gamma-Glutamyltransferase
- Liver and Gallbladder Ultrasonography

ABBREVIATIONS

- ALP = alkaline phosphatase
- CALP = corticosteroid isoenzyme of ALP

Suggested Reading

Bain PJ. Liver. In: Latimer KS, ed. *Duncan and Prasse's Veterinary Laboratory Medicine: Clinical Pathology*, 4th ed. Ames: Iowa State Press, 2003: 193–214.

Center SA. Diagnostic procedures for evaluation of hepatic disease. In: Guilford WG, Center SA, Strombeck DR, *et al.*, eds. *Strombeck's Small Animal Gastroenterology*. Philadelphia: WB Saunders, 1996: 130–188.

Willard MD, Tvedten DC. Gastrointestinal, pancreatic, and hepatic disorders. In: Willard MD, Tvedten H, eds. *Small Animal Clinical Diagnosis by Laboratory Methods*, 4th ed. St Louis: Saunders Elsevier, 2004: 208–246.

INTERNET RESOURCES

Cornell University, College of Medicine: Clinical Pathology Modules, Veterinary Clinical Chemistry—Alkaline phosphatase (AP, ALP, SAP), http://diaglab.vet.cornell.edu/clinpath/ modules/chem/alkphos.htm.

AUTHOR NAME

Perry J. Bain

BASICS

TYPE OF SPECIMEN
Blood

TEST EXPLANATION AND RELATED PHYSIOLOGY
Atopy is a genetically predisposed tendency to develop IgE-mediated allergy to environmental allergens. Although IgE is a primary mediator of atopy, other mechanisms may be involved in some atopic patients.

Allergen-specific serologic tests measure the amount of allergen-specific IgE present in serum. All commercially available allergen-specific serologic tests evaluate levels of allergen-specific IgE through ELISA. The procedure for performing an allergen-specific serologic test can be briefly summarized as follows: The allergen is bound to a substrate, the patient's serum containing allergen-specific IgE is incubated with the allergen, and a reagent is added to detect the allergen-IgE antibody complexes. Monoclonal antibodies, polyclonal antibodies, and recombinant IgE-receptor fragments are the 3 detection reagents that are currently in use. Different laboratories may use various types of allergen sources, substrates, and reagents.

INDICATIONS
• To select environmental allergens for allergen-specific immunotherapy (hyposensitization, desensitization). Other factors important in allergen selection include the patient's history, patient's environment, and knowledge of local flora.
• Allergen-specific serologic testing may be selected in some rare situations over intradermal allergy testing (intradermal skin testing). These situations include patients that cannot have their hair coats clipped for intradermal allergy testing and patients with severe skin disease over sites where an intradermal allergy test would typically be performed.

CONTRAINDICATIONS
• Allergen-specific serology should not be used to diagnose atopy. The diagnosis of atopy should be based on the patient's history, physical examination, and the clinician's exclusion of other causes for the clinical signs.
• Allergen-specific serology is currently not helpful for identifying food allergens in patients.

POTENTIAL COMPLICATIONS
None

CLIENT EDUCATION
• Glucocorticoids may affect allergen-specific IgE levels and, if possible, should be discontinued prior to the test.
• Allergen-specific serologic testing does not identify all allergens. A food trial followed by food challenges will be necessary to identify food allergens.
• Allergen-specific immunotherapy is a long-term therapy that is typically continued throughout a pet's life.

BODY SYSTEMS ASSESSED
Dermatologic

 SAMPLE

COLLECTION
5–6 mL of venous blood

HANDLING
• Collect the serum into a serum-separator tube or red-top tube.
• Separate the serum within 30 min of drawing the sample.

STORAGE
No refrigeration is required.

STABILITY
Serum containing IgE is stable at room temperature, with refrigeration, or with freezing.

PROTOCOL
None

 INTERPRETATION

NORMAL FINDINGS OR RANGE
• Low levels or absence of allergen-specific IgE
• Several different companies offer allergen-specific serologic testing. Each company employs different technologies to detect allergen-specific IgE in a patient's serum. Clinicians are advised to consult the reference range provided by the company. Values from one company's allergen-specific serologic test cannot be compared to those of another company.

ABNORMAL VALUES
Value above the company's reference range is considered consistent with an allergy to that environmental allergen. Results must always be interpreted within the context of the patient's history and environment.

CRITICAL VALUES
None

INTERFERING FACTORS
Drugs That May Alter Results or Interpretation
Drugs That Interfere with Test Methodology
None

Drugs That Alter Physiology
Glucocorticoids may affect serum allergen-specific IgE levels.

Disorders That May Alter Results
None

Collection Techniques or Handling That May Alter Results
The serum sample should not be heated: IgE is heat labile and is destroyed by heating to 56°C for 4 h.

Influence of Signalment

Species
Allergen-specific serologic tests have been studied less in cats than in dogs.

Breed
None

Age
The typical age of onset for atopic signs in dogs is 6 months to 3 years. If the onset of clinical signs does not fall within this range, other causes should especially be excluded prior to allergy testing.

Gender
None

Pregnancy
None

LIMITATIONS OF THE TEST
• Normal findings (lack of elevated allergen-specific IgE) can occur in atopic patients that have a non–IgE-mediated form of atopic disease. If no elevations in allergen-specific IgE are noted on serology, intradermal allergy testing is recommended to evaluate the cellular immunity of the skin.
• False positives can occur with allergen-specific serologic testing. Normal, nonallergic dogs can have elevated allergen-specific IgE levels. Some commercially available allergen-specific serologic tests may also detect nonrelevant immunoglobulins such as IgG.

Sensitivity, Specificity, and Positive and Negative Predictive Values
None

Valid If Run in a Human Lab?
No. The assays are species specific.

CLINICAL PERSPECTIVE
• Allergen-specific serologic test results should be interpreted based on the patient history and environment.
• If atopy is suspected but no positives are noted on the allergen-specific serologic test, intradermal allergy testing is recommended.

• Referral to a veterinary dermatologist should be considered for additional diagnostic workup and management of atopic dermatitis.

MISCELLANEOUS

ANCILLARY TESTS
None

SYNONYMS
Serologic allergy test

SEE ALSO
Blackwell's Five-Minute Veterinary Consult: Canine and Feline Topics
Atopic Dermatitis
Related Topics in This Book
Intradermal Testing

ABBREVIATIONS
None

Suggested Reading
DeBoer DJ, Verbugge MJ. Results of canine serum allergen specific IgE determinations performed by commercial laboratories on canine IgE-free samples and on samples from non-allergic dogs [Abstract]. *Vet Dermatol* 2005; 16: 195.
Patterson AP, Schaeffer DJ, Campbell KL. Reproducibility of a commercial in vitro allergen-specific assay for immunoglobulin E in dogs. *Vet Rec* 2005; 157: 81–85.

INTERNET RESOURCES
GREER Veterinary, Allergy testing and treatment for canine, feline, and equine, http://www.greerlabs.com/vet/vet.index.php
HESKA ALLERCEPT allergy assessment and treatment program, http://www.heska.com/allergy/index.asp

AUTHOR NAME
Kathy C. Tater

ALPHA-1 PROTEASE INHIBITOR

 BASICS

TYPE OF SPECIMEN
Feces

TEST EXPLANATION AND RELATED PHYSIOLOGY
Alpha-1 protease inhibitor (α_1-PI) is a plasma protein lost into the gut at about the same rate as albumin and other similarly sized plasma proteins. Since it is a proteinase inhibitor, it is resistant to degradation in the gut lumen by other proteinases and remains intact, thereby enabling assay. This provides a measure of general protein loss into the gut (PLE) and can aid in diagnosis of abnormal levels of protein loss.

INDICATIONS
To assess GI protein loss or PLE
- In animals with panhypoproteinemia or hypoalbuminemia, with or without chronic diarrhea
- In animals at risk for familial PLE

CONTRAINDICATIONS
The test is not validated for cats that are <1 year of age.

POTENTIAL COMPLICATIONS
None

CLIENT EDUCATION
- The fecal samples must be collected after normal defecation, not by manual collection, or the results will be altered.
- Samples that are not promptly frozen and kept frozen until analysis may cause false-negative results.

BODY SYSTEMS ASSESSED
Gastrointestinal

 SAMPLE

COLLECTION
- 3 fresh fecal samples, 1g each, on 3 consecutive days.
- Must be collected from naturally passed defecations

HANDLING
- Collect fecal samples as soon as possible after defecation into special preweighed fecal tubes available from the lab that performs the test.
- Freeze samples immediately after collection.

STORAGE
Samples must be kept frozen and delivered frozen to the lab.

STABILITY
- Significant degradation occurs if feces are kept at room temperature or refrigerated.
- Frozen samples are reportedly stable up for to 100 days.

PROTOCOL
None

 INTERPRETATION

NORMAL FINDINGS OR RANGE
- Dogs: 0.23–5.67 μg/g fecal material
- Cats: 0.04–1.6 μg/g fecal material

ABNORMAL VALUES
- Dogs: mean 3-day α_1-PI $\geq$ 9.4 μg/g feces or an individual sample $\geq$ 15.0 μg/g feces
- Cats: mean 3-day α_1-PI > 1.6 μg/g feces

CRITICAL VALUES
None

INTERFERING FACTORS
Drugs That May Alter Results or Interpretation
Drugs That Interfere with Test Methodology
None

Drugs That Alter Physiology
None known, although chronic NSAID use in humans affects GI mucosal permeability. One study in dogs did not support this.

Disorders That May Alter Results
None known in dogs and cats, although intestinal blood loss significantly increases α_1-PI levels in people without GI mucosal disease.

Collection Techniques or Handling That May Alter Results
- Feces should be collected manually because abrasion of the colon wall may increase α_1-PI levels.
- Special preweighed fecal tubes, supplied by the lab, must be used.
- Fecal samples should be frozen immediately after defecation. A delay in freezing feces will alter the results.

Influence of Signalment
Species
None

Breed
The test may identify familial PLE in soft-coated Wheaten terriers with subclinical protein loss.

Age
The test is not a valid measure of GI protein loss in cats that are <1 year of age because of highly variable α_1-PI levels.

Gender
None

Pregnancy
None

LIMITATIONS OF THE TEST
- α_1-PI levels may vary widely in consecutive fecal samples, so multiple, random samples must be assayed to improve diagnostic utility.
- Because protein loss into the gut is seen with a wide variety of causes, this test is probably not very specific.

Sensitivity, Specificity, and Positive and Negative Predictive Values
N/A

Valid If Run in a Human Lab?
No. The test is species specific, and ELISAs have been validated for use only in dogs and adult cats.

Causes of Abnormal Findings

High values	Low values
Inflammatory gastroenteropathies like inflammatory bowel disease	Not significant
Small intestinal bacterial overgrowth	
Intestinal lymphangectasia	
Familial PLE or PLN in soft-coated Wheaten terriers	
GI neoplasia	
GI foreign bodies	
Intussusceptions	
Infectious gastroenteritis	
GI hemorrhage(?)	
Possible de novo synthesis of α_1-PI in the GI mucosa(?)	

CLINICAL PERSPECTIVE

- The clinical utility of this test appears to be limited to screening for PLE in animals with either early disease or mild disease or as a noninvasive part of a multisystem workup for hypoalbuminemia or panhypoproteinemia.
- Recent information suggests that the level of fecal α_1-PI varies over the course of chronic intestinal disease and may not always be abnormal especially later in disease stages, contrary to the expectations that, as protein loss in the gut increased, so would the level of fecal α_1-PI.
- There is little information available about the test as a valid indicator of PLE in cats.

MISCELLANEOUS

ANCILLARY TESTS

- To exclude decreased protein production and PLN, liver function testing should be performed on patients with hypoproteinemia or hypoalbuminemia and their urine protein/creatinine ratio determined.
- Patients with hypoproteinemia, hypoalbuminemia, and/or chronic diarrhea who have abnormally high levels of fecal α_1-PI, but no evidence of PLN or hepatic dysfunction, should have GI biopsies to confirm a cause of PLE.

SYNONYMS

α_1-PI

SEE ALSO

Blackwell's Five-Minute Veterinary Consult: Canine and Feline Topics
- Exocrine Pancreatic Insufficiency
- Protein-Losing Enteropathy
- Small Intestinal Bacterial Overgrowth

Related Topics in This Book

- Cobalamin
- Folate
- Gastrointestinal Ultrasonography
- Pancreatic Ultrasound
- Trypsin-like Immunoreactivity

ABBREVIATIONS

- α_1-PI = alpha-1 protease inhibitor
- PLE = protein-losing enteropathy
- PLN = protein-losing nephropathy

Suggested Reading

Hall EJ, German AJ. Diseases of the small intestine. In: Ettinger SJ, Feldman EC, eds. *Textbook of Veterinary Internal Medicine*, 6th ed. St Louis: Saunders Elsevier, 2005: 1332–1377.

Melgarejo, T, Williams DA, Asem EK. Enzyme-linked immunosorbent assay for canine α_1-protease inhibitor. *Am J Vet Res* 1998; 59: 127–130.

Murphy KF, German AJ, Ruaux GC, *et al*. Fecal α_1-proteinase inhibitor concentration in dogs with chronic gastrointestinal disease. *Vet Clin Pathol* 2003; 32: 67–72.

Murphy KF, German AJ, Ruaux GC, *et al*. Fecal α_1-proteinase inhibitor concentration in dogs receiving long-term nonsteroidal anti-inflammatory drug therapy. *Vet Clin Pathol* 2003; 32: 136–139.

INTERNET RESOURCES

Texas A&M University, College of Veterinary Medicine, Gastrointestinal Laboratory, http://www.cvm.tamu.edu/gilab/.

AUTHOR NAME

Lisa Moses

AMBULATORY ELECTROCARDIOGRAPHIC MONITORING

 BASICS

TYPE OF PROCEDURE
Electrodiagnostic

PROCEDURE EXPLANATION AND RELATED PHYSIOLOGY
Arrhythmias and conduction disturbances can occur sporadically and therefore can easily be missed on a short lead II screening ECG. Because of the sporadic nature of many arrhythmias, long-term monitoring is often necessary to assess efficacy of therapy.

A *Holter monitor* is a device used to evaluate the cardiac electrical system for 24–48h in a home or in-hospital setting. A Holter monitor can be used to determine whether an arrhythmia is present, what the arrhythmia is, how frequently it occurs, and whether medication or disease progression has changed the arrhythmia. However if clinical signs do not occur while the patient is wearing the monitor, one may still not know with certainty whether an arrhythmia is responsible for the clinical signs.

An *event monitor* (aka *loop monitor*) is a device that can be used to evaluate a patient for an extended monitoring period (5–7 days); however, it stores only the most recent 1–2 min of electrical activity. If clinical signs (syncope, collapse) occur, the owner must activate a button on the machine to save the most current cardiac electrical activity (1–2 min), as well as the previous 30–60s. Therefore, an event monitor provides information on the cardiac electrical activity during and immediately preceding the episode. However, it does not provide a quantification of the daily electrical activity. Additionally, if the owner is not present to activate the monitor during the episode, the electrical activity associated with the episode will not be saved.

INDICATIONS
Holter Monitoring
- To identify and quantify arrhythmias
- To screen boxers for arrhythmogenic right ventricular cardiomyopathy (boxer cardiomyopathy), Doberman pinschers for dilated cardiomyopathy (DCM), and German shepherds for congenital idiopathic ventricular arrhythmias
- To monitor patients before and after treatment with antiarrhythmics

Event Monitoring
- To identify an arrhythmia that may be associated with intermittent clinical signs (syncope, exercise intolerance)
- To exclude a cardiac electrical event as a cause of the clinical signs

CONTRAINDICATIONS
- A small number of patients may find wearing the monitor stressful. If possible, any symptoms associated with congestive heart failure (dyspnea, tachypnea) should be addressed medically before placing the monitor.
- Optimally, a Holter monitor should be evaluated before and after starting ventricular antiarrhythmic therapy to accurately assess the benefits and potential adverse effects of treatment. However, do not postpone treatment in order to obtain a pretreatment monitor in cases with severe ventricular arrhythmias [rapid ventricular tachycardia, sustained ventricular tachycardia, frequent R on T (R wave of the VPC superimposed on the preceding T wave)].

POTENTIAL COMPLICATIONS
Adhesive tape is generally needed to adhere the electrodes to the skin. In rare cases, some patients may develop a local skin reaction to the tape and adhesive material.

CLIENT EDUCATION
- Shaving of the area prior to application of the electrodes is recommended to ensure clear ECGs. Owners who are concerned about shaving the area for cosmetic reasons should be advised that the electrodes may be applied without shaving, but the reading may be less accurate.
- Use of event monitor requires client interaction to activate the unit as close to the onset of clinical signs as possible.
- The owner should maintain a detailed activity and event log during the time a Holter monitor is worn. This is critical to be able to correlate any clinical findings with abnormalities present on the ECG.

BODY SYSTEMS ASSESSED
Cardiovascular

 PROCEDURE

PATIENT PREPARATION
Preprocedure Medication or Preparation
None

Anesthesia or Sedation
None

Patient Positioning
The patient should be standing during placement to ensure correct placement of the electrodes.

Patient Monitoring
None

Equipment or Supplies
- An event monitor or Holter monitor with a patient cable and electrodes
- 1-inch white tape
- 3-inch adhesive tape
- 3-inch self-adhesive bandage wrap
- Electrode gel

Techniques
Holter Monitor
- The specific technique will vary slightly, depending on the brand of monitor. Please consult the equipment brochure for specific instructions.
- Prepare as many parts of the setup as possible before involving the patient. The monitor is likely to have 2–7 electrodes. Set aside 2 pieces of white tape approximately 2 inches long for each electrode. Snap the ends of the patient cable to the electrodes.
- With the patient standing, shave a spot for each electrode approximately 2 × 1.5 inches. The locations of the electrodes on the animal will vary depending on the type of monitor, so please consult your equipment for specific instructions.
- Apply a small amount of electrode gel to each electrode. Too much gel will interfere with the ability of the electrodes to stick. Apply the electrodes to the shaved patches. After applying each one, place 2 pieces of the white tape over the sides of the electrode. Once all of the electrodes are attached, begin approximately 1 inch below the first electrode and place a strip of 3-inch-wide adhesive tape around the dorsal aspect of the patient to cover all of the electrodes and the white tape. In most cases, it is not necessary to encircle the patient completely, and we advise against placing the tape on the ventral aspect of the chest, because the tape can be very difficult to remove. Finish and cut the tape at least 1 inch below the last electrode. Next, take the 3-inch self-adhesive bandage wrap and wrap all of the way around the patient. Start at the top of the back and put a piece of white tape on the end so that it will stick to the underlying adhesive tape. Bundle the wires of the electrode cords and place another piece of white tape around the bundle. Coil the rest of the patient cable into a circle approximately 4 inches in diameter between the shoulder blades of the patient, leaving enough of the end of the cable so it reaches to the neck. Use the adhesive tape to cover the coil.

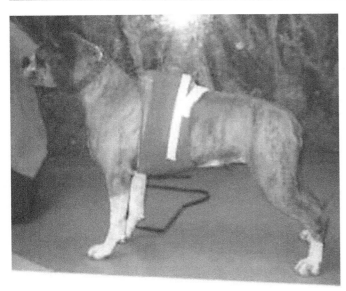

Figure 1

A boxer with a Holter monitor wrapped securely to its body.

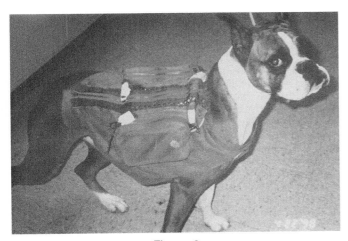

Figure 2

A boxer wearing a Holter vest.

- Plug the end of the patient cord into the monitor and secure the plug. Place the monitor on the back of the animal and cover the monitor with an additional layer of tape (Figure 1).
- Some clinicians prefer to place a vest over the final layer of adhesive tape and place the monitor into a pocket on the side of the vest. This may help secure the monitor and electrodes into a slightly tighter position (Figure 2). Vests may be purchased specifically for this use or may be created from durable, machine-washable material (see Internet Resources).
- While wearing the monitor we encourage the patient to participate in normal daily activity.

Event Monitor
- It is attached to the animal in a manner similar to the Holter unit, although the number of leads will vary.
- It must remain accessible to the owner.
- When the animal has a clinical event (e.g., syncope), the owner activates the memory feature by pressing a button on the unit that will preserve the ECG into memory for a preprogrammed time prior to pushing the button and then continue to record into memory for a preprogrammed time.

SAMPLE HANDLING
- Ship the Holter tape to site for analysis (see the Internet Resources section).
- Transmit the event-monitor recording over the phone to telemedicine consultant (see the Internet Resources section).

APPROPRIATE AFTERCARE
Postprocedure Patient Monitoring
While wearing the unit, ensure that the wrap is not too tight.

Nursing Care
N/A

Dietary Modification
N/A

Medication Requirements
N/A

Restrictions on Activity
- To obtain the most useful information about a patient, owners should be encouraged to allow the patient to pursue regular activities while wearing the monitor.
- Keep the ambulatory monitor dry, so allow no swimming, bathing, or extended periods in the rain.

Anticipated Recovery Time
N/A

 INTERPRETATION

NORMAL FINDINGS OR RANGE
- Interpretation will vary depending on the type of monitor (Holter vs event).
- The normal canine heart rate on a Holter monitor can range from 29 to 240 beats/min with an average rate of 52–86 beats/min. Periods of sinus arrhythmia are common. Occasional second-degree AV block, rare VPCs, and atrial premature complexes in geriatric animals can be normal variants. In most breeds, <25 VPCs in 24 h can be normal. In boxers, normal variation may be as high as 100 VPCs in 24 h.
- The normal feline heart rate on a Holter monitor has been reported to range from 68 to 294 beats/min, with an average heart rate of 114–202 beats/min. Periods of sinus arrhythmia are noted in most cats. VPCs are observed infrequently (generally <50).

ABNORMAL VALUES
- Interpretation will vary depending on type of monitor, species and clinical complaint.
- Advanced second-degree or complete AV block
- Prolonged periods of sinus arrest
- Frequent atrial or ventricular premature complexes
- Atrial fibrillation
- Ventricular tachycardia

CRITICAL VALUES
Ventricular tachycardia and complete AV block require immediate attention

INTERFERING FACTORS
Drugs That May Alter Results of the Procedure
Antiarrhythmic agents or drugs that alter autonomic tone (e.g., β blockers, digoxin, sympathomimetics, bronchodilators) affect heart rhythm.

Conditions That May Interfere with Performing the Procedure
None

AMBULATORY ELECTROCARDIOGRAPHIC MONITORING

Procedure Techniques or Handling That May Alter Results

• Failure to secure the electrodes sufficiently to a patient may allow a significant amount of motion artifact that may prevent an accurate reading. Free-moving cable wires or kinked patient cords also degrade ECG quality.

• Failure to shave the electrode area, particularly on animals with thick fur, can increase artifact.

• The results of a Holter monitor should be evaluated to determine the number of hours of artifact. Generally, we prefer no more than a total of 4h of artifact (20h of readable material).

Influence of Signalment on Performing and Interpreting the Procedure

Species
The procedure is often difficult to perform on cats and tiny dogs because of size of units and poor patient tolerability to procedure.

Breed
• Cocker spaniels have very pronounced sinus arrhythmia as a normal variant.
• Normal boxers may have up to 100 VPCs in 24h.
• The presence of VPCs is a risk factor in Doberman pinschers for developing DCM.

Age
Atrial premature complexes may be normal variants in geriatric patients.

Gender
None

Pregnancy
None

CLINICAL PERSPECTIVE

• Use of a Holter monitor answers these questions:
  • Is there an arrhythmia present today?
  • What and how frequent is the arrhythmia?
  • Has a drug or disease progression changed the arrhythmia?
• Use of an event monitor answers this question:
  • Is there a cardiac electrical reason for the clinical signs that occur while the monitor is being worn?
• Holter monitoring is useful in assessing the severity of a ventricular arrhythmia prior to initiating therapy and then monitoring the efficacy of that therapy. Due to normal fluctuations in frequency of VPCs, an 85% reduction in frequency is required to prove efficacy of antiarrhythmic therapy.
• In 1 study of Doberman pinschers with normal echocardiograms, all animals with >50 VPCs per 24 h, 94% with >10 VPCs per 24 h, and 94% with couplets or triplets of VPCs developed echocardiographic evidence of DCM within 1 year. However, it is important to note that not all Dobermans with VPCs develop cardiomyopathy, and the absence of VPCs on a 24-h Holter study does not rule out the subsequent development of DCM.
• In animals with frequent syncopal episodes, an event monitor is preferable to a Holter monitor for making a diagnosis because the event recording is timed with the clinical signs. In a study of 60 collapsing animals, 51 tracings (85%) were diagnostic, ruling out arrhythmias in 65% and ruling in arrhythmias in 35%.

MISCELLANEOUS

ANCILLARY TESTS
Echocardiography may be indicated if serious arrhythmias or frequent VPCs are detected.

SYNONYMS
• Event monitor

• Loop monitor
• Holter monitor

SEE ALSO
Blackwell's Five-Minute Veterinary Consult: Canine and Feline Topics
• Atrioventricular Block, Complete (Third Degree)
• Cardiomyopathy—Boxer
• Cardiomyopathy, Dilated—Dogs
• Sick Sinus Syndrome
• Syncope
• Ventricular Premature Complexes
• Ventricular Tachycardia

Related Topics in This Book
Electrocardiography

ABBREVIATIONS
• AV = atrioventricular
• DCM = dilated cardiomyopathy
• VPC = ventricular premature complex

Suggested Reading
Bright JM, Cali JV. Clinical usefulness of cardiac event recording in dogs and cats examined because of syncope, episodic collapse, or intermittent weakness: 60 cases (1997–1999). *J Am Vet Med Assoc* 2000; 216: 1110–1114.
Calvert CA, Jacobs GJ, Smith DD, *et al.* Association between results of ambulatory electrocardiography and development of cardiomyopathy during long-term follow-up in Doberman pinschers. *J Am Vet Med Assoc* 2000; 216: 34–39.
Calvert CA, Wall M. Results of ambulatory electrocardiography in overtly healthy Doberman pinschers with equivocal echocardiographic evidence of dilated cardiomyopathy. *J Am Vet Med Assoc* 2001; 219: 782–784.
Meurs KM, Spier AW, Wright NA, Hamlin RL. Use of ambulatory electrocardiography for detection of ventricular premature complexes in healthy dogs. *J Am Vet Med Assoc* 2001; 218: 1291–1292.
Miller RH, Lehmkuhl LB, Bonagura JD, Beall MJ. Retrospective analysis of the clinical utility of ambulatory electrocardiographic (Holter) recordings in syncopal dogs: 44 cases (1991–1995). *J Vet Intern Med* 1999; 13: 111–122.
Petrie JP. Practical application of Holter monitoring in dogs and cats. *Clin Tech Small Anim Pract* 2005; 20: 173–181.
Spier AW, Meurs KM. Evaluation of spontaneous variability in the frequency of ventricular arrhythmias in boxers with arrhythmogenic right ventricular cardiomyopathy. *J Am Vet Med Assoc* 2004; 224: 538–541.
Ware WA. Twenty-four hour ambulatory electrocardiography in normal cats. *J Vet Intern Med* 1999; 13: 175–180.

INTERNET RESOURCES
Alice King Chatham Medical Arts (AKCMA), http://www.akcma.com/home. Source for ambulatory ECG vests (search for "dog jacket with pocket").
Biomedical Systems, http://www.biomedsys.com. Source for ambulatory ECG monitors and interpretation.
Canine Holter Monitor Service, Veterinary Cardiac Genetics Lab, College of Veterinary Medicine, Washington State University, http://www.Holtermydog.com. Source for ambulatory ECG monitors and interpretation.
IDEXX Laboratories, http://www.idexx.com. Source for ambulatory ECG monitors and interpretation.

AUTHOR NAMES
Kathyrn M. Meurs and Allison Lamb

BASICS

TYPE OF SPECIMEN
Blood

TEST EXPLANATION AND RELATED PHYSIOLOGY
The ammonia (NH_3) level in plasma has been used to assess decreased hepatocellular function, shunting of portal blood flow to systemic circulation, and absence of normal urea cycle enzyme function. The overall level depends on dietary intake of protein, normal portal venous circulation, and presence of normally functioning hepatocytes with normal urea cycle enzyme pathways.

Ammonia is primarily a waste product of GI bacterial digestion of dietary protein. Other sources include enteric metabolism of ingested urea, exfoliated cellular debris, and pathologic bleeding into the alimentary canal. The liver receives the NH_3 via the portal vein and is the primary site of urea synthesis (Krebs-Henseleit cycle) from NH_3. This is the main route for elimination of NH_3 with a very high first-pass elimination. The resulting BUN is then excreted by the kidneys.

Small quantities of NH_3 are also derived from endogenous catabolism of skeletal muscle. The addition of NH_3 via renal ammoniagenesis is largely negated via normal urinary secretion. When the kidneys are contributing to the correction of metabolic alkalosis, NH_3 production and blood values may be increased because of NH_3 loss into the renal veins. Alternatively, with decreased renal function, NH_3 levels may rise because of decreased excretion. Muscle cells play a small role in clearance of blood NH_3.

Ammonia is considered to be one of many waste products of metabolism that increase when normal hepatic function or portal venous circulation is disrupted. In that sense, it is a marker for, and not the sole mediator of, hepatic encephalopathy. Symptoms of pure hyperammonemia (as may be seen with urea enzyme cycle deficiencies) are not the same as those of portosystemic shunting of blood or liver failure. The nervous system is affected by hyperammonemia, which causes abnormal function of the blood-brain barrier, impaired cerebral blood flow, abnormal neuronal excitability, deranged neurotransmitter metabolism, balance, interactions with neuroreceptors, and degenerative neuronal changes (if chronic).

A variety of test methods are used for determining plasma NH_3, including "wet" spectrophotometric methods (most laboratories), dry-reagent kits (e.g., VetTest Chemistry Analyzer, IDEXX Laboratories, Westbrook, Maine, USA; and Blood Ammonia Checker II, Menarini, Florence, Italy), and ion-selective electrodes.

INDICATIONS
• Screen for insufficiency of liver (hepatocellular) functional ability and/or total cell volume.
• Screen for portosystemic venous shunting (congenital or acquired).
• Screen for urea cycle enzyme deficiencies.

CONTRAINDICATIONS
• None for fasting NH_3 level
• Do not perform an ammonia-tolerance test if there are symptoms of encephalopathy.

POTENTIAL COMPLICATIONS
• None for fasting NH_3 level
• An ammonia-tolerance test can cause the following:
  • Vomiting
  • Encephalopathy or coma

CLIENT EDUCATION
• Results are most accurate after the patient has fasted for 12h.
• An ammonia-tolerance test may be necessary in Maltese and possibly other small terrier breeds that have mild to modest elevations in serum bile acids.

BODY SYSTEMS ASSESSED
• Hepatobiliary
• Cardiovascular

SAMPLE

COLLECTION
• 1–3 mL of arterial (preferred) or venous blood
• Consider submitting paired patient samples and a control sample from a healthy patient, so that specimens are handled similarly in order to help with test reliability.

HANDLING
• Lithium heparin anticoagulant is usually preferred.
• To chill the sample, place it immediately on ice.
• Separate the sample via a centrifuge (preferably refrigerated) within 15–30 min.
• Analyze the sample within 15–30 min of collection.

STORAGE
• None. One study showed that canine plasma needed to be analyzed within 30 min and could not be stored at any temperature for any length of time.
• Although other studies variably suggest that feline plasma may be processed then stored at $-2°C$ for 1–2 days, none have shown standard freezers or refrigeration temperatures to be acceptable for canine or feline samples.

STABILITY
Not stable. Altered values develop when samples are held beyond 30 min even when the samples have been properly chilled, all clots are prevented, and the plasma has been separated from RBCs.

PROTOCOL
An ammonium-tolerance test (ATT) may improve sensitivity.
• Oral ATT
  • Collect resting samples after the patient has fasted for 12 h.
  • Administer 100 mg/kg ammonium chloride as a dilute solution or in gelatin capsules. The dose should not exceed 20 mg/mL and a total dose of 3 g.
  • Collect the samples at 15 and 30 min after challenge.
• Rectal ATT
  • Administer a warm-water enema 12h prior to the test.
  • Collect a resting sample.
  • Administer 100 mg/kg ammonium chloride or 2 mL/kg 5% ammonium chloride by enema (a catheter with a high rectal placement).
  • Collect samples at 15 and 30 min after challenge.
• A modified oral ATT using a standardized meal may be more sensitive than a single fasting NH_3 level. This may reduce the degree of risk of the adverse side effects of a traditional oral ATT.
  • The meal should supply 33 kcal/kg, with a protein concentration of around 30.3% dry matter.
  • Collect samples before and 6 h after feeding.

INTERPRETATION

NORMAL FINDINGS OR RANGE
• *Maximum* normal fasting plasma values may vary depending on the test system or laboratory used.
  • Dogs: approximately 40–120 $\mu g/dL$
  • Cats: approximately 35–100 $\mu g/dL$
• ATT: Blood ammonia levels should not increase >2-fold.

AMMONIA

ABNORMAL VALUES
- Fasting ammonia: values above the reference range
- ATT: A 3- to 10-fold increase above baseline indicates ammonia intolerance consistent with hepatic insufficiency or a portosystemic vascular anomaly.

CRITICAL VALUES
Values of >400 $\mu g/dL$ are thought to be of increased immediate clinical significance.

INTERFERING FACTORS
Drugs That May Alter Results or Interpretation
Drugs That Interfere with Test Methodology
None

Drugs That Alter Physiology
Decreased level
- Antibiotics reduce bacterial intestinal flora that produce ammonia.
- Lactulose (oral or rectal)
- Cleansing or retention enemas [lactulose, lactose, neomycin, Betadyne (povidone iodine)]
- Low-protein diets

Increased level
- Blood transfusion: Stored blood products *may* have elevated ammonia levels.
- Parenteral amino acid solutions
- Narcotics
- Valproic acid
- Diuretics that enhance metabolic alkalosis and renal ammoniagenesis
- High-protein meals

Disorders That May Alter Results
- Hemolysis can cause spuriously high values because RBCs contain 3-fold more NH_3 than does plasma.
- Lipemia may alter the results of reflectance spectrophotometric methods.
- Reduction in skeletal muscle mass in debilitated patients may increase NH_3 level.

Collection Techniques or Handling That May Alter Results
- Natural oils from fingertips may increase NH_3.
- The proximity of the analyzer or reagents to ammonia- or ammonium-based disinfectants may alter the test results.
- Incomplete cooling of the sample may increase NH_3 concentration.
- Clotting of the sample may increase NH_3 concentration.
- Delay in separation of the RBCs from the plasma may increase NH_3 concentration.
- Prolonged venous occlusion while obtaining blood samples may increase the release of NH_3 from RBCs and cause transient changes in muscle metabolism that affect the NH_3 concentration.
- Exposure of an NH_3 test reagent to other test reagents in multitest chemistry analyzers

Influence of Signalment
Species
None

Breed
Because bile acid assays are unreliable in Maltese terriers, an ammonia-tolerance test may be necessary to detect liver disease or subclinical portosystemic vascular anomalies.

Age
None

Gender
None

Pregnancy
None

LIMITATIONS OF THE TEST
- Difficult sample-handling requirements are a major obstacle.
- Any values above the reference range may suggest an increased risk of symptoms but with poor correlation of symptoms to ammonia levels.
- Not all animals with hepatoencephalopathy have elevated NH_3.
- NH_3 levels are not consistently elevated with chronic liver parenchymal disease and rarely elevated with acute hepatic disease.

Sensitivity, Specificity, and Positive and Negative Predictive Values
- 80% of dogs with portosystemic vascular anomalies have elevated NH_3.
- 90% of cats with portosystemic vascular anomalies have elevated NH_3.
- Approximately 50% of dogs with chronic hepatitis have elevated NH_3.

Valid If Run in a Human Lab?
Yes.

Causes of Abnormal Findings

High values	Low values
Hepatic	Not applicable
Reduced hepatocellular mass of any cause: chronic hepatitis, cirrhosis, neoplasia, necrosis	
Disruption of normal hepatocellular function: vacuolar-metabolic disorders, hepatic lipidosis, decreased perfusion, hypoxia	
Portosystemic shunts	
Congenital	
Major vascular shunts	
Portal venous hypoplasia, microvascular dysplasia, noncirrhotic portal hypertension	
Portal vein atresia	
Hepatic arteriovenous fistula	
Acquired	
Cirrhosis	
Chronic hepatitis with fibrosis	
Metabolic alkalosis	
Hypokalemia (related to metabolic alkalosis)	
Renal dysfunction or urinary obstruction	

CLINICAL PERSPECTIVE
- Ammonia contributes to hepatic encephalopathy; however, ammonia concentrations are much higher in the brain than in the blood, and a clear correlation is not seen.
- Run plasma ammonia tests with a control sample.

MISCELLANEOUS
ANCILLARY TESTS
- Serum bile acid profile
- BUN and albumin (which are produced by the liver)
- BUN, creatinine, and urine specific gravity to exclude decreased renal excretion
- Hepatic ultrasound
- Hepatic biopsy
- Prothrombin time and partial thromboplastin time (coagulation factors produced by the liver)

SYNONYMS
NH_3

SEE ALSO

Blackwell's Five-Minute Veterinary Consult: Canine and Feline Topics

- Specific chapters on hepatitis
- Arteriovenous Fistula
- Arteriovenous Malformation of the Liver
- Hepatic Encephalopathy
- Hepatic Failure, Acute
- Hepatotoxins
- Portosystemic Shunting, Acquired
- Portosystemic Vascular Anomaly, Congenital

Related Topics in This Book

- Alanine Aminotransferase
- Angiography and Angiocardiography
- Bile Acids
- Liver and Gallbladder Ultrasonography
- Liver Biopsy

ABBREVIATIONS

- ATT = ammonium-tolerance test
- NH_3 = ammonia

Suggested Reading

Hitt ME, Jones BD. Effects of storage temperature and time on canine plasma ammonia concentrations. *Am J Vet Res* 1986; 47: 363–364.

Ogilvie GK, Engelking LR, Anwer MS. Effects of plasma sample storage on blood ammonia, bilirubin, and urea nitrogen concentrations: Cats and horses. *Am J Vet Res* 1985; 46: 2619–2622.

Walker MC, Hill RC, Guilford WG, *et al.* Postprandial venous ammonia concentrations in the diagnosis of hepatobiliary disease in dogs. *J Vet Intern Med* 2001; 15: 463–466.

INTERNET RESOURCES

Kogika MM, Matsuura S, Hagiwara MK, et al. Evaluation of prepandial and postprandial serum bile acids and plasma ammonia concentrations in healthy dogs, and the effects of frozen storage on plasma ammonia concentrations. Braz J Vet Res Anim Sci 1999;36(1), http://www.scielo.br/scielo.php?script = sci_arttext&pid = S1413–95961999000100005.

AUTHOR NAME

Mark E. Hitt

AMYLASE

BASICS

TYPE OF SPECIMEN
Blood

TEST EXPLANATION AND RELATED PHYSIOLOGY
Amylase, which is an enzyme that hydrolyzes starch and glycogen, arises from the pancreas and many other tissues, such as duodenum, kidney, lung, and spleen, and is cleared from the plasma by the kidneys.

Elevations of this enzyme in dogs are often associated with pancreatitis. After experimental induction of pancreatic inflammation, amylase levels rise and peak within 12–48 h and return to normal within 8–14 days. However, elevations are also seen with diseases of other amylase-producing tissues and with decreases in glomerular filtration rate (GFR). Pancreatitis in cats is not associated with increased amylase concentrations. Cats with pancreatitis may have decreased serum amylase concentrations.

The test performed in reference laboratories and some in-clinic analyzers most commonly uses spectrophotometry. Some in-clinic analyzers use a dry-reagent methodology. Different reagent methodologies include amyloclastic (measures the disappearance of starch in the reaction mixture), saccharogenic (measures the appearance of glucose and maltose), and chromogenic procedures. Maltase activity in normal canine serum adversely affects the saccharogenic method and should not be used for veterinary patients.

INDICATIONS
- Clinical signs suggestive of canine pancreatitis (vomiting, anorexia, abdominal pain, icterus)
- Nonseptic, inflammatory abdominal exudate

CONTRAINDICATIONS
None

POTENTIAL COMPLICATIONS
None

CLIENT EDUCATION
- Dogs should be fasted for most accurate results.
- Clients should know that amylase is a nonspecific test and can be associated with pancreatitis, as well as disease in other organs such as kidney or intestine.

BODY SYSTEMS ASSESSED
- Gastrointestinal
- Hepatobiliary
- Renal and urologic

SAMPLE

COLLECTION
- 1–2 mL of venous blood
- Abdominal fluid

HANDLING
- A red-top tube or serum-separator tube is preferred.
- A lithium heparin (green-top) tube is acceptable but not preferred.

STORAGE
Refrigerate or freeze.

STABILITY
- 1 week at room temperature
- At least 1 month at 2°–8°C (refrigerated)
- Years at −20°C (frozen)

PROTOCOL
None

INTERPRETATION

NORMAL FINDINGS OR RANGE
- Dogs: 371–1,503 IU/L
- Cats: 571–1,660 IU/L
- Reference intervals may vary, depending on the laboratory and assay.

ABNORMAL VALUES
Values above reference range

CRITICAL VALUES
None

INTERFERING FACTORS
Drugs That May Alter Results or Interpretation
Drugs That Interfere with Test Methodology
None

Drugs That Alter Physiology
Drugs that may induce pancreatitis include
- Glucocorticoids
- Antibiotics, such as metronidazole, sulfonamides, and tetracycline
- Diuretics, including furosemide and thiazides
- Other drugs, such as asparaginase and azothiaprine

Disorders That May Alter Results
None

Collection Techniques or Handling That May Alter Results
None

Influence of Signalment

Species
Elevated amylase can be suggestive of pancreatitis in dogs, but is an unreliable indicator of pancreatitis in cats.

Breed
None

Age
None

Gender
None

Pregnancy
None

LIMITATIONS OF THE TEST

• Amylase has poor sensitivity and specificity for the diagnosis of pancreatitis.
• Because amylase is produced in nonpancreatic tissues such as the kidney or intestine, diseases of these tissues may increase amylase activity.
• The level of amylase activity does not correlate with the severity of pancreatitis, and normal amylase levels can be seen in some patients with severe acute pancreatitis.

Sensitivity, Specificity, and Positive and Negative Predictive Values
N/A

Valid If Run in a Human Lab?
Yes—unless a saccharogenic test method is used, which will provide inaccurate test results for dogs.

Causes of Abnormal Findings

High values	Low values
Decreased GFR	Not significant
Severe dehydration	
Renal disease	
Urinary tract obstruction	
Pancreatitis	
Intestinal disease	
Hepatic disease	

CLINICAL PERSPECTIVE

• If a patient has high amylase values, additional workup is needed to exclude liver disease, intestinal disease, or decreased GFR.

• Amylase levels of >3-fold normal are less likely to be due nonpancreatic disease.
• Newer tests, such as canine pancreatic lipase immunoreactivity, offer greater sensitivity and specificity than does amylase for the diagnosis of this disorder.
• Abdominal fluid amylase levels of >2-fold serum amylase suggests pancreatitis, although bowel rupture is also possible.

MISCELLANEOUS

ANCILLARY TESTS
• Lipase, pancreatic lipase immunoreactivity, or trypsin-like immunoreactivity for confirmation of pancreatic disease
• BUN, creatinine, urinalysis for evaluation of renal function
• Liver enzymes
• Ultrasound of the pancreas

SYNONYMS
None

SEE ALSO
Blackwell's Five-Minute Veterinary Consult: Canine and Feline Topics
Pancreatitis
Related Topics in This Book
• Lipase
• Pancreatic Lipase Immunoreactivity
• Pancreatic Ultrasonography
• Trypsin-like Immunoreactivity

ABBREVIATIONS
GFR = glomerular filtration rate

Suggested Reading
Brobst DF. Pancreatic function. In: Kaneko JJ, Harvey JW, Bruss ML, eds. *Clinical Biochemistry of Domestic Animals*, 5th ed. San Diego: Academic, 1997: 353–366.
Steiner JM. Diagnosis of pancreatitis. *Vet Clin North Am Small Anim Pract* 2003; 33: 1181–1195.

INTERNET RESOURCES
Cornell University, College of Medicine: Clinical Pathology Modules, Veterinary Clinical Chemistry—Amylase, http://www.diaglab.vet. cornell.edu/clinpath/modules/chem/amylase. htm.

AUTHOR NAME
Denise Wunn

ANGIOGRAPHY AND ANGIOCARDIOGRAPHY

BASICS

TYPE OF PROCEDURE
Radiographic and/or fluoroscopic

PROCEDURE EXPLANATION AND RELATED PHYSIOLOGY
Angiography is the procedure whereby a radiopaque contrast media is injected into the lumen of the vasculature for radiographic observation. In angiocardiography, the contrast is injected into selected cardiac chambers, enabling visualization of chamber dimension, function, or communications between chambers of the heart or vessels. Angiography is used to diagnose cardiovascular abnormalities definitively when the cause or severity is not evident by routine examination, including echocardiography.

INDICATIONS
To identify congenital and acquired abnormalities of cardiac or vascular blood flow [e.g., patent ductus arteriosus (PDA), ventricular septal defect, atrial septal defect, pulmonic stenosis (PS), aortic stenosis (AS), aortic insufficiency, portosystemic shunt (PSS), pulmonary thromboembolism (PTE), arterial thromboembolism (ATE)].

CONTRAINDICATIONS
• Not recommended in animals with known adverse reactions to iodinated contrast media
• Increased risk in patients with severe cardiac disease, heart failure, or preexisting renal disease. In particular, angiographic studies are not recommended in severely debilitated animals or in cats with reduced left ventricular contractile function.

POTENTIAL COMPLICATIONS
• Injection of air bubbles into the left side of the heart can cause an air embolism, leading to acute myocardial infarction, cerebral accident, or death. Paradoxical embolism can also occur with right heart injections if right-to-left shunting is present.
• Cardiac or vascular perforation of the endocardium and myocardium can occur during catheter manipulation or secondary to rapid injection of the contrast bolus through an end-hole catheter.
• Cardiac tamponade secondary to ventricular rupture and pericardial effusion
• Hemorrhage, thrombosis, or hematoma formation at vascular access sites
• In patients with cardiac disease or congestive heart failure (CHF), the use of contrast agents may lead to complications such as transient hypotension, depressed cardiac function, arrhythmias, increased pulmonary capillary pressure, and/or worsening of heart failure, secondary to hyperosmolality of the contrast agents.
• Nephrotoxicity, especially in animals with preexisting renal compromise or dehydration
• Contrast agents may rarely cause allergic reactions such as fever, urticaria, laryngeal edema, or anaphylaxis.
• Infection
• Life-threatening arrhythmias secondary to catheter-induced ventricular irritability
• Catheter breakage or foreign body embolization

CLIENT EDUCATION
• The normal preanesthetic protocol should be observed.
• The animal can usually be discharged from the hospital the same day or next day, if there are no complications, depending on concurrent disease or procedures.
• The catheter insertion site may require bandaging with monitoring for infection or inflammation.
• If a cutdown procedure was performed for vascular access, then the sutures are removed in 7–10 days.

BODY SYSTEMS ASSESSED
• Cardiovascular
• Hepatobiliary

PROCEDURE

PATIENT PREPARATION
Preprocedure Medication or Preparation
• Nothing by mouth should be allowed after midnight on the day of the procedure.
• A CBC and a chemistry profile are recommended for mature or elderly patients.
• Avoid venipuncture at vascular access site prior to the procedure.
• Regular medications are continued.

Anesthesia or Sedation
• Most angiographic procedures require sedation or a light plane of anesthesia.
• Routine anesthetic medications are administered.

Patient Positioning
The animal is placed in the most appropriate position for opacification of desired structures: left lateral, right lateral, or dorsal recumbency may be most appropriate depending on the procedure.

Patient Monitoring
ECG, blood pressure, and oxygen saturation are monitored continuously.

Equipment or Supplies
• Fluoroscopic capability with image intensification to reduce radiation exposure to operator
• A movable radiographic table is desirable, enabling patient positioning to remain constant.
• Angiograms and angiocardiograms are recorded on videotape, 35-mm cinematic film, or digitally.
• Radiopaque contrast material—a low-osmolality contrast agent that is safer for patients with cardiac disease. For example, iohexol (Omnipaque 300; Amersham Health, Princeton, NJ) is water soluble with osmolality ≈3 times that of blood; iodine concentration = 300 mg/mL.
• A Luerlock syringe for angiography, with or without automated power injector
• A standard pack of surgical instruments for vascular access (cutdown procedure) and/or supplies for a percutaneous introducer sheath with hemostasis port
• Sterile towels and drapes
• A variety of sterilized catheters, guidewires, sheath introducers, and 3-way stopcocks
• Suture material and surgical blades
• A sterile bowl with warmed heparinized sterile saline (500 IU sodium heparin per 250 mL of normal saline), unless coil occlusion is planned
• Inhalation anesthesia and monitoring equipment
• A direct current defibrillator with internal and external paddles
• Emergency cardiac drugs in the event of cardiac emergency

TECHNIQUE
• Preanesthesia sedation, endotracheal intubation, and inhalation anesthesia with monitoring are established. A light anesthetic plane will usually suffice for angiographic studies.
• The area of catheter insertion is clipped, and sterilely prepped and draped.

For Selective Angiocardiography
• Vascular access is accomplished via percutaneous catheter insertion or surgical cutdown.

ANGIOGRAPHY AND ANGIOCARDIOGRAPHY

- All catheters and introducer sheaths are flushed with sterile heparinized saline.
- The use of a cardiac catheter with multiple side holes is recommended to prevent recoil during delivery of contrast and/or penetration of contrast into endocardium and myocardium.
- The catheter is guided via fluoroscopy to the desired vessel or cardiac chamber. Common locations include these:
  - Right ventricle—for PS
  - Main pulmonary artery (PA) or PA branches—to detect PTE
  - Left ventricle—for AS
  - Root of the aorta—to diagnose severity of aortic insufficiency
  - Aortic arch or thoracic aorta—to detect PDA
  - Distal aorta—to diagnose aortic or systemic thromboembolism
- A large bolus of radiographic iodinated contrast is rapidly injected with fluoroscopic visualization and recording. The angiogram can then be replayed as necessary (ideally in slow motion) for identification of morphology and cardiac function.
- Angiocardiography or ventriculography dosage: 400–440 mg iodine/kg of contrast per injection (or 1.3–1.5 mL/kg iohexol), injected over 1–2 s by using the smallest appropriate syringe. Large dogs are optimally injected by using an automated power injector.
- The maximum total dosage of contrast media per study should not exceed 1,000–1,200 mg iodine/kg (or 3.3–4.0 mL/kg iohexol).
- Care must be taken not to inject air, especially on the left side of the heart, where 1 small bubble can occlude a coronary or cerebral artery and lead to acute myocardial infarction or stroke.
- Catheters should be frequently flushed to prevent thrombus formation.

For Nonselective Angiography
- A large-bore (18–20 gauge or larger) IV catheter is placed, preferably in the jugular vein.
- A large bolus of contrast is rapidly injected IV over 1–2 s.
- Dose of contrast is typically 0.75–1.5 mL/kg. Alternatively, the desirable dose of iodine is 400–440 mg/kg per injection.
- Radiographic exposures are obtained 0.5–15.0 s after injection. Shorter times are needed for evaluation of the right heart and PA, whereas longer times are required for left heart evaluation, for larger animals, and for animals with heart failure or slow circulation times. The following are some suggested times for radiographic exposures after contrast injection into a jugular venous catheter:
  - Right atrium: 0.5–1.0 s
  - Right atrium, right ventricle, and PA: 1.0–2.5 s
  - Pulmonary vein, left atrium, and left ventricle: 3–5 s
  - Left ventricle and aorta: 5–7 s
  - Left ventricle and aorta with CHF: 8–12 s

SAMPLE HANDLING
N/A

APPROPRIATE AFTERCARE
Postprocedure Patient Monitoring
- If a cutdown was performed, catheters are removed and vessels are repaired or ligated.
- If a percutaneous sheath introducer or IV catheter was used, continuous pressure is applied for several minutes until hemostasis is assured; for arterial sites, continuous pressure is applied to the site for ≈20–30 min to assure hemostasis. Risk of life-threatening arterial bleeding from arterial sites leads some cardiologists to prefer surgical cutdown over percutaneous access.
- Bandaging can be applied as necessary to the neck or the peripheral catheter sites.
- Normal postanesthetic monitoring is performed.

Nursing Care
See the "Cardiac Catheterization" chapter.

Dietary Modification
None

Medication Requirements
None unless dictated by underlying condition

Restrictions on Activity
Leash walks are recommended only for 10–14 days after the procedure if an intervention was performed (e.g., coil occlusion).

Anticipated Recovery Time
Patients are usually discharged from the hospital 1–2 days following most procedures. Full recovery is anticipated within 1 week, although most animals appear to recover fully within 1–2 days.

 INTERPRETATION

NORMAL FINDINGS OR RANGE
Normal cardiovascular anatomy

ABNORMAL VALUES
Congenital cardiac malformation (e.g., PDA, atrial septal defect or ventricular septal defect with left to right or right to left shunting of blood, AS, PS, aorticopulmonary window, tetralogy of Fallot, arteriovenous fistula, PTE, ATE, PSS)

CRITICAL VALUES
None

INTERFERING FACTORS
Drugs That May Alter Results of the Procedure
None

Conditions That May Interfere with Performing the Procedure
- Metabolic abnormalities, electrolyte disturbances, preexisting renal disease, or infectious conditions may increase the risk of anesthesia or contrast reactions.
- CHF, uncontrolled arrhythmias
- Bleeding disorders and coagulopathies

Procedure Techniques or Handling That May Alter Results
- Adequate opacification of structures of interest, especially in dogs weighing >15–20 kg, can be difficult, especially without a pressure injector.
- Because of the effects of contrast dilution in nonselective angiography, it may be difficult to detect left-sided abnormalities in animals weighing >20 kg.
- Timing of postinjection exposures may be difficult to predict without fluoroscopy.

Influence of Signalment on Performing and Interpreting the Procedure
Species
For selective angiograms and angiocardiograms, the small vessels and hearts in cats and in dogs weighing <2.5 kg often require superior operator skill to perform the procedure successfully. Feline vessels are also prone to vasospasm, which can be partially attenuated with topical lidocaine administration on the vessel.

Breed
None

Age
None

Gender
None

Pregnancy
Prolonged exposure to radiation is not recommended for pregnant patients.

CLINICAL PERSPECTIVE
- Angiography is a good method for evaluating cardiovascular lesions or PSS (Figures 1–3).

ANGIOGRAPHY AND ANGIOCARDIOGRAPHY

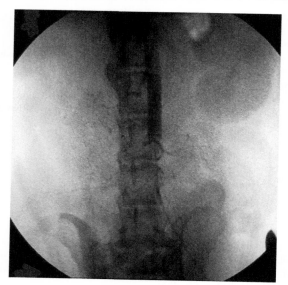

Figure 1

Angiogram of a dog with ATE. The dog, which had posterior paresis, lack of femoral arterial pulses, and signs suggestive of aortic thromboembolism, is in ventrodorsal recumbency, with a catheter placed in the distal aorta for injection of contrast material. Note the discrete lack of contrast in the distal aorta because of the presence of the thrombus.

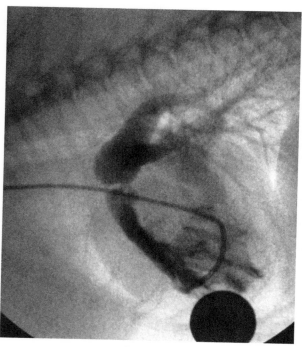

Figure 2

Angiocardiogram of a dog with severe valvular PS. With the dog in lateral recumbency, a catheter has been advanced through the jugular vein and right atrium and across the tricuspid valve into the right ventricle. Severe valvular PS is documented when contrast is injected into the right ventricle and flows past the stenotic valve and into the PA. Note the filling defect at the level of the pulmonic valve, resulting from valve thickening and valvular dysplasia, as well as the poststenotic dilation of the main PA. The right ventricular wall is also thickened.

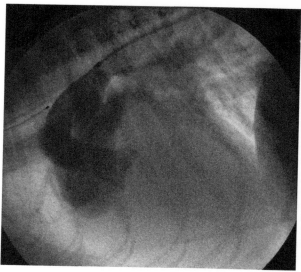

Figure 3

Angiogram from a dog with a large PDA. With the dog in lateral recumbency, a catheter has been inserted into the femoral artery and advanced into the aorta to the level of the PDA. The aortic root fills with contrast, and the PDA is visualized, documenting communication between the aorta and main PA. Note that the main PA also fills well with contrast.

- Nonselective angiography is most useful in identifying abnormalities of large veins, right heart structures, and right-to-left cardiac shunts, and to confirm thromboembolism.
- Selective angiocardiography is usually preferred for identification of complex cardiac malformations.
- Selective angiography and angiocardiography are included as part of therapeutic procedures for correction of defects such as PS, AS, PDA, and PSS (Figures 4–6).

MISCELLANEOUS

ANCILLARY TESTS

- If nonselective angiography yields inconclusive results, selective angiography or angiocardiography would be appropriate.
- PS, AS, PDA, and PSS are generally corrected via balloon valvuloplasty, coil embolization, or a surgical approach.

SYNONYMS

None

SEE ALSO

Blackwell's Five-Minute Veterinary Consult: Canine and Feline Topics

- Aortic Stenosis
- Aortic Thromboembolism
- Arteriovenous Fistula
- Arteriovenous Malformation of the Liver
- Atrial Septal Defect
- Atrioventricular Valvular Stenosis
- Patent Ductus Arteriosus
- Portosystemic Vascular Anomaly, Congenital
- Pulmonary Thromboembolism
- Pulmonic Stenosis
- Tetralogy of Fallot
- Ventricular Septal Defect

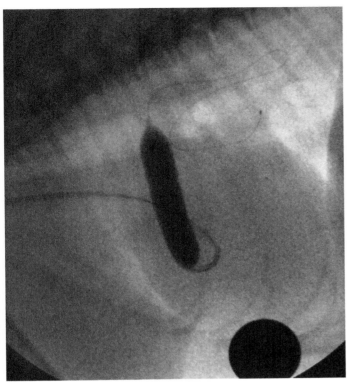

Figure 4

Balloon dilatation in a dog with PS (the same dog depicted in Figure 2). Contrast fills the fully inflated balloon dilatation catheter, which has been positioned over the stenotic region of the pulmonic valve. The catheter has been inserted into the jugular vein and advanced into the right ventricle, across the pulmonic valve, and into the PA, with the middle of the balloon placed at the stenotic region of the valve.

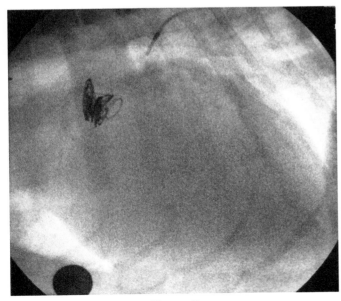

Figure 5

Radiographic view following deployment of several PDA coils. This radiographic view was obtained following placement of several coils within the PDA from the dog depicted in Figure 3.

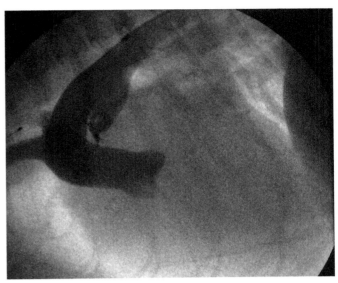

Figure 6

Angiogram from a dog with several coils occluding a PDA (the dog in Figures 3 and 5). This angiogram followed placement of a number of thrombogenic coils within the PDA. Note the lack of contrast in the main PA, indicating successful closure of the PDA by using the coil occlusion technique.

Related Topics in This Book
Cardiac Catheterization

ABBREVIATIONS
- AS = aortic stenosis
- ATE = arterial thromboembolism
- CHF = congestive heart failure
- PA = pulmonary artery
- PDA = patent ductus arteriosus
- PS = pulmonic stenosis
- PSS = portosystemic shunt
- PTE = pulmonary thromboembolism

Suggested Reading

Kittleson MD, Kienle RD. Cardiac catheterization. In: Kittleson MD, Kienle RD, eds. *Small Animal Cardiovascular Medicine*. St Louis: CV Mosby, 1998: 118–132.

Miller MS. Special diagnostic techniques for evaluation of cardiac disease. In: Goodwin JK, Tilley LP, eds. *Manual of Canine and Feline Cardiology*, 2nd ed. Philadelphia: WB Saunders, 1995: 119–123.

Morgan R. Nonselective angiography. In: Morgan R, ed. *Morgan's Handbook of Small Animal Practice*, 3rd ed. Philadelphia: WB Saunders, 1997: 35–36.

Suter PF. Special procedures for the diagnosis of thoracic disease. In: *Thoracic Radiography: A Text Atlas of Thoracic Diseases of the Dog and Cat*. Wettswil, Switzerland: Peter F. Suter, 1984: 63–71.

Wallack ST. Angiography: Dog and cat. In: *The Handbook of Veterinary Contrast Radiography*. Solana Beach, CA: San Diego Veterinary Imaging, 2003: 31–36.

Wise M. Non-selective angiocardiography in the normal dog and cat. *Vet Radiol* 1982; 23: 144–151.

INTERNET RESOURCES
None

AUTHOR NAMES
Barbara P. Brewer and John E. Rush

BASICS

TYPE OF SPECIMEN
Blood

TEST EXPLANATION AND RELATED PHYSIOLOGY
AGAP is a calculation used to help differentiate causes of metabolic acidosis and mixed acid-base disorders. It may be normal, increased, or decreased, depending on the underlying metabolic disorder. The AGAP is calculated by subtracting the sum of measured major serum anions (Cl^- and HCO_3^-) from the sum of measured major cations (Na^+ and K^+), using the formula $(Na^+ + K^+) - (Cl^- + HCO_3^-)$.

In addition to commonly measured serum electrolytes, there are minor cations and anions that are not typically measured but are important in regulating electroneutrality. These are called unmeasured cations (UC^+) and unmeasured anions (UA^-). In reality, there is no true anion "gap," because electrolytes, unmeasured cations, and unmeasured anions in serum must balance to preserve electroneutrality, such that $(Na^+ + K^+ + UC^+) = (Cl^- + HCO_3^- + UA^-)$. This formula is reduced to: $AGAP = UA^- - UC^+$ to denote that any numerical gap calculated is a result of changes in either UA^- or UC^+.

In metabolic acidosis, for every decrease in HCO_3^-, there must be an increase in Cl^- or UA^- to maintain electroneutrality. Hyperchloremic metabolic acidosis with a normal AGAP develops when HCO_3^- is replaced with Cl^- such that the resultant difference in $(UA^- - UC^+)$ is unchanged. A normochloremic metabolic acidosis with an increased AGAP develops when HCO_3^- is replaced by UA^- such that the difference in $(UA^- - UC^+)$ is increased, but the Cl^- concentration is unchanged.

Unmeasured cations include calcium and magnesium. Unmeasured anions include albumin, phosphates, sulfates, and organic acids (e.g., lactate, ketones, ethylene glycol metabolites). Clinically, in most cases, an increased AGAP metabolic acidosis (normochloremic) implies accumulation of organic acids; whereas, a normal AGAP metabolic acidosis (hyperchloremic) is usually associated with an increased chloride concentration.

As the total CO_2 measurement (TCO_2) represents for the most part the bicarbonate concentration in blood, the TCO_2 concentration can be substituted for measured bicarbonate (HCO_3^-) in the foregoing formulas.

INDICATIONS
To differentiate causes of metabolic (nonrespiratory) acidosis and mixed acid-base disorders

CONTRAINDICATIONS
None

POTENTIAL COMPLICATIONS
None

CLIENT EDUCATION
None

BODY SYSTEMS ASSESSED
- Endocrine and metabolic
- Gastrointestinal
- Renal and urologic
- Respiratory

SAMPLE

COLLECTION
AGAP is a calculation.

HANDLING
See specific chapters on sodium, chloride, potassium, and bicarbonate.

STORAGE
See specific chapters on sodium, chloride, potassium, and bicarbonate.

STABILITY
Long-term (>2 h) exposure of serum to room air artifactually increases the AGAP.

PROTOCOL
None

INTERPRETATION

NORMAL FINDINGS OR RANGE
- Dogs: 12–24 mEq/L
- Cats: 13–27 mEq/L
- Reference intervals may vary, depending on the laboratory and assay.

ABNORMAL VALUES
Values above reference interval

CRITICAL VALUES
Severely increased AGAP acidosis is most commonly associated with ethylene glycol intoxication.

INTERFERING FACTORS
Drugs That May Alter Results or Interpretation
Drugs That Interfere with Test Methodology
Bromide can artificially elevate chloride, decreasing the calculated AGAP.

Drugs That Alter Physiology
Several therapeutic agents (crystalloid fluids, diuretics, sodium bicarbonate) may blunt an increased AGAP, making the underlying medical condition seem less severe. Calculate the AGAP before therapy.

Disorders That May Alter Results
- Hypoalbuminemia and hyperglobulinemia reduce or mask the severity of an increased AGAP.
- Alkalosis and dehydration artificially increase the AGAP.

Collection Techniques or Handling That May Alter Results
Underfilling blood collection tubes can affect AGAP by causing a false decrease in serum TCO_2.

Influence of Signalment
Species
Cats have slightly higher AGAP than dogs.

Breed
None

Age
None

Gender
None

Pregnancy
None

LIMITATIONS OF THE TEST
• Poor correlation in numerous studies with the outcome or the severity of injury or illness.
• AGAP may be normal in critically ill patients with conditions typically associated with an increased gap acidosis if associated with concurrent hypoalbuminemia, hyperchloremia, or mixed acid-base disorders because this may blunt the AGAP increase and confound interpretation.
• A normal AGAP does not exclude metabolic acidosis caused by increased organic acids.

Sensitivity, Specificity, and Positive and Negative Predictive Values
Not available

Valid If Run in a Human Lab?
Yes.

Causes of Abnormal Findings

High values	Low values
Increased AGAP, normochloremic	Hypoalbuminemia
Lactic acidosis	IgG multiple
Uremic acidosis	myeloma
Ketoacidosis	Laboratory error
Ethylene glycol toxicity	
Salicylate toxicity	
Severe dehydration and decreased	
tissue perfusion	
Laboratory error	
Normal AGAP, hyperchloremic	
Small-bowel diarrhea	
Carbonic anhydrase inhibitors	
Ammonium chloride	
Parenteral amino acid solutions	
Chronic respiratory alkalosis	
Dilutional acidosis	
Renal tubular acidoses	
Atypical hypoadrenocorticism	

CLINICAL PERSPECTIVE
• Increased AG (normochloremic metabolic acidosis): usually associated with conditions causing lactic acidosis (e.g., exercise, shock, ischemic disorders), uremic acidosis (e.g., renal failure), ketoacidosis (e.g., diabetes ketoacidosis), ethylene glycol or salicylate toxicity, severe dehydration, and laboratory error (prolonged standing of serum).
• Normal AG (hyperchloremic metabolic acidosis): usually associated with conditions that result in chloride retention and bicarbonate loss (e.g., acute amall bowel diarrhea; administration of carbonic anhydrase inhibitors, ammonium chloride, or parenteral amino acids; chronic respiratory alkalosis; dilutional acidosis with use of saline crystalloid fluid; or renal tubular acidosis).

• Finding an elevated AGAP, regardless of serum bicarbonate concentration, suggests metabolic acidosis.
• With high AGAP metabolic acidosis, consider a mixed metabolic acid-base disorder if the AGAP change does not approximate the bicarbonate change.

MISCELLANEOUS
ANCILLARY TESTS
• Arterial blood-gas analysis to help define the acid-base disorder
• Specific tests based on suspected etiology (e.g., ethylene glycol, serum and urine glucose, serum and urine ketones)

SYNONYMS
AGAP

SEE ALSO
Blackwell's Five-Minute Veterinary Consult: Canine and Feline Topics
• Acidosis, Metabolic
• Ethylene Glycol Poisoning
• Lactic Acidosis

Related Topics in This Book
• Bicarbonate
• Blood Gases
• Chloride
• Ethylene Glycol
• Lactate
• Potassium
• Sodium
• Urine Ketones

ABBREVIATIONS
• TCO_2 = total CO_2 measurement
• UA^- = unmeasured anions
• UC^+ = unmeasured cations

Suggested Reading
DiBartola SP. Metabolic acid-base disorders. In: Dibartola SP, ed. *Fluid Therapy in Small Animal Practice*. Philadelphia: WB Saunders, 2000: 211–226.
DeMorais HSA, DiBartola SP. Mixed acid-base disorders. Part I: Clinical approach. *Comp Cont Educ Pract Vet* 1993; 15: 1619–1626.
Rose BD, Post TW. Metabolic acidosis. In: Rose BD, Post TW, eds. *Clinical Physiology of Acid-Base and Electrolyte Disorders*, 5th ed. New York: McGraw-Hill, 2001: 583–592.

INTERNET RESOURCES
None

AUTHOR NAME
Michael S. Lagutchik

ANTICOAGULANT PROTEINS

BASICS

TYPE OF SPECIMEN
Blood

TEST EXPLANATION AND RELATED PHYSIOLOGY
AT (formerly AT III) and protein C are plasma proteins critical for regulation of fibrin clot formation. AT inhibits the action of serine protease coagulation factors, particularly thrombin (factor IIa) and factors VIIa, IXa, Xa, and XIa, by irreversibly binding to the catalytic site of active factors. AT-factor complexes are then rapidly cleared from circulation. Endogenous and therapeutic heparin greatly enhances AT's anticoagulant effect.

Protein C is a vitamin K–dependent anticoagulant factor that neutralizes factors Va and VIIIa, which act as cofactors to coagulation. Protein C is converted to its active form at the surface of endothelial cells and requires protein S as its cofactor. In addition to its anticoagulant effect, protein C modulates inflammation and promotes fibrinolysis.

The lack of anticoagulant proteins is a risk factor for thrombosis. AT and protein C are both synthesized exclusively in the liver. Patients with hepatic failure can therefore acquire anticoagulant deficiencies. In addition, deficiencies of both proteins may develop secondary to increased consumption following systemic activation of coagulation and inflammation. AT deficiency may also develop in protein-losing syndromes. Protein C has a short plasma half-life of 6 h, and its activity falls rapidly in vitamin K–deficiency states. To date, hereditary deficiencies of these factors have not been identified in dogs or cats.

Functional, chromogenic tests are preferred over immunoassays that detect protein concentration. Results are often expressed as a percentage of activity in patient samples compared to a species-specific normal plasma pool considered to have 100% activity.

INDICATIONS
- Investigate the cause of thrombosis.
- Document a hypercoagulable state.
- Assess liver function.
- Diagnose DIC (AT).
- Noninvasively assess portal flow (protein C).
- Assess vitamin K deficiency (protein C).

CONTRAINDICATIONS
None

POTENTIAL COMPLICATIONS
None

CLIENT EDUCATION
None

BODY SYSTEMS ASSESSED
- Hemic, lymphatic, and immune
- Hepatobiliary

SAMPLE

COLLECTION
2.7 mL of venous blood

HANDLING
- Collect blood directly into 3.2% or 3.8% sodium citrate (blue-top tubes).
  - An exact ratio of blood to citrate (9 parts:1 part) is critical.
  - 2.7 mL of blood in 0.3 mL of citrate yields sufficient plasma for AT and protein C assays.
- Centrifuge and remove the supernatant plasma within 1 h of collection.
- Use plastic or additive-free siliconized glass tubes for storage and shipment.

STORAGE
- Store in a refrigerator pending assay within 4 h.
- Store in a freezer if assayed >4 h after collection.
- Ship overnight on cold packs.

STABILITY
Frozen (−20°C): 2 weeks

PROTOCOL
None

INTERPRETATION

NORMAL FINDINGS OR RANGE
These reference intervals are from the Comparative Coagulation Section of the Cornell University Animal Health Diagnostic Center; values from other laboratories may vary, depending on the assay.

AT
- Dogs: 65%–145%
- Cats: 75%–110%

Protein C
- Dogs: 75%–135%
- Cats: 65%–120%

ABNORMAL VALUES
Values below the reference range

CRITICAL VALUES
Not known

INTERFERING FACTORS
Drugs That May Alter Results or Interpretation
Drugs That Interfere with Test Methodology
High levels of oxyglobin may interfere with the results of colorimetric assays.

Drugs That Alter Physiology
- Heparin causes a progressive decrease in AT.
- Coumadin impairs synthesis of functional protein C.

Disorders That May Alter Results
Severe hemolysis may interfere with the results of colorimetric assays.

Collection Techniques or Handling That May Alter Results
- Inappropriate anticoagulant (heparin, EDTA) or a tube with clot activator
- Poor venipuncture technique, incomplete blood draw, or prolonged storage at room temperature may falsely decrease value.

Influence of Signalment
Species
None

Breed
None

Age
None

Gender
None

Pregnancy
None

ANTICOAGULANT PROTEINS

LIMITATIONS OF THE TEST
Sensitivity, Specificity, and Positive and Negative Predictive Values
None

Valid If Run in a Human Lab?
No. Interpretation of AT requires species-specific reference ranges. Human protein C assays require modification for dogs and cats.

Causes of Abnormal Values

AT deficiencies	Protein C deficiencies
Decreased synthesis	Decreased synthesis
Liver disease	Liver disease
Increased consumption	Vitamin K deficiency
DIC	Cholestasis
Heparin therapy	Coumadin therapy
Increased loss	Anticoagulant rodenticide
Protein-losing nephropathies	intoxication
Protein-losing enteropathies	Portosystemic shunting
	Increased consumption
	DIC
	Sepsis

CLINICAL PERSPECTIVE
- Low levels of plasma anticoagulant proteins increase the risk of pathologic thrombus formation.
- Measurement of AT can aid in the diagnosis of DIC. Laboratory criteria include abnormal coagulation assays (aPTT, PT, fibrinogen), low AT, high fibrin degradation products and D-dimer, falling or low platelet count, and schistocytosis.
- Low activity of both AT and protein C is often a sign of liver failure.
- Specific reduction of protein C may indicate vitamin K deficiency (accompanied by abnormal aPTT and/or PT) or portosystemic shunting.

MISCELLANEOUS

ANCILLARY TESTS
- Coagulation screening tests (aPTT, PT, fibrinogen)
- Fibrin breakdown products (D-dimer)
- Chemistry panel and urinalysis

SYNONYMS
- Antithrombin (AT)
- Antithrombin III (ATIII)
- Protein C

SEE ALSO
Blackwell's Five-Minute Veterinary Consult: Canine and Feline Topics
- Anticoagulant Rodenticide Poisoning
- Cirrhosis and Fibrosis of the Liver
- Disseminated Intravascular Coagulation
- Glomerulonephritis
- Hepatic Failure, Acute
- Hepatitis
- Hepatotoxins
- Portosystemic Shunting, Acquired
- Portosystemic Vascular Anomaly, Congenital
- Protein-Losing Enteropathy
- Proteinuria

Related Topics in This Book
- Partial Thromboplastin Time, Activated
- Prothrombin Time

ABBREVIATIONS
- aPTT = activated partial thromboplastin time
- AT = antithrombin
- DIC = disseminated intravascular coagulation
- PT = prothrombin time

Suggested Reading
de Laforcade AM, Shaw SP, Freeman LM, *et al.* Coagulation parameters in dogs with naturally occurring sepsis. J *Vet Intern Med* 2003; 17: 674–679.
Thomas JS, Green RA. Clotting times and antithrombin III activity in cats with naturally developing disease. *J Am Vet Med Assoc* 1998; 213: 1290–1295.
Toulza O, Center SA, Brooks MB, *et al.* Evaluation of plasma protein C activity for detection of hepatobiliary disease and portosystemic shunting in dogs. *J Am Vet Med Assoc*, 2006; 229: 1761–1771.

INTERNET RESOURCES
Cornell University, College of Veterinary Medicine, Department of Population Medicine and Diagnostic Sciences: Comparative coagulation, http://www.diaglab.vet.cornell.edu/coag/test/proteinC.asp.
Lab Tests Online, http://www.labtestsonline.org/understanding/analytes/antithrombin/test.html.
Massachusetts General Hospital, http://www.massgeneral.org/pathology/coagbook/CO000300.htm

AUTHOR NAME
Marjory Brooks

BASICS

TYPE OF SPECIMEN
Bait
Blood
Feces and/or stomach content
Tissue
Urine

TEST EXPLANATION AND RELATED PHYSIOLOGY
Anticoagulants, which are the most commonly used rodenticides, are categorized as short-acting first-generation, and relatively long-acting second-generation, compounds that may require single small ingestions. The predominant first-generation rodenticide is warfarin. Second-generation rodenticides include bromadiolone, brodifacoum, diphacinone, chlorophacinone, and pindone, among others. These products are often dyed blue-green.

Anticoagulant rodenticides inhibit hepatic vitamin K–epoxide reductases. Inhibition of these enzymes disables the mechanism of vitamin K recycling that is necessary for the formation of clotting factors II, VII, IX, and X. Clinical signs of anticoagulant exposure are delayed until clotting factors have been used up, usually 3–5 days after ingestion.

Common testing methods for anticoagulant rodenticides may involve high-performance liquid chromatography or gas chromatography/mass spectrometry. Individual laboratories may not test for all known anticoagulant rodenticide active ingredients.

There are a few commonly used rodenticides that do not act as anticoagulants. Active ingredients in these products may include cholecalciferol, bromethalin, strychnine, sodium fluoroacetate (compound 1080), and zinc phosphide.

INDICATIONS
• Known exposure to rodenticides
• Suspect material in feces or GI content (blue-green dye)
• Suspect bait material
• Unexplained coagulopathy

CONTRAINDICATIONS
Blood transfusion may mask presence of anticoagulants—collect blood before transfusion.

POTENTIAL COMPLICATIONS
Prolonged bleeding after sample collection if a coagulopathy is present

CLIENT EDUCATION
• Rodenticide toxicosis may be an emergency, and treatment should be initiated before identification of the rodenticide.
• Follow-up treatment depends on correct identification of the active ingredient involved.
• If possible, the client should bring in the labeled product that was the source of exposure.
• Anticoagulant rodenticide screens may not detect cholecalciferol, bromethalin, zinc phosphide, strychnine, or other rodenticide ingredients.

BODY SYSTEMS ASSESSED
Hemic, lymphatic, and immune

SAMPLE

COLLECTION
• 10 mL of whole blood in heparin
• 50 mL of urine

• 50 g of liver, stomach content, feces, or bait
• Call the laboratory to determine the best sample.

HANDLING
• Store samples in clean containers.
• Keep cold.
• Wrap solid material in foil.
• Urine, tissue, or GI content may be frozen.

STORAGE
• Refrigerate blood.
• Freeze urine, tissue, or GI content.

STABILITY
N/A

PROTOCOL
None

INTERPRETATION

NORMAL FINDINGS OR RANGE
Negative results

ABNORMAL VALUES
The detection of any rodenticide is significant and confirms exposure.

CRITICAL VALUES
None

INTERFERING FACTORS
Drugs That May Alter Results or Interpretation
Drugs That Interfere with Test Methodology
Warfarin or coumadin

Drugs That Alter Physiology
Many protein-bound drugs enhance the effects of anticoagulants.

Disorders That May Alter Results
Rodenticides may not be detectable in transfusion recipients.

Collection Techniques or Handling That May Alter Results
None

Influence of Signalment
Species
None

Breed
None

Age
None

Gender
None

Pregnancy
None

LIMITATIONS OF THE TEST
Sensitivity, Specificity, and Positive and Negative Predictive Values
None

Valid If Run in a Human Lab?
Yes.

CLINICAL PERSPECTIVE
• Determination of the active ingredient is critical for appropriate treatment because second-generation rodenticides are more potent and their action lasts longer. Some laboratories do not test for all compounds.
• Consumption of tissues from diphacinone-poisoned animals can cause secondary poisoning.

- Factor VII has the shortest half-life (6.2 h), so an elevated PT can be the first laboratory abnormality and shows up within 1–2 days after ingestion. At this point the intrinsic pathway is still operational and there may be no clinical signs or at most mild evidence of hemorrhage.
- As the other coagulation factors are used up, about 3–5 days after ingestion, laboratory tests will show an elevated aPTT. Platelet count will generally be in the normal to low-normal range. At this stage, hemorrhage will be unchecked.

MISCELLANEOUS

ANCILLARY TESTS
- Activated clotting time
- aPTT
- Protein induced in vitamin K antagonism (PIVKA) test
- PT

SYNONYMS
Rodenticide screen

SEE ALSO
Blackwell's Five-Minute Veterinary Consult: Canine and Feline Topics
Anticoagulant Rodenticide Poisoning

Related Topics in This Book
- Activated Clotting Time
- Partial Thromboplastin Time, Activated
- PIVKA Test
- Prothrombin Time

ABBREVIATIONS
- aPTT = activated partial thromboplastin time
- PT = prothrombin time

Suggested Reading
Means C. Anticoagulant rodenticides. In: Plumlee KH, ed. *Clinical Veterinary Toxicology*, 1st ed. St Louis: CV Mosby, 2003: 444–446.
Murphy MJ. Rodenticides. *Vet Clin North Am Small Anim Pract* 2002; **32**: 469–484.
Murphy MJ, Talcott PA. Anticoagulant rodenticides. In: Peterson ME, Talcott PA, eds. *Small Animal Toxicology*, 2nd ed. Philadelphia: WB Saunders, 2005: 563–577.

INTERNET RESOURCES
Beasley V. Toxicants that interfere with the function of vitamin K. In: Beasley V, ed. Veterinary Toxicology. Ithaca, NY: International Veterinary Information Service (IVIS), 1999, http://www.ivis.org/advances/Beasley/Cpt20/ivis.pdf.

AUTHOR NAME
Karyn Bischoff

ANTINUCLEAR ANTIBODY

BASICS

TYPE OF SPECIMEN
Blood

TEST EXPLANATION AND RELATED PHYSIOLOGY
Antinuclear antibodies (ANAs) are immunoglobulins directed against components of the cell nucleus (DNA, RNA, histones, and nonhistone proteins). The ANA test is used to detect the presence of ANAs in serum. Elevated concentrations of ANAs are most often associated with a diagnosis of SLE and SLE-related disorders. However, increased ANA levels may be found in animals with other immune-mediated disorders such as rheumatoid arthritis, Sjögren-like syndrome, and lymphocytic thyroiditis, as well as with chronic inflammatory and neoplastic disorders. Elevated ANA levels have also been detected in people and dogs with chronic infectious disease (viral, bacterial, protozoal, or fungal). Additionally, high ANA titers may be found in clinically healthy dogs or in particular dog breeds (e.g., German shepherds), or in animals receiving certain medical therapies. The majority of retrospective information about ANA testing is from canine patients. It is difficult to interpret elevated ANA titers in cats, because many healthy cats have been reported to have elevated titers. In general, ANA titers are usually much higher in animals affected with SLE than with other disorders. Because many variables are associated with a positive ANA test result, it is recommended that verification of the diagnosis of SLE not be based on a positive ANA test or high titer alone. It is advisable to interpret elevated ANA titers with cautious consideration of the patient's clinical history and potentially precipitating factors, and to corroborate the suspicion of SLE with appropriate clinical signs and other diagnostic results (see the Clinical Perspective section).

Most commercially available ANA tests employ indirect immunofluorescence to detect ANAs in the serum. The IFA assay is considered to be the most reliable assay. Tissue or cellular substrates of nucleated cells, such as mouse or rat liver (or occasionally kidney) cells or human epithelial cell cultures (e.g., HEp-2 cell line), are used in the test. A substrate slide is incubated with patient serum, and the patient's ANAs bind to the nuclear components on the slide. Species-specific fluoresceinated anti-IgG antibodies are added to the slide, and these antibodies detect the bound ANAs, producing positive nuclear staining. The ANA titer is obtained by serial dilutions of the patient's serum, the highest positive dilution reported. If positive, the pattern of nuclear staining is included in the results. Common patterns of nuclear fluorescence include *speckled*, *homogeneous* (diffuse), *nuclear rim* (peripheral), and *nucleolar* staining. In people, causal relationships between staining patterns, the presence of specific autoantibodies, and subsequent manifestations of clinical disease have been thoroughly researched and established, but unfortunately these cause-and-effect relationships have not been recognized in veterinary patients. Because the potential clinical effects of particular ANAs are not known, testing for individual autoantibodies in veterinary patients by using ELISA or Western blot is not recommended.

INDICATIONS
• Nonerosive inflammatory arthropathy or polyarthritis
• Dermatologic lesions (especially facial and mucocutaneous) unresponsive to antibiotic or antihistamine therapy
• Proteinuria
• Immune-mediated cytopenias
• Persistent lymphadenopathy
• Fever of unknown origin
• Thyroid dysfunction

CONTRAINDICATIONS
Concurrent or previous drug therapy that may cause false-negative or false-positive results (see the Interpretation section)

POTENTIAL COMPLICATIONS
None

CLIENT EDUCATION
None

BODY SYSTEMS ASSESSED
• Cardiovascular
• Dermatologic
• Endocrine
• Hemic, lymphatic, and immune
• Musculoskeletal

SAMPLE

COLLECTION
1–2 mL of venous blood

HANDLING
Collect the blood sample in a red-top tube or serum-separator tube.

STORAGE
Refrigerate for short-term storage, but freeze for long-term storage.

STABILITY
• Room temperature: 1 day
• Refrigerated (2°–8°C): 1 week
• Frozen (−20°C): 1 year

PROTOCOL
None

INTERPRETATION

NORMAL FINDINGS OR RANGE
Negative results (titer of <1:20)

ABNORMAL VALUES
• 1:20–1:80 = low positive titer
• >1:80 = high positive titer

CRITICAL VALUES
None

INTERFERING FACTORS
Drugs That May Alter Results or Interpretation
Drugs That Interfere with Test Methodology
None

Drugs That Alter Physiology
• Drugs that may cause a false-positive result include acetazolamide, aminosalicylic acid (aspirin), chlorothiazides, griseofulvin, hydralazine, methimazole, penicillin, phenylbutazone, phenytoin, procainamide, streptomycin, sulfonamides, and tetracyclines.
• Drugs that may cause a false-negative result include cytotoxic drugs (chemotherapy) and corticosteroids.

Collection Techniques or Handling That May Alter Results
None

Influence of Signalment
Species
None

Breed
• German shepherds may have elevated ANA titers without evidence of clinical disease.
• Canine breeds possibly genetically predisposed to SLE include Old English sheepdogs, Shetland sheepdogs, German shepherds, collies, beagles, Afghan hounds, Irish setters, and poodles.
• Siamese, Persian, and Himalayan cats may be predisposed to SLE.

Age
None

Gender
None

Pregnancy
None

LIMITATIONS OF THE TEST
Unfortunately, veterinary laboratories do not have a standardized protocol for performing ANA-IFA testing. Controls and procedures may differ. Cutoff values for a positive test may vary from lab to lab, depending on the types of substrate used, and there is an inherent subjectivity to the interpretation of nuclear staining patterns. Caution should be used when comparing test results from labs that use different protocols.

Sensitivity, Specificity, and Positive and Negative Predictive Values
The test is very sensitive but not specific, and therefore false positive results are common.

Valid If Run in a Human Lab?
No. The test requires species-specific reagents.

Causes of Abnormal Findings
These are the causes of elevated ANA titers in dogs and cats:

SLE
This is most common disorder associated with elevated ANA titers.

Dermatologic Diseases
- Pemphigus erythematosus
- Pemphigus vulgaris (titers tend to be lower than with pemphigus erythematosus)
- Discoid lupus
- Generalized demodicosis
- Fleabite allergy
- Plasma cell pododermatitis

Hematologic Diseases
- Immune-mediated hemolytic anemia
- Immune-mediated thrombocytopenia

Cardiopulmonary Disease
- Bacterial endocarditis
- Dirofilariasis

Miscellaneous Disorders
- Rheumatoid arthritis
- Lymphocytic thyroiditis
- Ulcerative autoimmune stomatitis
- Sjögren-like syndrome
- Bacterial infections (e.g., ehrlichiosis, anaplasmosis, bartonellosis)
- Protozoal infections (e.g., leishmaniasis)
- Cholangiohepatitis
- FIP
- FeLV
- Myasthenia gravis
- Certain neoplastic disorders (e.g., lymphoma)

CLINICAL PERSPECTIVE
- Patients with waxing-and-waning multisystemic clinical signs or fever of unknown origin should be evaluated for SLE or SLE-related disease.
- The presence of 2 or more symptoms supportive of autoimmune disease (e.g., nonseptic polyarthritis, dermatologic lesions, glomerulonephritis, immune-mediated hemolytic anemia, or immune-mediated thrombocytopenia) should increase clinical suspicion of SLE in the face of an elevated ANA titer.
- Biopsies of affected tissue (e.g., skin, synovium, kidney) may be necessary if the ANA titer is low positive or equivocal or if a false negative is suspected (e.g., previous steroidal therapy).
- Because of the high rate of false positives, ANA testing is not recommended in animals with a single site of immune-mediated disease (e.g., just IMHA or just polyarthritis).
- Multiple infectious diseases may exhibit clinical signs that mimic SLE (e.g., polyarthritis, thrombocytopenia, proteinuria) and may elevate the ANA titer. Ehrlichiosis, Rocky Mountain spotted fever, leishmaniasis, and bartonellosis should be ruled out through serology and/or PCR testing.

- The ANA test may be used to monitor response to immunosuppressive therapy (i.e., remission of clinical signs may be accompanied by a decrease in the elevation of the titer).

MISCELLANEOUS
ANCILLARY TESTS
- Coombs' test
- Lupus erythematosus (LE) cell test
- Rheumatoid factor
- Test for infectious disease titers (*Bartonella, Ehrlichia, Anaplasma,* Rocky Mountain spotted fever, leishmania)

SYNONYMS
ANA test

SEE ALSO
Blackwell's Five-Minute Veterinary Consult: Canine and Feline Topics
- Anemia, Immune-Mediated
- Lupus Erythematosus, Cutaneous (Discoid)
- Lupus Erythematosus, Systemic (SLE)
- Myasthenia Gravis
- Pemphigus
- Polyarthritis, Erosive, Immune-Mediated
- Polyarthritis, Nonerosive, Immune-Mediated
- Sjögren-like Syndrome
- Thrombocytopenia, Primary Immune-Mediated

Related Topics in This Book
- *Bartonella*
- Coombs' Test
- *Ehrlichia/Anasplama*
- Lupus Erythematosus Cell Preparation
- Rheumatoid Factor
- Rocky Mountain Spotted Fever

ABBREVIATIONS
- ANA = antinuclear antibody
- SLE = systemic lupus erythematosus

Suggested Reading
Day MJ. Systemic lupus erythematosus. In: Feldman BF, Zinkl JG, Jain NC, eds. *Schalm's Veterinary Hematology,* 5th ed. Ames, IA: Blackwell, 2006: 820–825.
Medleau L, Miller WH. Immunodiagnostic tests for small animal practice. *Compend Contin Educ Pract Vet* 1983; 5: 705–711.
Smith BE, Tompkins MB, Breitschwerdt EB. Antinuclear antibodies can be detected in dog sera reactive to *Bartonella vinsonii* subsp. *berkhoffi, Ehrlichia canis,* or *Leishmania infantum* antigens. *J Vet Intern Med* 2004; 18: 47–51.
Tizard IR. The systemic immunological diseases. In: *Veterinary Immunology: An Introduction,* 6th ed. Philadelphia: WB Saunders, 2000: 386–390.
Werner LL, Turnwald GH, Willard MD. Immunologic and plasma protein disorders. In: Willard MD, Tvedten H, eds. *Small Animal Clinical Diagnosis by Laboratory Methods,* 4th ed. Philadelphia: WB Saunders, 2004: 299–301.

INTERNET RESOURCES
Cornell University, College of Veterinary Medicine, Clinical Pathology Laboratory: Available test, http://www.diaglab.vet.cornell.edu/clinpath/test/immun/ana.asp.

AUTHOR NAME
Maria Vandis

AQUEOCENTESIS AND VITREOCENTESIS

 BASICS

TYPE OF PROCEDURE
Diagnostic sample collection

PROCEDURE EXPLANATION AND RELATED PHYSIOLOGY
Aqueocentesis and vitreocentesis involve aspiration of small amounts of aqueous humor or vitreous for diagnostic or therapeutic purposes. These techniques are indicated for severe or persistent anterior and posterior segment ocular disease to obtain specific diagnosis of inflammatory, infectious, or neoplastic disease. Subsequent treatment and prognosis will depend on diagnostic results. Aqueocentesis can also be used for emergency management of glaucoma that does not respond to medical therapy.

Since the sample size is small (0.1–0.5 mL), prioritization of the diagnostic test based on clinical suspicion is critical. Cytology (often concentrated with ultracentrifugation); aerobic, anaerobic, and fungal cultures; specific serologies; and PCR will provide the most useful information. To decrease the risk of complications, both aqueocentesis and vitreocentesis require general anesthesia.

INDICATIONS
• To provide a definitive diagnosis of inflammatory, infectious, or neoplastic processes within the eye. Examples include blastomycosis, cryptococcosis, prototheca, lymphoma, Voyt-Koyanagi-Harada–like (VKH) syndrome (aka uveodermatologic syndrome), and toxoplasmosis.
• Aqueocentesis can be used as a short-term measure to reduce severely elevated intraocular pressure in acute glaucoma cases that do not respond to medical management.

CONTRAINDICATIONS
• Coagulopathy

POTENTIAL COMPLICATIONS
• Corneal trauma or edema secondary to endothelial cell damage
• Hemorrhage (hyphema from iris vessels or bleeding from the posterior vessels)
• Traumatic cataract or lens subluxation
• Uveitis, with possible secondary glaucoma
• Endophalmitis, sterile or secondary to bacterial contamination
• Retinal detachment

CLIENT EDUCATION
• Animals should be fasted prior to anesthesia.
• Owners should be warned about potential complications.

BODY SYSTEMS ASSESSED
• Ophthalmic

 PROCEDURE

PATIENT PREPARATION
Preprocedure Medication or Preparation
• Pupillary dilation is recommended to enhance transpupillary visualization for vitreocentesis.

Anesthesia or Sedation
• General anesthesia (e.g., propofol or inhaled anesthetic) is required in order to decrease risk of complications and minimize patient movement.

Patient Positioning
• Lateral recumbency so that the needle can be comfortably inserted through the dorsolateral quadrant. The pars plana ciliaris is largest in

this quadrant and is the intended site of penetration for vitreocentesis in order to decrease the risk of complications.

Patient Monitoring
• As needed for anesthesia
• Monitor for signs of hemorrhage and increased inflammation.

Equipment or Supplies
• Aqueocentesis: 25- to 30-gauge needle, two 1-mL syringes with 3-way stopcock, and sterile saline for refilling the anterior chamber
• Vitreocentesis: 22- to 23-gauge needle, two 1-mL syringes with 3-way stopcock, and sterile saline for refilling the posterior segment
• Delicate conjunctival tissue forceps for anchoring the globe
• An eyelid speculum
• Head loupes for magnification may be helpful.

TECHNIQUE
• The patient is anesthetized.
• The eye and surrounding conjunctiva and eyelids are prepared with dilute povidone-iodine solution and sterile saline.
• The globe can be stabilized by grasping the bulbar conjunctiva with delicate tissue forceps.
• Aqueocentesis: A 25- to 30-gauge needle is tunneled through the sclera, entering 1–2 mm behind the limbus at an angle to penetrate the anterior chamber between the iris and the cornea. The angled tunnel decreases the risk of continued aqueous leakage when the needle is withdrawn. Once the needle enters the anterior chamber, a 0.1- to 0.2-mL sample is slowly withdrawn while the tip of the needle is visualized to avoid contact with the cornea, iris, or lens.
• Vitreocentesis: A 22- to 23-gauge needle is inserted ≈7 mm behind the limbus (through the pars plana ciliaris). Microscopic visualization though the pupil can help the surgeon avoid the lens anteriorly and the retina posteriorly. Once the needle is in place, 0.1–0.25 mL can be withdrawn.
• An equal amount of sterile saline can be injected into the eye to avoid increase prostaglandin production associated with sudden ocular hypotension. This is best achieved using two 1-mL syringes and a 3-way stopcock.
• As the needle is withdrawn, the forceps can be used to grasp and hold over the needle tract opening to decrease the chance of leakage.

SAMPLE HANDLING
Sterile transport to a laboratory

APPROPRIATE AFTERCARE
Postprocedure Patient Monitoring
Monitor for increased inflammation and possible increases in intraocular pressure associated with secondary glaucoma.

Nursing Care
None

Dietary Modification
None

Medication Requirements
• Topical steroids with antibiotics and atropine for anterior uveitis
• Systemic anti-inflammatory medications for posterior uveitis. Use systemic steroids with caution if an infectious disease process is a concern.
• Topical antiglaucoma medications (e.g., carbonic anhydrase inhibitors), as needed, for elevations in intraocular pressure

Restrictions on Activity
None

Anticipated Recovery Time
None

INTERPRETATION

NORMAL FINDINGS OR RANGE
- No cells should be present in the sample.
- Total protein concentration should be 21–37 mg/dL.
- Microbial cultures should be negative for bacterial or fungal growth.

ABNORMAL VALUES
- Protein concentrations of 40–65 mg/dL can be consistent with clinical aqueous flare.
- Protein concentrations as high as 600–2,000 mg/dL can be seen with severe disease or after intraocular surgery.
- Any bacterial growth on submitted cultures
- Any positive serologic test result
- Any inflammatory or neoplastic cells in the fluid

CRITICAL VALUES
- Positive confirmation of infectious agents or neoplastic cells

INTERFERING FACTORS
Drugs That May Alter Results of the Procedure
Preoperative antibiotics or anti-inflammatory medications might mask the disease process.

Conditions That May Interfere with Performing the Procedure
None

Procedure Techniques or Handling That May Alter Results
Contamination from extraocular tissues or poor tissue preparation

Influence of Signalment on Performing and Interpreting the Procedure

Species
None

Breed
None

Age
- Vitreocentesis will be easier in older patients because vitreous degenerates and liquefies with age. Alternatively, it may be necessary to use a larger-gauge needle to withdraw vitreous from a young patient.

Gender
None

Pregnancy
None

CLINICAL PERSPECTIVE
- Aqueocentesis and vitreocentesis are performed to definitely diagnose inflammatory, infectious, and neoplastic disease. Although the technique is simple, the requirement of general anesthesia and the risk of complications dictate that less invasive tests results, such as routine clinical pathologic tests and radiographs, be evaluated first.

MISCELLANEOUS

ANCILLARY TESTS
- Aerobic bacterial, anaerobic bacterial, and fungal culture and sensitivity
- Fluid protein and cytologic analysis
- Tests to evaluate for causative systemic disease should also include these:
  - Chest and abdominal radiographs
  - Lymph node aspiration
  - Abdominal ultrasound

SYNONYMS
- Hyalocentesis
- Paracentesis

SEE ALSO
Blackwell's Five-Minute Veterinary Consult: Canine and Feline Topics
- Anterior Uveitis—Cats
- Anterior Uveitis—Dogs
- Chorioretinitis
- Glaucoma
- Retinal Detachment

Related Topics in This Book
- Bacterial Culture and Sensitivity
- Fine-Needle Aspiration

ABBREVIATIONS
None

Suggested Reading
Gelatt KN, ed. *Veterinary Ophthalmology*, 3rd ed. Philadelphia: Lippincott Williams & Wilkins, 1990.

INTERNET RESOURCES
None

AUTHOR NAME
A. Brady Beale

ARTHROCENTESIS WITH SYNOVIAL FLUID ANALYSIS

BASICS

TYPE OF PROCEDURE
Diagnostic sample collection

PROCEDURE EXPLANATION AND RELATED PHYSIOLOGY
Joint disease can occur in 1 or multiple joints and is typically classified as being inflammatory and infectious, or inflammatory and noninfectious, or noninflammatory. As these categories are defined by synovial fluid and cell analyses, joint disease cannot be fully characterized without the aid of sample collection. Arthrocentesis is in essence a fine-needle aspirate of the joint space and is a safe, quick, and relatively easy procedure that can be performed in most clinical settings. The equipment needed is minimal and inexpensive, and the techniques are not difficult to learn. The information obtained from successful joint taps, coupled with a good history, physical examination, and appropriate ancillary diagnostics, is invaluable in attempting to differentiate among the various classes of joint disease. Correct identification of the disease process will then enable the clinician to offer the most appropriate form of treatment.

INDICATIONS
- Joint pain or distention
- Lameness or gait abnormality (once orthopedic or neurologic disease has been ruled out)
- Fever of unknown origin
- Undefined lethargy or nonspecific pain

CONTRAINDICATIONS
- Coagulopathy
- Severe thrombocytopenia ($<20,000/\mu L$)

POTENTIAL COMPLICATIONS
- Complications associated with sedation
- Iatrogenic joint infection
- Hemarthrosis

CLIENT EDUCATION
- Patients will need to be sedated.
- Patients will need to have multiple joints shaved.

BODY SYSTEMS ASSESSED
Musculoskeletal

PROCEDURE

PATIENT PREPARATION
Preprocedure Medication or Preparation
None

Anesthesia or Sedation
- General anesthesia is usually not required.
- Mild to moderate sedation is required.

Patient Positioning
Lateral recumbency with the selected joint(s) on the upper side

Patient Monitoring
- Standard for sedation protocol
- Assess for pain and adjust the level of sedation accordingly.

Equipment or Supplies
- Clippers
- Surgical scrub solution, alcohol, and gauze
- Sterile 3-mL syringes
- 22-Gauge 1-inch (25.4 mm) needles (for cats and small dogs)
- 22-Gauge $1\frac{1}{2}$-inch (38.1 mm) needles (may be needed for large dogs)

- 25-Gauge $\frac{6}{36}$-inch (15.9 mm) needles (for very small animals)
- Sterile gloves
- A culturette or culture transport vial
- Glass microscope slides
- EDTA tubes

TECHNIQUE
- Prior to starting the procedure, have all your equipment in place and familiarize yourself with the anatomy of the selected joint (Figures 1–5). Even when only 1 joint appears to be affected, it is recommended that at least 3 be sampled.
- Clip overlying hair and aseptically prepare the chosen joint.
- Put on sterile gloves.
- An assistant opens the syringe case and aseptically places the syringe on a sterile field (e.g., the open-glove package). The assistant then opens the needle case. Pick up the syringe and place it aseptically into the hub of the needle. Place pressure against the hub and then pull back as your assistant is removing the needle cap. This procedure will leave you holding a sterile needle and syringe.

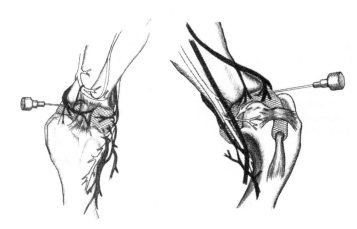

Figure 1

Schematic representation of landmarks for the shoulder joint.

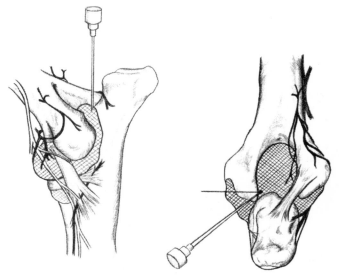

Figure 2

Schematic representation of landmarks for the elbow joint.

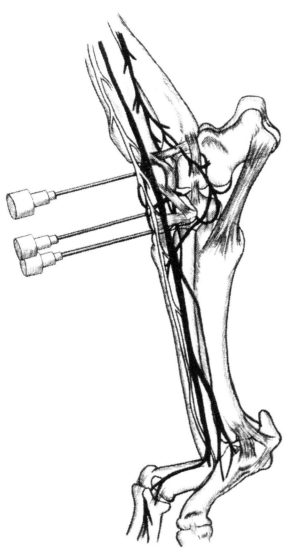

Figure 3

Schematic representation of landmarks for the carpal joint.

- Flex the joint by using the opposite hand that you will use for aspiration of the joint and palpate the appropriate landmarks for the specific joint to be tapped with the dominant hand.
- Holding the syringe, pass the needle through the skin, joint capsule, and synovial membrane and into the joint cavity. It is unlikely that you will be able to feel the needle penetrate each layer. Attempt to avoid articular cartilage, but if bone is encountered, you can pull back slightly and redirect the needle into the joint space.
- Gently aspirate. Unless the joint is severely distended, you may obtain only a few drops of fluid in the hub of the needle. As soon as fluid appears in the hub of the needle, release negative pressure and remove the needle from the joint. If the joint is significantly distended, a larger volume of fluid may be removed from the joint space. If blood is seen at any point in the procedure, immediately release pressure and remove the needle.
- A large amount of blood makes cytologic evaluation too difficult, and tapping a new joint space is advisable. A small amount of blood may be in the joint space as part of the disease process.

- The following discussion about individual joints is presented in order of increasing difficulty:

Carpal Joint
- You should be able to palpate the space between the radius and proximal carpal bones, the proximal carpal bones and distal carpal bones, and the carpal and metacarpal bones.
- With the hand you are not using for aspiration, flex the joint to achieve a maximum amount of open joint space. The most common joint space to be tapped is the radiocarpal joint. The larger the space, the easier it is to obtain a good sample.
- Holding the syringe, insert the needle from the cranial surface through the skin and joint capsule and into the joint space. Avoid the prominent accessory cephalic vein on the dorsal surface.

Stifle Joint
- This is large and may be approached from either the medial or lateral aspect.
- Flex the stifle joint to open the joint space.
- Insert the needle from the cranial aspect, lateral or medial to the patellar ligament. The needle should enter the joint approximately halfway between the patella and tibial tuberosity.
- Angle the needle toward the center of the joint. It may be helpful to apply digital pressure to the opposite side of the patellar ligament to cause joint fluid to collect toward your approach. A fat pad is present that may interfere with obtaining fluid. If fluid is not obtained initially, back up the needle, redirect, and aspirate.

Tarsal Joint
- Two small joint spaces can be tapped in the tarsus.
- One approach is to flex the joint slightly and palpate the cranial space between the tibia and tibiotarsal bone. Insert the needle from the cranial and lateral aspect and direct it medially. This joint is shallow, so you will not need to advance the needle very far.
- The second approach is from the distal aspect and is accomplished by flexing the tarsal joint more fully to open the space between the distal fibula, tibia, and calcaneus bones. Palpate this space and insert the needle from a caudolateral position. The needle should be advanced parallel to calcaneus distally and slightly medially.

Elbow
- Flex the elbow to an ≈45° angle. This opens the space between the humerus and the ulna.
- Insert the needle between the olecranon process and the lateral condyle of the humerus and advance it distally and slightly medially, following the cranial surface of the ulna.
- You may also attempt to insert the needle into this space from the lateral aspect by entering the joint between the ulna and the lateral condyle of the humerus.

Scapulohumeral Joint
- Flex the joint slightly to widen the space. Palpate the greater tubercle and the acromion process of the scapula.
- Approach the joint from the lateral aspect and insert the needle slightly cranial and distal to the acromion process and just caudal to the greater tubercle. The needle should be directed in a caudal-medial and slightly downward direction.
- The joint space can be approached also from a cranial direction. Insert the needle medial to the greater tubercle and ventral to the supraglenoid tubercle, angling it in a cranial-caudal direction.

SAMPLE HANDLING
- Joint fluid should be evaluated grossly for color and viscosity at the time of the tap. A change in the color or viscosity of the joint fluid can indicate disease or blood contamination.
- If the sample is contaminated with blood by a traumatic tap, the blood usually does not mix evenly, whereas blood from ongoing hemorrhage into the joint appears evenly distributed.
- The viscosity may be roughly estimated by ejecting 1 drop of the fluid onto a slide (without touching the needle to the slide) and

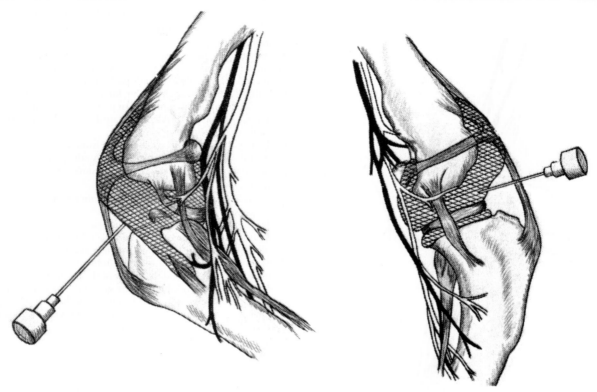

Figure 4

Schematic representation of landmarks for the stifle joint.

assessing the length of the resultant string that forms when the needle is withdrawn slowly from the slide [2.5 cm (≈1 inch) is considered normal]. A watery consistency that does not form a string is indicative of disease. The slide can then be used to prepare a smear for cytologic evaluation.
• Many taps yield only a few drops of fluid, and complete fluid analysis may be difficult. Slides should always be submitted for cytologic evaluation because determining the type of cells in the fluid is likely to be the most helpful piece of information in defining the disease process.
• If enough fluid can be obtained, a small amount of the sample should be placed in an EDTA tube for fluid analysis.
• Culture and microbial sensitivity testing should be on a sample from 1 joint, if possible. The probability of bacterial infection is greater in patients that have monoarthropathies and purulent-appearing joint fluid. Some clinicians advocate using enrichment broth because organisms infecting joints (especially *Mycoplasma*) can be difficult to culture. Communication with the microbiology laboratory is recommended if fastidious or slow-growing organisms, such as *Mycoplasma*, are to be successfully isolated.

APPROPRIATE AFTERCARE
Postprocedure Patient Monitoring
• Standard for sedation protocol
• Monitor for increased joint pain or swelling.
Nursing Care
None
Dietary Modification
• In some cases, a weight-reducing diet is recommended.
• Specific diets are available for dogs with joint disease.

Medication Requirements
Dependent on primary disease process
Restrictions on Activity
Dependent on primary disease process
Anticipated Recovery Time
Immediate after recovery from sedation

INTERPRETATION
NORMAL FINDINGS OR RANGE
See Table 1.

CRITICAL VALUES
None

INTERFERING FACTORS
Drugs That May Alter Results of the Procedure
None

Conditions That May Interfere with Performing the Procedure
• Coagulopathy
• Severe skin disease or infection

Procedure Techniques or Handling That May Alter Results
Traumatic tap with blood contamination

Influence of Signalment on Performing and Interpreting the Procedure
Species
• Feline chronic progressive polyarthropathy has been documented in male cats.

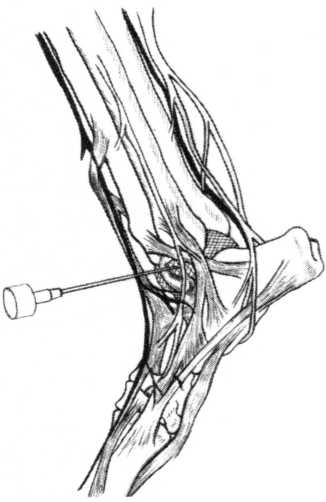

Figure 5

Schematic representation of landmarks for the tarsal joint.

• Bacterial L-form infection can cause a severe, erosive polyarthritis in cats.

• Calicivirus (both by natural infection and by vaccination) can cause a transient polyarthritis in young kittens.

Breed
• Arthrocentesis may be more difficult to perform in small-breed dogs.
• An erosive polyarthropathy has been documented in young greyhounds.
• Swollen hock syndrome occurs in sharpeis.

Age
None

Gender
None

Pregnancy
None

CLINICAL PERSPECTIVE
• Whenever joint disease is suspected, an accurate medical history and a thorough physical examination are extremely important. Along with standard questions, trauma and travel history, and drug and toxin

(e.g., anticoagulant) exposure should be addressed. The physical examination should include a thorough musculoskeletal and neurologic examination to help the clinician differentiate joint disease from primary orthopedic or neurologic problems. Although careful attention must be paid to evaluating joints for effusion and pain with flexion or extension, it is extremely important to note that significant joint disease can be present despite a lack of abnormalities found by joint palpation.

• Initial diagnostic testing that should be considered before joint taps are performed include a CBC, chemistry profile, urinalysis with a urine culture, and radiographs of affected and corresponding nonaffected joints. A coagulation panel can be submitted if hemarthrosis secondary to toxicity or inherited disease is suspected. Further studies, such as serologic testing for infectious disease and systemic testing for immune-mediated disease, should also be considered when appropriate historical or clinical signs are present. Blood cultures may also be performed to look for a systemic infectious cause of joint inflammation.

• Occasionally (especially in cats), fever and lethargy are the sole presenting signs in animals with polyarthritis.

• As cats and small dogs have smaller joints, it may be more difficult to obtain a good sample from these patients.

• Once an inflammatory process is defined, there is considerable overlap in cytologic findings between the specific causes of inflammation. In general, inflammatory disease is characterized by the presence of increased numbers of neutrophils and a variable increase in large, mononuclear cells in the joint fluid. Septic joints tend to have a very high number of neutrophils, which may also exhibit degenerative changes. Bacterial organisms are usually not seen; *Ehrlichia* sp. morulae are seen infrequently. Increased numbers of nondegenerate neutrophils are generally seen with an immune-mediated process. A more complete review of cytologic changes in joint disease can be found in the Suggested Reading section.

• Rheumatoid arthritis, an erosive disease of the distal joints in small dogs, is extremely rare. Radiographs are helpful in making this diagnosis. Rheumatoid factor analysis is not necessary in the majority of cases.

• Reactive polyarthritis may be seen secondary to systemic infectious disease, drugs, neoplasia, or any chronic inflammatory condition.

• With proper technique, significant complications are very rare.

MISCELLANEOUS

ANCILLARY TESTS
• Joint radiographs
• Infectious disease testing (Lyme, *Ehrlichia*, heartworm, leishmania, *Toxoplasma*)
• Antinuclear antibody serology
• Urine protein/creatinine ratio
• Rheumatoid factor

SYNONYMS
Joint tap

SEE ALSO
Blackwell's Five-Minute Veterinary Consult: Canine and Feline Topics
• Arthritis (Osteoarthritis)
• Arthritis, Septic
• Lameness
• Polyarthritis, Erosive, Immune-Mediated
• Polyarthritis, Nonerosive, Immune-Mediated
Related Topics in This Book
• Bacterial Culture and Sensitivity
• Fluid Analysis

ARTHROCENTESIS WITH SYNOVIAL FLUID ANALYSIS

Table 1   Abnormal values

Variable	Normal	Trauma or hemarthrosis	Degenerative arthropathy	Inflammatory arthropathy
Appearance	Clear to straw colored	Clear to red	Clear to yellow	Yellow to bloody, often hazy or cloudy
Protein	<2.5 g/dL	Variable	<2.5 g/dL	Often >2.5 g/dL
Viscosity	High	Decreased	Normal to decreased	Decreased
Nucleated cell count (cells/μL)	<3,000	Increased RBCs, nucleated count relative to blood	1,000–10,000	5,000 to >100,000
Neutrophils	<5%	Relative to blood	<10%	>10% to 100%
Mononuclear cells	>95%	Relative to blood	>90%	10% to <90%
Comments	Only a small amount of fluid should be present	Erythrophagia helps to confirm previous hemorrhage	Cells are typically macrophages and may be vacuolated.	Wide variation in nucleated cell count exists and depends on the specific disease process. Refer to cytology references for more specific information.

ABBREVIATIONS
None

Suggested Reading

Baker R, Lumsden JH. Synovial fluid. In: *Color Atlas of the Cytology of the Dog and Cat*. St Louis: CV Mosby, 2000: 209–221.

Crow SE, Walshaw SO. *Manual of Clinical Procedures in the Dog and Cat*. Philadelphia: JB Lippincott, 1987: 196–197.

Evans HE, deLahunta A, eds. *Guide to the Dissection of the Dog*. St Louis: Saunders Elsevier, 2000: 48–51 and 88–93.

MacWilliams PS, Friedrichs KR. Laboratory evaluation and interpretation of synovial fluid. *Vet Clin North Am Small Anim Pract* 2003; 33: 153–178.

Schrader SC. The use of the laboratory in the diagnosis of joint disorders of the dog and cat. In: Kirk RW, ed. *Current Veterinary Therapy XII*. Philadelphia: WB Saunders, 1995: 1166–1171.

Taylor SM. Joint disorders. In: Nelson RW, Couto CG, eds. *Small Animal Internal Medicine*. St Louis: CV Mosby, 2003: 1071–1092.

INTERNET RESOURCES
None

AUTHOR NAME
Karyn Harrell

BASICS

TYPE OF PROCEDURE
Endoscopic

PROCEDURE EXPLANATION AND RELATED PHYSIOLOGY
- Arthroscopy uses a fine-diameter telescope to examine the internal structure of a joint.
- The arthroscope and other instrumentation are inserted through a series of small incisions or portals through the skin and underlying soft tissue structures into the joint. The portals are often defined by their location or use (e.g., camera or scope portal, instrument portal, egress portal). There are usually three portals, and their use can be alternated during a given procedure.
- *Cannulas*, which are used to maintain the portals and protect the instruments, are metal or plastic tubes that are inserted through the portals.
- *Triangulation* refers to the technique whereby a hand instrument and the structure of interest are both viewed by the camera such that the procedure can be performed.
- The magnified image is transmitted through the arthroscope to a camera that is then connected to a viewing screen or monitor. The light from an external light source is transmitted along the arthroscope via fiber optics.
- Irrigation of the joint is important in order to maintain a clear field of view. It also distends the joint, improving visualization of the structures of interest, and acts to remove debris and contamination. Fluid often enters the joint via the arthroscopic cannula and exits via the egress (outflow) portal. Gravity or fluid pumps are used to deliver the fluid, depending on the joint and procedure. Lactated Ringer's solution is the fluid of choice, although 0.9% sodium chloride may also be used.
- The magnification combined with evaluation of the joint in a more natural environment enables diagnosis of early or discrete lesions or changes to the cartilage (e.g., erosion, eburnation, or chondromalacia), ligaments, tendons, and synovial villi.
- *Second-look arthroscopy* is the repeated evaluation of a joint to monitor response to treatment or progression of disease.
- The procedure is typically performed by a surgical specialist and not in general practice.

INDICATIONS
- The presence of joint disease is based on history, and physical/orthopedic examination, with or without radiographic changes.
- Diagnostic evaluation, therapeutic management, or both, of infectious, degenerative, traumatic, neoplastic, and developmental diseases. Common diseases and procedures for each joint are listed:
  - *Elbow*: canine elbow dysplasia [fragmented medial coronoid process (FCP), osteochondrosis of the humeral condyle, ununited anconeal process (UAP), and osteoarthritis]
  - *Shoulder*: osteochondritis dissecans (OCD) of the humeral head, diagnostic evaluation (e.g., biopsy), shoulder instability (e.g., tears of the glenohumeral ligament or subscapularis tendon), and bicipital tenosynovitis
  - *Carpus*: intra-articular fractures, joint instability (e.g., radial carpal joint involvement), and osteoarthritis
  - *Hip*: evaluation prior to triple pelvic osteotomy (TPO), osteoarthritis, and drain placement in septic arthritis
  - *Stifle*: OCD of the femoral condyles, diagnosis and debridement of cranial cruciate ligament tear, evaluation of the menisci, medial meniscal release, and partial or complete meniscectomy
  - *Tarsus*: osteoarthritis, joint instability, OCD of the talus (e.g., medial trochlear ridge)

CONTRAINDICATIONS
- Pyoderma; wounds in the surgical site
- Coagulation abnormalities or recent aspirin administration

POTENTIAL COMPLICATIONS
- Swelling of the soft tissues around the joint because of extravasation of fluid is common but usually resolves with postoperative bandaging.
- Loss of osteochondral fragment or other tissue that is being excised.
- Infection and neurovascular injuries are rare.
- Iatrogenic cartilage lesions develop, some of which are of little clinical significance.
- Other complications are related to the complex nature of arthroscopy in veterinary patients (i.e., limited visualization because of inappropriate positioning, difficulties inserting instruments or with achieving adequate joint distention). They decrease in frequency with experience.

CLIENT EDUCATION
- The procedure is performed by a surgical specialist in the referral facility.
- The procedure reduces postoperative morbidity (e.g., pain, joint scar tissue).
- Bandages placed at the time of surgery are usually removed within 24–48 h.
- In cases of cartilage lesions or joint instability, the procedure is not going to prevent the progression of, or reverse ongoing, osteoarthritic changes.

BODY SYSTEMS ASSESSED
Musculoskeletal

 PROCEDURE

PATIENT PREPARATION
Preprocedure Medication or Preparation
- Medications used are clinician dependent.
- Aspirin use should be avoided for 10–14 days before surgery.
- Patients should be fasted for 10–12 h before the procedure.
- Perioperative antibiotics (i.e., cefazolin) are often given.

Anesthesia or Sedation
General anesthesia is required.

Patient Positioning
Variable and dependent on the joint of interest

Patient Monitoring
As per typical general anesthesia cases

Equipment or Supplies
- Hair clippers
- Sterile preparation supplies
- A video camera and monitors
- A light source and cable
- A telescope
- Cannulas
- Specific arthroscopic instruments as needed for the procedure
- Irrigation supplies
- Surgical instruments
- Suture material
- A scalpel blade

TECHNIQUE
- After the patient is anesthetized, the joint of interest is aseptically prepared. The use of local analgesia, in the form of intra-articular blocks, nerve blocks, or epidural analgesia, is appropriate and clinician dependent. Depending on the joint and area of interest, the portal sites are identified. The joint is distended by inserting a needle and instill-

ing an amide local anesthetic or saline. A skin incision, corresponding to the site of arthroscope insertion, is made that extends through the subcutaneous tissue into the joint capsule. A trochar with cannula is placed, following the same path, to create the portal. The trochar is removed, and the arthroscope is placed through the cannula. The camera is then attached so that placement of subsequent portals can be visualized and iatrogenic injury minimized. Once correct placement of the arthroscope is confirmed, an egress site is established and fluid flow is begun. Lactated Ringer's solution or saline is used to distend the joint and clear of debris. Hand instruments, which may be powered (e.g., a electric shaver), are introduced through instrument portals, and the procedure is completed. The joint is lavaged, and the portal sites are closed with skin sutures only. A soft, padded bandage is often placed prior to the patient's recovery from anesthesia.

SAMPLE HANDLING
None

APPROPRIATE AFTERCARE
Postprocedure Patient Monitoring
As with any procedure requiring general anesthesia

Nursing Care
Monitor for bandage complications (e.g., slipping, swelling of toes)

Dietary Modification
None

Medication Requirements
They depend on clinician preference and the joint or surgical procedure performed. NSAIDs or opioids may be prescribed.

Restrictions on Activity
Most patients will have a bandage placed for 24–48 h postoperatively. During this time, activity is restricted to brief leash walks. After this, the level of activity will depend on the site and surgical procedure but can involve 10–14 days of exercise restriction.

Anticipated Recovery Time
Most animals will be completely recovered by 2–4 weeks postoperatively; this depends on the original cause of lameness and the arthroscopic procedure performed.

INTERPRETATION

NORMAL FINDINGS OR RANGE
Absence of any inflammation, cartilaginous or bony lesions

ABNORMAL VALUES
Variable and dependent on the joint being examined (see the Indications section)

CRITICAL VALUES
- Articular cartilage lesions
- Intra-articular fracture
- Evidence of infectious disease (i.e., septic arthritis)

INTERFERING FACTORS
Drugs That May Alter Results of the Procedure
- Aspirin or other anti-inflammatory medications that affect coagulation
- Intra-articular steroid injections or systemic steroid administration

Conditions That May Interfere with Performing the Procedure
- Superficial pyoderma over joint of interest
- Neoplasia of the skin or subcutaneous tissue overlying the joint of interest
- Any diseases or problems that would make the patient an unsuitable anesthetic candidate
- Intra-articular steroid injections or systemic steroid administration

Procedure Techniques or Handling That May Alter Results
Arthroscopy is a difficult procedure that has a steep learning curve. Inexperience may limit a clinician's ability to assess adequately all areas of a joint.

Influence of Signalment on Performing and Interpreting the Procedure
Species
In cats, because of size limitations, not all joints can be examined.

Breed
Smaller breeds are more difficult, and not all joints can be examined.

Age
None

Gender
None

Pregnancy
The procedure is not advised in pregnant patients because of the risks associated with general anesthesia.

CLINICAL PERSPECTIVE
- Arthroscopy is a minimally invasive surgical procedure that can be both a diagnostic and a therapeutic procedure.
- It carries a much lower morbidity than arthrotomy.
- Arthroscopy can be used in combination with other surgical techniques (e.g., arthroscopic assisted tibial plateau-leveling osteotomy) to decrease surgical and anesthetic time and patient morbidity.

MISCELLANEOUS

ANCILLARY TESTS
- Abnormal tissue should be submitted for cytologic or histopathologic evaluation.
- In cases where septic inflammation is suspected, samples should be submitted for aerobic and anaerobic culture and sensitivity testing.

SYNONYMS
None

SEE ALSO
Blackwell's Five-Minute Veterinary Consult: Canine and Feline Topics
- Antebrachial Growth Deformities
- Arthritis (Osteoarthritis)
- Arthritis, Septic
- Cruciate Ligament Disease, Cranial
- Elbow Dysplasia
- Hip Dysplasia
- Lameness
- Osteochondrosis
- Patellar Luxation
- Shoulder, Joint, Ligament, and Tendon Conditions

Related Topics in This Book
- General Principles of Endoscopy
- Arthrocentesis with Synovial Fluid Analysis
- Computed Tomography
- Magnetic Resonance Imaging
- Skeletal Radiography

ABBREVIATIONS
OCD = osteochondritis dissecans

Suggested Reading
Beale BS, Hulse DA, Schulz KS, Whitney WO. *Small Animal Arthroscopy.* Philadelphia: WB Saunders, 2003.

Radlinsky MA. Ancillary diagnostic techniques for the lame patient. *Vet Clin North Am* 2001; **31**: 181–192.

Rochat MC. Arthroscopy. *Vet Clin North Am* 2001; **31**: 761–787.

Van Bree HJJ, Van Ryssen B. Diagnostic and surgical arthroscopy in osteochondrosis lesions. *Vet Clin North Am* 1998; **28**: 161–189.

Van Ryssen B, Van Bree H, Whitney WO, Schulz KS. Small animal arthroscopy. In: Slatter D, ed. *Textbook of Small Animal Surgery,* 3rd ed. Philadelphia: WB Saunders, 2003: 2285–2306.

INTERNET RESOURCES

Gulf Coast Veterinary Specialists (GCVS): Canine arthroscopy, http://www.gcvs.com/surgery/arthroscopy.htm.

Storz (Karl Storz Veterinary Endoscopy): Canine arthroscopy, http://www.ksvea.com/small_arthro.html.

AUTHOR NAMES

Duane A. Robinson and Michael G. Conzemius

ASPARTATE AMINOTRANSFERASE

 BASICS

TYPE OF SPECIMEN
Blood

TEST EXPLANATION AND RELATED PHYSIOLOGY
Aspartate aminotransferase (AST) is an enzyme located in the cytosol and mitochondria of many cell types. The highest concentration of AST can be found in skeletal muscle, followed by liver and cardiac muscle. Therefore, increased serum AST levels most commonly indicate either hepatocellular or muscle injury (skeletal or cardiac). AST may be released from cells with either sublethal cell injury (leakage) or necrosis. With mild damage, only cytoplasmic AST is released, whereas severe tissue damage also results in release of mitochondrial enzyme. Thus, in animals with liver disease, significantly elevated AST levels suggest a leak of AST from both sites, and hence more severe damage, than a similar ALT level. The half-life of AST is approximately 5–12 h in dogs and 1–2 h in cats, with a return to normal levels in about 3–4 days after resolution of injury.

RBCs also contain significant AST, so serum levels may also increase with intravascular hemolytic disease. AST is also found in renal epithelial cells and brain tissue, but a leak of enzyme from these tissues is reflected in urine and cerebrospinal fluid, respectively.

INDICATIONS
- To test for hepatic disease
- To detect muscle injury and necrosis

CONTRAINDICATIONS
None

POTENTIAL COMPLICATIONS
None

CLIENT EDUCATION
None

BODY SYSTEMS ASSESSED
- Hepatobiliary
- Musculoskeletal
- Hemic, lymphatic, and immune

 SAMPLE

COLLECTION
0.5–2.0 mL of venous blood

HANDLING
- Plain red-top tube or serum-separator tube
- EDTA, sodium heparin anticoagulant, or lithium heparin anticoagulant are acceptable.
- Separate serum or plasma from cells within 8 h at room temperature or within 2 days at 2°–8°C (refrigerated).

STORAGE
Refrigerate or freeze serum or plasma for long-term storage.

STABILITY
- 1 day at room temperature
- 1 week at 2°–8°C (refrigerated)

PROTOCOL
None

 INTERPRETATION

NORMAL FINDINGS OR RANGE
- Dogs: 16–54 IU/L
- Cats: 12–42 IU/L
- Reference intervals may vary, depending on laboratory and assay used.

ABNORMAL VALUES
Values above the reference interval

CRITICAL VALUES
None

INTERFERING FACTORS
Drugs That May Alter Results or Interpretation
Drugs That Interfere with Test Methodology
- Metronidazole may artifactually depress AST activity as determined by NADH-coupled analytic methods. Interference is from similarity in absorbance peaks of NADH (340 nm) and metronidazole (322 nm).
- AST activity can be decreased by drugs that impair activation of vitamin B_6 to pyridoxal 5'-phosphate (P5P) (e.g., cephalosporin, cyclosporine, isoniazide). This effect can be avoided if P5P is added as an assay cofactor.

Drugs That Alter Physiology
- AST activity can be increased by a variety of hepatotoxic drugs (e.g., erythromycin, rifampin, sulfonamides, acetaminophen, caparsolate).
- Anticonvulsants may induce enzyme synthesis or possible hepatotoxicity.

Disorders That May Alter Results
- Marked lipemia may interfere with spectrophotometric assays.
- Low vitamin B_6 levels (idiopathic or after hemodialysis) may decrease AST activity, as this vitamin is an essential cofactor of the enzyme.

Collection Techniques or Handling That May Alter Results
In vitro hemolysis will increase CK measurements, which might alter interpretation of elevated AST.

Influence of Signalment
Species
None

Breed
None

Age
Higher levels are seen in neonatal kittens during the first 2 months of life.

Gender
None

Pregnancy
None

LIMITATIONS OF THE TEST
- Because of wide tissue distribution (muscle, erythrocytes), AST elevations are not specific for liver injury.
- It generally has high sensitivity for liver or muscle damage, but AST activity may be normal or only slightly increased with significant chronic disease associated with decreased hepatic mass.

Sensitivity, Specificity, and Positive and Negative Predictive Values
None

Valid If Run in a Human Lab?
Yes.

Causes of Abnormal Findings

High values	Low values
Hepatocellular injury or leakage	Hepatic atrophy (as in chronic congenital portosystemic shunts)
Inflammation (hepatitis)	
Toxin and drug reactions	
Hepatic or biliary neoplasia	Decreased P5P levels (if not added to assay)
Corticosteroid hepatopathy	
Hepatic lipidosis	
Hypoxia (anemia, cardiovascular disease)	
Pancreatitis	
Trauma	
Cirrhosis	
Liver flukes	
Copper storage disease	
Muscle injury and necrosis	
Trauma	
Overexertion	
Myositis	
Intravascular hemolysis	
Immune-mediated hemolytic anemia	
Oxidant damage	
Zinc	
Onions	
Acetaminophen (cats)	
Other oxidants	
RBC parasites	
In vitro hemolysis (artifact)	

CLINICAL PERSPECTIVE

- If AST is increased without increased CK and with no evidence of in vitro or in vivo hemolysis, hepatocellular injury is likely the cause.
- Increases in ALT provide supportive evidence of hepatocyte injury.
- If serum or plasma is significantly hemolyzed, an elevated AST level is at least partially due to intravascular hemolysis.

MISCELLANEOUS

ANCILLARY TESTS

- CK levels to rule in/out muscle necrosis as a possible cause of an increased AST level
- ALT to help confirm hepatocellular injury
- ALP or GGT may help detect any cholestatic component of liver disease.
- Serum bile acids or ammonia to assess hepatic function

SYNONYMS

- AST
- Serum glutamic oxaloacetic transaminase (SGOT)

SEE ALSO

Blackwell's Five-Minute Veterinary Consult: Canine and Feline Topics

- Hepatic Failure, acute
- Hepatic Lipidosis
- Hepatitus, chronic active
- Hepatitus, granulomatous
- Hepatitus, infectious canine
- Hepatitus, suppurative and hepatic abscess
- Hepatotoxins
- Myocardial Infarction
- Myocarditis
- Myopathy, Focal Inflammatory—Masticatory Muscle Myositis and Extraocular Myositis
- Myopathy, Generalized Inflammatory—Polymyositis and Dermatomyositis

Related Topics in This Book

- Alanine Aminotransferase
- Bile Acids
- Bilirubin
- Creatine Kinase

ABBREVIATIONS

- ALP = alkaline phosphatase
- CK = creatine kinase
- P5P = pyridoxal 5′-phosphate

Suggested Reading

Bain PJ. Liver. In: Latimer KS, ed. *Duncan and Prasse's Veterinary Laboratory Medicine: Clinical Pathology*, 4th ed. Ames: Iowa State Press, 2003: 193–214.

Center SA. Diagnostic procedures for evaluation of hepatic disease. In: Guilford WG, Center SA, Strombeck DR, et al., eds. *Strombeck's Small Animal Gastroenterology*. Philadelphia: WB Saunders, 1996: 130–188.

Tams T. 2002. Liver disease: Diagnostic evaluation. In: *Proceedings from the Atlantic Coast Veterinary Conference 2001*, Hillsborough, NJ, 14 October 2008.

Willard MD, Twedt DC. Gastrointestinal, pancreatic, and hepatic disorders. In: Willard MD, Tvedten H, eds. *Small Animal Clinical Diagnosis by Laboratory Methods*, 4th ed. St Louis: Saunders Elsevier, 2004: 208–246.

INTERNET RESOURCES

None

AUTHOR NAME

Perry J. Bain

BASICS

TYPE OF SPECIMEN
Blood

TEST EXPLANATION AND RELATED PHYSIOLOGY
Babesiosis is caused by intraerythrocytic protozoan parasites, transmitted by ticks. Hemolytic anemia is the most serious clinical consequence of infection, but thrombocytopenia can also occur. Babesiosis can present as either an acute or a chronic condition, and some animals can be asymptomatic carriers. Several available testing options are available:

PCR
Amplification of a specific piece of DNA from organism of interest: EDTA-anticoagulated whole blood is the sample of choice. Obtain samples *before* treatment, because treatment may reduce the number of organisms and result in false-negative test results.

IFA Assay and ELISA
Detection of antibodies against organism of interest. It may take >3 weeks for patient to develop an antibody titer.

Light Microscopy
Detection of *Babesia* organisms in RBCs in a thin peripheral blood smear. They can appear either as light blue, teardrop-shaped organisms with a dark purple nucleus (e.g., *Babesia canis*) or as fine rings with an eccentric purple nucleus (signet-ring shape; e.g., *Babesia gibsoni*). Parasitemia of infected animals can range from 0.0001% to >10% of RBCs. At least 8 genetically unique *Babesia* species or subspecies can infect dogs and 2 can infect cats, including *B. canis canis*, *B. c. vogeli*, *B. c. rossi*, *B. gibsoni*, *B. conradea*, *Theileria annae*, *B. felis* (feline), *B. c. presentii* (feline), and several unnamed, yet genetically unique, *Babesia* spp. Most laboratories test for only 2 canine species, and cross-reactivity is not always present. Knowledge of which species are tested for is important for both antibody and DNA testing.

INDICATIONS
- Anemia (typically regenerative)
- Thrombocytopenia
- Hyperglobulinemia
- Splenomegaly
- Icterus and pigmenturia
- Screening of blood donors or breeding animals

CONTRAINDICATIONS
None

POTENTIAL COMPLICATIONS
None

CLIENT EDUCATION
Results are available in 3–14 days; a negative test does not necessarily rule out infection

BODY SYSTEMS ASSESSED
Hemic, lymphatic, and immune

SAMPLE

COLLECTION
- 2 mL of venous blood
- Capillary blood (ear tip or toenail) for blood smears

HANDLING
- PCR: EDTA anticoagulant. Ship overnight on ice.
- IFA or ELISA: red-top tube. Ship overnight on ice.

- Microscopy: thin blood smears, unstained (fix with methanol if shipment delayed for >2 days). Ship at room temperature, no ice.

STORAGE
- PCR: refrigerator or freezer
- IFA or ELISA: refrigerator or freezer
- Microscopy: room temperature, protected from light

STABILITY
- IFA, ELISA, or PCR
  - Refrigeration (2°–8°C) for days
  - Frozen (−20° to −80°C) for months to years
- Microscopy: Unstained blood smears can be stored for days. Stained slides can be stored for years.

PROTOCOL
None

INTERPRETATION

NORMAL FINDINGS OR RANGE
- PCR: no *Babesia* DNA
- IFA or ELISA: no anti-*Babesia* antibodies
- Microscopy: no *Babesia* organisms identified

ABNORMAL VALUES
- PCR: The presence of *Babesia* DNA indicates infection.
- IFA or ELISA: The presence of anti-*Babesia* antibodies indicates exposure to *Babesia*.
- Microscopy: The identification of *Babesia* organisms in RBCs indicates infection.

CRITICAL VALUES
None

INTERFERING FACTORS
Drugs That May Alter Results or Interpretation
Drugs That Interfere with Test Methodology
None

Drugs That Alter Physiology
Antiprotozoal therapy (imidocarb dipropionate, atovaquone and azithromycin, clindamycin, etc.) may cause false-negative PCR test results and prevent microscopic identification of organism in RBCs.

Disorders That May Alter Results
None

Collection Techniques or Handling That May Alter Results
- Smears of *capillary* blood may improve organism recovery since infected RBCs may accumulate in these narrow vessels.
- *Babesia gibsoni* organisms are best observed on slides stained with a modified Wright's stain.
- The quality of the smear, stain, and slide reader all affect the sensitivity and specificity of microscopy.

Influence of Signalment
Species
None

Breed
- *Babesia gibsoni* in the United States is most commonly diagnosed in American pit bull terriers.
- *Babesia canis vogeli* in the United States is most commonly diagnosed in greyhounds.

Age
IFA or ELISA: Infected puppies may not have any detectable antibodies.

Gender
None

Pregnancy
None

LIMITATIONS OF THE TEST
- The absence of *Babesia* organisms in a blood smear and a negative PCR test result do not rule out infection.
- False-negative result may occur if lab does not test for the specific *Babesia* species or subspecies causing infection.

Sensitivity, Specificity, and Positive and Negative Predictive Values
- PCR
  - Sensitivity: for a single test, 82%; increasing to 100% with 2 consecutive tests run 1 month apart
  - Specificity: approaches 100% especially with appropriate positive and negative controls
  - Positive predictive value: near 100%
  - Negative predictive value: unknown
- IFA or ELISA: unknown
- Microscopy: unknown

Valid If Run in a Human Lab?
No.

CLINICAL PERSPECTIVE
- No test can completely rule out the presence of *Babesia*; interpret results in light of clinical signs. Response to treatment may be an appropriate challenge in some cases.
- PCR is only way to identify the *Babesia* species reliably.

MISCELLANEOUS

ANCILLARY TESTS
- CBC, biochemical profile, and urinalysis
- Coombs' test

- Tests for organisms (e.g., *Ehrlichia canis*, leishmania) that might cause anemia, thrombocytopenia, and/or hyperglobulinemia

SYNONYMS
None

SEE ALSO
Blackwell's Five-Minute Veterinary Consult: Canine and Feline Topics
Babesiosis

Related Topics in This Book
- Hemotrophic Mycoplasmas
- Red Blood Cell Count
- Red Blood Cell Morphology

ABBREVIATIONS
None

Suggested Reading
Birkenheuer AJ, Levy MG, Breitschwerdt EB. Development and evaluation of a seminested PCR for detection and differentiation of *Babesia gibsoni* (Asian genotype) and *B. canis* DNA in canine blood samples. *J Clin Microbiol* 2003; 41: 4172–4177.
Boozer AL, Macintire DK. Canine babesiosis. *Compend Contin Educ Pract Vet* 2005; 27: 33–42.

INTERNET RESOURCES
University of Georgia, College of Veterinary Medicine, Veterinary Clinical Pathology Clerkship Program: Cleveland CW, Peterson DS, Latimer KS. An overview of canine babesiosis, http://www.vet.uga.edu/vpp/clerk/Cleveland/.

AUTHOR NAME
Adam J. Birkenheuer

BACTERIAL CULTURE AND SENSITIVITY

 BASICS

TYPE OF SPECIMEN
Blood
Feces
Tissue
Urine

TEST EXPLANATION AND RELATED PHYSIOLOGY
Culture and sensitivity testing to aid in diagnosis of infection disease is 1 of the most common tests in the diagnostic laboratory. Proper specimen selection and collection are crucial to proper diagnosis. In addition, it is important to distinguish normal flora from infectious agents. After the specimen arrives at the laboratory, it is streaked on bacteriologic medium, a process used to isolate individual colonies for further diagnostics. The medium is then incubated either aerobically or anaerobically to allow sufficient growth so further testing can be performed both to help identify the bacteria and to perform susceptibility testing.

Different methodologies may be used to determine antimicrobial susceptibility. With Kirby-Bauer disk diffusion, a bacterial lawn is streaked onto an agar plate, and antimicrobial-impregnated disks are placed on the plate and incubated overnight. A zone of inhibition is measured in millimeters around each disk to determine whether the bacteria is susceptible or resistant to that antimicrobial. Some methodologies use doubling dilutions in micrograms per milliliter of the antimicrobials to determine susceptibility, reporting minimum inhibitory concentrations (MICs).

INDICATIONS
To identify bacteria causing infection and determine the most appropriate therapy

CONTRAINDICATIONS
None

POTENTIAL COMPLICATIONS
None

CLIENT EDUCATION
None

BODY SYSTEMS ASSESSED
Dependent on location of infection

 SAMPLE

COLLECTION
The sample depends on the site of potential infection.
- Swab the site (e.g., ear, discharge) by using a sterile swab. Swabs tipped with inert, nontoxic rayon are preferred.
- Fine-needle aspirate: Preparation of the aspiration site is important to prevent contamination of sample with normal flora.
- 0.5–1.0 mL of urine: Cystocentesis is the method of choice. Catheterized or voided urine is acceptable, but urine collected by either of these methods requires quantitative urine cultures for interpretation.
- 0.5–1.0 mL of effusion
- Material aspirated from the lesion (e.g., abscess)
- 4 mL of venous blood
- Feces
- Tissue biopsy
- Wash (tracheal wash, nasal flush, prostatic wash)

HANDLING
Remove surface exudate by wiping with sterile saline or 70% alcohol prior to any type of percutaneous aspiration.

Aerobic Culture
- Sterile swab: Swabs should be placed into some type of microorganism collection and transport container (e.g., BactiSwab, Remel, Lenexa, KS; BBL CultureSwab, Becton-Dickinson, Franklin Lakes, NJ; Fisherfinest Transport Swabs, Fisher HealthCare, Houston, TX). These containers typically consist of a round-bottomed sleeve designed to protect the sample. Some transport systems contain medium designed to enhance survival of any microorganisms present. Amies medium is often used, but other types of media that enhance survival of more fastidious bacteria are also available. When using a transport container that uses media, ensure that the swab is completely immersed in the culture medium.
- Submit fluids (urine, effusion, aspirated material, wash solutions) in a sterile tube. Plain red-top tubes are acceptable, but the use of serum-separator tubes or plastic red-top tubes with clot activator should be avoided.
- Biopsy: Place the sample in a sterile container and add several drops of sterile saline to keep the tissue moist.
- Catheter tip: 5 cm of the distal tip is placed into a sterile container for transport.

Anaerobic Culture
- Tissue or aspirates of deep material are always superior to superficial swab specimens.
- If a swab must be used, pass it deep into the base of the lesion.
- Biopsy: Place the sample in sterile container and add several drops of sterile saline to keep the tissue moist.
- If sample processing will be delayed by >2 h, place the sample into a specific anaerobic transport tube or vial. Anaerobic transport medium is a mineral salt-base soft agar with reducing agents designed to maintain an anaerobic environment for an extended period, maintaining viability of the more fastidious microorganisms. Some systems include a color indicator that assures the efficacy of the system by continuously monitoring the environment and changing color if the medium has become oxygenated.
- Swabs of material are plunged deep into the agar so that even though material at the top of the tube is exposed to oxygen, material at the bottom of the tube remains anaerobic.
- Transport fluids in an anaerobic transport vial. After cleaning the rubber stopper with alcohol, push the needle through the septum and inject the fluid on top of the anaerobic transport medium.
- Samples in anaerobic transport medium can generally be used for both aerobic and anaerobic cultures.

Fecal Culture
Use fecal transport medium when submitting for detection of *Salmonella*, *Shigella*, *Campylobacter*, and other fecal pathogens.

Mycoplasma Culture
Semen or mucus from respiratory tract can be submitted in a sterile container. Material can also be collected on a sterile swab and submitted in a microorganism transport container that contains Aimes transport medium without charcoal, although this is not an optimal method.

Blood Culture
- Wash the venipuncture site with antiseptic, followed by a sterile-water rinse.
- Apply tincture of iodine or povidone-iodine with sterile gauze pads and allow to dry.
- While the iodine is drying, remove the plastic cap covering each of 2 blood culture bottles and decontaminate each rubber stopper with 70% alcohol.
- Wipe the venipuncture site with sterile cotton balls or gauze pads soaked in 70% alcohol, removing the iodine.

- Draw 4 mL of blood.
- Change the needle, inoculate 2 mL into each of the blood culture bottles, and mix well.

STORAGE
- To increase viability of organisms and prevent overgrowth, refrigerate samples for routine aerobic culture until shipped.
- Specimens for anaerobic culture, blood culture, and fecal culture should be maintained at room temperature.

STABILITY
Aerobes
Refrigerate for ≈2 days.

Anaerobes
- Stable in an anaerobic transport tube for 1–2 days (depending on the organism)
- Stable in a red-top tube or standard microorganism collection and transport system (e.g., BactiSwab, BBL CultureSwab, Fisherfinest Transport Swabs) for ≤2 h
- Refrigeration decreases viability.

PROTOCOL
None

 INTERPRETATION

NORMAL FINDINGS OR RANGE
- No growth of bacteria in culture
- Growth of normal flora only, but no pathogenic organisms

ABNORMAL VALUES
- Growth of pathogenic organisms
- Kirby-Bauer microbial-susceptibility results for antimicrobials are reported as either susceptible or resistant.
- Some antimicrobial-susceptibility results are reported with an MIC, which is the lowest concentration in micrograms per milliliter that inhibits the growth of a given strain of bacteria. When using MICs to select an appropriate antimicrobial, 3 criteria are important:
  1. The MIC on the clinical microbiology report
  2. The antimicrobial's normal range used to establish susceptibility. The range is tested as serially doubling dilutions in micrograms per milliliter.
  3. The breakpoint of the antimicrobial: The dilution where the bacteria begin to show resistance.
- The breakpoint and the normal range differ by drug and bacterial species. Therefore, comparing antimicrobial MICs is based on differences between the breakpoint and the normal range for each antimicrobial. The further the MIC is from the breakpoint in its normal range, the more susceptible that organism is to the antimicrobial.

CRITICAL VALUES
None

INTERFERING FACTORS
Drugs That May Alter Results or Interpretation
Drugs That Interfere with Test Methodology
None

Drugs That Alter Physiology
Antibiotics

Disorders That May Alter Results
None

Collection Techniques or Handling That May Alter Results
- Specimens that are 2 days old may lose viability.
- An inappropriate collection tube:
  - The EDTA is bacteriostatic.

- The clot activator in serum-separator tubes and plastic red-top tubes may affect results.
- Samples for anaerobic cultures have limited viability if not transported in specific anaerobic transport tubes.

Influence of Signalment
Species
None

Breed
None

Age
None

Gender
None

Pregnancy
None

LIMITATIONS OF THE TEST
- *Mycobacterium* sp. and *Nocardia* sp. are more difficult to culture because extended incubation periods, aerobic incubation, and special medium are necessary for their isolation. Cultures for these organisms should be specifically requested.
- It is important to bear in mind that MIC is just 1 of the criteria used to select an antimicrobial. Antimicrobial selection also depends on the location of infection, what dose and route of administration will achieve adequate concentrations at the site of infections, and how long the infection needs to be treated.

Sensitivity, Specificity, and Positive and Negative Predictive Values
None

Valid If Run in a Human Lab?
Yes.

CLINICAL PERSPECTIVE
- In cultures from a mucosal surface (e.g., tracheal wash, nasal swab, vaginal discharge, urine collected by catheter or free catch), interpretation must consider the presence of normal flora.
  - Large numbers of a single microorganism in almost pure culture suggests a pathogenic process.
  - A mixture of ≥4 different organisms in light to moderate numbers suggests growth of normal flora.
  - Light growth from a sample submitted in enrichment broth suggests normal flora (or suppression of growth by antimicrobial therapy).
- Specific anaerobic transport containers are more expensive than routine microorganism collection and transport containers (and may not be provided gratis by diagnostic laboratories), but can be readily obtained from commercial distributors of microbiology supplies and improve the likelihood of documenting an anaerobic infection.
- Chances of documenting bacteremia are increased by submitting 2 sets of blood cultures collected from different venipuncture sites or from the same site 15–30 min apart.

 MISCELLANEOUS

ANCILLARY TESTS
Dependent on the site of infection
- Urinalysis if signs of urinary tract infection; biochemistry profile and leptospirosis titers if signs suggest renal failure
- Fluid analysis
- Radiography of chest or abdomen to identify the site of infection
- Fecal float and/or direct fecal smear if diarrhea is present

BACTERIAL CULTURE AND SENSITIVITY

SYNONYMS
- Aerobic culture
- Anaerobic culture
- Blood culture

SEE ALSO
Blackwell's Five-Minute Veterinary Consult: Canine and Feline Topics
- Abscessation
- Actinomycosis
- Endocarditis, Infective
- Nocardiosis
- Pneumonia, Bacterial
- Prostatitis and Prostatic Abscess
- Pyelonephritis
- Pyothorax
- Salmonellosis
- Sepsis and Bacteremia

Related Topics in This Book
Dermatophyte Culture

ABBREVIATIONS
MIC = minimum inhibitory concentration

Suggested Reading
Aucoin D. *Target: The Antimicrobial Reference Guide to Effective Treatment*, 2nd ed. Port Huron, MI: North American Compendiums, 2002.
Jones RL. Laboratory diagnosis of bacterial infections. In: Greene CE, ed. *Infectious Diseases of the Dog and Cat*, 3rd ed. St Louis: Saunders Elsevier, 2006: 267–273.
Mena E, Thompson FS, Armfield AY, *et al.* Evaluation of Port-A-Cul transport system for protection of anaerobic bacteria. *J Clin Microbiol* 1978; 8:28–35.

INTERNET RESOURCES
Becton Dickinson (BD) Diagnostic Systems, Product Center, http://www.bd.com/ds/productCenter/CT-PortACul.asp. Examples of anaerobic transport tubes/vials.

AUTHOR NAMES
Terri Wheeler and Joyce S. Knoll

BASICS

TYPE OF PROCEDURE
Radiographic

PROCEDURE EXPLANATION AND RELATED PHYSIOLOGY
BIPS are small (1.5 and 5 mm in diameter), solid radiopaque markers that are pilled or fed to dogs and cats and followed via abdominal radiographs as they transit through the GI tract. The passage of small, compared to larger, BIPS and speed of transit can be assessed radiographically and used to evaluate patients for GI obstruction and motility disorders. However, it should be noted that the use of BIPS to predict the transit of a meal (especially GE time) accurately is controversial. For most clinicians, the likely greatest potential application of BIPS is as a convenient alternative to liquid barium for the diagnosis of physical GI obstructions.

INDICATIONS
• Diagnosis of physical GI obstructions in stable patients with the following:
  • Acute vomiting
  • Chronic vomiting, diarrhea, anorexia, and constipation (rule out gastric outflow obstruction, partial bowel obstruction, colonic stricture)
• Diagnosis of GI motility disorders (delayed GE, adynamic ileus, gastric and intestinal dumping syndromes, colonic dysmotility) in patients with the following:
  • Chronic or recurrent gastric dilation
  • Chronic vomiting or diarrhea
  • Chronic or recurrent constipation

CONTRAINDICATIONS
• Compelling evidence of a GI obstruction on survey abdominal radiographs
• Poor gag reflex or a patient too weak to swallow
• A situation in which rapid diagnosis and intervention are critical (e.g., signs of shock)

POTENTIAL COMPLICATIONS
• Aspiration of BIPS
• Intra-abdominal foreign material or peritonitis if BIPS are administered to patients with a GI perforation

CLIENT EDUCATION
• The patient will be fasted for 24h prior to the administration of BIPS with food (chronic GI complaints).
• The procedure may take longer than 12–24 h.

BODY SYSTEMS ASSESSED
Gastrointestinal

PROCEDURE

PATIENT PREPARATION
Preprocedure Medication or Preparation
Remove retained feces by enema if BIPS are to evaluate constipation.

Anesthesia or Sedation
• Avoid the use of anesthetics and sedatives, if possible, because many drugs alter GI motility.
• Diazepam (0.1 mg/kg IV) can be used in cats to aid consumption of BIPS mixed in food without substantially altering GI transit.
• Acepromazine (0.1 mg/kg SC) can be used in fractious cats, with the appropriate normal reference intervals (i.e., cats given acepromazine) used to interpret results.

Patient Positioning
As needed for abdominal radiographs

Patient Monitoring
Observe for emesis of BIPS, which may result in a nondiagnostic study.

Equipment or Supplies
• One large capsule or 4 small capsules of BIPS (Medical I.D. Systems, Grand Rapids, MI).
• Both capsule options contain a total of ten 5-mm and thirty 1.5-mm BIPS.
• The BIPS manual with the normal reference intervals (Medical I.D. Systems)
• Prescription Diet d/d, i/d, or r/d (Hill's Pet Nutrition, Topeka, KS) if the BIPS are to be administered with food. The normal reference intervals for GI transit of fed BIPS are based on these diets.
• A pill-administering device and fish or vegetable oil as a lubricant, as needed to facilitate pilling
• Radiographic film and equipment

TECHNIQUE
BIPS Administration
• The same number of BIPS (10 large and 30 small) should be administered to all patients regardless of size.
• BIPS should be administered with the patient on an empty stomach to evaluate acute GI complaints where the primary interest is to rule out a physical GI obstruction. Pill-administrating devices and lubrication of the capsules with fish or vegetable oil may facilitate pilling in very small patients.
• BIPS should be administered with canned Prescription Diet d/d or i/d (dogs only) to evaluate chronic GI complaints where partial obstruction and motility disorders are differentials.
• BIPS should be administered with Prescription Diet r/d to evaluate chronic or recurrent constipation, or to increase the sensitivity of diagnosing a partial bowel obstruction where suspected.
• When given with food, patients should be fasted for 24 h and then fed approximately one-quarter of their maintenance energy requirements with the BIPS dispersed throughout the food. In cats, the large BIPS can be left within the split half of the gelatin capsules and buried in the food to facilitate consumption.

Radiographic Technique and Timing
• At least 2 radiographic views of the abdomen (standard lateral and ventrodorsal views) should be obtained at all time points to determine the location of BIPS within the gut.
• If it is unclear whether the BIPS are in the colon, an air enema (20 mL/kg) can be administered via a Foley catheter and the radiographs repeated.
• If BIPS are administered on an empty stomach (acute GI complaints), the first set of radiographs should be obtained at 6–24 h. If the patient is stable, these radiographs are usually taken in the morning after administration. Additional radiographs may be needed if the BIPS have not reached the colon or if bunching of the BIPS is detected without other signs of obstruction (rule out transient bunching).
• If BIPS are administered with Prescription Diet d/d or i/d (chronic GI complaints), a common protocol is to radiograph at 2 h if gastric dumping is a differential, 8 h to detect delayed GE, and at least 4–6 h later (12–14 h after administration) or the next morning if large BIPS have not yet reached the colon (to detect partial bowel obstruction).
• If BIPS are administered with Prescription Diet r/d to evaluate constipation, radiographs should be obtained at 24, 48, and 72 h.

Calculation of GE and Orocolic Transit (OCT) Times
• Note the time the radiographs were made after administration of BIPS.
• Count the number of small BIPS within the stomach, small intestine, and large intestine. Do not include BIPS of uncertain location.

BARIUM-IMPREGNATED POLYETHYLENE SPHERES (BIPS)

- Determine the percentage of small BIPS that have left the stomach and entered the large intestine and compare these percentages to the normal reference intervals provided by the manufacturer.
- Repeat the calculations for the large BIPS.

Calculation of Colonic Transit (CT) Time

- Note the time the radiographs were made after administration of BIPS.
- Count the number of small BIPS within the proximal large intestine (ascending and transverse colon) and distal large intestine (descending colon). Do not include BIPS of uncertain location and exclude BIPS caudal to the brim of the pelvis.
- Determine the percentage of small BIPS in the proximal and distal colon and compare these percentages to the normal reference intervals provided by the manufacturer.
- Repeat the calculations for the large BIPS.

SAMPLE HANDLING
None

APPROPRIATE AFTERCARE
Postprocedure Patient Monitoring
None

Nursing Care
None

Dietary Modification
None

Medication Requirements
None

Restrictions on Activity
None

Anticipated Recovery Time
Immediate

 INTERPRETATION

NORMAL FINDINGS OR RANGE

- BIPS should not form a persistent bunching pattern (focal accumulation).
- Large BIPS should have similar GI transit (slightly slower) than small BIPS, and both sizes should reach the colon after an adequate period has passed. Note that gastric retention of large BIPS (with normal GE time) may be seen normally in cats and small dogs or if the BIPS were not adequately dispersed in the meal.
- Normal reference intervals for GE, OCT, and CT of BIPS are provided by the manufacturer.

ABNORMAL VALUES

- Persistent bunching of BIPS associated with delayed GI transit (except for bunching orad to impacted feces) suggests a physical GI obstruction.
- Failure of large BIPS to reach the colon after an adequate period has passed compared to small BIPS suggests a partial GI obstruction.
- Prolonged GE or OCT of BIPS indicates abnormal motility, a GI obstruction, or both.
- Overly rapid GE or OCT of BIPS suggests a gastric or intestinal dumping syndrome (rare).
- Prolonged CT of BIPS indicates abnormal colonic motility, colonic obstruction, or both.

CRITICAL VALUES

Persistent bunching of BIPS (especially if bunched in a dilated loop of small bowel) and failure to reach the colon is highly suggestive of a physical bowel obstruction requiring surgical intervention.

INTERFERING FACTORS

Drugs That May Alter Results of the Procedure

- Anticholinergic drugs and opioids profoundly slow GI transit.
- Drugs with prokinetic activity (e.g., metoclopramide, cisapride, ranitidine, erythromycin) may hasten GI transit.
- Anesthetic drugs and sedatives commonly alter GI motility.

Conditions That May Interfere with Performing the Procedure
Frequent vomiting may result in a nondiagnostic study.

Procedure Techniques or Handling That May Alter Results
Inadequate dispersal of BIPS within the test meal may result in gastric retention of large BIPS (GE time should remain normal).

Influence of Signalment on Performing and Interpreting the Procedure

Species
- Cats can be difficult to pill, more likely to refuse consumption of large BIPS, and retain large BIPS within the stomach normally.
- There are separate reference intervals for the normal GI transit of BIPS in dogs and cats.

Breed
Toy-breed dogs may be difficult to pill and may retain large BIPS within the stomach normally.

Age
Puppies have more rapid GE than adult dogs.

Gender
The effect on GI transit of BIPS in dogs and cats is unknown.

Pregnancy
Although pregnancy alters GI motility in many species, the effect on GI transit of BIPS in dogs and cats is unknown.

CLINICAL PERSPECTIVE

- If the GI transit of BIPS is found to be normal, it is unlikely that a GI obstruction or motility disorder exists. Thus, BIPS are a cheap, convenient, and noninvasive way of ruling out these differentials.
- If the radiographic pattern (see the list below) or speed of transit of BIPS is found to be abnormal, further diagnostic tests or exploratory surgery should be considered.
- Unfortunately, BIPS cannot always differentiate physical GI obstructions from abnormal motility. Delayed GE and OCT are common both in patients with acute nonobstructive GI complaints (e.g., gastroenteritis, pancreatitis, peritonitis) and in patients with physical obstructions, and may prevent BIPS from forming the classic bunching pattern proximal to an obstruction.
- Common radiographic patterns of BIPS and their clinical significance:
  - Delayed GE of small and large BIPS indicates a physical obstruction to gastric outflow or depressed gastric or gastroenteric motility. It is important to note that this finding is common in patients with acute nonobstructive GI complaints and can also be seen with physical obstructions of the small bowel.
  - Gastric retention of large, but not small, BIPS (with prolonged GE time) is highly suggestive of a physical gastric outflow tract obstruction.
  - Delayed OCT with small intestinal bunching of BIPS is highly suggestive of a physical small bowel obstruction. If there is no evidence of small intestinal dilation associated with the bunching, radiographs should be repeated in 1–2 h to rule out transient bunching (most common at the ileocolic valve).
  - Delayed OCT without bunching of BIPS is most suggestive of depressed GI motility. As with delayed GE, this finding is common in patients with acute nonobstructive GI complaints, but can also occur secondary to a physical GI obstruction. A physical

obstruction cannot be excluded until the large BIPS reach the colon. If the large BIPS fail to reach the colon after an adequate period has passed, further diagnostic imaging or exploratory surgery should be considered.

MISCELLANEOUS

ANCILLARY TESTS
Further diagnostic imaging of the GI tract via abdominal ultrasound, endoscopy, or scintigraphy should be considered when the results of a BIPS study are abnormal.

SYNONYMS
Radiopaque markers

SEE ALSO
Blackwell's Five-Minute Veterinary Consult: Canine and Feline Topics
- Constipation and Obstipation
- Diarrhea, Chronic—Cats
- Diarrhea, Chronic—Dogs
- Gastric Motility Disorders
- Gastrointestinal Obstruction
- Vomiting, Acute
- Vomiting, Chronic

Related Topics in This Book
- General Principles of Radiography
- Abdominal Radiography

ABBREVIATIONS
- BIPS = barium-impregnated polyethylene spheres
- CT = colonic transit
- GE = gastric emptying
- OCT = orocolic transit

Suggested Reading
Guilford WG. Gastric emptying of BIPS in normal dogs with simultaneous solid-phase gastric emptying of a test meal measured by nuclear scintigraphy [Letter]. *Vet Radiol Ultrasound* 2000; 41: 381–383.
Guilford WG, Strombeck DR. Intestinal obstruction, pseudo-obstruction, and foreign bodies. In: Guilford WG, Center SA, Strombeck DR, et al., eds. *Strombeck's Small Animal Gastroenterology*, 3rd ed. Philadelphia: WB Saunders, 1996: 487–502.
Lester NV, Roberts GD, Newell SM, *et al.* Assessment of barium impregnated polyethylene spheres (BIPS) as a measure of solid-phase gastric emptying in normal dogs: Comparison to scintigraphy. *Vet Radiol Ultrasound* 1999; 40: 465–471.
Robertson ID, Burbidge HM. Pros and cons of barium-impregnated polyethylene spheres in gastrointestinal disease. *Clin Radiol* 2000; 30: 449–465.

INTERNET RESOURCES
Med I.D. Systems: BIPS products, http://www.medid.com/ bips_products.html. Includes BIPS manual and normal reference intervals.

AUTHOR NAME
Sally Bissett

BARTONELLA

BASICS

TYPE OF SPECIMEN
Blood
Tissue

TEST EXPLANATION AND RELATED PHYSIOLOGY
Bartonellosis is caused by small, Gram-negative bacteria capable of causing a long-lasting intraerythrocytic bacteremia and infection of endothelial cells. These bacteria are most often transmitted by arthropods such as fleas, sand flies, lice, and ticks.

Several species are infectious in cats (*Bartonella henselae, B. koehlerae, B. clarridgeiae, B. bovis, B. quintana*). Fever, lethargy, transient anemia, lymphadenopathy, neurologic dysfunction, or reproductive failure has been reported following experimental infections with *B. henselae* and *B. clarridgeiae*. Naturally occurring disease associated with infection is more difficult to define because of a high prevalence of apparently asymptomatic infections. Stomatitis, urinary tract disease, and uveitis have been reported in association with natural infections in cats.

Bartonella vinsonii (berkhoffii) is considered the most frequent *Bartonella* species to cause disease in dogs, although infection with other *Bartonella* species can also apparently occur. *Bartonella vinsonii (berkhoffii)* has been reported to cause endocarditis, particularly involving the aortic valve. *Bartonella vinsonii (berkhoffii)* or closely related *Bartonella* species may also contribute to development of cutaneous vasculitis, anterior uveitis, polyarthritis, meningoencephalitis, and immune-mediated hemolytic anemia. Thrombocytopenia is found in approximately half of the dogs with disease manifestations.

Several test options are available, but optimal testing techniques vary between dogs and cats, and care must be used when deciding which test is optimal for each patient.
• IFA assays, ELISAs, and Western blots all detect IgG antibodies against *Bartonella* organisms. These tests can be used when screening a patient for exposure. Positive results are consistent with previous exposure to *Bartonella*. Tests for antibody do not confirm a current infection in the blood and, depending on the case, confirmation with additional tests may be required. Cross-reactivity with organisms, such as *Coxiella, Chlamydia pneumoniae*, and other *Bartonella* sp., and nonreactivity can cause confounding results.
• Conventional PCR and real-time PCR techniques that amplify *Bartonella* DNA from blood and tissue samples can be used to diagnose infection. False-negative results are possible particularly when low numbers of circulating organisms are present, hence a negative result does not definitively rule out the presence of *Bartonella* in a patient. Real-time PCR enables quantification of DNA. When PCR is used, mispriming and sample contamination may produce false-positive results.
• In dogs, culturing *Bartonella* by using routine microbiologic techniques is often unsuccessful, and detectable growth may take 1–2 months. A recently described liquid medium preparation (*Bartonella-Alphaproteobacteria* growth medium) appears to be more sensitive for detection of *Bartonella* in dogs and is available from at least one diagnostic laboratory (North Carolina State Vector Borne Disease Diagnostic Laboratory). In cats, isolation of *Bartonella* via culture on blood agar plates is considered the gold standard. Since cats are only intermittently bacteremic, multiple cultures may be required in order to confirm an infection.
• *Bartonella* organisms are rarely appreciated in blood films of bacteremic cats, even though the organism can be cultured from the blood of many healthy and sick cats.

INDICATIONS
Bartonella testing should be pursued when clinical signs are consistent with an underlying disorder associated with the organism. Unfortu-

nately, our understanding of *Bartonella* and its pathologic effects on dogs and cats is preliminary.

Dogs
• Endocarditis, myocarditis, or arrhythmias
• Hepatitis (especially peliosis hepatic or granulomatous and lymphocytic hepatitis)
• Granulomatous lymphadenitis
• Epistaxis
• Granulomatous rhinitis
• Polyarthritis
• Thrombocytopenia
• Anemia
• Leukocytosis and eosinophilia

Cats
The high prevalence of *Bartonella* infections makes clinical associations with diseases difficult to confirm. The following conditions have been reported in cats with *Bartonella*:
• Endocarditis
• Stomatitis (suspect association)
• Lymphadenopathy (suspect association)
• Uveitis

CONTRAINDICATIONS
None

POTENTIAL COMPLICATIONS
None

CLIENT EDUCATION
• Culture may take up to 2 months. Serologic tests may take up to 2 weeks.
• Many animals have antibodies against *Bartonella* spp., and the association between these antibodies and disease is uncertain.
• Domestic cats are a major reservoir for human infections, with transmission through contamination by cat scratches with flea excrement or by cat bites. Although infections are usually localized and self-limiting, immunocompromised individuals are at risk for systemic and sometimes fatal infections. Susceptible individuals should practice flea and tick control, and avoid interactions with cats that result in scratches or bites, but thoroughly wash such injuries if they occur.

BODY SYSTEMS ASSESSED
• Cardiovascular
• Dermatologic
• Gastrointestinal
• Hemic, lymphatic, and immune
• Hepatobiliary
• Ophthalmic

SAMPLE

COLLECTION
• 2 mL of venous blood
• Biopsy of tissue from the representative lesion
• PCR can be performed on formalin-fixed paraffin-embedded tissues but is suboptimal.
• Tissue for PCR may be obtained via fine-needle aspiration or biopsy.

HANDLING
IFA
Place 2 mL in a serum-separated tube (red top) and ship overnight on ice.

PCR
• Aseptically collect blood into a plastic EDTA tube (purple top) and freeze it immediately.

- Dilute the tissue in sterile saline and freeze it.
- Ship the sample overnight on ice.

Culture
- Aseptically collect samples.
- Collect blood or fluid into a plastic EDTA tube and ship it overnight on ice.
- Wrap the tissue sample in saline-soaked sterile gauze and place it on ice for overnight shipment.

STORAGE
- IFA or ELISA: refrigerator or freezer
- PCR: refrigerator or freezer
- Culture: refrigerator or freezer (refer to instructions from your specific diagnostic laboratory)

STABILITY
IFA
- Refrigerated (2°–8°C): stable for days
- Frozen (−20° to −80°C): stable months to years

PCR
- Refrigerated (2°–8°C): days to weeks
- Frozen (−20° to −80°C): months to years. If DNA can survive in a dinosaur fossil for millions of years, it can live in your fridge for a few weeks.

Culture
For optimal results, samples should be sent immediately.

PROTOCOL
None

INTERPRETATION

NORMAL FINDINGS OR RANGE
- Animals that have not been exposed to *Bartonella* should not have detectable antibodies against *Bartonella* antigens. Normal dogs and cats that have been exposed to *Bartonella* may or may not have elevated antibody titers.
- Uninfected animals should be PCR negative, although a negative PCR result does not rule out infection.
- Uninfected animals should be culture negative, although a negative culture result does not rule out infection.

ABNORMAL VALUES
- IFA titers of ≥1:64 are considered seroreactive.
- Western blot results of 3+ or 4+ are considered seroreactive.
- Positive PCR results are consistent with a current infection.
- Growth of *Bartonella* via culture techniques is consistent with a current infection.

CRITICAL VALUES
None

INTERFERING FACTORS
Drugs That May Alter Results or Interpretation
Drugs That Interfere with Test Methodology
None

Drugs That Alter Physiology
- The use of immunosuppressive drugs such as steroids may increase the ability to diagnose infection by PCR and culture.
- The use of antibiotics such as azithromycin and doxycycline may decrease the ability to diagnose infection by PCR and culture.

Disorders That May Alter Results
None

Collection Techniques or Handling That May Alter Results
PCR contamination may affect results.

Influence of Signalment
Species
See the Indications section.

Breed
None

Age
None

Gender
None

Pregnancy
None

LIMITATIONS OF THE TEST
- IFA is of limited use in cats, given the large number of chronically infected healthy cats.
- 5%–12% of infected cats may be seronegative.
- Cross-reactivity of serologic testing can lead to confounding results.

Sensitivity, Specificity, and Positive and Negative Predictive Values
- IFA and electroimmunoassay for serum IgG in cats
  - Positive predictive value: 39%–46%
  - Negative predictive value: 89%–97%
- Sensitivity, specificity, and predictive values for IFA in dogs have not been clearly established.
- The true sensitivity, specificity, and predictive values of PCR and culture are unknown.

Valid If Run in a Human Lab?
No.

CLINICAL PERSPECTIVE
- Our knowledge of the full disease spectrum caused by *Bartonella* spp. in domestic animals is in its infancy.
- Some evidence suggests that *Bartonella* sp. infection might induce chronic immunosuppression that could predispose animals to secondary infections, resulting in a wide array of clinical manifestations.
- In most cases, clinical diagnosis must be assessed in conjunction with response to treatment. If there is not an appropriate response to treatment, clinicians should consider coinfection with other vector-borne diseases or an alternative diagnosis.

MISCELLANEOUS

ANCILLARY TESTS
- Blood culture to rule out bacteremia caused by traditional organisms
- Serologic assays or PCR for vectorborne diseases such as anaplasmosis (*Anaplasma phagocytophilum*), ehrlichiosis (*Ehrlichia canis, E. ewingii, E. canis*), or Rocky Mountain spotted fever.

SYNONYMS
None

SEE ALSO
Blackwell's Five-Minute Veterinary Consult: Canine and Feline Topics
- Bartonellosis
- Ehrlichiosis
- Endocarditis, Infective
- Rocky Mountain Spotted Fever
- Stomatitis
- Ticks and Tick Control

Related Topics in This Book
- Bacterial Culture and Sensitivity
- Echocardiography

- *Ehrlichia/Anaplasma*
- Rocky Mountain Spotted Fever

ABBREVIATIONS
None

Suggested Reading

Boulouis H, Chang C, Henn J, *et al.* Factors associated with the rapid emergence of zoonotic *Bartonella* infections. *Vet Res* 2005; 36: 383–410.

Guptill L. Bartonellosis. *Vet Clin North Am Small Anim Pract* 2003; 33: 809–825.

Henn J, Liu C, Kasten R, *et al.* Seroprevalence of antibodies against *Bartonella* species and evaluation of risk factors and clinical signs associated with seropositivity in dogs. *Am J Vet Res* 2005; 66: 688–694.

INTERNET RESOURCES

Breitschwerdt EB. Canine bartonellosis: An emerging infectious disease, http://www.yourgo2girl.com/projects/ac2006/smallanimal/s13.pdf.

Brunt J, Guptill L, Kordick DL, et al. American Association of Feline Practitioners 2006 Panel report on diagnosis, treatment and prevention of *Bartonella* spp. infections, http://www.aafponline.org/resources/guidelines/Bartonella_Panel_Report_2006.pdf.

AUTHOR NAMES

Michael W. Wood and Adam Birkenheuer

BASICS

TYPE OF SPECIMEN
Urine

TEST EXPLANATION AND RELATED PHYSIOLOGY
Bence-Jones proteins are a component of immunoglobulin, specifically unassociated κ or λ light chains, which are produced in excess by B-cell–derived clonal cell populations. Multiple myeloma and, rarely, extramedullary plasma cell tumors and chronic B-cell lymphocytic leukemia can produce Bence-Jones proteinuria. Multiple myeloma is a clonal proliferation of malignant plasma cells, typically arising in the bone marrow, that produces an immunoglobulin or component of immunoglobulin. Because of their small size (MW = 22,000–44,000), Bence-Jones proteins can pass easily from the blood through the normal glomerular fenestrations of the kidney into the urine. Bence-Jones proteins were named after the English physician Henry Bence-Jones, who described their ability to precipitate when urine is heated to $45°–70°C$ and then redissolve when urine is further heated to near boiling. Today, more reliable tests for detection of Bence-Jones proteinuria include urine protein electrophoresis, immunoelectrophoresis, and immunofixation electrophoresis. These sophisticated techniques are required to identify Bence-Jones proteins because the proteins are not detectable via urine protein dipsticks.

INDICATIONS
Clinical suspicion of multiple myeloma

CONTRAINDICATIONS
None

POTENTIAL COMPLICATIONS
None

CLIENT EDUCATION
- A negative test result does not exclude a diagnosis of multiple myeloma.
- A positive test result requires additional confirmatory testing.

BODY SYSTEMS ASSESSED
Hemic, lymphatic, and immune

 SAMPLE

COLLECTION
- 10 mL of urine
- Cystocentesis is preferred, with clean free-catch and catheterized samples acceptable.
- Early morning urine collection is preferred.

HANDLING
Transfer to a sterile plastic, leak-proof container or red-top tube. Do not submit the urine in syringe.

STORAGE
Refrigerate or freeze prior to shipping. Ship on ice packs.

STABILITY
- Room temperature: $\approx$2h
- Refrigerated (2°–8°C): 1 week
- Frozen (−18°C): 1 month

PROTOCOL
None

 INTERPRETATION

NORMAL FINDINGS OR RANGE
Negative for monoclonal proteins on urine protein electrophoresis

ABNORMAL VALUES
- Suggested by a monoclonal spike in β-protein or γ-protein regions on urine protein electrophoresis
- Confirmed by immunoelectrophoresis for κ or λ light chains

CRITICAL VALUES
None

INTERFERING FACTORS
Drugs That May Alter Results or Interpretation
Drugs That Interfere with Test Methodology
None

BENCE-JONES PROTEINS

Drugs That Alter Physiology
None

Disorders That May Alter Results
- Hemoglobin from hemorrhage or hemolysis may interfere with analysis.
- β_2-Microglobulin may interfere with analysis.
- Bacterial overgrowth may interfere with results.
- Marked proteinuria may result in a false-positive result.

Collection Techniques or Handling That May Alter Results
- Specimen not refrigerated promptly
- Delay in specimen processing; bacterial contamination

Influence of Signalment

Species
None

Breed
None

Age
None

Gender
None

Pregnancy
None

LIMITATIONS OF THE TEST
The heat-precipitation test is insensitive and nonspecific for detecting Bence-Jones proteins.

Sensitivity, Specificity, and Positive and Negative Predictive Values
N/A

Valid If Run in a Human Lab?
No. Species-specific antisera are required in order to identify dog and cat light and heavy chains.

Causes of Abnormal Findings

Positive results	Negative results
Multiple myeloma	Intermittent secretion of light chain
Extramedullary plasmacytoma	Light-chain concentration below limit of detection of the assay
Other B-cell–derived neoplasms such as chronic lymphocytic leukemia	Nonsecretory type of multiple myeloma (rare)
Chronic lymphoplasmacytic inflammation (rare)	False negative
	Delay in sample processing
	Sample not refrigerated
	Bacterial contamination
False positive	
Marked proteinuria	
β_2-Microglobulin interference	
Hemoglobin interference	

CLINICAL PERSPECTIVE
- Of the 4 following criteria, 2 are generally required for diagnosis of multiple myeloma:
  - Radiographic evidence of osteolytic bone lesions
  - >20% plasma cells in bone marrow aspirates or biopsy specimens
  - Monoclonal or biclonal gammopathy with serum electrophoresis
  - Bence-Jones proteinuria
- Animals with lytic bone lesions can become hypercalcemic.
- Of dogs and cats with multiple myeloma, >50% may have light-chain proteinuria. Reasons for a negative result in a Bence-Jones

protein test include (1) an intermittent secretion or concentration too low to be detected in a single urine sample, (2) myeloma cells that may be secreting intact immunoglobulin molecules rather than free light chains, and (3) nonsecretory types of multiple myeloma (rare) that do not produce Bence-Jones proteinuria.

• A positive Bence-Jones protein test result on urine electrophoresis can be confirmed and further characterized by more sensitive and specific techniques, such as immunoelectrophoresis and immunofixation electrophoresis. Immunofixation electrophoresis distinguishes between κ and λ light chains and identifies the heavy chains of IgA, IgM, and IgG, but cannot distinguish between free light chains (Bence-Jones proteins) and those associated with the intact immunoglobulins.

MISCELLANEOUS

ANCILLARY TESTS
• Chemistry profile to evaluate for hyperglobulinemia and hypercalcemia
• Serum protein electrophoresis to evaluate for monoclonal or biclonal gammopathy
• Radiography to evaluate for osteolytic lesions
• Bone marrow cytology and/or biopsy to evaluate for plasmacytosis
• Serum and/or urine immunoelectrophoresis or immunofixation electrophoresis

SYNONYMS
• Free immunoglobulin light chains
• M proteins
• Myeloma proteins
• Paraproteins

SEE ALSO
Blackwell's Five-Minute Veterinary Consult: Canine and Feline Topics
• Hypercalcemia
• Multiple Myeloma
Related Topics in This Book
• Globulins
• Immunoglobulin Assays
• Protein Electrophoresis
• Skeletal Radiography

ABBREVIATIONS
None

Suggested Reading
Bienzle D. Hematopoietic neoplasia. In: Latimer KS, Mahaffey EA, Prasse KW, eds. *Duncan and Prasse's Veterinary Laboratory Medicine Clinical Pathology*, 4th ed. Ames: Iowa State Press, 2003: 89–90.
Thrall MA, Weiser G, Jain N. Laboratory evaluation of bone marrow. In: Thrall MA, Baker D, Campbell T, et al., eds. *Veterinary Hematology and Clinical Chemistry*. Philadelphia: Lippincott Williams & Wilkins, 2004: 172–174.

INTERNET RESOURCES
University of Georgia, College of Veterinary Medicine, Veterinary Clinical Pathology Clerkship Program: Maczuzak M, Latimer KS, Krimer PM, Bain PJ. Canine multiple myeloma, http://www.vet.uga.edu/VPP/clerk/Maczuzak/index.php.

AUTHOR NAME
Patty J. Ewing

BICARBONATE

BASICS

TYPE OF SPECIMEN
Blood

TEST EXPLANATION AND RELATED PHYSIOLOGY
Blood pH is tightly controlled, and the carbonic acid–bicarbonate buffering system is one of the most important mechanisms by which pH is maintained. The simplified equation that demonstrates the role of bicarbonate is as follows: $H^+ + HCO_3^- \leftrightarrow H_2CO_3 \leftrightarrow H_2O + CO_2$, where H^+ is the hydrogen ion concentration, HCO_3^- is bicarbonate, H_2CO_3 is carbonic acid, H_2O is water, and CO_2 is dissolved carbon dioxide. The components of this system function through the law of mass action, and this concept clarifies how HCO_3^- buffers hydrogen ions.

Measurement of HCO_3^- is used to assess the acid-base balance of patients and to differentiate underlying type(s) and severity of acid-base disorders. Most blood-gas analyzers actually calculate HCO_3^- concentration by using the Henderson-Hasselbach equation and measurements of pH and PCO_2, as follows: $pH = 6.10 + \log[HCO_3^-]/0.03(PCO_2)$. In the past, chemistry analyzers determined $[HCO_3^-]$ by adding a strong acid to a blood sample and measuring the total amount of carbon dioxide generated through a colorimetric reaction, but these techniques have largely been replaced by enzymatic methods. This total carbon dioxide (TCO_2) content is the sum of the HCO_3^- concentration, carbamino compounds, and the dissolved CO_2 in blood. Because the latter 2 substances are present in extremely low quantities, TCO_2 provides an indirect estimate of HCO_3^- anion, and these terms are often used interchangeably. It is important not to confuse the $PaCO_2$ with TCO_2, because $PaCO_2$ represents that part of the acid-base system under respiratory control, whereas TCO_2/HCO_3^- represents that part under metabolic control.

Generally, HCO_3^- is controlled by body metabolism (especially the kidneys), and carbon dioxide is controlled by respiration. Simplistically, for pH to balance, an increase in 1 component of the acid-base equation (CO_2 or HCO_3^-) must be offset by a decrease in the opposite component. HCO_3^- is the principal buffer system for the extracellular fluid.

In general, HCO_3^- is decreased with primary metabolic acidosis or compensated respiratory alkalosis (metabolic response to balance the alkalosis induced by hypocapnia). Primary metabolic acidosis can be caused by addition of endogenous or exogenous acid (e. g., ethylene glycol, lactic acidosis, ketoacidosis) or failure to excrete acids properly as a result of renal failure. Both situations result in consumption of HCO_3^- to neutralize the acids and balance pH. Metabolic acidosis can also be caused by loss of HCO_3^- into the GI tract (e. g., diarrhea) or urine (proximal renal tubular acidosis—rare).

In general, HCO_3^- is increased with primary metabolic alkalosis or compensated respiratory acidosis (metabolic response to balance the acidosis induced by hypercapnia). Primary metabolic alkalosis can be caused by loss of acid or addition of alkali (e. g., administration of sodium bicarbonate). Acid is lost most often because hydrochloric acid is lost by vomiting. Loop diuretics, thiazide diuretics, and hypokalemia can cause renal loss of H^+ leading to metabolic alkalosis. Hypokalemia can be the result of increased secretion of aldosterone by either an adrenal tumor or hyperplastic adrenal glands or the result of refeeding syndrome. Refeeding syndrome can develop in malnourished patients fed a high carbohydrate load, with a profound, rapid decrease in serum phosphate, magnesium, and potassium as these 3 electrolytes move into cells.

INDICATIONS
- Evaluate the acid-base status.
- Differentiate the different acid-base imbalances.
- Assess the severity of acid-base imbalances.

CONTRAINDICATIONS
None

POTENTIAL COMPLICATIONS
None

CLIENT EDUCATION
None

BODY SYSTEMS ASSESSED
- Endocrine and metabolic
- Gastrointestinal
- Renal and urologic
- Respiratory

SAMPLE

COLLECTION
- Collect 1 mL of venous blood (best if collected anaerobically to prevent loss of CO_2).
- Arterial blood may be indicated as part of assessment of the patient's global acid-base status.

HANDLING
- Samples can be collected into the following:
  - A plain red-top tube or serum-separator tube
  - Sodium heparin or lithium heparin anticoagulant (green-top tube) is acceptable.
- Citrate and EDTA anticoagulant are not recommended.
- Minimize dead space in the specimen container by filling the tube adequately.
- Avoid repeated opening and closing of tube because this exposes the sample to room air and promotes diffusion of CO_2 out of the sample.
- Separate serum or plasma from cells within 2–4 h. Carbonic anhydrase in RBCs accelerates conversion of HCO_3^- to CO_2 which is lost into the dead space.

STORAGE
Refrigerate for short-term storage, and freeze for long-term storage.

STABILITY
- Room temperature: 1 day
- Refrigerated (4°–8°C): up to 3 days
- Frozen (−18°C): 1 month

PROTOCOL
None

INTERPRETATION

NORMAL FINDINGS OR RANGE
Dogs [HCO₃⁻]
- Arterial, 18–26 mEq/L
- Venous, 20–24 mEq/L

Cats [HCO₃⁻]
- Arterial, 14–22 mEq/L
- Venous, 20–23 mEq/L

Note

- For HCO_3^-, 1 mEq/L = 1 mmol/L
- TCO_2 is normally 1–2 mEq/L higher than the calculated $[HCO_3^-]$.

ABNORMAL VALUES

Generally, values that are >10% above or below the normal ranges for each species should cause concern.

CRITICAL VALUES

A severe decrease in $[HCO_3^-]$ (<11–12 mEq/L) implies a severe metabolic acidosis.

INTERFERING FACTORS

Drugs That May Alter Results or Interpretation

Drugs That Interfere with Test Methodology
None

Drugs That Alter Physiology

- Acetazolamide and ammonium chloride induce a metabolic acidosis with a decrease in $[HCO_3^-]$.
- Furosemide, thiazide diuretics, and sodium bicarbonate administration induce a metabolic alkalosis with an increase in $[HCO_3^-]$.
- Nephrotoxic drugs (e. g., aminoglycosides, amphotericin B) may lower $[HCO_3^-]$, inducing a metabolic acidosis.

Disorders That May Alter Results

Prolonged venous stasis will decrease pH and increase $[HCO_3^-]$.

Collection Techniques or Handling That May Alter Results

- Use of EDTA, oxalate, or fluoride anticoagulants
- Underfilling the tube (heparin or red-top tube) will decrease pH and $[HCO_3^-]$. CO_2 will diffuse out of sample into the dead space, resulting in a HCO_3^- [i.e., TCO_2] reduction and increased calculated AGAP. These changes may be mistaken for a metabolic acidosis.
- Failure to properly cap the sample or repeatedly opening the tube can also lead to loss of CO_2 and an artifactual decrease in HCO_3^- [i.e., TCO_2].
- Prolonged contact with the clot can cause as much as a 5% decrease in $[HCO_3^-]$.

Influence of Signalment

Species
Cats tend to have a slightly lower $[HCO_3^-]$ than dogs.

Breed
None

Age
None

Gender
None

Pregnancy
None

LIMITATIONS OF THE TEST

- Many factors influence HCO_3^- concentration, which can result in a lack of sensitivity for any given disease state.
- Multiple causes of changes in HCO_3^- (increases or decreases) are possible, thus limiting specificity.
- Abnormal HCO_3^- concentration does not imply a primary metabolic abnormality, because the change in HCO_3^- concentration may be an expected secondary response to respiratory disorders or may represent the presence of mixed acid-base disorders.

Sensitivity, Specificity, and Positive and Negative Predictive Values

N/A

Valid If Run in a Human Lab?

Yes.

Causes of Abnormal Findings

High values	Low values
Primary Metabolic alkalosis	Metabolic acidosis
Vomiting	Lactic acidosis
Diuretic therapy	Uremic acidosis
Hyperadrenocorticism	Ketoacidosis
Primary hyperaldosteronism	Diarrhea
Administration of alkali (e. g.,	Ethylene glycol intoxication
sodium bicarbonate, antacids,	Renal tubular acidosis
phosphate binders, citrate,	Hypoadrenocorticism
gluconate, acetate)	Drug intoxications (e. g.,
Compensated respiratory	salicylates)
acidosis	Dilutional acidosis
Refeeding syndrome	Administration of ammonium
	chloride, carbonic anhydrase
	inhibitors, or amino acid
	parenteral nutrition supplements
	Compensated respiratory alkaloses

CLINICAL PERSPECTIVE

- Increased $[HCO_3^-]$ is usually caused by metabolic alkalosis, most commonly caused by vomiting or diuretic therapy, but is also expected as a normal compensatory response to respiratory acidosis.
- Decreased $[HCO_3^-]$ is usually caused by metabolic acidosis, most commonly caused by acute small-bowel diarrhea, dilutional acidosis, lactic acidosis, uremic acidosis, ketoacidosis, or ethylene glycol toxicity. Decreased $[HCO_3^-]$ is also expected as a normal compensatory response to respiratory alkalosis.
- Shock can decrease HCO_3^- (metabolic acidosis) through accumulation of lactic acid as a by-product of decreased tissue perfusion.
- A decreased $[HCO_3^-]$ associated with a normal AGAP suggests $[HCO_3^-]$ loss (e. g., diarrhea).
- A decreased $[HCO_3^-]$ associated with an increased AGAP suggests the presence of an unmeasured acid (e. g., ketones, uremic acids, lactic acid, ethylene glycol metabolites).

MISCELLANEOUS

ANCILLARY TESTS

- Arterial blood-gas analysis is useful in defining the presence and extent of a concurrent respiratory disorder or a mixed acid-base disorder.
- Specific tests based on suspected etiology (e. g., ethylene glycol, serum and urine glucose, serum and urine ketones)

SYNONYMS

- Bicarb
- Total CO_2 (TCO_2)

SEE ALSO

Blackwell's Five-Minute Veterinary Consult: Canine and Feline Topics

- Acidosis, Metabolic
- Lactic Acidosis

Related Topics in This Book

- Anion Gap
- Blood Gases
- Chloride
- Ethylene Glycol

- Lactate
- Urine Ketones

ABBREVIATIONS

- AGAP = anion gap
- H^+ = hydrogen ion
- HCO_3^- = bicarbonate
- H_2CO_3 = carbonic acid
- $PaCO_2$ = arterial partial pressure of carbon dioxide
- PCO_2 = carbon dioxide tension
- TCO_2 = total carbon dioxide

Suggested Reading

DeMorais HSA, DiBartola SP. Mixed acid-base disorders. Part I. Clinical approach. *Comp Contin Educ Pract Vet* 1993; 15: 1619–1626.

DiBartola SP. Metabolic acid-base disorders. In: Dibartola SP, ed. *Fluid Therapy in Small Animal Practice.* Philadelphia: WB Saunders, 2000: 211–226.

Richey MT, McGrath CJ, Portillo E, *et al.* Effect of sample handling on venous PCO_2, pH, bicarbonate, and base excess measured with a point-of-care analyzer. *J Vet Emerg Crit Care* 2004; 14: 253–258.

Rose BD, Post TW. Metabolic acidosis. In: Rose BD, Post TW, eds. Clinical Physiology of Acid-Base and Electrolyte Disorders, 5th ed. New York: McGraw-Hill, 2001: 583–592.

Willard MD, Tvedten H. Electrolyte and acid-base disorders. In: Willard MD, Tvedten H, eds. *Small Animal Clinical Diagnosis by Laboratory Methods,* 4th ed. Philadelphia: WB Saunders, 2004: 117–134.

INTERNET RESOURCES

Cornell University, College of Medicine, Animal Health Diagnostic Center: Bicarbonate and anion gap, http://diaglab.vet.cornell.edu/clinpath/modules/chem/bicarbag.htm.

AUTHOR NAME

Michael S. Lagutchik

BASICS

TYPE OF SPECIMEN
Blood
  Urine

TEST EXPLANATION AND RELATED PHYSIOLOGY
Bile acids (BAs) are synthesized in the liver from cholesterol and secreted into bile, with a pool of BAs being stored in the gallbladder. The BAs, which function in the digestive tract as biologic detergents to help break down lipids, are largely recycled via enterohepatic recirculation rather than excreted. They are absorbed from the intestine and returned to the liver via the portal circulation. They are efficiently resorbed from the portal circulation and resecreted into the bile, with only a small amount passing into the systemic circulation in normal animals. Thus, BA measurements assess biliary excretion, portal circulation, and hepatic function. Serum BA levels may be increased in animals with hepatic insufficiency, cholestatic disease, or portosystemic shunts. This test is typically performed on paired samples, the first collected after withholding food and the second postprandially. The first sample should represent a baseline value, whereas the postprandial sample is effectively a challenge to assess hepatic uptake of a bolus of BAs released by the gallbladder contraction stimulated by feeding.

Most diagnostic laboratories use an enzymatic assay that spectrophotometrically quantifies total serum 3α-hydroxylated BAs. The VetScan point-of care analyzer (A baxis, Union City, CA) also uses this type of methodology to quantify serum bile acids An in-office competitive immunoassay test (IDEXX Snap Bile Acid Test; IDEXX Laboratories, Westbrook, ME) has become available that shows strong agreement with the enzymatic assay within the working range of 5–30 μmol/L. Snap test results of >25 μmol/L may warrant further quantification with the enzymatic assay.

Only small amounts of conjugated or sulfated (water soluble) BAs are present in the urine of normal animals. As urine BAs accumulate over a long time interval, transient increases in serum BAs might be detected by this test that might be missed by a single fasting blood test. The testing of urine BAs may also be more convenient than serum BAs, because fasting and postprandial samples are not needed (in theory, the urine should reflect both preprandial and postprandial levels), and postprandial serum lipemia would not be a problem (as it often is with serum BA tests). Urine BA measurements are typically expressed as a ratio with urine creatinine to adjust for variations in urine concentration. Testing may detect urine nonsulfated BAs, urine sulfated BAs, or both.

INDICATIONS
- Assessment of hepatic function
- Detection of cholestatic disease
- Screening for portosystemic shunt

CONTRAINDICATIONS
None

POTENTIAL COMPLICATIONS
None

CLIENT EDUCATION
None

BODY SYSTEMS ASSESSED
- Cardiovascular
- Hepatobiliary

SAMPLE

COLLECTION
0.5–2.0 mL of venous blood
  At least 1 mL of urine

HANDLING
- The blood sample can be collected into plain red-top tube or serum-separator tube.
- Urine can be a voided sample or collected by catheterization or cystocentesis.

STORAGE
Refrigerate for short-term storage, and freeze for long-term storage.

STABILITY
Stable for >3 days in refrigerated serum.

PROTOCOL
- The baseline sample is collected after fasting (8–12 h).
- The postprandial sample is collected 2 h after feeding:
  - Feed a maintenance diet (avoid low-fat, low-protein foods).
  - Feed at least 2 teaspoons of food to animals weighing <5 kg.
  - Feed about one-quarter can to larger animals.
  - Avoid overfeeding, because lipemia can compromise results.
  - Visually confirm meal consumption.

INTERPRETATION

NORMAL FINDINGS OR RANGE
Reference intervals may vary, depending on laboratory and assay.

Serum
- Dogs: 0–8 μmol/L, fasting; 0–30 μmol/L, 2 h postprandial
- Cats: 0–5 μmol/L, fasting; 0–15 μmol/L, 2 h postprandial

Urine
- Dogs: <7.3 μmol/mg creatinine (UNSBA + USBA)
- Cats: <4.4 μmol/mg creatinine (UNSBA + USBA)

ABNORMAL VALUES
Values above the reference interval

CRITICAL VALUES
None

INTERFERING FACTORS
Drugs That May Alter Results or Interpretation
Drugs That Interfere with Test Methodology
Treatment with ursodiol (a synthetic BA) will increase serum BA measurements.

Drugs That Alter Physiology
Cholestyramine binds BAs and prevents their resorption, decreasing blood levels.

Disorders That May Alter Results
- Gallbladder contraction can be unpredictable. Spontaneous gallbladder contraction (without feeding) may increase the fasting BA level. Alternately, incomplete contraction after feeding may result in a lower value than expected.
- Lipemia is a common problem with postprandial samples. Lipemia may increase BA measurement (spectrophotometry).
- Ileal disease (or resection) or other malabsorption disorders may decrease BA levels (decreased absorption).
- Small-bowel bacterial overgrowth can alter bacterial processing of BA, decreasing ileal absorption.

Collection Techniques or Handling That May Alter Results
- Hemolysis may decrease BA measurement.
- Heparin may decrease BA measurement.
- If lipid-clearing agents are employed to eliminate lipemia, these may decrease measured BAs.

Influence of Signalment
Species
None

BILE ACIDS

Breed
- Terrier breeds, including Yorkshire terriers, shih tzus, Maltese, bichon frises, Tibetan spaniels, and Havanese, are prone to microvascular dysplasia, which can increase serum BAs.
- Maltese dogs often have elevated postprandial serum BAs in the absence of hepatobiliary disease. An ammonia-tolerance test may be warranted to rule out microvascular dysplasia.

Age
None

Gender
None

Pregnancy
None

LIMITATIONS OF THE TEST
- Not all patients with liver disease have elevated BA.
- The level of BA elevation is not diagnostic for the type of liver disease or the prognosis.
- Postprandial BA levels are generally more sensitive than fasting BA for detection of hepatobiliary disease.

Sensitivity, Specificity, and Positive and Negative Predictive Values
Dogs: Serum BA
- Postprandial BA, >15 μmol/L
  - Sensitivity, 82%; specificity, 89%
- Fasting BA, >20 μmol/L
  - Sensitivity, 59%; specificity, 100%
- Postprandial BA, >25 μmol/L
  - Sensitivity, 74%; specificity, 100%

Cats: Serum BA
- Fasting BA, >15 μmol/L
  - Sensitivity, 54%; specificity, 96%
- Postprandial BA, >20 μmol/L
  - Sensitivity, 100%; specificity, 80%

Dogs: UNSBA + USBA/Creatinine
- Specificity, 100%; sensitivity, 61%
- Positive predictive value, 100%; negative predictive value, 18%

Cats: UNSBA + USBA/Creatinine
- Specificity, 88%; sensitivity, 85%
- Positive predictive value, 96%

Valid If Run in a Human Lab?
Yes—if the assay has been validated in animals. Not all methods provide accurate results. A valid radioimmunoassay is available, but these values cannot be compared to those obtained using an enzymatic assay.

Causes of Abnormal Findings

High values	Low values
Inflammation (hepatitis and/or cholangiohepatitis) Toxin and/or drug reactions Hepatic or biliary neoplasia Corticosteroid hepatopathy Hepatic lipidosis Pancreatitis Gallstones Cirrhosis Portosystemic shunt Hepatic microvascular dysplasia	No clinical significance

CLINICAL PERSPECTIVE
- The BA test is warranted in animals with a suspected vascular anomaly such as a portosystemic shunt, or as a test of liver function in an animal with equivocal enzyme elevations (e. g., slightly increased ALT). As a general rule, hepatic dysfunction and/or vascular anomaly is likely when resting or post-prandial bile acids are greater than 25 μmol/L (dog) and 20 μmol/L (cat).
- The BA test can be helpful in assessing liver function in animals treated with drugs that induce liver enzymes (e. g., glucocorticoids, phenobarbital), because the BA level is usually normal unless there is actual liver damage.
- The BA test is not warranted in animals with obvious liver disease (e. g., icteric but not anemic, large liver mass, markedly elevated ALT).
- Increased BA levels caused by cholestatic disease are typically associated with elevated ALP and/or GGT levels.
- Portosystemic shunts may cause marked BA elevations (particularly postprandial) with normal or mildly increased hepatic enzyme (ALT, AST, ALP) levels. The fasting BA level may be normal in animals with shunts unless significant hepatic atrophy has occurred.
- Because BAs are recirculated, little hepatic function is required in order to maintain BA levels. Therefore, decreased BA values are not observed in even profound hepatic insufficiency.
- Intestinal malabsorption, delayed gastric emptying, and changes in intestinal motility may cause the fasting BA level to be higher than the postprandial level.
- Patients with portosystemic shunts tend to have lower urine bile acids: creatinine ratios than patients with hepatocellular disease.
- The presence of ammonium biurate crystalluria suggests hyperammonemia and may warrant determination of BA levels to look for evidence of a portosystemic vascular anomaly.

MISCELLANEOUS
ANCILLARY TESTS
- ALT and/or AST to evaluate hepatocellular injury
- ALP and/or GGT to test for increased values that occur with cholestatic disease
- A test of ammonia level to evaluate hepatic function and portal circulation, which should be normal in cholestatic disease unless shunting and/or decreased hepatic function are also present
- Albumin and BUN levels may be decreased with loss of hepatic function (as in hepatic atrophy).

SYNONYMS
- BAs
- Bile salts
- Urine bile acids (UBAs)

SEE ALSO
Blackwell's Five-Minute Veterinary Consult: Canine and Feline Topics
- Hepatic Encephalopathy
- Hepatic Failure, acute
- Hepatic Lipidosis
- Hepatitus, chronic active
- Hepatitis, granulomatous
- Hepatitis, infectious canine
- Hepatitis, suppurative and hepatic abscess
- Hepatoportal Microvascular Dysplasia
- Hepatotoxins
- Portosystemic Shunting, Acquired
- Portosystemic Vascular Anomaly, Congenital

Related Topics in This Book
- Alanine Aminotransferase
- Alkaline Phosphatase
- Ammonia
- Aspartate Aminotransferase
- Gamma-Glutamyltransferase
- Liver and Gallbladder Ultrasonography
- Liver Biopsy

ABBREVIATIONS
- ALP = alkaline phosphatase
- BA = bile acid
- UNSBA = urine nonsulfated bile acids
- USBA = urine sulfated bile acids

Suggested Reading

Bain PJ. Liver. In: Latimer KS, ed. Duncan and Prasse's Veterinary *Laboratory Medicine: Clinical Pathology*, 4th ed. Ames: Iowa State Press, 2003: 193–214.

Balkman CE, Center SA, Randolph JF, *et al.* Evaluation of urine sulfated and nonsulfated bile acids as a diagnostic test for liver disease in dogs. *J Am Vet Med Assoc* 2003; 222: 1368–1375.

Center SA. Diagnostic procedures for evaluation of hepatic disease. In: Guilford WG, Center SA, Strombeck DR, *et al.*, eds. *Strombeck's Small Animal Gastroenterology*. Philadelphia: WB Saunders, 1996: 130–188.

Trainor D, Center SA, Randolph F, *et al.* Urine sulfated and nonsulfated bile acids as a diagnostic test for liver disease in cats. *J Vet Intern Med* 2003; **17**: 145–153.

Willard MD, Twedt DC. Gastrointestinal, pancreatic, and hepatic disorders. In: Willard MD, Tvedten H, eds. *Small Animal Clinical Diagnosis by Laboratory Methods*, 4th ed. St Louis: Saunders Elsevier, 2004: 208–246.

INTERNET RESOURCES
Antech Diagnostics: Serum bile acids testing, http://www.antechdiagnostics.com/clients/antechNews/2003/may03_02.htm.

AUTHOR NAME
Perry J. Bain

BILIRUBIN

 BASICS

TYPE OF SPECIMEN
Blood

TEST EXPLANATION AND RELATED PHYSIOLOGY
Bilirubin is a yellow pigment produced as a breakdown product of hemoglobin. The heme portion of the hemoglobin molecule is excreted as bilirubin. A small amount of bilirubin is also produced from the degradation of cytochromes and myoglobin. Bilirubin is initially produced (chiefly in macrophages) in an unconjugated non-water-soluble form. This is transported to the liver (bound to albumin in blood), where it is conjugated (made water soluble) by glucuronidation and excreted into bile. Conjugated bilirubin (C-bili) is sometimes referred to as *direct reading* bilirubin, whereas unconjugated bilirubin (U-bili) may be referred to as *indirect reading* bilirubin. Biliprotein (sometimes called delta bilirubin) is C-bili that is covalently bound to serum albumin. This form of bilirubin is cleared more slowly from the circulation than non-protein-bound C-bili, with a half-life of ≈2 weeks. Total bilirubin is a combination of the conjugated, unconjugated, and biliprotein forms.

Conventional wet-chemistry spectrophotometric methods measure C-bili and total bilirubin and, from these, U-bili can be calculated. Some dry-chemical methods (Vitros; Ortho-Clinical Diagnostics, Raritan, NJ) can measure C-bili, U-bili, and total bilirubin. From these values, biliprotein can be calculated.

Bilirubin levels in blood may be increased by increased erythrocyte breakdown (prehepatic icterus), decreased hepatic uptake, conjugation or excretion (hepatic icterus), or extrahepatic cholestasis (posthepatic icterus).

INDICATIONS
- Suspected hepatobiliary disease
- Suspected hemolytic disease

CONTRAINDICATIONS
None

POTENTIAL COMPLICATIONS
None

CLIENT EDUCATION
None

BODY SYSTEMS ASSESSED
- Hemic, lymphatic, and immune
- Hepatobiliary

 SAMPLE

COLLECTION
0.5–2.0 mL of venous blood

HANDLING
Collect into plain red-top tube or serum-separator tube.

STORAGE
- Protect from light.
- Refrigerate for short-term storage.
- Freeze for long-term storage.

STABILITY
- Bilirubin levels can decrease up to 50% if exposed to direct sunlight.
- Refrigerated (2°–8°C): >1 week if protected from light
- Frozen (−20°C): ≈3 months

PROTOCOL
None

 INTERPRETATION

NORMAL FINDINGS OR RANGE
- Dogs: 0.1–0.3 mg/dL
- Cats: 0.1–0.3 mg/dL
- Reference intervals may vary, depending on laboratory and assay.

ABNORMAL VALUES
Values above the reference range

CRITICAL VALUES
None

INTERFERING FACTORS
Drugs That May Alter Results or Interpretation
Drugs That Interfere with Test Methodology
Propranolol administration may increase bilirubin measurements.

Drugs That Alter Physiology
None

Disorders That May Alter Results
- Hemolysis may artifactually increase values.
- Lipemia may artifactually increase values.

Collection Techniques or Handling That May Alter Results
- Avoid the use of hemolysed samples.
- Exposure to ultraviolet light (including sunlight) will decrease bilirubin levels.

Influence of Signalment
Species
None

Breed
None

Age
None

Gender
None

Pregnancy
None

LIMITATIONS OF THE TEST
- Bilirubinuria typically precedes hyperbilirubinemia.
- Bilirubin is a relatively insensitive test for cholestasis. Enzyme increases (ALP, GGT) are typically more sensitive indicators of cholestatic disease.

Sensitivity, Specificity, and Positive and Negative Predictive Values
N/A

Valid If Run in a Human Lab?
Yes.

Causes of Abnormal Findings

High values	Low values
Prehepatic	Not significant
Accelerated RBC destruction (hemolysis)	
Immune-mediated hemolytic anemia	
Acetaminophen	
Zinc toxicity	
RBC parasites	
Hypophosphatemia	
Transfusion reactions	
Microangiopathic anemia	
Internal hemorrhage	
Hepatic	
Hepatitis or cholangiohepatitis	
Toxin or drug reactions	
Hepatic neoplasia	
Corticosteroid hepatopathy	
Hepatic lipidosis	
Cirrhosis	
Chronic portosystemic shunt (with the hepatic atrophy)	
Copper storage disease	
Posthepatic	
Gallbladder disease	
Bile peritonitis	
Biliary neoplasia	
Cholecystitis	
Pancreatitis	

CLINICAL PERSPECTIVE
- Markedly elevated bilirubin levels may be visually detected in sclera, nonpigmented skin, mucous membranes, or plasma as icterus or jaundice.
- The proportion of unconjugated and conjugated bilirubin may not be a reliable indicator of the cause of the icterus, because many hemolytic or hepatic diseases present as mixed conjugated-unconjugated hyperbilirubinemia.
- Prehepatic icterus should be accompanied by evidence of hemolysis (e. g., anemia, spherocytosis, Heinz bodies) or internal hemorrhage.
- Hepatic or posthepatic icterus should have increased levels of hepatocellular enzymes (ALT, AST), cholestatic enzymes (ALP, GGT), and/or indicators of hepatic insufficiency such as increased bile acids or ammonia.

- The proportion of biliprotein (delta bilirubin) increases with prolonged cholestasis. This can prolong the increase in serum bilirubin even after the inciting condition has been resolved.

MISCELLANEOUS
ANCILLARY TESTS
- CBC for evidence of hemolytic disease (e. g., anemia, spherocytosis)
- Testing of ALT to evaluate hepatocellular injury
- Evaluation of ALP and/or GGT to look for cholestatic disease
- Evaluation of ammonia or bile acids
- Hepatobiliary ultrasonography

SYNONYMS
- Bili
- Total bilirubin

SEE ALSO
Blackwell's Five-Minute Veterinary Consult: Canine and Feline Topics
- Anemia, Immune-Mediated
- Bile Duct Obstruction
- Bile Peritonitis
- Gallbladder Mucocele
- Hepatic Lipidosis
- Hepatitus, chronic active
- Hepatitis, granulomatous
- Hepatitis, infectious canine

Related Topics in This Book
- Alkaline Phosphatase
- Bile Acids
- Gamma-Glutamyltransferase
- Liver Biopsy
- Liver and Gallbladder Ultrasonography

ABBREVIATIONS
- ALP = alkaline phosphatase
- C-bili = conjugated bilirubin
- U-bili = unconjugated bilirubin

Suggested Reading
Bain PJ. Liver. In: Latimer KS, ed. *Duncan and Prasse's Veterinary Laboratory Medicine: Clinical Pathology,* 4th ed. Ames: Iowa State Press, 2003: 193–214.
Center SA. Diagnostic procedures for evaluation of hepatic disease. In: Guilford WG, Center SA, Strombeck DR, *et al.*, eds. *Strombeck's Small Animal Gastroenterology.* Philadelphia: WB Saunders, 1996: 130–188.
Willard MD, Twedt DC. Gastrointestinal, pancreatic, and hepatic disorders. In: Willard MD, Tvedten H, eds. *Small Animal Clinical Diagnosis by Laboratory Methods,* 4th ed. St Louis: Saunders Elsevier, 2004: 208–246.

INTERNET RESOURCES
Long Beach Animal Hospital: Liver disease, http://www.lbah.com/liver.htm.

AUTHOR NAME
Perry J. Bain

BLADDER TUMOR ANALYTE

BASICS

TYPE OF SPECIMEN
Urine

TEST EXPLANATION AND RELATED PHYSIOLOGY
Bladder tumors contain proteolytic enzymes that can degrade the basement membrane into fragments consisting of type IV collagen, fibronectin, laminin, and proteoglycans. When released into the urine, these fragments form complexes. The V-TBA test (Polymedco, Redmond, WA) contains human IgG attached to latex particles that recognize these basement membrane complexes and cause an agglutination reaction when enough of the basement membrane complexes are present. A color change differentiates positive from negative results.

INDICATIONS
Used as a screening test in dogs suspected of having TCC

CONTRAINDICATIONS
• Urine with glucosuria, proteinuria, pyuria, and hematuria
• Allow ample time for recovery after bladder trauma (e. g., surgery, biopsy) before running the test.

POTENTIAL COMPLICATIONS
Collection of urine via cystocentesis may increase the risk of tumor seeding along the needle tract if the patient has a transitional cell carcinoma.

CLIENT EDUCATION
This test is best used to screen healthy animals or as an adjunct to other diagnostics when TCC is suspected.

BODY SYSTEMS ASSESSED
Renal and urologic

SAMPLE

COLLECTION
• A minimum of 0.5 μL of urine supernatant
• Urine can be collected by free catch, nontraumatic catheterization, cystocentesis, or with mass aspiration. Only a small number of samples collected by catheterization have been evaluated.
• Collect the urine into a dry urine cup, *not* into foam or paper cups.

HANDLING
• Centrifuge the urine and transfer the supernatant into a clean tube.
• It is recommended that the urine not be heated or frozen.

STORAGE
• The test is best performed within 2 days of sample collection.
• If the test cannot be performed immediately, the urine should be refrigerated (2°–8°C) but be at room temperature before testing.

STABILITY
• Reasonable stability for 1 week at 2°–8°C
• Reasonable stability for 2 weeks at −20°C

PROTOCOL
None

INTERPRETATION

NORMAL FINDINGS OR RANGE
Negative test result

ABNORMAL VALUES
Positive test result

CRITICAL VALUES
None

INTERFERING FACTORS
Drugs That May Alter Results or Interpretation
Drugs That Interfere with Test Methodology
The effects of drug administration (piroxicam, other palliative or experimental drugs) on this test are unknown.

Disorders That May Alter Results
False-positive reactions can be caused by the following:
• Hematuria (>30–49 RBCs per high-power field)
• Proteinuria (4+)
• Pyuria (>30–40 WBCs per high-power field)
• Significant glucosuria (4+)

Collection Techniques or Handling That May Alter Results
Although a study concluded that urine supernatant could be refrigerated for 1 week or frozen for 2 weeks, a small number of their samples had varying results after storage.

Influence of Signalment
Species
None

Breed
None

Age
None

Gender
None

Pregnancy
None

LIMITATIONS OF THE TEST
• Numerous false-positive reactions because of hematuria, significant proteinuria, or glucosuria.
• False-negative reactions have been reported in 2 dogs with prostatic neoplasia, 1 dog with an intramural infiltrative TCC, and 1 dog with both an extensively metastatic neuroendocrine neoplasia and a TCC.
• Test specificity is low when trying to differentiate bladder tumor from other forms of lower urinary tract disease.

Sensitivity, Specificity, and Positive and Negative Predictive Values
• Manufacturer's findings
  • Sensitivity, 90%
  • Specificity, 78%
  • Positive predictive value, 64%
  • Negative predictive value, 95%
• Other studies found specificity as low as 35% when trying to differentiate dogs with neoplasia from dogs with other lower urinary tract disease.

Valid If Run in a Human Lab?
Yes.

Causes of Abnormal Findings

High values	Low values
TCC	Not significant
Lower urinary tract disease	
Urinary tract infection (cystitis)	
Postcystotomy	
Urethritis, ureterocele, urethral caruncle	
Urethral sphincter mechanism incompetence	
Bladder rhabdomyosarcoma	
Urethral spindle cell tumor	
Renal disease	
Idiopathic renal hemorrhage	
Glomerulonephritis	
Non–urinary tract diseases	
Diabetes	
Hyperadrenocorticism	
Mammary septal panniculitis	
Dental disease	

CLINICAL PERSPECTIVE

- Useful as a screening test in healthy, aged patients to rule out the presence of a TCC
- Helpful in conjunction with other diagnostics to help confirm a TCC in dogs suspected of having a bladder tumor
- The test should be used only if the urine shows no evidence of hematuria, marked glucosuria, or marked proteinuria.
- Urine pH (5.0–8.5), specific gravity (1.006–1.053), oil droplets (1–4+), bacteriuria, bilirubinuria, crystalluria (4+ amorphous, 3+ struvite, 2+ bilirubin, and 4+ ammonium biurate), sperm (4+), epithelial cells (0–20/high-power field), and granular or hyaline casts (0–1/high-power field) were found *not* to effect the V-BTA test.

 MISCELLANEOUS

ANCILLARY TESTS

- Ultrasonography to visualize a bladder mass
- Urinalysis with cytology
- Cytology of a mass aspirate
- Contrast cystography
- Surgical excision with biopsy

SYNONYMS

- Bladder tumor antigen
- Veterinary bladder tumor antigen test (V-BTA)

SEE ALSO

Blackwell's Five-Minute Veterinary Consult: Canine and Feline Topics

Transitional Cell Carcinoma, Renal, Bladder, Urethra

Related Topics in This Book

- Cystourethrography
- Cystourethroscopy
- Lower Urinary Tract Ultrasonography
- Urinalysis Overview
- Urine Glucose
- Urine Protein
- Urine Sediment

ABBREVIATIONS

TCC = transitional cell carcinoma
V-BTA = veterinary bladder tumor antigen test

Suggested Reading

Billet JPH, Moore AH, Holt PE. Evaluation of a bladder tumor antigen test for the diagnosis of lower urinary tract malignancies in dogs. *Am J Vet Res* 2002; 62: 370–373.

Borjesson DL, Christopher MM, Ling GV. Detection of canine transitional cell carcinoma using a bladder tumor antigen urine dipstick test. *Vet Clin Pathol* 1999;28:33–38.

Henry CJ, Tyler JW, McEntee MC, *et al.* Evaluation of a bladder tumor antigen test as a screening test for transitional cell carcinoma of the lower urinary tract in dogs. *Am J Vet Res* 2003; 64: 1017–1020.

INTERNET RESOURCES

Polymedco: V-BTA test, http://www.vetbta. com.

AUTHOR NAME

Karen Zaks

BLEEDING TIME

 BASICS

TYPE OF PROCEDURE
Function test

PROCEDURE EXPLANATION AND RELATED PHYSIOLOGY
The ability of a patient to form a platelet plug in response to vascular injury is the first step in preventing uncontrolled bleeding and is termed *primary hemostasis*. For this process to occur, both platelet number and function must be adequate. In addition, von Willebrand factor (vWf) is necessary for platelet adhesion to injured vessels and subsequent formation of a platelet plug.

Bleeding time (BT) is a direct patient assessment of platelet function in dogs and cats. The most common and well-standardized form of BT is the buccal mucosal bleeding time (BMBT). It is a fast and easy screening test that can be performed in any clinic and requires minimal equipment. A prolonged BMBT is supportive of von Willebrand disease (vWD) or a primary platelet function defect (congenital or acquired). As vWD is the most common congenital hemostatic disorder in dogs, a BMBT should be part of a standard hemostatic workup.

INDICATIONS
- Presurgical screening for breeds predisposed to vWD
- Patients exhibiting unexplained epistaxis, GI bleeding, or petechiation or ecchymosis with a normal platelet number

CONTRAINDICATIONS
Severe thrombocytopenia

POTENTIAL COMPLICATIONS
Prolonged bleeding from the test site

CLIENT EDUCATION
None

BODY SYSTEMS ASSESSED
Hemic, lymphatic, and immune

 PROCEDURE

PATIENT PREPARATION
Preprocedure Medication or Preparation
None

Anesthesia or Sedation
- Usually unnecessary in dogs
- Sedation is usually necessary for cats (a ketamine and valium combination will not interfere with test results).

Patient Positioning
- Lateral or sternal recumbency
- Sitting or standing

Patient Monitoring
None

Equipment or Supplies
- 1- to 2-inch (25.4–30.8 mm) muzzle gauze
- A spring-loaded lancet [e. g., Surgicutt bleeding time device (International Technidyne, Edison, NJ); Simplate II bleeding time device (Organon Teknika, Durham, NC)] (Figure 1)
- 4 × 4-inch gauze or filter paper
- A timer or watch with a second hand

TECHNIQUE
- Place the patient in a comfortable, quiet position.
- Fold the patient's upper lip upward and secure it with muzzle gauze.
- Pressure from the gauze should cause a mild to moderate vascular congestion in the upper lip.
- Place the lancet tightly against a flat portion of the upper lip, rostral to the muzzle gauze.
- Remove the safety tab and depress the trigger to release the blade (Figure 2).
- A standardized incision will have been made (1 mm deep by 5 mm wide) in the lip.
- Start timing at the moment the incision is made.
- Place the filter paper or gauze ≈0.5 cm below the incision to blot the blood that drains from this incision (Figure 3).
- Care must be taken in the blotting process to avoid touching the wound and dislodging the forming platelet plug.
- Repeat the blotting procedure every 10 s until new drops of blood are no longer seen on the filter paper.
- Record the time elapsed.
- Note that the Simplate device will make 2 cuts of equal length and depth. If using this device, an average of the 2 times is recorded.

SAMPLE HANDLING
N/A

APPROPRIATE AFTERCARE
Postprocedure Patient Monitoring
Monitor for prolonged bleeding. However, excessive bleeding from test site is usually not severe enough to cause a significant drop in RBC parameters, even in an animal with a coagulopathy.

Nursing Care
None

Dietary Modification
None

Medication Requirements
Usually none. If prolonged bleeding occurs, an epinephrine-soaked gauze or ice pack can be applied to the site.

Restrictions on Activity
If the BT is prolonged, the animal should remain inactive for 15–30 min after bleeding has stopped.

Anticipated Recovery Time
Immediate

 INTERPRETATION

NORMAL FINDINGS OR RANGE
- Dogs: Bleeding should stop entirely by 4 min (some sources believe 3 min is a more appropriate upper number).
- Cats: Bleeding should stop by $2^{1}/_{2}$–3 min.

ABNORMAL VALUES
- BMBTs above the accepted normal range are noteworthy.
- Results should be verified and the test repeated if they are initially abnormal.
- Prolonged BTs warrant further investigation.
- Certain underlying conditions can prolong the BMBT. These include thrombocytopenia ($<90,000/\mu$L), vasculitis, uremia, and hyperglobulinemia.

CRITICAL VALUES
- A BMBT of 5–10 min is considered a mild to moderate abnormality.
- Values of >10 min are considered to be indicative of severe disease.

INTERFERING FACTORS
Drugs That May Alter Results of the Procedure
The administration of aspirin (and other drugs that inhibit platelet function) will decrease platelet function and cause a prolonged BMBT.

Conditions That May Interfere with Performing the Procedure
None

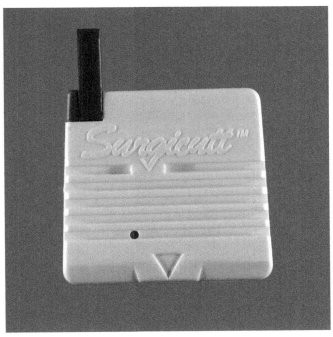

Figure 1

Surgicutt device for measuring BMBT.

Procedure Techniques or Handling That May Alter Results
- Gauze tied too tightly around the lip
- Use of a nonstandardized cutting instrument
- Blotting the incision itself instead of below the incision can dislodge the platelet plug and invalidate the results.

Influence of Signalment on Performing and Interpreting the Procedure
Species
- Slight variation between dogs and cats

Breed
- Numerous breeds of dogs are predisposed to vWD (common breeds include Doberman pinschers, Airedale terriers, golden retrievers,

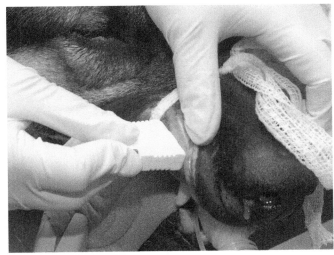

Figure 2

BMBT technique. Anesthesia is not required.

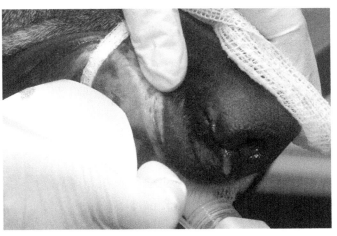

Figure 3

Use of filter paper to blot below the incision.

German shepherds, corgis, Shetland sheepdogs, German shorthaired pointers, Chesapeake Bay retrievers, Scottish terriers).
- Congenital platelet abnormalities are rare but exist in certain breeds of dogs and cats (otterhounds, bassett hounds, spitz, collies, Persian cats).
- The test result is valid in these cases, but further investigation is warranted.

Age
None

Gender
None

Pregnancy
None

CLINICAL PERSPECTIVE
- A complete CBC with a platelet count should be evaluated prior to the BMBT.
- A serum chemistry profile should also be assessed for uremia and evidence of other metabolic diseases.
- The results of tests of secondary hemostasis (coagulation panels) will be normal with primary platelet dysfunction and vWD (unless a predisposing infectious or metabolic disease is present).
- There have been reports of hypothyroidism exacerbating vWD, but this is not well documented.
- A careful history should be conducted to rule out the use of platelet-inhibiting drugs.
- References to a cuticle BT can also be found. This test is done by cutting 1 nail back short enough to cause bleeding and then monitoring the time it takes to stop bleeding. As this time is dependent on how far back the nail is cut and is difficult to standardize, this form of the test is not recommended.
- The most common reason to have a prolonged BMBT is vWD. As vWD can vary greatly in severity, it is important to pursue further testing to characterize this disease more fully.

 MISCELLANEOUS

ANCILLARY TESTS
- vWD analyses (factor levels, multimeric distribution, and DNA analysis are available)
- Platelet function analyses

- Ehrlichial disease testing
- Protein electrophoresis (if globulins are increased)

SYNONYMS
Buccal mucosal bleeding time

SEE ALSO
Blackwell's Five-Minute Veterinary Consult: Canine and Feline Topics
- Thrombocytopathies
- Von Willebrand Disease

Related Topics in this Book
- Anticoagulant Screen
- Coagulation Factors
- Partial Thromboplastin Time, Activated
- Platelet Count and Volume
- Platelet Function Tests
- Prothrombin Time
- Von Willebrand Factor

ABBREVIATIONS
- BMBT = buccal mucosal bleeding time
- BT = bleeding time
- vWD = von Willebrand disease
- vWf = von Willebrand factor

Suggested Reading
Boudreaux MK. Acquired platelet dysfunction. In: Feldman BF, Zinkl JG, Jain NC, eds. *Schalm's Veterinary Hematology*. Philadelphia: Lippincott Williams & Wilkins, 2000: 496–500.
Brooks M. Von Willebrand disease. In: Feldman BF, Zinkl JG, Jain NC, eds. *Schalm's Veterinary Hematology*. Philadelphia: Lippincott Williams & Wilkins, 2000:509–515.
Catalfamo JL, Dodds WJ. Hereditary and acquired thrombopathias. *Vet Clin North Am Small Anim Pract* 1988; 18: 185–193.
Couto CG. Disorders of Hemostasis. In: Nelson RW, Couto CG, eds. *Small Animal Internal Medicine*. St Louis: CV Mosby, 2003: 1185–1194.
Johnson GS, Turrentine MA, Kraus KH. Canine von Willebrand's disease: A heterogenous group of bleeding disorders. *Vet Clin North Am Small Anim Pract* 1988; 18: 195–229.

INTERNET RESOURCES
Cornell University, College of Veterinary Medicine: Hemostasis, http://www.diaglab.vet.cornell.edu/clinpath/modules/coags/coag.htm.

AUTHOR NAME
Karyn Harrell

BASICS

TYPE OF SPECIMEN
Blood

TEST EXPLANATION AND RELATED PHYSIOLOGY
Blood gases are used to evaluate the acid-base status of patients. Additionally, arterial samples may be used to evaluate the adequacy of oxygenation and ventilation. Venous blood samples are not adequate for evaluation of oxygenation.

Normal physiologic reactions within the body are designed to occur at a set pH value. For example, abnormally low vascular tone, as well as the development of a coagulopathy, may accompany acidosis. The major variables evaluated when assessing the acid-base status include the pH, HCO_3^-, PCO_2, and base excess (or deficit). Abnormalities within acid-base status are typically classified as acidosis, alkalosis, or mixed disorders. Each disorder may be caused by metabolic and/or respiratory abnormalities. The term *metabolic* implies a net gain or loss of HCO_3^-, whereas the term *respiratory* implies a net gain or loss of CO_2. The PCO_2 level and pH are inversely proportional, whereas there is a direct relationship between HCO_3^- level and pH.

When interpreting acid-base balance, evaluate pH first: Determine whether it is too high (alkalosis), too low (acidosis), or normal. Alkalosis is classified as metabolic if due to elevated HCO_3^- (>24 mmol/L) and respiratory if associated with a decreased PCO_2 (<36 mmHg). Acidosis is classified as metabolic if associated with a decreased HCO_3^- (<20 mmol/L), and respiratory if associated with an increased PCO_2 (>40 mmHg). With mixed acid-base disorders, 2 problems may either exacerbate the disorder (e. g., concurrent respiratory and metabolic acidosis) or mask the problem, producing a normal pH if the 2 disorders have opposite effects (e. g., concurrent metabolic acidosis and respiratory alkalosis).

Generally, development of an acid-base disturbance is accompanied by compensation by either the respiratory system or the renal system. This compensation attempts to return the pH to an overall normal range, but it is important to note that compensation is never completely successful. Some refer to compensation as either *secondary* or *adaptive*. Respiratory compensatory efforts will occur immediately, whereas metabolic compensation will not reach its full level for 2–3 days because maximum efficiency in renal handling of HCO_3^- requires time. In severe metabolic alkalosis, respiratory compensatory attempts will be limited by the hypoxemia that accompanies hypoventilation.

Hypoxemia is defined as a PaO_2 of <90 mmHg. Hypoxemia has 5 potential underlying pathologies: (1) low inspired-oxygen concentration, (2) ventilation-perfusion mismatch, (3) pure shunt, (4) diffusion impairment, and (5) hypoventilation. Hypoventilation will have a high PCO_2 value (>50 mmHg). Low inspired oxygen may occur at altitude or with anesthetic machine malfunction. Pure shunt includes cardiac defects (e. g., tetralogy of Fallot). Diffusion impairment includes diseases that thicken the alveolar-capillary membrane. Ventilation-perfusion (V/Q) mismatch reflects an altered balance between ventilated and perfused lung regions.

When assessing the oxygenation status of patients, it is prudent to consider not only the actual PaO_2 value but also to calculate the alveolar-arterial (A-a) gradient. The normal range is <15. The A-a gradient is calculated by subtracting the measured PaO_2 from the calculated ideal PAO_2 by using this formula: PAO_2 = [% inspired O_2 × (atmospheric − water-vapor pressure)] − ($PaCO_2$/0.8). For example, in room air at sea level, in normal dogs with a PaO_2 of 95 mmHg and a PCO_2 of 40 mmHg, the PAO_2 = [0.21(760 − 47)] − (40/0.8) = 150 − 50 = 100. The measured PaO_2 of 95 mmHg is subtracted from this value to get an A-a gradient of 5.

This formula is particularly useful if a patient is markedly hyperventilating or hypoventilating. For example, a dog with a PaO_2 of 84 and a PCO_2 of 22 is hyperventilating. However, calculation of the A-a gradient gives a value of 38.5, which is markedly elevated, suggesting that increased respiratory rate is compensating for primary lung disease. Conversely, in a dog with PaO_2 of 65 and a PCO_2 of 59, the A-a gradient is 11.25, which is normal, which indicates that hypoventilation, and subsequent hypoxemia, is caused by some disorder other than primary lung disease.

At increasing inspired-oxygen concentrations, the A-a gradient becomes more cumbersome and less accurate. Thus, if the concentration of inspired oxygen is directly known, the PaO_2/FiO_2 ratio may be calculated instead. The normal value for the PaO_2/FiO_2 is 100:0.21 or 476. In people and dogs, acute lung injury is said to exist at a ratio of <300 and acute respiratory distress syndrome at a ratio of <200.

INDICATIONS
- Assessment of acid-base balance
- Assessment of oxygenation (arterial samples only)

CONTRAINDICATIONS
- Avoid arterial collection when patients have severe coagulopathy.
- Avoid arterial collection when patients have cellulitis or open infection at the collection site.

POTENTIAL COMPLICATIONS
- Hematoma at the sampling site
- Collection of a venous sample instead of intended arterial sample and subsequent inappropriate patient-management decisions.

CLIENT EDUCATION
None

BODY SYSTEMS ASSESSED
- Cardiovascular
- Endocrine and metabolic
- Renal and urologic
- Respiratory

SAMPLE

COLLECTION
- Venous or arterial blood
- Typically, heparinized blood samples are analyzed. Self-filling syringes are commercially available and routinely used for arterial samples.

HANDLING
- Samples should be collected under anaerobic conditions for the most accurate PCO_2 and HCO_3^- values.
- Samples should be processed immediately to prevent altered values.
- Arterial samples exposed to room air will have an increased PaO_2 and decreased PCO_2.

STORAGE
If immediate analysis is not possible, samples may be stored on ice for 4–6 h.

STABILITY
For 4–6 h if kept on ice

PROTOCOL
None

BLOOD GASES

 INTERPRETATION

NORMAL FINDINGS OR RANGE
- pH, 7.36–7.44
- PCO_2, 36–40 mmHg
- HCO_3^-, 20–24 mEq/L (or mmol/L)
- Base excess, +/−4
- PO_2, 90–100 mmHg (at sea level)
- Reference intervals may vary, depending on sea level, laboratory, and assay.

ABNORMAL VALUES
Values above or below the reference range

CRITICAL VALUES
- pH, <7.2 or >7.5
- PCO_2, <20 or >55 mmHg
- PO_2, <60 (arterial sample)
- HCO_3^-, <13 or >33 mmol/L
- Base excess (or deficit), >12

INTERFERING FACTORS
Drugs That May Alter Results or Interpretation
Drugs That Interfere with Test Methodology
None

Drugs That Alter Physiology
Supplemental oxygen; bicarbonate infusions
Disorders That May Alter Results
None

Collection Techniques or Handling That May Alter Results
- Difficulty in arterial puncture may result in either a fully or partially deoxygenated (venous) sample.
- Prolonged storage at room temperature will affect results.
- Administration of excessive heparin will dilute the sample and may result in altered values.

Influence of Signalment
Species
Arterial blood-gas collection is very challenging in cats. Cats have a lower PCO_2 than other species.

Breed
Brachycephalic dogs may have a lower PaO_2, but this may reflect the relative difficulty restraining them for sampling.

Age
Whereas, in people, decreased PaO_2 accompanies aging, this has not been found to be true in dogs.

Gender
None

Pregnancy
Advanced pregnancy in humans may cause an altered respiratory pattern that produces respiratory alkalosis with a compensatory metabolic acidosis. PaO_2 is unchanged. This effect might be observed in late pregnancy in companion animals.

LIMITATIONS OF THE TEST
Sensitivity, Specificity, and Positive and Negative Predictive Values
N/A

Valid If Run in a Human Lab?
Yes.

Causes of Abnormal findings

Analyte	High values	Low values
HCO_3^-	Metabolic alkalosis High GI obstruction Profound hypokalemia	Metabolic acidosis Poor perfusion (lactic acidosis) Renal failure Diabetic ketoacidosis Ethylene glycol intoxication
PCO_2	Compensation for respiratory acidosis Respiratory acidosis Severe respiratory failure Cervical lesion Excessive analgesics Large dog placed in lateral recumbency Compensation for metabolic alkalosis	Compensation for respiratory alkalosis Respiratory alkalosis Panting Fever Pain Compensation for metabolic acidosis
PO_2	Not significant	Hypoxemia Pulmonary disease Edema Contusions Pneumonia Pleural space disease Pneumothorax Pleural effusion Diaphragmatic hernia Cardiovascular shunts (e. g., tetralogy of Fallot) Hypoventilation Pain Respiratory depressants Intracranial disease Cervical disease

CLINICAL PERSPECTIVE
- Determine whether appropriate compensation is occurring or if 2 disorders are present. Guidelines for compensation are the following:
  - Metabolic acidosis: Each 1-mEq/L decrease in HCO_3 will decrease PCO_2 by 0.7 mmHg.
  - Metabolic alkalosis: Each 1-mEq/L increase in HCO_3 will increase PCO_2 by 0.7 mmHg.
  - Respiratory acidosis
    - Acute: Each 1-mmHg increase in PCO_2 will increase HCO_3 by 0.15 mEq/L.
    - Chronic: Each 1-mmHg increase in PCO_2 will increase HCO_3 by 0.35 mEq/L.
  - Respiratory alkalosis
    - Acute: Each-1 mmHg decrease in PCO_2 will decrease HCO_3 by 0.25 mEq/L.
    - Chronic: Each 1-mmHg decrease in PCO_2 will decrease HCO_3 by 0.55 mEq/L.
- Severe acidosis is common with ethylene glycol intoxication.
- All assessments of oxygenation should include assessment of the CO_2 (PCO_2) and, if warranted, calculation of the A-a gradient.
- It is crucial to recognize that an arterial blood gas merely provides objective evidence as to degree of impairment, but it is not specific for the cause. For example, a dog with severe pulmonary contusions

and a dog with severe pulmonary edema may have indistinguishable blood-gas values.

MISCELLANEOUS

ANCILLARY TESTS
- Chemistry profile and urinalysis
- Ethylene glycol test
- Thoracic radiographs to look for cardiopulmonary disease

SYNONYMS
- Oxygen (O_2) saturation
- Partial pressure of carbon dioxide in blood (PCO_2)
- Partial pressure of oxygen in blood (PO_2)
- pH

SEE ALSO
Blackwell's Five-Minute Veterinary Consult: Canine and Feline Topics
- Acidosis, Metabolic
- Alkalosis, Metabolic
- Diabetes Mellitus with Ketoacidosis
- Ethylene Glycol Poisoning
- Hypoxemia

Related Topics in This Book
- Anion Gap
- Bicarbonate

- Lactate
- Thoracic Radiography

ABBREVIATIONS
- A-a gradient = alveolar-arterial gradient
- FiO_2 = fraction of inspired oxygen
- HCO_3^- = bicarbonate
- $PaCO_2$ = arterial partial pressure of carbon dioxide
- PaO_2 = arterial partial pressure of oxygen
- PAO_2 = alveolar partial pressure of oxygen

Suggested Reading
King LG, Anderson JG, Rhodes WH, Hendricks JC. Arterial blood gas tensions in healthy aged dogs. *Am J Vet Res* 1992; 53: 1744–1748.
Proulx J. Respiratory monitoring: Arterial blood gas analysis, pulse oximetry, and end-tidal carbon dioxide analysis. *Clin Tech Small Anim Pract* 1999; 14: 227–230.

INTERNET RESOURCES
Charlie's Clinical Calculators, MedCalc: acid-base calculator, http://www.medcalc. com/acidbase.html.
Colorado State University, College of Veterinary Medicine & Biomedical Sciences, Veterinary Emergency and Critical Care Medicine: Acid/base, blood gas interpretation [at high altitude], http://www.cvmbs.colostate.edu/clinsci/wing/fluids/bloodgas.htm.

AUTHOR NAME
Elizabeth Rozanski

BLOOD PRESSURE DETERMINATION: NONINVASIVE AND INVASIVE

BASICS

TYPE OF PROCEDURE
Blood Pressure measurement

PROCEDURE EXPLANATION AND RELATED PHYSIOLOGY
Blood pressure (BP) is determined by cardiac output and systemic vascular resistance. Maintaining BP is absolutely vital to maintaining organ perfusion and thereby organ function. Given the central role that BP plays, it is an important parameter to monitor.

Both elevated and decreased BP can be seen in small animal patients. Hypertension most commonly occurs secondary to concurrent diseases. Diseases that have been associated with increased BP include renal disease, hyperthyroidism, hyperadrenocorticism, hyperaldosteronism, diabetes mellitus, obesity, and pheochromocytoma. In people, essential (idiopathic) hypertension is the most common form of hypertension. Though rare in small animals, it does appear that older cats can be hypertensive without a disease being present known to elevate BP. Hypotension can occur with any disease that causes shock (e. g., anaphylaxis, trauma, hemorrhage, sepsis), as well as with the administration of certain medications (e. g., anesthetics, arterial vasodilators).

BP can be measured directly (also called invasively) or indirectly (noninvasively). The most common way to measure BP directly is by introducing a catheter into an artery and then connecting this catheter to an external pressure transducer. Less commonly, the pressure transducer is in the catheter (direct-tip catheter). Direct BP measurement does require expertise for proper placement of the catheter, as well as for obtaining reliable readings, and is generally not suited for routine use in awake patients.

Two main methodologies are used for indirect BP readings: Doppler and oscillometric. Doppler is well suited for use in cats and dogs, and readings can be obtained over a wide range of pressures. Unfortunately, it is rarely possible to get a diastolic reading, so Doppler will almost always provide incomplete BP information. Oscillometric devices record diastolic, systolic, and usually also mean arterial BP. They have been generally felt to be less accurate than Doppler, but newer units are very promising. Given that there is less preparation time involved in using oscillometric devices, they lend themselves well to screening exams.

INDICATIONS
• When signs of end-organ damage are present, such as retinal hemorrhage and/or detachment, cardiac hypertrophy of undetermined origin, or neurologic signs
• When diseases are present known to cause hypertension, such as renal disease, hyperthyroidism, and hyperadrenocorticism
• In critical care patients
• Anesthesia
• Administration of medications known to affect BP
• Geriatric patients, especially cats

CONTRAINDICATIONS
• Indirect BP: none
• Direct BP: Bleeding disorders would be a contraindication to direct BP measurement, given the risk of hemorrhage from an arterial venipuncture.

POTENTIAL COMPLICATIONS
Indirect BP
None

Direct BP
• Hemorrhage from the arterial puncture site
• Hematoma formation at the puncture site (can be extensive if the femoral artery is used)
• Pain related to venipuncture
• Thrombosis and potentially arterial thromboembolism
• Infection of the puncture site

CLIENT EDUCATION
None

BODY SYSTEMS ASSESSED
Cardiovascular

PROCEDURE

PATIENT PREPARATION
Preprocedure Medication or Preparation
None required for indirect measurement. With direct measurement, the site of arterial puncture should be clipped and sterilely prepared.

Anesthesia or Sedation
Generally not desirable. If direct BP readings are to be taken in a conscious patient, infiltration of local anesthetics can facilitate placement of the arterial line. Local anesthetic will also minimize arterial spasm in sedated or anesthetized patients.

Patient Positioning
• It is ideal to have the site where BP is being measured at the level of the heart.
• It is vital for oscillometric BP devices that the extremity is not bearing weight when the reading is taken.

Patient Monitoring
• None for indirect. With direct BP measurement, the patency of the catheter needs to be maintained and the area inspected for evidence of hemorrhage.

Equipment or Supplies
• Indirect BP measurement: oscillometric or Doppler device
• Direct BP measurement: direct-tip catheter pressure transducer or arterial catheter with external pressure transducer

TECHNIQUE
Indirect
Doppler (Figure 1)
• Clip the area where BP is to be measured (the area just below the metacarpal or metatarsal pads, ventral aspect of tail).
• Apply ultrasound gel to the transducer.
• Apply the cuff to the area above the transducer (the width of cuff should be 30%–40% of limb circumference) attached to the sphygmomanometer.
• Position the transducer so that a good arterial signal is obtained.
• Inflate the cuff until the signal is no longer audible and then slowly deflate the cuff until the signal returns. The pressure at which the signal returns is considered to be systolic pressure. Continue to deflate the cuff; in rare cases, a muffling of the signal can be heard that can be diastolic pressure.
• Repeat the measurement, but wait at least 15–30 min between readings.

Oscillometric
• Apply the cuff to appropriate site (between the elbow and the carpus, above the elbow, at the tail base, at the distal hind limb).

BLOOD PRESSURE DETERMINATION: NONINVASIVE AND INVASIVE

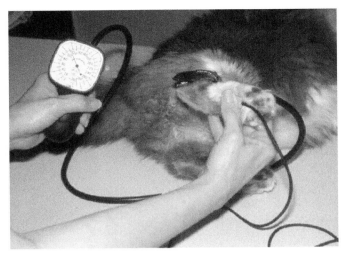

Figure 1

Doppler technique: Blood pressure is being measured just below the metatarsal pad.

- Activate the machine to start automatic inflation and measurement.
- Repeat the measurement.

Direct
- Clip and surgically prepare the puncture site. Common sites include the dorsal pedal (metatarsal) artery, femoral artery, and lingual artery.
- An over-the-needle catheter (usually 20–24 gauge) is inserted into the area where the artery is palpated. With the femoral artery, a small cutdown incision may facilitate this. Larger catheters are preferable, though not too large because these will occlude the artery.
- Once blood has flashed into the catheter, the needle is removed and the catheter capped. The catheter is flushed with heparinized saline (the addition of heparin to flush solutions is debatable in venous catheters but is important to maintain the patency of arterial catheters) and taped or sutured in place.
- The catheter is attached to noncompliant tubing that is filled with heparinized saline from a pressurized bag (pressure prevents blood from backing up into the arterial catheter).
- The tubing is attached to a calibrated pressure transducer. The pressure transducer is then attached to appropriate monitoring equipment.
- The tubing and catheter need to be flushed frequently to maintain patency.

SAMPLE HANDLING
N/A

APPROPRIATE AFTERCARE
Postprocedure Patient Monitoring
- Indirect: none
- Direct: Monitor the arterial puncture site for indications of hemorrhage. This is especially important if the femoral artery was used.

Nursing Care
- Indirect: none
- Direct: Apply a pressure bandage to the arterial puncture site, if possible.

Dietary Modification
N/A

Medication Requirements
N/A

Restrictions on Activity
None

Anticipated Recovery Time
None

INTERPRETATION

NORMAL FINDINGS OR RANGE
- Normal ranges will often depend on the method used to measure BP, age, breed, and, to some degree, operator factors (experienced vs novice).
- In a large epidemiologic study in dogs, the average value for BP was 133/75 measured with an oscillometric monitor (Bodey & Michell 1996).
- In cats, normal BP has been found to be 125/90 via direct methods.

ABNORMAL VALUES
- Hypertension is considered to be present in most cases where systolic BP is >150 and diastolic BP is >95 mmHg.

CRITICAL VALUES
- Critical hypotension is present with a mean arterial BP of <60 mmHg or a systolic pressure of <80 mmHg.
- Critical hypertension is present with a systolic BP of >180 mmHg and/or a diastolic BP of >120 mmHg. At BPs greater than 150/95 some degree of target organ damage is possible.

INTERFERING FACTORS
Drugs That May Alter Results of the Procedure
- Most anesthetics will alter BP. Generally, pressure is decreased; however, α_2-adrenergic agonists can cause an increase by increasing systemic vascular resistance.
- β Blockers, angiotensin-converting enzyme (ACE) inhibitors, nitroprusside, and calcium-channel blockers will decrease BP.
- Ocular medications can affect BP, as well. Timolol has been shown to decrease BP whereas phenylephrine can increase it.
- Adrenergic agents will often increase BP.

Conditions That May Interfere with Performing the Procedure
N/A

Procedure Techniques or Handling That May Alter Results
Indirect
- Anything that leads to patient stress can lead to white-coat hypertension and thereby inaccurate BP readings.
- Appropriate cuff size is important (the width of the cuff should be 30%–40% of limb circumference). Cuffs that are too large cause low readings, whereas cuffs that are too small cause falsely elevated readings.
- With Doppler, it is vital that enough time is taken between readings. There is a tendency with this device to get multiple readings in a short time in awake patients. This tends to result in a higher BP being determined. With time, BP tends to decrease as the patient becomes acclimated to the procedure.

BLOOD PRESSURE DETERMINATION: NONINVASIVE AND INVASIVE

Direct
- Contact of the catheter with the vessel wall will cause errors.
- Blood clots or air bubbles in the catheter and tubing will cause inaccurate readings.
- Inappropriate tubing (too compliant) can fail to transmit the pressure wave appropriately, damping the signal.
- Excessively long tubing or kinking of tubing will cause erroneous readings.
- Small catheters produce a limited dynamic response so that accurate measurements are not possible.

Influence of Signalment on Performing and Interpreting the Procedure
Species
Cat and dog normal ranges are similar.

Breed
No breed-related differences have been noted in cats. Among dogs, sighthounds tend to have higher BPs than other breeds and, on average, their systolic BP is 10–20 mmHg higher than other breeds. In some individuals that may mean that their normal BP is in the range that would be considered hypertensive.

Age
BP increases with age.

Gender
Males will have higher BPs than females; on average, the difference is <10 mmHg.

Pregnancy
Unknown

CLINICAL PERSPECTIVE
- There are many indications for BP measurement, to detect both hypotension and hypertension.
- In older animals, BP screening indicated as hypertension is most common in geriatric patients.
- For general practice, indirect methods are best suited for screening patients.
- Direct BP measurement is ideal where continuous BP measurement is needed, especially in very critical cases.

MISCELLANEOUS

ANCILLARY TESTS
If hypertension is found, appropriate laboratory tests are indicated to identify whether an underlying cause can be found.

SYNONYMS
None

SEE ALSO
Blackwell's Five-Minute Veterinary Consult: Canine and Feline Topics
- Hypertension, Systemic
- Hyperthyroidism
- Renal failure

Related Topics in This Book
None

ABBREVIATIONS
BP = blood pressure

Suggested Reading
Acierno MJ, Labato MA. Hypertension in dogs and cats. *Compend Contin Educ Pract Vet* 2004; 26: 336–345.
Bodey AR, Michell AR. Epidemiological study of blood pressure in domestic dogs. *J Small Anim Pract* 1996; 37: 116–125.
Carr AP. Measuring blood pressure in dogs and cats. *Vet Med* 2001; 96: 135–144.
Love L, Harvey R. Arterial blood pressure measurement: Physiology, tools and techniques. *Compend Contin Educ Pract Vet* 2006; 28: 450–461.
Waddell LS. Direct blood pressure monitoring. *Clin Tech Small Anim Pract* 2000; 15: 111–118.

INTERNET RESOURCES
None

AUTHOR NAME
Anthony P. Carr

BASICS

TYPE OF PROCEDURE
Diagnostic sample collection

PROCEDURE EXPLANATION AND RELATED PHYSIOLOGY
The procedure involves using a syringe with attached hypodermic needle and aspirating blood percutaneously through vessel wall and into syringe to the desired amount and withdrawal of needle-syringe combination. For arterial blood collection, a heparinized syringe with an attached needle is used.

INDICATIONS
To obtain a blood sample for test analysis

CONTRAINDICATIONS
- Severe coagulopathy
- If a patient struggles or stresses to the point where it can further injure itself or the restrainers

POTENTIAL COMPLICATIONS
- Complications are rare.
- Excessive bleeding can cause a hematoma in patients with a coagulopathy. A pressure wrap to the area should resolve this problem.
- Multiple venipunctures of the same vein and area could cause bruising, phlebitis, or thrombosis to the vein.

CLIENT EDUCATION
Clients should be warned that there might be an area of hair clipped at the site and a small bandage applied, which should remain in place for 1 h after the procedure.

BODY SYSTEMS ASSESSED
All

PROCEDURE

PATIENT PREPARATION
Preprocedure Medication or Preparation
- None
- For arterial blood collection, oxygen therapy should be discontinued for 5–10 min before sample collection if assessment of a patient breathing room air is desired.

Anesthesia or Sedation
- Generally no sedatives are required.
- If a patient is fractious, a mild sedative may be needed.

Patient Positioning
- Positioning for the procedure is vital for a positive outcome.
- For venous blood collection, the patient will need to be restrained as needed for the vein being accessed and the vein compressed proximal to the site of puncture. For jugular venipuncture, it is best to have the patient in a sitting position with the head held high and slightly turned to the opposite side. For saphenous venipuncture, the vein is best viewed with the patient in lateral recumbency. Cephalic veins are best used when the patient is in sternal recumbency with the leg extended.
- For arterial blood collection, the patient will need to be restrained in lateral recumbency with the bottom back leg held out by the restrainer, being careful not to compress the artery and disrupt arterial blood flow. If a patient's dyspnea worsens when in lateral recumbency, it may be necessary to perform this procedure with the patient standing or sitting.

Patient Monitoring
- None

- Dyspneic patients should be monitored closely for signs of increased dyspnea. If this occurs during the procedure, oxygen should be administered and the patient allowed to sit.

Equipment or Supplies
- An appropriately sized syringe, generally not larger than the amount of blood needed
- A needle: Use the smallest to cause the least trauma and pain to the patient but large enough to easily draw the volume of blood needed [e.g., 22 or 20 gauge × 1 inch (25.4 mm)].
- An alcohol swab
- Appropriate collection tubes in which to place blood
- A heparinized syringe for arterial blood collection (1- or 3-mL syringe with a 25-gauge needle). Draw heparin into syringe and then push all of the heparin back into the heparin vial, leaving just enough to coat the inside of the syringe.
- An arterial blood sampler (e.g., Micro ABG; Vital Signs, Towota, NJ) may also be used.

TECHNIQUE
Prior to patient restraint, gather all supplies needed.

Venous Blood Collection
Based on the amount of blood needed and the quality of the available veins, a vein will be selected by the venipuncturist. Typically, the jugular vein is used when more than 2 mL of blood is needed. An alternative to this is the lateral saphenous vein in dogs and the medial saphenous vein in cats, which works well if a patient is struggling. If a small amount of blood is needed (<2 mL), the cephalic vein is used. The patient should be restrained, preferably on an examination table. The site is swabbed with alcohol. The vein is compressed proximal to the site to allow the vein to engorge. The vein is palpated, the needle is advanced through the skin over the vein and then into the vein lumen, and the syringe plunger pulled back to aspirate the appropriate amount of blood. Compression of the vein is released. The syringe and needle are then withdrawn as a unit and blood placed into appropriate collection tubes. The restrainer applies pressure directly to the venipuncture site for a few seconds then checks the site; if there is still bleeding, a Band-Aid can be applied.

Arterial Blood Collection
If an arterial blood sampler is used, remove the syringe from the wrapper and pull the plunger back to the desired amount of blood needed (0.4 mL is more than enough for most blood-gas analyzers). Prepare the clay-instilled cap of the sampler by putting the base piece on it. Place the sampler or heparinized syringe within easy reach. The patient should be restrained with its bottom leg held out. The restrainer should put a hand behind the patient's hock to keep its leg extended. The preferred site is the pedal artery, which lies just medial to midline and usually is strongest just distal to the hock. Find the artery by palpation. You will need to arrange your hands so as to be able to keep a finger on the pulse with 1 hand and align the syringe and needle in the other hand with the artery. It is then just a matter of aligning where you feel the pulse with your syringe and needle. Once your needle has penetrated the skin, you need to place negative vacuum on the plunger of the syringe and attempt to puncture the arterial wall. A flash of blood back into the syringe will usually be seen after arterial puncture. Allow the syringe to fill to the amount of blood needed, withdraw the syringe and needle, and have the restrainer place pressure over the site for several minutes. A small pressure wrap may be needed. You then will need to seal off the needle from room air immediately to avoid having your results altered by room air mixing with the sample. A rubber stopper or cork works well for this. If you are using the preheparinized blood-gas sampler syringe, the syringe simply needs to have the plunger withdrawn to the amount of blood needed, and it will then fill by the arterial pressure once the artery is punctured.

BLOOD SAMPLE COLLECTION

SAMPLE HANDLING

- Venous samples should be placed into appropriate collection tubes immediately so that the blood is in the anticoagulant tubes before the clot tubes. Invert the tubes several times to mix the samples thoroughly with the anticoagulant. Send the tubes to lab as the test protocol describes.
- Arterial samples for blood-gas analysis will need to be assayed immediately.

APPROPRIATE AFTERCARE

Postprocedure Patient Monitoring
Remove the pressure wrap 1 h after the procedure.

Nursing Care
None

Dietary Modification
None

Medication Requirements
None

Restrictions on Activity
None

Anticipated Recovery Time
Immediate recovery is expected.

INTERPRETATION

NORMAL FINDINGS OR RANGE
None

ABNORMAL VALUES
None

CRITICAL VALUES
N/A

INTERFERING FACTORS

Drugs That May Alter Results of the Procedure
None

Conditions That May Interfere with Performing the Procedure
Coagulopathy

Procedure Techniques or Handling That May Alter Results
None

Influence of Signalment on Performing and Interpreting the Procedure

Species
Vein selection may vary between dogs and cats.

Breed
None

Age
None

Gender
None

Pregnancy
None

CLINICAL PERSPECTIVE

When performed skillfully by trained, experienced personnel, venipuncture for blood sampling is usually a quick, simple procedure that causes minimal discomfort to patients and can be a valuable diagnostic tool.

MISCELLANEOUS

ANCILLARY TESTS
Blood-gas analysis

SYNONYMS
- Arteriopuncture
- Venipuncture

SEE ALSO
Blackwell's Five-Minute Veterinary Consult: Canine and Feline Topics
Many
Related Topics in This Book
Many

ABBREVIATIONS
None

INTERNET RESOURCES
None

AUTHOR NAME
Robin Lazaro

BASICS

TYPE OF SPECIMEN
Blood

TEST EXPLANATION AND RELATED PHYSIOLOGY
Microscopic evaluation of a blood smear is an essential part of a CBC and an adjunct to the cell counts provided by a hematology analyzer. A blood smear scan can provide a rapid estimate of WBC and platelet numbers, supplying critical information in an emergency situation or serving as an important cross-check for the numerical results generated by an analyzer. Examination of a blood smear is important for identifying a variety of cells (e.g., basophils, bands, blasts) and morphologic findings (e.g., polychromasia, toxic neutrophils, reactive lymphocytes) that tend to be missed by any hematology analyzer's autodifferential feature.

Blood smears should be examined systematically with both a low-power (10×) scan and a more detailed assessment of RBCs, WBCs, and platelets at 100× magnification. Five types of leukocytes can be found in peripheral blood—neutrophils, lymphocytes, eosinophils, monocytes, and basophils—although basophils are uncommon in normal dogs and cats. Other types of hematopoietic cells, such as immature granulocytes or blasts, should also be identified if present. The percentage of each type of WBC should be determined, platelet numbers estimated, and RBC and WBC morphologic features assessed.

INDICATIONS
- To verify the accuracy of results from a hematology analyzer
- To aid in determining a cause of anemia
- For diagnosis of inflammation, hematopoietic neoplasia, bone marrow disease
- As part of a workup of coagulopathy through assessment of platelet numbers

CONTRAINDICATIONS
None

POTENTIAL COMPLICATIONS
None

CLIENT EDUCATION
A 12-h fast prior to sample collection can minimize artifacts caused by lipemia.

BODY SYSTEMS ASSESSED
Hemic, lymphatic, and immune

SAMPLE

COLLECTION
1 mL of venous blood

HANDLING
Blood can be immediately smeared or collected into anticoagulant:
- EDTA anticoagulant is preferred.
- Heparin can be used but does not prevent platelet clumping.

STORAGE
Store smears at room temperature, protected from humidity and light. It is best if they are permanently coverslipped.

STABILITY
- Unfixed (unstained) slides are stable for a few weeks.
- Alcohol-fixed, stained slides can be stable for years.

PROTOCOL
- At 10× magnification

- Scan the feathered edge for clumped platelets, microfilariae, mast cells, blasts, clumped leukocytes, or other abnormalities.
- Assess WBC numbers (decreased, normal, increased) in the body of smear: Estimated WBC count/μL = average number of cells per 10× field × 100. Evaluate at least 10 fields, including 1 field at the feathered edge and 1 near the butt of smear.
- At 50×–100× magnification
  - Perform a leukocyte differential count. WBCs are flattened out and most readily identified in the RBC monolayer just behind the feathered edge (Figure 1), while appearing smaller and darker in thicker portions of the smear. Zigzag across the smear monolayer, identifying at least 100 WBCs. Nucleated RBCs should be counted separately.
  - Evaluate RBC and WBC morphologic features.
  - Estimate platelet numbers by counting platelets in at least ten 100× fields.

INTERPRETATION

NORMAL FINDINGS OR RANGE
- RBCs are closely opposed to each other in the monolayer, with little overlap.
- Approximately 5–15 WBCs per 10× field, with a predominance of neutrophils
- Approximately 10–25 platelets per 100× field in the monolayer

ABNORMAL VALUES
- Tightly packed or widely separated RBCs
- WBC or platelet numbers above or below the reference range

CRITICAL VALUES
- Fewer than 1–3 neutrophils per 10× field suggests significant neutropenia and an animal at risk of infections.
- Fewer than 1–3 platelets per 100× field suggests significant thrombocytopenia and an animal at risk of bleeding.

INTERFERING FACTORS
Drugs That May Alter Results or Interpretation
Drugs That Interfere with Test Methodology
None

Drugs That Alter Physiology
- Glucocorticoids can cause leukocytosis, neutrophilia, and lymphopenia, with or without monocytosis.
- Epinephrine can cause a leukocytosis, neutrophilia, and lymphocytosis, with or without thrombocytosis.
- Heinz body formation is seen with acetaminophen, benzocaine, phenazopyridine, propofol, and vitamin K.
- Cytopenias can occur secondary to various chemotherapeutic agents, as well as chloramphenicol (feline), estrogen (canine), griseofulvin, methimazole (feline), phenobarbital, phenylbutazone (canine), and trimethoprim sulfa.

Disorders That May Alter Results
- Hemolysis can result in a thick pink background that distorts RBCs.
- Lipemia can cause RBCs to be smudged during preparation of the smear.
- Hyperglobulinemia can result in a thick blue background that distorts RBCs.

Collection Techniques or Handling That May Alter Results
- Using poorly mixed blood produces a thin smear, suggesting anemia.
- Using clotted blood can artificially decrease platelet, RBC, and WBC numbers.
- Blood that is more than 6–12 h old is more likely to have platelet clumps and distorted leukocytes. Parasites such as the hemotrophic mycoplasmas (previous name: *Hemobartonella*) can detach from RBC membranes over time.

BLOOD SMEAR MICROSCOPIC EXAMINATION

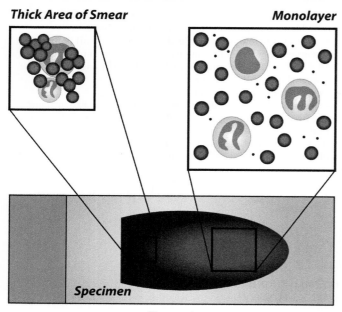

Thick Area of Smear

Monolayer

Specimen

Figure 1

This drawing of a blood smear illustrates how cell morphology is optimal in the monolayer just behind the feathered edge, where RBCs are evenly distributed. Cells in thicker areas, toward the back of the smear, are less flattened and appear smaller and darker and are more difficult to identify. The overlap of cells, in thicker portions of the smear, further obscures and distorts their morphologic features.

- Use of old stain or insufficient washing can produce a stain precipitate easily mistaken for bacterial cocci or RBC parasites.

Influence of Signalment

Species
- Canine RBCs have a prominent zone of central pallor and show little anisocytosis.
- Feline RBCs are small, lack obvious central pallor, and show mild anisocytosis.
- Canine eosinophils have round, variably sized granules, whereas feline eosinophils have smaller, rod-shaped granules. This distinction can occasionally be important for verifying the species of a mislabeled sample.
- Canine and feline basophils have indistinct granules distinct from those in other species.

Breed
- Low WBC numbers can be normal in greyhounds and the Belgian Tervuren.
- Low platelet numbers (4–10 per 100× field) can be normal in greyhounds.
- Some Cavalier King Charles spaniels have low numbers of extremely large platelets (approaching the size of an RBC).

Age
None

Gender
None

Pregnancy
None

LIMITATIONS OF THE TEST

Most accurate if performed by someone with experience interpreting blood smears

Sensitivity, Specificity, and Positive and Negative Predictive Values
N/A

Valid If Run in a Human Lab?
Yes—if technicians are appropriately trained in species specific findings.

Causes of Abnormal Findings

	High values	Low values
WBCs	Inflammation	Endotoxemia and/or sepsis
	Corticosteroid response	Overwhelming inflammation
		Drug toxicity
	Epinephrine response	Bone marrow disease (decreased
	Leukemia	production)
RBCs	Hemoconcentration	Blood loss
	Splenic contraction	Hemolysis
	Hypoxia	Bone marrow disease (decreased production)
Platelets	Iron deficiency	Immune-mediated destruction
	Inflammation	Tickborne diseases (ehrlichiosis,
	Myeloproliferative disorders	babesiosis, Rocky Mountain spotted fever)
	Epinephrine	Platelet consumption (e.g., thrombosis, hemorrhage)
		Bone marrow disease (decreased production)

CLINICAL PERSPECTIVE
- Wide spaces between RBCs in the monolayer suggest anemia.
- The absence of an RBC monolayer, or very narrow zone, suggests polycythemia.
- WBC estimates can be altered by changes in the hematocrit or changes in the thickness of the smear caused by variations in technique. A rule of thumb is this:
  - <5 WBCs per 10× field in the monolayer suggests leukopenia.
  - >20 WBCs per 10× field in the monolayer suggests leukocytosis.
  - The WBC estimate can appear artificially decreased if WBC are clumped or pushed out to the feathered edge.
- The presence of <10 platelets per 100× field in the monolayer suggests thrombocytopenia.
  - Each platelet corresponds to approximately 18,000–20,000/μL.
- The platelet estimate tends to appear artificially decreased when platelets are clumped.

MISCELLANEOUS

ANCILLARY TESTS
- RBC, WBC, and platelet counts
- Bone marrow aspirate and bone marrow biopsy
- Fine-needle aspiration and/or biopsy of peripheral and visceral lymphoid tissues in animals with large numbers of circulating blasts
- Immunophenotyping of circulating blasts

SYNONYMS
Peripheral blood smear evaluation

SEE ALSO
Blackwell's Five-Minute Veterinary Consult: Canine and Feline Topics
- Anemia, Nonregenerative
- Anemia, Regenerative
- Neutropenia

BLOOD SMEAR MICROSCOPIC EXAMINATION

- Pancytopenia
- Polycythemia
- Thrombocytopenia

Related Topics in This Book
- Complete Blood Count
- Heinz Bodies
- Platelet Count and Volume
- Red Blood Cell Count
- Red Blood Cell Morphology
- White Blood Cells: Basophils
- White Blood Cells: Eosinophils
- White Blood Cells: Lymphocytes
- White Blood Cells: Monocytes
- White Blood Cells: Neutrophils

ABBREVIATIONS
None

Suggested Reading

Cowell RL, Tyler RD, Meinkoth JH, eds. *Diagnostic Cytology and Hematology of the Dog and Cat*, 2nd ed. St Louis: CV Mosby, 1999.

Lassen ED, Weiser G. Laboratory technology for veterinary medicine. In: Thrall MA, ed. *Veterinary Hematology and Clinical Chemistry*. Philadelphia: Lippincott Williams & Wilkins, 2004: 3–21.

Mitzner BT. Why automated differentials fall short. *J Am Anim Hosp Assoc* 2001; **37**: 117–118.

INTERNET RESOURCES

AXIOM Veterinary Laboratories: Canine & feline haematology images, http://www.axiomvetlab.com/Some%20Useful%20Images.html.

AUTHOR NAME

Author Joyce S. Knoll

BLOOD SMEAR PREPARATION

BASICS

TYPE OF PROCEDURE
Diagnostic sample collection

PROCEDURE EXPLANATION AND RELATED PHYSIOLOGY
Examination of a blood smear is an integral part of a complete blood cell count. When examined by a trained technologist or pathologist, a blood smear can provide a large amount of information about RBCs, WBCs, and platelets. Preparation of a smear at the time of sample collection can provide a snapshot view of the patient's hematology status, minimizing the effects of sample deterioration, such as changes in leukocyte morphology and decreased platelet numbers. Hence, even samples sent to a diagnostic laboratory should include an air-dried smear of fresh blood.

Poorly prepared smears can either mask abnormalities or result in confusing artifacts. RBC and WBC morphologic features can be obscured by extremely thick smears, whereas changes in cell distribution on the smear due to uneven streaking can lead to serious errors in the differential count. Mastering the technique for preparing a good-quality blood smear takes some practice.

INDICATIONS
- When transport to a diagnostic laboratory delays sample processing
- An essential part of an in-house CBC

CONTRAINDICATIONS
Blood is clotted—results may be erroneous.

POTENTIAL COMPLICATIONS
None

CLIENT EDUCATION
None

BODY SYSTEMS ASSESSED
Hemic, lymphatic, and immune

PROCEDURE

PATIENT PREPARATION
Preprocedure Medication or Preparation
- Clean the venipuncture site with alcohol.
- Perform venipuncture and transfer blood into a tube containing EDTA (lavender top).

Anesthesia or Sedation
N/A

Patient Positioning
N/A

Patient Monitoring
N/A

Equipment or Supplies
- Clean glass slides
- Microhematocrit tubes (an optional way to transfer blood to slide)
- Wooden applicator sticks

TECHNIQUE
- Swirl a pair of applicator sticks in blood to check for blood clots.
- Place a drop of well-mixed blood at 1 end of a glass slide.
- Place a second glass slide at a 45° angle to the first slide, with the blood droplet positioned between the 2 slides (Figure 1). Avoid pressing down on the spreader slide.
- Smear thickness can be adjusted by changing the angle between the 2 slides. With samples from severely anemic animals, widening the angle between slides can help avoid making too thin a smear.
- Slide the top slide toward the drop of blood.
- When the spreader slide contacts the droplet, pause briefly, allowing blood to spread along the juncture between the 2 slides.

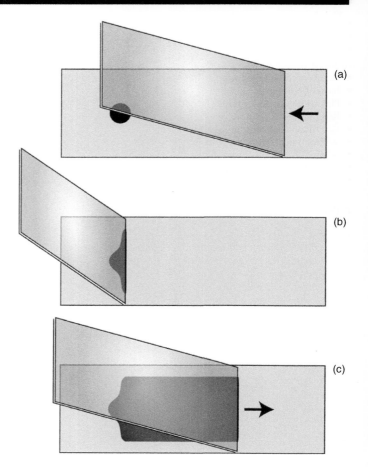

(a)

(b)

(c)

(d)

Figure 1

Proper technique for blood smear preparation.

- Move the spreader slide away from the drop of blood in a smooth, steady motion. The spreader slide should not be lifted until it has reached the far end of the lower slide.
- Allow the smear to air-dry and stain with some type of Romanovsky-type stain (e. g., Diff-Quick, Hema III, Giemsa, Wright stain).

SAMPLE HANDLING
- Air-dried blood smears can be stored several days at room temperature.
- Once fixed and stained, smears are stable for months to years if protected from light.
- A coverslip is needed for crisp resolution at 40-fold magnification. A temporary coverslip can be attached with a drop of immersion oil. Commercial mounting media can be used to attach a coverslip permanently, which also protects smears from scratches, dust, etc.

APPROPRIATE AFTERCARE
Postprocedure Patient Monitoring
N/A

Nursing Care
N/A

Dietary Modification
N/A

Medication Requirements
N/A

Restrictions on Activity
N/A

Anticipated Recovery Time
N/A

 INTERPRETATION

NORMAL FINDINGS OR RANGE
• A bullet-shaped blood smear that extends about one-third to two-thirds the length of the glass slide.
• The smear has a zone just behind the feathered edge in which RBCs are closely opposed to each other with little overlap (monolayer).

Causes of Abnormal Values

Common technique errors

Problem	Probable explanation(s)
Blunt rather than curved end	Spreader slide picked up prematurely
Smear covers entire slide and lacks feathered edge	1. Too large a drop of blood 2. Angle between 2 slides was too narrow
Lack of a monolayer— smear too thick	1. Too large a drop of blood 2. Angle between 2 slides too wide 3. Movement of spreader slide too fast
Striations running across smear ("chatter")	Movement of spreader slide not smooth—usually because slide was moved too slowly
Abnormally shaped smear	Corner of spreader slide lifted at some point
Jagged feathered edge	1. Dirty slide(s)—microscopic dust 2. Presence of large platelet clumps

CRITICAL VALUES
None

INTERFERING FACTORS
Drugs That May Alter Results of the Procedure
None

Conditions That May Interfere with Performing the Procedure
Marked polythemia may prevent preparing a smear with a monolayer and cause distorted leukocytes.

Procedure Techniques or Handling That May Alter Results
• Using poorly mixed blood can result in a thin smear suggesting anemia.
• Using clotted blood can result in artificially decreased platelet numbers.
• Platelets are more likely to be clumped in old blood (>6 h).
• Leukocyte morphologic features can be altered in old blood.
• A thick, squared-off feathered edge or the lack of a feathered edge can prevent recognition of platelet clumps or abnormal cells.

• Exposure of smears to formalin fumes produces a thick blue-green background and prevents accurate leukocyte identification.

Influence of Signalment on Performing and Interpreting the Procedure
Species
None

Breed
None

Age
None

Gender
None

Pregnancy
None

CLINICAL PERSPECTIVE
• Even precleaned slides can have glass chips on their surface, which should be wiped off.
• A smear of freshly collected blood may be needed to identify RBC parasites such as *Mycoplasma hemofelis*.
• A smear of freshly collected blood provides the most accurate platelet estimate.
• Capillary blood (e. g., from ear prick) can be helpful for finding RBC parasites such as *Babesia* sp.

 MISCELLANEOUS

ANCILLARY TESTS
None

SYNONYMS
Peripheral blood smear

SEE ALSO
Blackwell's Five-Minute Veterinary Consult: Canine and Feline Topics
None

Related Topics in This Book
• Blood Smear Microscopic Examination
• Platelet Count and Volume
• Red Blood Cell Count
• Red Blood Cell Morphology
• White Blood Cells: Basophils
• White Blood Cells: Eosinophils
• White Blood Cells: Lymphocytes
• White Blood Cells: Monocytes
• White Blood Cells: Neutrophils

ABBREVIATIONS
None

Suggested Reading
Thrall MA, ed. *Veterinary Hematology and Clinical Chemistry.* Philadelphia: Lippincott Williams & Wilkins, 2004: 9–15.
Walker D. Peripheral blood smears. In: Cowell RL, Tyler RD, Meinkoth JH, eds. *Diagnostic Cytology and Hematology of the Dog and Cat,* 2 nd ed. St Louis: CV Mosby, 1999: 254–283.

INTERNET RESOURCES
Research Animal Diagnostic Laboratory (RADIL), University of Missouri: RADIL standard operating procedure for making a blood smear, http://www.radil.missouri.edu/info/teaching/MakingBloodSmear.asp.

AUTHOR NAME
Joyce S. Knoll

BASICS

TYPE OF SPECIMEN
Blood

TEST EXPLANATION AND RELATED PHYSIOLOGY
Blood types, which are genetic markers on the surface of RBCs, are species specific and antigenic, which means that the immune system can recognize them and potentially produce antibodies against them. A set of 2 or more alleles at 1 gene locus makes up a blood group system. An individual lacking a given blood type may develop antibodies against it, either naturally (cats) or following sensitization via a mismatched transfusion (cats and dogs). Blood-typing methods are based on hemolytic or agglutination reaction in which a species-specific antiserum or chemical reagent is directed against specific RBC antigens.

Over 12 blood group systems have been recognized in dogs. It has not been determined whether all reported canine blood groups are serologically distinct. An international standardization was proposed for 7 blood groups, which have been referred to since then as DEA, for *d*og *e*rythrocyte *a*ntigen, followed by a number. A new canine blood type named *Dal*, lacking in some Dalmatians, has more recently been identified through discovery of its specific alloantibody. For each blood group, a dog may be either positive or negative, so an individual dog's RBCs can have several of these blood groups on their membranes. The DEA 1 system is an exception because it contains at least 2 subtypes: DEA 1.1 and DEA 1.2 (and perhaps a third one, DEA 1.3, described in Australia). An individual dog's RBCs can have only 1 of these subtypes on their membranes. RBCs may be DEA 1.1 positive or negative, but only DEA 1.1–negative cells can be DEA 1.2 positive.

Dogs do not have clinically significant naturally occurring alloantibodies; however, they may become sensitized after receiving a blood type–mismatched transfusion. It is widely recognized that the most antigenic and consequently clinically significant blood group in dogs is DEA 1.1. For this reason, blood typing for DEA 1.1 is desirable prior to transfusions to avoid sensitization, and this blood group antigen has been the main focus of commercially available blood-typing methods.

In cats, an AB blood group system has been defined that consists of 3 blood types: A, B and AB. The A allele is dominant over the B allele. Type AB is a rare third allele, which appears to be recessive to A but codominant to B. Although most cats are type A (>95% of domestic shorthairs), significant geographic and breed-associated differences have been found in the frequencies of these blood types. In contrast with dogs, cats possess naturally occurring alloantibodies against the blood type they are lacking. Of particular concern is the presence of very strong anti-A alloantibodies in all type B cats, such that transfusion of type A blood into a type B cat will produce a life-threatening acute transfusion reaction. Approximately a third of type A cats have weak anti-B alloantibodies, which may cause shortened survival of transfused B cells in type A cats, but tend to produce a relatively mild acute hemolytic reaction. A new blood type called *Mik*, identified outside of the feline AB blood group, was found to be capable of causing a hemolytic transfusion reaction.

DEA 1.1 and feline AB system blood-typing cards are available commercially as simple in-practice kits.
- The Rapid Vet-H canine and feline blood-typing cards (DMS Laboratories, Flemington, NJ) are easy to use in-house and provide results within 2 min. The animal blood type is indicated by visible RBC agglutination. It is important to remember that the level of agglutination depends on the amount of antigen expressed on RBC membranes.
- In the Alvedia Quick Test DEA 1.1 and Alvedia Quick Test A+B blood-typing kits (Alvedia, Villeur banne, France) RBCs migrate on a membrane and interact with monoclonal antibodies to produce a visible line that is simple to interpret. A second control line appears if the test was performed correctly. Results are stable and can be stored as part of the patient's record.
- Adapted from modern human blood-typing technique, a novel gel column technology (DiaMed AG, Cressier sur Morat, Switzerland) has also been introduced for canine (DEA 1.1) and feline blood typing and appears to be a reliable and rapid clinical laboratory method. This method is accurate and easy, but a specialized centrifuge is required. Gel cards can be easily photocopied or scanned for a permanent record of results.
- Typing services and/or polyclonal antisera are also available for DEA 1.1, 1.2, 3, 4, 5 and 7, and for the more recently described canine *Dal* and feline *Mik* blood types.

INDICATIONS
- Screening blood donors and recipients to assure blood compatibility
- Screening breeding cats to ensure blood-compatible mates and avoid neonatal isoerythrolysis

CONTRAINDICATIONS
None

POTENTIAL COMPLICATIONS
None

CLIENT EDUCATION
None

BODY SYSTEMS ASSESSED
Hemic, lymphatic, and immune

SAMPLE

COLLECTION
A 1- to 2-mL venous blood sample

HANDLING
EDTA anticoagulant

STORAGE
Refrigerate for short-term storage.

STABILITY
The physical integrity of RBCs is critical for correct results. Ideally, samples should be blood typed within 2–3 days of blood collection.

PROTOCOL
None

INTERPRETATION

NORMAL FINDINGS OR RANGE
- Dogs: ≈50% are positive for the DEA 1.1 system.

Canine blood types	% Positive	% Negative
DEA 1		
1.1	33–45	55–67
1.2	7–20	35–60*
DEA 3	5–10	90–95
DEA 4	87–98	2–13
DEA 5	12–2	78–88
DEA 7	8–45	55–92

*DEA 1.1–negative and DEA 1.2–negative dogs.

- Cats: Most are type A (>95% of domestic shorthairs); <5% are type B, and <1% are type AB.

ABNORMAL VALUES
None

CRITICAL VALUES
None

INTERFERING FACTORS
Drugs That May Alter Results or Interpretation
Drugs That Interfere with Test Methodology
Recent blood transfusion (packed RBCs or whole blood)

Drugs That Alter Physiology
None

Disorders That May Alter Results
- Severe anemia may cause false-negative results because the number of RBCs may be insufficient to agglutinate in response to antiserum.
- Autoagglutination, such as in immune-mediated hemolytic anemia, precludes typing by most methods because such blood samples will always appear positive.
- Marked rouleaux can be mistaken for a weak positive reaction with the Rapid Vet-H canine and feline blood-typing cards.

Collection Techniques or Handling That May Alter Results
Hemolysis of the blood may not allow blood typing, because the physical integrity of the RBCs is critical for correct results.

Influence of Signalment
Species
- Dogs: DEA 1.1, 1.2, 3, 4, 5, 6, 7 and 8, and *Dal*
- Cats: Feline AB blood groups (type A, B or AB) and *Mik*

Breed
- Dogs: Breed-associated differences in the frequency of blood types are possible but not described to date, with the exception of the lack of the *Dal* blood type in some Dalmatians.
- Cats: Significant geographic and breed-associated differences in the frequencies of these blood types have been found.

Breed	% Type A	% Type B
Abyssinian	84	16
Birman	82	18
British shorthair	64	36
Burmese	100	0
Cornish rex	67	33
Devon rex	59	41
Domestic shorthair USA	96–99	1–4
Exotic shorthair	73	27
Himalayan	94	6
Japanese bobtail	84	16
Maine coon	97	3
Norwegian forest	93	7
Persian	86	14
Scottish fold	81	19
Siamese	100	0
Sphinx	83	17

Age
None

Gender
None

Pregnancy
None

LIMITATIONS OF THE TEST
Sensitivity, Specificity, and Positive and Negative Predictive Values
N/A

Valid If Run in a Human Lab?
No.

CLINICAL PERSPECTIVE
- It is recommended to blood type canine blood donors and patients for at least DEA 1.1 prior to transfusion to limit sensitization by transfusion, because DEA 1.1 is recognized to be the most antigenic and clinically significant blood type.
- A canine patient negative for a given blood type can become sensitized and produce specific antibodies against this blood type if transfused with positive blood. A subsequent transfusion of positive blood may lead to an immediate hemolytic transfusion reaction. Such transfusion reactions have been documented against DEA 1.1, 4, and one common antigen.
- The sensitization (i.e., the production of antibodies in negative dogs) against DEA 4 or the *Dal* antigen is particularly challenging because finding compatible blood may be extremely difficult given the high prevalence of those blood types in the canine population.
- Because of naturally occurring alloantibodies, feline donors and recipients should always be blood typed prior to transfusion. As little as 1 mL of type A blood can lead to a fatal hemolytic transfusion reaction if given to a type B cat.
- Type A and AB kittens born to type B queens are at risk of developing neonatal isoerythrolysis caused by the presence of strong anti-A alloantibodies in the colostrum of type B queens. The disease is characterized by a severe hemolytic anemia and possible nephropathy, as well as other organ failures. To avoid neonatal isoerythrolysis, it is recommended to blood type breeding mates, particularly in breeds with a high incidence of type B cats.
- Any dogs and cats that have undergone transfusion >4 days earlier should be crossmatched to look for the presence of antibodies before receiving additional blood even when getting it from the same donor.

MISCELLANEOUS

ANCILLARY TESTS
Crossmatch

SYNONYMS
None

SEE ALSO
Blackwell's Five-Minute Veterinary Consult: Canine and Feline Topics
- Anemia, Nonregenerative
- Anemia, Regenerative
- Blood Transfusion Reactions

Related Topics in This Book
- Crossmatch
- Hematocrit
- Red Blood Cell Count
- Red Blood Cell Morphology

ABBREVIATIONS
DEA = dog erythrocyte antigen

Suggested Reading
Blais MC, Berman L, Oakley DA, Giger U. Canine Dal blood type: A red cell antigen lacking in some Dalmatians. *J Vet Intern Med* 2007; 21: 281–286.

Giger U. Blood typing and crossmatching to ensure compatible transfusions. In: Bonagura JD, ed. *Kirk's Current Veterinary Therapy*, 13th ed. Philadelphia: WB Saunders, 2000: 396–399.

Giger U, Gelens CJ, Callan MB, Oakley DA. An acute hemolytic transfusion reaction caused by dog erythrocyte antigen 1.1 incompatibility in a previously sensitized dog. *J Am Vet Med Assoc* 1995; 206: 1358–1362.

Griot-Wenk ME, Giger U. Feline transfusion medicine: Blood types and their clinical importance. *Vet Clin North Am Small Anim Pract* 1995; 25: 1305–1322.

Hale AS. Canine blood groups and their importance in veterinary transfusion medicine. *Vet Clin North Am Small Anim Pract* 1995; 25: 1323–1332.

Hohenhaus AE. Importance of blood groups and blood group antibodies in companion animals. *Transfus Med Rev* 2004; 18: 117–126.

Weinstein NM, Blais MC, Harris K, *et al.* A newly recognized blood group in domestic shorthair cats: The *Mik* red cell antigen. *J Vet Intern Med* 2007; 21: 287–292.

INTERNET RESOURCES

DiaMed Veterinary Diagnostics: Veterinary diagnostics, http://www.diamed.ch/products.aspx?mode=prod_group&id=22&navvis.

DMS Laboratories, http://www.rapidvet.com/.

Midwest Animal Blood Services: Laboratory testing, http://www.midwestabs.com/erythrocyte.htm.

Penn Veterinary Medicine: Feline AB and canine DEA 1.1 blood typing, http://w3.vet.upenn.edu/research/centers/penngen/services/transfusionlab/bloodtype.html.

AUTHOR NAME

Marie-Claude Blais

BASICS

TYPE OF PROCEDURE
Biopsy

PROCEDURE EXPLANATION AND RELATED PHYSIOLOGY
Bone lesions found on radiographic examination may have characteristic appearances, but a definitive diagnosis can not be made without direct examination of the structure and cell content of the affected region. Because bone is a structural tissue, it is often not appropriate to remove large portions because this will predispose it to fracture. Because the sample must therefore be small, the expectation may only be to determine the basic pathologic process (i.e., neoplasia vs inflammation). Again, because the sample must be small, it is important for the clinician to select a site that contains the primary pathology, and not just reactive tissue around, nor the necrotic tissue of the center of, the lesion.

In patients with suspected pathologic fracture, the primary process must be identified rapidly to plan appropriate therapy. Frozen section enables more complete evaluation but is often unavailable. If representative tissue is available, examination of roll preparations or squeeze smears may be sufficient to rule neoplasia in or out.

Specimens can be obtained via a closed technique using a large-bore needle (e.g., Jamshidi) or Michele trephine, or via an open technique with an osteotome, bone cutter, or saw.

INDICATIONS
- Determine the cause of lesions that are osteolytic, osteoproductive, or both.
- Identify a neoplastic process and, ideally, characterize its type and malignancy.
- Identify causative organisms in osteomyelitis (e.g., bacterial, fungal).
- Rule out neoplastic or infectious causes (e.g., cyst, avascular necrosis).

CONTRAINDICATIONS
- Patients receiving anticoagulant therapy are at higher risk for uncontrolled bleeding.
- If a lesion is likely neoplastic, and local surgical resection is being considered, biopsy may lead to seeding of the exit path of the needle or trephine.

POTENTIAL COMPLICATIONS
- Bleeding may occur if a major vessel is damaged by passage of the instrument or if the lesion is highly vascular.
- The bone may fracture if extensive osteolysis already exists or if a relatively large biopsy instrument weakens the bone.

CLIENT EDUCATION
- Bone biopsy will require heavy sedation or general anesthesia, so patients must be withheld from food for at least 12 h prior to the procedure.
- After the procedure, the patient will likely be painful or lame. Restricting activity for 1–2 weeks will help improve patient comfort and reduce the likelihood of fracture.

BODY SYSTEMS ASSESSED
Musculoskeletal

PROCEDURE

PATIENT PREPARATION
Preprocedure Medication or Preparation
Careful review of the lesion on radiographs and comparison to regional landmarks are necessary so that the biopsy will be located in the optimal position. In lesions that are lytic centrally and productive on the periphery, the ideal site to obtain tissue is in the intermediate zone. The central, lytic area may be necrotic, and the response around the edges may just be reaction to the expansile process.

Anesthesia or Sedation
Most biopsies can be performed with the patient under heavy sedation with or without local analgesia. Open biopsy of deep lesions may require general anesthesia.

Patient Positioning
This will vary depending on the location of the lesion. As some force may be needed to advance the biopsy instrument, techniques to prevent patient movement should be considered (e.g., manual support, limb ties, body taping).

Patient Monitoring
Heart and respiratory rates increase, or patient movement may indicate inadequate analgesia or anesthesia.

Equipment or Supplies
- Clippers
- Skin-preparation solutions (e.g., alcohol, chlorhexidine scrub)
- Sterile gloves
- A scalpel
- A Jamshidi needle (16 or 18 gauge) or Michele trephine (3- or 4-mm core diameter). The trephine will provide a larger specimen but also create a much larger defect than will the Jamshidi needle.
- 5 or 6 microscope slides
- Sterile curettes for culture, or transport medium jars
- 2 or 3 small jars of formalin
- Gauze sponges—4 × 4 inches
- Open surgical biopsy
  - Surgical drapes and instruments
  - Osteotome and mallet, or bone cutters or saw

TECHNIQUE
- Locate the site(s) and plan the direction of entry.
- Clip the hair over sufficient area to allow palpation of the lesion and identification of important regional landmarks.
- Prepare the skin.

Closed
- Perform a stab incision at the surface of the lesion.
- Drive the biopsy instrument into the lesion. In most instances, only 1 side is penetrated (Figure 1).
- Wiggle the instrument to break off the base of the core.
- Withdraw instrument. Place your thumb over top of instrument to create a vacuum in the needle to help hold the specimen.
- Culture the tip of the instrument, if indicated.
- Deliver the specimen.
- *Repeat.* Two specimens from different regions of the lesion will increase the diagnostic accuracy.

Open
- Use a surgical approach to the lesion.
- Excise the specimen with appropriate instrument(s).

SAMPLE HANDLING
- Culture: If infection is suspected, a portion of the specimen can be delivered sterile into transport medium.
- Cytology: A roll preparation can be used for cytologic evaluation. The core specimen is placed between 2 microscope slides and gently rolled. Rolling the sample too aggressively may disrupt the cellular architecture.
- Histopathologic evaluation: Place the sample in formalin.

APPROPRIATE AFTERCARE
Postprocedure Patient Monitoring
Maintain pressure on the site until hemorrhage has stopped.

Nursing Care
Assess the level of patient discomfort, and administer analgesic medications as required.

Dietary Modification
None

Medication Requirements
Analgesic medications may be necessary for 12–48 h, depending on the extent of the biopsy.

BONE BIOPSY

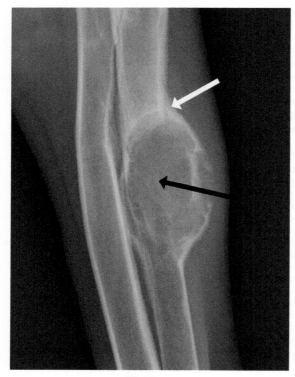

Figure 1

Careful assessment of the structure of the lesion is necessary so that tissue representative of the pathologic process is sampled. Bone on the periphery (*white arrow*) will likely be reactive and not contain the primary pathology. Tissue from the center of a large, lytic lesion (*black arrow*) may be necrotic.

Restrictions on Activity
Limited for 1–2 weeks. Longer restriction may be needed if fracture risk is high.

Anticipated Recovery Time
Ranges from 1 day to 2 weeks, depending on size of the biopsy sample.

 INTERPRETATION

NORMAL FINDINGS OR RANGE
Normal bone tissue and marrow

ABNORMAL VALUES
- Neoplasia
  - Malignant, primary—osteosarcoma, chondrosarcoma, synovial cell sarcoma
  - Malignant, metastatic—osteosarcoma, adenosarcoma, multiple myeloma
  - Benign—paraosteal osteoma, tumoral calcinosis, multiple cartilaginous exostoses, dystrophic calcification
- Infection: bacterial or fungal osteomyelitis
- Avascular necrosis: reparative tissue peripherally, absence of viable osteocytes

CRITICAL VALUES
Iatrogenic fracture while advancing the biopsy instrument

INTERFERING FACTORS
Drugs That May Alter Results of the Procedure
None

Conditions That May Interfere with Performing the Procedure
None

Procedure Techniques or Handling That May Alter Results
- Centrally located specimens may contain just necrotic material.
- Peripherally located specimens may contain just reactive bone.

Influence of Signalment on Performing and Interpreting the Procedure
Species
None

Breed
None

Age
None

Gender
None

Pregnancy
None

CLINICAL PERSPECTIVE
- The closed approach should be used for more superficial lesions and where the likelihood is high of obtaining diagnostic tissue.
- An open approach should be used for deep or small lesions or for lesions from which it is felt little tissue may be retrieved.

 MISCELLANEOUS

ANCILLARY TESTS
- Thoracic radiographs for metastasis evaluation
- A thorough orthopedic examination for other sites and for suitability of the patient for amputation

SYNONYMS
None

SEE ALSO
Blackwell's Five-Minute Veterinary Consult: Canine and Feline Topics
- Chondrosarcoma, Bone
- Fibrosarcoma, Bone
- Hemangiosarcoma, Bone
- Osteomyelitis
- Osteosarcoma

Related Topics in This Book
- Bacterial Culture and Sensitivity
- Bone Marrow Aspirate and Biopsy
- Bone Marrow Aspirate Cytology: Microscopic Evaluation

ABBREVIATIONS
None

Suggested Reading
Chun R. Common malignant musculoskeletal neoplasms of dogs and cats. *Vet Clin North Am Small Anim Pract* 2005; 35: 1155–1167.
Powers BE, LaRue SM, Withrow SJ, *et al.* Jamshidi needle biopsy for diagnosis of bone lesions in small animals. *J Am Vet Med Assoc* 1988; 193: 205–210.

INTERNET RESOURCES
WebMD, Information and Resources: Bone biopsy, http://www.webmd.com/a-to-z-guides/Bone-Biopsy.

AUTHOR NAME
Simon C. Roe

BASICS

TYPE OF PROCEDURE
Diagnostic sample collection

PROCEDURE EXPLANATION AND RELATED PHYSIOLOGY
Cytologic examination of samples collected via bone marrow aspiration (BMA) is an important step in assessing the presence or absence, quantity, and ratio of precursors of the RBC, platelet, and WBC lines in patients with increases or decreases in peripheral blood cell counts. Cytologic examination is also an important part of staging patients with hematologic and certain other malignancies, where evidence of bone marrow involvement is associated with a higher stage of disease. Histologic examination of samples collected via bone marrow biopsy (BMB) provides additional information regarding tissue architecture within the bone marrow and is an important step in evaluating primary bone marrow disorders, such as aplastic anemia, nonregenerative anemia, myelodysplasia and myelofibrosis.

Poorly prepared smears or inadequately harvested core biopsy samples can make interpretation difficult.

INDICATIONS
- BMA
  - To identify cell types, quantity, and ratio of precursor cells within the bone marrow (e.g., when peripheral cytopenias are noted)
  - To identify the presence of suspected infectious agents
  - To assess marrow involvement in neoplastic conditions
- BMA provides information on the cell types present but no information on bone marrow structure and may therefore be less useful for identifying structural bone marrow diseases. Therefore, BMB is indicated for animals with suspected structural bone marrow abnormalities (aplastic anemia, nonregenerative anemia, myelodysplasia, myelofibrosis).

CONTRAINDICATIONS
None

POTENTIAL COMPLICATIONS
Hemorrhage is a risk but not expected to be clinically significant, since bleeding will occur primarily into bone marrow.

CLIENT EDUCATION
- The procedure has minimal risk.
- Mild discomfort associated with the procedure can be alleviated through the use of a local anesthetic, heavy sedation, or light anesthesia.

BODY SYSTEMS ASSESSED
Hemic, lymphatic, and immune

PROCEDURE

PATIENT PREPARATION
Preprocedure Medication or Preparation
Hair clipping and aseptic skin preparation are indicated prior to BMA or BMB.

Anesthesia or Sedation
Local anesthesia (lidocaine) in conjunction with heavy sedation or light anesthesia

Patient Positioning
- Palpate the desired site of sample collection (amenable locations include the head of the humerus, iliac crest, and trochanteric fossa) and position the animal accordingly.

- *Humerus*: Lateral recumbency with the patient's foreleg rotated externally and extended caudally 45°, keeping the leg parallel to the table or floor
- *Iliac crest*: On the sternum or belly with the patient's legs extended forward, rounding the lumbosacral area
- *Trochanteric fossa*: Lateral recumbency

Patient Monitoring
- Monitoring for adequate analgesia and level of sedation
- Monitoring for bleeding at the aspiration or biopsy site

Equipment or Supplies
- A sterile scrub
- Sterile gloves
- Sterile 4 × 4-inch gauze
- A no. 11 blade
- 1 mL of 2% lidocaine

Bone Marrow Aspiration
- A Rosenthal or Illinois BMA needle
- A 6- or 12-mL syringe
- EDTA solution (if available)
- A watchglass (if available)
- Pipette or hematocrit tubes (if available)
- Glass slides

Bone Marrow Biopsy
- A Jamshidi infant needle or pediatric BMB needle
- A 6- or 12-mL syringe
- A jar containing 10% buffered formalin for sample

TECHNIQUE
- BMA or BMB generally requires 2 people: 1 to position the animal, monitor sedation or anesthesia, and assist with sample handling, and the other to collect the sample.
- Clip an approximately 5-cm² area and perform a surgical scrub. After surgical preparation of the site, infiltrate the area with 0.5–1.0 mL of local anesthetic (e.g., 2% lidocaine), making sure to also block the periosteum. Follow with a final surgical scrub.
- Make a small stab incision with the 11 blade.

Bone Marrow Aspiration
Insert the bone marrow needle through the stab incision made in the skin and subcutaneous tissues. Position the needle on the periosteum. Holding the instrument closely between the thumb and index finger and within the closed palm, begin to rotate the instrument back and forth with gentle pressure until it is solidly within the marrow cavity. Care must be taken to keep the needle and instrument in line; avoid rocking the needle during its advancement. Firm adequate placement can be determined by the ability to move the limb by moving the inserted instrument gently side to side. Once positioned in the marrow cavity, the cap and stylet are removed and a 6- or 12-mL syringe (containing 0.5 mL of EDTA, if available) is attached to the instrument and used to aspirate with negative pressure. As soon as marrow is seen within the syringe, negative pressure is released to minimize dilution or contamination of the sample with peripheral blood. The syringe is then detached and its contents emptied in single small drops onto a series of glass slides, placing 1 drop per slide (alternatively, the contents may be emptied into a watchglass containing 0.5–1.0 mL of EDTA). Working quickly to avoid clotting of the sample, the bone marrow drops are smeared onto each of the slides (see the "Fine-Needle Aspiration" chapter for slide preparation technique). Alternatively, if a watchglass containing EDTA is used, individual bone marrow particles may be collected using a pipette or hematocrit tube, transferred to the slides, and the sample then smeared along the length of the slide; this technique reduces the risk of clotting prior to slide preparation.

Bone Marrow Biopsy
Insert the biopsy instrument through the stab incision made in the skin and subcutaneous tissues. Position the needle on the periosteum.

Hold the instrument so that the plastic handle rests in the palm and the needle extends between the index and middle fingers. Close the fingers over the plastic handle and palm and begin to rotate the instrument back and forth with gentle pressure until it penetrates the outer cortex and enters the marrow cavity. Once securely positioned within through the outer cortex, the stylet is removed and the needle is advanced 1–2 cm within the marrow by continuing to rotate the instrument back and forth with gentle pressure. At this point, a core of bone marrow should be lodged within the hollow needle. To break off the core within the needle and ensure it is removed along with the instrument, sharply twist the instrument several times in a clockwise direction, followed by several twists in a counterclockwise direction, and then firmly rock the instrument in a circular motion in 1 direction and then the other. Finally, attach a 6- or 12-mL syringe to the end of the instrument and apply a single burst of negative pressure. The instrument can then be removed from the bone by rotation and steady traction. Once the instrument is removed, use the "shepherd's crook" inserted retrograde though the needle to push the bone marrow core biopsy gently out through the top of the instrument and place the sample in formalin.

SAMPLE HANDLING
- *BMA*: Air-dried samples can be stored at room temperature, though samples should be fixed and stained as soon after collection as possible (within 3–7 days) for optimal assessment of cellular morphology.
- *BMB*: Collected samples should be placed in 10% buffered formal for submission to the histopathology laboratory.
- A peripheral blood sample should be collected and submitted at the time of either BMA or BMB.

APPROPRIATE AFTERCARE
Postprocedure Patient Monitoring
- Monitor for evidence of mild superficial hemorrhage at the BMA or BMB site.
- Monitor for evidence of discomfort at the BMA or BMB site.

Nursing Care
None

Dietary Modification
None

Medication Requirements
None

Restrictions on Activity
None

Anticipated Recovery Time
Immediate

INTERPRETATION

NORMAL FINDINGS OR RANGE
Bone marrow should be evaluated by a trained pathologist. Factors assessed include cellularity (normal range, 25% fat and 75% cells to 75% fat and 25% cells; varies according to age), evaluation of megakaryocyte series (normal range, approximately 4–50 megakaryocytes per spicule), evaluation of erythrocyte series (abundance, proportions, morphology), evaluation of granulocytic series (abundance, proportions, morphology), evaluation of myeloid/erythroid ratio (normal range, 0.75:1 to 2:1), examination for organisms (e.g., *Histoplasma capsulatum*, *Leishmania donovani*, *Toxoplasma gondii*, *Cytauxzoon felis*, *Ehrlichia* spp.), and examination for erythrophagocytosis, plasmacytosis, iron-containing pigments, neoplastic cell infiltration, and myelofibrosis.

ABNORMAL VALUES
- Decreased overall cellularity
- Increases or decreases in megakaryocyte numbers

- Abnormal numbers, proportions, or morphology of erythrocyte or granulocyte series
- Presence of infectious organisms
- Evidence of erythrophagocytosis, plasmacytosis, or decreased iron-containing pigments
- Neoplastic cell infiltration

CRITICAL VALUES
None

INTERFERING FACTORS
Drugs That May Alter Results of the Procedure
- Administration of immunosuppressive therapies (as for suspected immune-mediated cytopenias) prior to sample collection may alter interpretation.
- Administration of corticosteroids or other chemotherapeutic agents prior to sample collection may alter the presence or number of neoplastic cells.

Conditions That May Interfere with Performing the Procedure
None

Procedure Techniques or Handling That May Alter Results
- Inadequate sample collection
- Excessive aspiration with BMA may lead to dilution or contamination of the sample with peripheral blood.

Influence of Signalment on Performing and Interpreting the Procedure
Species
None

Breed
Some breed-related variability; for example, increased hematocrit, mild thrombocytopenia, mild leukopenia may be seen in greyhounds.

Age
Normal bone marrow cellularity decreases with age: Samples from juvenile, adult, and geriatric animals contain approximately 25% fat and 75% cells, 50% fat and 50% cells, and 75% fat and 25% cells, respectively.

Gender
None

Pregnancy
None

CLINICAL PERSPECTIVE
Cytologic examination of samples collected via BMA is an important step in assessing the presence or absence, quantity, and ratio of precursors of the RBC, platelet, and WBC lines in patients with increases or decreases in peripheral blood cell counts. Assessment can support a diagnosis of immune-mediated cytopenias and be used to provide information on prognosis and predicted time to recovery following initiation of treatment. Cytologic examination is also an important part of staging patients with hematologic and certain other malignancies, where evidence of bone marrow involvement is associated with a higher stage of disease. Histologic examination of samples collected via BMB provides additional information regarding tissue architecture within the bone marrow and is an important step in evaluating primary bone marrow disorders, such as aplastic anemia, nonregenerative anemia, myelodysplasia, and myelofibrosis.

MISCELLANEOUS

ANCILLARY TESTS
A CBC should be performed in conjunction with BMA and BMB.

SYNONYMS
None

SEE ALSO

Blackwell's Five-Minute Veterinary Consult: Canine and Feline Topics
- Anemia, Aplastic
- Anemia, Immune-Mediated
- Anemia, Nonregenerative
- Myelodysplastic Syndromes
- Myeloproliferative Disorders
- Thrombocytopenia

Related Topics in This Book
- Bone Marrow Aspirate Cytology: Microscopic Evaluation
- Fine-Needle Aspiration

ABBREVIATIONS
- BMA = bone marrow aspiration
- BMB = bone marrow biopsy

Suggested Reading
Cowell RL, Tyler RD, Meinkoth JH. *Diagnostic Cytology and Hematology of the Dog and Cat.* St Louis: CV Mosby, 1999.

INTERNET RESOURCES
None

AUTHOR NAME
Laurel E. Williams

BONE MARROW ASPIRATE CYTOLOGY: MICROSCOPIC EVALUATION

BASICS

TYPE OF SPECIMEN
Tissue

TEST EXPLANATION AND RELATED PHYSIOLOGY
Since bone marrow is the major hematopoietic organ of the body, examination of it aids in evaluating a multitude of hematologic disorders, such as underlying diseases that decrease or increase the numbers of cells in peripheral circulation. The most common indication for microscopic bone marrow evaluation is a peripheral blood abnormality that cannot be readily explained by a good medical history or by physical examination, chemistry profile, and/or other diagnostic procedures. In addition, bone marrow evaluation may aid in monitoring disease progression and/or response to therapy, determination of disease prognosis, and staging of certain neoplasms. Finally, body iron stores can be estimated, particularly if special stains are used, and occult infectious agents may be identified. A CBC collected within 24 h of marrow collection is an absolute requirement for appropriate interpretation of findings.

In young animals, active hematopoiesis occurs throughout the skeleton in both the long bones (e.g., humerus, femur) and flat bones (e.g., ribs, pelvis). However, the hematopoietic activity of long bones regresses with maturity such that active hematopoiesis in normal adult animals is restricted to the flat bones and extremities of the long bones (e.g., proximal humerus or femur); the central area of the long bones is composed predominantly of adipose tissue. Furthermore, hematopoietic regions of adult animals contain a higher percentage of fat as compared to these areas in young animals. Thus, knowledge of the age-related anatomic distribution of hematopoietic tissue is invaluable to practitioners collecting their own samples so that an appropriate, representative specimen may be collected.

Active hematopoietic tissue is extremely vascular and the spaces between vascular sinuses are filled with hematopoietic cells. The hematopoietic areas are bordered by the endothelium lining the vascular sinuses and are given structural scaffolding by adventitial cells. Hematopoietic tissue is predominantly composed of megakaryocyte, erythrocyte, granulocyte, and monocyte cell precursors in various stages of maturation. Low numbers of resident macrophages, lymphocytes, plasma cells, and mast cells, as well as a variable amount of adipose tissue, are also normally present.

Collection of both aspirates and core biopsy specimens is technically simple. Aspirate and core biopsy specimens are often collected as part of the same procedure, although, in some instances, an aspirate alone may yield sufficient information. Collection of an aspirate is easier, faster, and less expensive than a biopsy. Aspirated specimens also enable detailed analysis of cell populations, individual cell identification, and morphologic evaluation and are more amenable to cytochemical staining and immunocytochemistry. However, aspirates do not preserve architecture and may not be representative of the marrow as a whole. Myelofibrosis, regardless of the cause and, to a certain extent, the severity, often exfoliates poorly and may yield an insufficient specimen, so a core biopsy is crucial in these instances. Core biopsies have a longer turnaround time and are more expensive, but their utility lies in the preservation of tissue architecture and more accurate impression of overall cellularity. Additionally, cell arrangement, necrosis, infiltrative patterns, myelofibrosis, absolute megakaryocyte numbers, and quantification of iron stores can be better assessed in a core biopsy sample.

Depending on the practitioner's discretion, the aspirate may be evaluated in house or sent to a pathologist. Practitioners who are reasonably comfortable with cytology may attempt a subjective in-house examination. Clarification by a boarded pathologist always remains a viable option if uncertainty exists. Prior to laboratory submission, a slide should be stained to assess whether it contains an adequate number of well-preserved hematopoietic unit particles or spicules. Spicules grossly appear as fatty streaks on unstained preparations and as intensely staining blue areas on stained preparations. If the slide is satisfactory, the stained and, preferably, additional unstained slides may then be sent to a diagnostic laboratory.

INDICATIONS
- Peripheral blood abnormalities
  - Unexplained, persistent decreases in cell numbers, including nonregenerative or poorly regenerative anemia, leukopenia, or thrombocytopenia
  - Unexplained, persistent elevations in cell numbers
  - Atypical cells in peripheral blood
- Clinical staging of malignancy
- Unexplained hyperproteinemia or monoclonal gammopathy
- Unexplained hypercalcemia
- Fever of unknown origin, especially in searching for occult disease, including infectious agents
- Assessment of body iron stores
- Suspicion of osteomyelitis or infiltrative or proliferative bone marrow disease as may or may not be suggested by diagnostic imaging
- A bone marrow core biopsy is indicated when repeated aspiration attempts, particularly if different sites are sampled, fail to obtain adequate marrow samples.

CONTRAINDICATIONS
None

POTENTIAL COMPLICATIONS
None

CLIENT EDUCATION
None

BODY SYSTEMS ASSESSED
Hemic, lymphatic, and immune

SAMPLE

COLLECTION
Marrow from wing of ilium or proximal humerus or femur, prepared onto carefully labeled standard-sized glass microscope slides

HANDLING
Transport in an appropriate protective slide container

STORAGE
Store at room temperature, protected from light. Avoid its exposure to extreme temperatures, humidity, and formalin fumes.

STABILITY
- Stained slides are stable for months to years.
- Unstained slides are stable for 1 week or more.

PROTOCOL
- Subjective evaluation of the marrow begins with a low-power (4×–10×) magnification of overall cellularity, megakaryocyte numbers, and iron content.
  - Evaluate cellularity: Identify large, intact particles and compare the proportion of darkly staining, blue-to-purple material (hematopoietic tissue) to the proportion of colorless adipose tissue within the particle to determine a rough percentage. Particles of normal adult animals are composed of one-third to two-thirds cells, with the remainder being composed of fat. Estimates of cellularity will be inaccurate if the number of particles on the slide is low.

BONE MARROW ASPIRATE CYTOLOGY: MICROSCOPIC EVALUATION

• Assess megakaryocytes: Approximately 2–7 megakaryocytes are normally associated with each particle, although the exact number varies by species and the technique used to make the cytologic preparation. Megakaryocytes are the largest of the hematopoietic cells and are easily seen at low-power magnification. Mature megakaryocytes should predominate; they have abundant pale basophilic cytoplasm with fine magenta granules and 8 or more nuclei fused into a dense, lobulated mass.

• Assess iron stores: A few small clumps of brown to black material per particle representing iron stored in the form of hemosiderin are routinely identified in the bone marrow of normal dogs. Prussian blue reaction should be used to confirm the presence or absence of iron. Stainable iron is usually absent in normal bone marrow from healthy cats.

• At high power (50×–100× magnification), attempt a general assessment of cell distribution [myeloid/erythroid (M/E)ratio].

   • Erythroid precursors appear as smaller, darker cells. They generally have darker basophilic cytoplasm and round nuclei with condensed chromatin.

   • Myeloid precursors are larger and paler with light blue cytoplasm that may contain magenta primary granules or secondary granules with a round, indented, or U-shaped nucleus. Secondary granules can be eosinophilic, basophilic, or nonstaining (i.e., in neutrophil precursors).

   • In healthy animals, there are approximately equal numbers of erythroid and myeloid precursors that should be overwhelmingly predominated by the more mature precursor stages.

• Other cells, such as macrophages, lymphocytes, plasma cells, and mast cells, are normally found in low numbers.

• If any single type of cell appears to predominate, or if unusual morphologies are encountered, evaluation by a board-certified pathologist is recommended.

INTERPRETATION

NORMAL FINDINGS OR RANGE
• Cellularity (adults): 33%–66% hematopoietic cells, with the remaining percentages being adipose tissue
• Megakaryocytes: 2–7 megakaryocytes per spicule; highly variable depending on the technique used to prepare the slide
• M/E ratio: 0.75–2.53 (dogs) and 1.21–2.16 (cats)

ABNORMAL VALUES
Values above or below the reference ranges

CRITICAL VALUES
None

INTERFERING FACTORS
Drugs That May Alter Results or Interpretation
Drugs That Interfere with Test Methodology
None

Drugs That Alter Physiology
Some drugs have been associated with toxic effects on hematopoietic cells, including diethylstilbestrol, phenylbutazone, chloramphenicol (especially cats), sulfadiazine, methimazole, albendazole, phenobarbital, and griseofulvin.

Disorders That May Alter Results
• Poorly cellular aspirates may occur with hypocellular marrow, stromal reactions (e.g., myelofibrosis), and neoplasms resulting in myelophthisis (e.g., mesenchymal neoplasms).
• Chronic blood loss anemia may lead to megakaryocytic hyperplasia even though the animal has a normal platelet count.

Collection Techniques or Handling That May Alter Results
• Inappropriate collection site (i.e., an area not actively involved in hematopoiesis)
• An insufficient number of particles
• Excessive pressure when preparing cytologic slides or delayed collection (>30 min) after animal's death may result in lysed cells.
• Delayed processing
• Clotted aspirates will have a reduced number of cells and skewed differential cell counts.

Influence of Signalment
Species
• Cats normally lack stainable iron, regardless of their age.
• Subtle variations in differential cell percentages (e.g., cats may have slightly more numerous lymphocytes than dogs)

Breed
None

Age
• Young animals have active hematopoietic tissue throughout long and flat bones. Adult animals exhibit the most active hematopoiesis in their flat bones and the extremities of their long bones. The central area of long bones contains abundant adipose tissue and very little active hematopoietic tissue.
• Older dogs often have abundant stainable iron, whereas younger dogs do not.

Gender
None

Pregnancy
None

LIMITATIONS OF THE TEST
Sensitivity, Specificity, and Positive and Negative Predictive Values
N/A

Valid If Run in a Human Lab?
Yes.

CLINICAL PERSPECTIVE
Cytologic findings must be interpreted in light of the medical history, clinical findings, CBC, and results from other diagnostic tests and procedures. A bone marrow aspirate cannot be adequately interpreted without a concurrent CBC, particularly with regard to assessment of the M/E ratio.

MISCELLANEOUS

ANCILLARY TESTS
• Concurrent CBC (obtained within the last 24 h)
• Blood film for morphologic assessment of circulating blood cells
• Concurrent bone marrow aspirate and bone marrow core biopsy sample

Causes of Abnormal Values

Marrow component	High values (hyperplasia)	Low values (hypoplasia)
Iron stores	Hemolysis Previous blood transfusions Anemia of inflammatory disease Parenteral iron supplementation	Iron deficiency

Overall cellularity	Proliferative response to peripheral demand (see specific lineages)
	  Anemia and/or hypoxemia (erythroid hyperplasia)
	  Purulent inflammation (granulocytic hyperplasia)
	  Thrombocytopenia (megakaryocytic hyperplasia)
	Neoplasia, primary or metastatic
	  Acute lymphoblastic leukemia
	  Acute myeloid leukemia
	  Lymphoma, stage V
	  Multiple myeloma
	  Malignant histiocytosis
	  Mastocytosis
		Generalized hypoplasia/aplasia
		  Certain antibiotics (e.g., trimethoprim-sulfadiazine, cephalosporins, chloramphenicol)
		  Exogenous or endogenous estrogens (dogs and ferrets)
		  Anticonvulsants (e.g., phenobarbital)
		  Phenylbutazone (dogs)
		  Griseofulvin (cats)
		  Thiacetarsamide, meclofenamic acid, quinidine (a possible cause in dogs)
		  Albendazole
		  Chemotherapy
		  Radiation
		  Myelonecrosis (may have degenerate cells)
		  Myelofibrosis
		  Canine parvovirus infections (erythroid and myeloid hypoplasia)
		  FeLV infection (especially with feline parvovirus infection)
		  Severe *Ehrlichia canis* infection
		  Primary immune-mediated destruction of hematopoietic precursor cells
		  Idiopathic

Erythrocytes	Effective erythroid hyperplasia in response to anemia and/or hypoxemia
	Ineffective erythroid hyperplasia
	  Severe iron deficiency
	  Folate deficiency
	  Certain myeloproliferative and myelodysplastic disorders
	  Congenital dyserythropoiesis
	  Immune-mediated hemolytic anemia in which metarubricytes and reticulocytes are targeted (dogs)
	Response to Epo treatment
	Renal or other Epo-secreting neoplasms
		Selective erythroid hypoplasia
		  Parvovirus vaccination?
		  Gray collies with cyclic hematopoiesis (followed by erythroid hyperplasia)
		  Chloramphenicol (especially in cats)
		  Lymphoid malignancy
		  Immune mediated, targeting early erythroid precursors
		  Immune mediated, associated with recombinant Epo therapy
		  FeLV type C infection
		  Dogs with idiopathic myelofibrosis
		  Anemia of inflammatory disease (concomitant granulocytic hyperplasia)
		  Endocrinopathies (e.g., hypothyroidism, hypoadrenocorticism, hypopituitarism, hypoandrogenism; usually does not increase M/E ratio)
		  Chronic renal disease (usually does not increase M/E ratio)

Neutrophils	Effective granulocytic hyperplasia
	  Proliferative response to purulent inflammation (granulocytic hyperplasia)
	  Dogs with β_2-integrin adhesion molecule deficiency
	  Gray collies with cyclic hematopoiesis
	  Early estrogen toxicity (with concomitant erythroid and megakaryocytic aplasia)
	Ineffective neutrophilic hyperplasia
	  Myelodysplastic disorders
	  Acute myelocytic leukemia
	  Neutropenic cats with FeLV and/or FIV infection
	  Dogs given anticonvulsants that have a peripheral neutropenia
	  Infectious agent in marrow
	    Leishmaniasis
	    Histoplasmosis
	Response to G-CSF treatment
	Paraneoplastic neutrophilia
		Selective neutrophilic hypoplasia
		  Azathioprine (cats)
		  Griseofulvin (cats with dermatophyte infections; risk increased in FIV-positive cats)
		  Methimazole (reported in cats)
		  Recombinant G-CSF from another species (similar to recombinant Epo–induced anemia)
		  Canine and feline parvovirus infection (concurrent erythroid hypoplasia)
		  Gray collies with cyclic hematopoiesis (followed by neutrophilic hyperplasia)
		  FeLV-induced cyclic hematopoiesis
		  Immune mediated

(Continued)

BONE MARROW ASPIRATE CYTOLOGY: MICROSCOPIC EVALUATION

Marrow component	High values (hyperplasia)	Low values (hypoplasia)
Eosinophils	Parasitic disease (especially nematode and fluke infestation) Inflammation of organs rich in mast cells (skin, lung, intestine, uterus) IgE-mediated allergic hypersensivity reactions Eosinophilic granulomas Hypereosinophilic syndrome Eosinophilic leukemia Myelodysplastic disorders Mast cell and other tumors (uncommon to rare)	
Basophils	Usually associated with same disorders causing eosinophilia Dirofilariasis (dogs and cats) Lymphomatoid granulomatosis Basophilic leukemia Myelodysplastic disorders	
Megakaryocytes	Primary and secondary immune-mediated thrombocytopenia Ongoing intravascular coagulation Hypersplenism Vascular injury Infections (e.g., early *Ehrlichia canis*) and toxicoses causing platelet destruction Thrombocythemia	Selective megakaryocytic hypoplasia Immune mediated Drug induced: hypoplasia usually generalized, but megakaryocytes may be specifically decreased [e.g., dapsone (in dogs) and ribavarin (in cats, concomitant erythroid hypoplasia possible)] Meclofenamic acid Phenylbutazone Trimethoprim-sulfadiazine Chemotherapy

- FeLV and FIV assays
- *Ehrlichia* spp. titer
- Serum urea nitrogen and/or serum creatinine concentration to evaluate renal function
- Immunofluorescent assay for antibodies to hematopoietic cells
- Immunocytochemistry, immunophenotyping, and cytochemical stains to determine clonality and lineage of abnormal cells identified in marrow
- Perl's staining for iron stores, which form dark blue prussian blue pigment

SYNONYMS
None

SEE ALSO
Blackwell's Five-Minute Veterinary Consult: Canine and Feline Topics
- Anemia, Aplastic
- Anemia, Nonregenerative
- Ehrlichiosis
- Feline Leukemia Virus Infection (FeLV)
- Leukemia, Acute Lymphoblastic
- Lymphoma—Cats
- Lymphoma—Dogs
- Mast Cell Tumors

Related Topics in this Book
- Complete Blood Count
- Ferritin
- Iron and Total Iron-Binding Capacity

ABBREVIATIONS
- Epo = erythropoietin
- FeLV = feline leukemia virus
- FIV = feline immunodeficiency virus
- G-CSF = granulocyte–colony–stimulating factor
- M/E ratio = myeloid/erythroid ratio

Suggested Reading
Grindem CB, Neel JA, Juopperi TA. Cytology of bone marrow. *Vet Clin North Am Small Anim Pract* 2002; **32**: 1313–1374.
Harvey JW. *Atlas of Veterinary Hematology: Blood and Bone Marrow of Domestic Animals*. Philadelphia: WB Saunders, 2001.

INTERNET RESOURCES
None

AUTHOR NAME
Rebekah G. Gunn-Christie and John W. Harvey

BONE SCAN

BASICS

TYPE OF PROCEDURE
Nuclear medicine

PROCEDURE EXPLANATION AND RELATED PHYSIOLOGY
Skeletal scintigraphy is used as an aid to determine the site or sites of increased skeletal turnover. The radiopharmaceuticals used for bone scintigraphy bind to exposed areas of inorganic matrix in areas that are actively remodeling with both osteoblastic and osteoclastic activity. The radiopharmaceutical delivery depends on blood flow to a given region, and areas of suspected vascular compromise can be evaluated.

INDICATIONS
• Localize areas of increased bone turnover.
• Detect bone metastatic lesions.
• Detect areas of soft tissue or bone with vascular compromise.
• Determine the clinical significance of multiple radiographic lesions to determine areas of increased bone turnover that might then be correlated to clinical findings and lameness. A positive bone scan, however, does not necessarily equate with pain localization.

CONTRAINDICATIONS
None

POTENTIAL COMPLICATIONS
• Radiopharmaceutical decay within a patient that requires emergent surgery for an unrelated reason. Appropriate handling of all blood and urine, as well as, allowing for radioactive decay of contaminated surgical instruments prior to washing and sterilizing are required.

CLIENT EDUCATION
• Use of a radiopharmaceutical requires clients to be aware of potential radiation hazard once their animal has been released from the hospital.
• Clients should avoid prolonged contact with their animal over the next 48 h because the bound radiopharmaceutical continues to decay and is excreted by the kidneys into the urine.
• Technetium 99m (^{99m}Tc) has a physical half-life of 6.02 h and decays by isomeric transition with a 140-keV γ photon.

BODY SYSTEMS ASSESSED
• Musculoskeletal
• Respiratory

PROCEDURE

PATIENT PREPARATION
Preprocedure Medication or Preparation
• The patient should be well hydrated.
• Aged animals should be given fluids for a full 4 h prior to the scan to ensure that they are well hydrated. Decreased renal function, as can occur with age, can impact methylene diphosphonate (MDP) clearance from the soft tissues, and signal (bone) to noise (background soft tissue) decreases. Image quality will be improved when an animal is fully hydrated.
• An indwelling IV catheter should be placed in a limb that is not considered to be the affected limb or area in question.

Anesthesia or Sedation
Typically, sedation is required for the bone phase because imaging may last up to 1 h.

Patient Positioning
Lateral recumbency over the gamma camera.

Patient Monitoring
None is required during the procedure unless the patient is tranquilized.

Equipment or Supplies
• A gamma camera with an appropriate computer connection for acquisition and processing.
• A Geiger-Müeller survey meter for postprocedure monitoring.
• A radiopharmacy or designated "hot" laboratory for preparation of the radiopharmaceutical [^{99m}Tc-MDP or ^{99m}Tc-hydroxymethylene diphosphonate (HDP)] or where a local radiopharmacy may deliver a unit dose of the radiopharmaceutical.
• *Note*: Anyone using radioisotopes or radionuclides needs clearance and appropriate licensing from the individual state radiation protection and environmental safety departments.

TECHNIQUE
• The bone scan can be divided into 3 phases. Each phase has specific imaging requirements and acquisition parameters (see Table 1).
• For the vascular phase, typically the distal extremities (elbow and distal stifle) are imaged and a palmar/caudal or dorsal/cranial image of the affected and contralateral limbs is acquired simultaneously. The image acquisition consists of a dynamic data set that is acquired during the initial 90 s of circulation of the radiopharmaceutical after injection. Areas that lack normal blood supply will be photopenic (lack γ photons), and areas that have increased blood supply will have increased numbers of γ photons compared with the contralateral limb. The vascular phase (delivery) is critical for uptake of the radiopharmaceutical.
• The radiopharmaceutical will rapidly equilibrate with the extracellular fluid space (interstitial space) and will start to be excreted by the kidneys immediately.
• For the soft tissue phase, the static images are evaluated by direct comparison of affected limb and the contralateral limb. Areas of increased radiopharmaceutical uptake will be secondary to increased inflammatory changes within the area, as well as breakdown of local normal capillary beds, that are caused by the disease process.
• For the bone-phase images, static images will be acquired after a certain period to allow for the background soft tissues to clear and the signal (bone uptake) to noise (soft tissue uptake) to improve. Clearance depends on several factors, including age of the patient, renal status, and vascular integrity of the region of interest. Older patients will clear more slowly than young, immature patients. Patients with renal compromise will clear more slowly than dogs and cats with normal renal function.
• The lateral images of the right and left sides should be directly compared. Areas of increased radiopharmaceutical uptake should be described as to the area of uptake, degree of uptake (mild, moderate, or severe relative to surrounding bone), focal or multifocal, and pattern of uptake (e.g., linear fissure vs entire diaphyseal uptake). Dorsal or cranial (palmar/plantar/caudal) images can be obtained with both limbs in the field of view for direct comparison.
• Areas of increased radiopharmaceutical turnover are commonly seen in degenerative joint disease, fractures (healed or healing), an area of active bone turnover (physis/metaphysis), and neoplasia (primary or metastatic) or infection. The changes are sensitive (will allow for the detection of lesions before they become apparent on radiographs) but are nonspecific.

SAMPLE HANDLING
• As urine and blood will be radioactive, any blood or urine samples that are needed for tests should be obtained prior to the injection of the radiopharmaceutical.
• The patient and all related blood and urine products will have completely decayed to background by 5 days (10 physical half-lives) after IV injection of the radiopharmaceutical.

Table 1	The 3 phases of a bone scan			
Imaging phase	Time to image after injection	Acquisition parameters	Matrix	Positioning
Vascular phase	Simultaneous with injection	Dynamic frame mode; 1 s/frame for 90 s	128 × 128 × 16	Reformat to 2–4 s/frame and review in dynamic cine mode.
Soft tissue	3–5 min after injection	Static frame mode; 60 s/image	256 × 256 × 16	Compare limb with suspected lameness to contralateral limb.
Bone phase	2–4 h after injection	Static frame mode; 60 s/image	256 × 256 × 16	Compare limb with suspected lameness to contralateral limb.

APPROPRIATE AFTERCARE
Postprocedure Patient Monitoring
Postprocedural patient monitoring consists of determining when the radiopharmaceutical has decayed to the appropriate background levels for release criteria that will be specific to the individual's nuclear medicine license.

Nursing Care
None

Dietary Modification
None

Medication Requirements
None

Restrictions on Activity
A patient's confinement in a radiation-restricted area and that patient's release back to the general public will depend on postmonitoring exposure levels and the license requirements that the radiation safety officer of the license has preestablished with the state and appropriate regulatory authorities.

Anticipated Recovery Time
N/A

INTERPRETATION
NORMAL FINDINGS OR RANGE
• Normally, ^{99m}Tc-MDP will bind to the hydroxyapatite crystal of the inorganic matrix of mineralized bone. This binding is called *chemisorption*. The normal microenvironment of the cortical and cancellous bone is such that proteins cover the surfaces of the organic matrix (collagen fibers) and inorganic matrix unless active remodeling is taking place. In the case of active remodeling, the inorganic matrix is exposed and MDP competitively binds to the matrix. Increased blood flow to an area may increase the skeletal binding of MDP by severalfold; however, it is active remodeling that will significantly increase the binding of MDP. Normal findings would include radiopharmaceutical accumulation in the kidneys and urinary bladder.
• Young animals: The physis and metaphysis will have significant increases of MDP binding and appear as highly active linear bands.
• Mature animals: The diaphysis of the long bones will have the least amount of uptake. The epiphyses will have the most uptake because of the thicker areas of subchondral bone at the joint surfaces.
• Old animals: As renal function decreases, this can impact MDP clearance from the soft tissues, and the signal (bone) to noise (background soft tissue) ratio decreases.
• If ^{99m}Tc-MDP is injected SC, there can be lymphatic uptake and regional lymph node uptake on the side of injection. However, it has been reported that lymph nodes with metastases of bone tumors will also take up the radiopharmaceutical.

ABNORMAL VALUES
• Focal areas of increased uptake within the long bones, ribs, or vertebrae can be secondary to trauma (fracture), healing or healed fracture, infection, neoplasia (primary or metastatic), or panosteitis (dogs).

• Focal areas of decreased uptake ("cold" spots) can be secondary to lack of blood supply or to focal areas of avascular bone segments (comminuted fractures or avascular necrosis of the femoral head). In addition, it has been reported in human medicine that multiple myeloma will cause multifocal cold spots throughout the skeleton. This is not the case in veterinary medicine and in the author's experience; multiple myeloma will appear as multifocal hot spots.
• Any area of dystrophic mineralization will serve as a source that can bind MDP or HDP. This has been shown in calcinosis cutis and pulmonary mineralization in dogs that have Cushing's disease.
• Primary bone tumors that have metastasized to other soft tissue structures (e.g., lungs, kidneys) and are actively laying down new bone will actively take up MDP.
• Multifocal areas of increased radiopharmaceutical uptake that show a severe degree of uptake. This indicates a systemic process that is polyostotic, such as fungal septicemia and osteomyelitis or bone metastatic disease.

CRITICAL VALUES
None

INTERFERING FACTORS
Drugs That May Alter Results of the Procedure
None anticipated. The possibility of editronate administration causing competitive inhibition of ^{99m}Tc-MDP has yet to be investigated in dogs and cats.

Conditions That May Interfere with Performing the Procedure
None

Procedure Techniques or Handling That May Alter Results
• Poor radiolabel with IV injection of either sodium pertechnetate or technetium dioxide will result in an invalid study.
• Ensuring that the gamma camera has been appropriately maintained, has been photopeaked to 140 keV, and is functioning normally will greatly enhance image acquisition. A low-energy all-purpose or low-energy high-resolution collimator should be used for acquisition.

Influence of Signalment on Performing and Interpreting the Procedure
Species
No major species differences have been noted.

Breed
• No major breed differences have been noted.
• Familiarity with breed-associated juvenile orthopedic disease or canine-related juvenile orthopedic disease would be beneficial.

Age
There is increased radiopharmaceutical uptake noted at the level of the physes and metaphyses with age.

Gender
None

Pregnancy
• None
• ^{99m}Tc-MDP has been shown to be excreted in the milk in actively lactating dogs and cats.

BONE SCAN

CLINICAL PERSPECTIVE

Bone scans can be useful in the following situations:
- Evaluation of patients with lameness that cannot be localized to a specific joint
- Evaluation for bone metastases
- Evaluation for bone sepsis or bone healing within an area that may lack a normal blood supply from a comminuted fracture
- Evaluation of dogs or cats with multifocal bone lesions to see areas of increased turnover
- Evaluation of total hip prosthesis for infection
- Evaluation of dogs with juvenile orthopedic disease (e.g., a fragmented medial coronoid process)
- Evaluation for pulmonary mineralization in dogs with Cushing's disease

MISCELLANEOUS

ANCILLARY TESTS

Survey skeletal radiographs are required of the anatomic areas where increased radiopharmaceutical uptake is identified.

SYNONYMS
- Blood-pool imaging
- Bone imaging
- Bone scintigraphy
- Musculoskeletal scintigraphy

SEE ALSO
Blackwell's Five-Minute Veterinary Consult: Canine and Feline Topics
- Chondrosarcoma
- Osteomyelitis
- Osteosarcoma

- Panosteitis
- Pulmonary Mineralization

Related Topics in this Book
Skeletal Radiography

ABBREVIATIONS
- HDP = hydroxymethylene diphosphonate
- MDP = methylene diphosphonate

Suggested Reading

Berry CR, Ackerman N, Monce K. Pulmonary mineralization in four dogs with Cushing's syndrome. *Vet Radiol Ultrasound* 1994; 35: 10–16.

Forrest LJ, Thrall DE. Bone scintigraphy for metastasis detection in canine osteosarcoma. *Vet Radiol Ultrasound* 1994; 35: 124–130.

Goggin JM, Hoskinson JJ, Carpenter JW, *et al.* Scintigraphic assessment of distal extremity perfusion in 17 patients. *Vet Radiol Ultrasound* 1997; 38: 211–220.

Lamb CR. Non-skeletal distribution of bone-seeking radiopharmaceuticals. *Vet Radiol Ultrasound* 1990; 31: 246–253.

Lamb CR, Schelling SH, Berg J. Lymph node uptake of ^{99m}Tc-MDP during bone scintigraphy in dogs. *Vet Radiol Ultrasound* 1989; 30: 268–271.

Poteet B. Small animal skeletal scintigraphy. In: Daniel GB, Berry CR, eds. *Textbook of Veterinary Nuclear Medicine.* Harrisburg, PA: American College of Veterinary Radiology, 2006.

INTERNET RESOURCES
American College of Veterinary Radiology (ACVR), http://www.acvr.org.
Radiological Society of North America (RSNA), http://www.rsna.org.
Society of Nuclear Medicine (SNM), http://www.snm.org.

AUTHOR NAMES
Anthony Pease and Clifford R. Berry

BASICS

TYPE OF PROCEDURE
Electrodiagnostic

PROCEDURE EXPLANATION AND RELATED PHYSIOLOGY
The brain-stem auditory evoked response (BAER) is a graphic recording of the evoked response in brain-stem activity elicited by an auditory stimulus. The test is performed by providing a repetitive auditory stimulus to 1 ear while providing a masking noise to the other ear. The sounds are transmitted by earphones placed in the ear canal. The evoked potentials are recorded from subdermal scalp electrodes; because these potentials are relatively small, the waveforms are averaged to eliminate extraneous electrical activity. A normal BAER consists of 4–5 highly reproducible, time-locked waves obtained within 10 ms of the stimulus and represent activation of structures along the auditory pathway in the brain stem. The first large wave (wave I) is generated by action potentials in the cochlear division of the vestibulocochlear nerve (cranial nerve VIII). Subsequent waves are generated by brain-stem nuclei and tracts that comprise the auditory pathway, including the cochlear nucleus, rostral olivary nucleus, lateral lemniscus, and caudal colliculus.

The BAER is an objective, noninvasive method of assessing the functional integrity of the inner ear and cochlear nerve, as well as the auditory pathways within the brain stem. In addition, disease of the external or middle ear can be evaluated to a limited extent, particularly in cases in which the disease limits the transmission of normal sound waves to the receptors in the inner ear.

INDICATIONS
- To screen animals for congenital deafness
- To assess for acquired deafness
- To evaluate brain-stem function

CONTRAINDICATIONS
None

POTENTIAL COMPLICATIONS
None

CLIENT EDUCATION
- As a test for hearing, the BAER evaluates each ear for the expected response to auditory stimulation, and animals with unilateral deafness can be identified. Animals with unilateral hearing loss may appear clinically normal to their owner.
- Partial hearing loss is more difficult to assess and is often not recognized. Similarly, a BAER cannot discriminate an animal's ability to hear only certain frequencies or tones, because these characteristics of the stimulus are not varied during testing.

BODY SYSTEMS ASSESSED
Nervous

PROCEDURE

PATIENT PREPARATION
Preprocedure Medication or Preparation
None

Anesthesia or Sedation
Animals that object to either the electrodes being placed subdermally on the scalp or the earphones inserted into the ear canals can be sedated for the procedure. Neither sedation nor anesthesia will affect the test results.

Patient Positioning
- The animal is placed in sternal recumbency.
- If the animal is not heavily sedated or anesthetized for the procedure, its head should be gently restrained to prevent the animal's movement from dislodging the earphones or electrodes. Excessive movement will also cause electrical interference, and the elicited responses will not be averaged into the final waveform. This prolongs the time required to perform the test.

Patient Monitoring
None

Equipment or Supplies
- An electrodiagnostic unit capable of performing BAER, which also has the auditory stimulator and transducer needed to create the audible clicks
- Scalp electrodes
- Specially designed, disposable tubal insert earphones

TECHNIQUE
- The earphones are placed securely in the external ear canals.
- Subdural electrodes are placed at specific sites on the scalp; the recording electrode is placed at the vertex, the reference electrode at the mastoid just rostral to the base of the ear, and the ground electrode on the dorsal midline of the midcervical region.
- A 70- to 90-decibel click stimulus is applied to the test ear at a rate of 10 Hz while a masking noise of 30–40 decibels less than the test stimulus is applied to the opposite ear. Typically, 500–1,000 repetitions are averaged to produce the final waveform.

SAMPLE HANDLING
N/A

APPROPRIATE AFTERCARE
Postprocedure Patient Monitoring
None

Nursing Care
None

Dietary Modification
None

BRAIN-STEM AUDITORY EVOKED RESPONSE

Medication Requirements
None

Restrictions on Activity
None

Anticipated Recovery Time
None

 ## INTERPRETATION

NORMAL FINDINGS OR RANGE

A BAER is evaluated with respect to the number of waveforms present, as well as the latency and relative amplitude of the waveforms. The BAER normally results in 4–5 waveforms; expected latencies for each of the generated waveforms have been established for dogs and cats. As a general rule, wave I appears at a latency of approximately 1 ms, with each successive peak occurring at <1-ms intervals (Figure 1).

ABNORMAL VALUES

• When used as an assessment of hearing, the absence of any identifiable waveforms (a flat line) is indicative of deafness in the ear being tested.

• An increase in the latency of all waveforms and an increase in the stimulus intensity necessary to obtain a detectable response are suggestive of conductive hearing loss. This disturbance of transmission through the external or middle ear can be caused by otitis externa, tympanic membrane rupture, otitis media, or disease of the bony ossicles.

• Increased latency between waveform peaks is indicative of a brain-stem lesion causing delayed conduction along the auditory pathway. Similarly, a ratio of wave V amplitude to wave I amplitude of <0.5 indicates brain-stem disease. However, brain-stem disease can be present without alterations in the BAER if the auditory pathways are not involved in the disease process.

• An animal with a severe, irreversible brain lesion compatible with brain death will have complete loss of all waves or a preservation of wave I with an absence of all subsequent waves.

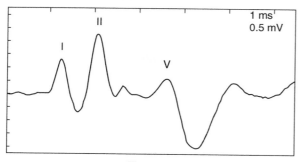

Figure 1

Normal BAER recording from a dog.

CRITICAL VALUES

None

INTERFERING FACTORS

Drugs That May Alter Results of the Procedure
None

Conditions That May Interfere with Performing the Procedure
None

Procedure Techniques or Handling That May Alter Results
None

Influence of Signalment on Performing and Interpreting the Procedure

Species
None

Breed
None

Age
• Studies have demonstrated that the BAER thresholds mature in dogs and cats by approximately 3 weeks of age.
• Hereditary deafness associated with the white or merle coat color is due to cochlear agenesis or early degeneration. Animals of predisposed breeds can be screened for congenital deafness as early as 5–6 weeks of age. If the results of initial screening are equivocal, it is recommended that the test be repeated in 1 month.

Gender
None

Pregnancy
None

CLINICAL PERSPECTIVE

• BAER testing is most commonly performed to screen for deafness in certain breeds of dogs that are predisposed to hereditary hearing loss, the most notable of which is the dalmatian. Hearing loss in these animals can be unilateral or bilateral.

• In a specialty-practice setting, BAER testing may be used as a tool to evaluate animals for brain-stem disease. This is most commonly performed in animals with vestibular disease, where differentiation of central from peripheral vestibular disease is important from diagnostic and prognostic standpoints.

• BAER testing can also be used to assess prognosis in animals with severe brain disease that has caused a comatose state. In these animals, an absence of waveforms is suggestive of irreversible brain injury. However, this assessment can be performed only in animals known to have normal hearing.

 ## MISCELLANEOUS

ANCILLARY TESTS

• A thorough otoscopic exam should be performed in any animal with an abnormal BAER (particularly when the animal fails to respond to a normal stimulus intensity or the latency of all waveforms is increased)

to determine whether debris in the ear canal, severe canal stenosis, or rupture of the tympanic membrane is contributing to the hearing loss.
• Animals with evidence, based on BAER testing, of brain-stem disease should undergo imaging of the brain and possible analysis of cerebrospinal fluid to assess for potential causes of the dysfunction.

SYNONYMS
• BAER
• Brain-stem auditory evoked potential

SEE ALSO
Blackwell's Five-Minute Veterinary Consult: Canine and Feline Topics
• Deafness
• Otitis Externa and Media
• Otitis Media and Interna
Related Topics in This Book
None

ABBREVIATIONS
BAER = brain-stem auditory evoked response

Suggested Reading
Eger CE, Lindsay P. Effects of otitis on hearing in dogs characterized by brainstem auditory evoked response testing. *J Small Anim Pract* 1997; 38: 380–386.
Fischer A, Obermaier G. Brainstem auditory-evoked potentials and neuropathologic correlates in 26 dogs with brain tumors. *J Vet Intern Med* 1994; 8: 363–369.
Holliday TA, Nelson HJ, Williams DC, Willits N. Unilateral and bilateral brainstem auditory-evoked response abnormalities in 900 Dalmatian dogs. *J Vet Intern Med* 1992; 6: 166–174.
Steiss JE, Cox NR, Hathcock JT. Brain stem auditory-evoked response abnormalities in 14 dogs with confirmed central nervous system lesions. *J Vet Intern Med* 1994; 8: 293–298.

INTERNET RESOURCES
Strain GM. Deafness in dogs & cats. Louisiana State University School of Veterinary Medicine, http://www.lsu.edu/deafness/deaf.htm.

AUTHOR NAME
Karen R. Muñana

BRAIN ULTRASONOGRAPHY

 BASICS

TYPE OF PROCEDURE
Ultrasonographic

PROCEDURE EXPLANATION AND RELATED PHYSIOLOGY
Ultrasound examination of the brain requires an acoustic window through the skull. Dogs with hydrocephalus often have a persistent bregmatic fontanel that enables imaging of the brain. In these cases, an ultrasound examination is a quicker, less expensive, and more available screening tool than computed tomography (CT) or magnetic resonance imaging (MRI). Ultrasound images of the brain have relatively poor anatomic detail compared to those with CT and especially MRI. Ultrasound imaging of the brain in patients with a closed fontanel may be accomplished through the temporal window or foramen magnum, although these acoustic windows provide a more limited view of the brain in many cases. A portion of the skull can be removed surgically to provide a window for ultrasound; however, this invasive technique requires anesthesia. For these cases, CT and MRI, which are less invasive, provide a more complete evaluation of the brain than ultrasound will provide. Ultrasound is excellent for distinguishing fluid versus soft tissue, enabling straightforward identification of hydrocephalus, cysts, and abscesses. Intraoperative ultrasound of the brain is used mainly to aid surgical dissection by identifying nonpalpable and nonvisible lesions. Ultrasound is used postoperatively to evaluate the completeness of removal of a lesion or look for evidence of complications.

INDICATIONS
- Suspected hydrocephalus
- Intraoperative location of brain tumor, cyst, abscess, or hemorrhage

CONTRAINDICATIONS
Atlantoaxial instability is a contraindication for ultrasound imaging of the brain through the foramen magnum. Hyperflexion of the head is required for imaging through the foramen magnum and could cause severe injury to the spinal cord if concurrent atlantoaxial instability is present. To assess for possible atlantoaxial subluxation in toy-breed dogs, survey radiographs should be made prior to this ultrasound procedure.

POTENTIAL COMPLICATIONS
Excess pressure by the ultrasound probe could potentially injure the brain tissue. Judicious use of the ultrasound probe will prevent this complication.

CLIENT EDUCATION
- The use of ultrasound to image the brain is safe, fast, and economical in screening for hydrocephalus in an animal with an open fontanel.
- CT or MRI of the brain is often necessary for a complete evaluation of the brain following ultrasound.
- Intraoperative ultrasound localization of a brain lesion can reduce the amount of dissection and palpation of the brain tissue, therefore reducing trauma to the brain.
- Intraoperative brain ultrasound assists in identifying all abnormal tissue for removal.

BODY SYSTEMS ASSESSED
Nervous

 PROCEDURE

PATIENT PREPARATION
Preprocedure Medication or Preparation
None

Anesthesia or Sedation
- This is required only if necessary for a surgical procedure or to assist in keeping the patient still during the ultrasound examination.
- Sedation is more often required for imaging through the foramen magnum to enable sufficient flexing of the atlanto-occipital joint for imaging.

Patient Positioning
- Patients with an open bregmatic fontanel can often be imaged with them standing or sitting.
- Lateral recumbency is used in some cases, depending on the temperament of the patient.

Patient Monitoring
No special monitoring is needed for use of ultrasound.

Equipment or Supplies
- A real-time B-mode ultrasound scanner with a high-frequency transducer
- A transducer with a small footprint (contact with skin area) and sector image. This allows the ultrasound beam to get through the opening in the skull and widen out to image more of the brain. A high-resolution linear array transducer may be used but will present a more restricted view of the brain.
- The transducer frequency should be ≥7 MHz for the best resolution.
- Ultrasound gel for imaging through the skin surface
- Intraoperative ultrasound
  - Normal saline solution or sterile acoustic gel to couple the transducer with the surface of the brain
  - A sterile sleeve for a transducer, if the transducer is used intraoperatively

TECHNIQUE
Imaging Through the Open Bregmatic Fontanel
- Clip or part the hair, if thick, over the fontanel. If the hair is fine, thin, or both, the transducer may be coupled sufficiently to the skin without the hair being clipped.
- Place sufficient ultrasound gel on the skin surface of ultrasound transducer, and place the transducer directly over the open fontanel.
- Adjust the depth and gain to produce the best image of the brain.
- Obtain sagittal and transverse views of the brain by sweeping slowly from side to side in the sagittal plane and rostral to caudal in the transverse plane.

Imaging Through the Temporal Window
- Clip or part the hair and apply acoustic gel to the skin.
- The temporal window is located just dorsal to the juncture of the zygomatic arch, with the temporal bone at the juncture of the parietal and temporal bones, where the bone can be thin enough to enable imaging through this window.
- The exact location and quality of view obtained through this window vary.
- Transverse and dorsal views of the brain are obtained through this window.

Imaging Through the Foramen Magnum
- Clip the hair and clean the skin centered on the midline occipital region of the head.
- The patient is placed in lateral recumbency, and its head is hyperflexed.
- Apply ultrasound gel to the skin surface or transducer.
- Place the ultrasound transducer on the patient's skin sagittal to the head, and point the transducer toward its nose.
- Generally, only sagittal images are obtained from this acoustic window.
- One advantage of this window is the ability to evaluate the blood flow in the basilar artery with Doppler.

- This view does not enable imaging of the brain rostral to the interthalamic adhesion but enables imaging of the proximal cervical spinal cord.

Intraoperative Imaging
- Place a sterile sleeve over the transducer and cord.
- Fill the brain case with normal saline and image through the fluid or place the transducer *gently* on the surface of the brain by using saline flush or sterile gel to allow sonic coupling of the transducer and brain surface.
- The exact positioning of the transducer will depend on the location and size of the surgical opening in the skull. However, brain images should be obtained in at least 2 different planes. Do not agitate the saline solution by shaking it or by filling the brain case rapidly because this produces microbubbles in the solution that, throughout the fluid, produce numerous hyperechoic foci that can interfere with imaging if present in sufficient numbers.

SAMPLE HANDLING
N/A

APPROPRIATE AFTERCARE
Postprocedure Patient Monitoring
None

Nursing Care
Clean acoustic gel from the skin surface following the procedure.

Dietary Modification
None

Medication Requirements
None

Restrictions on Activity
None

Anticipated Recovery Time
Immediate

INTERPRETATION

NORMAL FINDINGS OR RANGE
- The normal brain tissue is relatively hypoechoic, with some echogenic surfaces are observable that reveal the brain anatomy.
- The lateral ventricles should be observed as anechoic fluid filled structures in both hemispheres and can be imaged in both the transverse and the sagittal planes.
- The normal ultrasound anatomy of the brain has been described (see Hudson et al. 1989).
- Normal lateral ventricular height measured caudal to the interthalamic adhesion has a normal mean of 0.15 cm.

ABNORMAL VALUES
- Hydrocephalus is considered present if the height of the lateral ventricules measured caudal to the interthalamic adhesion is >0.35 cm.
- A ventricle/mantle ratio of >0.25 indicates hydrocephalus. The height of the lateral ventricle measured caudal to the interthalamic adhesion is divided by the cerebral mantle thickness at the same level. The cerebral mantle thickness is measured from the roof of the lateral ventricle to the dorsal brain surface.
- A ventricle/hemisphere ratio of >0.19 indicates hydrocephalus. The width of the lateral ventricle is divided by the hemispheric width measured from the third ventricle (midline) to the lateral surface of the brain.
- The sizes of the lateral ventricles in hydrocephalus do not correlate well with clinical signs, with some patients having occult hydrocephalus (no clinical signs).

- Most brain neoplasms appear as echogenic or mixed echogenic and hypoechoic masses in the relatively hypoechoic brain tissue.
- The sonographic appearance of abscesses and hemorrhage varies, depending on the age of the lesion.
- Fluid with swirling echogenic material may indicate an exudate or hemorrhage. However, some cerebrospinal fluid in the ventricles may have sufficient protein content to show swirling material in the fluid. A sample of the fluid must be obtained for definitive diagnosis.

CRITICAL VALUES
None

INTERFERING FACTORS
Drugs That May Alter Results of the Procedure
None

Conditions That May Interfere with Performing the Procedure
A closed bregmatic fontanel, small foramen magnum, or thick bone in the temporal window requires surgical removal of bone to provide an acoustic window in order to image the brain. In these cases, it is advisable to consider alternative imaging such as CT or MRI to evaluate the brain.

Procedure Techniques or Handling That May Alter Results
Artifact and acoustic shadowing from a very small opening in the skull or the use of a linear array transducer may not provide a sufficient image to reasonably assess the condition of the brain.

Influence of Signalment on Performing and Interpreting the Procedure
Species
None

Breed
Brachycephalic breeds may have slightly larger lateral ventricles without clinical signs as a breed variation.

Age
The brain of mature dogs and cats with a closed fontanel cannot be imaged by this means and must be imaged through the temporal window, through the foramen magnum, or by surgically removing a portion of the skull.

Gender
None

Pregnancy
None

CLINICAL PERSPECTIVE
- Ultrasound is an easy, safe, and inexpensive means of evaluating the brain for hydrocephalus when an open bregmatic fontanel is present.
- The lateral ventricular size does not always correlate with clinical signs in mild to moderate enlargement.
- CT and MRI are the techniques of choice for presurgical imaging of the brain for most diseases except as stated previously for hydrocephalus.
- Ultrasound can be very useful intraoperatively for locating lesions in the brain. However, surgery of the brain requires specialized training and knowledge in neurosurgery and is usually best referred to a specialist to provide the optimal outcome for patients.

MISCELLANEOUS

ANCILLARY TESTS
A thorough neurologic examination is required to correlate with ultrasound findings.

SYNONYMS
- Cranial ultrasound
- Transcranial ultrasound

BRAIN ULTRASONOGRAPHY

SEE ALSO
Blackwell's Five-Minute Veterinary Consult: Canine and Feline Topics
Hydrocephalus

Related Topics in this Book
- General Principles of Ultrasonography
- Computed Tomography
- Magnetic Resonance Imaging

ABBREVIATIONS
- CT = computed tomography
- MRI = magnetic resonance imaging

Suggested Reading

Hudson JA, Cartee RE, Simpson ST, *et al.* Ultrasonographic anatomy of the canine brain. *Vet Radiol* 1989; 30: 13–21.

Hudson JA, Simpson ST, Buxton DF, *et al.* Ultrasonographic diagnosis of canine hydrocephalus. *Vet Radiol* 1990; 31: 50–58.

Saito M, Olby NJ, Spaulding KA, *et al.* Identification of arachnoid cysts in the quadrigeminal cistern using ultrasonography. *Vet Radiol* 2001; 42: 435–439.

Saito M, Olby NJ, Spaulding KA, *et al.* Relationship among basilar artery resistance index, degree of ventriculomegaly, and clinical signs in hydrocephalic dogs. *Vet Radiol* 2003; 44: 687–694.

Spaulding KA, Sharp NJH. Ultrasonographic imaging of the lateral cerebral ventricles in the dog. *Vet Radiol* 1990; 31: 59–64.

INTERNET RESOURCES
None

AUTHOR NAME
George A. Henry

BASICS

TYPE OF PROCEDURE
Diagnostic sample collection

PROCEDURE EXPLANATION AND RELATED PHYSIOLOGY
BAL is a technique for collecting fluid for diagnostic purposes from the small airways, alveoli, and, in some cases, the interstitium. The procedure is typically performed during bronchoscopy, enabling visual examination of the airways and directed lavage of specific lung lobes. Also, BAL can be performed without a bronchoscope. A sufficient volume of sterile saline is instilled into the lungs to fill alveoli. The saline, along with cells and epithelial lining fluid from the lung, is then retrieved by suction. The volume of fluid retrieved is adequate for analysis by cytologic, microbiologic, or other techniques.

INDICATIONS
• To obtain specimens from dogs or cats undergoing bronchoscopy for the evaluation of cough, increased respiratory efforts, abnormal thoracic radiographs, or other signs of lung disease
• To obtain specimens from dogs or cats with signs of respiratory disease in which other less invasive procedures (such as tracheal wash, or transthoracic lung aspiration of a solid mass adjacent to the body wall) are unlikely to, or have failed to, provide a sufficient specimen from the lungs. Often such patients have diffuse interstitial lung disease as assessed by thoracic radiography.

CONTRAINDICATIONS
• Inability to provide oxygen supplementation for up to several hours following BAL. BAL causes transiently decreased pulmonary function (see the Potential Complications section). However, since this procedure is indicated for only patients with lung disease, clinical judgment must be used to determine which patients are candidates for BAL. Those patients without increased respiratory efforts at rest in room air are generally good candidates. Those patients with increased respiratory efforts while receiving supplemental oxygen therapy are poor candidates. The capability of supporting the patient with more prolonged oxygen supplementation and possibly positive pressure ventilation during recovery may allow for BAL of moderately compromised patients.
• Any contraindication for general anesthesia

POTENTIAL COMPLICATIONS
• Pulmonary function is transiently decreased following BAL, which decreases oxygenation of blood. The compromise is particularly severe during the first minutes following the procedure, with mild to moderate compromise persisting during the first few hours and minimal compromise for up to 2 days. Hypoxemia generally responds to oxygen supplementation.
• In patients with emphysema, cysts, or bulla, pneumothorax could occur from rupture due to BAL or positive pressure ventilation.
• Complications related to general anesthesia

CLIENT EDUCATION
• Don't feed the animal the morning of the procedure.
• Potential benefit must be weighed with potential risk, along with consideration of other diagnostic options, on a case-by-case basis.

BODY SYSTEMS ASSESSED
Respiratory

PROCEDURE

PATIENT PREPARATION
Preprocedure Medication or Preparation
• Withhold food as for any general anesthetic procedure.
• Atropine
• For cats, a bronchodilator

• Preoxygenate for 5–10 min before BAL.

Anesthesia or Sedation
• For bronchoscopic BAL, follow the anesthetic protocol as for bronchoscopy.
• For nonbronchoscopic BAL in dogs, administer hydromorphone premedication followed by propofol titrated to enable intubation.
• For nonbronchoscopic BAL in cats, administer ketamine and valium IV to enable intubation. Drip injectable lidocaine onto the larynx to facilitate intubation.

Patient Positioning
• For bronchoscopic BAL, sternal recumbency
• For nonbronchoscopic BAL in dogs, dorsal recumbency
• For nonbronchoscopic BAL in cats, lateral recumbency, placing the side most affected radiographically in the down position

Patient Monitoring
• Pulse oximetry is ideal.
• Mucous membrane color and capillary refill time
• Respiratory rate and effort
• Heart rate and rhythm

Equipment or Supplies
• Sterile 0.9% sodium chloride solution (saline)
• 35-mL syringes
• A laryngoscope
• An anesthetic machine with bag for delivery of oxygen immediately following BAL

For Bronchoscopic BAL
• Routine bronchoscopic equipment
• A sterile endotracheal tube if the patient is sufficiently large for a scope to be passed through an endotracheal tube

For Nonbronchoscopic BAL in Dogs
• A syringe adapter
• A 16 French polyvinyl chloride stomach tube, modified by cutting both ends, leaving a length slightly longer than the distance from estimated position of the end of a positioned endotracheal tube to the last rib. The syringe adapter is placed in 1 end. The other end is tapered slightly by use of a sterilized, metal, handheld pencil sharpener or by shaving with a scalpel blade.
• A sterile endotracheal tube if the patient is sufficiently large for a feeding tube to be passed through an endotracheal tube

For Nonbronchoscopic BAL in Cats
• A sterile endotracheal tube
• A syringe adapter

TECHNIQUE
Regardless of technique used, a good BAL specimen is characterized by the presence of visible foam. The foam forms because surfactant is present in the sample and is indicative of a deep lung specimen. The total retrieved volume from the first bolus instilled is variable, but from the subsequent boluses it is ideally >50%. Retrieval of much lower volumes should cause one to assess the technique being used, such as the position of the bronchoscope or lavage catheter. If only negative pressure is obtained during suctioning to retrieve BAL fluid, the airway mucosa may be being suctioned into the bronchoscope or catheter. This can occur from being lodged in too small of an airway or because the patient has chondromalacia (such as with chronic bronchitis). Suctioning efforts may need to be less vigorous in such cases, or the scope or catheter withdrawn slightly or repositioned in another bronchus. All patients should be positioned in sternal recumbency and administered 100% oxygen for at least 5–10 min after the procedure. They should be given several deep breaths (or sighs) with the anesthetic bag to help open atelectatic areas of lung.

For Bronchoscopic BAL
Following bronchoscopic examination of the airways, the scope is passed into the lobe to be lavaged until the scope is gently lodged against the airway walls. Saline is instilled through the biopsy channel of the bronchoscope and then immediately retrieved by suction using the same syringe. Air is eliminated from the syringe, and further suctioning is attempted until no further fluid is obtained. With the scope in the same

position, the procedure is repeated. For most dogs, when a pediatric bronchoscope of 4.8-mm outer diameter is used, 2 boluses are instilled in each position sampled with a volume of 25 mL each. The volume per bolus is decreased in small dogs. If sufficient volume is not recovered from the lower instilled volumes, additional boluses are instilled while the patient is in the same position. For cats, 5 boluses of 10 mL each are used. To increase the sensitivity of the procedure, lavage can be performed in more than one lobe.

For Nonbronchoscopic BAL in Dogs
The modified feeding tube is used as the lavage catheter. Ideally, it is passed through a sterile endotracheal tube that has been positioned with minimal contamination by the oropharynx. In dogs for which the endotracheal tube would be too small to pass the feeding tube, the feeding tube is passed directly through the larynx into the trachea. To minimize contamination, care should be taken to avoid touching the end of the tube against the oral or pharyngeal mucosa. The modified feeding tube is passed down the airways until resistance is felt. The tube is withdrawn a few centimeters and again passed down the airways until the tube is convincingly lodged within an airway and not abutting an airway division. A syringe adapter is placed on the proximal end of the tube, maintaining sterility at all times. Syringes are prepared in advance containing 25 mL of saline and 5 mL of air. A saline bolus is instilled, followed by the air (achieved by holding the syringe upright so that the air is instilled after the saline), and immediately withdrawn by suction using the same syringe. Air is eliminated from the syringe, and suction is repeated until no additional fluid is retrieved. The procedure is repeated with a second bolus. A third bolus may be needed if a sufficient specimen is not obtained. Saline volumes per bolus should be decreased for small dogs, but be prepared to instill multiple boluses to retrieve sufficient return.

For Nonbronchoscopic BAL in Cats
A sterile endotracheal tube is positioned as cleanly as possible, minimizing contamination from the oropharynx. To achieve this, the larynx is anesthetized by dripping lidocaine on the mucosa and a laryngoscope is used. The cuff is inflated to create an airtight seal. To avoid tracheal tears, use a sufficiently large endotracheal tube and fill the cuff only as much as necessary (<3 mL of air). A saline bolus is instilled at a volume of 5 mL/kg body weight. The volume may be decreased for very obese cats or compromised patients. The saline is immediately withdrawn using the same syringe. Air is eliminated from the syringe, and suction is repeated until no additional fluid is retrieved. The procedure is repeated with a second bolus. A third bolus may be needed if a sufficient specimen is not obtained.

SAMPLE HANDLING
- Specimens are submitted for cytologic evaluation and microbial culture.
- Cytologic examination should include total nucleated cell and differential cell counts, as well as qualitative assessment. The return from the first bolus has a relatively great contribution from the larger airways than subsequent boluses. Unless one is particularly interested in distinguishing among these results, the returned fluid samples from all boluses from a particular site are combined for cytologic analysis. Fluid from individual lung lobes is evaluated separately by cytology.
- Fluid for submission for cytology should be refrigerated and analyzed as soon as possible (ideally, the same day). If prompt submission is not possible, slides should be made and submitted along with the fluid.
- Slides must be prepared with a concentrating technique such as cytocentrifugation or sedimentation. If there is mucus visible in the specimen, a squash preparation of the mucus may improve the likelihood of visualizing infectious agents. Squash preparations are not adequate for cell counting and morphology.
- Bacterial culture is indicated in all patients. Samples for mycoplasmal and fungal cultures should be submitted in select patients. Specimens from individual lobes can be combined for microbial culture.
- Fluid for culture should be placed in appropriate storage media, generally provided by the microbiology laboratory.

APPROPRIATE AFTERCARE
Postprocedure Patient Monitoring
- Oxygen saturation
- Respiratory rate and effort
- Mucous membrane color
- Heart rate and rhythm

Nursing Care
Routine postanesthetic care

Dietary Modification
None

Medication Requirements
Oxygen supplementation, as needed

Restrictions on Activity
Cage rest until fully recovered

Anticipated Recovery Time
Pulmonary function will generally have returned to near prelavage levels within a few hours of the procedure. Complete recovery in healthy dogs, based on pulmonary function tests and histopathology, occurs within 2 days.

INTERPRETATION

NORMAL FINDINGS OR RANGE
- Reported ranges for cell counts in healthy dogs and cats vary with the methodology used. Even using 1 method, it is not possible to completely standardize the technique or control the volume of fluid retrieved. Therefore, reference ranges should be used for guidance only. Absolute counts may be more representative of the cells in the lung than relative counts, in some cases.
- The values provided are approximations only.
- Total nucleated cell counts in healthy dogs and cats are generally $<500/\mu L$.
- The majority of cells in health are alveolar macrophages.
- Neutrophils are generally <15% of nucleated cells.
- Eosinophils are generally <15% of nucleated cells in dogs. Apparently healthy cats can have a higher percentage of eosinophils in BAL fluid (rarely >50%). Increased eosinophil counts in cats must be interpreted cautiously, in conjunction with clinical signs.
- Mast cells are rarely seen.

ABNORMAL VALUES
- Inflammation is identified by the presence of increased numbers of a specific cell type (e.g., eosinophilic or neutrophilic inflammation).
- Cells are evaluated for evidence of intracellular pathogens, activation, degeneration, and criteria of malignancy.
- Slides are examined for pathogenic organisms. Careful scrutiny of the entire slide is indicated. There may be as few as 1 fungal, protozoan, or parasitic organism on an entire slide. The absence of pathogens does not rule out their presence in the lung.
- Growth of bacteria in culture may be indicative of infection, normal tracheal bacteria, or contamination. Growth of bacteria from patients with BAL cytology supportive of infection is considered to be significant. Generally, bacteria causing infection will grow on media that are inoculated directly with BAL fluid. Growth of bacterial from BAL fluid only after being incubated in enrichment broth is less likely to indicate infection. However, if the patient has recently received antibiotics, low bacterial numbers may represent actual infection.

CRITICAL VALUES
None

INTERFERING FACTORS
Drugs That May Alter Results of The Procedure
Current or recent administration of antibiotics can interfere with the diagnosis of bacterial infection. Bacterial numbers can be sufficiently lowered as to be undetectable cytologically. Growth of organisms in culture may be prevented even with antibiotics that have not successfully eliminated the infection in vivo. Most antibiotics should, ideally, be discontinued for at least 1 week prior to BAL. Fluoroquinolones should be discontinued for at least 2 weeks. Antibiotics that sustain prolonged tissue

concentrations (such as azithromycin) could possibly affect results for even longer.

Conditions That May Interfere with Performing the Procedure
Bronchomalacia may interfere with retrieval of fluid as a result of the airway wall collapsing around the catheter or biopsy channel during suction.

Procedure Techniques or Handling That May Alter Results
Modification of any aspect of the procedure may influence results. Consistency in technique should be practiced.

Influence of Signalment on Performing and Interpreting the Procedure

Species
The recommended procedure is different for dogs and cats, as already described in the Technique section. Cytology from healthy dogs and cats is also slightly different, as already described in the Normal Findings or Range section.

Breed
None known

Age
None known

Gender
None known

Pregnancy
Risks of anesthesia or hypoxemia

Clinical Perspective
- BAL is indicated in nearly all patients that are undergoing bronchoscopy.
- BAL provides a high-quality cytologic specimen representing processes within the small airways, the alveoli and, in some cases, the interstitium.
- BAL provides a specimen of sufficient volume for microbiologic cultures.
- BAL is less invasive and less expensive than thoracotomy.
- Alternative techniques for collecting cytologic specimens from the lung include tracheal wash and transthoracic lung aspiration. Tracheal wash is generally sufficient if bronchoscopy is not indicated and clinical signs and radiographs suggest predominantly airway disease or bronchopneumonia. Transthoracic lung aspiration is generally sufficient if a mass can be sampled directly with ultrasound guidance.
- BAL provides a cytologic specimen, not a tissue specimen. As such, the specimen may not represent the underlying disease process. Lung biopsy may be needed for a definitive diagnosis.
- BAL should not be performed unless the veterinarian is prepared to provide necessary supportive care for respiratory compromise.

MISCELLANEOUS

ANCILLARY TESTS
If results are not diagnostic, thoracotomy or thoracoscopy and lung biopsy may be indicated.

SYNONYMS
BAL

SEE ALSO
Blackwell's Five-Minute Veterinary Consult: Canine and Feline Topics
- Cough
- Pneumonia, Interstitial

Related Topics in This Book
- General Principles of Endoscopy
- Bronchoscopy
- Thoracoscopy
- Tracheal Wash
- Ultrasound-Guided Mass or Organ Aspiration

ABBREVIATIONS
BAL = bronchoalveolar lavage

Suggested Reading
Hawkins EC. Bronchoalveolar lavage. In: King LG, ed. *Textbook of Respiratory Disease in Dogs and Cats*. Philadelphia: WB Saunders, 2004: 118–128.
Hawkins EC. Diagnostic tests for the lower respiratory system. In: Nelson RW, Couto CG, eds. *Small Animal Internal Medicine,* 3rd ed. St Louis: CV Mosby, 2003: 255–286.
Hawkins EC, Berry CR. Use of a modified stomach tube for bronchoalveolar lavage in dogs. *J Am Vet Med Assoc* 1999; 215: 1635–1639.
Hawkins EC, DeNicola DB. Collection of bronchoalveolar lavage fluid in cats, using an endotracheal tube. *Am J Vet Res* 1989; 50: 855–859.
Hawkins EC, DeNicola DB, Plier ML. Cytological analysis of bronchoalveolar lavage fluid in the diagnosis of spontaneous respiratory tract disease in dogs: A retrospective study. *J Vet Intern Med* 1995; 9: 386–392.

INTERNET RESOURCES
None

AUTHOR NAME
Eleanor C. Hawkins

BASICS

TYPE OF PROCEDURE
Endoscopic

PROCEDURE EXPLANATION AND RELATED PHYSIOLOGY
- Bronchoscopy is an endoscopic examination of the large and small airways, including the trachea, carina, and bronchi (main stem, lobar, and segmental bronchi).
- Flexible instruments can also evaluate subsegmental bronchi and smaller airways.

INDICATIONS
- Coughing, wheezing, panting, exercise intolerance, and noisy breathing
- Symptoms localized to the respiratory tree that are not easily explained by more conventional and less invasive methods
- Unexplained airway or parenchymal radiographic lesions

CONTRAINDICATIONS
- Any condition for which general anesthesia is relatively or absolutely contraindicated
- Severe upper or lower airway obstruction or collapse requires very close supervision during and immediately following anesthesia.
- Most patients undergoing bronchoscopy have some degree of hypoxemia with or without airway obstruction.

POTENTIAL COMPLICATIONS
- Cough
- Stridor
- Hypoxemia
- Hemoptysis
- Pneumonia
- Respiratory distress
- Death

CLIENT EDUCATION
- General recommendations for general anesthesia
- Increased cough may occur for 12–24h following the procedure.
- Patients usually return home the same day as the procedure.
- The risk of significant postprocedural complications is usually related to the anesthetic event in a respiratory-compromised patient rather than the procedure itself.

BODY SYSTEMS ASSESSED
Respiratory

PROCEDURE

PATIENT PREPARATION
Preprocedure Medication or Preparation
- IV catheterization
- Some patients may require sedation prior to anesthesia.
- Some feline patients may require bronchodilator therapy (inhaled albuterol, 2 puffs 30 min prior to anesthesia induction).

Anesthesia or Sedation
- Propofol for canine patients (2–6 mg/kg IV for induction; 0.1–0.2 mg/kg IV/min to maintain anesthesia)
- Propofol or ketamine-diazepam (e.g., Valium) combinations for feline patients
- Isoflurane or sevoflurane gas anesthesia for prolonged procedures
- Supplemental oxygen by face mask for 5–10 min prior to beginning the procedure. If patients are not intubated, supplemental oxygen can be administered through the biopsy channel of the bronchoscope.

- Patients with upper airway obstruction may require postprocedural sedation.

Patient Positioning
Dorsal recumbency and mouth gag

Patient Monitoring
- Pulse oximetry
- Electrocardiography
- Respiration depth and rate
- Routine evaluation of anesthesia

Equipment or Supplies
- Laryngoscope
- Endotracheal tube (shortened)
- Bronchoscope(s)
- Light source (for bronchoscope)
- Suction machine and tubing
- Angled connector for gas anesthetic
- Camera and monitor (optional)
- Suction trap (optional)
- Cytocentrifuge (optional, to process cellular samples)
- Culture swabs
- Biopsy forceps
- Guarded microbiology brush
- Cytology brush
- Oral gag
- Formalin jar

TECHNIQUE
- Thorough and complete bronchoscopy can be performed in <10 min. The patients can be evaluated by using injectable, short-term anesthetic drugs.
- When more prolonged procedures are planned, patients can be intubated with a shortened endotracheal tube. Anesthesia is maintained in these cases by use of isoflurane or sevoflurane.
- A oral gag is placed, and the bronchoscope is introduced into the respiratory tree.
- The larynx, trachea, carina, and bronchi (main stem, 7 lobar, variable segmental, and subsegmental bronchi) are evaluated in terms of size, lumen integrity, mucosal shape, secretions, erythema and vascularity.
- Secretions can be obtained for cytology and culture by using a guarded microbiology brush with or without cytology brush.
- Perform bronchoalveolar lavage by wedging the distal end of the bronchoscope into a specific bronchus (depends on radiographic findings). Sterile saline is instilled through the biopsy channel of the bronchoscope and retrieved by gentle hand suction into a suction cup or the syringe used to instill the saline. This may be repeated as needed (1 mL/kg body weight may be instilled in each of 1–4 total lavages, although 2–3 lavages of 5–20 mL each is usually sufficient). *Distilled water or nonisotonic water should never be used for this procedure because use of these fluids can cause life-threatening hypoxemia and/or bronchoconstriction.*
- Extensive suction of the nonretrieved fluid is not recommended because suction induces hypoxemia.
- The bronchial mucosa is biopsied using standard biopsy forceps and mucosal biopsy techniques. Lung parenchyma may be obtained via transbronchial biopsy techniques. The latter is performed only by very sophisticated operators skilled in this technique.
- The procedure is finished and the bronchoscope withdrawn.

SAMPLE HANDLING
- Biopsy material is placed in formalin and handled in routine fashion.
- Guarded culture swabs are clipped into a sterile and appropriate microbiology container.
- Specific handling and media are required for semiquantitative cultures and mycoplasma.

APPROPRIATE AFTERCARE
Postprocedure Patient Monitoring
Patients are monitored after anesthesia in standard fashion. Particular emphasis should be placed on respiratory rate and effort.

NURSING CARE
Standard postanesthetic care is routine.

DIETARY MODIFICATION
N/A

MEDICATION REQUIREMENTS
• Individual patients may require sedation with or without cough suppression after anesthesia and bronchoscopy.
• Buprenorphine may be safely used in this setting.
• Furosemide (1 mg/kg IV) can be used to facilitate lung clearance of injected BAL fluid.

RESTRICTIONS ON ACTIVITY
• Activity should be restricted based on anesthetic protocol and postanesthetic recovery time.
• Restrictions are determined on a patient-by-patient basis.

ANTICIPATED RECOVERY TIME
Most patients can be returned to their owner within 2–3h of completion of a routine bronchoscopy.

 INTERPRETATION

NORMAL FINDINGS OR RANGE
• Normal airway mucosa is pink. Submucosal vessels are easily seen but do not protrude onto the surface of the mucosa. All airways from trachea to subsegmental bronchi are round. The dorsal tracheal membrane appears as a thin strip of tissue at a 12 o'clock position and does not protrude into the airway lumen. Tracheal cartilage is easily seen. Canine airways have minimal airway mucus. Feline healthy airways have relatively more white mucus distributed intermittently and randomly.
• Many patients have commensal bacterial flora within their respiratory tract. Positive bacterial cultures that require growth in enrichment media (thioglycolate, etc.) usually exist at $\leq 10^3$ colony-forming units/mL. This represents colonization rather than infection.
• Alveolar macrophages account for >80% of the cells obtained by BAL. They do not represent granulomatous inflammation.
• Eosinophils may be recovered in large numbers in BAL fluid from normal and healthy cats.
• Light accumulations of lymphocytes and plasma cells within bronchial mucosa are common in tissues from healthy dogs and cats.

ABNORMAL VALUES
• Airway mucosa may be pale or erythematous. Airway mucus may be abundant. Focal accumulations of mucus represent mucus plugging or pneumonia. Submucosal vessels may be difficult to see (edema) or more prominent (inflammation). Multiple airway lumen may be narrow or oblong (bronchoconstriction or bronchomalacia) or dilated (bronchiectasis). The dorsal tracheal membrane may protrude into the lumen of the trachea.
• Positive bacterial cultures grown on primary culture plates usually represent true airway and/or lung infection.
• Neutrophil counts of >10% of the differential cell count may represent sterile inflammation (bronchitis). Intracellular bacteria represent true infection. Eosinophil counts of >5% of the differential count in dogs may represent allergic or parasitic disease. Even higher numbers of eosinophils in feline BAL fluid may be normal. Neoplastic cells or fungal elements may be found cytologically.

• Cells found in bronchial mucosal biopsy samples often parallel the BAL cytologic findings. However, BAL cytology may not reflect specific cellular elements within diseased lung tissue.

CRITICAL VALUES
• Foreign bodies
• Tracheal damage or rupture
• Endobronchial bleeding

INTERFERING FACTORS
Drugs that May Alter Results of the Procedure
• Corticosteroids
• Antibiotics and/or antifungals

Conditions that May Interfere with Performing the Procedure
• Inadequate anesthesia
• Profound airway and/or tracheal collapse
• Profound laryngeal paralysis and/or collapse

Procedure Techniques or Handling That May Alter Results
• Airway culture material should be placed into appropriate culture media soon after collection.
• Airway cytologic material should be processed into cellular samples (slides) within 30 min.
• Distilled water should not be used to dilute cytologic material (cell lysis occurs).

Influence of Signalment on Performing and Interpreting the Procedure
Species
• The feline species is prone to life-threatening bronchoconstriction.
• Appropriate methods to prevent this complication in the cats should precede the procedure in susceptible individuals (e.g., albuterol inhalation).

Breed
Certain dog breeds, including huskies, malamutes, and other "snow dogs" may have a particular form of eosinophilic bronchitis.

Age
A patient's age may affect the particular anesthetic protocol chosen, as well as the length of time used to perform the procedure.

Gender
N/A

Pregnancy
Specific anesthetic protocols should be chosen to minimize the risk to both the bitch and the fetus.

CLINICAL PERSPECTIVE
• Bronchoscopy is the least invasive method of obtaining material from the respiratory tract for cytology and biopsy.
• For purposes of obtaining material for culture, a transtracheal wash does not require general anesthesia and may be the preferred technique.
• Bronchoscopy is a relatively straightforward procedure in medium-sized to large dogs. In cats and dogs weighing <15 lb, the bronchoscope may occlude $\geq 50\%$ of the tracheal lumen. For this reason, bronchoscopy in these animals should be performed only by persons well trained for this procedure.

 MISCELLANEOUS

ANCILLARY TESTS
• Computed tomography
• Open lung biopsy
• Thorascopic lung biopsy
• Ultrasound-guided lung aspiration

BRONCHOSCOPY

SYNONYMS

None

SEE ALSO

Blackwell's Five-Minute Veterinary Consult: Canine and Feline Topics

- Bronchitis, Chronic (COPD)
- Pneumonia, Aspiration
- Pneumonia, Bacterial
- Pneumonia, Eosinophilic
- Pneumonia, Fungal
- Pneumonia, Interstitial
- Tracheal Collapse

Related Topics in This Book

None

ABBREVIATIONS

BAL = bronchoalveolar lavage

Suggested Reading

King LG, ed. *Textbook of Respiratory Disease in Dogs and Cats*. St Louis: Saunders Elsevier, 2005.

Tams TR, ed. *Small Animal Endoscopy*, 2nd ed. St Louis: Saunders Elsevier, 1999.

INTERNET RESOURCES

None

AUTHOR NAME

Philip Padrid

BASICS

TYPE OF SPECIMEN
Blood

TEST EXPLANATION AND RELATED PHYSIOLOGY
Domestic dogs and wild *Canidae* are the definitive host for *Brucella canis* infection. They are much less susceptible to *Brucella abortus* and *Brucella suis*. Cats are quite resistant to *B. canis* but can be infected experimentally. Human cases have been reported, but compared to *Brucella abortus* and *Brucella melitensis* infection, people are relatively resistant to *B. canis*.

Brucella canis, a small, aerobic, Gram-negative coccobacillus, readily crosses mucous membranes. The most common routes of infections are conjunctival and oronasal. Therefore, given the same exposure, neutered and "virgin" animals may become infected, as well as sexually intact animals. Venereal transmission also occurs. The greatest numbers of organisms are shed in aborted material and postabortion vaginal discharge, which readily contaminate the environment. Large numbers are shed in semen, particularly during the first 6–8 weeks of infection. Organisms are also shed in urine, especially in male urine, and in milk. Tissue macrophages and other phagocytic cells carry the organisms to lymphoid tissue, bone marrow, and the reproductive tract, where they multiply. They persist in mononuclear phagocytes, bone marrow, lymph node, spleen, and prostate. Persistence of the organisms in the prostate is thought to explain the greater number of organisms recovered from the urine of infected males than from females. Clinical signs are epididymitis and/or orchitis and infertility in males, and abortion and early embryonic death in females. Early embryonic death may be mistaken for failure to conceive. Fever is uncommon. Lymphadenopathy is transient. Scrotal dermatitis is occasionally seen. Otherwise, infected animals are healthy. *Brucella canis* may infect nonreproductive organs, most notably the eye and intervertebral disk. In such cases, there are clinical signs associated with uveitis and diskospondylitis, respectively. Meningoencephalitis and glomerulonephropathy are much less common.

Antibody response to *B. canis* infection begins within weeks of infection, but may not be detectable until 8–12 weeks after inoculation, depending on the test methodology. Antibodies to cell wall (somatic) LPS antigens of *B. canis* cross-react with many other organisms, including *Pseudomonas*, *Staphylococcus*, *Bordetella bronchiseptica*, *Actinobacillus equuli*, and *Brucella ovis*. Therefore, all the serologic tests using cell wall LPS antigens have high false-positive rates, some as high as 60%. Antibodies to the less mucoid variant (M−) of *B. canis* have less cross-reactivity. The addition of 2-mercaptoethanol (2-ME) eliminates the less specific reactions of IgM antibodies, but false positives are still common. Internal cytoplasmic protein antigen (CPAg), on the other hand, is unique to the *Brucella* organisms. Therefore, serologic tests using CPAg are highly specific for *Brucella* infection. Obtaining CPAg uncontaminated by LPS for use in serologic testing is technically difficult.

Serologic tests for *B. canis* infection include 2-ME RSAT (D-Tec CB canine brucellosis antibody test; Synbiotics, San Diego, CA); 2-ME TAT; AGID using cell wall (LPS) antigen; AGID using CPAg; ELISA using LPS or CPAg; and IFA using LPS. Unfortunately, laboratory reagents and methods have not been standardized for any of these tests except 2-ME RSAT and 2-ME TAT. Availability of the standardized reagents for 2-ME TAT is sporadic. Therefore, the *reliability of test results and the accuracy of interpretation are extremely variable among laboratories* (see the Interpretation section).

INDICATIONS
- A screening test to detect *B. canis* infection in dogs
- Routine, prebreeding, and prepurchase evaluation of normal animals
- Routine part of the evaluation of infertility in male and female dogs
- Evaluation of symptomatic animals and animals suspected to have been exposed

CONTRAINDICATIONS
None

POTENTIAL COMPLICATIONS
None

CLIENT EDUCATION
Brucella canis is a zoonotic organism. Laboratory personnel and veterinarians handling infected specimens, and owners of infected dogs, are at greatest risk. The actual prevalence in people is unknown because *B. canis* is not detected by the typical methods used to detect *B. abortus*, *B. melitensis*, and *B. suis*, which are much more virulent in people. Biohazard precautions should be taken when handling specimens from suspect animals. Owners should be informed about the potential risks to the health of family members and other dogs in the household. All people exposed to infected and suspect animals should practice good hygiene.

BODY SYSTEMS ASSESSED
Reproductive

SAMPLE

COLLECTION
2–3 mL of venous blood

HANDLING
- Harvest 1–3 mL of serum from cells and place it in a sterile tube.
- Hemolysis will interfere with some assays.

STORAGE
- Refrigerate if the assay will be run within 3 days.
- Store frozen (−20°C) if >3 days before assay.

STABILITY
- Can be stored for days at 2°–8°C (refrigeration)
- Can be stored for months to years at −20° to −80°C (freezer)
- Maintain appropriate temperature during transport.
- Prevent thawing of frozen samples.

PROTOCOL
- Handling the RSAT kit
  - Reagents must be at room temperature when the test is performed.
  - Store the kit in a refrigerator. Do not leave it at room temperature for extended periods.
  - The 2-ME must be kept refrigerated, in the dark, and tightly capped.
- The RSAT uses *B. ovis* for the antigen. The test has 2 steps. When the result of the first step is negative, the test is complete and the result is negative. When the result of the first step is positive, 2-ME is added as the second step. When the result of the second step is also positive, the result is positive. When the result of the first step is positive and that of the second step is negative, the result should be considered probably negative. In this situation, a confirmatory test could be performed at the time, or the RSAT could be repeated in 1 month. The New York State (NYS) Diagnostic Laboratory at Cornell University has developed a RSAT using the M− variant of *B. canis* for the antigen. This M− RSAT has fewer false-positive results. It is not commercially available for in-house use or use by other laboratories.

BRUCELLOSIS SEROLOGY

INTERPRETATION

NORMAL FINDINGS OR RANGE
Negative results

ABNORMAL VALUES
* Positive results
* Interpretation of TAT titers varies among laboratories. Titers of 1:50–1:100 should be considered suspect. Titers of ≥1:200 should be considered positive.
* False-positive results are very common and occur in *all* assays (RSAT, TAT, AGID, and IFA) using cell wall LPS antigens. Positive results must be confirmed by other methods.

CRITICAL VALUES
None

INTERFERING FACTORS
Drugs That May Alter Results or Interpretation
Drugs That Interfere with Test Methodology
None

Drugs That Alter Physiology
Current and recent antibiotic therapy will cause titers to decline and negative results.

Disorders That May Alter Results
None

Collection Techniques or Handling That May Alter Results
Hemolysis will cause false-positive results in some agglutination assays.

Influence of Signalment
Species
Canine. Cats are resistant to infections.

Breed
None

Age
Any age, but most commonly diagnosed in adults. Infected neonates usually do not survive.

Gender
* Intact and neutered animals are equally susceptible, given equal exposure.
* Clinical signs in intact males are epididymitis, orchitis, and infertility.
* Clinical signs in intact females are abortion and early embryonic death. Early embryonic death may be mistaken for failure to conceive.

Pregnancy
Spontaneous abortion is the classic clinical sign.

LIMITATIONS OF THE TEST
* False-negative results are expected.
  * Early in infection (<8–12 weeks)
  * In chronic infection (>6 months to 2 years)
  * As a result of recent or current antibiotic therapy
* Serologic tests are screening only. The definitive diagnosis requires organism identification. See the Ancillary Tests section.

Sensitivity, Specificity, and Positive and Negative Predictive Values
N/A

Valid If Run in a Human Lab?
No. Accuracy and reliability vary greatly even among veterinary diagnostic labs.

CLINICAL PERSPECTIVE
* Because it is highly sensitive, the RSAT is excellent for screening animals for *B. canis* infection. Animals with negative test results are

Test	Antigen	Comments
RSAT	Cell wall from *B. ovis*	Fast, easy, preferred screening test; in-house or lab Highly sensitive False positives common; must confirm by other methods False negatives uncommon
TAT	Cell wall	Semiquantitative titer False positives similar to RSAT; 2-ME somewhat more specific Longer time before titers become positive
AGID	Cell wall	Very sensitive False positives; complex procedure
AGID	CPAg	Complex procedure Most specific serologic test but least sensitive Available through NYS Diagnostic Laboratory
RSAT	Cell wall from M– *B. canis*	More specific than other RSAT Available through NYS Diagnostic Laboratory
ELISA	Cell wall or CPAg	Good results but limited availability Complex procedure
IFA	Cell wall	May be less sensitive than 2-ME TAT Despite its availability and use by several diagnostic labs, specificity and sensitivity have not been thoroughly evaluated

unlikely to have the disease unless the test was performed soon after exposure, or was performed on dogs with chronic infection or dogs that had recent antibiotic therapy. When recent exposure is suspected, blood culture is a better screening test than is serology, because bacteremia is present 2–4 weeks after infection and persists for many months.
* The RSAT and other serologic tests are sensitive but not specific for *B. canis* infection. False-positive results are very common. Positive results must be confirmed. Meanwhile, appropriate measures should be taken to prevent spread of the disease should *B. canis* infection be confirmed. Antibiotic therapy must not be initiated in the individual or other dogs in the kennel until samples for confirmatory tests have been obtained because doing so will cause cultures and serologic test results to become negative.
* AGID using purified CPAg is confirmatory. However, this assay requires a lab with expertise, such as the NYS Diagnostic Laboratory. The AGID (CPAg) is specific for *Brucella* infection. It is possible, though unlikely, that the *Brucella* is one other than *B. canis*.
* When the clinical findings are classic for *B. canis*, such as third-trimester abortion, the opportunity to submit specimens for culture should not be missed while awaiting serologic results.

MISCELLANEOUS

ANCILLARY TESTS
Confirm positive results of serologic tests by using cell wall LPS antigen. Culture is the gold standard, but PCR is also useful. Submit the following:
* Blood
* Postabortion vaginal discharge
* Semen

SYNONYMS
Brucella canis

SEE ALSO

Blackwell's Five-Minute Veterinary Consult: Canine and Feline Topics
- Abortion, Spontaneous, and Pregnancy Loss—Dogs
- Brucellosis
- Diskospondylitis
- Epididymitis/Orchitis
- Infertility, Female
- Infertility, Male— Dogs
- Spermatozoal Abnormalities

Related Topics in this Book
- Relaxin
- Semen Analysis
- Semen Collection

ABBREVIATIONS

- AGID = agar gel immunodiffusion
- CPAg = cytoplasmic protein antigen
- LPS = lipopolysaccharide
- M− = the less mucoid strain of *Brucella canis*
- 2-ME = 2-mercaptoethanol
- RSAT = rapid slide agglutination test
- TAT = tube agglutination test

Suggested Reading

Greene CE, Carmichael LE. Canine brucellosis. In: Greene CE, ed. *Infectious Diseases of the Dog and Cat,* 3rd ed. St Louis: Saunders Elsevier, 2006: 369–381.

Johnson CA. Genital infections and transmissible venereal tumor. In: Nelson RW, Couto CG, eds. *Small Animal Internal Medicine.* St Louis: CV Mosby, 2003: 936–938.

Johnston SD, Root Kustritz MV, Olson PN. *Canine and Feline Theriogenology.* Philadelphia: WB Saunders, 2001: 319–321.

INTERNET RESOURCES

Shin SJ, Carmichael L. Canine brucellosis caused by *Brucella canis*. In: Carmichael LE, ed. Recent Advances in Canine Infectious Diseases. Ithaca, NY: International Veterinary Information Service (IVIS), 1999, http://www.ivis.org/advances/infect_dis_carmichael/shin/ivis.pdf.

AUTHOR NAME

Cheri A. Johnson

BUFFY COAT PREPARATIONS

 BASICS

TYPE OF SPECIMEN
Blood

TEST EXPLANATION AND RELATED PHYSIOLOGY
The buffy coat is an off-white layer immediately above the column of packed RBCs in a centrifuged sample of whole blood. The buffy coat consists predominantly of leukocytes. A narrow white layer of platelets is just above the buffy coat, but usually platelets can be observed as a separate layer only with magnification. The leukocyte count can be estimated by observing the height of the buffy coat. During intense regeneration, reticulocytes may be in the buffy coat, which then appears red tinged. The buffy coat is used to prepare smears of concentrated leukocytes, most often in looking for circulating mast cells, neoplastic cells, or infectious agents. Buffy coat smears contain numerous leukocytes and platelets. Polychromatophilic cells may be present in buffy coat smears of animals with regenerative anemia.

INDICATIONS
- Mast cell tumor staging
- Hematopoietic neoplasia
- Detection of some infectious agents, e.g., *Leishmania* spp., *Hepatozoon* spp., *Ehrlichia* spp., *Anaplasma phagocyctophilum*, *Trypanosoma* spp., and *Histoplasmosis capsulatum*
- Cell concentration for DNA-based assays for infectious agents, e.g., *Mycobacterium* spp.
- May be helpful to concentrate leukocytes for cytochemical staining of neoplastic cells

CONTRAINDICATIONS
None

POTENTIAL COMPLICATIONS
None

CLIENT EDUCATION
None

BODY SYSTEMS ASSESSED
Hemic, lymphatic, and immune

 SAMPLE

COLLECTION
2 mL of venous blood

HANDLING
Collect into EDTA anticoagulant

STORAGE
- Process the sample within several hours of collection or store the blood in refrigerator.
- Store the buffy coat smears at room temperature and protected from light.

STABILITY
- EDTA-anticoagulated blood
  - Several hours at room temperature
  - 1 day at 2°–8°C (refrigerated)
- Smears are stable for years, especially if protected by a permanent coverslip. After several years, the stain may begin to fade.

PROTOCOL
- Buffy coat smear preparation: method 1
  - Fill a Wintrobe tube with EDTA blood and centrifuge at 300 g for 15 min.
  - Remove plasma with a pipette, leaving a small amount just above the buffy coat.
  - Transfer the remaining plasma and the buffy coat to a clean test tube and mix the sample gently.
  - Place 1 drop of resuspended buffy coat onto several clean glass slides.
  - Spread the buffy coat with another glass slide by a push or pull technique to prepare the smear.
- Buffy coat smear preparation: method 2
  - Fill a microhematocrit tube to 75% of its length with blood, sealing 1 end with clay.
  - Centrifuge the sample in a microhematocrit centrifuge according to the manufacturer's directions.
  - Break the hematocrit tube along the line between the buffy coat and the top of the packed RBC column.
  - Place 1 drop of buffy coat on a clean glass slide and spread the buffy coat by using a second glass slide. With this method, there is a possibility of exposure to glass shards and blood, and there is less volume for smear preparation.
- Stain buffy coat smears with Wright or Wright-Giemsa stain.
- Attach a glass coverslip with permanent mounting media if smears are going to be archived.
- Examine stained buffy coat smears microscopically using a 10× or 20× scanning objective and a 40×, 50×, or 100× objective.
- A wet preparation of a buffy coat smear may be used to detect motile *Trypanosoma* trypomastigotes or *Dirofilaria* microfilaria. Alternately, with low magnification, *Dirofilaria* microfilaria may be visualized moving in the plasma just above the buffy coat in the hematocrit tube.

 INTERPRETATION

NORMAL FINDINGS OR RANGE
No mast cells, neoplastic cells, or infectious agents

ABNORMAL VALUES
The presence of mast cells, neoplastic cells, or infectious agents

CRITICAL VALUES
None

INTERFERING FACTORS
Drugs That May Alter Results of the Procedure
Drugs That Interfere with Test Methodology
None

Drugs That Alter Physiology
None

Disorders That May Alter Results
Disorders other than mast cell neoplasia associated with increased numbers of circulating mast cells include regenerative anemia, inflammatory or allergic disorders, and gastric torsion.

Collection Techniques or Handling that May Alter Results
- Some commercial quick stains do not stain mast cell granules adequately.
- Leukocyte morphology is poorly preserved in blood that is stored improperly.
- Leukocytes may stain poorly in samples that have been exposed to formalin fumes.

Influence of Signalment

Species
None

Breed
None

Age
None

Gender
None

Pregnancy
None

LIMITATIONS OF THE TEST
Sensitivity, Specificity, and Positive and Negative Predictive Values
N/A

Valid If Run in a Human Lab?
Yes.

Causes Of Abnormal Findings
- Infectious agents
  - *Trypanosoma* trypomastigotes
  - Morulae of *Ehrlichia* spp. and *Anaplasma* spp. in monocytes, lymphocytes, neutrophils, or platelets
  - *Leishmania* trypomastigotes in leukocytes
  - *Hepatozoon* gametocytes in leukocytes
  - *Histoplasma* yeasts in leukocytes
- Mast cells
  - Allergic disorders
  - Gastric torsion
  - Inflammation
  - Mast cell neoplasia
  - Regenerative anemia
- Neoplastic hematopoietic cells

CLINICAL PERSPECTIVE
- Dogs with nonneoplastic disorders, especially acute inflammatory disorders, may have >1,000 mast cells per buffy coat smear.
- Dogs with mast cell neoplasia that have increased numbers of circulating mast cells might have a poorer prognosis, but data to support this have not been reported.
- Buffy coat smears are not necessary to detect neoplastic cells in most cases of acute or chronic lymphoid or myeloid leukemia.

 MISCELLANEOUS

ANCILLARY TESTS
- Cytologic evaluation of organs or tissues for diagnosis of mast cell tumors and hematopoietic neoplasia
- Serology and DNA-based assays are more sensitive for the diagnosis of some infectious agents.

SYNONYMS
None

SEE ALSO
Blackwell's Five-Minute Veterinary Consult: Canine and Feline Topics
- Ehrlichiosis
- Hepatozoonosis
- Histoplasmosis
- Leishmaniasis
- Mast Cell Tumors

Related Topics in This Book
- Blood Smear Microscopic Examination
- *Ehrlichia/Anaplasma*
- Fine-Needle Aspiration
- Skin Biopsy

ABBREVIATIONS
None

Suggested Reading
Green CE. *Infectious Diseases of the Dog and Cat,* 3rd ed. Philadelphia: WB Saunders, 2006: 212–222, 579, 679–680, 709.
Lassen ED. Laboratory evaluation of plasma and serum proteins. In: Thrall MA, ed. *Veterinary Hematology and Clinical Chemistry.* Philadelphia: Lippincott Williams & Wilkins, 2004: 401–412.
Willard MD, Tvedten H. *Small Animal Clinical Diagnosis by Laboratory Methods,* 4th ed. St Louis: Saunders Elsevier, 2004: 18–19.

INTERNET RESOURCES
None

AUTHOR NAME
Maxey L. Wellman

BASICS

TYPE OF SPECIMEN
Blood

TEST EXPLANATION AND RELATED PHYSIOLOGY
Vitamin D is derived either from the metabolism of cholesterol or from dietary sources. Cholesterol is altered by UV irradiation in the skin to vitamin D_3 (cholecalciferol), which is then converted by 25-hydroxylase in hepatocytes to *calcidiol* (25-hydroxycholecalciferol). Calcidiol is converted by 1α-hydroxylase in renal tubular cells to *calcitriol* (1,25-dihydroxycholecalciferol). Calcitriol promotes increased serum calcium concentrations by stimulating intestinal absorption, bone resorption, and proximal renal tubular resorption. Insufficient renal mass, as seen in chronic renal failure, may result in inadequate synthesis of calcitriol. Activated macrophages may also produce 1α-hydroxylase. Production of calcitriol by macrophages is seemingly unregulated and may lead to increased serum calcitriol with granulomatous diseases.

Laboratories can measure both calcitriol and calcidiol. Measurement of calcidiol may provide a better indication of overall vitamin D status from nutrition and UV irradiation for 2 reasons: calcidiol has a longer serum half-life (approximately 3 weeks, compared to approximately 4–6h for calcitriol). In addition, calcidiol production is not regulated and depends primarily on substrate concentration (dietary consumption and UV exposure).

INDICATIONS
Diagnosis of vitamin D deficiency or toxicity

CONTRAINDICATIONS
None

POTENTIAL COMPLICATIONS
None

CLIENT EDUCATION
Question clients about their animal's diet and possible exposure to vitamin D–containing substances.

BODY SYSTEMS ASSESSED
Endocrine and metabolic

SAMPLE

COLLECTION
1–2 mL of venous blood

HANDLING
- Collect the sample into a plain red-top tube or serum-separator tube.
- Ship the serum overnight with a cold pack.

STORAGE
Store at −20°C (frozen)

STABILITY
- Room temperature: up to 3 days
- Frozen (−20°C): up to 2 years

PROTOCOL
None

INTERPRETATION

NORMAL FINDINGS OR RANGE
Results vary among assay methods and laboratories, so use laboratory-specific reference ranges, if possible.

Published Canine Reference Intervals
- Calcitriol: vary from 20–50 pg/mL to 22–106 pg/mL
- Calcidiol: vary from 60–215 nmol/L to 73–461 nmol/L

Published Feline Reference Intervals
- Calcitriol: 20–40 pg/mL
- Calcidiol: 65–170 nmol/L

ABNORMAL VALUES
Values above and below the reference interval

CRITICAL VALUES
None

INTERFERING FACTORS
Drugs That May Alter Results or Interpretation
Drugs That Interfere with Test Methodology
Calcitriol analogs used therapeutically to minimize renal secondary hyperparathyroidism will cross-react with some calcitriol assays. After initiation of therapy, monitor patients by serial measurement of serum calcium, phosphate, and plasma PTH, rather than by measurement of calcitriol.

Drugs That Alter Physiology
None

Disorders That May Alter Results
None

Collection Techniques or Handling That May Alter Results
Some references recommend avoiding exposure to light. One study reports that sample stability was affected by exposure to UV light and repeated freezing and thawing.

Influence of Signalment
Species
Normal ranges are slightly lower in cats than in dogs.

Breed
None

Age
Slightly higher in 10- to 12-week-old puppies and kittens than in adults: puppies, 60–120 pg/mL; kittens, 20–80 pg/mL.

Gender
None

Pregnancy
None

LIMITATIONS OF THE TEST
Sensitivity, Specificity, and Positive and Negative Predictive Values
N/A

Valid If Run a in Human Lab?
Yes.

Causes of Abnormal Findings

High values	Low values
Vitamin D toxicosis	Vitamin D deficiency
Cholecalciferol rodenticides (calcipotriol)	Dietary deficiency
Antipsoriasis cream (tacalcitol)	Intestinal disease with malabsorption (loss of fat-soluble vitamins)
Increases also seen with the following:	Decreases also seen with the following:
Granulomatous disease (calcitriol is increased, calcidiol is not)	Renal failure
HHM as seen with lymphoma and anal sac adenocarcinoma	HHM as seen with lymphoma and anal sac adenocarcinoma
Primary hyperparathyroidism	Hyperphosphatemia
Hypophosphatemia	Hypomagnesemia

CLINICAL PERSPECTIVE

• Measuring vitamin D metabolites can aid in the diagnosis of vitamin D toxicosis, but does not appear clinically useful in distinguishing causes of hypercalcemia.

• Decreased calcitriol may support diagnosis of vitamin D deficiency, but low calcitriol concentration is found in a variety of more common etiologies, which must first be excluded.

• Dogs with chronic renal failure usually have normal to low calcitriol concentration regardless of whether their serum calcium concentrations are low, normal, or high.

• Serum calcium concentration is usually high with all causes of increased calcitriol.

• Serum calcium concentration varies with causes of low calcitriol (dependent on primary etiology).

• Serum PTH will be increased with primary hyperparathyroidism or chronic renal failure and decreased with vitamin D toxicosis, HHM, or granulomatous disease.

• Serum PTH-rp is increased with HHM.

 MISCELLANEOUS

ANCILLARY TESTS

• Chemistry profile, including calcium and phosphate
• PTH and PTH-rp

SYNONYMS

• 1,25-Dihydroxycholecalciferol
• Vitamin D

SEE ALSO

Blackwell's Five-Minute Veterinary Consult: Canine and Feline Topics

• Anal Sac Disorders
• Hypercalcemia
• Lymphoma—Dogs
• Renal Failure, Acute Uremic
• Renal Failure, Chronic
• Vitamin D Toxicity

Related Topics in This Book

• Calcium
• Parathyroid Hormone
• Parathyroid-Related Protein
• Phosphorus

ABBREVIATIONS

• HHM = humoral hypercalcemia of malignancy
• PTH = parathyroid hormone
• PTH-rP = parathyroid hormone–related protein
• UV = ultraviolet

Suggested Reading

Hauser BB, Reusch CE. Serum levels of 25-hydroxycholecalciferol and 1,25-dihydroxycholecalciferol in dogs with hypercalcaemia. *Vet Res Commun* 2004; 28: 669–680.

Rosol TJ, Nagode LA, Couto CG, et al. Parathyroid hormone (PTH)–related protein, PTH, and 1,25-dihydroxyvitamin D in dogs with cancer-associated hypercalcemia. *Endocrinology* 1992; 131: 1157–1164.

Schenck PA, Chew DJ, Nagode LA, Rosol TJ. Disorders of calcium: Hypercalcemia and hypocalcemia. In: DiBartola SP, ed. *Fluid, Electrolyte, and Acid-Base Disorders in Small Animal Practice,* 3rd ed. St Louis: Saunders Elsevier, 2006: 122–194.

INTERNET RESOURCES

Michigan State University, Diagnostic Center for Population and Animal Health: Medicine offers measurement of serum vitamin D, http://www.animalhealth.msu.edu.

AUTHOR NAMES

Deanna M.W. Schaefer and M. Judith Radin

CALCIUM

BASICS

TYPE OF SPECIMEN
Blood

TEST EXPLANATION AND RELATED PHYSIOLOGY
Calcium is an important structural constituent of bone and is required for coagulation, neuromuscular excitability, skeletal muscle contraction, and cardiovascular function. Ca homeostasis is controlled by interactions of PTH, calcitonin, and vitamin D with the intestine, bone, kidneys, and parathyroid glands. The effect of PTH is to increase Ca concentrations in the face of hypocalcemia by causing increased release of Ca from bone, increased intestinal absorption, and increased renal tubule resorption. Vitamin D promotes intestinal absorption of Ca and may facilitate actions of PTH on bone. In response to hypercalcemia, calcitonin decreases Ca by inhibiting effects of PTH on bone.

In blood, total Ca occurs as bound and free forms in roughly equal proportions. Of the bound Ca, ≈40% is protein bound (primarily to albumin) and 10% is complexed with citrate, phosphates, lactate, and other anions. Free Ca or iCa, which makes up the remaining 50% portion in blood, is the physiologically active form. Acid-base status affects the amount of Ca bound to the anionic sites on proteins. In acidosis, more Ca becomes unbound, increasing the iCa concentration. Alkalosis increases Ca binding to proteins causing a decreased iCa concentration.

The protein concentration, especially albumin, affects total Ca concentration. With hypoalbuminemia, the total Ca concentration is lowered. Hyperalbuminemia has the opposite effect. Formulas that correct total Ca concentration for albumin or total protein concentration have been used for dogs. The relationship is similar for cats but not as strong. However, some authors advise that these formulas be used cautiously because they may not be accurate for different systems and methods that are used to determine Ca, albumin, and total protein concentrations; they may not fully correct for differences between Ca binding to albumin vs globulins; they do not take into account changes in complexed calcium or acid-base effects; they do not consider differences between puppies and adult dogs; and they are only an estimate of the corrected Ca concentration.

Routine chemistry profiles provide a total Ca concentration determined colorimetrically. Determination of iCa requires special instrumentation using ion-specific electrodes for Ca. Many instruments capable of measuring iCa also measure pH and can adjust the measured Ca for a pH of 7.4.

INDICATIONS
• Total Ca concentration is a part of a routine biochemistry profile.
• If available, iCa may be a better assessment of Ca balance in animals with hyperproteinemia or hypoproteinemia, renal disease, acid-base imbalances, or hyperparathyroidism.
• Signs suggestive of hypocalcemia, such as facial rubbing, muscle twitching, or tetany or seizures
• Animals that are PU/PD, weak, or have a cardiac arrhythmia

CONTRAINDICATIONS
None

POTENTIAL COMPLICATIONS
None

CLIENT EDUCATION
None

BODY SYSTEMS ASSESSED
• Cardiovascular
• Endocrine and metabolic
• Gastrointestinal
• Musculoskeletal

• Neuromuscular
• Renal and urologic
• Reproductive

SAMPLE

COLLECTION
1–3 mL of venous blood

HANDLING
• The sample can be collected into the following:
  • A plain red-top tube or serum-separator tube (total Ca)
  • A sodium heparin, or lithium heparin, anticoagulant is also acceptable.
• For iCa, samples need to be collected anaerobically, placed on ice, and delivered to the laboratory immediately or stored in a tightly sealed container to maintain anaerobic conditions. Avoid the use of serum-separator tubes.
• Anticoagulants, which chelate Ca (e.g., EDTA, citrate) or cause precipitation of Ca (e.g., oxalate), are not acceptable.

STORAGE
Total Ca
Refrigerate for short-term storage.
iCa
• Heparinized whole blood should be analyzed immediately.
• If there is a delay, the sample should be tightly capped to maintain anaerobic conditions and be put on ice.
• Serum or plasma stored in an airtight container can be refrigerated or frozen.

STABILITY
Total Ca
• Room temperature: ≈1 week
• Refrigerated (2°–8°C): ≈3 weeks
• Frozen (−20°C): ≈1 year. However, coprecipitation of Ca with lipids or fibrin (from plasma) may occur with frozen samples, and plastic or glass may adsorb Ca during storage.
iCa
When maintained under anaerobic conditions (i.e., in an airtight container), iCa concentration in serum or plasma is stable for the following periods:
• Room temperature: ≈3 days
• Refrigerated (−4°C): ≈1 week
• Frozen (−20°C): ≈6 months

PROTOCOL
None

INTERPRETATION

NORMAL FINDINGS OR RANGE
Reference intervals may vary among laboratories, instrumentation, and methodology.
Total Ca
• Dogs: 9.0–11.5 mg/dL (2.25–2.88 mmol/L)
• Cats: 8.0–11.5 mg/dL (2.00–2.88 mmol/L)
iCa
• Dogs: 4.6–5.5 mg/dL (1.15–1.38 mmol/L)
• Cats: 4.5–5.5 mg/dL (1.13–1.38 mmol/L)

ABNORMAL VALUES
Total Ca
• Dogs: <9.0 or >11.5 mg/dL

- Cats: <8.0 or >11.5 mg/dL

iCa
- Dogs: <4.6 or >5.5 mg/dL
- Cats: <4.5 or >5.5 mg/dL

CRITICAL VALUES
- Total Ca of <7 mg/dL can lead to clinical signs of tetany.
- Total Ca of >16 mg/dL can lead to acute renal failure, cardiac toxicity, and possibly soft tissue mineralization.
- When the [total Ca] × [phosphorus] product is 60–70 or greater, there is an increased risk of soft tissue mineralization.

INTERFERING FACTORS
Drugs That May Alter Results or Interpretation
Drugs That Interfere with Test Methodology
- Administration of fluorides and oxalate may cause Ca precipitation.
- Administration of acetaminophen, cefotaxime, chlorpropamide, or hydralazine can cause artificial increases in Ca.

Drugs That Alter Physiology
- A wide variety of drugs or substances potentially cause decreases in Ca, including albuterol, anticonvulsants, asparaginase, aspirin, cisplatin, citrate, mithramycin, diuretics (furosemide), EDTA, fluoride, gastrin, glucagon, glucocorticoids, glucose, insulin, isoniazide, magnesium salts, phenobarbital (long term), phosphate-containing enemas and IV phosphate administration (potassium phosphate), and tetracycline (in pregnancy).
- Drugs or substances that potentially cause increases in Ca include alkaline antacids and antacids with Ca, aluminum hydroxide, anabolic steroids and androgens, Ca salts and parenteral Ca administration, cholecalciferol rodenticides, danazol, dienestrol, diethylstilbestrol, diuretics [chronically administered (chlorthalidone, ergocalciferol, furosemide, thiazides)], estrogen, hydrochlorothiazide, excess oral phosphate binders, propranolol, progesterone, testosterone, theophylline, vitamin A (acute intoxication), and vitamin D.

Disorders That May Alter Results
- Total Ca is falsely increased by lipemia and hemolysis (formation of a hemoglobin-chromogen complex), but iCa is unaffected.
- Total Ca is decreased by marked bilirubinemia.

Collection Techniques or Handling That May Alter Results
- Prolonged occlusion (i.e., 2–3 min) of the vessel during phlebotomy may mildly increase Ca.
- Use of an inappropriate anticoagulant
- Carbon dioxide loss because of nonaerobic sample handling can change the iCa concentration.

Influence of Signalment
Species
None

Breed
None

Age
Puppies between 6–24 weeks of age have slightly higher serum Ca concentrations (1–2 mg/dL) than adults.

Gender
None

Pregnancy
Small-breed female dogs are at increased risk of hypocalcemia during the first 3 weeks postpartum, while nursing a litter.

LIMITATIONS OF THE TEST
Sensitivity, Specificity, and Positive and Negative Predictive Values
N/A

Valid If Run in a Human Lab?
Yes.

Causes of Abnormal Findings

High values	Low values
Hypercalcemia of malignancy: lymphoma, anal sac adenocarcinoma, multiple myeloma, various carcinomas	Hypoalbuminemia: hypoproteinemia, protein-losing enteropathy, protein-losing glomerulopathy
Hyperalbuminemia: dehydration	Ethylene glycol toxicosis
Acidosis: increased iCa	Alkalosis: low iCa
Renal: chronic renal failure (more common), familial renal disease (Lhasa apso), acute renal failure (uncommon)	Renal: acute and chronic renal failure, urethral obstruction (especially cats)
Hypoadrenocorticism	Pancreatitis: acute, necrotizing
Primary hyperparathyroidism	Hypoparathyroidism
Hypervitaminosis D: calciferol rodenticides, excess dietary supplementation	Eclampsia (dogs) (puerperal tetany)
Osteolytic bone lesions: osteomyelitis, neoplasia (osteosarcoma, lymphoma, carcinoma, myeloma)	Dietary imbalance: Ca deficient, hypovitaminosis D, excess phosphorus (nutritional secondary hyperparathyroidism)
Granulomatous disease: blastomycosis	Intestinal malabsorption syndromes (dogs)
Schistosomiasis	Thyroid surgery: thyroidectomy
Factitious: lipemia, postprandial	Factitious: sample run on EDTA, citrate, or oxalate plasma
Hypertrophic osteodystrophy (dogs)	Tumor-lysis syndrome
Iatrogenic: excessive Ca supplementation, oral phosphate binders	Iatrogenic: after bicarbonate administration, phosphate infusions, or phosphate enemas; transfusion with citrated blood products
Idiopathic hypercalcemia (cats)	
Age: young large-breed dog <1 year	Hypomagnesemia: rare
Plant toxicity: jasmine (*Cestrum* sp.), *Solarum* sp.	Soft tissue trauma, rhabdomyolysis
Hypervitaminosis A	Drugs (see the section Drugs That May Alter Results or Interpretation)
Drugs (see the section Drugs That May Alter Results or Interpretation)	

CLINICAL PERSPECTIVE
- In many instances, total Ca concentration is adequate for disease recognition and management. However, for certain diseases, such as renal disease or hyperparathyroidism, or when there are abnormalities in protein concentrations or the acid-base balance, iCa measurement may be a better assessment of the Ca status.
- In conditions associated with abnormal PTH secretion or secretion of parathyroid hormone–related protein, there may be inverse changes in Ca and phosphorus concentrations.
- One of the most common causes of hypercalcemia is the hypercalcemia associated with malignancy.
- A common cause of hypocalcemia is hypoalbuminemia, which is usually not clinically significant.

MISCELLANEOUS
ANCILLARY TESTS
- A serum chemistry profile (especially albumin, total protein, phosphorus concentrations)
- An imaging technique to look for neoplasia

CALCIUM

- Blood-gas analysis
- PTH and parathyroid hormone–related protein levels as workup for hypercalcemia of malignancy
- Urinary fractional excretion of Ca

SYNONYMS
None

SEE ALSO
Blackwell's Five-Minute Veterinary Consult: Canine and Feline Topics
- Hypoalbuminemia
- Hypercalcemia
- Hypocalcemia
- Hyperparathyroidism
- Hypoparathyroidism
- Hyperparathyroidism, Renal Secondary
- Lymphoma—Cats
- Lymphoma—Dogs
- Polyuria and Polydipsia
- Renal Failure, Acute Uremia
- Renal Failure, Chronic
- Vitamin D Toxicity

Related Topics in This Book
- Albumin
- Calcitriol
- Magnesium
- Phosphorus

ABBREVIATIONS
- Ca = calcium
- iCa = ionized calcium
- PTH = parathyroid hormone, parathormone
- PU/PD = polyuria/polydipsia

Suggested Reading

Feldman EC, Nelson RW. Hypercalcemia and primary hyperparathyroidism. In: Feldman EC, Nelson RW, eds. *Canine and Feline Endocrinology and Reproduction, 3rd ed.* St Louis: Saunders Elsevier, 2004: 660–715.

Feldman EC, Nelson RW. Hypocalcemia and primary hypoparathyroidism. In: Feldman EC, Nelson RW, eds. *Canine and Feline Endocrinology and Reproduction, 3rd ed.* St Louis: Saunders Elsevier, 2004: 716–742.

Nelson RW, Turnwald GH, Willard MD. Endocrine, metabolic, and lipid disorders. In: Willard MD, Tvedten H, eds. *Small Animal Clinical Diagnosis by Laboratory Methods, 4th ed.* St Louis: Saunders Elsevier, 2004: 165–207.

Rosol TJ, Chew DJ, Nagode LA, Schenck P. Disorders of calcium. In: DiBartola SP, ed. *Fluid Therapy in Small Animal Practice.* Philadelphia: WB Saunders, 2000: 108–162.

INTERNET RESOURCES
None

AUTHOR NAME
Karen E. Russell

BASICS

TYPE OF PROCEDURE
Radiographic (fluoroscopic)

PROCEDURE EXPLANATION AND RELATED PHYSIOLOGY
Cardiac catheterization is the procedure in which a catheter is passed directly into selective positions within the heart or great vessels of a living organism. The catheter can be inserted into a vessel percutaneously or via direct vascular exposure (vascular cutdown). Common vessels used for cardiac catheterization include the jugular vein, carotid artery, femoral artery, and femoral vein, depending on which chambers or vessels are to be assessed. The catheter can then be used to measure intravascular pressure, obtain samples for oximetry data, or perform angiography.

INDICATIONS
• Diagnostic catheterization is performed to confirm the presence or assess the severity of anatomic or physiologic lesions. Echocardiography has become the gold standard for assessing most cardiac diseases, though complex congenital cardiac defects occasionally require the more exhaustive evaluation enabled by cardiac catheterization.
• Intracardiac pressure is measured to quantify the severity of cardiac defects (e.g., pulmonic stenosis, aortic stenosis). Intracardiac pressure is measured prior to and following any therapeutic procedures (e.g., balloon valvuloplasty) to evaluate postprocedural hemodynamic improvements.
• Angiocardiography provides a more complete anatomic characterization of cardiac abnormalities via injection of radiopaque contrast material.
• Oximetry and blood-gas sampling are useful in detection of left-to-right and right-to-left intracardiac shunting of blood.
• Placement of temporary and permanent pacemakers improves bradycardic rhythm disturbances such as complete heart block, persistant atrial standstill, and sick sinus syndrome.
• In cases of severe heartworm disease (caval syndrome), adult worms can be extricated from the right atrium (RA) or right ventricle (RV) via cardiac catheterization, reducing worm burden prior to adulticide treatment.
• Pulmonary capillary wedge pressure can be measured.
• Cardiac output can be determined via the thermodilution method through cardiac catheterization.

CONTRAINDICATIONS
• Metabolic abnormalities, infectious conditions, or drug toxicities, which may increase anesthetic risk or dispose patients toward increased ventricular irritability

• Decompensated cardiac conditions, including congestive heart failure (CHF), increase patient risk.
• A history of uncontrolled ventricular arrhythmia, which may lead to the induction of potentially life-threatening arrhythmias
• Bleeding disorders (coagulopathies) may disrupt hemostasis at vascular access sites, leading to excessive blood loss, thrombosis, or hematoma formation.
• Dehydrated animals or those with significant preexisting renal disease are at increased risk of contrast-induced reactions.
• A history of prior adverse reactions to contrast media should be considered a relative contraindication.

POTENTIAL COMPLICATIONS
• Life-threatening ventricular arrhythmias
• Arrhythmia may interfere with the interpretation of hemodynamic and angiographic data.
• Hemorrhage, thrombosis, or hematoma formation at vascular access sites
• Allergic/anaphylactic reactions or azotemia following administration of radiopaque contrast media
• Cardiac or vascular perforation
• Infection

CLIENT EDUCATION
• Cardiac catheterization requires anesthesia, and standard anesthetic risks and procedures should be discussed.
• The risks and potential complications of the procedure should be explained.
• In cases of therapeutic procedures, factors that might preclude procedure completion should be discussed. For example, balloon valvuloplasty is contraindicated if an anomalous left coronary artery is detected.

BODY SYSTEMS ASSESSED
Cardiovascular

PROCEDURE

PATIENT PREPARATION
Preprocedure Medication or Preparation
• Record a complete medical history and perform physical cardiovascular exams, including echocardiography and ECG.
• Evaluate a CBC and chemistry profile for mature or elderly individuals.
• Continue regularly prescribed medications.
• Allow no food or water on the day of procedure.

CARDIAC CATHETERIZATION

- Administer flea treatment, if necessary to decrease the risk of surgical site contamination.
- Evaluate PCV and total solids, and perform an Azostix test on the day of the procedure.
- If the jugular vein or carotid artery are to be used as the site of catheter introduction, no jugular blood should be sampled prior to the procedure.
- Antibiotic prophylaxis (i.e., cefazolin, 20 mg/kg) is often administered at the beginning of the procedure and every 2 h until ≈4 h after the procedure.

Anesthesia or Sedation
- Standard preanesthetic protocol, followed by inhalation anesthesia, to immobilize and desensitize the patient
- Equipment for positive pressure ventilation and oxygen administration should be available.

Patient Positioning
Patients are generally positioned in right or left lateral recumbency, depending on the surgeon's preference.

Patient Monitoring
ECG, peripheral blood pressure, and oxygen saturation are monitored continuously.

Equipment or Supplies
- A multichannel physiologic recorder is required for the measurement of intracardiac pressure. The instrument must be calibrated to an appropriate range of pressures.
- Fluoroscopic guidance, using image intensification to reduce radiation exposure to the operator, is employed during catheter placement and positioning.
- A movable radiograph table is desirable so that patients may remain in a constant position.
- Angiograms are recorded on videotape or stored digitally.
- A standard pack of sterile surgical instruments is necessary for vascular access (cutdown). Surgical instruments that might be used for emergency thoracotomy should be available.
- A wide variety of sterilized catheters, guidewires, and sheath introducers, as well as any specialized equipment necessary for the particular procedure (e.g., pacing lead and pulse generator, transdermal pacing electrodes, balloon catheters (Figure 1), embolization coils (Figure 2), pressure tubing).
- Appropriate suture material, as well as surgical blades (nos. 10 and 11)
- A sterile bowl with warmed saline for flushing catheters. Heparin is added for all procedures except those involving placement of embolization divises (e.g., thrombogenic coils or Amplatz devise).
- A direct-current defibrillator (with a cardiac pacing function for cardiac pacemaker placement)
- Drugs for cardiac emergencies and cardiopulmonary resuscitation

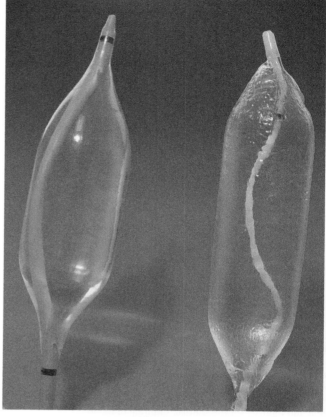

Figure 1

Two catheters used for balloon dilation of congenital defects such as pulmonic or aortic stenosis. The balloon catheter on the *left* is an older, more rigid type, whereas the balloon catheter on the *right* is a newer, low-profile balloon catheter.

TECHNIQUE
- A light anesthetic plane, sufficient to keep the patient immobilized and desensitized, will usually suffice, except during deep dissection of the neck musculature to access the carotid artery.
- The area of catheter insertion is clipped and sterilely draped.
- Vascular access is obtained either via incision and surgical cutdown or a percutaneous catheter introducer system (modified Seldinger technique).

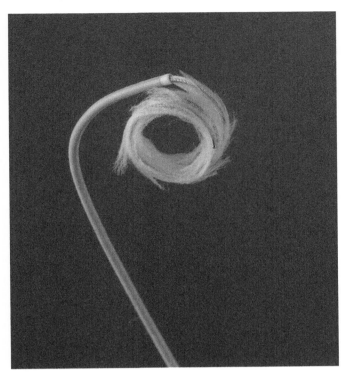

Figure 2

PDA coil. Shown is a 4 French catheter with an embolization coil partially extruded. The coils are made of steel embedded with Dacron fibers, which promote thrombus formation and subsequent PDA occlusion.

- All catheters and introducer sheaths are flushed with sterile saline to avoid administration of air bubbles and to prevent thrombus formation.
- In the surgical cutdown procedure, a small incision is made over the vessel, and the vessel is isolated. A loose ligature (i.e., 2–0 silk) or bulldog clamp is placed around the vessel proximally and distally to the catheter insertion site for hemostasis control. A small venotomy or arteriotomy is made using vascular scissors or a no. 11 blade, tightening the silk proximally as necessary to provide hemostasis. The catheter is inserted through the puncture site and advanced under fluoroscopic guidance to the desired intracardiac or intravascular location.

- A percutaneous (Seldinger) catheter introducer system is often preferred for vascular access to the jugular vein, femoral artery, or femoral vein. The vessel is located via digital palpation, and a vascular cannula with stylet or an 18-gauge thin-walled needle is inserted into the vessel. The stylet is removed, and a flexible guidewire is inserted through the cannula or needle into the vessel. The needle is removed, leaving the wire in place. An end-hole catheter, with or without vascular dilator, is then threaded over the guidewire into the vessel, the guidewire and vascular dilator are removed, and the catheter is flushed with saline. An introducer sheath with hemostasis port is used to facilitate catheter exchanges and reduce blood loss.
- A wide variety of radiopaque catheters and guidewires are available, depending on the specific purpose and vessel used. Inflatable balloon-tip catheters (Berman angiographic or balloon wedge) facilitate catheter placement into the RV and pulmonary artery (PA). Pigtail catheters minimize trauma and enable easier passage through the aortic valve. Catheters that are used for dogs and cats usually range in size from 4 to 8 French outside diameter and from 50 to 120 cm long. The largest catheter that can be easily inserted and manipulated is usually preferred, especially if angiographic studies are planned.
- For pressure measurement, the catheter is advanced into the desired chamber or vessel and is connected to pressure tubing, which is connected to a pressure transducer and calibrated physiologic recorder. Three-way stopcocks are placed at all catheter and tubing connections. All catheters and tubing are flushed to eliminate air bubbles. Pressures are recorded for baseline readings, as well as at appropriate intervals, and during any therapeutic interventions to assess postprocedural hemodynamic improvement.
- Angiography and angiocardiography are used to visualize cardiovascular regions of interest. Radiopaque contrast material is injected through the catheter for evaluation of cardiac morphology by fluoroscopy. Pressure injectors can be used to facilitate rapid delivery of a bolus of contrast.
- Oximetry/blood-gas sampling can be used to assess shunt fraction and severity of shunt defects. Blood samples are obtained from appropriate vessels or chambers in animals with atrial septal defect, ventricular septal defect, or more complicated defects. Left-to-right, right-to-left, and bidirectional shunting can be quantified based on oxygen saturation in cardiac and vascular regions of interest.
- Temporary and permanent pacemaker pacing leads are placed via cardiac catheterization in cases of bradycardic rhythm disturbances (e.g., third-degree AV block, persistent atrial standstill). Certain tachyarrhythmias can also be managed with a multifunction pacemaker or implantable cardioverter-defibrillator; however, the latter has yet to be widely adopted for use in veterinary patients.

• Coil embolization and Amplatz canine duct occluder (ACDO) devises have become an increasingly popular, minimally invasive alternatives to thoracotomy for the correction of PDA and certain congenital portosystemic shunts. A catheter is inserted via femoral artery into the ductus, and coils are advanced via a guidewire through the catheter and deployed into the PDA. For portosystemic shunts, catheter access is via the jugular vein, and coils, often after placement of a caval stent, are placed directly into the shunting vessel.

• Endomyocardial biopsy can be used for endomyocardial tissue sampling. The bioptome is advanced through a long sheath introducer to the desired region, the jaws are opened and advanced gently into the endocardial surface under fluoroscopic guidance, and then the jaws are closed and the bioptome is withdrawn.

• In cases of severe heartworm infestation (especially caval syndrome), alligator-style forceps or other specially designed catheters (e.g., Ishihara heartworm forceps) can be advanced into the RA and RV to remove adult heartworms, reducing worm burden prior to adulticide treatment.

• Cardiac output can be measured via cardiac catheterization through the use of a Swan-Ganz thermodilution catheter and cardiac output computer.

• Pulmonary venous and left atrial pressures can be estimated via insertion of a balloon wedge catheter into the PA and pulmonary circulation. When the end-hole catheter is wedged into a small pulmonary vessel, regional pulmonary flow is occluded, and the catheter measures pressure transmitted from the pulmonary capillaries, which is an estimation of left atrial pressure.

SAMPLE HANDLING

• For oximetry, samples are collected in sterile heparinized syringes and directly analyzed using a blood-gas analyzer and/or oximeter.

• Endomyocardial biopsy samples are submitted in formalin for histopathology.

APPROPRIATE AFTERCARE
Postprocedure Patient Monitoring

• If a percutaneous sheath introducer was used, this is removed, and continuous pressure is applied for several minutes until hemostasis is assured. For arterial sites, continuous pressure is applied to the site for ≈20–30 min to assure hemostasis. Serious or life-threatening arterial bleeding from the femoral arterial site leads some cardiologists to prefer surgical cutdown over percutaneous access.

• If surgical vascular access was obtained, catheters are removed and vessels are repaired or ligated.

• If the neck was used, it should be bandaged.

• Standard postanesthetic monitoring is conducted until the animal has recovered fully.

• Once the patient is fully awake, water should be offered to compensate for the diuretic effect of contrast medium. Animals that do not drink within the first few hours should receive IV fluids.

• Regular medications are continued, and additional doses of antibiotic may be administered postprocedurally, depending on routine practice of the attending veterinarian.

Nursing Care

• Incision is monitored continually for bleeding over the first 1–4 h, especially after arterial catheterization, with additional application of digital pressure, as needed.

• Temperature, pulse, and respiration are checked every hour until parameters are within normal limits.

• The animal is kept clean and warm in an intensive care unit (ICU) setting.

• When the patient has recovered fully from anesthesia, water is introduced slowly.

• Regular medications, as well as analgesic medications if necessary, are administered.

• After catheterization, continuous ECG monitoring is often performed for 24 h to check for catheter-induced arrhythmia secondary to irritation of the endocardium by the catheter tip.

Dietary Modification
None, unless CHF is present

Medication Requirements

• None unless dictated by an underlying condition

• Sedation may be required to prevent coil or pacing lead dislodgment in the immediate postoperative period.

Restrictions on Activity
Mildly restricted activity (leash walks only) is recommended for 2–3 weeks after the procedure. In pacemaker cases, a harness rather than a collar is recommended for the remainder of the animal's life.

Anticipated Recovery Time
Patients are usually discharged from the hospital 1–2 days after the procedure. Full recovery is anticipated in ≈2 weeks, although many animals appear to recover fully within 24–48 h.

INTERPRETATION
NORMAL FINDINGS OR RANGE
In animals with normal cardiac structures and function, normal intracardiac pressures (see the table), arterial oxygen tension (>80 mmHg), arterial oxygen saturation (>90%), and venous oxygen tension

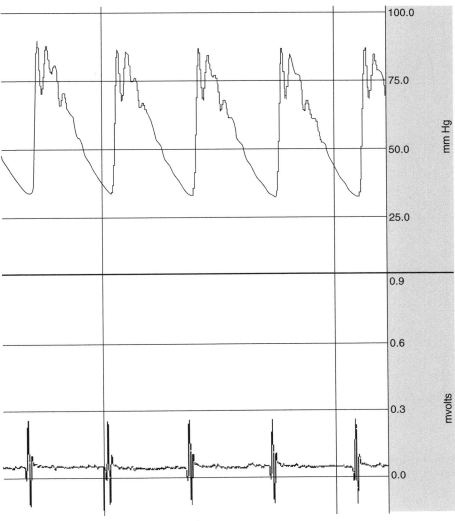

Figure 3

Arterial pressure tracing from a dog with PDA. Systemic arterial blood pressure measured in the aorta, and ECG recordings of an anesthetized dog with PDA prior to coil embolization. The *top* graph shows a wide aortic pulse pressure with a systolic blood pressure of ≈85 mmHg and a diastolic pressure of ≈32 mmHg. The *bottom* tracing depicts the simultaneous ECG recording.

(>40 mmHg), as well as the absence of shunting of blood, would be expected.

Cardiac chamber or vessel	Normal cardiac pressures	
	Systole	Diastole
Right atrium	4–6	0–4
Right ventricle	15–30	0–5
Pulmonary artery	15–30	5–15
Pulmonary wedge	6–12	4–8
Left atrium	5–12	<8
Left ventricle	95–150	<10
Aorta	95–150	70–100

ABNORMAL VALUES

Values outside the normal range are often seen with pulmonic stenosis with or without an anomalous coronary artery, aortic or subaortic stenosis, PDA, mitral stenosis, tricuspid stenosis, ventricular septal defect, or atrial septal defect with either left-to-right or right-to-left shunting, aorticopulmonary window, tetralogy of Fallot, AV fistula, persistent left or right cranial vena cava, pulmonary hypertension, or myocarditis.

CRITICAL VALUES

Critical cardiac compromise may be seen with the following conditions:

• Cardiac tamponade secondary to ventricular rupture and pericardial effusion

• Life-threatening arrhythmias as a result of catheter-induced ventricular irritability

• Migration of an embolization coil into the distal aorta and vasculature

• Anaphylactic shock reaction after injection of radiopaque contrast material (very rare)

• Catheter breakage and foreign body embolization

CARDIAC CATHETERIZATION

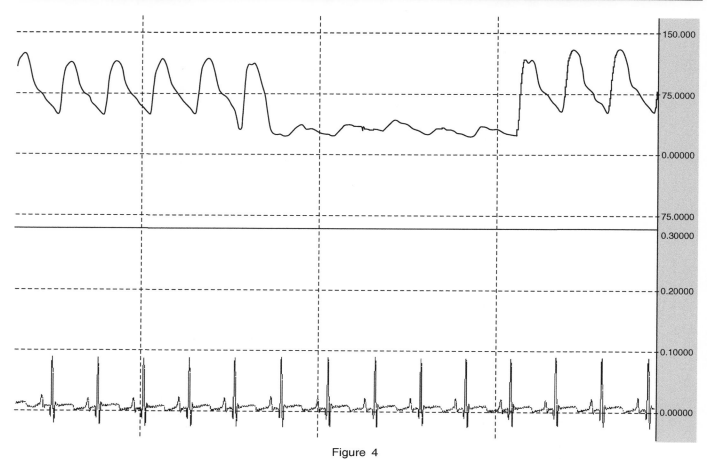

Figure 4

Aorta and PA pressure tracing from a dog with PDA. Pressure and ECG recordings of a dog with PDA, as the catheter is advanced from the aorta into the PDA body (*left side* of the tracing; pressure, ≈118/73 mmHg), then into the PA (*middle* of the tracing; pressure, ≈36/24 mmHg), and then pulled back into the PDA (*right side* of the tracing).

INTERFERING FACTORS
Drugs That May Alter Results of the Procedure
• Anesthetic choice may alter blood pressure, and the use of inhalant anesthesia often leads to systemic pressures of 80–100 mmHg.
• Heparin administration may hamper thrombus formation.

Conditions That May Interfere with Performing the Procedure
• Metabolic abnormalities, electrolyte disturbances, or infectious conditions
• CHF
• Uncontrolled ventricular arrhythmias
• Bleeding disorders and coagulopathies
• Pronounced cardiac remodeling or anatomic defect that hampers catheter manipulation

Procedure Techniques or Handling That May Alter Results
• Arrhythmia can alter pressure and angiographic findings.
• Overhydration with saline or contrast media can precipitate acute CHF, especially in patients with compromised cardiac function.
• Improper sample collection may yield invalid oximetry findings.
• Improper calibration (calibration requires operator skill and experience) or malfunction of the physiologic recorder will cause intracardiac pressures to be reflected inaccurately.
• Lack of adequate catheter supplies and a skilled team (i.e., surgeon, assistant, cardiology technician, anesthesia support, and radiology technician)

Influence of Signalment on Performing and Interpreting the Procedure
Species
Superior operator skill is often required to perform cardiac catheterization successfully in the small vessels and the heart of cats and of dogs weighing <2.5 kg. Cats are also prone to vasospasm, which can be partially attenuated with topical lidocaine administration on the vessel.

Breed
None

Age
None

Gender
None

Pregnancy
Prolonged exposure to fluoroscopy (radiation) is not recommended in pregnant patients.

CLINICAL PERSPECTIVE
• Cardiac catheterization can provide a definitive diagnosis in cases where the diagnosis is still in question after standard testing.
• A less invasive and less risky alternative to thoracotomy is found through cardiac catheterization in the treatment of stenotic valvular lesions (balloon valvuloplasty) and PDA (coil embolization or ACDO).

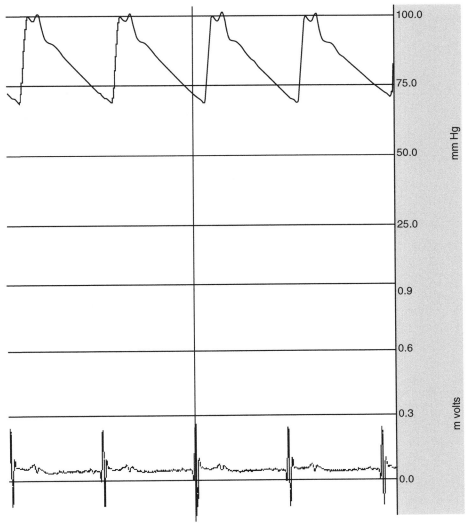

Figure 5

Arterial pressure tracing from a dog with PDA after coil occlusion. Systemic arterial blood pressure, measured in the aorta, and ECG recordings, of the same dog depicted in Figure 3, after deployment of coils into the PDA. The *top* graph shows an increase in blood pressure and a more normal aortic pulse pressure of ≈100/70 mmHg after PDA coil embolization. The ECG recording is on the *bottom* graph.

• Pacemaker implantation eliminates clinical signs and reduces the risk of sudden death in animals that require cardiac pacing (AV block, atrial standstill, sick sinus syndrome) persistent.
• Cardiac catheterization is a valuable tool for quantifying hemodynamic data and/or response to therapy (e.g., oximetry, pulmonary capillary wedge pressure, calculation of cardiac output).
• Extraction of heartworms from the right heart in cases of severe infestation decreases the risk of heartworm adulticide by reducing worm burden prior to treatment.

MISCELLANEOUS

ANCILLARY TESTS
• Computed tomographic angiography
• Periprocedural ultrasonography using transesophageal echocardiography

SYNONYMS
None

SEE ALSO
Blackwell's Five-Minute Veterinary Consult: Canine and Feline Topics
• Aortic Stenosis
• Arteriovenous Fistula
• Atrial Septal Defect
• Atrial Standstill
• Atrioventricular Block, Complete (Third Degree)
• Carnitine Deficiency
• Heartworm Disease—Dogs
• Patent Ductus Arteriosus
• Pulmonic Stenosis
• Sick Sinus Syndrome
• Tetralogy of Fallot
• Ventricular Septal Defect

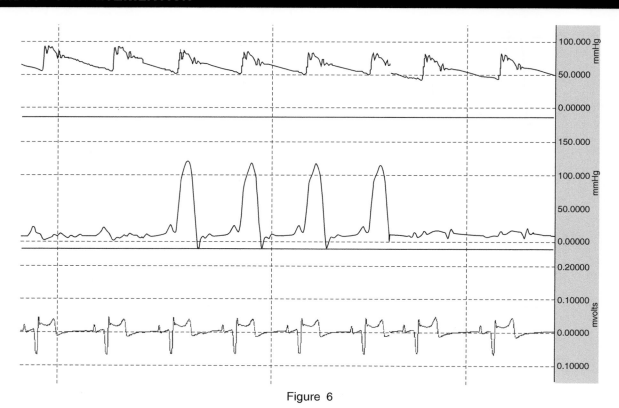

Figure 6

Pressure tracings and ECG recording of an anesthetized dog with pulmonic stenosis and tricuspid regurgitation. The *top* tracing reflects aortic pressure (≈88/50 mmHg) obtained from a catheter in the aorta. The *middle* graph reflects serial pressures recorded from the RA (≈20/4 mmHg; *left side* of the graph), RV (≈121/12 mmHg; *middle* of the graph), and PA (≈20/8 mmHg; *right side* of the graph), as the catheter was advanced from the RA to RV and then into the PA. High RV systolic pressure is secondary to pulmonic stenosis, and there is a gradient of ≈100 mmHg across the stenotic pulmonic valve. The high RA pressure is likely caused by high RV pressure coupled with tricuspid regurgitation.

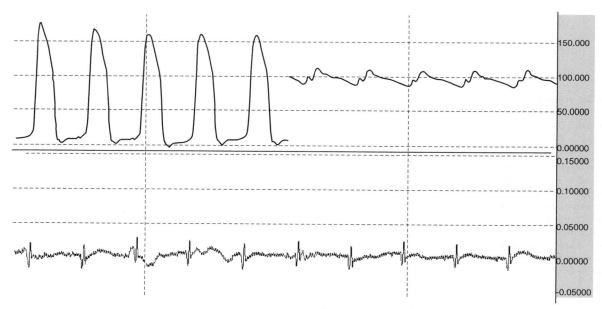

Figure 7

Pressure and ECG recordings of an anesthetized dog with subaortic stenosis. The *top* graph shows a recording of left ventricular pressure (≈159/10 mmHg; *left side* of the graph) and aortic pressure (≈114/90 mmHg; right side of the graph) as a catheter was pulled from the left ventricle into the aorta. The higher systolic pressure in the left ventricle is secondary to subaortic stenosis, with an estimated peak pressure gradient of nearly 50 mmHg. Note the narrowed arterial pulse-pressure difference of <30 mmHg, which is the graphical representation of the weak arterial pulses typically present in dogs with subaortic stenosis. The *bottom* graph shows a simultaneous ECG recording.

Related Topics in This Book
- Angiography and Angiocardiography
- Blood Gases

ABBREVIATIONS
- ACDO = Amplatz canine duct occluder
- AV = atrioventricular
- CHF = congestive heart failure
- PA = pulmonary artery
- PDA = patent ductus arteriosus
- RA = right atrium
- RV = right ventricle

Suggested Reading

Kittleson MD, Kienle RD. Cardiac catheterization. In: Kittleson MD, Kienle RD, eds. *Small Animal Cardiovascular Medicine.* St Louis: CV Mosby, 1998: 118–132.

Miller MS. Special diagnostic techniques for evaluation of cardiac disease. In: Miller MS, Tilley LP, eds. *Manual of Canine and Feline Cardiology,* 2nd ed. Philadelphia: WB Saunders, 1995: 119–123.

Wallack ST. Angiography: Dog and cat. In: *The Handbook of Veterinary Contrast Radiography.* Solana Beach, CA: San Diego Veterinary Imaging, 2003: 31–36.

INTERNET RESOURCES
None

AUTHOR NAMES

Barbara P. Brewer and John E. Rush

CARNITINE

BASICS

TYPE OF SPECIMEN
Blood
Tissue
Urine
Seminal fluid

TEST EXPLANATION AND RELATED PHYSIOLOGY
L-carnitine (β-hydroxy-γ-trimethylaminobutyric acid) is a small, water-soluble molecule, obtained primarily from dietary animal protein and endogenous synthesis in the liver by use of the essential precursor amino acids lysine and methionine. Although carnitine is classified as an amino acid derivative, it is not an α-amino acid and the amino group is not free. As a result, carnitine is not used for protein synthesis.

Carnitine is found in the body either as free carnitine, short-chain acylcarnitine, or long-chain acylcarnitine. Acylcarnitine indicates carnitine bound to a fatty acid. Total carnitine is the sum of all the individual carnitine fractions. Normally, the free carnitine fraction is higher than either the short-chain or the long-chain acylcarnitine fractions.

Cardiac and skeletal muscles are significant storage sites for carnitine and contain 95%–98% of the carnitine in the body. Carnitine is concentrated in these tissues by an active membrane transport mechanism. The heart cannot synthesize carnitine and depends on transport of carnitine from the circulation into cardiac muscle.

The normal heart obtains 60% of it total energy production from oxidation of long-chain fatty acids. Carnitine functions as a cofactor of several important enzymes necessary for transport of long-chain fatty acids from the cytosol into the mitochondrial matrix. Once inside the mitochondria, fatty acids undergo β-oxidation to generate energy [adenosine triphosphate (ATP)]. Another important function of carnitine is its buffering capacity, which modulates the intramitochondrial acyl-CoA/CoA ratio. This is important because the buildup of acyl-CoA derivatives in mitochondria inhibits oxidative metabolism, and these derivatives can act as detergents at high concentrations. Carnitine also has a role in detoxification in mitochondria by facilitating removal of short-chain and medium-chain organic acids. Carnitine supplementation has also been used in therapeutic weight-loss diets for both dogs and cats to spare lean body mass during a weight-loss program. In addition, carnitine supplementation has been shown to be beneficial in the management of hepatic lipidosis in cats. In humans, spermatozoa require L-carnitine for maturation. Carnitine supplementation has shown to be beneficial in people with idiopathic asthenospermia (defective sperm motility). The epididymides of dogs produce carnitine, and dogs with obstructive azoospermia may be distinguished from those with aspermatogenesis (secretory azoospermia) by measuring seminal carnitine concentration.

Potential causes of carnitine deficiency include decreased carnitine synthesis, decreased dietary intake, intestinal malabsorption, increased renal loss (such as with cystinuria), abnormally increased esterification of free carnitine, and membrane transport defects.

Carnitine deficiency is classified as either (1) plasma carnitine deficiency, characterized by low concentrations of free plasma carnitine; (2) systemic carnitine deficiency, characterized by low concentrations of free plasma and tissue carnitine; (3) myopathic carnitine deficiency, characterized by low free myocardial carnitine concentrations in the presence of normal and sometimes elevated plasma carnitine concentrations; or (4) carnitine insufficiency, characterized by a ratio of esterified carnitine to free carnitine that exceeds 0.4 in the presence of normal concentrations of free carnitine. Plasma carnitine deficiency alone is not a well-documented state and is included to account for the fact that only plasma carnitine is often tested in veterinary medicine.

In dogs, carnitine deficiency has been associated primarily with dilated cardiomyopathy (DCM) and lipid-storage myopathies; however, carnitine deficiency has also been associated with ceroid lipofuscinosis in dogs. In experimental studies, carnitine deficiency has been associated with cardiac ischemia and ventricular arrhythmias in dogs. Carnitine deficiency has not been reported in cats, perhaps because cats are true carnivores and, as a result, consume diets high in animal protein sources, which are good dietary sources of carnitine.

INDICATIONS
- DCM in dogs
- Lipid-storage myopathy in dogs
- Ceroid lipofuscinosis in dogs
- Cystinuria in dogs
- Differentiate azoospermia from aspermatogenesis as a cause of male infertility in dogs.

CONTRAINDICATIONS
None

POTENTIAL COMPLICATIONS
An endomyocardial biopsy to evaluate cardiac muscle carnitine levels may perforate the heart or cause arrhythmias or hemorrhage.

CLIENT EDUCATION
- Collect blood after an overnight fast. Do not withhold water.
- Detection of a low plasma carnitine concentration can be helpful in diagnosing carnitine deficiency. However, a normal plasma carnitine concentration does not rule out the myopathic form of carnitine deficiency, which is the most common form of carnitine deficiency in dogs with DCM. Endomyocardial biopsy is needed to rule out the myopathic form of carnitine deficiency.
- L-carnitine is expensive to administer, especially if obtained through a health food store. It is more economical to buy it in bulk. Any purchase from a health food store should have the U.S. Pharmacopeia (USP) verification on the label to ensure the purity of the product.

BODY SYSTEMS ASSESSED
- Cardiovascular
- Hepatobiliary
- Musculoskeletal
- Renal and urologic

SAMPLE

COLLECTION
- Venous blood, >3 mL
- Urine, ≥5 mL
- Cardiac muscle, approximately 2–4 mg (the typical size sample obtained with endomyocardial biopsy forceps)
- Skeletal muscle, 2–4 mg
- Seminal fluid, ≥0.5 mL

HANDLING
Plasma Carnitine
- Use a heparinized (green top) tube or a syringe coated with heparin.
- If collecting blood in a non–heparin-coated syringe, remove the rubber stopper from the green-top tube to reduce the risk of hemolyzing the sample.
- If using a heparin-coated syringe, remove the needle from the vein and draw an additional 1 mL of air into the syringe for mixing space in the syringe.
- Immediately place the sample on wet ice.

- Centrifuge the sample (by using a refrigerated centrifuge, if available) within 30 min of obtaining the sample.
- Immediately separate plasma from cells and immediately freeze (in a −70°C freezer, if available). Be careful to avoid contaminating the plasma with cells from the buffy coat. If sample is hemolyzed, consider drawing a new sample.
- Ship the sample on dry ice to the laboratory by overnight express mail.

Urine Carnitine
- For dogs, 24-h urine collection is required for assessing urine carnitine concentrations (see the Protocol section).
- Pool the entire 24-h urine sample, mix thoroughly, and transfer an aliquot (≥5 mL) into a plastic tube.
- Freeze immediately.

Cardiac Muscle Carnitine
Obtain sample tissue from the right ventricle by an endomyocardial biopsy technique. Immediately blot the sample with gauze to remove blood, wrap the sample in foil, and snap-freeze it in liquid nitrogen.

Skeletal Muscle Carnitine
Obtain sample tissue from the cranial tibial muscle by a percutaneous biopsy technique. Immediately blot the sample with gauze to remove blood, wrap the sample in foil, and snap-freeze it in liquid nitrogen.

Shipment
Samples should be frozen immediately after being obtained, and shipped on dry ice by overnight express.

STORAGE
All samples should be stored frozen in an ultracold freezer (−70°C).

STABILITY
- Very unstable at room temperature (2°–8°C)
- Samples are stable for years when stored in an ultracold (−70°C) freezer.

PROTOCOL
24-Hour Urine Carnitine Sample
- Catheterize and empty the urinary bladder and record the time to the nearest minute.
- Place the dog in an individual metabolism cage. All voided urine should be collected in a plastic container surrounded by dry ice in an insulated box.
- If the dog is housebroken and unlikely to urinate voluntarily in cage, a regular cage can be used. Catheterize and empty the dog's urinary bladder at least every 8 h. Immediately freeze all collected urine until the end of the collection.
- At the end of the collection, empty the urinary bladder by catheterization and record the time to the nearest minute.
- Briefly thaw and pool all urine collected during the 24-h collection period. Mix it thoroughly and record the total volume of urine.
- Screen the urine samples for blood contamination by using a reagent strip. If blood is present, repeat collection after 24 h, provided blood is no longer present in urine.

Cardiac Muscle Carnitine Sample
Cardiac muscle biopsies are generally limited to research and referral practices and are performed while dogs are under general anesthesia and monitored by continuous ECG and indirect blood pressure oscillometry. Cardiac muscle biopsy samples are obtained from the right ventricle by a percutaneous endomyocardial biopsy technique. After collection, immediately blot the sample with gauze to remove blood, wrap the sample in foil, and snap-freeze it in liquid nitrogen.

Skeletal Muscle Carnitine Sample
Skeletal muscle biopsies are generally limited to research and referral practices and must be obtained while dogs are under general anesthesia or very heavy sedation. See the "Muscle and Nerve Biopsy" chapter for more details on this procedure. Once the biopsy sample is obtained, it

is immediately blotted with gauze to remove blood, wrapped in foil, and snap-frozen in liquid nitrogen.

Seminal Carnitine Sample
Semen is collected by manual stimulation of the penis through a collecting funnel. Collect the first 2 fractions of semen, and stop collection as soon as clear prostatic fluid appears, to minimize dilution of the sample with prostatic fluid. Immediately centrifuge the semen sample, transfer the supernatant into a plastic vial, and freeze it in an ultracold (−70°C) freezer until assayed. Ship the sample on dry ice to the laboratory by overnight express mail.

 INTERPRETATION

Normal Findings or Range
ABNORMAL VALUES
Values below the reference range

CRITICAL VALUES
None

INTERFERING FACTORS
Drugs that May Alter Results or Interpretation
Drugs That Interfere with Test Methodology
None

Drugs That Alter Physiology
- In cardiac tissue, doxorubicin (Adriamycin) inhibits carnitine palmitoyltransferase 1 and 2 dose-dependently, reduces carnitine levels in cardiac myocytes, and causes DCM.
- In some studies in people and rodents, choline supplementation reduces urinary excretion of carnitine and promotes tissue carnitine accretion, particularly in skeletal muscle. In other studies, choline supplementation decreases carnitine synthesis by competing with the enzyme that converts lysine into carnitine.
- Pivalic acid–containing antibiotics, such as cefetamet pivoxil and pivampicillin, induce carnitine deficiency in people and in some animal models, including dogs, by forming excessive tissue levels of pivaloylcarnitine ester. These esters are readily released from tissues and subsequently lost in urine at a rate that exceeds carnitine synthesis.
- In people, long-term administration of total parenteral nutrition can result in carnitine deficiency. It is not known whether this occurs in dogs or cats.
- Administration of androgens and estrogen can affect carnitine levels.
- Only L-carnitine should be administered as a supplement. D-carnitine (the other optical isomer) renders mammalian L-carnitine–containing enzyme systems inactive and should not be administered. D-carnitine is no longer available in the United States.

Disorders That May Alter Results
Hematuria may falsely elevate urine carnitine levels.

Collection Techniques or Handling That May Alter Results
- Plasma carnitine falsely increased by hemolysis or contamination with cells from the buffy coat
- An increased ester carnitine concentration caused by failure to place the plasma carnitine sample immediately on wet ice and centrifuge within 30 min
- Failure to snap-freeze cardiac and skeletal muscle biopsy samples in liquid nitrogen within 10 s of collection can increase the ester carnitine fraction.
- Failure to blot off excess blood from cardiac and skeletal muscle biopsy samples prior to freezing may result in blood contamination of the results.

Influence of Signalment
Species
Carnitine deficiency reported in dogs but not cats

CARNITINE

Feline values	Plasma free carnitine	Plasma ester carnitine	Plasma total carnitine
Males ($n = 9$)	3.9–18.3 μmol/L	0–5.8 μmol/L	5.0–22.2 μmol/L
Females ($n = 4$)	5.0–33.8 μmol/L	0–11.6 μmol/L	5.2–44.4 μmol/L

Canine values	Free carnitine	Ester carnitine	Short-chain acylcarnitine	Long-chain acylcarnitine	Total carnitine
Plasma (μmol/L)	9–36	N/A	<7	N/A	12–40
Urine (nmol/kg/24 h)	1,097–6,742	N/A	1,10–2,537	0–144	1,519–9,050
Cardiac muscle (nmol/mg NCP)	3.5–11.5 or	<5			4.5–14.0 or
Skeletal muscle (nmol/mg NCP)	0.94–9.8* 2.2–15.4	N/A	0.05–2.7* 0.1–4.1	0–0.66 0.05–0.81	1.78–12.4* 4.3–18.3
Seminal fluid (nmol/mL) Intact	N/A	N/A	N/A	N/A	256–1,636
Castrated	N/A	N/A	N/A	N/A	4–24

*Reference range from 18 healthy adult beagles.

Breed
- An association between carnitine deficiency and DCM has been demonstrated in the following:
  - Boxers
  - American cocker spaniels
  - Breeds that develop cystine or urate urolithiasis
- An association between carnitine deficiency and myopathy has been demonstrated in the following:
  - Labrador retrievers: lipid storage myopathy
  - Cocker spaniels: lipid storage myopathy
  - Rottweilers: juvenile-onset distal myopathy
  - Tibetan terriers: ceroid lipofuscinosis

Age
- Cats
  - Free and total plasma carnitine levels are higher in intact adult cats than in intact kittens.
  - Ester plasma carnitine levels are the same or higher in intact kittens than in intact adult cats.
- Dogs: The effect of age on canine carnitine levels is unknown.

Gender
- Androgens contribute to regulation of plasma and tissue carnitine levels in rats and people. Neutering female rats increases plasma carnitine, whereas estrogen administration decreases plasma carnitine.
- In a study that used very small numbers of cats (9 intact male cats; 4 intact female cats), female cats had higher plasma and liver carnitine levels than did male cats (Jacobs et al. 1990) (table above).
- Unpublished work by the author has not found any difference in carnitine levels between adult neutered male dogs and adult spayed female dogs (table above).

Pregnancy
Unknown

LIMITATIONS OF THE TEST
In dogs, determination of urine protein/carnitine ratios and determination of urine fractional excretion of carnitine are unreliable methods of assessing urine carnitine concentrations. Whether the same is true in cats is not known.

Sensitivity, Specificity, and Positive and Negative Predictive Values
N/A

Valid If Run in a Human Lab?
Yes—if appropriate mehodology is used (radioisotopic or radioenzymatic assay).

Causes of Abnormal Findings

High values	Low values
Mishandling of sample can increase ester carnitine fraction	Breed predilection
Chronic kidney disease	Cystine or urate urolithiasis
Endotoxemia increases free plasma carnitine concentration (dogs)	Protein-restricted diet
Myocardial damage—leakage from myocytes	Vegetarian or boiled-meat diet
	Fanconi syndrome (humans)
	Hemodialysis (humans)

CLINICAL PERSPECTIVE
- L-carnitine is a very safe substance to administer. The only reported side effect of administering very high doses of carnitine in dogs is diarrhea.
- L-carnitine supplementation is indicated in the following:
  - American cocker spaniels, boxers, and dogs with cystine or urate urolithiasis that develop DCM
  - Dogs that develop DCM while consuming a protein-restricted diet, a boiled-meat diet, or a vegetarian diet
  - Dogs with lipid storage myopathies or ceroid lipofuscinosis
- Cats with hepatic lipidosis
- L-carnitine supplementation is beneficial in sparing lean body mass in dogs or cats consuming a therapeutic weight-loss diet.
- Dogs with obstructive azoospermia may be distinguished from those with aspermatogenesis (secretory azoospermia) by measuring seminal carnitine concentration. If the carnitine concentration is low in the supernatant of a semen sample obtained after complete ejaculation, there is a high probability of bilateral blockage of the excurrent ducts.

MISCELLANEOUS
ANCILLARY TESTS
- Echocardiography in dogs with heart disease

- Muscle biopsy using either oil red O or Sudan black for histopathology
- Ejaculation (male dogs)

SYNONYMS
None

SEE ALSO
Blackwell's Five-Minute Veterinary Consult: Canine and Feline
Topics
- Cardiomyopathy, Dilated—Cats
- Cardiomyopathy, Dilated—Dogs
- Carnitine Deficiency
- Hepatic Lipidosis
- Obesity

Related Topics in This Book
- Echocardiography
- Muscle and Nerve Biopsy
- Taurine

ABBREVIATIONS
- CoA = coenzyme A
- DCM = dilated cardiomyopathy
- NCP = noncollagenous protein

Suggested Reading

Ibrahim WH, Bailey N, Sunvold GD, Bruckner GG. Effects of carnitine and taurine on fatty acid metabolism and lipid accumulation in the liver of cats during weight gain and weight loss. *Am J Vet Res* 2003; 64: 310–315.

Jacobs G, Keene B, Cornelius LM, Rakich P. Plasma, tissue, and urine carnitine concentrations in healthy adult cats and kittens. *Am J Vet Res* 1990; 51: 1345–1348.

Keene BW, Panciera DP, Atkins CE, *et al.* Myocardial L-carnitine deficiency in a family of dogs with dilated cardiomyopathy. *J Am Vet Med Assoc* 1991; 201: 647–650.

Olson PN, Behrendt MD, Amann RP, *et al.* Concentration of carnitine in the seminal fluid of normospermic, vasectomized, and castrated dogs. *Am J Vet Res* 1987; 48: 1211–1215.

Pion PD, Sanderson SL, Kittleson MD. Effectiveness of taurine and levocarnitine in dogs with heart disease. *Vet Clin North Am Small Anim Pract* 1998; 28: 1495–1514.

INTERNET RESOURCES
None

AUTHOR NAME
Sherry Lynn Sanderson

CATHETER-ASSISTED STONE RETRIEVAL

BASICS

TYPE OF PROCEDURE
Diagnostic sample collection

PROCEDURE EXPLANATION AND RELATED PHYSIOLOGY
Use of large-bore catheters to retrieve urocystoliths is safe and rapid. In many patients, anesthesia is not required.

INDICATIONS
• To remove small uroliths (<2 mm in diameter) from the urinary bladder
• Small uroliths can be analyzed to accurately determine the composition of remaining uroliths too large to remove by catheter retrieval or other noninvasive procedures.

CONTRAINDICATIONS
None

POTENTIAL COMPLICATIONS
• Urinary tract infection
• Transient hematuria
• Transient pollakiuria

CLIENT EDUCATION
• Catheter urolith retrieval is usually performed without general anesthesia.
• In fractious animals and cats, general anesthesia is recommended.
• Catheter-assisted stone retrieval may facilitate urethral obstruction in patients with uroliths of sufficient size to obstruct the urethra.

BODY SYSTEMS ASSESSED
Renal and urologic

PROCEDURE

PATIENT PREPARATION
Preprocedure Medication or Preparation
None

Anesthesia or Sedation
• Catheter retrieval can be performed in many patients without anesthesia.
• Urethral anesthesia can be achieved with intraurethral instillation of local anesthetic agents (e.g., carbocaine, lidocaine).
• The use of general anesthesia should be considered in cats and fractious dogs.

Patient Positioning
Left or right lateral recumbency

Patient Monitoring
None

Equipment or Supplies
• Flexible urinary catheters (typically soft flexible 8 French catheters)
• Sterile physiologic solutions (e.g., normal saline, lactated Ringer's solution)
• A large-volume syringe (20–60 mL)
• A sterile water-soluble lubricant

TECHNIQUE
• Anesthetize the patient, if necessary. If general anesthesia is not necessary, instill a local anesthetic into the urethra.
• Although not essential, cut the tip of the catheter to create an open end. Avoid creating sharp edges.
• Measure catheter insertion length necessary for the catheter tip to reside in the bladder neck.

• Cleanly pass the catheter through the urethra ostium, positioning the tip of the catheter in the bladder neck.
• Use the urinary catheter to fill the urinary bladder with the sterile physiologic solution. The bladder should not contain more than the volume of the syringe.
• With the patient in lateral recumbency, position your hand below the urinary bladder.
• Agitate the bladder up and down to disperse uroliths in it.
• While agitating the bladder, use the syringe to evacuate the bladder contents by gradually pulling the syringe plunger to create negative pressure in the urinary catheter.
• Separate the uroliths from the fluid. Filter the contents of the syringe through a fine mesh or filter paper to collect very small uroliths.
• Repeat the procedure until a sufficient number of uroliths (i.e., 2–8) have been removed for quantitative analysis.
• When all uroliths in an animal are <2 mm in diameter, this procedure can render the patient stone free.

SAMPLE HANDLING
Submit uroliths for quantitative mineral analysis.

APPROPRIATE AFTERCARE
Postprocedure Patient Monitoring
If a patient also has uroliths of sufficient size to obstruct the urethra, care must be taken to inform clients to monitor urine voiding. Signs of urethral obstruction should be verified and corrected.

Nursing Care
None

Dietary Modification
None. (Appropriate urolith management may require dietary management.)

Medication Requirements
Administer a prophylactic antimicrobial agent for 3–5 days.

Restrictions on Activity
None

Anticipated Recovery Time
Postprocedural hematuria and dysuria are unlikely. If present, they should resolve in less than 1–4 h.

INTERPRETATION

NORMAL FINDINGS OR RANGE
N/A

ABNORMAL VALUES
N/A

CRITICAL VALUES
N/A

INTERFERING FACTORS
Drugs That May Alter Results of the Procedure
N/A

Conditions That May Interfere with Performing the Procedure
Urethral tumors or urethral strictures may impede catheter passage.

Procedure Techniques or Handling That May Alter Results
N/A

Influence of Signalment on Performing and Interpreting the Procedure
Species
None

Breed
None

Age
None

Gender
The smaller urethral diameter of male cats and small male dogs will impede the passage of large-bore catheters.

Pregnancy
None

CLINICAL PERSPECTIVE
• This procedure is best suited to obtain a sample of uroliths for quantitative analysis.
• The size of the urethra of the male cat will allow collection of only the smallest urocystoliths.

MISCELLANEOUS

ANCILLARY TESTS
If the procedure is unsuccessful, the mineral composition of uroliths can be predicted on the basis of crystalluria, the radiographic appearance of uroliths, and breed and gender of the patient.

SYNONYMS
None

SEE ALSO
Blackwell's Five-Minute Veterinary Consult: Canine and Feline Topics
• Urolithiasis, Calcium Oxalate
• Urolithiasis, Calcium Phosphate
• Urolithiasis, Cystine
• Urolithiasis, Struvite—Cats
• Urolithiasis, Struvite—Dogs
• Urolithiasis, Urate
• Urolithiasis, Xanthine

Related Topics in This Book
• Urolith Analysis
• Voiding Urohydropropulsion

ABBREVIATIONS
None

Suggested Reading
Crow SE, Walshaw SO. *Manual of Clinical Procedures in the Dog, Cat, and Rabbit, 2nd ed.* Philadelphia: Lippincott-Raven, 1997:124.
Lulich JP, Osborne CA. Catheter-assisted retrieval of urocystoliths from dogs and cats. *Am J Vet Med Assoc* 1992; 201: 111–113.

INTERNET RESOURCES
None

AUTHOR NAMES
Jody Lulich and Carl Osborne

CENTRAL VENOUS PRESSURE

 BASICS

TYPE OF PROCEDURE
Pressure measurement

PROCEDURE EXPLANATION AND RELATED PHYSIOLOGY
Central venous pressure (CVP) is a measurement of the intravascular pressure within the intrathoracic vena cava. CVP measurements reflect venous return, venous compliance, and right ventricular function. CVP can be used as an indirect measure of central venous volume and of right atrial and right ventricular end-diastolic pressures. Clinical techniques for measuring CVP include the use of a calibrated manometer or an electronic pressure transducer. The manometer technique, described herein, remains the most commonly used technique in veterinary medicine and is technically simple to perform.

INDICATIONS
• Monitoring fluid therapy in any critically ill patient
• Guiding resuscitation in hypovolemic patients
• Monitoring fluid therapy in patients at risk for volume overload, including the following:
  • Patients undergoing diuresis for renal failure
  • Patients requiring fluid therapy that have preexisting heart disease
  • Patients in congestive heart failure

CONTRAINDICATIONS
Central venous catheter placement and therefore CVP measurement are contraindicated in patients at risk for hemorrhage (coagulopathy, severe thrombocytopenia).

POTENTIAL COMPLICATIONS
• Complications associated with CVP measurement are primarily related to the complications associated with placement and maintenance of a central venous catheter and can include hemorrhage, catheter-associated infection/sepsis, vascular irritation or phlebitis, and thromboemboli or air emboli.
• Cardiac arrhythmias can be associated with a CVP catheter with a tip that is inadvertently placed in the heart.

CLIENT EDUCATION
N/A

BODY SYSTEMS ASSESSED
Cardiovascular

 PROCEDURE

PATIENT PREPARATION
Preprocedure Medication or Preparation
• CVP measurement requires the placement of a central venous catheter. Central venous catheters may be placed aseptically in the jugular, femoral, or lateral saphenous veins.
• General anesthesia is rarely required for central venous catheter placement though sedation and/or a local block may be necessary.
• The tip of the central venous catheter should be placed in the intrathoracic cranial vena cava just cranial to the right atrium for jugular catheter placement or in the intrathoracic caudal vena cava for lateral saphenous and femoral vein catheters. Correct placement of a CVP catheter can be confirmed by visualization of the radiopaque catheter on a lateral thoracic radiograph.
• Correct placement of a CVP catheter can be suggested by visualization of fluctuations in the manometer meniscus during CVP readings. With a properly placed and patent CVP catheter, small fluctuations in the meniscus will coincide with heartbeats, and slightly larger fluctuations will coincide with respiratory excursions. If these fluctuations are not observed, it may indicate an improperly placed catheter or a catheter occlusion. Very

large fluctuations coinciding with the heart rate may indicate that the catheter has been mistakenly placed in the heart.

Anesthesia or Sedation
Sedation may be required for central venous catheter placement. Administration of combinations of opioids and benzodiazepines is recommended.

Patient Positioning
Lateral recumbency or sternal recumbency

Patient Monitoring
N/A

Equipment or Supplies
• A fluid-extension set
• A sterile 250-mL bag of 0.9% sodium chloride
• A fluid-administration set
• A manometer
• A 3-way stopcock

TECHNIQUE
• A fluid bag with a fluid-administration set is connected to a 3-way stopcock. A manometer and a fluid-extension set are connected to the other 2 ports of the 3-way stopcock. The fluid-administration set and fluid-extension set should be filled with 0.9% by allowing fluid to flow from the bag of 0.9% sodium chloride with the stopcock in the off position to the manometer.
• After the fluid-administration set and fluid-extension set are filled with saline, the extension set is connected to the patient's central venous catheter port. With the stopcock still in the off position to the manometer, the fluid is allowed to flow into the patient's central venous catheter, effectively flushing the catheter and ensuring that it is patent.
• The stopcock is then turned off to the patient, and the manometer is held vertically. It is allowed to fill to three-quarters full with the sterile saline solution. Care is taken *not* to allow fluid to flow over the top of the manometer because this can contaminate the sterile system.
• After the manometer is filled, the fluid-administration set should be clamped (there is no fluid flow in the system) and the zero reference point must be determined. The *zero reference point* is an imaginary horizontal line drawn from the level of the right atrium to the manometer. The manometer should be held vertically with the stopcock resting on the table or cage floor to ensure that it does not move while the zero reference point is being established or while CVP readings are being taken. The external anatomic landmark for measuring the zero reference point is the manubrium in laterally recumbent patients and the scapulohumeral joint or point of the shoulder in sternally recumbent patients.
• After the zero reference point has been determined, the stopcock is turned off to the fluid-administration set and fluid bag. This allows the water column within the manometer to equilibrate with the pressure at the tip of the CVP catheter. The meniscus of the manometer is then read to obtain the equilibrium value. The equilibrium value *minus* the zero reference point is the CVP reading.
• For example, if the zero reference point = 5 cm H_2O and the equilibrium point = 15 cm H_2O, then the CVP = 10 cm H_2O (15 cm H_2O − 5 cm H_2O).

SAMPLE HANDLING
N/A

APPROPRIATE AFTERCARE
The central venous catheter should be capped with a sterile injection cap and flushed with heparinized saline to maintain patency after each reading.

Postprocedure Patient Monitoring
N/A

Nursing Care
• The patency of the central venous catheter must be maintained for serial monitoring.
• A sterile dressing or bandage must be maintained over the central venous catheter insertion site.

Dietary Modification
N/A

Medication Requirements
None

Restrictions on Activity
N/A

Anticipated Recovery Time
N/A

 INTERPRETATION

NORMAL FINDINGS OR RANGE
The normal reference range is 2–10 cm H_2O.

ABNORMAL VALUES
- CVP readings of <2 cm H_2O suggest hypovolemia.
- Decreasing trends in CVP measurement may indicate hemorrhage, fluid loss, or decreasing intrathoracic pressure.
- CVP readings of >10 cm H_2O may suggest volume overload.
- Pericardial effusion or other causes of right-sided heart failure may be associated with high CVP readings.
- Increasing trends in CVP readings may indicate impending fluid overload and increasing intravascular volume, as well as possible increasing intrathoracic pressure, intra-abdominal pressure, and decreasing cardiac function.

CRITICAL VALUES
CVP readings of <2 cm H_2O suggesting hypovolemia require immediate fluid resuscitation and clinical evaluation of the patient for other indicators of shock and underlying causes of hypovolemia.

INTERFERING FACTORS
Drugs That May Alter Results of the Procedure
- Administration of vasopressors (dopamine, vasopressin, norepinephrine) can increase CVP readings.
- Administration of vasodilators (nitroprusside, acepromazine) can decrease CVP readings.

Conditions That May Interfere with Performing the Procedure
Wounds that inhibit the placement of a central venous catheter may preclude CVP monitoring.

Procedure Techniques or Handling That May Alter Results
- Partial or complete occlusions of the cranial vena cava, central venous catheter or extension set can alter CVP results (they usually increase). Occlusions of the catheter may be intraluminal or extraluminal occlusions (kinking). A catheter can kink anywhere along its length, though the most common site is at the insertion.
- Patients on positive pressure ventilation may have high CVP results that do not truly reflect intravascular volume and right ventricular function but are caused by the positive pressure ventilator breaths. These high CVP values may be compounded by the addition of positive end-expiratory pressure (PEEP) or continuous positive airway pressure (CPAP).
- Because of the recirculation of the regurgitant blood within the right cardiac chambers in patients with tricuspid regurgitation, CVP measurements may not reflect volume changes or right ventricular end-diastolic pressure.
- CVP may be increased in patients with increased intra-abdominal pressure or with the application of external hind-limb and/or abdominal counterpressure.
- CVP results may be erroneous if the zero reference point is not measured appropriately.
- Serial CVP readings should be recorded in with the patients in the same recumbent position (i.e., right lateral, left lateral, or sternal).

Influence of Signalment on Performing and Interpreting the Procedure
Species
N/A

Breed
N/A

Age
N/A

Gender
N/A

Pregnancy
N/A

CLINICAL PERSPECTIVE
- A single CVP measurement, unless it is very low or very high, may be of little value, and the trend of change in serial CVP measurements is more important than any single reading.
- CVP measurements should be interpreted in conjunction with other cardiovascular measurements (e.g., blood pressure) and physical perfusion parameters (e.g., heart rate, mucous membrane color, capillary refill time, pulse quality).

 MISCELLANEOUS

ANCILLARY TESTS
If CVP results are abnormal, then other tests should be performed to help assess hydration and perfusion, including evaluation of packed cell volume and total solids, measurement of direct or indirect blood pressure, and evaluation of lactate, urine output, and physical perfusion parameters.

SYNONYMS
None

SEE ALSO
Blackwell's Five-Minute Veterinary Consult: Canine and Feline Topics
- Renal Failure, Acute Uremia
- Shock, Cardiogenic
- Shock, Hypovolemic
- Shock, Septic

Related Topics in This Book
Blood Pressure Determination: Noninvasive and Invasive

ABBREVIATION
CVP = central venous pressure

Suggested Reading
Darovic GO, Kumar A. Monitoring central venous pressure. In: Darovic GO, ed. *Hemodynamic Monitoring: Invasive and Noninvasive Clinical Application*, 3rd ed. Philadelphia: WB Saunders, 2002: 177–190.
de Laforcade AM, Rozanski EA. Central venous pressure and arterial blood pressure measurements. *Vet Clin North Am Small Anim Pract* 2001; 31 1163–1174.
Marino PL. Central venous pressure and wedge pressure. In: Marino PL, ed. *The ICU Book*, 2nd ed. Baltimore: Williams & Wilkins, 1998: 166–177.
Riel DL. Jugular catheterization and central venous pressure. In: Ettinger SJ, Feldman EC, eds. *Textbook of Veterinary Internal Medicine*, 6th ed. Philadelphia: WB Saunders, 2005: 293–294.

INTERNET RESOURCES
None

AUTHOR NAMES
Lee V. Herold and Marla Lichtenberger

CEREBROSPINAL FLUID TAP

BASICS

TYPE OF PROCEDURE
Diagnostic sample collection

PROCEDURE EXPLANATION AND RELATED PHYSIOLOGY
CSF is an ultrafiltrate of plasma that bathes the brain and spinal cord. It is produced primarily by the choroid plexus in the ventricular system of the brain and travels caudally into the central canal of the spinal cord. CSF is absorbed by the arachnoid villi, which are specialized arachnoid cells that project into the venous sinuses that surround the brain. Because CSF is in direct contact with the nervous tissue, changes in the fluid reflect disease processes within the central nervous system (CNS). Whether a pathologic process will cause CSF abnormalities depends on the nature and extent of the lesion, as well as on the proximity of the lesion to the ventricular system and subarachnoid space.

INDICATIONS
CSF analysis is an important component of the diagnostic evaluation of any patient with CNS disease.

CONTRAINDICATIONS
• Increased ICP secondary to mass lesions or inflammatory brain disease, because of the increased risk of brain herniation. Insertion of the spinal needle into the subarachnoid space creates a pressure gradient and can cause the brain structures to shift caudally along this gradient. With herniation of the cerebellum through the foramen magnum, respiratory centers and pathways within the brain stem can be compressed, which can cause respiratory arrest.
• Thrombocytopenia (platelet count, $<50,000$ cells/μL) because of the increased risk of hemorrhage into the subarachnoid space

POTENTIAL COMPLICATIONS
• Trauma to neural tissue because of improper advancement of the needle
• Hemorrhage
• Infection

CLIENT EDUCATION
• General anesthesia is required.
• Food should be withheld on the day of the procedure.
• CSF taps are invasive procedures with inherent risks; however, in most instances the potential risks are far outweighed by the diagnostic benefits of obtaining a fluid sample.

BODY SYSTEMS ASSESSED
Nervous

PROCEDURE

PATIENT PREPARATION
Preprocedure Medication or Preparation
If the procedure is to be performed in an animal with a suspected increase in ICP, the osmotic diuretic mannitol (0.5–1.0 g/kg, IV over 15–20 min) may be administered immediately prior to the tap.

Anesthesia or Sedation
• General anesthesia is required.
• The use of anesthetic agents, such as ketamine and halothane, that increase ICP should be avoided in animals with intracranial disease.
• Animals with a suspected increase in ICP should be hyperventilated to maintain a carbon dioxide partial pressure of 30–35 mmHg.

Patient Positioning
Lateral recumbency. Right lateral recumbency is the preferred position for right-handed individuals and left lateral recumbency for left-handed individuals.

Patient Monitoring
Monitor for airway patency during a cisternal tap because the neck is flexed during positioning. Use of a guarded endotracheal tube will minimize this risk.

Equipment or Supplies
• Hair clippers
• A sterile scrub
• Sterile gloves
• A spinal needle: 22 gauge, $1\frac{1}{2}$ inches (38.1 mm) for cisternal tap; 22 gauge $2\frac{1}{2}$–$3\frac{1}{2}$ inches (63.5–88.9 mm) for lumbar tap
• A sterile tube (free of additives) or a syringe in which to collect fluid

TECHNIQUE
General Comments
• Fluid is most commonly collected from the cerebellomedullary cistern (CMC) (cisternal tap), because that is the easiest location from which to obtain an adequate sample for analysis. Fluid is more difficult to obtain from the lumbar site, and there is an increased chance of blood contamination.
• 1 mL of CSF per 5 kg of body weight can be safely removed from an animal.

Cisternal Tap
• The skin in the area is clipped and aseptically prepared.
• The head is flexed at a right angle to the vertebral column, with the nose held parallel to the table surface.

• The cranial margins of the wings of the atlas and the external occipital protuberance are palpated. An imaginary line is drawn from 1 wing of the atlas to the other, at the cranial margins. Another line is drawn from the external occipital protuberance caudally along midline. The CMC is located at the point where these lines intersect.

• The needle is inserted on midline perpendicular to the neck. Once the skin has been penetrated, the stylet can be withdrawn from the needle. The needle is advanced very slowly, a few millimeters at a time, and the hub of the needle observed for fluid. A slight increase in resistance may be observed just before penetration into the CMC.

• If the needle hits bone, the needle tip should be redirected slightly cranially or caudally toward the CMC. If this is not successful, the needle should be withdrawn and the procedure restarted.

• If blood is obtained, the needle has typically been directed lateral to the intended space. The needle should be withdrawn and the procedure repeated.

Lumbar Tap
Collection of fluid at the level of the L5-L6 intervertebral space:
• The skin in the area is clipped and aseptically prepared.
• The pelvic limbs are held cranially to flex the lumbar spine and open up the interarcuate space.
• The ilial wings are palpated. The dorsal spine palpated on midline just cranial to the ilial wings is that of L6.
• The needle is positioned on midline, at the caudal aspect of the L6 dorsal spine, and advanced cranially at a 30°–45° angle from an imaginary line drawn perpendicular to the spine.
• After the needles passes through the interarcuate ligament and enters the spinal canal, the tail or pelvic limbs often twitch. The needle is advanced until bone is hit at the floor of the spinal canal, the stylet is withdrawn, and fluid is collected. If fluid is not immediately obtained, the needle should be backed out slowly until CSF flow is evident.

SAMPLE HANDLING
• CSF should be analyzed within 30–60 min of collection, because the low-protein environment causes cellular instability. If analysis within this time frame is not possible, the sample should be preserved. Autologous serum added to a final concentration of ≈10% has been shown to provide sufficient preservation to enable analysis for up to 2 days after collection. If this is done, a second aliquot of nonpreserved CSF should also be obtained for determination of protein concentration and total cell count.
• CSF should always be submitted for evaluation, regardless of whether it visually appears normal, because the cell count or protein concentration must be markedly increased before the sample will appear cloudy.

APPROPRIATE AFTERCARE
Postprocedure Patient Monitoring
None

Nursing Care
None

Dietary Modification
None

Medication Requirements
None

Restrictions on Activity
None

Anticipated Recovery Time
None apart from the time required to recover from general anesthesia

INTERPRETATION
NORMAL FINDINGS OR RANGE
Normal CSF is clear and colorless. Routine analysis includes RBC count, WBC count, protein determination, and cytologic evaluation. Normal values are RBCs, $0/\mu L$; WBCs, $0–5/\mu L$, with lymphocytes predominating; and protein, 0–25 mg/dL (cisternal) and 0–45 mg/dL (lumbar).

ABNORMAL VALUES
• An increase in RBC count is due to either iatrogenic blood contamination or hemorrhage in the subarachnoid space. Previous hemorrhage may cause xanthochromia (yellow fluid), because of the presence of bilirubin that arises from breakdown of hemoglobin in the sample. Erythrophagocytosis may be observed on cytology.
• An increase in nucleated cell count in the CSF is referred to as *pleocytosis*. A *leukocytic* pleocytosis in the absence of hemorrhage is indicative of local inflammation. The predominant cell population helps to characterize the inflammation further and suggests potential etiologies.
 • A *lymphocytic* pleocytosis is seen most commonly with viral infections, the necrotizing encephalitides, ehrlichiosis, or CNS lymphoma.
 • A *neutrophilic* pleocytosis is most common with bacterial infections and steroid-responsive meningitis. The neutrophils may appear degenerate with bacterial disease. Neutrophils may also predominate with FIP, fungal disease, or Rocky Mountain spotted fever, as well as with meningiomas and vascular lesions of the CNS.

CEREBROSPINAL FLUID TAP

• An *eosinophilic* pleocytosis is typically associated with parasitic migration, protozoal infections, cryptococcosis, protothecosis, lymphoma and uncommonly, rabies infection. This pattern is also characteristic of an idiopathic, steroid responsive eosinophilic meningoencephalitis of dogs and cats.

• A *mixed-cell* pleocytosis, with a variable number of lymphocytes, large mononuclear cells, and neutrophils, is seen with GME, as well as in fungal, protozoal, rickettsial, and chronic bacterial infections.

• An elevation in CSF protein concentration is caused by either intrathecal antibody production or breakdown of the blood-CSF barrier and extravasation of serum protein into the subarachnoid space. An increase in CSF protein with a normal leukocyte count is called albuminocytologic dissociation, and is seen most commonly with neoplastic, degenerative and vascular disorders.

CRITICAL VALUES
None

INTERFERING FACTORS
Drugs That May Alter Results of the Procedure
• Prior treatment with corticosteroids may decrease the CSF WBC count in animals with CNS inflammatory disease.
• Previous antibiotic treatment in animals with a bacterial infection may alter the number and type of leukocytes present in the CSF.

Conditions That May Interfere with Performing the Procedure
None

Procedure Techniques or Handling That May Alter Results
Delays in sample analysis, particularly analysis of an unpreserved sample, can cause erroneous cytologic results because cellular disintegration makes the cell types difficult to identify.

Influence of Signalment on Performing and Interpreting the Procedure
Species
None

Breed
None

Age
None

Gender
None

Pregnancy
None

CLINICAL PERSPECTIVE
• CSF analysis is an integral part of the diagnostic evaluation of animals with CNS disease and is the primary means of confirming the presence of CNS inflammation.

• In animals with signs of intracranial disease, CSF is typically performed after the brain is imaged, in order to identify mass lesions that potentially increase the risk of the procedure. In certain instances, a CSF tap may still be recommended in an animal with a mass lesion to provide additional diagnostic information. In these cases, precautions should be taken (i.e., administration of mannitol or hyperventilation during anesthesia) to decrease the intracranial pressure and minimize the risks.

• If a myelogram is planned in the evaluation of an animal with spinal disease, CSF should be collected prior to myelography, because injection of the contrast agent into the subarachnoid space incites an inflammatory response.

• If inflammation is present in the CSF, further testing should be performed to attempt to identify the cause. If no underlying infectious cause can be found, a noninfectious, inflammatory cause such as GME, the necrotizing encephalitides, or steroid responsive meningitis should be suspected.

• Bear in mind that normal CSF can be obtained in an animal with CNS inflammatory disease, particularly if the focus of inflammation is deep within the parenchyma at a distance from the ventricular system and subarachnoid space, or if corticosteroids have been previously administered.

MISCELLANEOUS
ANCILLARY TESTS
• If CSF pleocytosis is identified, potential causes for the inflammation should be pursued. Serum and CSF samples should be submitted for serologic tests and a CSF sample submitted for PCR to evaluate for viral, rickettsial, protozoal, and fungal disease. CSF should be submitted for aerobic and anaerobic culture in cases where a bacterial infection is suspected.

• If CSF protein concentration is increased, protein electrophoresis can be performed to characterize the pattern of protein elevation.

SYNONYMS
• CSF tap
• Spinal tap

SEE ALSO

Blackwell's Five-Minute Veterinary Consult: Canine and Feline Topics

- Encephalitis
- Meningitis/Meningoencephalomyelitis/Meningomyelitis, Bacterial
- Meningoencephalomyelitis—Eosinophilic
- Meningoencephalomyelitis—Granulomatous
- Steroid-Responsive Meningitis-Arteritis—Dogs

Related Topics in This Book

Fluid Analysis

ABBREVIATIONS

- CMC = cerebellomedullary cistern
- CNS = central nervous system
- CSF = cerebrospinal fluid
- GME = granulomatous meningoencephalomyelitis
- ICP = intracranial pressure

Suggested Reading

Bienzle D, McDonnell JJ, Stanton JB. Analysis of cerebrospinal fluid from dogs and cats after 24 and 48 hours of storage. *J Am Vet Med Assoc* 2000; 216: 1761–1764.

Cellio BC. Collecting, processing, and preparing cerebrospinal fluid in dogs and cats. *Compend Contin Educ Pract Vet* 2001; 23: 786–792.

Chrisman CL. Cerebrospinal fluid analysis. *Vet Clin North Am Small Anim Pract* 1992; 22: 781–810.

INTERNET RESOURCES

None

AUTHOR NAME

Karen R. Muñana

BASICS

TYPE OF SPECIMEN
Blood

TEST EXPLANATION AND RELATED PHYSIOLOGY
Chloride (Cl) is the principal anion in the extracellular fluid compartment. Homeostasis of Cl is primarily regulated by the kidneys, but the GI system has a minor role. Dietary Cl is absorbed in the jejunum and distal colon in conjunction with Na, and Cl is also absorbed in the ileum. Facilitated Cl transport in the ileum and colon is a driving force for Na and water reabsorption. In the kidneys, 50%–60% of filtered Cl is reabsorbed in the proximal tubules. Cl also is reabsorbed in the distal nephron under the influence of aldosterone, and is actively reabsorbed in the thick ascending limb of the loop of Henle.

Cl usually accompanies Na and is needed to maintain electrical neutrality. Changes in serum Cl often parallel changes in serum Na and both respond proportionally to alterations in free body water. Cl also plays an important role in maintenance of the blood buffer system and acid-base balance. Changes in Cl generally oppose those of serum HCO_3 such that hyperchloremia is associated with metabolic acidosis, whereas hypochloremia is associated with metabolic alkalosis.

It may be diagnostically helpful to correct the serum Cl for the serum Na concentration. If the corrected Cl value is abnormal, this indicates a change in Cl independent of Na:
- Dogs: Cl (corrected) = Cl (measured) × 146/Na (measured)
- Cats: Cl (corrected) = Cl (measured) × 156/Na (measured)

Most laboratories measure Cl by using ion-selective electrodes (i.e., direct or indirect potentiometry), but other titration methods (e.g., colorimetry) and dry-reagent methods may also be available.

INDICATIONS
- GI signs
- Polyuria and polydipsia
- Acid-base derangements
- Monitoring of therapy with diuretics, parenteral nutrition, Na or Cl salt–containing medications or fluids

CONTRAINDICATIONS
None

POTENTIAL COMPLICATIONS
None

CLIENT EDUCATION
None

BODY SYSTEMS ASSESSED
- Endocrine and metabolic
- Gastrointestinal
- Renal and urologic

SAMPLE

COLLECTION
0.5–1.0 mL of venous blood

HANDLING
Collect the sample in a red-top tube or a serum-separator tube.

STORAGE
- Refrigerate for short-term storage.
- Freeze the serum or plasma for long-term storage.

STABILITY
- Room temperature: 1 day
- Refrigerated (2°–8°C): 1 week
- Frozen (−20°C): 1 year

PROTOCOL
None

INTERPRETATION

NORMAL FINDINGS OR RANGE
- Dogs: 107–113 mEq/L
- Cats: 117–123 mEq/L
- Cats: 117–123 mEq/L
- Reference intervals may vary, depending on the laboratory and assay.

ABNORMAL VALUES
Values above or below the reference intervals

CRITICAL VALUES
None

INTERFERING FACTORS
Drugs That May Alter Results or Interpretation
Drugs That Interfere with Test Methodology
Drugs containing halides (e.g., potassium bromide) may cause pseudohyperchloremia. Halides are measured as Cl by ion-selective electrodes.

Drugs That Alter Physiology
- Loop and thiazide diuretics and sodium bicarbonate may cause hypochloremia.
- Acetazolamide, ammonium chloride, glucocorticoids, and drugs that diminish renal concentrating ability (e.g., amphotericin) may cause hyperchloremia.

Disorders That May Alter Results
- In a lipemic sample, pseudohyperchloremia may be diagnosed if a non–ion-selective colorimetric assay is used, but using a non–ion-selective titrimetric method may cause pseudohypochloremia.
- Hyperproteinemia may cause pseudohypochloremia if a titrimetric method is used.
- Hyperviscosity may alter results if samples are diluted prior to analysis (i.e., by indirect potentiometry).

Collection Techniques or Handling That May Alter Results
None

Influence of Signalment
Species
None

Breed
None

Age
None

Gender
None

Pregnancy
None

LIMITATIONS OF THE TEST
Sensitivity, Specificity, and Positive and Negative Predictive Values
N/A

Valid If Run in a Human Lab?
Yes.

Causes of Abnormal Findings

High values	Low values
Pseudohyperchloremia	**Pseudohypochloremia**
Sample evaporation	Dilutional artifact
Potassium bromide therapy	Lipemia and
Lipemia (colorimetric method)	hyperproteinemia
	(titrimetric methods)
Normal corrected Cl	**Normal corrected Cl**
(concurrent hypernatremia)	**(concurrent hyponatremia)**
Hemoconcentration	GI loss
Pure water loss (diabetes	Third-space loss (ascites,
insipidus)	uroabdomen)
Hypotonic fluid loss (e.g.,	Urinary loss
diabetes mellitus)	Renal failure
	Hypoadrenocorticism
	Ketonuria
	Edematous conditions
	Burns
Corrected hyperchloremia	**Corrected hypochloremia**
Excessive loss of Na (and	Excessive loss of Cl relative
HCO$_3$) relative to Cl (e.g.,	to Na
small-bowel diarrhea)	Vomiting Cl-rich stomach
Excessive gain of Cl relative	contents
to Na	Thiazide or loop diuretics
Therapy with Cl-containing	Hyperadrenocorticism
salts	Cavitary effusion
Parenteral nutrition	Congestive heart failure
Fluid therapy with 0.9% NaCl	Chronic respiratory
or hypertonic saline	acidosis
Salt poisoning	Therapies containing high Na
Renal retention of Cl	concentration relative
Renal failure	to Cl
Renal tubular acidosis	Na-containing antibiotics
Hypoaldosteronism	Sodium bicarbonate
Ketoacidotic diabetes	
mellitus	
Potassium-sparing diuretics	
(amiloride, spironolactone)	
Acetazolamide	
Chronic respiratory alkalosis	
(decreased renal retention	
of HCO$_3$)	

CLINICAL PERSPECTIVE

• Elevated Cl, following correction for serum Na, is most often associated with small-bowel diarrhea and a hyperchloremic metabolic acidosis.

• Decreased Cl, following correction for serum Na, is often associated with an upper GI obstruction with loss and/or sequestration of HCl and metabolic alkalosis.

MISCELLANEOUS

ANCILLARY TESTS

• Na, potassium, HCO$_3$
• Blood-gas analysis, anion gap
• Urine fractional excretion of Cl

SYNONYMS

Cl

SEE ALSO

Blackwell's Five-Minute Veterinary Consult: Canine and Feline Topics

• Diarrhea, Acute
• Diarrhea, Antibiotic Responsive
• Diarrhea, Chronic—Cats
• Diarrhea, Chronic—Dogs
• Gastrointestinal Obstruction
• Renal Tubular Acidosis

Related Topics in This Book

• Bicarbonate
• Blood Gases
• Potassium
• Sodium

ABBREVIATIONS

• Cl = chloride
• HCO$_3$ = bicarbonate
• Na = sodium

Suggested Reading
de Morais HA. Disorders of chloride. In: Dibartola SP, ed. *Fluid Therapy in Small Animal Practice*, 2nd ed. Philadelphia: WB Saunders, 1992: 73–82.
Manning AM. Electrolyte disorders. *Vet Clin North Am Small Anim Pract* 2001; 31: 1300–1303.

INTERNET RESOURCES

Cornell University, College of Veterinary Medicine, Clinical Pathology Modules, Routine Blood Chemistry: Electrolytes, Interpretation of Serum Chloride Results, http://diaglab.vet.cornell.edu/clinpath/modules/chem/chloride.htm

AUTHOR NAME

Maria Vandis

BASICS

TYPE OF SPECIMEN
Blood

TEST EXPLANATION AND RELATED PHYSIOLOGY
Cholesterol is a type of lipid derived from triglycerides found primarily in tissues of animal origin. It is an important constituent of cell membranes and is a crucial precursor of numerous molecules such as steroid hormones, vitamin D, and bile salts. Digestion and intestinal absorption of animal-based diets contribute to some of the body's cholesterol, but the majority is synthesized by hepatocytes. Accordingly, cholesterol serves as an important measure of hepatic synthetic function.

Cholesterol is water insoluble; therefore, most cholesterol in plasma is packaged in lipoproteins that were synthesized by hepatocytes. Serum cholesterol concentration represents the total cholesterol concentration; reacting cholesterol molecules originate from hydrolyzed lipoproteins, predominantly cholesterol-rich low-density lipoprotein (LDL) and high-density lipoprotein (HDL) molecules. Cholesterol is usually determined via a series of enzymatic reactions with a resultant color change that is measured spectrophotometrically.

Disorders of lipoprotein metabolism are frequently multifactorial and involve excess hepatic synthesis, defective lipolysis, or defects in clearance or cellular uptake of lipoproteins. Lipolysis of lipoproteins occurs on the luminal surface of capillary endothelial cells and is catalyzed by lipoprotein lipase under the control of insulin. Lipoprotein remnants are removed by the liver and any remaining cholesterol is recycled into lipoproteins, excreted in bile, or degraded into bile acids.

Hyperlipidemia (or *hyperlipoproteinemia*) is an increase in plasma lipids (cholesterol and/or triglycerides) and may be either primary or secondary. *Primary hyperlipidemia* is associated with a hereditary derangement of lipoprotein metabolism and is rare. *Secondary hyperlipidemia* is much more common and is associated with numerous diseases, especially certain endocrinopathies and nephrotic syndrome. Hypocholesterolemia is most commonly associated with portosystemic shunts.

INDICATIONS
- Hyperlipidemia
- Suspect endocrinopathy
- Suspect hepatic disease
- Suspect nephrotic syndrome

CONTRAINDICATIONS
None

POTENTIAL COMPLICATIONS
Postvenipuncture bleeding if hepatic coagulation factor synthesis is decreased.

CLIENT EDUCATION
The patient must fast for 12 h.

BODY SYSTEMS ASSESSED
- Endocrine and metabolic
- Hepatobiliary
- Renal and urologic

SAMPLE

COLLECTION
1 mL of venous blood

HANDLING
A plain red-top, serum-separator tube, or heparin (green-top tube)

STORAGE
Refrigerate or freeze the serum for long-term storage.

STABILITY
- 1 day at room temperature
- Refrigerated (2°–8°C): 1 week
- Frozen: 3 months at −20°C; several years at −70°C

PROTOCOL
None

INTERPRETATION

NORMAL FINDINGS OR RANGE
- Dogs: 133–367 mg/dL (3.45–9.50 mmol/L)
- Cats: 70–229 mg/dL (1.8–5.9 mmol/L)
- Reference intervals may vary, depending on laboratory and assay.

ABNORMAL VALUES
Values above or below the reference range

CRITICAL VALUES
None

INTERFERING FACTORS
Drugs That May Alter Results or Interpretation
Drugs That Interfere with Test Methodology
None

Drugs That Alter Physiology
- IV heparin (promotes secretion of lipoprotein lipase and hepatic lipase)
- Corticosteroids may cause an increase via multiple mechanisms.

Disorders That May Alter Results
- Hemolysis and hyperproteinemia artifactually increase reflectance spectrophotometry results.
- Bilirubin and ascorbic acid negatively interfere with enzymatic assays.

Collection Techniques or Handling That May Alter Results
- Iatrogenic hemolysis
- In nonfasted samples, a postprandial cholesterol increase may be mistaken for metabolic disease.

Influence of Signalment
Species
None

Breed
None

Age
Increases with age

Gender
None

Pregnancy
None

LIMITATIONS OF THE TEST
Sensitivity, Specificity, and Positive and Negative Predictive Values
N/A

Valid If Run in a Human Lab?
Yes.

Causes of Abnormal Findings

High values	Low values
Primary hyperlipidemia	Decreased production
Idiopathic hyperlipidemia of miniature schnauzers	Congenital portosystemic vascular anomalies
Idiopathic hyperchylomicronemia	Hepatic failure
Lipoprotein lipase deficiency	Maldigestion/exocrine pancreas insufficiency
Hypercholesterolemia of briards	Malabsorption/protein-losing enteropathy (especially lymphangiectasia)
Increased production	
Postprandial hyperlipidemia	Severe malnutrition
Protein-losing nephropathy (nephrotic syndrome)	Other, unknown, or multiple mechanisms
Decreased lipoprotein clearance	Hypoadrenocorticism
Hypothyroidism	
Protein-losing nephropathy	
Other, unknown, or multiple mechanisms	
Diabetes mellitus (marked)	
Hyperadrenocorticism (mild)	
Exogenous corticosteroids (moderate)	
Acute (necrotizing) pancreatitis	
Obstructive cholestasis (rare)	

CLINICAL PERSPECTIVE
• If hypercholesterolemia is associated with significant renal proteinuria, consider nephrotic syndrome.
• If hypercholesterolemia is associated with alopecia or polyuria-polydipsia, rule out endocrinopathies.
• With a portosystemic shunt, hypocholesterolemia may be the only abnormality in a chemistry profile.
• Significantly higher cholesterol levels are seen in obese animals; the cholesterol concentration decreases with weight loss.

MISCELLANEOUS
ANCILLARY TESTS
• Full chemistry panel for hepatic, renal, and pancreatic function
• Urinalysis to check for proteinuria, glucosuria, and ketonuria
• Thyroid function tests
• Liver function tests

SYNONYMS
None

SEE ALSO
Blackwell's Five-Minute Veterinary Consult: Canine and Feline Topics
• Amyloidosis
• Diabetes Mellitus without Complication—Cats
• Diabetes Mellitus without Complication—Dogs
• Diabetes with Hyperosmolar Coma
• Diabetes with Ketoacidosis
• Glomerulonephritis
• Hyperadrenocorticism (Cushing's Disease)—Cats
• Hyperadrenocorticism (Cushing's Disease)—Dogs
• Hypothyroidism
• Nephrotic Syndrome
• Pancreatitis
• Portosystemic Vascular Anomaly, Congenital
Related Topics in This Book
• Albumin
• Bile Acids
• Glucose
• Glucose Curve
• Triglycerides
• Urea Nitrogen

ABBREVIATIONS
None

Suggested Reading
Evans EW, Duncan JR. Proteins, lipids, and carbohydrates. In: Latimer KS, Mahaffey EA, Prasse KW, eds. *Duncan and Prasse's Veterinary Laboratory Medicine*. Ames: Iowa State Press, 2003: 162–192.
Stockham SL, Scott MA. Lipids. In: Stockham SL, Scott MA, eds. *Fundamentals of Veterinary Clinical Pathology*, 2nd ed., Ames: Iowa State Press, 2008: 763–782.

INTERNET RESOURCES
Cornell University, College of Medicine: Clinical Pathology Modules, Veterinary Clinical Chemistry—Cholestrol, http://www.diaglab.vet.cornell.edu/clinpath/modules/chem/cholest.htm.

AUTHOR NAMES
Rebekah Gray Gunn-Christie and J. Roger Easley

COAGULATION FACTORS

BASICS

TYPE OF SPECIMEN
Blood

TEST EXPLANATION AND RELATED PHYSIOLOGY
Coagulation factors are plasma proteins that interact to catalyze the transformation of soluble fibrinogen to form an insoluble fibrin clot. The factors circulate in plasma as proenzymes or pro-cofactors but are rapidly activated at sites of blood vessel and tissue injury. In vivo, coagulation factors assemble on membrane surfaces to form active enzyme complexes that amplify and sustain the generation of thrombin (factor IIa). Thrombin converts fibrinogen to fibrin, has key roles in platelet activation, and has both positive and negative regulatory effects on coagulation and fibrinolysis.

Coagulation factors are designated by Roman numerals, assigned in the order of their characterization, and with the subscript "a" denoting an active form. Fibrinogen (factor I) is a glycoprotein composed of polypeptide chains. Upon cleavage by thrombin, the fibrinogen chains polymerize and are ultimately cross-linked (by factor XIII) to form a stable fibrin meshwork. Most coagulation factors are serine protease enzymes whose specific substrates are inactive coagulation factors. Fibrinogen and all the serine protease factors are synthesized exclusively in the liver. To assume an active conformation, a subgroup of these factors (factors II, VII, IX, and X) require vitamin K–dependent γ-carboxylation after synthesis. Factors V and VIII are cofactors that are needed to catalyze the activity of factors X and IX, respectively.

Coagulation protein deficiencies typically manifest as deep tissue hemorrhage and hematoma formation, and prolonged hemorrhage from sites of surgery or trauma. In most cases, factor deficiencies develop secondary to an underlying disease process and will resolve as the disease is treated. Although less common, hereditary factor deficiencies such as hemophilia do occur in dogs and cats. Bleeding diatheses caused by deficiencies of fibrinogen and factors II, VII, VIII, IX, X, and XI have been reported in dogs and cats.

Functional factor assays (coagulant activity assays) are usually performed in assay systems that measure the time for in vitro clot formation with end point based on detection of a fibrin clot. The clinical severity of a bleeding tendency depends on a patient's residual factor activity and on the deficient factor's role in supporting in vivo hemostasis.

INDICATIONS
• Ancillary tests to define the cause of abnormal coagulation screening tests (activating clotting time, APTT, PT)
• Definitive diagnosis of inherited and acquired coagulation factor deficiencies
• Monitoring response to transfusion therapy

CONTRAINDICATIONS
None

POTENTIAL COMPLICATIONS
None

CLIENT EDUCATION
Coagulation factor deficiencies often cause severe bleeding. Factor deficiencies most often develop secondary to an underlying disease process and will resolve as the disease is treated. Those patients with hereditary factor deficiencies often require periodic transfusion. Propagation of the traits can be prevented through genetic counseling and selective breeding.

BODY SYSTEMS ASSESSED
Hemic, lymphatic, and immune

SAMPLE

COLLECTION
2.7 mL of venous blood

HANDLING
• Collect blood directly into 3.2% or 3.8% sodium citrate anticoagulant (blue-top tubes).
  • An exact blood to citrate ratio (9 parts:1 part) is critical.
  • 2.7 mL of blood in 0.3 mL of citrate yields sufficient plasma (approximately 1.0–1.5 mL) for coagulation factor analyses.
• Centrifuge the whole blood and remove the plasma within 1 h of collection.
• Store the plasma in plastic or additive-free siliconized glass tubes.

STORAGE
• Store the plasma in a refrigerator pending assay within 4 h.
• Store the plasma in a freezer pending shipment or if assay is >4 h after collection.
• Ship the same day or overnight on cold packs.

STABILITY
For 2 weeks at −20°C (frozen)

PROTOCOL
None

INTERPRETATION

NORMAL FINDINGS OR RANGE
• Factor activity results are usually reported as the percentage of a same-species standard plasma. Factor activities of ≥50% (of the standard) are normal for most assay systems.
• Canine fibrinogen: 147–470 mg/dL
• Feline fibrinogen: 75–270 mg/dL
• Reference ranges are from the Comparative Coagulation Section of the Cornell University Animal Health Diagnostic Center. Values may vary depending on the laboratory and assay.

ABNORMAL VALUES
• Factor activities of ≤50% (of the standard)
• Fibrinogen levels above or below the reference range

CRITICAL VALUES
• Factor activity of <20% is a risk factor for abnormal bleeding after surgery or injury. A combined deficiency of multiple factors exacerbates clinical severity.
• Factor activity of <5% is a risk factor for spontaneous hemorrhage.
• Clinical severity of the bleeding tendency varies for different factors.
• Factor XII deficiency is common in cats but does not cause a bleeding tendency.

INTERFERING FACTORS
Drugs That May Alter Results or Interpretation
Drugs That Interfere with Test Methodology
None

Drugs That Alter Physiology
• Coumadin treatment causes low activities of vitamin K–dependent factors (factors II, VII, IX, X).

• Heparin therapy inhibits all serine protease factors (through enhanced antithrombin activity).
• Plasma expanders (e.g., dextrans, hetastarch) can impair activity of factor VIII–von Willebrand factor complex.

Disorders That May Alter Results
High fibrinogen often accompanies systemic inflammatory conditions. Marked elevations in fibrinogen may decrease the sensitivity of coagulant activity assays.

Collection Techniques or Handling That May Alter Results
• Poor venipuncture technique and failure to draw blood directly into anticoagulant are common sources of artifact.
• Sodium citrate must be used as the anticoagulant. Artifactual factor deficiencies result from the use of heparin (green-top tube), EDTA (purple-top tube), excess or inadequate citrate anticoagulant, plain glass (e.g., red top) tubes, or tubes containing a serum separator with clot activator.

Influence of Signalment
Species
None

Breed
• Factor VII deficiency: beagle, husky, Klee Kai, deerhound; DSH
• Factor VIII deficiency (hemophilia A) is the most common hereditary factor deficiency, which is found in purebred and mixed-breed dogs and cats. Mild to moderate hemophilia may be propagated widely within a breed. Mild hemophilia A (factor VIII activity, 5%–15%) has been reported in German shepherds and recently in golden retrievers.
• Factor X deficiency: cocker spaniel, Jack Russell terrier; DSH
• Factor XI deficiency: springer spaniel, Kerry blue terrier; DSH
• Factor XII deficiency: a common factor deficiency in DSH and domestic longhair (DLH) cats and reported in Siamese and Himalayan cats

Age
• Severe congenital coagulation factor deficiency (<1% of normal activity) can result in death shortly after birth or in the neonatal period due to hemorrhage.
• In surviving neonates, signs of coagulopathy generally appear before 6 months of age. Moderate factor deficiencies (5%–10% factor activities) manifest as prolonged bleeding after routine procedures such as vaccination, tail docking, dewclaw removal, ear cropping, and castration or ovariohysterectomy.

Gender
None

Pregnancy
None

LIMITATIONS OF THE TEST
Sensitivity, Specificity, and Positive and Negative Predictive Values
N/A

Valid If Run in a Human Lab?
No. Factor activity assays should be performed using same-species standards and require species-specific reference ranges. Human fibrinogen assays can be adapted for canine and feline plasmas.

Causes of Abnormal Values

Acquired factor deficiencies

Disease condition	Abnormal screening test results	Deficient factors
Liver failure	aPTT, PT, TCT, fibrinogen	All factors & fibrinogen
Vitamin K deficiency (anticoagulant rodenticide, cholestasis, coumadin therapy)	aPTT, PT	Factors II, VII, IX, X
Fulminant or hemorrhagic DIC	aPTT, PT, TCT, fibrinogen	All factors & fibrinogen
Snakebite envenomation	aPTT, PT, TCT, fibrinogen	Fibrinogen (may affect other factors)
Heparin therapy	aPTT, TCT	Factors II, IX, X, XI, XII

Hereditary factor deficiencies

Factor	Abnormal screening test results	Comments
Fibrinogen (factor I)	aPTT, PT, TCT, fibrinogen	Autosomal trait: DSH
Prothrombin (factor II)	aPTT, PT	Autosomal trait: rare
Factor V	aPTT, PT	No reported animal cases
Factor VII	PT	Autosomal trait: beagle, husky, Klee Kai, deerhound; DSH
Factor VIII	aPTT	Hemophilia A is the most common factor deficiency, X-linked trait: many breeds and mixed
Factor IX	aPTT	Hemophilia B, X-linked trait: many breeds and mixed
Factor X	aPTT, PT	Autosomal trait: cocker spaniel, Jack Russell terrier; DSH
Factor XI	aPTT	Autosomal trait: springer spaniel, Kerry blue terrier; DSH
Factor XII	aPTT	Hageman trait, autosomal, no bleeding diathesis: common in cats

CLINICAL PERSPECTIVE
• Acquired disease conditions cause combined deficiencies of multiple coagulation factors. In contrast, hereditary factor deficiencies almost invariably affect a single factor.

COAGULATION FACTORS

• The coagulopathy of liver disease is multifactorial, resulting from impaired vitamin K absorption, compromised hepatic factor synthetic capacity, and impaired fibrin polymerization.

• Factor VII has a short plasma half-life, rendering this factor sensitive to vitamin K–deficient states. Mild or early vitamin K deficiency can be detected through specific factor VII analyses. Most patients with clinically evident hemorrhage because of vitamin K deficiency will have marked deficiency of all vitamin K–dependent factors (factors II, VII, IX, X).

• High and low factor activities may be found in patients with DIC caused by concomitant activation and depletion of coagulation factors. Low factor activities with hypofibrinogenemia are an indication for transfusion of DIC patients with signs of hemorrhage or requiring invasive procedures.

• Acquired factor VIII deficiency (caused by development of anti–factor VIII antibodies) is a rare autoimmune coagulopathy in people. Although factor VIII autoantibodies have not been reported in animals, alloantibodies directed against factor VIII and factor IX have developed in canine hemophilia A and B patients after multiple transfusions.

• Acquired factor X deficiency is a rare complication of multiple myeloma in people and is presumably due to adsorption of factor X to amyloid fibrils. This coagulopathy has not yet been documented in animals.

• Hemophilia A (factor VIII deficiency) is the most common hereditary factor deficiency in dogs and cats. Hemophilia A (or B) should be suspected in any young male with recurrent signs of abnormal bleeding, especially hemarthrosis, hematoma formation, and prolonged bleeding from minor wounds.

MISCELLANEOUS

ANCILLARY TESTS
Coagulation screening tests (e.g., aPTT, PT, TCT, fibrinogen)

SYNONYMS
Clotting factor assays

SEE ALSO
Blackwell's Five-Minute Veterinary Consult: Canine and Feline Topics
• Coagulation Factor Deficiency
• Coagulopathy of Liver Disease
• Von Willebrand Disease

Related Topics in This Book
• Fibrinogen
• Partial Thromboplastin Time, Activated
• PIVKA Test
• Platelet Count and Volume
• Platelet Function Tests
• Prothrombin Time
• Von Willebrand Factor

ABBREVIATIONS
• APTT = activated partial thromboplastin time
• DIC = disseminated intravascular coagulation
• DSH = domestic shorthair
• PT = prothrombin time
• TCT = thrombin clotting time

Suggested Reading
Brooks M. Hereditary bleeding disorders in dogs and cats. *Vet Med* 1999; 94: 555–564.
Brooks MB. Coagulopathies and thrombosis In: Ettinger SJ, Feldman EC, eds. *Textbook of Veterinary Internal Medicine: Diseases of the Dog and Cat*, 5th ed. Philadelphia: WB Saunders, 2000: 1829–1841.
Mischke R. Activated partial thromboplastin time as a screening test of minor or moderate coagulation factor deficiencies for canine plasma. *J Vet Diagn Invest* 2000; 12: 433–437.

INTERNET RESOURCES
Lab Tests Online: Coagulation factors, http://www.labtestsonline.org/understanding/analytes/coagulation_factors/test.html.
Wikipedia: Coagulation, http://en.wikipedia.org/wiki/Coagulation#The_coagulation_cascade.

AUTHOR NAME
Marjory Brooks

BASICS

TYPE OF SPECIMEN
Blood

TEST EXPLANATION AND RELATED PHYSIOLOGY
Cobalamin is a water-soluble vitamin and an important cofactor for a variety of biochemical reactions. Cobalamin uptake from the small intestine can be affected by several factors and can therefore be used as an indirect marker for GI disease. Serum cobalamin may yield information on the site and cause of intestinal disease. Cobalamin is usually abundant in commercial canine and feline diets, making a dietary insufficiency unlikely. However, patients that are fed an exclusively vegetarian diet will likely develop cobalamin deficiency unless their food is supplemented.

Dietary cobalamin is tightly bound to dietary protein. After digestion of these dietary proteins in the stomach by pepsin and hydrochloric acid, cobalamin is released and immediately bound to R protein, a protein secreted in saliva and gastric juice. Pancreatic enzymes (i.e., trypsin) digest R protein, again releasing cobalamin. Intrinsic factor, which in dogs and especially cats is mainly produced in the pancreas, binds to cobalamin and serves as a transporter at the distal small intestine, where the cobalamin–intrinsic factor complexes are absorbed by specific receptors located exclusively in the ileal mucosa. Cobalamin that is not in complex with intrinsic factor is not readily absorbed, even if provided at high doses.

The major disease processes that interfere with cobalamin uptake are EPI, distal or diffuse small-intestinal disease, and excess bacterial use of cobalamin in canine small-intestinal bacterial overgrowth. As the exocrine pancreas is the only source of intrinsic factor in cats and the main source for intrinsic factor in dogs, EPI is commonly associated with cobalamin deficiency in dogs and cats, and should be ruled out in patients with GI signs and a decreased serum cobalamin concentration. Any long-standing and severe intestinal diseases (e.g., inflammatory bowel disease, lymphoma, or fungal disease) affecting the ileum may reduce expression of or damage cobalamin receptors, leading to cobalamin malabsorption, depletion of body stores of cobalamin, and ultimately a reduced serum cobalamin concentration.

Most reference laboratories measure serum cobalamin by using a competitive chemiluminescence assay (Immulite; DPC-Siemens, Los Angeles, CA). However, serum cobalamin can also be measured by radioimmunoassays that have been validated for use in dogs and cats.

INDICATIONS
Assessment of GI function

CONTRAINDICATIONS
None

POTENTIAL COMPLICATIONS
None

CLIENT EDUCATION
The patient should be fasted (ideally, at least 12 h).

BODY SYSTEMS ASSESSED
Gastrointestinal

SAMPLE

COLLECTION
1–2 mL of venous blood

HANDLING
- Collect the serum into a red-top or serum-separator tube.
- Separate the serum from the blood clot and transfer the serum into new tube. Do *not* submit unseparated serum to laboratory.
- Ship the serum with an ice pack to the laboratory.

STORAGE
Refrigeration of the sample is recommended.

STABILITY
- Room temperature: a few days
- Freezer (−20°C): at least 6–8 weeks

PROTOCOL
None

COBALAMIN

INTERPRETATION

NORMAL FINDINGS OR RANGE
- Dogs: 252–908 ng/L
- Cats: 290–1,500 ng/L
- Reference ranges are from the GI Laboratory at Texas A&M University. Values may vary depending on the laboratory and assay.

ABNORMAL VALUES
Below the reference range

CRITICAL VALUES
None

INTERFERING FACTORS
Drugs That May Alter Results or Interpretation
Drugs That Interfere with Test Methodology
Recent parenteral administration (<4 weeks) of cobalamin will increase serum cobalamin concentrations.

Drugs That Alter Physiology
None

Disorders That May Alter Results
None

Collection Techniques or Handling That May Alter Results
None

Influence of Signalment
Species
None

Breed
Chinese sharpeis, border collies, and giant schnauzers are predisposed to cobalamin deficiency.

Age
Neonatal puppies (up to 8–13 weeks) have lower serum cobalamin concentrations than adult dogs.

Gender
None

Pregnancy
None

LIMITATIONS OF THE TEST
Sensitivity, Specificity, and Positive and Negative Predictive Values
N/A

Valid If Run in a Human Lab?
Yes—if a laboratory has validated the assay for dogs and cats and has established species-specific reference ranges.

Causes of Abnormal Findings

High values	Low values
No known clinical significance for increased serum cobalamin concentrations in dogs and cats	Distal or diffuse small-intestinal disease involving ileum (e.g., inflammatory bowel disease, lymphoma, fungal disease)
Recent parenteral administration of cobalamin	Small-intestinal bacterial overgrowth EPI

CLINICAL PERSPECTIVE
- In patients with a subnormal serum cobalamin concentration, serum trypsin-like immunoreactivity should always be measured to rule out EPI.
- Subnormal serum cobalamin concentrations may lead to GI disease and systemic complications (i.e., immunodeficiency, central or peripheral neurologic disease, but rarely anemia), and patients should receive parenteral cobalamin supplementation.
- Cobalamin deficiency on a cellular level may even occur when serum cobalamin concentration is in the low end of the normal range (<350 ng/L), and parenteral cobalamin supplementation should also be considered in these patients.

MISCELLANEOUS

ANCILLARY TESTS
- Assay the serum folate concentration.
- Evaluate the serum trypsin-like immunoreactivity.
- Determine the concentration of serum pancreatic lipase immunoreactivity.

SYNONYMS
- B_{12}
- Vitamin B_{12}

SEE ALSO
Blackwell's Five-Minute Veterinary Consult: Canine and Feline Topics
- Cobalamin Malabsorption
- Exocrine Pancreatic Insufficiency
- Protein-Losing Enteropathy
- Small Intestinal Bacterial Overgrowth

Related Topics in This Book
- Folate
- Gastrointestinal Ultrasonography

- Pancreatic Lipase Immunoreactivity
- Pancreatic Ultrasonography
- Trypsin-like Immunoreactivity

ABBREVIATIONS
EPI = exocrine pancreatic insufficiency

Suggested Reading

Ruaux CG, Steiner JM, Williams DA. Early biochemical and clinical responses to cobalamin supplementation in cats with signs of gastrointestinal disease and severe hypocobalaminemia. *J Vet Intern Med* 2005; 19: 155–60.

Simpson KW, Fyfe J, Cornetta A, *et al.* Subnormal concentrations of serum cobalamin (vitamin B_{12}) in cats with gastrointestinal disease. *J Vet Intern Med* 2001; 15: 26–32.

INTERNET RESOURCES
Texas A&M University, College of Veterinary Medicine, Gastrointestinal Laboratory: Serum cobalamin (vitamin B_{12}) and folate, http://www.cvm.tamu.edu/gilab/assays/b12folate.shtml.

AUTHORS NAMES
Jan S. Suchodolski and Jörg M. Steiner

BASICS

TYPE OF PROCEDURE
Endoscopic

PROCEDURE EXPLANATION AND RELATED PHYSIOLOGY
Colonoscopy is the procedure in which the colon and rectum are directly evaluated by using either a rigid or flexible endoscope. The procedure is most often used in the diagnosis of chronic large-bowel diarrhea caused by infiltrative disorders such as inflammatory bowel disease, fungal disease, or colonic tumors. The procedure may also be used to evaluate colonic or rectal strictures caused by fibrosis or tumors.

INDICATIONS
- Chronic large-bowel diarrhea unresponsive to symptomatic treatment
- Hematochezia
- Dyschezia
- Excess fecal mucus
- Change in feces shape
- Constipation
- Chronic vomiting

CONTRAINDICATIONS
- Coagulopathies if a biopsy is contemplated
- Megacolon with colonic muscular atrophy

POTENTIAL COMPLICATIONS
Colonic perforation

CLIENT EDUCATION
- Withhold food for 36–48 h before the procedure.
- Advise of risks of general anesthesia (flexible colonoscopy) and sedation (rigid colonoscopy).

BODY SYSTEMS ASSESSED
Gastrointestinal

 PROCEDURE

PATIENT PREPARATION
Preprocedure Medication or Preparation
- Multiple fecal examinations to rule out parasite infection (parasites associated with large-bowel diarrhea include hookworms, whipworms, *Giardia* and, in cats, *Tritrichomonas*)
- Fecal cytology for *Clostridium* spores or a test for clostridial enterotoxin
- Culture feces if pathogens are suspected (*Salmonella* or *Campylobacter* infection is rare)
- Fast dogs and cats for 36–48 h. Allow free water access.
- Careful digital rectal examination. Sedation or anesthesia is required for digital rectal examination in cats, and this is usually done immediately prior to the procedure.
- For rigid colonoscopy, patients can be prepared with multiple plain warm-water enemas until the effluent is clear. The use of soapy and hypertonic solutions should be avoided because they induce colonic hyperemia, which may mask colonic lesions. Phosphate enemas are contraindicated.
- Enemas are also desirable in flexible colonoscopy both prior to the administration of an oral colonic lavage solution and again the morning of the procedure until the effluent is clear.
- For flexible colonoscopy, the whole colon needs to be cleaned of fecal material by the oral administration of colonic lavage solutions, which cleanses the entire colon by causing an osmotic diarrhea.

- Commercially available solutions include polyethylene glycol plus electrolytes (e.g., GoLYTELY and Colyte). These are given via a gastric or nasoesophageal tube. The optimal dose is 80 mL/kg in 2 divided doses ≈2 h apart on the evening before the procedure.
- A dose of metoclopramide (0.5–1.0 mg/kg IM or SC) can be administered 30 min before administration of the colonic lavage solution to facilitate gastric emptying and reduce the risk of vomiting and aspiration pneumonia.
- Cats do not tolerate gastric intubation, and in this species the colonic lavage solution is better administered via a nasoesophageal tube. The dose is 80 mL/kg administered over a 4-h period. Metoclopramide is also indicated.
- The colonic lavage solution is administered again on the morning of the procedure ≈2 h before anesthesia is induced.
- Enemas may be contraindicated in patients with rectal disease, because the passage of the enema tube may be too painful. In these patients, administration of magnesium citrate solutions may be appropriate. These are hyperosmotic, however, and patients need to be well hydrated. The bottle should be opened and allowed to degas for at least 2 h before administration via stomach tube.

Anesthesia or Sedation
- Dogs undergoing rigid colonoscopy can sometimes be examined with only minimal restraint. The animal is held in the standing position by an assistant with 1 arm around the neck and another under and around the abdomen. Useful drugs include acepromazine (dogs or cats) and ketamine (cats).
- General anesthesia is required for flexible colonoscopy.
- Use of narcotic preanesthetic medications should be avoided because they initially stimulate aboral contractions of the small intestine that propel intestinal content into the proximal colon.

Patient Positioning
- For rigid colonoscopy, patients are either restrained in the standing position or kept in right lateral recumbency. This prevents any fluid from the proximal colon draining via gravity into the distal colon.
- For flexible colonoscopy, patients are placed in left lateral recumbency. This allows proximal colonic fluid to drain into the distal colon and facilitates examination of the proximal part of the organ.
- Patients can be placed on a tilt table with the head slightly lowered to prevent drainage of ileal or proximal colonic fluid during rigid endoscopy.

Patient Monitoring
- Routine anesthetic monitoring
- The plane of anesthesia may need to be deepened because air is insufflated into the proximal colon, and the colonoscope is maneuvered around the splenic and hepatic flexures into the proximal colon. Tension on colonic mesentery usually causes heart rate to increase.

Equipment or Supplies
Rigid Colonoscopy
- Stainless-steel human colonoscopes of a length and diameter appropriate for the patient
- Each colonoscope comes with an obturator that is used to facilitate insertion. Most colonoscopes have a cold-light supply.
- Rigid colonoscopes also come with a suction tube to remove fluid and debris, an insufflation bulb for air insufflation to distend the colon, and a pair of biopsy forceps. Biopsy forceps with an angled tip are best.
- The colonoscope has a hinged, but airtight, lens that is kept closed during air insufflation and advancement but that is opened to allow biopsy.

Flexible Colonoscopy
- Flexible endoscopes are of 2 types: (1) fiberoptic endoscopes or (2) video endoscopes, the latter containing a video chip at the end for transmitting video images.

- There are a variety of manufacturers of endoscopes for the veterinary market. Refurbished human fiberoptic endoscopes are also sometimes available.
- Most flexible endoscopes have a working length of 1 m and are marketed as gastroscopes. The outside diameter is critical for upper GI endoscopy, but less so for colonoscopy. Endoscopes with a working length 1 m and a diameter of 9.8 mm to 1.0 cm are appropriate for cats and dogs weighing up to 20–25 kg. For larger dogs, a colonoscope with a working length of 1.5 m is required. Some veterinary endoscopes combine a working length of 1.5 mm and a diameter of 9 mm, which is ideal.
- Given the choice, an endoscope with the largest biopsy channel should be selected. In most instruments, this is 2.8 mm.
- A selection of biopsy forceps is usually available. Forceps with elongated jaws are preferred and should have a serrated cutting edge.

TECHNIQUE
Rigid Colonoscopy
- A careful digital rectal examination is first performed. A thorough 360° palpation of the rectal mucosa is essential, as is lateral pressure, to test the pelvic diaphragm for weaknesses that may be associated with a rectal diverticulum or perineal hernia.
- The obturator is inserted into the endoscope and then well lubricated and passed blindly through the anus into the rectum.
- The obturator is removed and the window closed.
- The colonoscope is then advanced under direct observation through the window with air insufflation to distend the colon.
- Insufflation is continued until the colon is distended.
- The colonoscope should never be blindly advanced, and the tip should always be kept in the center of the lumen.
- The normal colonic mucosa should be pink, with submucosal vessels often visible under the surface. These vessels are an important criterion of normality.
- Air may escape through the anus during insufflation. If this prevents examination of the mucosa, an assistant should apply pressure around the area.
- Suction should be applied to remove liquid or debris. For this, the window has to be opened and the suction tube manually inserted. The window must be closed and air insufflated again before the instrument is advanced.
- The colonoscope should be advanced to its full length or to the splenic flexure, whichever comes first.
- Biopsy samples should be taken of any lesion or, if no lesion is visible, about every 5 cm. For this, the window is opened and the mucosa allowed to collapse. The biopsy instrument is inserted and the mucosa grasped gently. Gentle traction is then applied to tent the mucosa and stretch it away from the muscularis. The biopsy forceps are then firmly closed and the instrument withdrawn. The forceps should *never* be closed with forward pressure because this may cause colonic perforation. Mild bleeding is routine.
- Do not reinsufflate air after biopsy because that may rupture the colon.
- The colonoscope is withdrawn ≈5 cm and the process repeated. Multiple biopsy samples should always be taken, even of normal-appearing mucosa.

Flexible Colonoscopy
- The endoscope controls should be manipulated to ensure that there is 4-way deflection and that the air and water channels are functioning.
- The tip and first 15–20 cm of the endoscope are lubricated and the tip inserted into the rectum through the anus. Sometimes this can be facilitated, especially in brachycephalics, if it is inserted at the same time a gloved, lubricated finger is inserted into the rectum.
- Air is then insufflated and the endoscope advanced under direct observation.

- In general, biopsy samples should be taken as the instrument is withdrawn. It is preferable sometimes, however, to biopsy specific lesions as the instrument is advanced, because repeated movements of the endoscope may cause artifact. Biopsy specimens should be taken from the ascending, transverse, and descending colon. Biopsy is facilitated if the mucosa is partially collapsed. A minimum of 10–15 biopsy samples should be taken. Diagnosis is facilitated in tumors if a deep biopsy is taken. This means that the biopsy should be repeated at the same site to obtain a deeper sample.
- The canine colon and the feline colon are in the rough shape of a question mark, with 2 distinct bends encountered as the endoscope is advanced. The first is the splenic flexure where the descending colon transitions into the transverse colon. The second is the hepatic flexure, where the transverse colon transitions into the ascending colon.
- Passage of the endoscope past the 2 flexures requires knowledge of colonic anatomy and the confidence to advance the tip of the endoscope blindly around the bend as it is advanced and air is insufflated. The colonic mucosa will cover the tip for a short distance (1–3 cm) as it is advanced, causing a red out. If this persists, the endoscope should be withdrawn slightly and the process repeated.
- The transverse colon is short in cats, and both flexures may be passed simultaneously.
- The proximal (ascending) colon contains a slight protuberance with a central depression, the ileocolonic sphincter. Adjacent to this is an opening into the blind pouch of the cecum. This may be entered inadvertently without the sphincter being seen. If this occurs and the endoscope cannot be advanced, then it should be withdrawn a few centimeters and the process repeated.
- If appropriate, biopsy forceps can be passed through the ileocolonic sphincter and the ileum blindly biopsied. In a small percentage of patients, the endoscope can be passed through the sphincter and the distal ileum can be directly examined.
- Rectal lesions can sometimes be evaluated more effectively if the colonoscope is retroflexed and the lesion viewed from above. This maneuver is possible only in dogs weighing more than ≈15 kg. The biopsy forceps should be passed through the endoscope before the endoscope is retroflexed.

SAMPLE HANDLING
- Retrieve the sample from the jaws of the biopsy forceps with a 25-gauge needle and place the sample on a piece of filter paper or on a sponge in a histopathology cassette. The mucosal side should be uppermost. This can be accomplished by manipulation with an additional needle.
- Place the sample in formalin and label appropriately for the pathologist.

APPROPRIATE AFTERCARE
Postprocedure Patient Monitoring
Clients should be warned that the first feces passed after endoscopy may contain small amounts of blood.

Nursing Care
None

Dietary Modification
None

Medication Requirements
If the colon is markedly inflamed, symptomatic treatment with sulfasalazine can be initiated (25–40 mg/kg every 8 h in dogs and 20 mg/kg every 12 h in cats) for 5–7 days or until the biopsy report is received.

Restrictions on Activity
None

Anticipated Recovery Time
- Patients may be released to the owner the same day.
- 12–24 h

COLONOSCOPY

INTERPRETATION

NORMAL FINDINGS OR RANGE

Under the normal colonic mucosa, which is reddish pink, may be seen the submucosal blood vessels, an important criterion of normality. The mucosa is quite resilient and does not bleed when rubbed. The colon will exhibit longitudinal folds, which disappear with air insufflation. Occasional circular propagating or segmental contractions will be noticed.

ABNORMAL VALUES

Any deviation from the foregoing is abnormal. A longitudinal area of hyperemia 10–20 cm from the anus may indicate overvigorous enema tube insertion. Inflamed mucosa may bleed when rubbed with the tip of the endoscope. Other abnormalities include masses (usually polyps), strictures (e.g., adenocarcinoma or scar tissue), ulceration, and parasites (e.g., *Trichuris* spp.).

CRITICAL VALUES

Distention of the abdomen with air suggests colonic perforation. Abdominal radiographs confirm it. These patients need immediate exploratory laparotomy.

INTERFERING FACTORS

Drugs That May Alter Results of the Procedure
- Soapy water enemas induce colonic hyperemia and mucosal artifact.
- Phosphate enemas damage the colon and cause hyperphosphatemia.

Conditions That May Interfere with Performing the Procedure
- Megacolon with colonic muscle atrophy
- Colonic stricture

Procedure Techniques or Handling That May Alter Results
None

Influence of Signalment on Performing and Interpreting the Procedure

Species
None

Breed
- The boxer breed may have histiocytic ulcerative colitis. This is enrofloxacin responsive.
- German shepherds are predisposed to rectal adenocarcinoma.

Age
Suspect adenocarcinoma in old dogs with rectal stricture.

Gender
None

Pregnancy
None

CLINICAL PERSPECTIVE

- The most important aspect of colonoscopy is to obtain multiple biopsy samples and to work with a good pathologist. Read the biopsy report and treat the patient accordingly.
- Some patients with large-bowel diarrhea may respond to dietary manipulation alone.
- Colonic or rectal strictures may be caused by either chronic inflammation or a tumor. If the rectum is fixed and rigid at rectal examination and cannot be moved from side to side, then the dog is more likely to have a rectal adenocarcinoma.
- Rectal strictures can be treated by balloon dilation and anti-inflammatory drugs (e.g., sulfasalazine).
- Skill levels can be enhanced if the veterinarian takes an endoscopy course.
- Equipment life can be preserved if the proper cleaning and storage techniques are used.

MISCELLANEOUS

ANCILLARY TESTS
Colonic biopsy

SYNONYMS
None

SEE ALSO
Blackwell's Five-Minute Veterinary Consult: Canine and Feline Topics
- Colitis and Proctitis
- Colitis, Histiocytic Ulcerative

Related Topics in This Book
General Principles of Endoscopy

ABBREVIATIONS
None

Suggested Reading
Richter K. Endoscopic evaluation of the colon. In: McCarthy TC, ed. *Veterinary Endoscopy for the Small Animal Practitioner*. St Louis: Saunders Elsevier, 2005: 323–356.
Willard M. Colonoscopy. In: Tams TR, ed. *Small Animal Endoscopy*. St Louis: CV Mosby, 1999: 217–245.

INTERNET RESOURCES
None

AUTHOR NAME
Colin F. Burrows

BASICS

TYPE OF SPECIMEN
Blood

TEST EXPLANATION AND RELATED PHYSIOLOGY
A CBC includes a battery of hematology tests that provide a large amount of information about the peripheral blood. This is a relatively inexpensive, readily obtained screening test that can provide evidence of inflammation, anemia, a coagulopathy, or hematopoietic neoplasia. Many of the tests are performed by an automated hematology analyzer, with additional information provided through microscopic evaluation of a blood smear (see the "Blood Smear Microscopic Examination" chapter). Components of a CBC are discussed separately (see specific chapters for details) and include the following:

1. RBC count and RBC morphologic features
2. WBC count, leukocyte differential count, and WBC morphologic features
3. Neutrophil and band counts
4. Lymphocyte count
5. Monocyte count
6. Eosinophil count
7. Basophil count
8. Hemoglobin concentration
9. Hematocrit (or PCV)
10. RBC indices (MCH, MCHC, and MCV)
11. Platelet count and/or estimate

Several types of hematology instruments, specifically designed for analysis of veterinary samples, are now commercially available. These instruments provide rapid, accurate results and are less labor intensive than manual methods. The simplest models provide only cell counts (RBC, WBC, and platelets), whereas more expensive instruments provide more information, including a partial or complete differential count, identifying and quantifying the different leukocytes.

Most analyzers designed for in-office use rely on impedance technology. They count cells as the cells are drawn between a pair of electrodes. Because cells are poor electrical conductors, they introduce resistance as they pass through the electrical field, each producing a voltage pulse proportional to their size. Cell types are distinguished from one another primarily by their size differences. RBCs are lysed before WBCs are counted. The blood hemoglobin concentration is determined spectrophotometrically.

The quantitative buffy coat (QBC) Vet Autoread (IDEXX Laboratories, Westbrook, ME) uses density-gradient centrifugation to separate and count cells (QBC analysis). Variable cell density causes blood cells to sort into individual layers when blood is spun in a hematocrit tube. A molded cylindrical float is used to expand the WBC and platelet layers of the buffy coat, and acridine orange, coating the tube, stains nucleoproteins, lipoproteins, glycosamines, and other cellular substances. These cellular components fluoresce when subjected to ultraviolet light, and the variable degree of fluorescence is used to distinguish cellular subtypes further. The width of the different buffy coat layers is measured in a special electro-optical analyzer that measures the fluorescence emitted by the cells in the tube. The width of each band correlates with the number of each cell type. Hematocrit, platelet mass, total leukocyte count, and the counts of the neutrophil, eosinophil, and lymphocyte/monocyte subpopulations are automatically computed.

Several more sophisticated instruments rely on laser-based flow cytometer, using differences in light scatter to identify, count, and size cells. Some of these analyzers further incorporate peroxidase staining of RBC hemoglobin and leukocyte granules to aid in cell identification.

With all hematology analyzers, microscopic blood smear evaluation is recommended as a cross-check to verify the accuracy of the WBC and platelet counts generated by the analyzer, to verify a differential count, and to rule out the presence of platelet clumps. Automated instruments differ in their capability of performing differential cell counts, but even the most expensive analyzer generally cannot identify abnormal cell types such as immature granulocytes (bands), neoplastic blasts, and mast cells. Nucleated RBCs will often be included in the total leukocyte counts. A microscopic exam is also needed to identity additional important abnormalities such the spherocytosis or Heinz bodies or the presence of blasts, mast cells, microfilariae, or RBC parasites.

INDICATIONS
- Part of a general workup of any sick patient
- Part of a prophylactic screen of any geriatric patient

CONTRAINDICATIONS
None

POTENTIAL COMPLICATIONS
None

CLIENT EDUCATION
None

BODY SYSTEMS ASSESSED
Hemic, lymphatic, and immune

SAMPLE

COLLECTION
1–3 mL of venous blood

HANDLING
EDTA is the anticoagulant of choice.

STORAGE
- Refrigeration is recommended for short-term storage of blood.
- Stained smears should be protected from light.

STABILITY
- Whole blood
  - Several hours at room temperature
  - Refrigerated (2°–8°C): 1–2 days
- Stained smears are stable for many years, especially when protected from light and humidity.

LIMITATIONS OF THE TEST
Valid If Run in Human Lab?
Yes—if validated instrumentation is used, and trained personnel look at the animal blood smears.

MISCELLANEOUS

SYNONYMS
- CBC
- CBC and Diff

ABBREVIATIONS
QBC = quantitative buffy coat

Suggested Reading
Knoll JS. Clinical Automated Hematology Systems. In: Feldman BF, Zinkl JG, Jain NC, eds. *Schalm's Veterinary Hematology*, 5th ed. Ames, IA: Blackwell, 2001: 3–11.
Weiss DJ. Application of flow cytometric techniques to veterinary clinical hematology. *Vet Clin Pathol* 2002; **31**: 72–82.

INTERNET RESOURCES
Tvedten H. Diagnostic power of graphical reports from hematology analyzers. In: Proceedings of the 26th Congress of the World Small Animal Veterinary Association, Vancouver, 2001, http://www.vin.com/VINDBPub/SearchPB/Proceedings/PR05000/PR00041.htm.

AUTHOR NAME
Joyce S. Knoll

COMPUTED TOMOGRAPHY

BASICS

TYPE OF PROCEDURE
Radiographic

PROCEDURE EXPLANATION AND RELATED PHYSIOLOGY
CT and MRI are competitive and complementary imaging modalities that produce cross-sectional images of the patient that may be used to make a diagnosis or plan surgery. Whereas MRI is preferable because of its superior soft tissue contrast (i.e., ability to differentiate different tissue types), CT is preferable for evaluating some bone lesions, in situations when shorter imaging time is desirable (e.g., trauma evaluation), or when a sensitive test for gas, hemorrhage, or intracranial calcification is needed. Some common clinical CT examinations are sinonasal, temporal (ear) region, myelography, thoracic, abdominal, and elbow.

INDICATIONS
• CT is used extensively for planning radiation therapy.
• CT is used to guide biopsies.

CONTRAINDICATIONS
None, unless there are medical contraindications for general anesthesia

POTENTIAL COMPLICATIONS
Adverse reaction to contrast medium

CLIENT EDUCATION
General anesthesia will be required.

BODY SYSTEMS ASSESSED
All

PROCEDURE

PATIENT PREPARATION
Preprocedure Medication or Preparation
As for general anesthesia

Anesthesia or Sedation
• General anesthesia is required unless the patient is comatose.
• Sedation may be adequate only with some of the newer (faster) CT scanners.

Patient Positioning
Variable

Patient Monitoring
As for general anesthesia

Equipment or Supplies
• Appropriate contrast media if needed for study
• CT scanner and associated equipment

TECHNIQUE
• The patient is anesthetized or otherwise restrained.
• Images are made as is appropriate for the individual scanner and particular study.
• IV contrast is administered if indicated for individual study.

SAMPLE HANDLING
Images currently may be printed or stored digitally.

APPROPRIATE AFTERCARE
Postprocedure Patient Monitoring
As for general anesthesia

Nursing Care
None

Dietary Modification
None

Medication Requirements
None

Restrictions on Activity
None

Anticipated Recovery Time
As for general anesthesia

INTERPRETATION

NORMAL FINDINGS OR RANGE
The goals of the examination and the technique used to obtain images vary with the type of animal, suspected disease, and equipment. It is more effective not to consider CT as a global imaging method but rather as many individual types of examination (e.g., sinonasal CT, thoracic CT). Normal findings relate to the normal anatomic appearance of the various structures, and normal variability for breed, age, and image display (windows) need to be considered.

ABNORMAL VALUES
• For sinonasal CT, there are 3 common patterns: (1) destructive sinorhinopathy with mass effect, (2) destructive sinorhinopathy without mass effect, and (3) nondestructive sinorhinopathy. The term *destructive* refers to the presence of bone lysis. In pattern 1, the lysis often applies to the facial bones, and in pattern 2 the lysis frequently applies to the nasal conchae. In dogs, CT pattern 1 most likely is caused by nasal carcinoma, pattern 2 most likely is caused by aspergillosis, and pattern 3 is nonspecific (e.g., allergic, immune-mediated, infectious rhinitis or sinusitis, or a foreign body). More definitive tests (e.g., histology) often are performed to confirm the CT diagnosis. In cats, *Cryptococcus* should be added to the differential list for pattern 1, and lymphoma should be added for patterns 1 and 3. CT also may be used to evaluate the extent of other facial (nonnasal) tumors and dental disease.
• For temporal region CT, a major goal is to determine the extent of the disease: Does the disease extend into the middle or inner ear, does the lesion involve only the tympanic cavity or also the tympanic bulla (bulla osteitis), is the cause of vestibular signs central or peripheral, what are the boundaries of a mass, and does a polyp extend into the nasopharynx? Some abnormal signs include increased fluid or soft tissue within normal gas-filled structures, soft tissue mass, soft tissue mineralization, bone lysis, and increased thickness of the tympanic bulla.
• For CT myelography, distortion, thinning, and displacement of the ring of contrast material may be detected in compressive spinal cord disease. CT also is more sensitive than radiography for detecting bone lysis, or malformation or fracture of the articular processes. CT may be used for surgical planning to determine the site, including side, and extent of the lesion.
• Thoracic or abdominal CT is performed when further evaluation of a lesion is needed such that there is no superimposition of structures as during radiography. Cross-sectional imaging is useful for differentiating the extent of lesions and planning surgery (e.g., defining whether a mass encircles or erodes into the caudal vena cava). CT also is more sensitive for detecting certain lesions such as pulmonary nodules or bone lysis. IV or oral contrast studies also may be performed.
• Musculoskeletal CT is used because of improved imaging of certain structures (e.g., medial coronoid process), better contrast resolution (ability to differentiate tissue types), and cross-sectional imaging (no superimposition of structures). Also, CT may be more sensitive than radiography for small, nondisplaced fractures. Radiography, however, has better spatial resolution (ability to differentiate adjacent structures as different structures). Because of its high sensitivity for intracranial hemorrhage and short scanning time, CT is especially useful for evaluating acute head trauma.

CRITICAL VALUES
None

INTERFERING FACTORS
Drugs That May Alter Results of the Procedure
None

Conditions That May Interfere with Performing the Procedure
• Patients must remain still; otherwise motion artifact will adversely affect image quality.
• Since patients must remain still during the examination, any situation that would preclude general anesthesia or sedation (unless a patient is comatose) may interfere with performing CT.
• Metal implants or foreign bodies may cause substantial artifact that destroys image quality.
• If the patient is known to have had an adverse reaction to contrast medium, then contrast studies should be avoided unless necessary.

Procedure Techniques or Handling That May Alter Results
• Once the image is obtained, the window and level may be adjusted to preferentially display certain tissues. It often is helpful to look at images in multiple windows to obtain the maximum information.
• Inappropriate acquisition parameters may hinder critical evaluation of structures.

Influence of Signalment on Performing and Interpreting the Procedure
Species
None

Breed
The range of normal anatomic variation is vast.

Age
None

Gender
None

Pregnancy
The veterinarian might want to consider the necessity of exposing fetuses to ionizing radiation.

CLINICAL PERSPECTIVE
None

 MISCELLANEOUS

ANCILLARY TESTS
None

SYNONYMS
• CAT (computed axial tomography) scan
• CT scan

SEE ALSO
Blackwell's Five-Minute Veterinary Consult: Canine and Feline Topics
• Aspergillosis
• Elbow Dysplasia
• Intervertebral Disc Disease, Cervical
• Intervertebral Disc Disease, Thoracolumbar
• Nasal and Nasopharyngeal Polyps
• Rhinitis and Sinusitis
• Squamous Cell Carcinoma, Nasal and Paranasal Sinuses

Related Topics in This Book
General Principles of Radiography

ABBREVIATIONS
• CT = computed tomography
• MRI = magnetic resonance imaging

Suggested Reading
None

INTERNET RESOURCES
ACR RSNA (American College of Radiology and Radiological Society of North America), RadiologyInfo: Computed tomography (CT)—body, http://www.radiologyinfo.org/en/info.cfm?pg=bodyct&bhcp=1.
eMedicineHealth: CT scan, http://www.emedicinehealth.com/ct_scan article_em.htm.
NetDoctor.co.uk: CT scan, http://www.netdoctor.co.uk/health_advice/examinations/ctgeneral.htm.

AUTHOR NAME
Peter V. Scrivani

CONJUNCTIVAL SCRAPING AND CYTOLOGY

BASICS

TYPE OF PROCEDURE
Diagnostic sample collection

PROCEDURE EXPLANATION AND RELATED PHYSIOLOGY
The conjunctiva is the highly vascularized mucous membrane that covers the inner aspect of the eyelids (palpebral conjunctiva), the anterior aspect of the sclera (bulbar conjunctiva), and the entire third eyelid. The portions of the conjunctiva meet at the fornices, where the conjunctiva adheres loosely to the underlying tissue. Nonkeratinized, stratified squamous epithelium constitutes the surface of the conjunctiva, with the substantia propria consisting of vessels, nerves, loosely arranged connective tissue, and cellular components (e.g., immune cells, goblet cells). The functional anatomy and composition of the conjunctiva physically protect the globe, as well as enable free movement, provide immunologic protection, and produce the mucin layer of the tear film.

Diseases of the conjunctiva rapidly cause chemosis (associated with the extensive vascular supply), hyperemia, and ocular discharge. Chronicity may result in epithelial keratinization, as well as chronic mucoid to mucopurulent discharge. Disease processes may include infectious conjunctivitis (bacterial, viral, fungal, rickettsial, or parasitic), noninfectious conjunctivitis (allergic, follicular hyperplasia, or secondary to keratoconjunctivitis sicca), traumatic injury, neoplasia, and nonneoplastic mass infiltration (granuloma, cyst, or associated with episcleritis).

Scraping the conjunctival surface to obtain cells and microorganisms enables cytologic analysis, as well as culture and IFA assay. Appropriate, and possibly multiple, stains may therefore be necessary for thorough assessment; biopsy may also be indicated.

INDICATIONS
- Ocular discharge (mucoid, purulent)
- Ocular redness
- Ocular pain (blepharospasm, rubbing)
- Conjunctival mass or hyperplasia

CONTRAINDICATIONS
The presence of significant corneal disease, which may lead to rupture of the globe due to manipulation during the scraping procedure

POTENTIAL COMPLICATIONS
- Self-limiting blood-tinged ocular discharge
- Mild ocular discomfort

CLIENT EDUCATION
None

BODY SYSTEMS ASSESSED
Ophthalmic

PROCEDURE

PATIENT PREPARATION
Preprocedure Medication or Preparation
Rinse the ocular surface to remove debris or discharge.

Anesthesia or Sedation
- Topical anesthetic may be used if necessary, but is generally not necessary.
- Sedation generally is not necessary.

Patient Positioning
Sternal recumbency, sitting, or standing

Patient Monitoring
None

Equipment or Supplies
- A Kimura spatula or Bard-Parker scalpel blade
- Glass slides
- Appropriate stains for cytology (e.g., Wright-Giemsa, modified Wright-Giemsa, Gram)

TECHNIQUE
- After flushing of the ocular surface with eye wash, open the eyelids to expose the portion of conjunctiva to be sampled. If the entire conjunctival surface is involved, scraping is most easily performed on the lower eyelid; if a focal area is involved, obtain a sample from that area.
- The edge of the sterile Kimura spatula or the blunt edge of the scalpel blade (the edge of which would be situated closest to the scalpel blade handle) is scraped across the conjunctiva multiple times in the same direction until a small drop of fluid and cells accumulates on the edge of the instrument.
- Transfer the drop to a glass slide and gently spreading the drop around the slide to create a thin film.
- Repeat sample collection and place the samples on additional slides.

SAMPLE HANDLING
- Allow the samples to dry on the slides prior to staining.
- Stain the slides with the appropriate stain (e.g., modified Wright-Giemsa for quick, general screening; Gram stain for detection of bacteria).
- Leave 1–2 slides unstained to allow for further staining or submission to a laboratory, if necessary.

APPROPRIATE AFTERCARE
Postprocedure Patient Monitoring
None

Nursing Care
None

Dietary Modification
None

Medication Requirements
As indicated by results of cytology

Restrictions on Activity
None

Anticipated Recovery Time
Normal ocular comfort and appearance immediately to within 1 day

INTERPRETATION

NORMAL FINDINGS OR RANGE
- Sheets of nonkeratinized epithelial cells with large, round, homogeneous nuclei and abundant cytoplasm, possibly with melanin granules
- Small numbers of bacteria may be present.
- WBCs are rare.

ABNORMAL VALUES
- Neutrophils with or without intracellular bacteria may indicate bacterial or viral conjunctivitis.
- Eosinophils may indicate hypersensitivity disorder, parasitic infestation, or eosinophilic conjunctivitis/keratoconjunctivitis.
- Lymphocytes, plasma cells, or both may indicate reactive hyperplasia, allergic, or chronic conjunctivitis.
- An abnormal cell population (other than nonkeratinized epithelial cells) with or without mitotic figures may indicate neoplastic infiltration.

CRITICAL VALUES
Expect to find nonkeratinized epithelial cells in sheets with consistent cellular morphology, as well as small numbers of bacteria.

INTERFERING FACTORS
Drugs That May Alter Results of the Procedure
None

Conditions That May Interfere with Performing the Procedure
Significant corneal disease may result in rupture of globe if excessive pressure is applied to the conjunctival surface.

Procedure Techniques or Handling That May Alter Results
Inappropriate stains may not enable detection of specific cell types or microorganisms.

Influence of Signalment on Performing and Interpreting the Procedure
Species
- Certain infectious agents are more common in individual species (e.g., herpesvirus in cats, distemper virus in dogs).
- Neoplasia is rare in dogs and cats.
- Eosinophilic conjunctivitis or keratoconjunctivitis may be a distinct clinical entity in cats, whereas detection of eosinophils in dogs may indicate allergic disease.

Breed
None

Age
Puppies and kittens frequently experience infectious conjunctivitis (e.g., herpesvirus or *Chlamydophila* in cats, *Staphylococcus* in dogs).

Gender
None

Pregnancy
None

CLINICAL PERSPECTIVE
- Conjunctival scraping is indicated in cases of conjunctivitis that are nonresponsive to previous therapy (antibiotics, anti-inflammatory agents).

- Cytology should be performed in conjunction with culture, as well as possibly IFA assay or biopsies.
- Interpretation of results should be based on thorough assessment of multiple stained slides, as well as on the clinical presentation of the patient.

MISCELLANEOUS

ANCILLARY TESTS
- Conjunctival biopsy
- Conjunctival culture
- Fluorescein dye test
- Schirmer tear test

SYNONYMS
None

SEE ALSO
Blackwell's Five-Minute Veterinary Consult: Canine and Feline Topics
- Conjunctivitis—Cats
- Conjunctivitis—Dogs

Related Topics in This Book
- Fluorescein Dye Test
- Schirmer Tear Test

ABBREVIATIONS
None

Suggested Reading
Gelatt KN, ed. *Veterinary Ophthalmology*, 3rd ed. Philadelphia: Lippincott Williams & Wilkins, 1999.

INTERNET RESOURCES
None

AUTHOR NAME
Alison Clode

BASICS

TYPE OF SPECIMEN
Blood

TEST EXPLANATION AND RELATED PHYSIOLOGY
The Coombs' test detects erythrocyte surface antigen–associated antibody and/or complement and is most often used to aid in the diagnosis of IMHA. Antibody and/or complement may be bound to antigens on RBC membranes because of primary (idiopathic) or secondary causes (e.g., drug exposures, infections, neoplasia, and other immune disorders) of IMHA. The test is performed by first washing the patient's erythrocytes with phosphate-buffered saline to remove any unbound proteins. Dilutions of species-specific antiglobulin (e.g., goat anti–canine Ig) are then added to the patient's washed RBCs. Some laboratories use a single polyvalent antiserum containing multiple types of antiglobulin (e.g., goat anti–canine IgG, IgM, and complement component 3), whereas others use multiple isotypes of monovalent antisera, each containing only a single antiglobulin type. Erythrocytes and antisera are allowed to incubate, and then samples are assessed for agglutination. If sufficient amounts of antibody and/or complement are present on RBCs, these structures will be cross-linked by species-specific antiglobulin, causing agglutination.

INDICATIONS
- Suspected cases of IMHA
- Anemia of unknown etiology (regenerative or nonregenerative)

CONTRAINDICATIONS
Autoagglutination: If suspected, this should be confirmed by a direct saline agglutination test. If true autoagglutination exists (rather than rouleaux), then RBC clumps will fail to disperse when the sample is mixed with saline, and a Coombs' test is not indicated. Both *auto*agglutination and agglutination in a Coombs' test result from cross-linking of antibody adherent to RBC membranes; therefore, autoagglutination provides the same information as a positive Coombs' test.

POTENTIAL COMPLICATIONS
None

CLIENT EDUCATION
A negative Coombs' test result does not rule out the possibility of IMHA.

BODY SYSTEMS ASSESSED
Hemic, lymphatic, and immune

SAMPLE

COLLECTION
1 mL of venous blood

HANDLING
Collect the sample into an EDTA tube and transport it on ice packs.

STORAGE
Refrigerate the sample until it is shipped.

STABILITY
Analyze the sample within 1 day for the most accurate results.

PROTOCOL
None

INTERPRETATION

NORMAL FINDINGS OR RANGE
Negative (no agglutination)

ABNORMAL VALUES
Any agglutination is considered abnormal and constitutes a positive result.

CRITICAL VALUES
None

INTERFERING FACTORS
Drugs That May Alter Results or Interpretation
Drugs That Interfere with Test Methodology
None

Drugs That Alter Physiology
Previous immunosuppressive therapy may lead to false-negative results because of decreased antibody and complement binding to RBCs and ultimately decreased antibody production.

Disorders That May Alter Results
None

Collection Techniques or Handling That May Alter Results
- Clotted samples, or samples collected in anticoagulants other than EDTA, may produce false-positive Coombs' test results.
- Excessive delay before processing may cause false-negative results.

Influence of Signalment
Species
- Dogs: IMHA is the most common cause of hemolytic anemia.
- Cats: IMHA can occur but is less common.

Breed
A higher incidence of IMHA has been reported in cocker spaniels, Old English sheepdogs, English springer spaniels, poodles, and miniature schnauzers.

Age
Middle-aged dogs are typically most affected by IMHA.

Gender
Studies suggest a higher incidence of IMHA in female dogs.

Pregnancy
None

LIMITATIONS OF THE TEST
Sensitivity, Specificity, and Positive and Negative Predictive Values
Reported sensitivity values vary, but many are around 67%.
Valid If Run in a Human Lab?
No. Reagents are species specific (e.g., goat anti–canine Ig).

Causes of Abnormal Findings

Positive test results	Negative test results
IMHA (primary or secondary to foreign antigen) Previous blood transfusion Collection of blood in anticoagulant other than EDTA	Absence of IMHA Previous immunosuppressive therapy Low numbers of RBC surface antigen–associated antibody and/or complement Inadequate dilutions of antiglobulin (prozone effect) Elution of erythrocyte surface antigen–associated antibody or complement during cell washing or from excessive delay before testing Use of inappropriate reagents (reagents are species specific) Reagents that do not contain all antibody isotypes

CLINICAL PERSPECTIVE

• Because of the test's relatively low sensitivity, negative Coombs' test results are common in patients that present and progress like IMHA cases.
• Interpret a positive Coombs' test result with caution in the absence of other supporting evidence for IMHA.
• IMHA is best diagnosed based on a combination of laboratory data (i.e., CBC, Coombs' test, serum chemistry evaluation, and urinalysis) along with physical exam and history.
• Many labs report Coombs' test results as either positive or negative, but some report a titer for positive results. Titers, however, do not correlate with the severity of disease (i.e., higher titers are not necessarily associated with more severe disease).
• Coombs' tests performed at 4°C are controversial and often overused and overinterpreted. Healthy/normal animals may have cold-reacting autoagglutinins. In animals with suspected cold agglutinin disease, a positive Coombs' test is more clinically significant if the test was performed at room temperature than if run at 4°C since these extremely low temperatures are not seen physiologically. While the extremities can become colder than core body temperature, they never achieve temperatures as low as 4°C.

MISCELLANEOUS

ANCILLARY TESTS
• The direct saline agglutination test is used to rule out rouleaux and confirm autoagglutination caused by RBC surface antigen–associated antibody and/or complement.
• CBC: Marked spherocytosis suggests the presence of RBC surface antigen–associated antibody and/or complement even without a positive Coombs' test result.

SYNONYMS
• Direct antiglobulin test (DAT)
• Direct Coombs' test

SEE ALSO
Blackwell's Five-Minute Veterinary Consult: Canine and Feline Topics
• Anemia, Aplastic
• Anemia, Immune-Mediated
• Anemia, Nonregenerative
• Anemia, Regenerative
Related Topics in This Book
• Hematocrit
• Red Blood Cell Count
• Red Blood Cell Morphology

ABBREVIATIONS
• Ig = immunoglobulin
• IMHA = immune-mediated hemolytic anemia

Suggested Reading
Ettinger SJ, Feldman EC. *Textbook of Veterinary Internal Medicine: Diseases of the Dog and Cat, vol 2*, 6th ed. St Louis: Saunders Elsevier, 2005: 1899–1900.
Feldman BF, Zinkl JG, Jain NC. *Schalm's Veterinary Hematology*, 5th ed. Philadelphia: Lippincott Williams & Wilkins, 2000: 172–174.
Lassen D, Weiser G. Laboratory technology for veterinary medicine. In: Thrall MA, ed. *Veterinary Hematology and Clinical Chemistry*. Philadelphia: Lippincott Williams & Wilkins, 2004: 20–21.

INTERNET RESOURCES
None

AUTHOR NAME
Jed Overmann

CORTISOL

BASICS

TYPE OF SPECIMEN
Blood

TEST EXPLANATION AND RELATED PHYSIOLOGY
Cortisol is the major glucocorticoid secreted by the adrenal cortex. Most plasma cortisol is bound to plasma proteins. About 10% of circulating cortisol is free and metabolically active. This hormone affects metabolism of carbohydrates, proteins, and lipids, stimulating gluconeogenesis and causing a peripheral insulin resistance, inhibiting glucose transport into cells. It also has anti-inflammatory effects, in part because of effects on circulating leukocytes.

Cortisol secretion is controlled by classic negative feedback loops. Cortisol is secreted in response to ACTH from the anterior pituitary. ACTH secretion itself is controlled by the hypothalamic peptide corticotropin-releasing hormone. Rising levels of blood cortisol inhibit corticotropin-releasing hormone secretion from the hypothalamus, decreasing ACTH secretion, which, in turn, shuts off adrenal cortisol secretion. The result is pulsatile secretion of cortisol. The episodic release of cortisol results in an extremely broad reference range, and animals with both hyperadrenocorticism and hypoadrenocorticism often have cortisol levels that fall within the normal range. In addition, basal cortisol levels can be elevated by stress of transport, hospitalization, phlebotomy, or by severe acute or chronic illness.

Basal cortisol levels provide limited information regarding adreno-cortical function. However, cortisol is measured as part of a variety of stimulation and suppression tests that provide information regarding adrenocortical function in suspected cases of hyperadrenocorticism and hypoadrenocorticism.

INDICATIONS
Part of
- ACTH stimulation test
- Low-dose dexamethasone suppression test
- High-dose dexamethasone suppression test

CONTRAINDICATIONS
None

POTENTIAL COMPLICATIONS
None

CLIENT EDUCATION
- Basal levels of cortisol alone provide limited information regarding adrenocortical function.
- Atypical hyperadrenocorticism may require measurement of other steroid hormones.
- Samples collected after a 12-h fast are preferred.

BODY SYSTEMS ASSESSED
Endocrine and metabolic

SAMPLE

COLLECTION
1–2 mL of venous blood

HANDLING
- Choice of the collection tube depends on the assay: Some labs use serum (red-top tube), whereas others use plasma (EDTA or heparin). Check with the lab before submitting the sample.
- Centrifuge and separate the serum or plasma from the blood cells within 1 h.
- Remove the serum or plasma and store it in a transport tube (not in a serum-separator tube).
- Refrigerate or freeze the serum or plasma and transport it with cold packs in an insulated container.

STORAGE
Refrigerate the sample for short-term storage but freeze it for long-term storage.

STABILITY
- Refrigerated (2°–8°C): 5 days
- Frozen (−20°C): up to 2 months

PROTOCOL
None

INTERPRETATION

NORMAL FINDINGS OR RANGE
- Dogs: 0.6–6.0 µg/dL (16.6–166.0 nmol/L)
- Cats: 0.6–5.0 µg/dL (16.6–138.0 nmol/L)
- Reference intervals may vary, depending on the laboratory and assay.

ABNORMAL VALUES
Values above or below the reference range

CRITICAL VALUES
None

INTERFERING FACTORS
Drugs That May Alter Results or Interpretation
Drugs That Interfere with Test Methodology
- Prednisone or prednisolone (or structurally related steroids) will cross-react in the cortisol assay, falsely elevating the results.
- Dexamethasone does not interfere with the cortisol assay.

Drugs That Alter Physiology
- The blood cortisol concentration is decreased by anticonvulsant therapy, which can increase the liver metabolism of cortisol.
- Chronic glucocorticoid therapy can cause adrenal atrophy and subsequently a decreased cortisol level.
- Cortisol concentration is decreased by the administration of progestins such as megestrol acetate.
- Estrogen can increase the plasma cortisol level by increasing protein binding.

Disorders That May Alter Results
- Stress and nonadrenal illness

Collection Techniques or Handling That May Alter Results
- Nonfasting sample: grossly lipemic
- Delayed separation of serum: excessive hemolysis
- Storage in a serum-separator tube
- Inappropriate use of anticoagulant (assay dependent)

Influence of Signalment
Species
None

Breed
None

Age
None

Gender
None

Pregnancy
Cortisol levels are elevated during pregnancy.

LIMITATIONS OF THE TEST
Basal levels alone provide limited information about adrenocortical function.

Sensitivity, Specificity, and Positive and Negative Predictive Values
N/A

Valid If Run in a Human Lab?
No. The test should be validated for dogs and cats.

Causes of Abnormal Findings

High values	Low values
Hyperadrenocorticism	Hypoadrenocorticism
Stress	Iatrogenic hyperadrenocorticism
Nonadrenal illness	Improper handling and/or storage
Drugs: prednisone, prednisolone, or other related steroids	Progestins
Elevated estrogen/estrus	
Improper handling and/or storage	

CLINICAL PERSPECTIVE
- Adrenocortical function tests (i.e., ACTH stimulation or dexamethasone suppression tests) are required for definitive diagnosis of hyperadrenocorticism.
  - Dogs with hyperadrenocorticism often have basal cortisol levels that fall within the reference interval.
  - Stress and nonadrenal illness can elevate basal cortisol levels.
- When screening for hypoadrenocorticism
  - A cortisol value of <1 μg/dL in dogs with suspected Addison's disease can be definitive if clinical signs are supportive.
  - A cortisol value of >5 μg/dL excludes a diagnosis of hypoadrenocorticism.
  - Cortisol values of >1 μg/dL and <5 μg/dL are inconclusive.

MISCELLANEOUS

ANCILLARY TESTS
None

SYNONYMS
None

SEE ALSO
Blackwell's Five-Minute Veterinary Consult: Canine and Feline Topics
- Hyperadrenocorticism (Cushing's Disease)—Cats
- Hyperadrenocorticism (Cushing's Disease)—Dogs
- Hypoadrenocorticism (Addison's Disease)

Related Topics in This Book
- ACTH Stimulation Test
- Cortisol/Creatinine Ratio
- High-Dose Dexamethasone Suppression Test
- Low-Dose Dexamethasone Suppression Test

ABBREVIATIONS
ACTH = adrenocorticotropic hormone

Suggested Reading
Feldman EC, Nelson RW. Hyperadrenocorticism (Cushing's syndrome). In: Feldman EC, Nelson RW, eds. *Feline and Canine Endocrinology and Reproduction*, 3rd ed. St Louis: Saunders Elsevier, 2004: 252–357.
Ferguson DC, Hoenig M. Endocrine system. In: Lattimer KS, Mahaffey EA, Prasse KW, eds. *Duncan and Prasse's Veterinary Laboratory Medicine: Clinical Pathology*, 4th ed. Ames: Iowa State Press, 2003: 270–303.
Herrtage ME. Hypoadrenocorticism. In: Ettinger SJ, Feldman EC, eds. *Textbook of Veterinary Internal Medicine*, 6th ed. Philadelphia: WB Saunders 2004: 1612–1622.
Reusch CE. Hyperadrenocorticism. In: Ettinger SJ, Feldman EC, eds. *Textbook of Veterinary Internal Medicine*, 6th ed. Philadelphia: WB Saunders 2004: 1592–1611.

INTERNET RESOURCES
None

AUTHOR NAME
Janice M. Andrews

CORTISOL/CREATININE RATIO

 BASICS

TYPE OF SPECIMEN
Urine

TEST EXPLANATION AND RELATED PHYSIOLOGY
The urine cortisol/creatine ratio is a screening test for hyper-adrenocorticism (HAC), a clinical disorder characterized by physical manifestations resulting from excessive glucocorticoids. HAC is a common disorder in middle-aged to older dogs but is relatively rare in cats. Naturally occurring HAC is induced by either a functional adrenal cortical tumor or an ACTH-secreting pituitary adenoma (PDH), which produces bilateral adrenal cortical hypertrophy. PDH is the most common form of HAC in both dogs and cats. Iatrogenic HAC occurs secondary to administration of excessive corticosteroids and is seen almost exclusively in dogs. The clinical signs associated with canine HAC, such as polyuria, polydipsia, abdominal distention, and poor hair coat, may be observed with many disorders. In addition, changes in the minimum database are not unique to HAC. Cats commonly present with a history of poorly regulated diabetes mellitus.

Once HAC is suspected, definitive diagnosis and determination of the primary cause require a series of lengthy, expensive tests. A urine cortisol/creatinine ratio can serve as a simple, rapid screening test to determine whether further adrenal function testing is indicated. Unlike a determination of basal blood cortisol concentrations, which provides a "snapshot" of cortisol secretion at a single time point, urinary cortisol excretion parallels total daily cortisol production, which is increased in patients with acquired HAC. Dividing urine cortisol by creatinine standardizes cortisol excretion to the rate of creatinine excretion and thus accounts for differences in urine specific gravity. The urine cortisol/creatinine ratio (UCCR) is a very sensitive test for the diagnosis of HAC—virtually all patients with HAC will have an increased UCCR. However, the UCCR is not very specific. Patients without HAC but undergoing stress or other illness will also have an increased UCCR. The use of the UCCR alone to monitor mitotane therapy and in combination with dexamethasone suppression to differentiate between PDH and adrenal tumors is described in the literature, but it has not gained wide acceptance for these purposes.

Urine cortisol is measured by radioimmunoassay or ELISA. Ratios should be calculated by using molar concentrations of cortisol and creatinine (i.e., nmol/L). Results may be abbreviated in the following manner: a UCCR of 34×10^{-6} may be reported as 34.

INDICATIONS
Screening test for HAC in dogs and cats

CONTRAINDICATIONS
None

POTENTIAL COMPLICATIONS
None

CLIENT EDUCATION
- Avoid stressful situations prior to collecting a morning urine sample.
- Refrigerate the urine until delivery to the clinic.
- Test results may be increased in many diseases, including HAC.
- If the UCCR is increased, further testing will be required to reach a definitive diagnosis of HAC.

BODY SYSTEMS ASSESSED
Endocrine and metabolic

 SAMPLE

COLLECTION
1–2 mL of urine collected by any method

HANDLING
- Collect the urine into a clean container.
- Ship the sample on cold packs.

STORAGE
Refrigerate or freeze the sample.

STABILITY
- Room temperature: 2 days
- Refrigerated (4°C): 1 week
- Frozen (−20°C): at least 1 month

PROTOCOL
Urine can be collected on 2 consecutive days and mixed in equal volumes.

 INTERPRETATION

NORMAL FINDINGS OR RANGE
Reference values are laboratory, method, and species specific and depend on how the ratio is calculated and reported.
- Dogs: $<13 \times 10^{-6}$
- Cats: $<36 \times 10^{-6}$

ABNORMAL VALUES
- Dogs: $>13 \times 10^{-6}$. Values are usually $>30 \times 10^{-6}$ in dogs with HAC.
- Cats: $>36 \times 10^{-6}$. Results between 13×10^{-6} and 36×10^{-6} are considered borderline and may be seen in cats with HAC.

CRITICAL VALUES
None

INTERFERING FACTORS
Drugs That May Alter Results or Interpretation
Drugs That Interfere with Test Methodology
Cortisol, prednisolone, 11-deoxycortisol, prednisone, cortisone, and corticosterone cross-react with the cortisol assay.

Drugs That Alter Physiology
- Corticosteroids (all types and formulations)
- Progestins

Disorders That May Alter Results
None

Collection Techniques or Handling That May Alter Results
Storage at room temperature for >2 days

Influence of Signalment
Species
The UCCR is used almost exclusively in dogs, owing to the higher incidence of HAC in this species.

Breed
None

Age
None

Gender
None

Pregnancy
An increased UCCR is anticipated, depending on the stage of gestation.

LIMITATIONS OF THE TEST

Sensitivity, Specificity, and Positive and Negative Predictive Values in Dogs
- At a cutoff of $>60 \times 10^{-6}$ and disease prevalence of 46%
  - Positive predictive value, 87%
  - Negative predictive value, 100%
- As prevalence falls, the negative predictive value remains high, but the positive predictive value falls.

Valid If Run in A Human Lab?
Yes.

Causes of Abnormal Findings

High values	Low values
PDH	No lower limit of normality
Functional adrenal cortical tumor	
Physiologic stress	
Nonadrenal illness	

CLINICAL PERSPECTIVE
- The UCCR is a rapid, simple screening test but is never definitive for HAC.
- Physiologic stress and nonadrenal illness may also increase the UCCR.
- If the UCCR is increased, further diagnostic tests are required to reach a definitive diagnosis of HAC.

MISCELLANEOUS

ANCILLARY TESTS
- ACTH stimulation test to confirm HAC
- Low-dose dexamethasone suppression test to confirm HAC
- High-dose dexamethasone suppression test may distinguish between PDH and an adrenal tumor

- Endogenous ACTH determination to distinguish PDH from adrenal tumor
- Ultrasonographic examination of the adrenal glands

SYNONYMS
None

SEE ALSO
Blackwell's Five-Minute Veterinary Consult: Canine and Feline Topics
- Hyperadrenocorticism (Cushing's Disease)—Cats
- Hyperadrenocorticism (Cushing's Disease)—Dogs

Related Topics in This Book
- ACTH Assay
- ACTH Stimulation Test
- Adrenal Ultrasonography
- High-Dose Dexamethasone Suppression Test
- Low-Dose Dexamethasone Suppression Test

ABBREVIATIONS
- ACTH = adrenocorticotropic hormone
- HAC = hyperadrenocorticism
- PDH = pituitary-dependent hyperadrenocorticism
- UCCR = urine cortisol/creatinine ratio

Suggested Reading
Feldman EC, Nelson RW. Canine Hyperadrenocorticism and Hyperadrenocorticism in Cats. *In: Canine and Feline Endocrinology and Reproduction*, 4th ed. St Louis: Saunders Elsevier, 2004.
Jensen AL, Iversen L, Koch J, *et al.* Evaluation of the urinary cortisol:creatinine ratio in the diagnosis of hyperadrenocorticism in dogs. *J Small Anim Pract* 1997; **38**: 99–102.

INTERNET RESOURCES
Bruyette D. Feline adrenal disease. In: Scherk M, ed. 26th Congress of the World Small Animal Veterinary Association (WSAVA), Vancouver, 2001, http://www.vin.com/VINDBPub/SearchPB/Proceedings/PR05000/PR00106.htm.
Zwicker K, Bain PJ, Rakich PM, Latimer KS. Canine hyperadrenocorticism, diabetes mellitus, or both? University of Georgia, College of Veterinary Medicine, Veterinary Clinical Pathology Clerkship Program, http://www.vet.uga.edu/vpp/clerk/Zwicker.

AUTHOR NAME
Kristen R. Friedrichs

CREATINE KINASE

BASICS

TYPE OF SPECIMEN
Blood

TEST EXPLANATION AND RELATED PHYSIOLOGY
Creatine kinase (CK) is a cytoplasmic enzyme found within skeletal muscle, cardiac muscle, smooth muscle, the brain, and nerves. It is involved in the transfer of phosphate from creatine phosphate to adenosine triphosphate (ADP) to form ATP. CK is a dimer and 4 isoenzymes exist that have variable tissue distribution. Three isoenzymes are composed of *M* (muscle) and *B* (brain) subunits. Creatine kinase 1 (CK-1 or CK-BB) predominates in the brain, with CK-2 (CK-MB) and CK-3 (CK-MM) in cardiac and skeletal muscle. A unique dimer (CK-Mt) is found in the mitochondria of many tissues. Though CK-1 is present in cerebrospinal fluid, it is not present in the serum of healthy animals or animals with neurologic disease or injury to the central nervous system. Muscle damage, both cardiac and skeletal, causes this enzyme to leak into the serum.

CK activity increases rapidly after muscle damage. Peak levels occur at 6–12 h, and the magnitude of increase is somewhat proportional to the degree of muscle damage. However, because of its short half-life, CK activity decreases within 24–48 h following cessation of injury. Therefore, CK is an excellent measure of acute muscle damage. AST is also present in muscle and can sometimes increase with muscle injury. The increase lags behind the increases in CK, thus evaluating the patterns of enzyme activity abnormalities can help in the estimation of when the muscle was injured. For example, elevation of only CK indicates acute injury, whereas increases in both CK and AST denote ongoing or recent muscle injury.

CK activity can be assessed via several types of assays. Most laboratories rely on a kinetic assay that measures CK activity on a substrate. Storage at any temperature inactivates the enzyme, but addition of acetylcysteine reactivates the enzyme. Electrophoresis or immunologic assays can be used to measure CK isoenzymes.

INDICATIONS
- Detection of skeletal muscle injury
- Detection of cardiac muscle injury

CONTRAINDICATIONS
None

POTENTIAL COMPLICATIONS
None

CLIENT EDUCATION
None

BODY SYSTEMS ASSESSED
- Musculoskeletal
- Cardiovascular

SAMPLE

COLLECTION
0.5–1.0 mL of venous blood

HANDLING
- Serum-separator tube or plain red-top tube
- Sodium heparin anticoagulant or lithium heparin anticoagulant is acceptable.

STORAGE
- Refrigerate or freeze the serum for long-term storage.
- Avoid exposing the serum to bright light, which can cause falsely decreased activity.

STABILITY
- Room temperature: 2 days
- Refrigerated (2°–8°C): 1 week
- Frozen (−15° to −25°C): 1 month

PROTOCOL
None

INTERPRETATION

NORMAL FINDINGS OR RANGE
- Dogs: 48–364 IU/L
- Cats: 41–448 IU/L
- Reference intervals may vary, depending on the laboratory and assay.

ABNORMAL VALUES
Values above the reference interval

CRITICAL VALUES
None

INTERFERING FACTORS
Drugs That May Alter Results or Interpretation
Drugs That Interfere with Test Methodology
Dipyrone administration decreases values.

Drugs That Alter Physiology
- Corticosteroid administration can increase values.
- Insulin administration can activate CK and increase values.
- Streptokinase administration can increase CK activity from subsequent reperfusion injury.
- Amphotericin B administration can increase values because of muscle damage caused by severe hypokalemia.
- Drugs that can cause immune-mediated polymyositis, increasing CK activity, include penicillin, D-penicillamine, sulfonamides, and phenytoin.

Disorders That May Alter Results
Hemolysis can falsely increase CK.

Collection Techniques or Handling That May Alter Results
IM injections administered prior to sampling can increase CK.

Influence of Signalment
Species
Cats have relatively less CK than other species. Therefore, even small elevations in CK activity are important diagnostically.

Breed
None

Age
Young puppies have a higher CK level than adult dogs.

Gender
None

Pregnancy
None

LIMITATIONS OF THE TEST
Sensitivity, Specificity, and Positive and Negative Predictive Values
N/A

Valid If Run in a Human Lab?
Yes.

Causes of Abnormal Findings

High values	Low values
Traumatic muscle injury	Not clinically significant
Physical trauma	
IM injection	
Postoperative injury	
Infectious and/or inflammatory	
muscle disease	
Masticatory myositis (dogs)	
Immune-mediated polymyositis	
Hepatozoon sp.	
Neospora caninum	
Toxoplasma gondii	
Sarcocystis sp.	
Miscellaneous muscle disease	
Seizures	
Saddle thrombus	
Strenuous exercise	
Dirofilariasis	
Bacterial endocarditis	
Metabolic muscle disease	
Exertional rhabdomyolysis (racing	
greyhounds)	
Hyperthyroidism (cats)	
Hypothyroidism (dogs)	
Malignant hyperthermia (dogs)	
Anorexia (cats)	
Inherited/congenital muscle disease	
Musculodystrophy	
Hypokalemic myopathy in Burmese cats	
Myotonia (dogs)	
Phosphofructokinase deficiency (dogs)	

CLINICAL PERSPECTIVE

- Elevations in CK are indicative of muscle damage, with the magnitude of increase somewhat proportional to the severity of the injury.
- Because of its short half-life, CK activity declines rapidly after muscle injury resolves.
- Measurement of AST in conjunction with CK can help estimate when the insult occurred.
- Measurement of CK-MB may help identify CK increases caused by heart disease. However, CK-MB level appears to be somewhat less specific than troponin for heart disease, and the necessary species-specific immunoassays for CK-MB are not commercially available for dogs and cats.

MISCELLANEOUS

ANCILLARY TESTS
- AST determination
- 2M antibody test for masticatory muscle myositis
- Muscle biopsy
- Troponin evaluation

SYNONYMS
- CK
- Creatine phosphokinase (CPK)

SEE ALSO
Blackwell's Five-Minute Veterinary Consult: Canine and Feline Topics
- Myocardial Infarction
- Myocarditis
- Myopathy, Focal Inflammatory—Masticatory Muscle Myositis and Extraocular Myositis
- Myopathy, Generalized Inflammatory—Polymyositis and Dermatomyositis
- Specific chapters on noninflammatory myopathies

Related Topics in This Book
- Angiography and Angiocardiography
- Aspartate Aminotransferase
- Cardiac Catheterization
- Masticatory Muscle Myositis (2M Antibody Assay)
- Troponins, Cardiac Specific

ABBREVIATIONS
- CK-BB = creatine kinase 1: a dimer composed of 2 B protomers
- CK-MB = creatine kinase 2: a hybrid isoenzyme
- CK-MM = creatine kinase 3: a dimer composed of 2 M protomers
- CK-Mt = creatinine kinase composed of mitochondrial dimers

Suggested Reading
Bender HS. Muscle. In: Latimer KS, Mahaffey EA, Prasse KW, eds. *Veterinary Laboratory Medicine Clinical Pathology*, 4th ed. Ames: Iowa State Press, 2003: 260–269.
Lassen ED. Laboratory detection of muscle injury. In: Thrall MA, ed. *Veterinary Hematology and Clinical Chemistry*. Philadelphia: Lippincott Williams & Wilkins, 2004: 417–420.
Stockham SL, Scott MA. *Fundamentals of Veterinary Clinical Pathology*. Ames: Iowa State Press, 2002: 452–453.

INTERNET RESOURCES
None

AUTHOR NAME
Jennifer Steinberg

BASICS

TYPE OF SPECIMEN
Blood
Fluid
Urine

TEST EXPLANATION AND RELATED PHYSIOLOGY
Creatinine (CRT) is formed by the spontaneous conversion of muscle creatine into a ring structure. CRT is cleared from the body almost entirely by renal excretion through glomerular filtration. The amount of CRT produced daily is relatively constant and, in general, less influenced by extrarenal factors than is urea nitrogen. In some species, however, colonic bacteria can catabolize CRT and thus affect the serum CRT concentration.

The methodology for CRT measurement differs with the type of chemistry analyzer. With dry-reagent slides (e.g., VetTest, IDEXX Laboratories, Portland, ME; Vitros, Ortho-Clinical Diagnostics, Raritan, NJ), CRT is hydrolyzed to creatine. Subsequent reactions generate H_2O_2, which reacts with an indicator dye. The rate of change in the reflection density is proportional to the CRT concentration. On analyzers that employ wet-reagent methods, CRT reacts with picric acid to form a colored complex (Jaffe reaction). The rate of formation of the colored complex is proportional to the CRT concentration. In older assays, non-CRT chromogens (i.e., glucose, proteins, ketones) caused a positive interference. Conversion to kinetic assays has reduced this interference.

Increased CRT concentration (azotemia) can result from any disorder that causes decreased glomerular filtration rate (GFR) and/or decreased renal blood flow. It is important to interpret the CRT concentration in the context of the urine specific gravity (SG). With prerenal azotemia, the urine should be maximally concentrated. If the azotemia is renal in origin the SG falls within the isosthenuric range. Postrenal azotemia is generally associated with hyposthenuria. With worsening azotemia, extrarenal CRT excretion increases.

INDICATIONS
- Component of the minimum database
- To evaluate renal function in clinically ill patients
- Diagnosis of uroabdomen
- Calculation of GFR and electrolyte fractional excretion rates
- In urine, CRT measurement is used to correct other analyte levels for SG variability.

CONTRAINDICATIONS
None

POTENTIAL COMPLICATIONS
None

CLIENT EDUCATION
None

BODY SYSTEMS ASSESSED
Renal and urologic

SAMPLE

COLLECTION
1–2 mL of venous blood

HANDLING
- Plain red-top tube or serum-separator tube
- Sodium or lithium heparin anticoagulant (green-top tube) is acceptable.

- Centrifuge and remove serum and/or plasma from cellular material within 4 h of collection.

STORAGE
Refrigerate or freeze the serum for long-term storage.

STABILITY
Serum/Plasma
- Room temperature: 1–5 days
- Refrigerated (2°–8°C): <1 month
- Frozen (−18°C or less): indefinitely

Urine
- Room temperature: <3 days
- Refrigerated (2°–8°C): <5 days
- Frozen (−18°C or less): indefinitely

PROTOCOL
None

INTERPRETATION

NORMAL FINDINGS OR RANGE
- Dogs: 0.6–2.0 mg/dL (53.0–176.8 μmol/L)
- Cats: 0.9–2.2 mg/dL (79.6–194.5 μmol/L)
- Reference intervals may vary, depending on the laboratory and assay.

ABNORMAL VALUES
Values above the reference interval

CRITICAL VALUES
None

INTERFERING FACTORS
Drugs That May Alter Results or Interpretation
Drugs That Interfere with Test Methodology
- Lidocaine: increases values (dry chemistries)
- Nitrofurantoin: increases values (Jaffe reaction)
- Cefoxitin: increases values (Jaffe reaction)
- Dobutamine: decreases values
- Proline from hyperalimentation fluids: increases values

Drugs That Alter Physiology
Nephrotoxic drugs such as aminoglycoside antibiotics, amphotericin B, cisplatin, phenylbutazone, polymyxin B, cephalosporins (occasionally), and sulfamethoxazole (occasionally)

Disorders That May Alter Results
- Rhabdomyolysis may increase CRT production slightly.
- Cachexia/muscle wasting may decrease CRT concentration.

Collection Techniques or Handling That May Alter Results
None

Influence of Signalment
Species
None

Breed
Sighthounds (e.g., greyhounds) have a higher CRT.

Age
Kittens that are <2 months of age have higher CRT concentrations than adults.

Gender
None

Pregnancy
Elevated cardiac output can increase GFR and lower CRT.

LIMITATIONS OF THE TEST
- It is a relatively insensitive measure of renal function: CRT does not increase until GFR is reduced to <25% of normal.

• Increased CRT is not specific for renal disease and can be influenced by extrarenal disease.

Sensitivity, Specificity, and Positive and Negative Predictive Values
N/A

Valid If Run in a Human Lab?
Yes.

Causes of Abnormal Findings

High values	Low values
Prerenal	Increased GFR/renal blood flow
Decreased GFR/renal blood flow	Pregnancy
Hypovolemia: decreased blood volume; dehydration	Hyperthyroidism
Cardiac insufficiency	Cachexia
Shock	Not usually clinically significant
Increased CRT production (mild increase)	
Red-meat consumption	
Increased protein catabolism (possible)	
Renal	
Acute and chronic renal failure	
Inflammation/infection: glomerulonephritis, pyelonephritis; tubulointerstitial nephritis, leptospirosis, hemolytic uremic syndrome	
Toxins: ethylene glycol, aminoglycosides, hypercalcemia; myoglobin; phenylbutazone, cisplatin, plants (e.g., Easter lily, grapes, raisins), heavy metals	
Amyloidosis	
Hydronephrosis	
Congenital hypoplasia or aplasia	
Postrenal	
Lower urinary tract obstruction	
Leakage of urine from the urinary tract: bladder rupture, urethral trauma, ureteral or renal pelvic obstruction	

CLINICAL PERSPECTIVE
• With hypersthenuric urine [SG, >1.030 (dogs) or >1.035 (cats)], think prerenal azotemia (decreased renal perfusion).

• With isosthenuric urine (SG, 1.008–1.012) or minimally concentrated (1.012–1.030), think primary renal disease.
• When an abdominal fluid CRT is ≥2-fold, the simultaneous blood level is confirmatory for uroabdomen.

MISCELLANEOUS
ANCILLARY TESTS
• Blood/serum urea nitrogen
• Urinalysis, including SG
• Urinary fractional excretion
• Urine protein/creatinine ratio

SYNONYMS
None

SEE ALSO
Blackwell's Five-Minute Veterinary Consult: Canine and Feline Topics
• Azotemia and Uremia
• Renal Failure, Acute Uremia
• Renal Failure, Chronic
• Nephrotoxicity, Drug-Induced

Related Topics in This Book
• Glomerular Filtration Rate
• Urea Nitrogen
• Urine Gamma-Glutamyltransferase/Creatinine Ratio
• Urine Protein/Creatinine Ratio
• Urine Specific Gravity

ABBREVIATIONS
• CRT = creatinine
• GFR = glomerular filtration rate
• SG = specific gravity

Suggested Reading
Braun JP, Lefebvre AD, Watson DJ. Creatinine in the dog: A review. *Vet Clin Pathol* 2003; 32: 162–179.
Fettman MJ, Rebar A. Laboratory evaluation of renal function. In: Thrall MA, ed. *Veterinary Hematology and Clinical Chemistry*. Philadelphia: Lippincott Williams & Wilkins, 2004: 307–328.

INTERNET RESOURCES
None

AUTHOR NAME
Jennifer Steinberg

BASICS

TYPE OF SPECIMEN
Blood

TEST EXPLANATION AND RELATED PHYSIOLOGY
A blood crossmatch is performed to detect serologic incompatibility between a possible blood donor and recipient. In contrast with blood typing, which recognizes antigens on RBC membranes, a crossmatch evaluates plasma for the presence of antibodies. A major crossmatch, which is of greatest clinical significance, tests for alloantibodies in patient plasma against donor RBCs. The minor crossmatch looks for alloantibodies in donor's plasma against patient's RBCs. This is of lesser concern because the donor's plasma volume is small, particularly in packed RBC products, and is markedly diluted in recipients. A tube crossmatching procedure is most often used, with antibodies indicated by subsequent hemolysis or hemagglutination. A novel gel column technology (DiaMed AG, Cressier sur Morat, Switzerland) appears to be promising for crossmatching in dogs and cats.

INDICATIONS
Screening blood donors and recipients to assure blood compatibility

CONTRAINDICATIONS
None

POTENTIAL COMPLICATIONS
None

CLIENT EDUCATION
None

BODY SYSTEMS ASSESSED
Hemic, lymphatic, and immune

SAMPLE

COLLECTION
- 1–2 mL of venous blood from donor and recipient
- A segment from the tubing of the donor blood bag can be used.

HANDLING
- Collect the patient's (and possible donor's) blood into EDTA.
- Stored donor cells are often in citrated phosphate dextrose or citrated phosphate dextrose acetate-1 anticoagulant and cell preservative.

STORAGE
Refrigerate the sample for short-term storage.

STABILITY
- Whole blood in EDTA: crossmatch within 48–72 h of blood collection.
- Properly preserved donor blood: stable for 4–5 weeks after collection if stored at 4°C.

PROTOCOL
1. Centrifuge blood (1000 g for 5 min). Remove the plasma from each sample with a pipette, and transfer the sample to clean, properly labeled tubes. Note any hemolysis.
2. Wash RBCs 3 times with saline: Resuspend 0.25 mL of RBCs in 2–4 mL of saline. Centrifuge for 1min, remove the supernatant, repeat the procedure twice, and remove the supernatant.
3. Resuspend 0.10–0.25mL of washed RBCs in ≈4.5mL saline to obtain a 3%–5% RBC suspension.
4. For each donor, prepare 3 tubes labeled major, minor, and recipient control. Add to each tube 2 drops (50 μL) of plasma and 1 drop (25

μL) of RBC suspension as follows:
   Major: recipient plasma + donor RBCs
   Minor: donor plasma + recipient RBCs
   Control: recipient plasma + recipient RBCs
5. Mix gently and incubate for 15–20 min at 37°C.
6. Centrifuge for 15s.
7. Reading the results: Examine the supernatant for hemolysis. Gently resuspend the RBC button by tapping tube and examine for agglutinating clumps. Grade positive hemagglutination reactions as 1+ (fine), 2+ (small), 3+ (large), or 4+ (1 large agglutinate).
8. If macroscopic agglutination is not observed, examine a drop of resuspended RBCs for microscopic agglutination (100× or 400×). This is of questionable importance.
9. A positive reaction in the control tube indicates autoantibodies, which complicate the interpretation of other tubes.

INTERPRETATION

NORMAL FINDINGS OR RANGE
Compatible crossmatch: the absence of hemolysis or hemagglutination

ABNORMAL VALUES
Incompatible crossmatch: the presence of hemolysis or hemagglutination

CRITICAL VALUES
None

INTERFERING FACTORS
Drugs That May Alter Results or Interpretation
Drugs That Interfere with Test Methodology
None

Drugs That Alter Physiology
Hydroxyethyl starch solution (hetastarch) can lead to rouleaux, which can be mistaken for agglutination. Rouleaux can be distinguished from true agglutination if RBC clusters disperse with the addition of saline.

Disorders That May Alter Results
Autoagglutination, such as in immune-mediated hemolytic anemia, precludes crossmatching because such samples always appear incompatible.

Collection Techniques or Handling That May Alter Results
Severe hemolysis may preclude crossmatch testing.

Influence of Signalment
Species
- Dogs: A crossmatch is not necessary prior to first transfusion. Since dogs do not have significant naturally occurring alloantibodies, the initial crossmatch between 2 dogs that have never received a blood transfusion should be compatible.
- Cats: The initial blood crossmatch before the first transfusion may already be incompatible because of naturally occurring alloantibodies in cats. Because of strong naturally occurring anti-A alloantibodies, one might be able to predict the blood type of a feline patient based on crossmatch results and knowledge of the donor's blood type.

Breed
- Dogs: none
- Cats: Because of the increased prevalence of type B cats in certain breeds (e. g., Abyssinian, Devon rex, exotic shorthair), A-B incompatibility is more frequently encountered in those breeds.

Age
None

Gender
None

Pregnancy
- Dogs: Unlike women, bitches do *not* become sensitized to RBC antigens, and subsequently produce alloantibodies, during gestation.
- Cats: unknown

LIMITATIONS OF THE TEST
- A compatible crossmatch does not prevent sensitization or delayed transfusion reactions. It simply indicates that currently there are no significant antibodies against the RBCs.
- Crossmatching provides no information about leukocyte or platelet compatibility and, in some cases, may not be sensitive enough to detect anti-RBC antibodies.

Sensitivity, Specificity, and Positive and Negative Predictive Values
N/A

Valid If Run in a Human Lab?
Yes.

CLINICAL PERSPECTIVE
Any dogs and cats that have been given a previous transfusion should be crossmatched before they receive additional blood even when the same donor is being used. Alloantibodies can develop within 4 days and may last for many years.

 MISCELLANEOUS

ANCILLARY TESTS
Blood typing

SYNONYMS
None

SEE ALSO
Blackwell's Five-Minute Veterinary Consult: Canine and Feline Topics
Blood Transfusion Reactions
Related Topics in This Book
Blood Typing

ABBREVIATIONS
None

Suggested Reading
Blais MC, Berman L, Oakley DA, Giger U. The canine Dal blood type: A red cell antigen lacking in some Dalmatians. *J Vet Intern Med* 2007; 21: 281–286.
Giger U. Blood typing and crossmatching to ensure compatible transfusions. In: Bonagura JD, ed. *Kirk's Current Veterinary Therapy*, 13th ed. Philadelphia: WB Saunders, 2000: 396–399.
Hale AS. Canine blood groups and their importance in veterinary transfusion medicine. *Vet Clin North Am Small Anim Pract* 1995; 25: 1323–1331.
Hohenhaus AE. Importance of blood groups and blood group antibodies in companion animals. *Transfus Med Rev* 2004; 18: 117–126.

INTERNET RESOURCES
None

AUTHOR NAME
Marie-Claude Blais

BASICS

TYPE OF PROCEDURE
Diagnostic sample collection

PROCEDURE EXPLANATION AND RELATED PHYSIOLOGY
- Cystocentesis is the gold standard for sterile collection of urine for urinalysis and urine culture.
- Urinalysis is part of the minimum database when evaluating ill dogs and cats or when performing routine health screens. Urine culture should be performed in animals with clinical signs of lower urinary tract disease (e.g., pollakiuria, dysuria), in animals with active urine sediment, or in animals with diseases known to predispose them to urinary tract infections (e.g., diabetes mellitus, hyperadrenocorticism, renal failure).

INDICATIONS
- Routine collection of urine samples for urinalysis or urine culture
- Immediate relief of bladder overdistention in animals with urethral obstruction

CONTRAINDICATIONS
- Coagulopathy
- Pregnancy
- Suspected or confirmed transitional cell carcinoma
- Severe and diffuse cutaneous disease of caudal abdomen (e.g., severe pyoderma, pemphigus complex)

POTENTIAL COMPLICATIONS
- Seeding of transitional cell carcinoma tumor cells into the abdomen or along the needle track
- Transient hematuria (rare)
- Iatrogenic urinary tract infection (very rare)
- Bladder rupture (very rare)

CLIENT EDUCATION
None

BODY SYSTEMS ASSESSED
Renal and urologic

PROCEDURE

PATIENT PREPARATION
Preprocedure Medication or Preparation
- Typically, none is required.
- In rare cases, where urine is required for urinalysis or culture, but frequent voiding or recent urination has hampered urine collection, a single dose of a diuretic or isotonic fluids can be administered. This is primarily used in dysuric animals where urine is required for culture. Urine specific gravity cannot be interpreted under these conditions; differential diagnoses should be considered prior to increasing urine output artificially.

Anesthesia or Sedation
None is needed in most patients.

Patient Positioning
- For cystocentesis, the bladder is best palpated and isolated while the patient is in lateral recumbency (dogs and cats) or standing (dogs).
- Blind cystocentesis is performed with the patient in dorsal recumbency.

Patient Monitoring
None

Equipment or Supplies
- A 6- to 12-mL syringe
- A 22-gauge needle [usually 1½ inches (38.1 mm)]
- Ethanol

TECHNIQUE
- The bladder should be palpated prior to attempting cystocentesis. The bladder is normally present in the caudal abdomen; with increased urine volumes the bladder will move cranially, toward the ventral body wall.
- If the bladder can be palpated and contains enough urine to attempt cystocentesis, the bladder isolation technique should be used. In those dogs where the bladder is not easily palpated, the blind aspiration technique can be attempted. This technique is more commonly associated with complications and is less likely to be successful.
- Attach the needle to the syringe.

Bladder Isolation Technique
- Restrain the patient in lateral recumbency. In some dogs, the bladder is more easily palpated with the patient standing.
- The individual palpating the bladder should isolate the bladder between their hands, with the fingers spread slightly.
- Spray ethanol over the region isolated.
- Clean or spray the cystocentesis site with ethanol.
- This routine cleaning procedure likely provides minimal disinfection but is nonetheless considered standard practice.
- The bladder should be palpated and isolated with 1 hand. Once the bladder is isolated, the needle should be inserted without applying negative pressure.
- Alternatively, an assistant can attempt cystocentesis by inserting the needle and syringe between the fingers of the person who has isolated the bladder. This allows the bladder to be isolated by using 2 hands and may be easier in dogs. The individual palpating the bladder should guide the assistant as to how far to insert the needle.
- Once the needle has been inserted to the appropriate depth, the syringe plunger should be slowly drawn back, creating negative pressure. Negative pressure should not be applied until the person performing the procedure believes the bladder has been entered, as early aspiration increases the chance of contamination by GI tract content.
- When the desired volume of urine has been collected, negative pressure should be released and the syringe and needle removed.

Blind Aspiration Technique
- Restrain the patient in dorsal recumbency with the rear limbs extended.
- Spray ethanol over the caudal ventral abdomen.
- The needle is inserted at the site where alcohol pools. Alternatively, the bladder position can be estimated by determining where lines drawn between the last 2 sets of nipples theoretically cross (Figure 1). In male dogs, move the prepuce and penis to the side to enable insertion of the needle and syringe on the midline plane. The needle should be directed caudally at an approximately 30°–45° angle.
- Once the needle has been inserted to the appropriate depth, the plunger of the syringe should be slowly drawn back, creating negative pressure. If urine is not obtained, release negative pressure and then reposition the needle cranially or caudally, or alter the depth of needle insertion. Do not maintain negative pressure while repositioning the needle. Complete withdrawal and switching to a new needle is advocated by some clinicians (to prevent seeding of GI tract content), but no studies have evaluated which technique is safer.
- If GI tract content or blood is seen in the needle hub, release the negative pressure and then withdraw the needle and syringe. A fresh needle and syringe should be used if blind cystocentesis is reattempted.
- When the desired volume of urine has been collected, negative pressure should be released and the syringe and needle withdrawn.

SAMPLE HANDLING
- Samples collected for urinalysis should be analyzed immediately, if possible, because refrigeration for later analysis can alter some dipstick and sediment findings.

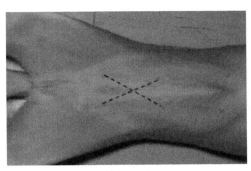

Figure 1

A female dog in dorsal recumbency, with *dotted lines* drawn between the last 2 sets of nipples. In the blind aspiration cystocentesis technique, the needle should be inserted where the lines cross and the needle directed caudally at an approximately 30°–45° angle.

- Urine samples collected for culture should be refrigerated or placed into bacteriostatic transport containers until plated onto appropriate media. The amount of urine to be submitted varies among diagnostic laboratories, but many microbiologists require at least 5 mL because this may increase the likelihood of isolation of infectious agents.

APPROPRIATE AFTERCARE
Postprocedure Patient Monitoring
None
Nursing Care
None
Dietary Modification
None
Medication Requirements
None
Restrictions on Activity
None
Anticipated Recovery Time
Immediate

INTERPRETATION
NORMAL FINDINGS OR RANGE
N/A

ABNORMAL VALUES
N/A

CRITICAL VALUES
N/A

INTERFERING FACTORS
Drugs That May Alter Results of the Procedure
- A number of drugs affect urinalysis findings. A thorough medical history is required for proper interpretation of results.
- Antibiotics may inhibit growth of bacteria if urine is submitted for culture.

Conditions That May Interfere with Performing the Procedure
- Cystocentesis may be difficult at times of low bladder urine volume (e.g., immediately after voiding; in pollakiuric patients). Urinary catheterization using sterile technique will allow small amounts of urine to be collected.
- Bladder rupture

Procedure Techniques or Handling That May Alter Results
- Improper or delayed handling of urine after collection affects urinalysis results.
- Urine samples may be contaminated inadvertently with GI tract content if aspiration is performed prior to the needle entering the bladder. Partially digested food, feces, and bacteria cause a false-positive active urine sediment and positive urine culture.

Influence of Signalment on Performing and Interpreting the Procedure
Species
See the "Urinalysis Overview" chapter for details regarding interpretation in dogs and cats. Some differences of note include these:
- Cat urine is typically more concentrated than dog urine, although the reference ranges in normal animals overlap significantly.
- Dogs may normally have a small amount of bilirubinuria, whereas bilirubinuria in cats is always a pathologic finding.
- Cats typically have more acidic urine than dogs; however, urine pH is significantly influenced by diet.
- Fat droplets are common in feline urine but rare in canine urine.

Breed
None

Age
- Neonatal puppies (<3 weeks old) have more dilute urine than pediatric or adult dogs.
- Transient proteinuria and glucosuria have been reported in neonatal puppies, although this is not a consistent finding in all studies.

Gender
Male dogs may have higher concentrations of urine bilirubin than female dogs.

Pregnancy
None

CLINICAL PERSPECTIVE
Cystocentesis should be considered the standard method for urine collection in all small-animal patients:
- Unlike in cystocentesis, urine samples collected by catheterization or midstream free catch may be contaminated by microorganisms and inflammatory cells normally found in the distal urethra, prepuce, and vaginal vault. Results of urine sediment examination or culture from urine samples not collected by cystocentesis must be interpreted with caution, and there is a higher risk of artifactual bacterial contamination.
- Palpation and isolation of the bladder by an assistant, rather than a blind attempt at urine collection in animals in ventral recumbency, significantly increase the success of urine collection and decrease the likelihood of contamination by GI content.
- Comparison of urinalysis findings from cystocentesis and free-catch midstream urine samples may assist in differentiating urethral or genital disease from bladder or upper urinary tract disease.
- Although cystocentesis of animals that may have transitional cell carcinoma of the urinary bladder may seed tumor cells into the abdomen or along the needle track, cystocentesis should still be routinely performed in dogs and cats unless a bladder mass has been confirmed by diagnostic imaging studies.

MISCELLANEOUS
ANCILLARY TESTS
- Urethral catheterization
- Urinalysis
- Urine culture

CYSTOCENTESIS

SYNONYMS
Bladder tap

SEE ALSO
Blackwell's Five-Minute Veterinary Consult: Canine and Feline Topics
None
Related Topics in This Book
- Bacterial Culture and Sensitivity
- Urethral Catheterization
- Urinalysis Overview

ABBREVIATIONS
None

SUGGESTED READING
None

INTERNET RESOURCES
None

AUTHOR NAME
Barrak M. Pressler

BASICS

TYPE OF PROCEDURE
Function test

PROCEDURE EXPLANATION AND RELATED PHYSIOLOGY
Cystometrogram

This procedure records pressure within the urinary bladder during filling and voiding (if voiding is stimulated). Pressure measurements are graphed against the volume of media (fluid or carbon dioxide gas) infused. In normal animals, the recorded pressures should be low in the empty bladder and remain low during most of the filling phase, because the urinary bladder muscle is highly compliant. Sensation of pressure and the urge to urinate increase only when the bladder is stretched sufficiently to stimulate stretch receptors in the bladder wall. As a normal threshold volume is approached, the pressure rises more rapidly and leads to urinary bladder contraction. A normal urinary bladder contraction should create high-pressure recordings and persist long enough to empty the bladder. Ideally urethral pressure is recorded concurrently with bladder pressures to ensure that urethral pressure is high during filling and low during voiding.

Urethral Pressure Profile

• This procedure records intraurethral pressure along the length of the urethra.

• Urethral pressure is compared to resting urinary bladder pressure and to normal animals of the same species and gender.

INDICATIONS
Cystometrogram

• To determine degree of atony in neurogenic disorders of voiding

• To detect bladder overactivity (detrusor instability) or poor bladder compliance in animals with refractory urinary incontinence

• To determine bladder function in animals with incomplete voiding, chronic urinary tract infection, or detrusor-urethral dyssynergia

Urethral Pressure Profile

• To evaluate animals with refractory urinary incontinence

• To determine concurrent functional disorders in animals with ectopic ureters or other congenital urogenital abnormalities

• To help localize position or length of urethral obstruction

• To document functional urethral obstruction or urethrospasm

• To document response to treatment (e.g., medications, bulking agents)

CONTRAINDICATIONS
• Active urinary tract infection
• Urinary bladder rupture
• Significant hematuria

POTENTIAL COMPLICATIONS
Cystometrogram

• Hematuria (common)
• Iatrogenic urinary tract infection
• Ascending pyelonephritis (with vesicoureteral reflux)
• Vesicoureteral reflux
• Urinary bladder rupture (rare)
• Air embolism (rare)

Urethral Pressure Profile

• Iatrogenic urinary tract infection
• Urethral trauma or tear (rare)

CLIENT EDUCATION
• Advise clients that sedation may be necessary.
• Advise clients that urethral catheterization is necessary.
• Advise clients of the possibility of iatrogenic urinary tract infection or inflammation.
• Advise clients of the possibility of urogenital irritation, hematuria, pollakiuria, or dysuria lasting <1 day.

BODY SYSTEMS ASSESSED
Renal and urologic

PROCEDURE

PATIENT PREPARATION
Preprocedure Medication or Preparation

• Allow animals to void normally.
• Provide adequate restraint for aseptic, atraumatic urethral catheterization.

Anesthesia or Sedation

Urethral Pressure Profile

• None preferred
• Propofol or light inhalant, if needed
• Xylazine has been historically used; reference ranges are available for this drug.
• General anesthesia is required for microtransducer methods; reference ranges are available.

CYSTOMETRY AND URETHRAL PRESSURE MEASUREMENT

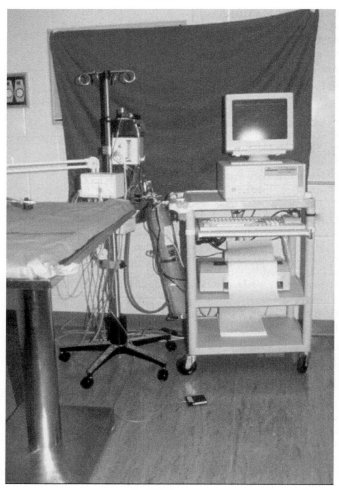

Figure 1

Janus System (Lifetech, Stafford, TX) computer software-based urodynamic system. Measurements can be made using the automated software package.

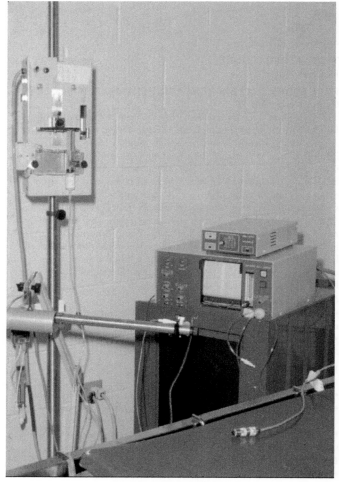

Figure 2

Older analog recorder (Lifetech, Stafford, TX) that provides printout pressure recordings for 1 or more channels. Measurements are made manually based on the recording.

Cystometrogram
- None preferred; however, the procedure may be uncomfortable for some animals.
- Medetomidine or xylazine interferes least with results.

Patient Positioning
Lateral recumbency with appropriate restraint

Patient Monitoring
- Monitor for discomfort during bladder filling.
- Monitor placement of urinary catheter.
- Monitor parameters for sedation or anesthesia (if either are needed).

Equipment or Supplies
- Appropriate specialized urodynamic catheters (ideal)
- Supplies needed for urethral catheterization
- Sterile saline or water for infusion
- Syringes

TECHNIQUE
Cystometrogram
- After urinary catheterization and bladder emptying, the ports of a double-lumen catheter are connected to a pressure-transducer line and fluid infusion line, respectively.
- Sterile water or saline is infused at 5–20 mL/min, depending on the size of the patient.
- Pressures are recorded during filling.
- Filling is stopped when a detrusor contraction is observed or when intravesicular pressure reaches 30–40 cm of water.
- Analysis of filling volume, compliance, threshold volume, and pressure can be completed either by urodynamic software system packages (Figure 1) or manually (Figure 2).

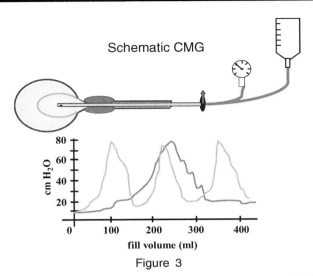

Schematic CMG

Figure 3

Schematic representation of the setup and results for a cystometrogram (CMG). The bladder is slowly filled with fluid as intravesicular pressures are recorded by a transducer. In the graph, the *solid line* is a schematic representation of a relatively normal filling and contraction study, whereas the multiple pressure spikes are examples of involuntary, unstable contractions (e.g., detrusor instability). Illustration courtesy of Dr. Julie Fischer.

• *Leak point pressure* can also be determined after moderate filling of the bladder. A large blood pressure cuff placed around the caudal abdomen is inflated until urine leakage is observed.

Urethral Pressure Profile
• Often completed after CMG
• Ideally a UPP catheter with multiple small pressure ports is used.
• Other catheters can be used, including a triple-lumen urodynamic catheter that enables simultaneous measurement of bladder and urethral pressures, along with fluid infusion.
• The UPP catheter port, or 1 lumen of the double-lumen catheter, is connected to a pressure transducer.
• Fluid is infused through a separate lumen or by using a stopcock at a low infusion rate (2 mL/min).

• Pressures are recorded as the catheter is withdrawn slowly (usually at 0.5–1.0 mm/s).
• Analysis of maximal urethral pressure, maximal urethral closure pressure, and functional profile length can be completed by either urodynamic software system packages or manually.

SAMPLE HANDLING
N/A

APPROPRIATE AFTERCARE
Postprocedure Patient Monitoring
• Monitor recovery from sedation or anesthesia (if either are needed).
• Monitor for urinary tract inflammation (mild discomfort or pollakiuria may be observed for 1–2 days).
• Monitor for urinary tract infection with follow-up urine culture (5–7 days after the procedure).

Nursing Care
None

Dietary Modification
None

Medication Requirements
The use of periprocedural antimicrobials (e.g., amoxicillin for 3 days) should be considered in animals with anatomic or functional compromise of urogenital host defenses.

Restrictions on Activity
None

Anticipated Recovery Time
Immediate, unless sedation or anesthesia is required

INTERPRETATION

NORMAL FINDINGS OR RANGE
• Ranges vary based on the machine used, sedation, and method.
• See the Suggested Reading section for more information.

ABNORMAL VALUES
Cystometrogram
This can detect involuntary bladder contractions, poor capacity or compliance, or weak or absent detrusor function (Figure 3).

CYSTOMETRY AND URETHRAL PRESSURE MEASUREMENT

Urethral Pressure Profile
- This can detect poor urethral closure pressure, urethral spasm, or areas of high urethral resistance (Figure 4).
- Ranges vary based on the machine used, sedation, and method.
- See the Suggested Reading section for more information.

CRITICAL VALUES
None

INTERFERING FACTORS
Drugs That May Alter Results of the Procedure
- Sedatives or anesthetics
- α-Adrenergic agonists
- Anticholinergic agents
- Cholinergic agents

Conditions That May Interfere with Performing the Procedure
- Urinary tract infection or inflammation
- Inability to place the urethral catheter

Procedure Techniques or Handling That May Alter Results
- Incorrect placement of urinary catheterization
- Technical errors
- Air bubbles in pressure lines
- Improper positioning of the patient, transducers, or lines

Influence of Signalment on Performing and Interpreting the Procedure
Species
UPP shapes vary with species and have been described for dogs, cats, and horses.

Breed
Filling rates vary based on animal size.

Age
Pediatric patients usually have higher urethral pressures and smaller bladder capacity than adults.

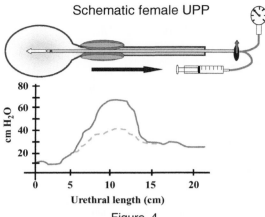

Schematic female UPP

Figure 4

Schematic representation of the setup and results of a urethral pressure profile (UPP) in a female dog. The urinary catheter is withdrawn through the urethra as pressures are recorded by a transducer. In the graph, the *solid line* represents a fairly normal curve, whereas the *dashed line* is consistent with urethral incompetence. Illustration courtesy of Dr. Julie Fischer.

Gender
UPP shapes and measurements vary between males and females.

Pregnancy
None

CLINICAL PERSPECTIVE
- Urodynamic tests can be useful for evaluation of unusual micturition disorders in dogs and cats. Integrated equipment and software for the procedures are limited to referral centers (veterinary teaching hospitals).

CYSTOMETRY AND URETHRAL PRESSURE MEASUREMENT

- Urodynamic procedures adapted for small animals are most useful for the evaluation of urinary incontinence.
- In the absence of urodynamic evaluation, urinary bladder and urethral function can be reasonably assessed based on medical history and physical examination findings, neurologic examination, careful observation of urination, urinary bladder expression, and measurement of residual volume.

MISCELLANEOUS

ANCILLARY TESTS

For proper interpretation and use, results must be combined with clinical signs, results of imaging studies, and observational findings.

SYNONYMS

- Cystometrogram
- Cystometrography
- Urethral pressure profile

SEE ALSO

Blackwell's Five-Minute Veterinary Consult: Canine and Feline Topics

- Ectopic Ureter
- Incontinence, Urinary
- Urinary Retention, Functional

Related Topics in This Book

- Cystourethroscopy
- Urethral Catheterization
- Urinalysis Overview

ABBREVIATIONS

- CMG = cystometrogram
- UPP = urethral pressure profile

Suggested Reading

Fischer JR, Lane IF. Incontinence and urine retention. In: Elliott J, Grauer G, eds. *BSAVA Manual of Canine and Feline Nephrology and Urology,* 2nd ed *(British Small Animal Veterinary Association series).* Ames, IA: Blackwell, 2007: 26–40.

Goldstein RE, Westropp JL. Urodynamic testing in the diagnosis of small animal micturition disorders. *Clin Tech Small Anim Pract* 2005; **20**: 65–72.

Lorenz MD, Kornegay J. *Handbook of Veterinary Neurology,* 4th ed. St Louis: Saunders Elsevier, 2004.

INTERNET RESOURCES

None

AUTHOR NAME

India F. Lane

CYSTOURETHROGRAPHY

BASICS

TYPE OF PROCEDURE
Radiographic

PROCEDURE EXPLANATION AND RELATED PHYSIOLOGY
Cystourethrography is the process of retrograde distention of the urethra and urinary bladder using sterile, iodinated (ionic or nonionic) contrast medium, room air (but see the Contraindications section), or soluble gas (i.e., carbon dioxide or nitrous oxide) to define the lumen and the wall. An alternative to this procedure is to distend the urinary bladder following IV administration of sterile, iodinated contrast medium, with manual compression of the urinary bladder, to induce voiding and opacify the urethra. In general, this is only a morphologic study and provides little physiologic information except subjective information on urethral sphincter competence once the urinary bladder is distended after iodinated contrast medium is administered IV (see also the "Excretory Urography" chapter). The author prefers a combined procedure that includes *both* the sequential contrast cystogram studies (pneumocystogram, double-contrast cystogram, and positive contrast cystogram) and either a retrograde urethrogram (which is more predictable) or a voiding urethrogram.

INDICATIONS
- To locate, assess and, as necessary, determine the continuity of the urethra and urinary bladder in any patient with lower urinary tract clinical signs, particularly in patients with acute trauma
- To define any abnormal contents of the urinary bladder or urethra (e. g., uroliths, polyps, masses, foreign bodies)
- To assess the causes of hematuria, pyuria, stranguria, and pollakiuria
- To assess the relationship between the urinary bladder, the urethra, and their surrounding structures (e.g., compressed or distorted bladder or urethra, retroflexed bladder, herniated bladder, urethrorectal fistula)
- To assess the urethra for leaks, particularly in the presence of retroperitoneal fluid
- To assess the urinary bladder for leaks, particularly in the presence of peritoneal fluid
- Determine focal, regional, or diffuse urinary bladder wall thickness
- To assess the prostate gland indirectly by using the prostatic portion of the urethra as an indicator of prostatic status

CONTRAINDICATIONS
- The use of room air in any patient with visible hematuria can produce a systemically fatal air embolism.
- Retrograde catheterization if there has been recurrent lower or upper urinary tract infections
- Aggressive bladder or urethral distention in a patient with recent bladder or urethral surgery
- Bladder compression to induce voiding in a patient with recent bladder or urethral surgery

POTENTIAL COMPLICATIONS
- Air embolism, which is potentially fatal
- Iatrogenic (e.g., catheter induced or overdistention induced) urethral or bladder trauma
- Introduction of urinary tract infections, which are potentially antibiotic resistant

CLIENT EDUCATION
- The animal should not have any food for at least 18 h prior to the procedure unless it is an emergency procedure.
- The animal should have a cleansing, tepid water enema at least 2 h before the procedure unless it is an emergency procedure.
- There is limited, although not insignificant, risk of an iatrogenic complication (e.g., bladder or urethral tear, urothelial excoriation) as a result of the catheterization and filling aspects of the procedure.

BODY SYSTEMS ASSESSED
Renal and urologic

PROCEDURE

PATIENT PREPARATION

Preprocedure Medication or Preparation
- Withhold food for at least 18 h prior to nonemergency procedures.
- Administer a cleansing, tepid water enema at least 2 h before nonemergency procedures.

Anesthesia or Sedation
Contrast cystourethrography is best performed with sedation or anesthesia to assure adequate positioning and limit the likelihood of patient motion that may cause lower urinary tract trauma. This should be limited to those patients that do not have physiologic contraindications to sedation or anesthesia.

Patient Positioning
Right recumbent and dorsally recumbent (VD) views are indicated before contrast-medium administration and sequentially thereafter. Various studies can be performed using a single catheterization. Where applicable, opposite recumbent (e.g., left or DV recumbent) or oblique views may facilitate bladder wall, bladder lumen, or trigone assessment.

Patient Monitoring
General observation of the patient well-being as would be expected in any patient under sedation or anesthesia

Equipment or Supplies
- Sodium-based, ionic (diatrizoate or iothalamate) or nonionic (iopamidol or iohexol) iodinated contrast media. Verify the iodine concentration to facilitate dilution to the appropriate concentrations (in milligrams of iodine/mL) for the uses defined in the Technique section.
- A flexible catheter that has sufficient tensile rigidity to allow retrograde catheterization without undue trauma as needed for urine evacuation and subsequent instillation of various contrast media
- A balloon catheter (Foley, Swan-Ganz) as necessary to prevent leakage during retrograde study of either the urethral or bladder
- The appropriate size of the catheters will depend on the patient.
- An otoscope with a 1- to 1½-inch (25.4–38.1 mm) small-bore cone is quite helpful in locating the external urethral orifice, particularly in small, fat, female dogs and most female cats.
- Radiographic facilities capable of creating adequate abdominal views
- Materials to harvest samples, as needed (e.g., culture equipment, microscope slides, coverslips)
- Syringes the size of which will depend on the volume to be used
- Sterile, water-soluble lubricant material to facilitate catheterization
- A 3-way stopcock
- A source of carbon dioxide or nitrous oxide for the pneumocystogram or double-contrast cystogram if the patient has gross hematuria. Always use a syringe filled with the gas via the 3-way stopcock and manually inject the patient. Never distend the urinary bladder directly from the compressed gas source.
- Appropriate, noninjurious antiseptic cleansing materials and disposable gauze or swabs to cleanse the urogenital area prior to any attempts to catheterize (e.g., topical chlorhexidine (Hibiclens) or dilute iodine solutions suitable for surgical preparation)
- A solution containing an approximately appropriate concentration of iodine, such as sterile diatrizoate or iothalamate, for positive contrast studies

TECHNIQUE
Make survey radiographs to be sure the patient has been adequately prepared and the radiographic techniques are adequate.

Cystography, Positive or Negative (Gas Based) and Double Contrast

- After emptying the bladder, distend the urinary bladder (via aseptic retrograde catheterization of the urethra → bladder) until palpably turgid (usually 3–5 mL/lb of body weight). This applies to either positive (use 150 mg/mL of iodine) or negative (usually use room air unless contraindications are present) contrast studies.
- Double-contrast *puddleogram* studies. Perform a negative contrast study as in the preceding paragraph, but follow air or gas with 1–3 mL of positive contrast media (use 150 mg/mL of iodine).
- The optimal sequence for full-contrast cystographic study is pneumocystogram → double-contrast cystogram → drainage → positive contrast cystogram using a single catheterization incident.
- Radiographic views and filming sequence: Make a lateral and VD view centered on the bladder and urethral regions immediately after administration. Make an oblique or DV view and opposite lateral views to clarify attached versus free filling defects.

Retrograde and Distention Retrograde Positive Contrast Urethrography

Best performed during the same imaging session as the contrast cystogram because the procedures are complementary.

Routine Retrograde Urethrogram

- Place the tip of a preferably open-ended catheter in the distal urethra. This is often much easier with a 4–7 French balloon (Swan-Ganz or Foley) catheter. Administer 5–20 mL (depending on the patient's size) of a solution containing ≈200 mg/mL of iodine.
- Make lateral or VD/DV radiographs individually, making the exposure at the end of, but before completion of, the volume to be injected. *Note*: Each view requires a separate injection so beware of overdistention if the bladder is full and the urethrogram is repeated multiple times.

Distention Retrograde Urethrocystogram (Generally Preferred to Routine)

- Distend the urinary bladder (via aseptic retrograde catheterization of the urethra → bladder) until the bladder is palpably turgid (usually 3–5 mL/lb of body weight) of a solution containing ≈150–200 mg/mL of iodine.
- Or perform a retrograde urethrogram immediately following the positive contrast phase of the cystogram.
- Then, catheterize the distal urethra with a 4–7 French balloon catheter (Swan-Ganz or Foley preferred, but an open-ended catheter will do, if necessary) and administer 5–20 mL (depending on the patient's size) of a solution containing ≈200 mg/mL of iodine.
- Make lateral or VD/DV radiographs individually, making the exposure at the end of, but before completion of, the volume to be injected. *Note*: Each view requires a separate injection so beware of overdistention if the bladder is full and the urethrogram is repeated multiple times.
- *Beware* of overdistending the catheter balloon because this can cause urethral pressure necrosis!
- *Beware* of overdistending the bladder with the balloon catheter in place as the bladder can be ruptured more easily than with a simple (nonballoon) catheter because there is no exit for the pressure!

Voiding Urethrography

- Distend the urinary bladder (via aseptic retrograde catheterization of the urethra → bladder) until the bladder is palpably turgid (usually 3–5 mL/lb of body weight) of a solution containing ≈150–200 mg/mL of iodine.
- Or perform a retrograde urethrogram immediately following the positive contrast phase of the cystogram.
- Apply pressure to bladder via a wooden or plastic spoon or equivalent until voiding is observed. Make the radiograph during active voiding. Keep your hands out of the primary X-ray beam!
- This procedure is not highly predictable.

SAMPLE HANDLING
None

APPROPRIATE AFTERCARE
Postprocedure Patient Monitoring

- Be sure the patient recovers promptly and completely from the sedation or anesthesia.
- Monitor any procedure-induced hematuria, further evaluate with urinalysis and, as necessary, submit a urine sample for culture and sensitivity testing, and treat with an appropriate antibiotic if hematuria persists for more than 1 or 2 voidings after removal of the catheter.
- Be sure the patient can urinate voluntarily once recovered from the sedation or anesthesia.
- Monitor for any evidence of procedure-induced urinary tract infection and treat as necessary.

Nursing Care
None

Dietary Modification
None

Medication Requirements
Antibiotics as necessary

Restrictions on Activity
None

Anticipated Recovery Time
Only as long as it takes to recover from the sedation or anesthesia

 INTERPRETATION

NORMAL FINDINGS OR RANGE
The size of the canine or feline bladder at survey radiography is quite variable and depends on previous medical history, including hydration and urine production, acute or chronic outflow obstruction, neurologic disorders, and training-based urinary retention. The palpable turgidity of the bladder can be assessed to determine whether the bladder is overdistended either as a preexisting condition or as a result of the contrast study. At moderate distention, the bladder wall is usually no more than 1–2 mm thick, with smooth serosal and mucosal borders. The urinary bladder should be evenly distensible, with an oval shape with smooth external and internal contours. Any variation in the bladder outline that affects its symmetry should be explainable by apposition to an adjacent normal organ (e.g., colon) or considered potentially abnormal and evaluated further. Similarly, the urethra should have a smooth luminal surface, at worst a mildly tortuous course (e.g., as occurs with abdominal press during the contrast study), and gradually tapering contours. In addition, the urethra should be on or very near the midline unless there is notable deviation of the bladder. Neither the urethra nor the bladder has any normal areas of mineralization in either the wall or the lumen in dogs or cats (Figure 1).

ABNORMAL VALUES
Intramural
Diffuse thickening of the urinary bladder wall (defined by contrast cystography) is usually a function of infection. However, regional wall thickening can be caused by trauma (occasionally depending on history), infection (uncommon), or neoplasia (most common). Diffuse mucosal irregularity is usually a function of infection, whereas regional or focal mucosal irregularities can be caused by trauma (uncommon), infection (polypoid lesions or urachal diverticula), or neoplasia (most common). Differentiation of inflammation from neoplasia is not specifically possible by use of imaging alone (histopathology or cytology is required), but sessile masses (broad based against the bladder wall) are more likely to be malignant, whereas polypoid masses (pedunculated or on a stock away from the wall) are more likely to be inflammatory. Normally, the urinary bladder and urethra do not leak,

CYSTOURETHROGRAPHY

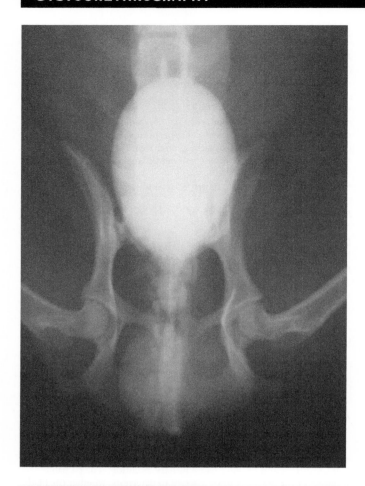

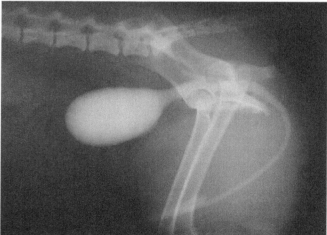

Figure 1

Ventrodorsal (**top**) and right lateral (**bottom**) views of a normal male canine positive contrast retrograde urethrocystogram. *Note*: The retrograde distention technique in normal male dogs results in the prostatic portion of the urethra appearing wider than the remaining urethral segments (e.g., membranous or penile).

and positive contrast studies are the procedures of choice for detecting leakage.

Intraluminal

Objects occupying space in the lumen are referred to as *filling defects* because they usually cause areas of no or incomplete filling (black holes) by iodinated contrast medium with either double-contrast or positive contrast cystourethrographic techniques. These filling defects are defined as *free* (i.e., they move with gravity to the deepest point of the bladder [often the geographic center on recumbent views] or move with contrast injection. Free intraluminal filling defects can be uroliths, blood clots, bubbles (which usually migrate to the periphery of the contrast pool on double-contrast studies), matrix plugs, sloughed mucosa (ulcerative cystitis), or fragments of tumor. By comparison, *attached* filling defects maintain a more or less fixed relationship with a region of the mucosal surface and do not move with gravity or contrast-medium flow. Attached filling defects are usually tumors (sessile) or inflammatory or neoplastic polyps (pedunculated) but can be hematomas or scars. Masses of any sort found primarily in the bladder trigone are most likely neoplastic. Be aware that positive contrast medium in more diluted mixtures than that defined above can mask struvite or oxalate uroliths, depending on the iodine concentration. Also, always check kidney status with trigonal masses (hydronephrosis). Urethral filling defects are judged by shape: Smooth with contours following the lumen are probably bubbles, irregular and focal filling defects are probably uroliths, and regional luminal or mural irregularities are usually tumors, but beware of posttrauma scarring, stricture formation, and pyogranulomatous urethritis. Always confirm findings with cytology or histology.

Extramural

A partially distended bladder can be distorted easily by regional organs or masses or both. However, care must be taken to ensure that wall or luminal distortions are indeed caused by regional influences instead of intramural disease. If there is a doubt, different positioning or more distention is indicated to minimize equivocation.

Remember

Contrast cystography is very useful for identifying bladder location (retroflexion, hernia) and for distinguishing the bladder from other caudal abdominal fluid-filled cavities defined by ultrasound, such as paraprostatic cysts, segmental uterine fluid distention, and intersex anomalies.

CRITICAL VALUES
None

INTERFERING FACTORS
Drugs That May Alter Results of the Procedure
None

Conditions That May Interfere with Performing the Procedure
- Urethral obstruction that cannot be relieved
- Contraindication for sedation in all but the most depressed patients

Procedure Techniques or Handling That May Alter Results
- Iatrogenic overdistention
- Rupture of the bladder or urethra
- Iatrogenic catheter trauma or perforation
- *Beware* of contrast-medium effects on urinalysis results probably for at least 24 h, including false increases in urine specific gravity and some interference with the culturing success of some microorganisms.

Influence of Signalment on Performing and Interpreting the Procedure
Species
Catheter size and availability

Breed
None

Age
None, provided the patient can endure the physiologic effects of sedation

Gender
None

Pregnancy
Radiation effects on first-trimester fetuses can be problematic, so this procedure is, therefore, a risk-benefit judgment for pregnant patients.

CLINICAL PERSPECTIVE
Contrast cystography provides morphologic information (size, shape, location, surface characteristics) on the urinary bladder and the urethra. Although somewhat similar information can be garnered from bladder ultrasound, intrapelvic urethral ultrasound is not rewarding with generally available transducers. In addition, contrast cystography requires a commitment to sedation and appropriate distention, limiting equivocation and interpretive error. This can be mimicked by ultrasound procedures, but only if the bladder is already full or deliberately distended. Contrast cystourethrography provides little information on sphincter function unless there is apparent morphologic distortion directly associated with the sphincter region.

 MISCELLANEOUS

ANCILLARY TESTS
Excretory urography

SYNONYMS
* Contrast cystogram
* Cystourethrogram

SEE ALSO
Blackwell's Five-Minute Veterinary Consult: Canine and Feline Topics
None

Related Topics in This Book
* General Principles of Radiography
* Cystometry and Urethral Pressure Measurement
* Cystourethroscopy
* Excretory Urography
* Lower Urinary Tract Ultrasonography
* Urethral Catheterization

ABBREVIATIONS
* DV = dorsal ventral
* VD = ventral dorsal

Suggested Reading
Burk RL, Feeney DA. The abdomen. In: Small Animal Radiology and Ultrasonography, 3rd ed. Philadelphia: WB Saunders, 2003: 355–427.
Johnston GR, Walter PA, Feeney DA. Diagnostic imaging of the urinary tract. In: Osborne CA, Finco DR, eds. *Canine and Feline Nephrology/Urology.* Baltimore: Williams & Wilkins, 1995: 230–276.
Park RD, Wrigley RH. The urinary bladder. In: Thrall DE, ed. *Textbook of Veterinary Diagnostic Radiology,* 4th ed. Philadelphia: WB Saunders, 2002: 571–587.
Weichselbaum RC, Feeney DA, Jessen CR, *et al.* In vitro evaluation of contrast medium concentrations and depth effects on the radiographic appearance of specific canine urolith mineral types. *Vet Radiol Ultrasound* 1998; 39: 396–411.

INTERNET RESOURCES
University of Minnesota: Veterinary radiology, http://www.cvm.umn.edu/vetrad/.

AUTHOR NAME
Daniel A. Feeney

BASICS

TYPE OF PROCEDURE
Endoscopic

PROCEDURE EXPLANATION AND RELATED PHYSIOLOGY
In this procedure, fiber optics within either rigid or flexible endoscopes are used to visualize structures of the male and female lower urinary tract, including the urethra, bladder, and ureteral openings. The techniques described can also assess the caudal reproductive tract of female dogs and cats. Transurethral retrograde endoscopy is the most common cystourethroscopy technique. In female dogs and cats, rigid and semirigid endoscopes of various sizes are used. In male dogs, the use of flexible endoscopes is necessary. In male cats, semirigid endoscopes can be used. Occasionally, in dogs and cats, a transabdominal or perineal approach via incisions is necessary because either a flexible endoscope is unavailable or the urethra is too small for retrograde cystourethroscopy.

INDICATIONS
• Suspected anatomic abnormalities, including urachal diverticula, ectopic ureters, vaginal septae, and urethroceles
• Recurrent or persistent urinary tract infections
• Suspected mass lesions, obstructions, and strictures
• Micturition disorders, including pollakiuria, stranguria, incontinence, and urine-stream abnormalities
• Hematuria
• Urine cellular atypia
• Stone retrieval or lithotripsy
• Urethral endoscopic injections
• Lower urinary tract biopsy samples, and cellular and sterile fluid collection
• Cystoscopy-guided stricture reduction via balloon
• Vaginal and vulvar discharge
• Vaginitis
• Breeding difficulties

CONTRAINDICATIONS
• Cystoscopy is an elective procedure and should be used in patients that are otherwise healthy or have been stabilized medically.
• Recent urinary tract surgery or trauma may predispose patients to extravasation of urine and instilled fluid.

POTENTIAL COMPLICATIONS
• Most complications can be avoided by using proper technique.
• Potential complications include these:
  • Iatrogenic urinary tract infection
  • Iatrogenic hematuria
  • Iatrogenic cystitis
  • Iatrogenic urethritis
  • Urethral adhesion formation
  • Urethral stricture
  • Extravasation of urine if muscularis is compromised
  • Bladder overdistention causing postprocedural dysuria

CLIENT EDUCATION
• Patients must be fasted for a minimum of 12 h prior to the procedure.
• Other diagnostics, including radiographic contrast studies, abdominal radiographs, and abdominal ultrasound, may be warranted before or after the procedure.
• The cystoscopic findings may warrant additional surgical intervention (i.e., larger surgical biopsies, tumor debulking).
• Complications are rare, but patients infrequently suffer from dysuria and hematuria after the procedure.
• Rarely, patients may be uncomfortable after the procedure.

• As with any diagnostic tool, normal findings are common despite patient clinical signs.

BODY SYSTEMS ASSESSED
• Renal and urologic
• Reproductive

 PROCEDURE

PATIENT PREPARATION
Preprocedure Medication or Preparation
• Patients should be fasted 12 h prior to the procedure.
• A preanesthetic biochemical panel with a CBC should be evaluated particularly in geriatric patients.
• Ideally, to ensure that a representative sample is obtained, urine for urinalysis and culture should be obtained prior to the procedure.
• An external genitalia and rectal exam should be performed in both the awake and the standing, as well as the sedated, recumbent animal.
• In females, the perivulvar area should be clipped of hair and the skin prepared with a povidone-iodine (Betadine) solution that can be rinsed off with sterile saline after a 5-min contact time.
• In males, the penile sheath should be flushed. The penis must be manually extruded and cleaned with a povidone-iodine solution and remain extruded during the procedure.
• A single periprocedural dose of antibiotics (i.e., a cephalosporin) should be administered.

Anesthesia or Sedation
• Opioids can be used during premedication.
• General anesthesia is necessary during the procedure.

Patient Positioning
• Patients may be in right, left, or dorsal recumbency, provided that the endoscopist maintains consistency between exams.
• Caution should be used to position the animal such that fluids used for bladder distention during the procedure are drained away from the patient.
• Patients can be adjusted during the procedure, provided that sterile technique is maintained and instruments are external when the adjustment is made.

Patient Monitoring
• Proper anesthetic monitoring should be used at all times.
• Caution must be used to ensure that patients are not wet during the procedure, because body temperature will decrease rapidly.

Equipment or Supplies
• Equipment varies depending on the patient.
• Female patients require rigid endoscopes with the following:
  • A telescope (a 30° tip angle is most common) for producing images
  • A sheath to protect the mucosa and telescope. A fluid and biopsy channel is optimal.
  • A bridge with a biopsy port, fluid or gas instillation port, and fluid drainage port are optimal.
• Instrumentation should be gas or liquid sterilized.
• Flexible cystoscopes are available for use in male dogs.
• A light source
• A sterile fluid source, such as a 0.9% sodium chloride
• A drainage bucket
• A drainage line
• A camera is optional, but necessary for projection and recording of images, as well as adjusting picture quality.
• An optional sterile camera sleeve
• Optional sterile towels with towel clamps
• Other optional items include biopsy forceps, stone-retrieval devices, lithotripsy, and cautery instruments.

- Sterile lubricant
- Povidone-iodine solution and sterile saline for patient preparation. Do not use povidone-iodine scrub solution.
- Sterile gloves

TECHNIQUE

- Liberally apply lubricant to the entire sheath.
- Attach the fluid source to bridge and fill the channel with fluid.
- The fluid bag should be hung no higher than 60 cm above the bladder. To help prevent bladder overdistention, do not use a pressure bag. The bladder should also be intermittently palpated during the procedure and pressure relieved, as necessary.
- Attach the drainage line from the bridge and extend it into the drainage bucket.
- With male dogs, an assistant's aid is necessary to extrude the penis. To introduce the nontapered flexible endoscope into the urethra, a gauze sponge frequently is needed to grasp the mucosa at the end of the penis, stabilize the tip, and enable endoscope introduction. Once inside the urethra, the fluid should then be used to distend the urethra.
- With female dogs, an assistant should initially part the vulva while the rigid endoscope is introduced into the vestibule while being held at a dorsal angle. Once the endoscope is inside, the assistant should apply caudal and slightly dorsal traction on the vulva while pinching it closed to create space within it. Fluid then should be used to fill the vestibule and vagina.
- Within the vestibule, the cingulum and urethral opening should be visualized within the same camera view for orientation and to note anatomic abnormalities.
- The endoscope enters the urethra, with the endoscopist cognizant of the tip angle and the shape of the sheath tip.
- Within the urethra, the endoscope should slide freely. If the scope drags, ensure that the fluids have distended the urethra, that the endoscope was adequately lubricated, and finally that the endoscope is of appropriate size. Ideally, the urethra is examined before the endoscope enters the bladder, because iatrogenic changes to the mucosa can occur.
- The normal urethra has a dorsal urethral membrane that can be used for orientation. The size of this membrane frequently varies.
- In male dogs, the ischial arch can be difficult to traverse with the flexible endoscope. Caution must be used to ensure that the endoscope is not too large. Adequate lubricant and fluid distention of the urethra should be ensured. Telescoping of the urethral mucosa is a sign that the endoscope diameter is too large.
- When the endoscope enters the bladder, sterile urine samples can be obtained, but these will be diluted by saline.
- The entire bladder should then be inspected systematically. Bladder mucosa examination should be performed in a moderately distended bladder with no folds or corrugations. Frequently, the urine within the bladder must be drained and replaced with sterile saline for adequate visualization. Starting at the apex, concentric circles should be made with the endoscope until the entire mucosa is examined.
- After mucosal examination, the bladder can be drained of fluid and the collapsed mucosa visualized. Vessels typically will become less visible.
- Backing the endoscope to the entrance of the bladder, fluids should then be used to distend the bladder. In the trigone, the ureteral papillae will initially appear as C-shaped slits on small masses of tissue. As the bladder distends, these masses will flatten; however, the slits should still be visible in direct opposition to each other on either side of dorsal midline. Urine jets from the ureteral papillae must be visualized to complete the exam. The frequency of the jets can be widely variable.
- Instilling a small air bubble into the bladder may help with orientation, enabling one to determine the up side. Manipulation of the bladder by palpation may also be used to examine the bladder successfully.
- Biopsy, stone retrieval, lithotripsy, and urethral submucosal injections should be preformed only after the exam is complete.

- The endoscope then enters the vagina and traverses to the level of the precervix. Mucosa is examined and can be strikingly different in an intact vs spayed female. Fluid collection for cytology or culture can be obtained at this point.

SAMPLE HANDLING

- If not previously obtained, a sterile urine sample should be collected for culture.
- Cystoscopic biopsy instruments collect very small tissue samples. Samples must be large enough not to fall through the mesh screen within the biopsy tray when fixation occurs.
- If the urine is highly cellular or if tissue exfoliates well, cytologic analysis of a urine sediment is recommended.
- A squash preparation made from a small biopsy sample may be used to obtain a cytologic diagnosis.
- If agar block cytology is available, this technique may enable assessment of the small samples.

APPROPRIATE AFTERCARE

Postprocedure Patient Monitoring
Monitor for hematuria, pollakiuria, and stranguria.

Nursing Care
None required. This is an outpatient procedure.

Dietary Modification
None specifically related to the procedure

Medication Requirements
- Antibiotics should be administered for 5 days after the procedure if sterility was broken or if periprocedural antibiotics were not given.
- Nonsteroidal anti-inflammatory medications can be given; however, they are not necessary for most procedures.

Restrictions on Activity
None

Anticipated Recovery Time
Anesthetic dependent

INTERPRETATION

NORMAL FINDINGS OR RANGE

- The benefit of cystourethroscopy is the ability to assess the lower urinary tract for anatomic abnormalities and diseases that affect the urinary tract mucosa. Technique and equipment are vital to proper interpretation of endoscopic findings, and hence watching and performing procedures are necessary to understand what is normal.
- On either side of the urethral papilla in female dogs, in bilateral recesses, are small openings that should not be mistaken for pathology.
- In females, the urethral mucosa is homogeneous throughout. Small blood vessels should be seen in the mucosa. Additional openings or tissue seen in the distended urethra are abnormal.
- In males, the mucosa of the urethra changes at the level of the prostate and glandular openings can be visualized.
- The proximal urethra increases subtly in diameter and opens directly into the bladder.
- In the bladder, blood vessels should be easily seen under the mucosa. They should not be tortuous or protrude from the mucosa.
- The ureteral papillae will initially appear as C-shaped slits on small mounds of tissue. As the bladder distends, the mounds will flatten; however, the slits should remain visible.
- Bands of tissue (frenulums) traversing the vaginal opening can be seen occasionally in normal females.
- Fibrous tissue encircling the vagina may be normal in some patients.
- Intact female dogs appear to have more folds within their vagina. If in estrus, female dogs may also have a prominence of tissue, originating from the urethral papilla, that can have a mass appearance.

CYSTOURETHROSCOPY

• Air bubbles sometimes reflect images and can be mistaken for pathologic processes such as calculi. Fat droplets may be seen floating in the urine of cats.

ABNORMAL VALUES

• Bands of tissue that distort the urethral opening are considered pathogenic. Large bands may be associated with ectopic ureters.

• A mucosa that has submucosal petechiations and prominent tortuous vasculature, is friable, and easily ulcerates or bleeds may be consistent with an inflammatory condition such as cystitis, urethritis, or vaginitis. Small raised nodules or polyps can also be seen secondary to chronic inflammation in the lower urinary tract.

• Proliferative urethritis appears as tissue proliferation.

• The appearance of transitional cell carcinomas may vary considerably and may initially appear as fimbriated, vascular masses and progress to white, irregular masses in the urethra or smooth, flat, raised lesions within the bladder. Polypoid-looking masses should not be disregarded. Location cannot be used to make a diagnosis because tumors can be located in the body of the bladder; however, the trigone and urethra are the most common locations for transitional cell carcinoma in dogs.

• Other neoplasms may present as mass lesions or may provide only subtle changes such as mucosal thickening or bladder wall stiffening.

• Ectopic ureters, urachal remnants, and other anatomic abnormalities can be identified by the distortion of normal anatomy. Ectopic ureteral openings can be found anywhere within the lower urinary tract.

• Cystic calculi and other debris may be seen after the bladder is flushed with urine, particularly if the original urine was highly concentrated.

• Urethral strictures, mucosal trauma, and abscesses can be visualized.

• Renal hematuria can be identified and localized by watching urine jets emerging from the ureteral papillae.

• Ureteroceles can sometimes be identified via cystoscopy.

CRITICAL VALUES

The procedure should be performed only in stable animals.

INTERFERING FACTORS

Drugs That May Alter Results of the Procedure
None

Conditions That May Interfere with Performing the Procedure
None

Procedure Techniques or Handling That May Alter Results
Samples should be kept in an isotonic solution or buffered formalin.

Influence of Signalment on Performing and Interpreting the Procedure

Species
In female cats, a semirigid endoscope may need to be used. The capability of these endoscopes to bend can make a complete examination of the bladder difficult. The lack of a sheath makes biopsy and adequate visualization difficult. Frequently, in female cats that cannot be examined adequately with a semirigid endoscope, male cats, and small male dogs, a transabdominal approach using rigid endoscopes is necessary.

Breed
Endoscope selection is frequently breed size dependent.

Age
No influence

Gender
Female dogs and large female cats are best examined by using a rigid endoscope. Male dogs can be examined with a flexible endoscope. Most male cats, very small male dogs, and some female cats need to be examined by using rigid endoscopes and a transabdominal approach.

Pregnancy
No influence

CLINICAL PERSPECTIVE

• Bladder distention with carbon dioxide instead of saline has been used in cases where a large amount of bleeding continuously obscures the view.

• When pathology is generalized within the bladder, larger blind biopsy samples can be obtained by passing a biopsy instrument through the sheath that remains in the bladder after the telescope has been removed.

MISCELLANEOUS

ANCILLARY TESTS

• Computed tomography
• Cystometry
• Cystourethrography
• Electrocautery or select mass resection
• Excretory urography
• Lithotripsy
• Magnetic resonance imaging
• Prostatic massage
• Stricture dilation
• Traumatic urethral catheterization
• Ureteral catheterization
• Urethral pressure profile
• Urethral submucosal bulking-agent injections
• Vaginography
• Voiding hydropropulsion

SYNONYMS

• Cystoscopy
• Endouroscopy

SEE ALSO

Blackwell's Five-Minute Veterinary Consult: Canine and Feline Topics
• Dysuria and Pollakiuria
• Ectopic Ureter
• Hematuria
• Incontinence, Urinary
• Lower Urinary Tract Infection
• Pyuria
• Transitional Cell Carcinoma, Renal, Bladder, Urethra
• Urolithiasis

Related Topics in This Book
• General Principles of Endoscopy
• Computed Tomography
• Cystometry and Urethral Pressure Measurement
• Cystourethrography
• Excretory Urography
• Magnetic Resonance Imaging
• Prostatic Wash
• Urethral Catheterization
• Vaginography
• Voiding Urohydropropulsion

ABBREVIATIONS

None

Suggested Reading
Messer J, Chew D, McLoughlin M. Cystoscopy: Techniques and clinical applications. *Clin Tech Small Anim Pract* 2005; 20: 52–64.

INTERNET RESOURCES

None

AUTHOR NAME

Michael W. Wood

BASICS

TYPE OF SPECIMEN
Blood

TEST EXPLANATION AND RELATED PHYSIOLOGY
D-dimer is a specific FDP, yielded by plasmin-mediated lysis of cross-linked fibrin. During coagulation, factor XIII is activated by thrombin. Activated FXIII, in the presence of calcium, creates bridges between fibrin molecules, producing cross-linked fibrin. This fibrin is insoluble and integrates with platelets, forming a stable clot or thrombus. D-dimer is created when the end-terminal sections (D-domain) of adjacent fibrin molecules are cross-linked by activated FXIII. This cross-linking alters the conformation of the fibrin D-domains, creating a novel antigen referred to as D-dimer. This antigen/epitope is exposed when plasmin cleaves cross-linked fibrin during fibrinolysis (Figure 1). This antigen is only present in cross-linked fibrin and can be detected by monoclonal antibodies that react specifically with this antigen in human samples.

Plasmin is a nonspecific enzyme, degrading coagulation factors, fibrinogen, soluble fibrin, and cross-linked fibrin. However, different degradation products are released when plasmin cleaves fibrinogen and/or soluble fibrin or cross-linked fibrin (Figure 1). Proteolysis of fibrinogen/soluble fibrin releases FDPs (fragments X, Y, D and E), whereas cleavage of cross-linked fibrin yields cross-linked fragments (X-oligomers), the smallest of which is D-dimer, covalently linked to fragment E. Therefore, D-dimer indicates both thrombin and plasmin generation and is specific for fibrinolysis. In contrast, FDPs can be produced by plasmin-mediated lysis of fibrinogen or fibrin and does not always require thrombin generation. Thus, it is not as specific for fibrinolysis as is D-dimer.

D-dimer is measured by using microplate ELISA or membrane ELISA (i.e., immunofiltration), or by using immunoturbidometric or latex agglutination assays. All assay formats rely on specific monoclonal antibodies against the human D-dimer epitope. Latex agglutination assays, which are easy to perform and readily available, provide semi-quantitative results. Immunoturbidometric procedures for D-dimer are now supplanting latex agglutination in veterinary diagnostic laboratories. Immunoturbidometry yields quantitative results and is more sensitive than latex agglutination but requires specialized equipment. Unfortunately, a canine-specific point-of-care immunofiltration assay is no longer available.

INDICATIONS
• Specific marker of fibrinolysis: This indicates the generation of thrombin (produces cross-linked fibrin via factor XIIIa) and plasmin (to release cross-linked degradation products containing D-dimer).
• Antemortem marker of overt thrombosis: *Cross-linked* fibrin can be lysed only after coagulation has been initiated to form a clot.
• Ancillary diagnostic test for DIC
• Indirect marker of hypercoagulability: Hypercoagulability is defined as pathologic activation of the coagulation cascade (and thrombin) without overt clot formation. It is considered a prothrombotic state; i.e., the animal is predisposed to developing thrombi.

CONTRAINDICATIONS
None

POTENTIAL COMPLICATIONS
None

CLIENT EDUCATION
None

BODY SYSTEMS ASSESSED
Hemic, lymphatic, and immune

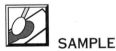

SAMPLE

COLLECTION
1–3 mL of venous blood

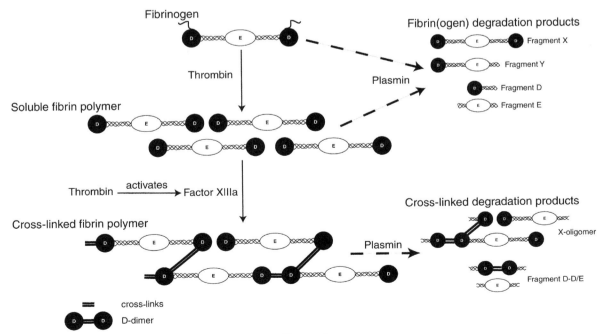

Figure 1

Schematic illustrating the formation of various degradation products created during the process of fibrinolysis, including FDPs and D-dimers.

HANDLING

The choice of tube depends on the type of assay. Check with the lab for its preference.

• The Serum must be collected into a special FDP-collection tube that contains fibrinolysis inhibitors. D-dimers may bind to clot, artificially decreasing the measured concentration.

• Plasma: citrate, heparin, or EDTA. Citrate is the preferred anticoagulant.

STORAGE

• Refrigerate the sample for short-term storage.
• Freeze the sample for long-term storage.

STABILITY

• Refrigerated (2°–8°C): 1 day, based on human data but may be longer in animals
• Frozen (−20°C or less): 3 months, based on human data but may be longer in animals

PROTOCOL

None

INTERPRETATION

NORMAL FINDINGS OR RANGE

• Dogs: <0.25 μg/mL (<250 ng/mL)
• Cats: <0.25 μg/mL (<250 ng/mL)
• Reference intervals may vary, depending on the assay.

ABNORMAL VALUES

Values above reference interval

CRITICAL VALUES

None

INTERFERING FACTORS

Drugs That May Alter Results or Interpretation

Drugs That Interfere with Test Methodology
None

Drugs That Alter Physiology
• Fibrinolytic drugs (e.g., streptokinase and tissue plasminogen activator) will increase D-dimer concentration by inducing clot lysis.

Disorders That May Alter Results

• Neutrophil proteases (elastase, cathepsin G) released in inflammatory states in human patients may cause a false positive (due to fibrinolysis) or false negative (due to degradation of D-dimer).

• Rarely, monoclonal gammopathies in human patients have been associated with a false-positive reaction for D-dimer.

• Extravascular coagulation with subsequent fibrinolysis (e.g., hemorrhage into tissue or body cavities) may increase D-dimer concentration.

• Any condition associated with fibrin formation and breakdown, physiologic (e.g., wound healing) or pathologic (e.g., neoplasia), can increase D-dimer concentration.

• Liver disease may increase D-dimer concentration by decreased clearance.

Collection Techniques or Handling That May Alter Results

Failure to collect blood into an FDP-collection tube will falsely increase D-dimer concentration in serum samples (in vitro fibrinolysis will not be inhibited).

Influence of Signalment

Species
None

Breed
None

AGE
• Concentrations may be high in neonates.
• Concentrations increase with age in humans.

Gender
None

Pregnancy
Increased in humans

LIMITATIONS OF THE TEST

• Some clinically healthy dogs and cats can have high D-dimer values with latex agglutination assays. The cause of this is not known (could be false positives).

• Results from different assays are not directly comparable, because of different sensitivity and antibody reactivity.

Sensitivity, Specificity, and Positive and Negative Predictive Values

Diagnosis of DIC
• Sensitivity: 77%–100%
• Specificity: 47%–95%
• Although D-dimer is a sensitive test for DIC, DIC should not be diagnosed based on high D-dimer alone, because any cause of thrombosis or fibrinolysis may increase the concentration. D-dimer results should be interpreted in conjunction with clinical and laboratory findings to achieve a diagnosis of DIC.

Diagnosis of Thrombosis
• Thrombosis is indicated by a D-dimer value of >0.25 μg/mL.
• Sensitivity: 83%–100%
• Specificity: <50%
• Limited studies in clinically ill dogs suggest that D-dimer is a sensitive test for thrombosis in animals, including pulmonary thromboembolism. However, test specificity is low because increased concentrations are seen in dogs with conditions associated with activation of coagulation and fibrinolysis (e.g., liver disease, hemorrhage), without documentation of thrombosis.

Marker of Hypercoagulability
• The sensitivity and the specificity of D-dimer for detection of hypercoagulable (prothrombotic) states in animals with various diseases (e.g., neoplasia, heart disease) are unknown.
• A D-dimer assay should not be the sole test for this purpose, but can be used together with other markers of thrombin generation (e.g., thrombin-antithrombin complexes).

Valid If Run in a Human Lab?

Yes—as long as validated assays are used. Different assays for D-dimer use antibodies with different specificities for human D-dimer. Not all of these antibodies cross-react with canine or feline D-dimer; therefore, only certain assays can be used in these species.

CLINICAL PERSPECTIVE

• The highest D-dimer values (>1 μg/mL) are seen in dogs with documented thrombosis or DIC. Therefore, the higher the D-dimer value is, the more likely it is that the patient has DIC or thrombosis. However, a D-dimer value of <1 μg/mL does not exclude these conditions.

• D-dimer appears to be more sensitive than plasma or serum FDPs for diagnosis of DIC and thrombosis.

• In most laboratories, D-dimer has replaced FDP testing for detection of fibrinolysis and diagnosis of DIC.

• D-dimer assays have not been validated in cats; however, high concentrations are seen in cats with DIC (e.g., secondary to feline infectious peritonitis virus infection) and cardiomyopathy (including those with acute aortic thromboembolism), suggesting the test may be useful in this species.

Causes of Abnormal Findings

High values	Low values
Thrombosis	Chronic thrombosis
DIC	Hyperadrenocorticism, chronic
Hyperadrenocorticism,	corticosteroid therapy
corticosteroid therapy	(human patients)
Protein-losing nephropathy or	
enteropathy	Localized thrombosis
Neoplasia	Arterial thromboembolism in
Amyloidosis	cats
Vasculitis	
Physiologic coagulation and	
fibrinolysis	
Wound healing	
Surgery	
Pathologic coagulation and	
fibrinolysis (without documented	
thrombi); i.e., hypercoagulable	
states	
Neoplasia	
Heart failure	
Liver disease	
Acute and chronic renal failure	
Feline cardiomyopathy	
Extravascular fibrinolysis	
Hemorrhage into body cavities or	
tissues; e.g., trauma	
Fibrinolytic therapy	
Streptokinase	
Tissue plasminogen activator	

MISCELLANEOUS

ANCILLARY TESTS
- Platelet count
- Hemostasis testing (prothrombin time, activated partial thromboplastin time, antithrombin activity)
- FDP assay

SYNONYMS
- Cross-linked fibrin D-dimer
- D-di
- Fibrin D-dimer
- Fragment D-dimer

SEE ALSO
Blackwell's Five-Minute Veterinary Consult: Canine and Feline Topics
- Cirrhosis and Fibrosis of the Liver
- Disseminated Intravascular Coagulation
- Hepatic Failure, Acute
- Hepatitis, Chronic Active
- Protein-Losing Enteropathy
- Proteinuria

Related Topics in This Book
- Anticoagulant Proteins
- Fibrin Degradation Products
- Partial Thromboplastin Time, Activated
- Prothrombin Time

ABBREVIATIONS
- DIC = disseminated intravascular coagulation
- FDP = fibrin(ogen) degradation product

Suggested Reading

Bedard C, Lanveschi-Pietersma A, Dunn M. Evaluation of coagulation markers in the plasma of healthy cats and cats with asymptomatic hypertrophic cardiomyopathy. *Vet Clin Pathol* 2007; **36**: 167–172.

Griffin A, Callan MB, Shofer FS, Giger U. Evaluation of a canine D-dimer point-of-care test kit for use in samples obtained from dogs with disseminated intravascular coagulation, thromboembolic disease, and hemorrhage. *Am J Vet Res* 2003; **64**: 1562–1569.

Monreal L. D-dimer as a new test for the diagnosis of DIC and thromboembolic disease [Editorial]. *J Vet Intern Med* 2003; **17**: 757–759.

Nelson OL, Andreasen C. The utility of plasma D-dimer to identify thromboembolic disease in dogs. *J Vet Intern Med* 2003; **17**: 830–834.

Stokol T, Brooks M, Erb H, Mauldin GE. D-dimer concentrations in healthy dogs and dogs with disseminated intravascular coagulation. *Am J Vet Res* 2000; **61**: 393–398.

INTERNET RESOURCES
Cornell University, College of Veterinary Medicine: Hemostasis, http://www.diaglab.vet.cornell.edu/clinpath/modules/coags/coag.htm.

AUTHOR NAME
Tracy Stokol

DENTAL RADIOGRAPHY

 BASICS

TYPE OF PROCEDURE
Radiographic

PROCEDURE EXPLANATION AND RELATED PHYSIOLOGY
The osseous structures surrounding teeth (i.e., alveolar bone) and jaws (i.e., mandibles, maxillae) frequently need evaluation for various pathologic conditions. Intraoral radiographs provide additional information on bone loss (i.e., extent and pattern) and other changes (e. g., neoplastic, traumatic) to enable practitioners to decide on appropriate therapy.

INDICATIONS
- Ideal: full-mouth radiographs on every patient, each dental visit
- Survey: Assess the normal anatomy; use as a baseline.
- Tooth abnormalities: Assess size, structure, variation in number (i.e., absence or multiple).
- Periodontal disease: Assess the extent and nature of periodontal bone loss.
- Endodontic disease: Assess pulpal vitality—the canal width and the presence of periapical bone loss.
- Acquired diseases: Assess caries and tooth resorption.
- Trauma: Evaluate the extent of osseous and dental damage.
- Neoplasia: Evaluate the extent of osseous involvement.

CONTRAINDICATIONS
Limit radiographic exposure in pregnant animals.

POTENTIAL COMPLICATIONS
Because a complete oral examination, including periodontal probing, necessitates general anesthesia, appropriate measures should be taken to prevent anesthetic complications.

CLIENT EDUCATION
- Appropriate preanesthetic considerations should be discussed with the owner.
- A complete oral examination, including intraoral radiography, will often reveal lesions not previously anticipated during the procedure, so the owner must be available for contact to discuss appropriate therapeutic choices.

BODY SYSTEMS ASSESSED
Gastrointestinal

 PROCEDURE

PATIENT PREPARATION
Preprocedure Medication or Preparation
Preanesthetic regimen, to include appropriate antimicrobial and pain medication, as indicated

Anesthesia or Sedation
General anesthesia is required, with a cuffed endotracheal tube.

Patient Positioning
Operator preference—lateral recumbency vs dorsal or ventral

Patient Monitoring
Appropriate monitoring, as for any general anesthetic procedure

Equipment or Supplies
Radiographic Unit
Although standard units may be used with intraoral films and proper positioning of patients, the convenience of a dental unit is a great advantage.

Films
- Intraoral films: common sizes, nos. 2 and 4 (Figure 1)

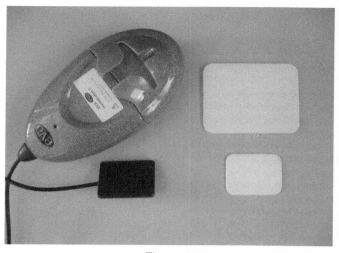

Figure 1

Commonly used intraoral films: sizes no. 4 (occlusal) and no. 2 (periapical).

- A digital sensor

Developing
- A rapid dental developer and fixer in a chairside developer
- Digital capabilities decrease the need for developing; a computer system must be available to the area.
- A viewbox
- A computer (for digital)

TECHNIQUE
- For intraoral films, the patients must be given general anesthesia, and all considerations should be met (e. g., preoperative diagnostics, patient monitoring and support).
- Positioning of the film within the oral cavity and positioning of the radiographic beam can be challenging.
- Always place the flat or white surface toward radiographic beam.
  - The lead coating on the back side of the film prevents backscatter but will be visible if the film is placed incorrectly.
  - The embossed dot on the film: The convexity faces the beam; the concavity (i.e., dimple) faces the inside the mouth.
- Place the film so the image of roots will be captured, not the crown.

Parallel Technique
- Place the intraoral film or sensor just lingual and parallel to the mandibular premolars and molars. Place the diagonal of the film across the position of the roots, with a corner sticking into the intermandibular space (Figure 2).
- Aim the radiographic beam perpendicular to both the film and the teeth.

Shadow Technique (Modified "Bisecting-Angle" Technique)
- Position the film as close to the tooth to be imaged as possible—you need to evaluate the roots, not the crown.
- If you aim the beam perpendicular to the film (Figure 3).
  - On the film, this would result in a tooth shadow or image that would be too short (like the shadow of a tree at noon).
- If you aim the beam perpendicular to tooth root(s) (Figure 4).
  - On the film, this would result in a tooth shadow or image that would be too long (like the shadow of a tree at daybreak).
- Split the difference—come halfway in-between the 2 positions (Figure 5).
  - The resulting shadow will be a compromise between the foreshortened and elongated images, with the image the approximate length of the tooth itself.

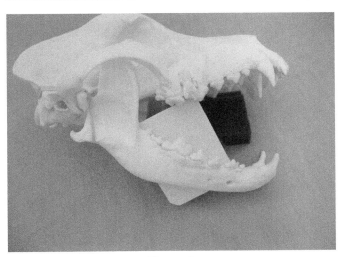

Figure 2

Parallel placement of an intraoral film to image the mandibular premolars and molars, as demonstrated on this dog skull. Note the corner is pushed into the intermandibular space.

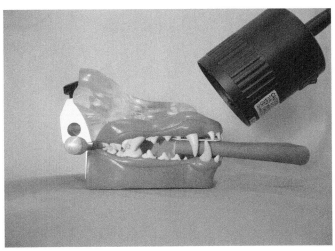

Figure 4

If the beam were aimed perpendicular to the teeth (roots), the images would be elongated.

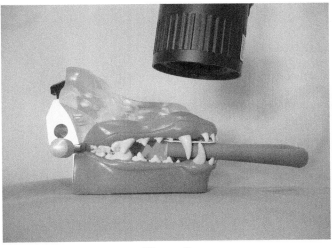

Figure 3

In imaging these maxillary incisors and canines, if the beam were aimed perpendicular to the film, the images would be foreshortened.

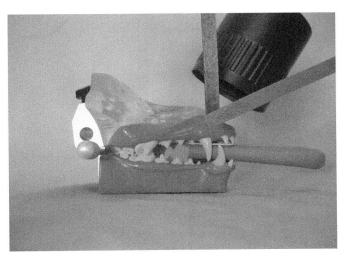

Figure 5

By splitting the difference between the 2 positions, the images will be closer to the actual size of the structures, minimizing distortion. The radiographic aid is placed with a stick perpendicular to the film and a stick is perpendicular to the tooth (root). The beam is aimed midway between the 2 sticks.

- In the images, a positioning device was made of 2 tongue depressors. A blue portion is aimed perpendicular to the film, and the red portion is aimed perpendicular to the tooth root. The X-ray beam or source is then positioned midway between the 2.
- When positioning the beam, ensure that it is aimed directly over the tooth (i.e., maxillary fourth premolar) or at midline (i.e., mandibular or maxillary incisors and canines for symmetry).
- Adjust the beam (laterally or obliquely for canines or mesially or distally for premolars) to "move" the superimposed apices away from each other.
- Hints
  - Maxillary incisors and canines of most dogs and cats (not brachycephalic breeds): Align the flat end of a positioning device (blue) to be parallel to the ventral fold of the nares (or haired portion of muzzle just under the nares) (Figure 6). In many cases, this will closely

approximate the correct beam alignment. Position the beam initially based on the nares and confirm the angle.
  - The use of intraoral film of the maxillary premolars in cats can be challenging.
- With a small feline mouth gag in place, adjust the head so the downside maxillary teeth are flat against the towel on the table and place the film outside of the mouth, slightly dorsal in relation to the teeth.
- Aim the beam from above, at a slightly oblique angle, so the image of the downside maxillary premolars will be projected on the film beneath (follow the beam), and the upside maxillary teeth will not be superimposed (Figure 7). Note or mark the film as extraoral for later identification purposes.

DENTAL RADIOGRAPHY

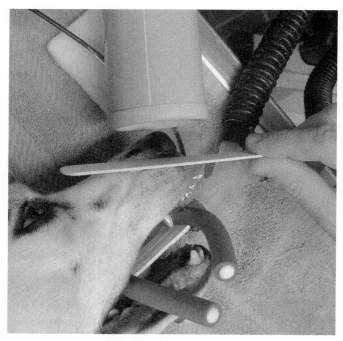

Figure 6

In most dogs (not brachycephalic) and even some cats, by aiming the beam perpendicular to the ventral aspect of the nasal fold, the positioning will be adequate (approximates the split-the-difference position).

Developing Films
• Films can be developed in an automatic processor and taped to the lead edge of a larger film but can be lost within the unit.
• Small containers with rapid developing and fixing solutions and water can be placed in the darkroom for hand dipping.
• Dental automatic processors can be used.
• A chairside developer with rapid developing and fixing solutions can easily be used at the dental area.
  • Film and clip are carried into the chamber, and the lid is secured, the film packet opened, and the film removed from packet and clip attached to the edge of the film.
  • The film is agitated in the developer.
    • Time depends on temperature and the strength of solution.
    • Spot develop: Observe developing changes through a safety top; when there is no further color change, advance to the water rinse and then fixer.
  • Fix at least twice as long as the developing time. If indistinct images or green discoloration result, fix longer.
  • Rinse thoroughly! Precipitates may form after drying if not completely rinsed.
  • Store in envelopes, mount the radiographs once they are completely dry.

SAMPLE HANDLING
None, other than radiographic film process as described in technique section

APPROPRIATE AFTERCARE
Postprocedure Patient Monitoring
Appropriate for general anesthesia
Nursing Care
None
Dietary Modification
None

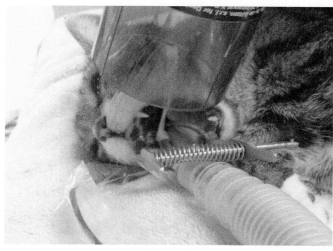

Figure 7

Another method of imaging the maxillary premolars in cats. Place the film or sensor below the head (extraoral) to image the downside premolars. Use a mouth gag and turn the head slightly oblique to avoid superimposition of the upside premolars. The film should be placed slightly dorsal to the position of the teeth, since an oblique film will be taken. Aim the beam across the head, aligning the beam with the teeth so the image will be captured on the film.

Medication Requirements
None
Restrictions on Activity
None
Anticipated Recovery Time
None. Recovery is immediate.

INTERPRETATION

NORMAL FINDINGS OR RANGE
• Reading films
  • Look at films with the dot coming out toward you.
  • This will be a view of the facial surfaces (i.e., vestibular, labial, buccal), as if you were doing an oral exam.
  • *Note*: Digital radiographs are taken and viewed from this orientation.
• Determine whether the image is of the maxilla or mandible and position the roots accordingly (i.e., mandibular roots pointing downward, maxillary roots pointing upward).
• Identify teeth—premolar vs molar—to determine nose to tail orientation.
  • From there, you can determine whether the image is of the right or left side (Figure 8).
  • Use of a panoramic dental chart or skull may help in determining this.
• *Exception*: Extraoral film taken of feline maxillary premolars—right and left—will be opposite as compared to an intraoral film (Figure 9).

ABNORMAL VALUES
Periodontal Disease
Assess the Extent
• Estimate the percentage of attachment loss to determine the stage of periodontal disease.
• Extensive bone loss may alert you to compromised jaw strength if extractions are planned.

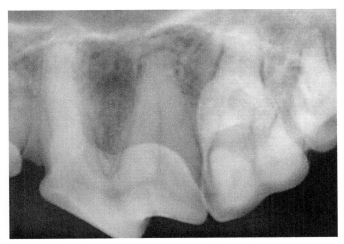

Figure 8

Reading a radiograph. (1) Find the dot: Place the film so you are looking with the dot coming out toward you. The surface of the film now facing you is the facial surface. (2) Identify whether the image is of the maxillary or mandibular, and adjust film so the roots point accordingly. (3) Determine which is the rostral extent and which is the caudal extent of the film. (4) Determine left or right. This film is maxillary, front to back—from left to right—fourth premolar to first molar, or left maxillary fourth premolar and first molar.

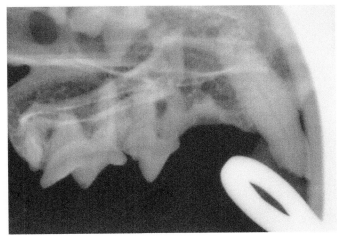

Figure 9

Feline right maxillary premolars. An extraoral film is read just the opposite: Right and left will be reversed as compared to an intraoral film.

Assess the Pattern of Bone Loss
• Crestal bone loss: loss of osseous height or flattening in-between teeth or in furcation. One of the indicators of initial periodontal bone loss.
• Horizontal bone loss: a pattern of bone loss across several roots or teeth in a flattened or scalloped loss. If accompanied by gingival recession, this will result in root or furcation exposure or both.
• Vertical bone loss: a pattern of bone loss extending down the axis of a root or roots that often is associated with a deep infrabony pocket. If the loss extends to periapical region, pulp can be compromised.

Endodontic Disease
• Periapical bone loss likely indicates extension of pulpal infection into the periapical region.

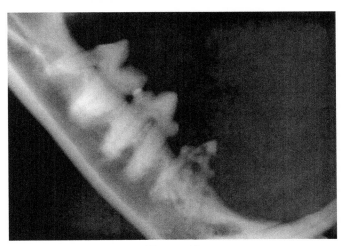

Figure 10

An odontoclastic lesion of feline teeth needs to be assessed radiographically, often in the presence of root resorption with indistinguishable root, periodontal ligament space, and alveolar bone.

• Canal width: Disproportionate canal width (larger) as compared to a similar tooth may indicate the pulp is nonvital (the dentin is no longer being deposited).

Tooth Resorption (Primarily Cats)
• Evaluate distinctions between tooth, periodontal ligament space, and bone.
• In true odontoclastic lesions, often the root structure is difficult to distinguish from surrounding bone, and no distinct periodontal ligament space is visible (Figure 10).
• In some cases where periodontal disease and attachment loss (i.e., gingiva, bone) have exposed roots, there can be resorption, but the remaining root structure is intact, distinguishable from surrounding bone, and even separated from it by an intact periodontal ligament space.

Operative Evaluation
Preextraction
• Evaluate the integrity of the periodontal ligament space: Its absence may indicate resorption or ankylosis, so typical extraction with periodontal ligament elevation may not be possible.
• Evaluate any abnormalities such as extra roots, abnormally shaped roots (dilacerated), or compromised bone.

Trauma
• Intraoral films can target specific areas of traumatic damage.
• Sometimes full skull radiographs provide a broader picture of the extent of damage.

Neoplasia
Any suspicious lesion should be radiographed and biopsied.

CRITICAL VALUES
None

INTERFERING FACTORS
Drugs That May Alter Results of the Procedure
None

Conditions That May Interfere with Performing the Procedure
The presence of foreign bodies or metal-containing prophy pastes may show as foreign objects.

Procedure Techniques or Handling That May Alter Results
Improper angulation will distort the image.

DENTAL RADIOGRAPHY

Influence of Signalment on Performing and Interpreting the Procedure

Species
None

Breed
None

Age
None

Gender
None

Pregnancy
- Appropriate considerations for general anesthesia
- Protect the patient and avoid excessive exposure to radiation.

CLINICAL PERSPECTIVE
Intraoral radiography is essential in evaluating oral or dental disease in conjunction with other assessments (e. g., probing, examination).

MISCELLANEOUS

ANCILLARY TESTS
A complete oral examination, including probing

SYNONYMS
Intraoral radiology

SEE ALSO
Blackwell's Five-Minute Veterinary Consult: Canine and Feline Topics
Multiple dental topics

Related Topics in This Book
- General Principles of Radiography
- Gingival Sulcus Measurement

Suggested Reading
DeForge DH, Colmery BH. *Atlas of Veterinary Dental Radiology.* Ames: Iowa State University Press, 2000.
Holmstrom SE, Frost Fitch P, Eisner ER. *Veterinary Dental Techniques,* 3rd ed. Philadelphia: WB Saunders, 2004.
Wiggs RB, Lobprise HB. *Veterinary Dentistry: Principles and Practice.* Philadelphia: Lippincott-Raven, 1997.

INTERNET RESOURCES
None

AUTHOR NAME
Heidi B. Lobprise

BASICS

TYPE OF SPECIMEN
Tissue

TEST EXPLANATION AND RELATED PHYSIOLOGY
Dermatophytes are fungi that grow in the keratinized layers of hair, skin, and nails. Symptoms are variable in dogs and cats and include alopecia, both localized and diffuse, scaling, and crusting. Most animals recover after treatment; however, immunodeficient animals can have severe disseminated dermatophyte infections. Many animals can also be asymptomatic carriers of dermatophytes and infect other animals or infect people. *Microsporum canis* is seen most frequently and accounts for ≈90% of infections in cats. Other common dermatophytes in small animals include *Trichophyton mentagrophytes* and *Microsporum gypseum*.

Diagnosis is based on using specialized dermatophyte media to culture fungus from hair, skin scrape or, rarely, skin biopsy sample. Identification of genus and species is based on macroscopic examination of the color of the surface and reverse side of fungal colonies, and microscopic examination of hyphae, macroconidia, and microconidia. For in-clinic screening, there is the Dermatophyte Test Media (DTM; Remel, Lenexa, KS), which includes a fungal nutrient, bacterial and saprophytic inhibitors, and a phenol red indicator. Colonies usually appear within 5–7 days after inoculation. Dermatophytes produce alkaline metabolites, which turn phenol in DTM agar red as soon as growth appears. Positive DTM cultures can be sent to a reference laboratory for organism identification. Diagnosis should not be based solely on a DTM red color change, because this can lead to a false-positive diagnosis of dermatophytosis.

INDICATIONS
- Apruritic to pruritic alopecia
- Cats: miliary dermatitis and almost any other dermatitis
- Dogs: folliculitis, furunculosis, and most cases of alopecia

CONTRAINDICATIONS
None

POTENTIAL COMPLICATIONS
None

CLIENT EDUCATION
Zoonotic potential

BODY SYSTEMS ASSESSED
Dermatalogic

SAMPLE

COLLECTION
Material can be collected several ways:
- Pluck the hair from around infected area or pluck the hairs that fluorescence apple green when viewed under a Wood's lamp.
- Scrap the skin of infected area. Use a sterile blade to collect material from infected nails.
- Use a sterile toothbrush to brush around infected areas.
- A skin biopsy sample can be sent to the lab for culturing (rare).

HANDLING
- If sending material to a reference lab:
  - Submit plucked hair in an envelope to keep the hair dry and free of moisture.
  - Submit a skin scrape sample in a plain red-top tube, sterile container, or a sterile swab (e.g., BD CultureSwab; Becton-Dickinson, Franklin Lakes, NJ).
  - Submit a sterile toothbrush in a sterile container.
  - Submit a skin biopsy sample in sterile saline.
- Inoculate DTM by gently pressing the hair, toothbrush bristles, or material from the skin scrape into agar.
- If sending positive DTM cultures to a reference lab, check for special shipping requirements.

STORAGE
Store materials in a dark place at room temperature and send to them to the lab within 1 day to prevent bacterial overgrowth.

STABILITY
Two days at room temperature

PROTOCOL
DTM cultures
- Inoculate the dermatophyte culture material with hair or material from the skin scrape.
- Incubate at room temperature for up to 2 weeks.
- Check the culture daily for growth: the surrounding medium turns red.
- Examine the gross appearance of the fungal colony.
- Prepare a thin smear of material from the colony and examine the material microscopically (either stained with lactophenol cotton blue or unstained), looking at features of hyphae and macroconidia to identify genus and species of dermatophyte (see the table in this chapter).

DERMATOPHYTE CULTURE

INTERPRETATION

NORMAL FINDINGS OR RANGE
Negative culture

ABNORMAL VALUES
Dermatophytes are diagnosed on the basis of colony morphology, hyphae, macroconidia, and microconidia.

CRITICAL VALUES
None

INTERFERING FACTORS

Drugs That May Alter Results or Interpretation
Drugs That Interfere with Test Methodology
None

Drugs That Alter Physiology
Steroids can worsen clinical dermatophytosis.

Disorders That May Alter Results
None

Collection Techniques or Handling That May Alter Results
None

Influence of Signalment
Species
Microsporum canis is seen in 90% of cats.

Breed
More common in long-haired cats

Age
Often seen in puppies and kittens

Gender
None

Pregnancy
Subclinical queens and bitches can become symptomatic during pregnancy.

LIMITATIONS OF THE TEST
• Some false negatives: Some dermatophyte species are difficult to culture.
• Bacterial and saprophytic fungal overgrowth is common.
• The microscopic exam is critical because saprophytic fungi can turn DTM agar red, potentially causing a false-positive interpretation.

Sensitivity, Specificity, and Positive and Negative Predictive Values
N/A

Valid If Run in a Human Lab?
Yes.

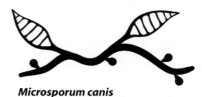

Microsporum canis

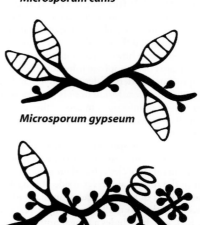

Microsporum gypseum

Trichophyton mentagrophytes

Figure 1

Microscopic appearance of common dermatophytes found in dogs and cats.

Causes of Abnormal Findings

Identifying features of common dermatophytes in dogs and cats		
	Gross appearance of the colony	Hyphae and conidia (see Figure 1)
Microsporum canis	Top: white, fluffy with yellowish pigment around edges Reverse side: deep yellow to tan	Septate hyphae with numerous macroconidia Macroconidia usually have >6 compartments
Microsporum gypseum	Top: cottony white center Reverse side: yellow to brownish	Septate hyphae Conidia with rounded edges and <6 compartments
Trichophyton mentagrophytes	Top: buff to white Reverse side: tan to brown	Septate hyphae Cigar-shaped conidia with clusters of conidiophores

CLINICAL PERSPECTIVE

• Although cats can present with classic circular alopecia, they are likely to have dermatophysis throughout the hair coat. Some cats are extremely pruritic, whereas others are not. Scaling can be multifocal to diffuse. Clinical signs can vary from a miliary dermatitis to alopecia and scaling that may appear symmetrical, or circular, on the inner and outer pinnae.

• Dogs usually develop focal lesions of alopecia with folliculitis, and furunculosis with scales and crusts. Some dogs develop a nodular lesion (kerion).

• Histopathologic evaluation of a lesion can demonstrate the presence of a fungus but cannot specifically identify it.

MISCELLANEOUS

ANCILLARY TESTS

• Wood's lamp
  • This can result in overdiagnosis because epidermal scales and sebum often produce fluorescence.
  • Not all pathogenic dermatophytes show fluorescence.
• Skin biopsy

SYNONYMS

Ringworm culture

SEE ALSO

Blackwell's Five-Minute Veterinary Consult: Canine and Feline Topics
• Alopecia—Cats
• Alopecia—Dogs
• Dermatophytosis

Related Topics in This Book
• Skin Biopsy
• Skin Surface and Otic Cytology
• Wood's Lamp Examination

ABBREVIATIONS

DTM = Dermatophyte Test Media

Suggested Reading

DeBoer JD, Moriello KA. Cutaneous fungal infections. In: Greene C, ed. *Infectious Diseases of the Dog and Cat*, 3rd ed. St Louis: Saunders Elsevier, 2005: 550–569.

Larone DH. Medically Important Fungi: A Guide to Identification, 3rd ed. Washington, DC: ASM, 1995.

Scott DW, Miller WH, Griffin CE, eds. *Muller and Kirk's Small Animal Dermatology*, 6th ed. Philadelphia: WB Saunders, 2001: 336–422.

INTERNET RESOURCES

None

AUTHOR NAME

Terri Wheeler

DESMOPRESSIN RESPONSE TEST

BASICS

TYPE OF PROCEDURE
Function test

PROCEDURE EXPLANATION AND RELATED PHYSIOLOGY
In normal animals, ADH, also known as arginine vasopressin, is produced in the hypothalamus and then stored and released from the posterior pituitary in response to increasing osmolality and decreasing blood volume. ADH then travels in the vasculature to the kidneys and, at the level of the nephron, binds to receptors on cells of the collecting ducts to promote water reabsorption. The result is total body water retention and increasing urine concentration.

Although many diagnostic tests are readily available for the identification of common causes of polyuria and polydipsia, some of the rarer causes require specific function tests to diagnose. To assess the renal responsiveness to ADH, a synthetic analog of vasopressin, called desmopressin, can be administered and the subsequent response monitored. Desmopressin has similar activity to endogenous ADH on the kidneys, with a longer-lasting effect and minimal direct hypertensive effect.

INDICATIONS
To distinguish central diabetes insipidus (CDI) from primary nephrogenic diabetes insipidus (NDI) and psychogenic polydipsia

CONTRAINDICATIONS
A relative contraindication exists for patients that have not been evaluated for other common causes of polyuria and polydipsia because it may delay a proper diagnosis.

POTENTIAL COMPLICATIONS
• Allergic reaction to the synthetic vasopressin analog
• Conjunctival inflammation occasionally occurs with conjunctival application.
• Hypervolemia or water intoxication. This is a particular concern in patients that retain water in response to desmopressin but also have altered thirst regulation and continue to drink large quantities of water (occasionally psychogenic polydipsic dogs and rarely those with CDI).

CLIENT EDUCATION
• Medication used for the testing can be costly and is also the primary long-term therapy for CDI.
• The animal must receive all of the medication as prescribed for accurate interpretation of the results.
• Additional testing may be required to determine the underlying etiology.

BODY SYSTEMS ASSESSED
• Endocrine
• Renal and urologic

PROCEDURE

PATIENT PREPARATION
Preprocedure Medication or Preparation
• With the desmopressin response test, the owner should determine an average 24-h water intake (if not already determined). This is done by providing water in previously measured bowls, refilling as often as needed so as not to restrict the total volume, and recording the volume of water consumed by the patient over a 24-h period. This process is repeated for 2 more 24-h periods, and then the volumes for the 24-h periods are averaged. Normal water consumption is <60 mL/kg/day, and abnormal is >100 mL/kg/day, with volumes in between being in a gray zone.

• The owner should avoid changing the patient's diet, particularly avoiding foods with a high salt content or extreme protein restriction during the test.

Anesthesia or Sedation
None

Patient Positioning
None

Patient Monitoring
• As the testing is performed in the home environment, the owner should be instructed on observing mentation changes, which might suggest water intoxication.
• The owner should also observe signs of polyuria and polydipsia in order to aid in determination of the success of the trial.

Equipment or Supplies
• Desmopressin acetate. This medication is available in one of three forms: intranasal spray, injection, or oral tablets. No veterinary products exist, so human formulations are used in an extralabel fashion by veterinarians and require a prescription. The trade name is DDAVP (Rhone-Poulenc Rorer, Collegeville, PA), although generics may be available for some forms. The intranasal preparation is available in 2.5- and 5-mL bottles at a concentration of 100 μg/mL. Although this can be administered effectively intranasally in dogs and cats, it appears far easier to administer this form into the conjunctival sac and achieve similar responses. One drop is $\approx$5 μg. The injectable desmopressin is available in either 4- or 15-μg/mL strengths; however, because of the cost, many veterinarians have used the intranasal preparation successfully for SC administration. While the intranasal formulation is not considered sterile and should thus not be used for IV administration, standard aseptic technique should be used when desmopressin is administered by injection. Also available are 0.1- and 0.2-mg oral tablets, with the 0.1 mg being approximately equivalent to a 5-μg dose of intranasal desmopressin. As the bioavailability of the oral formulation appears substantially less than that of the intranasal formulation for humans, preference for the latter exists in the desmopressin trial. Should the oral formulation be used and the expected response is not apparent, repeat testing with the intranasal formulation is recommended.
• A clean container for urine collection if a urine sample is going to be obtained prior to return to the veterinary hospital
• A calibrated refractometer

TECHNIQUE
• The owner begins administering desmopressin at a dose of 1–4 drops of the intranasal preparation (1 drop for cats) into the conjunctival sac every 12 h for 5–7 days. Alternatives include using the oral medication at a dose of 0.05–0.2 mg orally every 8 h or having the owner administer the intranasal solution SC at a dose of 5 μg twice daily. (It may be better tolerated in some cats than conjunctival administration.)
• The owner continues to offer food and water as before the trial. Although water consumption in general is not restricted, caution should be taken to ensure that the animal does not consume extremely large amounts of water immediately after desmopressin administration.
• A repeat 24-h water-intake measurement should be determined by the owner on about days 5–7. Although some animals may have a response faster than 5–7 days, the longer period allows for greater resolution of possible concurrent medullary washout.
• Additionally, at the end of the trial period, while the patient is still receiving medication, its urine should be collected either by the owner or the veterinarian about 2–4 h after the morning dose for measurement of urine specific gravity and osmolality.

SAMPLE HANDLING
Urine collected at home by the owner should be stored in an airtight container and refrigerated until brought to the veterinarian for testing.

APPROPRIATE AFTERCARE

Postprocedure Patient Monitoring
None

Nursing Care
None

Dietary Modification
None

Medication Requirements
To control clinical signs in patients with CDI, administration of DDAVP may need to be continued after the trial.

Restrictions on Activity
None

Anticipated Recovery Time
N/A

INTERPRETATION

NORMAL FINDINGS OR RANGE
Animals that have a decrease in water consumption by $\geq$50% are considered to have an ADH response. This could include normal animals as well as animals with varying degrees of central diabetes insipidus.

ABNORMAL VALUES
• A lack of change in water consumption or a urine specific gravity of <1.008 following the desmopressin response test suggests an ADH-unresponsive disorder, which would be consistent with NDI or psychogenic polydipsia (due to the lack of impact of desmopressin on thirst centers).
• An increase in urine specific gravity to between 1.008 and 1.020 is considered a partial response, and an increase in urine specific gravity to >1.020 is considered a complete response and consistent with CDI.
• Patients with hyperadrenocorticism tested with a desmopressin response test also may show increases in their urine specific gravity similar to those in dogs with partial or complete CDI.

CRITICAL VALUES
None

INTERFERING FACTORS

Drugs That May Alter Results of the Procedure
• Concurrent administration of heparin may decrease the effectiveness of desmopressin.
• Concurrent administration of fludrocortisone may enhance the effectiveness.

Conditions That May Interfere with Performing the Procedure
Conditions known to causes polyuria and polydipsia—including renal failure, hypercalcemia, hypokalemia, pyelonephritis, liver insufficiency, diabetes mellitus, pyometra (and prostatitis), primary renal glycosuria, hyperthyroidism, hyperadrenocorticism, and hypoadrenocorticism—all can cause abnormal results and should be treated and controlled prior to evaluating patients with a desmopressin response test.

Procedure Techniques or Handling That May Alter Results
Desmopressin solutions should be refrigerated. Failure to do so may lead to inactive medication and lack of response.

Influence of Signalment on Performing and Interpreting the Procedure

Species
None

Breed
None

Age
Renal development continues after birth for several weeks in both puppies and kittens. Although their urine-concentrating ability by 2 months of age approaches that of adults, caution should used in diagnosing partial central diabetes insipidus in immature animals with a urine specific gravity of >1.015 to <1.030 following a desmopressin response test, because maximal concentrating ability may not be reached until 3–4 months of age.

Gender
None

Pregnancy
The safety of desmopressin use in pregnant animals has not been established.

CLINICAL PERSPECTIVE
• The desmopressin response test is relatively simple.
• Several routinely available diagnostics should be performed to identify the cause of polydipsia and polyuria in patients prior to undertaking a desmopressin response test such that the remaining differentials include CDI, primary NDI, and psychogenic polydipsia.
• Performing a modified water-deprivation test prior to or following the desmopressin response test may be required to distinguish psychogenic polydipsia from NDI.
• Due to the relatively common occurrence of hyperadrenocorticism in dogs and the potential for misdiagnosis as partial CDI based on the desmopressin response test, a thorough evaluation for typical or atypical hyperadrenocorticism ideally should be performed prior to initiation of a desmopressin response test or, less optimally, after the desmopressin response test, if the results are consistent with partial CDI.

MISCELLANEOUS

ANCILLARY TESTS
• Modified water-deprivation test
• Pituitary imaging (magnetic resonance imaging or computed tomography)
• Random plasma and urine osmolality evaluation

SYNONYMS
• DDAVP trial
• Desmopressin trial

SEE ALSO
Blackwell's Five-Minute Veterinary Consult: Canine and Feline Topics
• Diabetes Insipidus
• Hyposthenuria
• Polyuria and Polydipsia

Related Topics in This Book
Water-Deprivation Test, Modified

ABBREVIATIONS
• ADH = antidiuretic hormone
• CDI = central diabetes insipidus
• DDAVP = brand name of desmopressin
• NDI = nephrogenic diabetes insipidus

Suggested Reading
Feldman EC, Nelson RW. Water metabolism and diabetes insipidus. In: Feldman EC, Nelson RW, eds. *Canine and Feline Endocrinology and Reproduction*, 3rd ed. Philadelphia: WB Sanders, 2004: 2–44.

DESMOPRESSIN RESPONSE TEST

Nichols R: Clinical use of the vasopressin analogue DDAVP for the diagnosis and treatment of diabetes insipidus. In: Bonagura JD, ed. *Kirk's Current Veterinary Therapy XIII: Small Animal Practice.* Philadelphia: WB Saunders, 2000: 325–326.

INTERNET RESOURCES
None

AUTHOR NAME
Nathan L. Bailiff

BASICS

TYPE OF SPECIMENS
Blood
Tissue
Urine

TEST EXPLANATION AND RELATED PHYSIOLOGY
Canine distemper virus (CDV) is highly contagious and causes a multisystemic disease that commonly affects the respiratory, GI system and central nervous system (CNS). It remains 1 of the most important viral diseases of dogs, producing high morbidity and mortality in unvaccinated populations worldwide. Antemortem diagnosis is not straightforward and requires an understanding of disease pathogenesis. Initial respiratory infection rapidly spreads to regional lymph nodes within 24 h. After the first week, further spread to the CNS and epithelial tissues (skin, GI, respiratory, genitourinary, exocrine, and endocrine glands) depends on the virulence of the virus strain, the dog's age and immune status. There are a variety of tests available to aid in diagnosing this infection.

Identification of Viral Antigen
The sensitivity of these tests is highly dependent on timing in relation to the onset of clinical signs. Viral particles/antigen can be found in circulating leukocytes early in the course of infection, often before the onset of clinical signs. From the onset of clinical signs, CDV antigen may disappear from the conjunctiva and genital epithelium within days to 1 week. CDV antigen may be detected for longer in macrophages and lower respiratory tract epithelium.

Light Microscopy
In the early stages of disease, cytoplasmic viral inclusion bodies may be detected in small numbers of circulating lymphocytes and occasional monocytes, neutrophils and erythrocytes. Inclusions are large (up to 3 μm) round to oval, and vary in color from blue-gray to purple. Inclusions can be easier to see with Diff-Quick as compared to Wright stain. Evaluation of buffy coat preparations may improve the chance of finding cells with inclusions. Depending on clinical signs and stage of infection, intracytoplasmic inclusions may be found in some epithelial cells (conjunctiva, urinary bladder) or occasionally in cells found in CSF.

Immunofluorescence Assay/ELISA
Direct immunofluorescence assays (dIFAs) can be used to detect CDV antigen in cytological smears prepared from conjunctiva, tonsils, genital or respiratory epithelium, whole blood, buffy coat, Cerebrospinal Fluid (CSF), urine sediment or bone marrow. These tests are highly specific and more reliable than routine light microscopy, but sensitivity depends on clinical signs and stage of infection and they are most useful in dogs with acute distemper. They are often unhelpful in cases where clinical onset is delayed or in chronic encephalitis. Bench top ELISA kits to detect CDV antigen have also been developed for in-clinic use.

Histopathology and Immunohistochemistry (IHC)
Histologic examination reveals intranuclear and intracytoplasmic eosinophilic inclusion bodies in numerous tissues. Biopsies from footpads, nasal mucosa or skin from the dorsal neck have been used to reliably diagnose Canine distemper (CD). In general, IHC demonstration of CDV antigen is superior to reliance on detection of cellular inclusion bodies, but in cases of chronic distemper, viral antigens are not always detected. For postmortem diagnosis collection of lungs, spleen, eyes, tonsils, stomach, small intestines, liver, urinary bladder and brain is recommended for immunohistochemical detection of CDV antigen within formalin-fixed paraffin-embedded tissue.

Measurement of Anti-CDV Antibodies in Serum and CSF
Demonstration of anti-CDV Ab in serum alone is of limited value for diagnosing CD, although titers of neutralization Abs do correlate with protection from infection. Increases in serum anti-CDV IgM occur in many dogs in the early stages of acute disease (81%) but also occur in dogs up to 3 weeks after first vaccination. Anti-CDV IgG is detected in vaccinated dogs as well as those naturally infected with CDV making interpretation difficult. However, increased anti-CDV Ab in CSF compared with serum may be helpful in diagnosing chronic forms of CD.

Identification of Viral RNA
Various methods have been used to detect CDV RNA, the most recently real-time reverse transcriptase–PCR (qRT-PCR). RNA detection is highly specific and a valuable antemortem test for CD in acute and chronic cases. Assay sensitivity depends on the sample used, collection technique, stage of disease, method of nucleic acid extraction, primers and PCR method. In acute cases, buffy coat or conjunctival swab is most useful while urine, whole blood, serum, or CSF can be used in chronic cases. In some studies, RT-PCR of urine has been more sensitive than serum or whole blood and equally sensitive to CSF in detecting CDV, even in neurologic forms of disease. Tissue sections including footpads, CNS and bladder can also be used to detect CDV nucleic acid. CDV has been detected in the blood of clinically normal puppies up to 10 days after vaccination with a modified live vaccine, so care needs to be taken in the interpretation of results from these patients.

Viral Isolation
Tissues can be cultured in canine blood lymphocytes or pulmonary macrophages and examined for cytopathic effects of CDV. Culture is unsuccessful with chronic distemper or vaccine induced encephalitis. This is generally a research tool, not commercially available.

INDICATIONS
To support a diagnosis of CD suggested by clinical presentation, signalment, and history

Peracute Form
Fever and sudden death

Acute Form
- Fever
- Severe leucopenia
- Conjunctivitis
- Respiratory disease: coughing due to catarrhal inflammation of larynx, bronchi, tonsils
- GI disease: severe vomiting, watery diarrhea
- CNS disease: behavioral changes, local myoclony, tonic-clonic spasms, ataxia, paresis

Subacute Neurologic Form
- Encephalitis with convulsions and seizures
- May follow from acute manifestations or appear after subclinical infection
- Surviving dogs have CNS sequelae (e.g., nervous ticks or involuntary leg movements)

Late Form, Seen in Old Dogs
- May occur without history of earlier acute or subacute disease
- Encephalitis with slow progressive loss of neurologic function
- Hard-pad disease: hyperkeratosis of footpads and nose

CONTRAINDICATIONS
None

POTENTIAL COMPLICATIONS
None

CLIENT EDUCATION
Widespread vaccination has significantly reduced the incidence of CD although cases still occur in unvaccinated dogs and occasionally in vaccinated dogs. Unvaccinated dogs or ferrets in the same household as an affected dog are potentially at greater risk. The virus is fragile in the environment, lasting only a few hours at room temperature (20°C) and is susceptible to common household disinfectants.

BODY SYSTEMS ASSESSED
- Dermatologic
- Gastrointestinal
- Hemic, lymphatic, and immune
- Nervous
- Ophthalmic
- Respiratory

SAMPLE

COLLECTION
- 1–2 mL of venous blood
- 3–5 mL of urine collected by any method
- Mucus and fluid collected by tracheal wash or bronchoalveolar lavage
- 0.3–1 mL of CSF
- Tissue biopsy (e.g., footpad, haired skin of dorsal neck, nasal mucosa)
- Tissue smears (e.g., conjunctiva, tonsils, genital or respiratory epithelium, urine sediment or bone marrow)

HANDLING
- Light microscopy
  - Collect the blood into EDTA for leukocyte evaluation.
  - Prepare the blood smear at the time of collection if analysis will be delayed.
  - Process the CSF as soon as possible.
- Serology: Collect the blood or CSF into plain tubes or serum-separator tubes.
- dIFA: Air-dry smears of tissue and fix them in acetone for 5 min.
- Histopathology: Fix biopsied tissue in 10% buffered formalin.
- RT-PCR: Collect the samples aseptically, immediately freeze them to minimize their degradation: CDV RNA is prone to degradation from enzymes in environment and on our hands. Ship the samples on ice.
  - Place the tissue in sterile saline and then freeze it.
  - Collect the urine into plain red-top tube.
  - Collect the blood into tubes containing EDTA.

STORAGE
- Routine light microscopy
  - Refrigerate the blood and/or urine.
  - To preserve the CSF, mix an aliquot with an equal volume of the dog's serum (double the resulting cell count to correct for the dilution factor). Use remaining CSF for protein and anti-CDV Ab measurement.
  - Store the smears at room temperature, protected from light and humidity.
- Serology: Refrigerate or freeze the serum.
- PCR: Refrigerate or freeze the sample.
- dIFA: Refrigerate the slides.
- Histopathology and IHC: Store the tissue in 10% buffered formalin. For IHC, process the tissue within 12 h.

STABILITY
- Routine light microscopy
  - Refrigerated blood and CSF (stabilized with serum) are stable for ≈1–2 days.
  - Stained smears are stable for months to years.
- Serology and PCR
  - Refrigerated (4°C) serum: several days
  - Frozen (−20°C): months to years
- IHC: ≤12 h in formalin
- dIFA: fixed smears, 3–5 days if refrigerated

INTERPRETATION

NORMAL FINDINGS OR RANGE
- Uninfected animals should be negative for viral antigen by all methods.
- Positive IgG Ab titers are seen in healthy vaccinated dogs.
- Positive IgM Ab titers are seen for ≈3 weeks after vaccination.

ABNORMAL VALUES
- Viral antigen detected by any method is consistent with a current infection.
- Serology

- A high IgM titer
- A convalescent IgG Ab titer that is 4-fold greater than the acute titer
- A CSF Ab titer that is greater than the serum Ab titer

CRITICAL VALUES
None

INTERFERING FACTORS
Drugs That May Alter Results or Interpretation
Drugs That Interfere with Test Methodology
None

Drugs That Alter Physiology
Vaccination can increase Ab titers. Modified live vaccine can cause a transiently positive PCR assay result.

Disorders That May Alter Results
None

Collection Techniques or Handling That May Alter Results
- Ab titers in CSF significantly contaminated with peripheral blood may reflect serum levels.
- Decreased IHC sensitivity with prolonged tissue fixation in formalin

Influence of Signalment
Species
Dogs

Breed
None

Age
Unvaccinated dogs 3–6 months of age are most susceptible as maternal Abs wane. However, all immunonaive dogs are potentially susceptible to CDV.

Gender
None

Pregnancy
None

LIMITATIONS OF THE TEST
Sensitivity, Specificity, and Positive and Negative Predictive Values
RT-PCR sensitivity depends on sample type and handling, stage of disease, choice of primers, and nucleic acid extraction method.
- Overall sensitivity: 54%–100%
- Urine reported to have 100% sensitivity and high specificity (assuming stringent methods)
- CSF: 88%–92%
- Serum: 54%–86%
- Whole blood: 88%
- Buffy coat: 63%

Valid If Run in a Human Lab?
No.

CLINICAL PERSPECTIVE
- Selection of sample sites should reflect the clinical presentation. Dogs with epithelial manifestations of disease should have these sites tested, whereas sampling epithelial sites of dogs with only neurologic signs is unrewarding (with the exception of urine).
- A negative result does not exclude a diagnosis of CD.
- The sensitivity of diagnostic tests is influenced by the manifestation and duration of clinical illness, as well as by the sample handling and transport. Consultation with the intended laboratory for sample requirements is essential.

MISCELLANEOUS

SYNONYMS
- Canine distemper (CD)
- Canine distemper virus (CDV)

SEE ALSO

Blackwell's Five-Minute Veterinary Consult: Canine and Feline Topics

Canine Distemper

Related Topics in This Book

None

ABBREVIATIONS

- Ab = antibody
- CD = canine distemper
- CDV = canine distemper virus
- CNS = central nervous system
- CSF = cerebrospinal fluid
- dIFA = direct immunofluorescence assay
- IHC = histopathology and immunohistochemistry
- RT-PCR = reverse transcriptase–polymerase chain reaction

Suggested Reading

Greene CE, Appel MJ. Canine distemper. In: Greene CE, ed. *Infectious Diseases of the Dog and Cat.* St Louis: Saunders Elsevier, 2006: 25–41.

Saito TB, Alfieri AA, Wosiacki SR, *et al.* Detection of canine distemper virus by reverse transcriptase–polymerase chain reaction in the urine of dogs with clinical signs of distemper encephalitis. *Res Vet Sci* 2006; **80**: 116–119.

INTERNET RESOURCES

Auburn University, College of Veterinary Medicine, Molecular Diagnostics: Canine distemper virus, http://www.vetmed.auburn.edu/index.pl/canine_distemper_virus.

University of California–Davis, Lucy Whittier Molecular & Diagnostic Core Facility, http://www.vetmed.ucdavis.edu/vme/taqmanservice/.

AUTHOR NAME

Jacqueline M. Norris

ECHOCARDIOGRAPHY

 BASICS

TYPE OF PROCEDURE
Ultrasonographic

PROCEDURE EXPLANATION AND RELATED PHYSIOLOGY
• Echocardiographic (Echo) modalities include 2-dimensional (2-D), M (motion)-mode, and Doppler Echo.
• 2-D Echo is used to qualitatively assess the heart (e.g., valves, motion) and pericardial space (e.g., effusion, neoplasia).
• M-mode Echo provides quantitative information in systole and diastole (e.g., wall thicknesses, chamber dimensions) and enables indices of myocardial function to be calculated.
• Doppler Echo identifies blood-flow direction, velocity, and turbulence, and enables noninvasive quantitative analysis of even mild valvular regurgitation, valvular stenosis, and shunts.
• M-mode, 2-D, and Doppler are used in concert to diagnose cardiac disease and monitor response to therapy. Their utility depends on accurate assessment of the patient's medical history, physical examination, thoracic radiographs, and the results of other diagnostic tests.

INDICATIONS
• Cats with murmurs after secondary disease is ruled out (e.g., hypertension, hyperthyroidism)
• Large-breed dogs with murmurs
• Cocker spaniels (both American and English) with murmurs
• Congenital heart disease
• Radiographic evidence of cardiomegaly or an abnormal cardiac silhouette
• Gallop rhythms not caused by fluid overload
• Unexplained arrhythmias (no trauma and no metabolic abnormalities)
• Muffled heart sounds or other suggestions of pericardial effusion
• Pleural effusion (e.g., chylous, transudate, modified transudate)
• Congestive heart failure (CHF) *after* stabilization
• Suspected pulmonary hypertension
• Polycythemia

CONTRAINDICATIONS
Animals in CHF should be stabilized with thoracocentesis, diuretics, vasodilators, oxygen, or any other drugs needed (e.g., antiarrhythmics) prior to Echo.

POTENTIAL COMPLICATIONS
Respiratory arrest may occur if dyspneic animals in CHF are restrained in lateral recumbency.

CLIENT EDUCATION
• Echo is not a complete test but complements thoracic radiography, electrocardiography, blood pressure measurement, and blood tests (e.g., total thyroxine) to assess cardiovascular function.
• Shaving the axillary and left apical regions of the thorax is necessary for optimal coupling of the transducer to the chest wall and imaging.
• Puppies and kittens require sedation (rarely, general anesthesia) for adequate Doppler examination.

BODY SYSTEMS ASSESSED
Cardiovascular

 PROCEDURE

PATIENT PREPARATION
Preprocedure Medication or Preparation
• Animals are shaved over the left and right axillary regions and the left cardiac apex.
• Coupling gel placed between the skin and transducer eliminates air pockets.

• Use of an Elizabethan collar on cats protects the assistant from being bitten.
• ECG electrode patches are placed on the metacarpal and metatarsal pads and secured with tape.

Anesthesia or Sedation
• Adult dogs and cats rarely need sedation.
• Puppies and adult dogs requiring sedation can be administered acepromazine (0.03 mg/kg IM) and buprenorphine (0.007 mg/kg IM) 20 min prior to Echo.
• Fractious cats may be administered acepromazine (0.1 mg/kg SC) and butorphanol (0.25 mg/kg SC) 20–30 min prior to the procedure.
• Cats with hypertrophic diseases should *not* be administered ketamine or tiletamine, because heart rate and myocardial oxygen demand increase and may precipitate arrhythmias or CHF.
• Hypotensive animals should not be sedated.
• Occasionally, kittens or fractious cats will need to be administered inhalation anesthetics for a thorough Echo examination.

Patient Positioning
Right and left lateral recumbency, using a table designed for Echo

Patient Monitoring
None unless the patient is sedated or anesthetized.

Equipment or Supplies
• A Doppler Echo machine with transducer appropriate to the size of the animal
• An Echo table
• Transducer coupling gel
• ECG electrode pads

TECHNIQUE
• The animal is held in lateral recumbency over the cutout in the Echo table. An assistant pulls the patient's bottom leg forward to move the triceps mass out of the way. Transducer coupling gel is applied to the thorax over the apex beat of the heart for imaging.
• Some cats and small dogs may be imaged while being held on the examiner's lap.
• Standard long-axis and short-axis views are obtained from both the right and left sides of the chest.

SAMPLE HANDLING
N/A

APPROPRIATE AFTERCARE
Postprocedure Patient Monitoring
N/A (unless sedated)

Nursing Care
N/A

Dietary Modification
N/A

Medication Requirements
N/A

Restrictions on Activity
N/A

Anticipated Recovery Time
N/A (unless sedated)

 INTERPRETATION

NORMAL FINDINGS OR RANGE
• Published tables are available for wall thickness and chamber dimensions correlated to body weight in dogs (Boon 2000) (see Table 1).
• There are published reports regarding the effects of breed and age variation on dogs' Echo parameters, but information is limited. Some of the reported breed normal values are listed in Table 2.
• Wall thickness and chamber dimensions for cats are published as a range for the species, with no correlation to body weight. Until more specific information is available, clinicians should interpret the results in light of

Table 1   Normal canine echocardiographic values*

	Weight (kg)										
Parameter	3	5	7	10	15	20	25	30	35	40	50
$LVID_d$ (mm)	24.6 (6.2)	27.4 (5.2)	30.0 (4.5)	32.7 (3.5)	37.1 (2.4)	41.4 (2.2)	44.8 (2.9)	48.3 (3.9)	51.7 (5.0)	54.8 (6.1)	60.7 (8.3)
$LVID_s$ (mm)	13.6 (5.5)	16.0 (4.7)	17.9 (4.0)	20.6 (3.1)	24.3 (2.1)	28.0 (2.0)	31.0 (2.5)	33.9 (3.4)	36.9 (4.5)	39.6 (5.4)	44.6 (7.4)
$LVPW_d$ (mm)	5.0 (2.1)	5.4 (1.7)	5.7 (1.5)	6.2 (1.2)	6.8 (0.8)	7.4 (0.7)	7.9 (1.0)	8.4 (1.3)	8.9 (1.7)	9.3 (2.0)	10.2 (2.8)
$LVPW_s$ (mm)	7.2 (1.7)	7.9 (1.6)	8.4 (1.4)	9.2 (1.3)	10.2 (1.1)	11.3 (1.1)	12.1 (1.2)	13.0 (1.3)	13.8 (1.5)	14.5 (1.7)	16.0 (2.2)
IVS_d (mm)	5.8 (2.1)	6.2 (1.7)	6.5 (1.5)	7.0 (1.2)	7.6 (0.8)	8.2 (0.7)	8.7 (0.9)	9.2 (1.3)	9.7 (1.7)	10.2 (2.0)	11.0 (2.7)
IVS_s (mm)	9.8 (2.6)	10.2 (2.2)	10.4 (2.0)	10.9 (1.7)	11.5 (1.2)	12.3 (1.1)	13.0 (1.5)	13.9 (2.3)	14.6 (2.6)	15.4 (3.5)	—
LA (mm)	12.7 (5.3)	14.0 (4.5)	15.0 (3.8)	16.3 (3.0)	18.3 (2.0)	20.2 (1.9)	21.8 (2.4)	23.3 (3.3)	24.8 (4.3)	26.2 (5.2)	28.8 (7.1)
Ao (mm)	13.8 (3.6)	15.3 (3.0)	16.4 (2.6)	18.1 (2.0)	20.4 (1.4)	22.8 (1.3)	24.6 (1.6)	26.4 (2.2)	28.3 (2.9)	30.0 (3.5)	33.1 (4.8)

*Fractional shortening, 28%–40%; and mitral valve E point to septal separation, <5–6 mm. Mean value given, ±SD in parentheses.
$LVID_d$, left ventricular (LV) internal dimension at end diastole; $LVID_s$, LV internal dimension at end systole; $LVPW_d$, LV posterior wall at end diastole; $LVPW_s$, LV posterior wall at end systole; IVS_d, interventricular septum at end diastole; IVS_s, interventricular septum at end systole; LA, left atrium (systole); and Ao, aortic root (diastole).
From Ware WA. Diagnostic tests for the cardiovascular system. In: Nelson RW, Couto CG, eds. Essentials of Small Animal Internal Medicine. St Louis: CV Mosby, 1992. Data from Bonagura JD, O'Grady MR, Herring DS. Echocardiography: Principles of interpretation. Vet Clin North Am Small Anim Pract 1985;15:1177–1194.

the body weight (e.g., a small cat with a diastolic wall thickness at the upper limit of the reference range may actually have cardiac hypertrophy). Some reported normal values for cats are presented in Table 3.
• Obesity complicates interpretation of Echo measurements, and estimated lean body weight correlated to the reference range may be appropriate.

ABNORMAL VALUES
See the Normal Findings or Range section.

CRITICAL VALUES
• Critical values vary with the species, breed, and size of the animal.

Table 2   Normal canine M-mode echocardiography values for eight different breeds

Mensural	Miniature poodle[1] (n = 20)*	English cocker spaniel[2] (n = 12)[†]	Pembroke Welsh corgi[1] (n = 20)*	Afghan hound[1] (n = 20)*	Golden retriever[1] (n = 20)*	Greyhound[3] (n = 16)[†]	Deerhound[5] (n = 21)[†]	Irish wolfhound[4] (n = 100)[†]
Weight (kg)	3 (1.4–9)	12.2 ± 2.2	15 (8–19)	23 (17–36)	32 (23–41)	20.7–32.5	41.3 ± 4.9	>50
Heart rate (beats/min)	150 (100–200)	—	120 (80–160)	120 (80–140)	100 (80–140)	—	125.7 ± 30	—
LVPWD (mm)	5 (4–6)	7.9 ± 1.1	8 (6–10)	9 (7–11)	10 (8–12)	12.1 ± 1.7	10.0 ± 1.8	9.5 ± 2.1
LVPWS (mm)	8 (6–10)	—	12 (8–13)	12 (9–18)	15 (10–19)	15.2 ± 2.2	15.3 ± 2.2	15.0 ± 3.3
LVD (mm)	20 (16–28)	33.8 ± 3.3	32 (28–40)	42 (33–52)	45 (37–51)	44.1 ± 3.0	51.2 ± 5.0	53.9 ± 5.2
LVS (mm)	10 (8–16)	22.2 ± 2.8	19 (12–23)	28 (20–37)	27 (18–35)	32.5 ± 3.5	34.0 ± 5.1	35.2 ± 4.8
FS (%)	47 (35–57)	34.3 ± 4.5	44 (33–57)	33 (24–48)	39 (27–55)	25.4 ± 6.3	33.5 ± 5.8	35.2 ± 4.9
EPSS (mm)	0 (0–2)	—	2 (0–5)	4 (0–10)	5 (1–10)	—	7.8 ± 1.6	7.4 ± 1.5
RV_d (mm)	4 (2–9)	—	10 (6–14)	10 (5–20)	13 (7–27)	—	22.6 ± 5.7	26.7 ± 5.3
IVS_d (mm)	5 (4–6)	8.2 ± 1.3	8 (6–9)	10 (8–12)	10 (8–13)	10.6 ± 1.7	9.1 ± 2.2	8.0 ± 1.9
IVS_s (mm)	8 (6–10)	—	12 (10–14)	13 (8–18)	14 (10–17)	13.4 ± 2.5	14.6 ± 4.1	13.7 ± 3.4
AOD (mm)	10 (8–13)	—	18 (15–22)	26 (20–34)	24 (14–27)	—	29.6 ± 3.7	30.5 ± 4.0
LAS (mm)	12 (8–18)	—	21 (12–24)	26 (18–35)	27 (16–32)	—	28.4 ± 3.9	33.7 ± 5.9

*Median (range).
[†]Mean ± standard deviation.
LVPWD, left ventricular (LV) posterior wall dimension at end diastole; LVPWS, LV posterior wall thickness at end systole; LVD, LV chamber dimension at end diastole; LVS, LV chamber dimension at end systole; FS, percent fractional shortening; EPSS, E-point septal separation; RV_d, right ventricular chamber dimension at end diastole; IVS_d, interventricular septal thickness at end diastole; IVS_s, interventricular septal thickness at end systole; AOD, aortic root at end diastole; and LAS, left atrium at end systole.

References:
1. Morrison SA, Moise NS, Scarlett JM, Mohammed H. Effect of breed and body weight on echocardiographic values of four breeds of dogs of differing weight and somatotype. J Vet Intern Med 1992;6:220–224.
2. Gooding JP, Robinson WF, Mews GC. Echocardiographic assessment of left ventricular dimensions in clinically normal English cocker spaniels. Am J Vet Res 1986;47:296–300.
3. Page A, Edmunds G, Atwell RB. Echocardiographic values in the greyhound. Aust Vet J 1993;70:361–364.
4. Vollmar A. Kardiologische Untersuchungen beim Irischen Wolfshund unter besonderer Berücksichtigung des Vorhofflimmerns und der Echokardiographie. Kleintierpraxis 1996;41:397–408.
5. Vollmar A. Kardiologische Untersuchungen beim Deerhound: Referenzwerte für die Echodiagnostik. Kleintierpraxis 1998;43:497–508.

ECHOCARDIOGRAPHY

Table 3   Normal feline echocardiographic values

Parameter	Range (unsedated)* (n = 30)	Range (sedated with ketamine)† (n = 30)
$RVID_d$ (mm)	2.7–9.4	1.2–7.5
$LVID_d$ (mm)	12.0–19.8	10.7–17.3
$LVID_s$ (mm)	5.2–10.8	4.9–11.6
SF (%)	39.0–61.0	30–60
$LVPW_d$ (mm)	2.2–4.4	2.1–4.5
$LVPW_s$ (mm)	5.4–8.1	—
IVS_d (mm)	2.2–4.0	2.2–4.9
IVS_s (mm)	4.7–7.0	—
LA (mm)	9.3–15.1	7.2–13.3
Ao (mm)	7.2–11.9	7.1–11.5
LA/Ao	0.95–1.65	0.73–1.64
EPSS (mm)	0.17–0.21	—
PEP(s)	—	0.024–0.058
LVET(s)	0.10–0.18	0.093–0.176
PEP/LVET	—	0.228–0.513
Vcf (circumf/s)	2.35–4.95	2.27–5.17

*Data from Jacobs G, Knight DH. M-mode echocardiographic measurements in nonanesthetized healthy cats: Effects of body weight, heart rate, and other variables. Am J Vet Res 1985;46:1705–1413.
†Data from Fox PR, Bond BR, Peterson ME. Echocardiographic reference values in healthy cats sedated with ketamine hydrochloride. Am J Vet Res 1985;46:1479–1484.
$RVID_d$, right ventricular internal dimension at end diastole; $LVID_d$, left ventricular (LV) internal dimension at end diastole: $LVID_s$, LV internal dimension at end systole; SF, shortening fraction; $LVPW_d$, LV posterior wall at end diastole; $LVPW_s$, LV posterior wall at end systole; IVS_d, interventricular septum at end diastole; IVS_s, interventricular septum at end systole; LA, left atrium (systole); Ao, aortic root (end diastole); EPSS, E point to septal separation; PEP(s), preejection period (seconds); LVET(s), left ventricular ejection time (seconds); and Vcf(circumf/s), velocity of circumferential fiber shortening.

• In cats, a septal or left posterior wall thickness in diastole of >6 mm is often used as a criterion for hypertrophic cardiomyopathy after systemic hypertension, hyperthyroidism, and dehydration are ruled out.

INTERFERING FACTORS

Drugs That May Alter Results of the Procedure
• Administration of ketamine may increase heart rate, increase wall thicknesses, and decrease ventricular chamber dimension and fractional shortening (FS) in cats.
• Most tranquilizers and anesthetic agents will slow heart rate and decrease FS to some degree.

Conditions That May Interfere with Performing the Procedure
• A patient's excessive panting prevents adequate visualization of the heart. Avoid the administration of oxymorphone or other drugs that cause panting.
• Poor imaging may be due to excessive obesity, pneumothorax, hyperinflation caused by chronic lung disease, or animals with a ventrodorsally compressed chest conformation.

Procedure Techniques or Handling That May Alter Results
• An inappropriate transducer frequency, a frame rate that is too slow, or a large transducer footprint may limit the ability to visualize the heart adequately.
• Oblique planes of imaging or nonstandard views will result in erroneous measurements.

Influence of Signalment on Performing and Interpreting the Procedure

Species
Reference ranges are published for cats and dogs.

Breed
• There are published reference ranges for greyhounds, Alaskan sled dogs, Irish wolfhounds, miniature poodles, Pembroke Welsh corgies, Afghan hounds, golden retrievers, and Maine coon cats.
• In dogs, recent analysis of breed-specific data (other than for sighthounds, which were few in number) did not shown significant differences in Echo measurements among breeds.
• Large-breed dogs tend to have lower normal ranges for FS than do small-breed dogs.

Age
• Changes in the growth of the heart, relative to body weight, were measured by M-mode Echo in English pointers during their first year of life.
• FS and the ratio of left atrial to aortic diameter decreased slightly, but significantly, as body weight increased.

Gender
None

Pregnancy
None

CLINICAL PERSPECTIVE
• Management of dogs or cats with cardiac disease is more likely to depend on sequential radiographs, blood work, ECG, or blood pressure measurement than repetitive Echo. (An exception is pressure-overload disease.)
• Whereas Echo is indicated to determine the etiology of a murmur or to assess cardiac function, chest radiographs are indicated to monitor CHF and response to treatment or to determine the etiology of a cough (e.g., heart vs lung disease).

MISCELLANEOUS

ANCILLARY TESTS
Thoracic radiographs, ECG, Doppler measurement of blood pressure, determination of total thyroxine level, and other blood tests

SYNONYMS
• Cardiac ultrasound
• Doppler echo

SEE ALSO
Blackwell's Five-Minute Veterinary Consult: Canine and Feline Topics
• All chapters on congenital cardiac diseases
• Atrioventricular Valve Endocardiosis
• Cardiomyopathy—Boxer
• Cardiomyopathy, Dilated—Cats
• Cardiomyopathy, Dilated—Dogs
• Cardiomyopathy, Hypertrophic—Cats
• Cardiomyopathy, Hypertrophic—Dogs
• Cardiomyopathy, Restrictive—Cats
• Endocarditis, Infective
• Endomyocardial Diseases—Cats

Related Topics in This Book
None

ABBREVIATIONS
• 2-D = 2-dimensional
• CHF = congestive heart failure
• Echo = echocardiography or echocardiographic
• FS = fractional shortening

Suggested Reading
Boon JA. *Handy Reference Veterinary Echocardiography.* Jackson, WY: Teton NewMedia, 2000.
Boon JA. *Manual of Veterinary Echocardiography.* Philadelphia: Williams & Wilkins, 1998.

Cote E. Echocardiography: Common pitfalls and practical solutions. *Clin Tech Small Anim Pract* 2005; **20**: 156–163.

Moise NS, Fox PR. Echocardiography and Doppler imaging. In: Fox PR, Sisson D, Moise NS, eds. *Textbook of Canine and Feline Cardiology*, 2nd ed. Philadelphia: WB Saunders, 1999: 130–171.

Sahn DJ, DeMaria A, Kisslo J, Weyman A. Recommendations regarding quantitation in M-mode echocardiography: Results of a survey of echocardiographic measurements. *Circulation* 1978; **58**: 1072–1083.

Thomas WP. Two-dimensional, real-time echocardiography in the dog. *Vet Radiol* 1984; **25**: 50–64.

INTERNET RESOURCES

E-chocardiography Journal: Echocardiographic images, http://www2.umdnj.edu/≈shindler/imgndx.html.

University of California–Davis, William R. Pritchard Veterinary Medical Teaching Hospital: Case studies in small animal cardiovascular medicine, http://www.vmth.ucdavis.edu/Cardio/cases/cases.htm.

Veterinary Information Network, http://www.vin.com/. Search for "echo cases."

AUTHOR NAME

Rosemary A. Henik

EHRLICHIA/ANAPLASMA

BASICS

TYPE OF SPECIMEN
Blood
Tissue

TEST EXPLANATION AND RELATED PHYSIOLOGY
Members of the family Anaplasmataceae are obligate intracellular Gram-negative bacteria that naturally infect a variety of wild and domestic animal species. Transmission is usually through ticks but may also occur via blood transfusions. The family Anaplasmataceae contains 4 genera of which the *Ehrlichia*, *Anaplasma* and, to a lesser extent, *Neorickettsia* genera are the most common cause of disease in dogs and cats. New genetic analysis has resulted in reclassification and nomenclature changes of some family members.

Most of these organisms cause a nonspecific multisystemic disorder with primary complaints being fever, lethargy, vomiting, diarrhea, and anorexia, with or without hemorrhagic tendencies. Some patients present with uveitis and/or retinal petechiae, polymyositis, polyarthritis, and central nervous system signs. These organisms are less host specific than originally thought, and cross-reactivity is common.

There are several available testing options for these organisms:

PCR
PCR is the amplification of a specific (hopefully) piece of DNA from the organism of interest. Since *Ehrlichia* and *Anaplasma* species live in WBCs or platelets (*A. platys*), EDTA-anticoagulated whole blood is the sample of choice for *Ehrlichia* and *Anaplasma* PCR testing. Aspirated bone marrow can also be analyzed. Obtain samples *before* treatment, because treatment may reduce number of organisms and result in false-negative test results.

IFA and ELISA
These are used to detect specific (hopefully) antibodies against the organism of interest. Serum is the typical sample tested for antibodies. Antibodies can be detected in other biologic samples such as synovial fluid and cerebrospinal fluid. IDEXX Laboratories (Portland, ME) offers 2 in-office assays that provide a rapid screen for antibodies to *E. canis* (Snap 3DX and Snap 4DX) and *A. phagocytophilum* (Snap 4DX). It may take a patient up to 3 or more weeks to develop antibodies potentially hindering diagnosis of acute disease.

Light Microscopy
• *Ehrlichia* and *Anaplasma* organisms may be observed in Romanovsky-stained (e.g., Wright, Diff-Quick) peripheral blood smears. They are 0.2- to 1.0-μm basophilic short rods to pleomorphic coccobacilli found singly or as clusters within host membrane-lined cytoplasmic vacuoles known as *morulae*. The different organisms preferentially infect certain blood cells, including neutrophils and eosinophils (*A. phagocytophilum*, *E. ewingii*), lymphocytes and monocytes (*E. canis*, *E. chafeensis*), and platelets (*A. platys*). The number of circulating organisms is often below the limit of light-microscopic detection. Buffy coat smears may improve the chances of organism recovery.
• Dogs are susceptible to infection by at least 5 different *Ehrlichia* and *Anaplasma* species: *E. canis*, *E. ewingii*, *E. chafeensis*, *A. platys*, and *A. phagocytophilum*. This may affect test interpretation because most laboratories only test for 1 or 2 species and cross-reactivity is not always present. Knowledge of which species are tested for is important for both antibody and DNA testing.

INDICATIONS
• Fever
• Thrombocytopenia
• Anemia (typically nonregenerative)
• Leukopenia and/or neutropenia
• Lymphocytosis
• Hyperglobulinemia (occasionally monoclonal)
• Splenomegaly
• Lymphadenopathy
• Epistaxis
• Polyarthritis
• Meningoencephalitis
• Uveitis and/or chorioretinitis
• Glomerulonephritis

CONTRAINDICATIONS
None

POTENTIAL COMPLICATIONS
None

CLIENT EDUCATION
• It can take 3- to 14-days to get results
• Negative results do not rule out infection.

BODY SYSTEMS ASSESSED
• Gastrointestinal
• Hemic, lymphatic, and immune
• Musculoskeletal
• Nervous
• Ophthalmic
• Renal and urologic

SAMPLE

COLLECTION
• 2 mL of venous blood for PCR (EDTA) or IFA/ELISA (serum)
• Bone marrow: 0.5–2.0 mL of aspirated EDTA anticoagulated bone marrow for PCR
• 0.5 mL synovial fluid for IFA/ELISA/PCR
• 0.5 mL cerebrospinal fluid for IFA/ELISA/PCR

HANDLING
• PCR: purple-top tube, on ice, overnight shipping
• IFA/ELISA: red-top tube, on ice, overnight shipping
• Snap test: red-top or purple-top tube
• Light microscopy: blood smears, unstained (fixed with methanol if not sent within 1–2 days); no ice

STORAGE
• PCR: refrigerator or freezer
• IFA/ELISA: refrigerator or freezer
• Light microscopy: room temperature

STABILITY
PCR
• Refrigerated (2°–8°C): days to weeks
• Frozen (−20° to −80°C): months to years. If DNA can survive in a dinosaur fossil for millions of years, it can live in your fridge for a few weeks.

IFA/ELISA
• Refrigerated (2°–8°C): stable for days
• Frozen (−20° to −80°C): stable for months to years

Light Microscopy
Unstained blood smears can be stored for days. Stained slides can be stored for years, especially if coverslipped and protected from light.

PROTOCOL
None

INTERPRETATION

NORMAL FINDINGS OR RANGE
- PCR: no *Ehrlichia* or *Anaplasma* DNA present
- IFA/ELISA: no anti–*Ehrlichia/Anaplasma* antibodies present
- Microscopy: no *Ehrlichia* or *Anaplasma* organisms identified

ABNORMAL VALUES
PCR
The presence of *Ehrlichia* or *Anaplasma* DNA in the sample indicates infection. The absence of *Ehrlichia* and/or *Anaplasma* DNA in the sample does not completely rule out infection.

IFA/ELISA
The presence of anti–*Ehrlichia/Anaplasma* antibodies indicates exposure to *Ehrlichia* and/or *Anaplasma* antigens; check with the laboratory for specific details about what titer is considered clinically significant. Active infection is suggested by comparing an acute and convalescent sample and documenting seroconversion; i.e., a 4-fold rise in antibody titer.

Light Microscopy
The identification of *Ehrlichia* or *Anaplasma* organisms in the WBCs or platelets indicates infection. The absence of *Ehrlichia* and *Anaplasma* organisms in the sample does not rule out infection in patients.

CRITICAL VALUES
None

INTERFERING FACTORS
Drugs That May Alter Results or Interpretation
Drugs That Interfere with Test Methodology
None

Drugs That Alter Physiology
Antibiotics with efficacy against *Ehrlichia* or *Anaplasma* may result in false-negative PCR and microscopy results.

Disorders That May Alter Results
None

Collection Techniques or Handling That May Alter Results
None

Influence of Signalment
Species
Dogs appear more likely than cats to be infected with *Ehrlichia* and *Anaplasma* species.

Breed
German shepherds have been overrepresented in several studies.

Age
None

Gender
None

Pregnancy
None

LIMITATIONS OF THE TEST
- The absence of *Ehrlichia* and *Anaplasma* organisms or DNA does not rule out infection.
- IDEXX Snap tests provide only a positive or negative result. The color intensity does not correlate with the antibody titer and cannot be used to look for a rising titer as evidence of active infection.

Sensitivity, Specificity, and Positive and Negative Predictive Values
PCR
The analytical sensitivity of most assays is quite good (5–50 organisms per reaction), but clinical sensitivities are widely unknown. Specificity approaches 100% when a lab runs controls and uses both screening and confirmatory assays. The positive predictive value is near 100%. The negative predictive value is unknown.

IFA/ELISA
True sensitivity, specificity and predictive values are largely unknown. There is typically a good correlation (≥90%) between IFA and ELISA. Cross-reactivity between *Ehrlichia* and *Anaplasma* species is unpredictable so false-positive and false-negative test results are possible.

IDEXX Snap 4DX
- *Anaplasma phagocytophilum* (compared to Western blot): sensitivity, 99.4%; specificity approaches 100%
- *Ehrlichia canis* (compared to Western blot): sensitivity, 98.9%; specificity approaches 100%
- *Anaplasma phagocytophilum* assay is reported to cross-react with *A. platys*.

Light Microscopy
Unknown

Valid If Run in a Human Lab?
No.

CLINICAL PERSPECTIVE
- No tests for *Ehrlichia* and *Anaplasma* are 100% sensitive or specific.
- Test results must be interpreted in light of clinical signs and response to treatment. If ehrlichiosis or anaplasmosis is highly suspected to be clinical in a seronegative dog, serology should be reevaluated in 2–3 weeks or a PCR assay should be performed.
- A similar constellation of clinical signs can be seen with Lyme disease and Rocky Mountain spotted fever. Coinfection, with several tickborne agents, is common. Systemic lupus erythematosus can also have a similar clinical presentation and is often diagnosed only after these infections have been ruled out.
- Infected blood cells are most likely to be seen in peripheral blood smears early in *Ehrlichia* and *Anaplasma* infection. PCR test results at this point should be positive, but, because of the time required to generate antibodies, IFA and/or ELISA results may be negative.
- Many animals are subclinically infected with *Ehrlichia* or have undergone spontaneous clearance of the organism.
- Some sources suggest declining antibody titers can be used to monitor response to treatment.

MISCELLANEOUS

ANCILLARY TESTS
- CBC with platelet count
- Buffy coat preparation
- Rocky Mountain spotted fever titer and/or PCR test
- Lyme test: preferably the quantitative assay for C6 antibodies available through IDEXX Laboratories (Portland, ME) or C6 assay included in the IDEXX Snap 3DX or Snap 4DX (see the "Lyme Disease Serology" chapter).
- Antinuclear antibody titer
- Joint radiographs and arthrocentesis

SYNONYMS
- *Anaplasma phagocytophilum* (formerly *Ehrlichia equi*)
- *Anaplasma platys* (formerly *Ehrlichia platys*)
- *Ehrlichia canis*
- *Ehrlichia chafeensis*
- *Ehrlichia ewingii*
- Granulocytic ehrlichiosis
- Monocytic ehrlichiosis
- Tropical canine pancytopenia

SEE ALSO
Blackwell's Five-Minute Veterinary Consult: Canine and Feline Topics
- Ehrlichiosis
- Lyme Disease
- Polyarthritis, Nonerosive, Immune-Mediated
- Rocky Mountain Spotted Fever
- Thrombocytopenia

Related Topics in This Book
- Arthrocentesis with Synovial Fluid Analysis
- Blood Smear Microscopic Examination
- Buffy Coat Preparations
- Lyme Disease Serology
- Platelet Count and Volume
- Rocky Mountain Spotted Fever
- White Blood Cells: Neutrophils

ABBREVIATIONS
None

Suggested Reading

Neer TM, Breitschwerdt EB, Greene RT, Lappin MR. Consensus statement on ehrlichial disease of small animals from the Infectious Disease Study Group of the ACVIM. *J Vet Intern Med* 2002; 16: 309–315.

INTERNET RESOURCES
McQuiston JH, McCall CL, Nicholson WL. Ehrlichiosis and related infections [Zoonosis update]. J Am Vet Med Assoc 2008, http://www.avma.org/reference/zoonosis/znehrlichiosis.asp.
Payne PA. New information sheds more awareness on canine ehrlichiosis. DVM Newsmagazine, June 1, 2003, http://www.dvmnews.com/dvm/New-information-sheds-more-awareness-on-canine-ehr/ArticleLong/Article/detail/60050.

AUTHOR NAME
Adam J. Birkenheuer

BASICS

TYPE OF PROCEDURE
Electrodiagnostic: heart electrical activity measurement

PROCEDURE EXPLANATION AND RELATED PHYSIOLOGY
The electrocardiogram (ECG, EKG) is an important tool. (Figure 1 illustrates common examples.) This technique does not require any sedation or anesthesia, is noninvasive and, once the basics are understood, interpretation is straightforward in most cases. If a challenging strip defies interpretation, specialists may be engaged by transtelephonic ECG to assist with interpretation if the results of a good physical examination, a database, and a medical history are available. Laboratory results are also important to have in hand before interpretation because clues may be gleaned from such studies that help to narrow interpretation. If a pleural or abdominal effusion is present, it is tested, and thoracic radiographs (at least 2 views) are also desirable as a concurrent test.

A diagnosis results when the interpretation includes physiologic changes, etiology, and obvious alterations in anatomic features, cardiac and blood pressure status, and assignment of prognosis.

The procedure consists of the capture of the electrical fields generated by the pumping heart. Waveforms are simply the recording of the electrical activity of the heart. Depolarization and repolarization generate these recordable changes. The concept of a lead is important to understand. Each lead gives us a little more information about the heart, but lead II is the basic lead from which we start our analysis. Each lead is a single plane of measurement of the function of the electrical activity of the heart. By setting up a positive and negative surface electrode setting, we may see the energy paths and analyze them. If energy is traveling away from the positive electrode, a negative orientation of the wave occurs, and if the net direction of the electrical energy impulse is toward the positive electrode, a positive deflection occurs. If the impulses are at perpendicular, an isoelectric deflection occurs.

- Each cardiac cycle will initiate with an impulse that originates in the *sinoatrial (SA) node*, which is located in the right atrium. An impulse will travel through the myocardium of the atria, resulting in depolarization. This event generates the *P wave* on the tracing. The tracing is recorded when the atrium contracts, not when the original SA node fires, because the latter event is too small to trigger a recordable event.
- As the impulse moves through the *atrioventricular (AV) node*, which is near the base of the right atrium, the *PR interval* is generated.
- Conduction is a bit slow to the ventricles, which is why we see the flat section. Of course, from a pathophysiologic perspective, this means the atrium may finish contracting before the ventricles contract—a very important synchronization.
- Once through the atrioventricular node, the conduction speed increases and the electrical activity fires through the bundle of His, the bundle branches, and the Purkinje system.
- Rapid, widespread depolarization of the ventricles then occurs. This leads to the *QRS complex* being recorded. Subsequent ventricle contraction then occurs.
- The *Q wave* is the interventricular septum depolarization and thus is the first negative deflection. The Q wave may not always be easy to isolate on tracings.
- The *R portion* is the ventricular myocardium depolarizing and the impulse traveling from the endocardium to the epicardium. It is a positive deflection and the most prominent waveform on the ECG.
- The *S wave* is the basal ventricle posterior wall and interventricular septum activating. It is the first negative deflection following the R wave.
- The repolarization of the ventricles is recorded as the *T wave*.
- As repolarization occurs, the *ST segment* is generated.

INDICATIONS
If one wishes to elucidate a cardiac arrhythmia or infer the status of the myocardium or the direct environment (as in pericardial effusion), then the ECG will be helpful. Tracings of the electrical activity of this organ may be affected either by physiologic or pathologic processes. Trying to isolate the etiology, diagnosis, and prognosis will lead us to use the ECG in these situations:
- Arrhythmias such as tachycardia and bradycardia
- Dyspnea, cyanosis, syncope, or seizures
- Shock, acute emergency, or severe illness, such as pyometra, gastric dilatation and volvulus syndrome (GDV or bloat), uremia, pancreatitis, and toxic insults
- Electrolyte disturbances (especially potassium) or in chronic diuretic administration
- Perisurgical monitoring (e.g., for anesthetic agent toxicity or depth of anesthesia) or preoperative assessments in geriatric patients
- An abnormal radiographic appearance of the heart or great vessels on radiographs (e.g., chamber enlargement pattern, especially right ventricular), which calls for supportive diagnostics, such as echocardiography
- Murmurs
- Diagnostic procedures, such as pericardiocentesis
- Routine health monitoring of senior or chronically ill patients where prognosis may be affected by cardiac function
- Pericarditis with low-amplitude signatures
- Elevations in vagal tone: nervous system, respiratory system, GI system
- Pharmacologic monitoring for agents with known cardiotoxicity (e.g., quinidine, digitalis, β blockers)

CONTRAINDICATIONS
None

POTENTIAL COMPLICATIONS
One needs to be sensitive to animals in a state of dyspnea to ensure this technique is not applied to their detriment.

CLIENT EDUCATION
- Inform clients that this is not a stand-alone test but interpreted in the context of the patient's medical history, clinical signs, and other database findings.
- Let them know that this is just a snapshot and that repeat ECG and Holter monitoring may be required to understand the problem more fully, especially with paroxysmal tachycardias and with blocks.

BODY SYSTEMS ASSESSED
Cardiovascular

PROCEDURE

PATIENT PREPARATION
Preprocedure Medication or Preparation
- The number of leads measured depends on the equipment.
- Three bipolar leads is minimum, and 3 additional unipolar leads are usual.
- This type of procedure does require a quiet, calm environment (and animal) in order to optimize results. Distraction during the test may produce spurious results, so care should be taken to let the animal settle in before measurement begins.
- An experienced technician or veterinarian should run the test and, ideally, serial tests should be conducted and interpreted by the same individuals to help maintain consistency.
- Turn off fluorescent bulbs or electrical equipment (especially in older equipment) in the room, do not cross your limbs, and avoid contact with metal surfaces.
- Before recording begins, clips must be effectively placed. The right arm (RA) and left arm (LA) electrodes are best clipped to the proximal olecranon area or even halfway down the radius. The right leg (RL) and left leg (LL) electrodes are clipped over the patella ligament. Before applying a clip, remember to apply conductive gel or 70% isopropyl alcohol. The advantage of the latter is that it does not get gummed up in long hair. For longer term (e.g., intraoperative) monitoring, gel is better because alcohol evaporates too quickly. The precordial chest (V lead) electrode is applied for precordial unipolar chest leads.

ELECTROCARDIOGRAPHY

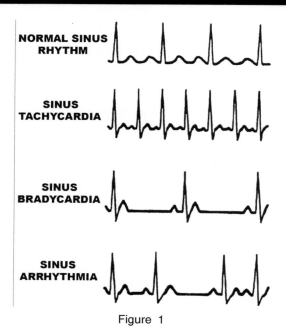

Figure 1

Common examples of electrocardiograms.

- Muscle tremors may produce artifacts. Common movements are also a problem in recording because they lead to vibrations along the baseline. Purring can also produce this problem. A hand placed gently on the animal's chest wall may help to reduce its shivering.
- A wandering baseline is often caused by respiratory-cycle movements because contact at the skin-clip interface can be poor. A patient's panting or coughing may also cause the same thing. To resolve this issue, gently hold the muzzle closed for 4 s.

Anesthesia or Sedation
- Anesthesia is not required, and sedation is rarely required.
- Pediatric patients may require snug restraint to enable testing.
- If ketamine is used with diazepam for sedation, arrhythmias may be masked.

Patient Positioning
- Since reference levels originate from the right lateral recumbent position, that position would be ideal, but, realistically, if a pet is recalcitrant or dyspneic, any position that minimizes tremors, shivering, panting, or struggling will do. As an alternative, standing is preferred to sitting if right lateral recumbency is too stressful.
- Hands must be used to hold the limbs apart to help keep interference to a minimum, and the forelimbs should be perpendicular. A second choice for recording is standing or sternal recumbency, whereas sitting is the last choice.

Patient Monitoring
Careful observation may identify sudden dyspnea or cyanosis. The sudden development of these abnormalities may indicate destabilization.

Equipment or Supplies
- ECG equipment is relatively inexpensive and ranges from transtelephonic sets to integrated computer oscillometric recorders that can print and upload to the computerized patient record directly.
- A blanket or soft pad for the table
- An ECG recording machine. The ECG apparatus should meet the requirements of the Committee on Electrocardiography of the American Heart Association. The amplifier is tied to a strip recorder, either on a computer screen or an oscilloscope, or by a stylus on wax paper. At a minimum, single-channel capture and an oscilloscope should be available. Three-channel equipment enables more detailed capture and analysis by enabling the tester to record 3 leads simultaneously.
- Contact gel or 70% isopropyl alcohol
- Clippers if the hair is too thick to provide close clip contact.

- A printer or a computer or transtelephony device, depending on where the results are to be sent or how they are to be recorded
- Separate the cables so they do not overlap. Usually, this is a set of 5 wires. Alligator clips are usually used for animals. Plate clips are better for electrical sensitivity but are more easily displaced by struggling animals. The alligator clips, which should be copper, should be filed and bent so they pinch less. With very small animals, placing a plate inside the clip may help maintain the patient's comfort without loss of efficiency.
- Once everything is attached, turn on the machine. An older one that requires warm-up should be warmed up before the patient is positioned.
- For those using a stylus, a hand may be needed to steady it in the center.
- Run the standardization marker for sensitivity and increase to 50 speed before you start to record.
- Switch leads to obtain 4-s segments approximately, with the goal to record a minimum of 4 good complexes for rhythm disturbances. Repeat as needed to cover available leads for the system.
- Finally, record a long strip of lead II for full rhythm assessment.
- A break will be needed if precordial leads are to be recorded, because the electrodes will need to be repositioned. Turn off the machine, turn it back on, and run the standardization again before recording.
- Turn off the record switch, turn off the machine, and clean the gel from the hair coat after gently removing the clips.
- For transtelephonic ECG, the portable preamplifier converts electrical signals into tones that can be sent over a phone line. Position the animal, attach 2 electrodes (moistened for good contact) to the forelimbs near the elbow, and then call the transtelephonic service.

SAMPLE HANDLING
- Sensitivity controls how tall the complexes are, with 1 mV being standard. This means 10 small boxes (1 cm) equals 1 mV.
- Change to 2 mV to increase the size of the complexes represented and to 0.5 mV to reduce the height of tall complexes.
- A marker must be done at the start of each strip to record the lead sensitivity. Newer models do this automatically.
- Position the baseline recording in the center of the paper strip for recording.
- Record at least 5–6 complexes for each lead and record a long strip especially if watching for arrhythmias. Check the polarity: If the R waves are not positive in lead I, check the hookup to see if it is still negative, which is abnormal for lead I.
- Placement of the grounding is not critical except that it should be far away as possible.
- For intraoperative monitoring, a patient's position is not critical.

APPROPRIATE AFTERCARE
Postprocedure Patient Monitoring
None

Nursing Care
None

Dietary Modification
None

Medication Requirements
None

Restrictions on Activity
None

Anticipated Recovery Time
None

INTERPRETATION

NORMAL FINDINGS OR RANGE
The findings can be divided into heart rate (HR), rhythm, analysis of complexes and intervals, electrical axis, and chest leads. (*See an ECG text guide for interpretation details.*) Abnormalities in rhythm, complexes and intervals, and waveforms, and disturbances in impulse conduction and mean electrical axis (MEA) can occur.

Canine	Feline

Canine

Rate
70–160 beats/min for adult dogs
60–140 beats/min for giant breeds
Up–180 beats/min for toy breeds
Up–220 beats/min for puppies

Rhythm
Normal sinus rhythm
Sinus arrhythmia
Wandering SA pacemaker

Measurements (lead II, 50 mm/s, 1 cm = 1 mV)
P wave
Width maximum, 0.04 s (2 boxes wide)
Width maximum, 0.05 s ($2^1/_2$ boxes wide) in giant breeds
Height maximum, 0.4 mV (4 boxes tall)
PR interval: Width, 0.06–0.13 s (3–$6^1/_2$ boxes)
QRS complex
Width maximum, 0.05 s ($2^1/_2$ boxes) in small breeds
Width maximum, 0.06 s (3 boxes) in large breeds
R-wave height*
Maximum, 3 mV (30 boxes) in large breeds
Maximum, 2.5 mV (25 boxes) in small breeds
ST segment
No depression, $\leq$0.2 mV (2 boxes)
No elevation, $\leq$0.15 mV ($1^1/_2$ boxes)
T wave
Can be positive, negative, or biphasic
Not greater than one-fourth amplitude of R wave
Amplitude range ±0.05–1.0 mV ($^1/_2$–10 boxes) in any lead
QT interval
Width, 0.15–0.25 s ($7^1/_2$–$12^1/_2$ boxes) at normal heart rate
Varies with heart rate (faster rates have shorter QT intervals and vice versa)

Electrical axis (frontal plane): +40° to +100°
Precordial chest leads (values of special importance)
CV_5RL (rV_2): T wave, positive; R wave, $\leq$3 mV (30 boxes)
CV_6LL (V_2): S wave, $\leq$0.8 mV (8 boxes); R wave, $\leq$3 mV (30 boxes)*
CV_6LU (V_4): S wave, $\leq$0.7 mV (7 boxes); R wave, $\leq$3 mV (30 boxes)*
V_{10}: negative QRS complex, T wave negative except in Chihuahuas

Feline

Rate
Range, 120–240 beats/min
Mean, 197 beats/min

Rhythm
Normal sinus rhythm
Sinus tachycardia (physiologic reaction to excitement)

Measurements (lead II, 50 mm/s, 1 cm = 1 mV)
P wave
Width maximum, 0.04 s (2 boxes wide)
Height maximum, 0.2 mV (2 boxes tall)
PR interval
Width, 0.05–0.09 s ($2^1/_2$–$4^1/_2$ boxes)
QRS complex
Width maximum, 0.04 s (2 boxes)
R-wave height maximum, 0.9 mV (9 boxes)
ST segment: no depression or elevation
T wave
Can be positive, negative, or biphasic; most often positive
Amplitude maximum, 0.3 mV (3 boxes)
QT interval
Width, 0.12–0.18 s (6–9 boxes) at normal heart rate
(range 0.07–0.20 s, $3^1/_2$–10 boxes)
Varies with heart rate (faster rates have shorter QT intervals and vice versa)

Electrical axis (frontal plane): 0 to ±160° (not valid in many cats)
Precordial chest leads
CV_6LL (V_2): R wave, <1 mV (10 boxes)
CV_6LU (V_4): R wave, $\leq$1 mV (10 boxes)

*Not valid for thin, deep-chested dogs <2 years of age.

CRITICAL VALUES
N/A

INTERFERING FACTORS
• Environmental interference, interpretation error, interpretation without a proper minimum database, or overinterpretation
• The ECG does not assess the heart itself, just the electrical activity of the myocardium, so an animal with advanced congestive heart failure (CHF) may have a normal ECG.
• Since not all abnormalities are present all of the time, serial studies or Holter monitors may be needed.
• Breed and conformation may affect the tracings and interpretation.

Drugs That May Alter Results of the Procedure
Sedation with tranquilizers such as ketamine and valium

Conditions That May Interfere with Performing the Procedure
Electrical interference, stress, dyspnea, or an uncooperative patient

Procedure Techniques or Handling That May Alter Results
A wandering baseline caused by movement, not adjusting the millivoltage or speed, improper patient position, contact with a metal surface, crossed wires or legs, or electrical interference

Influence of Signalment on Performing and Interpreting the Procedure
Species
Interpretations of tracings are specific to species.

Breed
Clip placement is affected in deep-chested breeds.

Age
Young dogs

Gender
None

Pregnancy
None

CLINICAL PERSPECTIVE
In summary, the utility of an ECG requires a thorough understanding of the technique and the meaning of the deflections on the final waveforms and the rate and rhythm changes. Knowing your equipment, taking care to minimize stress, and developing a proper database of information against which to compare your results before making an interpretation are important.

MISCELLANEOUS

ANCILLARY TESTS
• Holter monitoring
• Pericardiocentesis

ELECTROCARDIOGRAPHY

- Radiography
- Thoracocentesis
- Ultrasound

SYNONYMS
None

SEE ALSO
Blackwell's Five-Minute Veterinary Consult: Canine and Feline Topics
Cardiology topics
Related Topics in This Book
None

ABBREVIATIONS
SA = sinoatrial

Suggested Reading
Smith FWK, Tilley LP, Miller MS. Electrocardiography. In: Brichard SJ, Sherding RG, eds. *Manual of Small Animal Practice,* 3rd ed. St Louis: Saunders Elsevier, 2006.
Tilley LP. Essentials of Canine and Feline Electrocardiography. *Interpretation and Treatment,* 3rd ed. Ames, IA: Blackwell, 1992.
Tilley LP, Smith FWK, Oyama M, Sleeper M, eds. *Manual of Canine and Feline Cardiology,* 4th ed. St Louis: Saunders Elsevier, 2008.

INTERNET RESOURCES
VetGo Cardiology: Veterinary clinical cardiology, http://www.vetgo.com/cardio.

AUTHOR NAME
Larry P. Tilley

BASICS

TYPE OF PROCEDURE
Electrodiagnostic

PROCEDURE EXPLANATION AND RELATED PHYSIOLOGY
Electroencephalography (EEG) is the recording of electrical activity from the brain. Several electrodes are applied to the scalp, connected to a series of amplifiers, and the output is displayed graphically, either on a monitor (digital EEG) or on paper (analog EEG). The cortex is the source of the electrical activity but is influenced by structures, such as the thalamus, located deep within the brain. Patterns vary with the level of consciousness. Arousal and REM sleep show low-voltage, high-frequency activity, whereas the predominate pattern in slow-wave sleep (SWS) is high voltage and low frequency.

Just as the frequency of seizures can vary in a patient, the EEG findings can also be variable and, at times, completely normal. To improve the likelihood of epileptiform discharges occurring in the EEG, activation techniques can be used. Both sleep and sleep deprivation are useful diagnostic tools in human epilepsy. A period of sleep deprivation prior to the procedure may increase the chance that the patient will sleep during the recording. Thus, as most animals probably do not sleep well in unfamiliar surroundings, an overnight stay in the hospital the evening before a recording is strongly recommended.

INDICATIONS
- Seizure disorders
- EEG is also helpful in diagnosing sleep disorders.
- EEG aids in determining the level of cortical function in comatose patients.
- EEG (with ECG) can also help differentiate between syncope and seizures.

CONTRAINDICATIONS
- Sedation is usually indicated. Patients that are unlikely to tolerate these drugs may not be good candidates for the procedure.
- Electrode placement may be stressful, particularly for cats and toy breeds. Patients that cannot tolerate stress may not be good candidates for the procedure.

POTENTIAL COMPLICATIONS
- An adverse reaction to sedation is possible.
- Needle electrodes are normally used, so there is a very slight chance of infection.
- Rarely, seizures do occur during the procedure.

CLIENT EDUCATION
- Sleep deprivation is thought to increase the probability of epileptiform activity in the EEG. An overnight stay in the hospital the evening before a recording is recommended.
- EEGs may be performed immediately before imaging (magnetic resonance imaging or computed tomography) or cerebrospinal fluid taps.

BODY SYSTEMS ASSESSED
- Cardiovascular
- Nervous

PROCEDURE

PATIENT PREPARATION
Preprocedure Medication or Preparation
The animal should be fasted overnight if it is to be anesthetized after the EEG.

Anesthesia or Sedation
- With the exception of obtunded patients, sedation is routinely used.
- In dogs, a narcotic and tranquilizer combination such as meperidine (5 mg/kg SC) and acepromazine (0.1 mg/kg IV) works well.
- For cats, medetomidine (10–20 μg/kg IM) plus butorphanol (0.1 mg/kg IM) can be used in addition to physical restraint via cat bag.
- The use of general anesthesia should be avoided prior to or during this procedure.

Patient Positioning
- To minimize artifact, patients should be as relaxed as possible.
- Most medium-sized to large dogs are placed in right lateral recumbency.
- Sternal recumbency is typically used for small dogs and for cats.

Patient Monitoring
- An ECG is recorded simultaneously.
- Patients are observed continuously throughout the procedure.

Equipment or Supplies
- A system specifically designed for EEG is standard, though research polygraphs have also been used for this purpose (digital or analog).
- Needle electrodes are generally used to record the EEG, electro-oculogram, and ECG.
- Additional equipment is required for photic stimulation (an activation technique involving light flashed at various repetition rates) and video monitoring.

TECHNIQUE
- Once the patient is positioned, the electrodes are placed SC (Figure 1).
- Electrode impedance is checked and electrodes replaced as needed.
- A calibration signal is applied.
- Recording of the EEG begins.
- For optimal recording, the sensitivity can be adjusted as needed (20–150 μV/cm).
- Recording lengths vary depending on the reason for performing the EEG and the level of patient compliance.
- Sleep will increase the occurrence of epileptiform events. Thus, sleep should be included in all EEGs recorded from seizure patients.
- For sleep disorders, a period of REM sleep should also be included.
- Photic stimulation may be performed at the end of the recording.
- Synchronized video monitoring can be helpful in identifying artifact and correlating clinical signs with EEG events.
- In digital systems, special software can be used to analyze the EEG for epileptiform events.

SAMPLE HANDLING
N/A

APPROPRIATE AFTERCARE
Postprocedure Patient Monitoring
- Intermittent assessment via recording of temperature, pulse, and respirations and assessment of the patient's level of consciousness
- Observe the patient for seizures.

Nursing Care
No additional care is needed.

Dietary Modification
Food and water should be withheld until the patient is bright and alert.

Medication Requirements
- No additional medication is required, unless a reversal agent is desired for the sedative that was administered.
- A seizure protocol should be in place.

Restrictions on Activity
- Occasionally, patients are nonambulatory.
- Once sedation has worn off, no restrictions are indicated.

Anticipated Recovery Time
In most cases, a few hours

ELECTROENCEPHALOGRAPHY

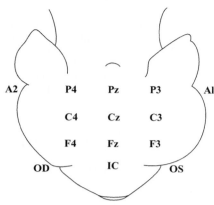

Figure 1

EEG electrode placement for cats and small dogs.

 INTERPRETATION

NORMAL FINDINGS OR RANGE
- Background activity should be symmetrical and appropriate for a state of arousal or sleep.
- Normal transient events, such as sleep spindles, should be present during SWS.

ABNORMAL VALUES
- Epileptiform activity, consisting of spikes, sharp waves, multiple spike–sharp wave complexes, or spike-and-wave discharges (Figure 2)
- Background asymmetry

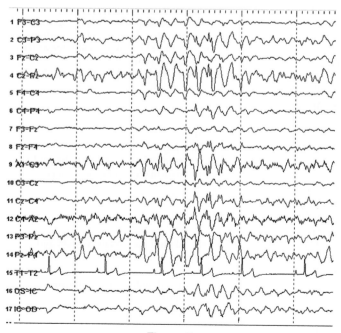

Figure 2

Epileptiform discharge recorded from a 6-year-old shih tzu with a history of collapsing episodes and left pelvic limb paddling.

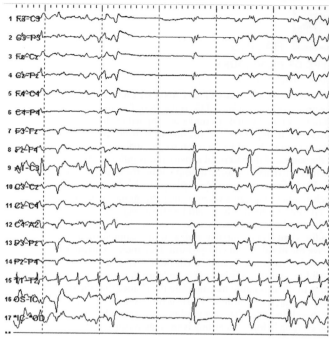

Figure 3

Burst suppression pattern associated with isoflurane anesthesia in a young research cat.

- Altered background activity (i.e., a high voltage, low-frequency pattern during arousal)
- REM sleep onset after little or no preceding SWS (a pattern suggestive of narcolepsy)

CRITICAL VALUES
- Continuous epileptiform activity indicates that the patient is in status epilepticus.
- An isoelectric or extremely low-voltage pattern is seen in cerebral death.
- Burst suppression, a pattern of alternating isoelectric periods and high-amplitude discharges, is associated with a grave prognosis and often precedes the aforementioned pattern (Figure 3).

INTERFERING FACTORS
Drugs That May Alter Results of the Procedure
- Barbiturates or most general anesthetics induce slowing of background activity and can lead to burst suppression or isoelectric patterns (which are reversible with discontinuation of the offending agent).

Conditions That May Interfere with Performing the Procedure
- Excessive noise or activity nearby may prevent the patient from going to sleep.
- Recordings from animals that are tense or panting are usually nondiagnostic because the EEG is obliterated by artifact.
- In comatose patients, monitoring equipment may cause electrical interference, which is especially problematic in patients with minimal cortical activity where the sensitivity needs to be increased.

Procedure Techniques or Handling That May Alter Results
- Electrode placement must be symmetrical because a signal recorded from electrodes that are too closely spaced will be erroneously attenuated.
- High electrode impedance will result in poor EEG quality.
- Securing electrode cables is necessary to minimize artifact.

- In analog systems, all amplifiers need to be accurately calibrated, and the pens must function properly.

Influence of Signalment on Performing and Interpreting the Procedure

Species
- Seizures, associated with intracranial or extracranial causes, are frequently reported in dogs but are rare in cats.
- Sleep disorders are also more common in dogs than cats.

Breed
- Idiopathic (presumably inherited) epilepsy occurs in a number of dog breeds (see the first entry in the Internet Resources section).
- Developmental anomalies, such as hydrocephalus and lissencephaly, are seen in toy breeds.
- An inherited form of narcolepsy occurs in Doberman pinschers, Labrador retrievers, and dachshunds. Acquired narcolepsy has been reported in several dog breeds and a few cats (see the second entry in the Internet Resources section).
- As recordings are from the scalp but the neurons generating the potentials are at a distance, skull and overlying muscle thickness will affect the signal (amplitudes will decrease as thickness increases).

Age
- The onset of idiopathic epilepsy is in young dogs, whereas symptomatic or cryptogenic epilepsy can occur at any age.
- Likewise, familial narcolepsy is apparent in young dogs, but acquired narcolepsy is variable.

Gender
In some canine studies, males had a slightly higher incidence of epilepsy than females.

Pregnancy
In epileptic humans, this condition is known to make it more difficult to control seizures.

CLINICAL PERSPECTIVE

In patients with a skull fracture or an open fontanel, amplitudes will be higher in the region of the defect (referred to as a *breach rhythm* in the case of the human alpha rhythm appearing at sites other than the posterior area where it normally occurs).

MISCELLANEOUS

ANCILLARY TESTS
- Cerebrospinal fluid tap
- Chemistry panel
- Magnetic resonance imaging or computed tomography
- Neurologic examination

SYNONYMS
EEG

SEE ALSO

Blackwell's Five-Minute Veterinary Consult: Canine and Feline Topics
- Seizures (Convulsions, Status Epilepticus)—Cats
- Seizures (Convulsions, Status Epilepticus)—Dogs
- Syncope

Related Topics in This Book
- Bile Acids
- Cerebrospinal Fluid Tap
- Computed Tomography
- Distemper
- Electrocardiography
- Glucose
- Glucose Curve
- Magnetic Resonance Imaging
- Urea Nitrogen

ABBREVIATIONS
- EEG = electroencephalography
- REM = rapid eye movement
- SWS = slow wave sleep

Suggested Reading
Binnie CD, Stefan H. Modern electroencephalography: Its role in epilepsy management. *Clin Neurophysiol* 1999; 110: 1671–1697.
Holliday TA, Williams DC. Interictal paroxysmal discharges in the electroencephalograms of epileptic dogs. *Clin Tech Small Anim Pract* 1998; 13: 132–143.
Hughes JR. *EEG in Clinical Practice,* 2nd ed. Boston: Butterworth-Heinemann, 1994.
Noachtar S, Binnie C, Ebersole J, *et al.* A glossary of terms most commonly used by clinical electroencephalographers and proposal for the report form for the EEG findings. *Electroencephogr Clin Neurophysiol Suppl* 1999; 52: 21–41.
Pedley TA. Interictal epileptiform discharges: Discriminating characteristics and clinical correlations. *Am J EEG Technol* 1980; 20: 101–119.

INTERNET RESOURCES
Holliday TA, Williams C. Clinical electroencephalography in dogs (1999). Vet Neurol Neurosurg J 1999;1, http://www.vin.com/VNNJ/Journal.plx?AID = 1471081.
International Veterinary Information Service (IVIS), http://www.ivis.org/advances/Vite/berendt/chapter_frm.asp?LA = 1.
International Veterinary Information Service (IVIS), http://www.ivis.org/advances/Vite/braund29/chapter_frm.asp?LA = 1.

AUTHOR NAME
Diane Colette Williams

ELECTROMYOGRAPHY

BASICS

TYPE OF PROCEDURE
Electrodiagnostic

PROCEDURE EXPLANATION AND RELATED PHYSIOLOGY
Electromyography is a means of assessing the electrical activity in resting or contracting muscles. However, because of the difficulty in persuading veterinary patients to contract a muscle in a controlled fashion while a needle is inserted into it, in veterinary medicine EMG is typically used to assess resting skeletal muscles. In normal resting muscle, apart from a short burst of insertional activity elicited when the needle is introduced into, or moved within, the muscle, there should be electrical silence. However, when a myofiber loses its nerve supply, it becomes spontaneously electrically active, producing fibrillation potentials and positive sharp waves that can be detected by EMG. Insertional activity is often prolonged, reflecting increased excitability, and bursts of activity called *complex repetitive discharges* may occur. Similar patterns of electrical activity can be seen in myopathies, and some myopathies (e.g., myotonia) produce distinctive electrical discharges (*myotonic discharges*). In most cases, EMG is not a definitive diagnostic test, but is used to confirm the presence, and map the extent, of pathology.

INDICATIONS
- Evaluation of muscle atrophy or hypertrophy
- Evaluation of animals with elevated creatine kinase
- Evaluation of animals with *lower motor neuron paresis* (weakness characterized by decreased to absent muscle tone and spinal reflexes)
- Evaluation of exercise intolerance or weakness of unknown etiology
- Evaluation of animals with unexplained megaesophagus or laryngeal paralysis

CONTRAINDICATIONS
- None unless anesthesia is contraindicated
- If an animal that has recently suffered an injury to nerves is being evaluated, denervation potentials will not appear until 7 days after the injury.

POTENTIAL COMPLICATIONS
- Use of contaminated EMG needle electrodes could cause infection.
- Routine complications of anesthesia or sedation are possible.
- If the patient being evaluated has megaesophagus, regurgitation, or both, the risk of aspiration pneumonia is increased during anesthesia or sedation.

CLIENT EDUCATION
- In preparation for anesthesia, food should be withheld from 10 p.m. the night before the procedure.
- Clients must understand that the results are rarely diagnostic of a particular disease, but help to identify the involvement of nerves and muscle and to localize the problem to certain nerves and muscles.

BODY SYSTEMS ASSESSED
Neuromuscular

PROCEDURE

PATIENT PREPARATION
Preprocedure Medication or Preparation
None

Anesthesia or Sedation
- This procedure is performed most reliably with patients under general anesthesia. There are no specific requirements with respect to anesthetic agent.

- If general anesthesia cannot be performed, EMG can be attempted with patients under sedation. However, voluntary contractions of muscles elicited by inserting the EMG needle complicate interpretation in sedate animals.

Patient Positioning
Any position that enables access to the muscles being investigated is acceptable. If possible, the patient should be placed on a nonmetal surface to decrease electrical interference. Sometimes it is necessary to turn off overhead lights and unplug other electrical equipment in the room to decrease 60-cycle interference.

Patient Monitoring
Routine anesthesia monitoring (heart rate, respiratory rate, blood pressure, pulse oximeter)

Equipment or Supplies
- An electrophysiologic machine that can perform EMGs
- Concentric or monopolar EMG needle electrodes with associated leads. Surface electrodes can also be used.
- A ground needle and lead
- Alcohol or iodine wipes to clean the needles while working

TECHNIQUE
- The muscles assessed depend on the presenting problem. For example, if an animal has unilateral thoracic limb lameness, the examination will concentrate on this limb. If the animal has a more generalized problem, appendicular (proximal and distal) and axial muscles will be examined.
- The ground needle is placed SC over the spine in the LS region when the pelvic limb is examined and at the cervicothoracic junction when the thoracic limb is examined.
- If using a concentric needle electrode, the needle is inserted into the muscle being examined and held in place for a few seconds to ensure the insertional activity fades quickly and to detect the presence of spontaneous activity. The needle is moved to several different places in the muscle belly and, once satisfied that the muscle is electrically silent or that any abnormality detected is repeatable, the next muscle is tested.
- If 2 monopolar needle electrodes are used, 1 is placed in the muscle belly being examined and the other is used to test the muscle in a radius of 1–2 cm from the first needle.
- EMG machines enable examiners both to see and to hear the electrical discharges and to record a tracing for the patient's record. Many machines include a data table in which the findings for each muscle are recorded.
- The order in which muscles are tested is not important, but the examiner must be thorough. In a complete examination, many people start with the interosseous muscles in the pelvic limb and work up the leg, along the paraspinal muscles, and then from distal to proximal up the thoracic limb. The study is completed with the cervical paraspinal muscles, the muscles of mastication, and the tongue. In specific cases, the laryngeal muscles and muscles of facial expression may be assessed.

SAMPLE HANDLING
N/A

APPROPRIATE AFTERCARE
Postprocedure Patient Monitoring
The patient's vital parameters should be monitored while it is recovering from anesthesia.

Nursing Care
None is needed specific to this diagnostic procedure.

Dietary Modification
None

Medication Requirements
None

Restrictions on Activity
None

Anticipated Recovery Time
There are no lasting effects from this procedure other than the time needed to recover from anesthesia or sedation.

INTERPRETATION

NORMAL FINDINGS OR RANGE
- Normal muscle is electrically silent when not contracting.
- Insertion of the needle into the muscle produces a burst of insertional activity that should last a few hundred milliseconds.
- End-plate spikes and miniature end-plate potentials can be detected in normal muscle, particularly around the motor point of the muscle.
- Motor-unit action potentials may be detected if the muscle contracts during the examination.

ABNORMAL VALUES
- Spontaneous electrical activity in muscle that is not actively contracting is abnormal.
- Fibrillation potentials, positive sharp waves, and complex repetitive discharges indicate either that the muscle is denervated or that there is a myopathy (Figure 1).

- Increased insertional activity indicates increased excitability and can be found with either a myopathy or chronic neuropathy.
- Myotonic discharges are diagnostic for myotonia.
- Giant motor-unit potentials may be detected in muscle that has been reinnervated following nerve injury.

CRITICAL VALUES
None

INTERFERING FACTORS
Drugs That May Alter Results of the Procedure
None

Conditions That May Interfere with Performing the Procedure
If end-stage fibrotic muscle is evaluated, the results may not reflect the true pathology.

Procedure Techniques or Handling That May Alter Results
Interpretation of EMG findings is specialized and requires training and experience.

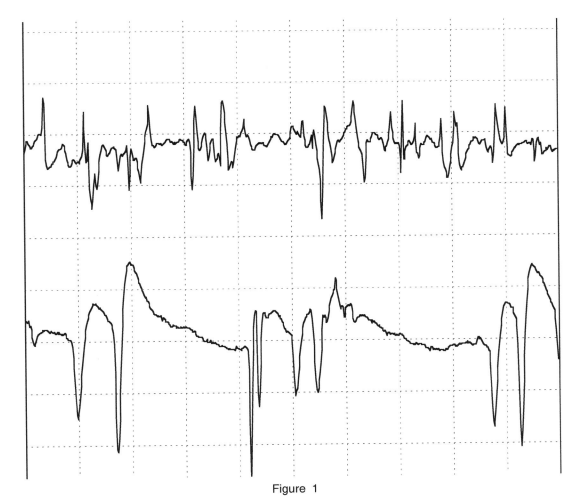

Figure 1

EMG recording from the triceps muscle of a dog. The *top trace* shows multiple fibrillation potentials (small-amplitude biphasic or triphasic waves). These small waves represent a single myofiber action potential passing the needle electrode. The *bottom trace* shows several positive sharp waves. These larger waveforms start with a positive deflection (*down* is positive) and are thought to be generated by an action potential from myofibers stopping adjacent to the needle electrode. *One box* represents 100 μV in the vertical axis and 10 ms in the horizontal axis.

ELECTROMYOGRAPHY

Influence of Signalment on Performing and Interpreting the Procedure

Species
None

Breed
None

Age
None

Gender
None

Pregnancy
None

CLINICAL PERSPECTIVE

• EMG is a useful screening test to identify denervation or a myopathy.

• If the results of EMG are abnormal, the clinician must be prepared to move on to evaluate the nerve with nerve conduction studies and to obtain nerve and muscle biopsy samples.

• Although it is optimal to perform an EMG with patients under general anesthesia, a quick screening EMG can be performed in a animal that is sedated and will often provide enough information to enable the clinician to determine the next step. For example, in an animal with chronic lameness in 1 limb, a quick EMG that shows fibrillation potentials in the muscles of the affected limb would lead the clinician to perform magnetic resonance imaging of that limb and the associated spinal cord segments.

• It is important to remember that the results of EMG will be normal in an animal that has just suffered a nerve injury: Electrical evidence of denervation will take ≈7 days to develop.

• Normal EMG findings do not rule out a myopathy. Muscle that is severely atrophied and replaced with fibrotic tissue may be electrically silent. These muscles can be identified by their appearance and by reduced or absent insertional activity.

MISCELLANEOUS

ANCILLARY TESTS

• If the EMG findings are abnormal, a nerve conduction study is indicated.

• If the findings of the nerve conduction study are normal, a muscle biopsy is performed.

• If both EMG findings and nerve conduction velocity are abnormal, nerve and muscle biopsies are usually performed.

SYNONYMS
EMG

SEE ALSO

Blackwell's Five-Minute Veterinary Consult: Canine and Feline Topics

• Megaesophagus
• Myopathy, Focal Inflammatory—Masticatory Muscle Myositis and Extraocular Myositis
• Myopathy, Generalized Inflammatory—Polymyositis and Dermato-myositis
• Myopathy, Noninflammatory—Endocrine
• Myopathy, Noninflammatory—Hereditary Labrador Retriever
• Myopathy, Noninflammatory—Hereditary Myotonia
• Myopathy, Noninflammatory—Hereditary X-Linked Muscular
• Myopathy, Noninflammatory—Metabolic

Related Topics in This Book

• Creatine Kinase
• Electroneurography
• Muscle and Nerve Biopsy

ABBREVIATIONS

EMG = electromyography

Suggested Reading

Kimura J. *Electrodiagnosis in Diseases of Nerve and Muscle: Principles and Practice.* Oxford: Oxford University Press, 2001.

Lorenz MD, Kornegay JN. *Handbook of Veterinary Neurology.* Philadelphia: WB Saunders, 2004.

Poncelet L. Electrophysiology. In: Platt S, Olby N, eds. *BSAVA Manual of Canine and Feline Neurology,* 3rd ed. Ames, IA: Blackwell, 2004: 54–69.

INTERNET RESOURCES

Steiss JE. Electrodiagnostic evaluation. In: Vite CH, ed. Braund's Clinical Neurology in Small Animals: Localization, Diagnosis and Treatment. Veterinary Neurology and Neurosurgery (IVIS), http://www.ivis.org/advances/Vite/toc.asp.

AUTHOR NAME
Natasha Olby

BASICS

TYPE OF PROCEDURE
Electrodiagnostic

PROCEDURE EXPLANATION AND RELATED PHYSIOLOGY
Nerve conduction studies involve stimulating a peripheral nerve to elicit a muscle contraction that is recorded as a compound muscle action potential (CMAP). The nerve is stimulated at different sites along the nerve to produce a CMAP. The latency of the CMAP is measured for each site (Figure 1). The distance between these sites, and the latency difference, are used to calculate the nerve conduction velocity (NCV). The NCV and the amplitude and area of the CMAP provide information on the segment of peripheral nerve being tested. Abnormalities in myelination decrease velocity and cause dispersion of the waveform, while loss of axons decreases the CMAP amplitude and area. Both axonal pathology and demyelination can cause conduction block and complete inability to elicit a CMAP.

INDICATIONS
- Evaluation of animals with lower motor neuron paresis in 1 or more legs (weakness characterized by decreased to absent muscle tone and spinal reflexes)
- Evaluation of animals with muscle atrophy
- Evaluation of animals with exercise intolerance
- Evaluation of animals with laryngeal paralysis

CONTRAINDICATIONS
None unless anesthesia is contraindicated

POTENTIAL COMPLICATIONS
- Contaminated needle electrodes can cause local infection.
- Careless placement of the needles can cause bleeding.
- Routine complications of anesthesia or sedation are possible.
- If the patient being evaluated has megaesophagus, regurgitation, or both, the risk of aspiration pneumonia during anesthesia is increased.

CLIENT EDUCATION
- Food should be withheld from 10 p.m. the night before the procedure in preparation for anesthesia.
- Clients must understand that the results are rarely diagnostic of a particular disease, but help to identify the involvement of nerves and to localize the problem to certain nerves.
- The nerve conduction study may indicate the need for a nerve or muscle biopsy.

BODY SYSTEMS ASSESSED
Nervous

PROCEDURE

PATIENT PREPARATION
Preprocedure Medication or Preparation
None

Anesthesia or Sedation
- Electroneurography requires general anesthesia.
- The use of neuromuscular blocking agents, such as atracurium, must be avoided.

Patient Positioning
The patient is placed in lateral recumbency and turned halfway through the procedure to enable evaluation of both sides of the body.

Patient Monitoring
- Routine anesthesia monitoring is necessary (heart rate, respiratory rate, blood pressure, and pulse oximetry).

- It is particularly important not to allow patients to become hypothermic: Rectal or esophageal temperature should be monitored regularly.

Equipment or Supplies
- An electrophysiologic machine that can perform nerve conduction studies
- Monopolar needle electrodes and leads to record from muscle and to stimulate the nerve. Surface electrodes can be used, in place of needle electrodes, to record the CMAP.
- A ground needle and lead
- A tape measure
- Alcohol or iodine wipes to clean the needles while working

TECHNIQUE
- Several different nerves can be tested. Typically, the sciatic-tibial nerve and the ulnar nerve are evaluated.
- The recording electrodes (active and reference) are placed ≈1 cm apart in the interosseous muscles of the limb being tested.
- The ground electrode is placed SC over the dorsum of the carpus or tarsus.
- The nerve is stimulated at the most distal stimulation point first (medial to the accessory carpal bone for the ulnar nerve and the neurovascular bundle just proximal to the hock for the tibial nerve). The stimulating electrodes are placed ≈1 cm apart adjacent to the nerve.
- Once a CMAP is produced, the strength of the stimulus is increased until the size of the CMAP does not increase further. The stimulus intensity is then increased by another 50% to ensure that supramaximal stimulation is used.
- Leaving the stimulating needles in place, new needles are placed at the next site to be stimulated (medial to the olecranon for the ulnar nerve and behind the lateral fabella for the tibial nerve). This is done in the same manner as previously described.
- A third, more proximal site can be stimulated for the sciatic-tibial nerve at the level of the sciatic notch.
- The distance is measured between the distal stimulating electrodes at each site and entered into the electrophysiologic machine. The NCV (in meters per second) between these sites is automatically calculated by the machine. Most machines will also automatically calculate the amplitude and the area of the CMAP.
- Skin temperature is monitored and recorded at the time each nerve is assessed because temperature does affect NCV.
- There are protocols published describing the stimulation sites and normal values for nerves less commonly evaluated, including the vagus, the facial nerve, the radial nerve, and the femoral nerve.

SAMPLE HANDLING
N/A

APPROPRIATE AFTERCARE
Postprocedure Patient Monitoring
The patient's vital parameters should be monitored while it recovers from anesthesia.

Nursing Care
None needed specific to this diagnostic procedure

Dietary Modification
None

Medication Requirements
None

Restrictions on Activity
None

Anticipated Recovery Time
There are no lasting effects of this procedure other than the time needed to recover from anesthesia or sedation.

ELECTRONEUROGRAPHY

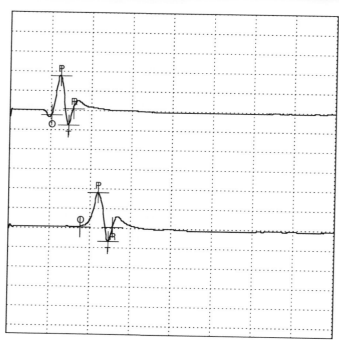

Figure 1

A nerve conduction study from the ulnar nerve of a dog. The *top trace* shows a CMAP following stimulation of the ulnar at the carpus. The *bottom trace* was generated by stimulating the ulnar nerve at the level of the elbow. The further away the stimulation site is from the recording site, the greater the latency of the CMAP. The CMAP is also slightly wider (i.e., lasts longer) with a smaller amplitude than the CMAP generated by stimulating at the carpus. This effect is known as *physiologic temporal dispersion* and reflects the different conduction velocities of different axons within the nerve; the greater the distance traveled, the greater the difference in time taken for action potentials in axons that conduct at different speeds to arrive at the neuromuscular junction. *One box* represents 5000 μV in the vertical axis and 3 ms in the horizontal axis. O, origin; P, peak; T, trough; and R, return.

INTERPRETATION

NORMAL FINDINGS OR RANGE
- It should be possible to elicit a muscle twitch and CMAP for each nerve tested.
- Each laboratory will have slightly different sets of normal ranges for NCV and CMAP amplitude, depending on the machine that is used and technical factors.
- NCV differs among nerves, nerve stimulation sites (proximal versus distal), age, limb length, and species.
- NCV in dogs usually is >50 m/s for the tibial nerve and >60 m/s in the ulnar nerve. In cats, NCV is usually 20–30 m/s faster.

ABNORMAL VALUES
- Inability to elicit a CMAP or muscle twitch indicates complete conduction block.
- Decreased NCV indicates demyelination in the region of nerve tested.
- Decreased CMAP amplitude and area indicates axonal loss. Increased CMAP amplitude and area indicates reinnervation of the muscle being tested, suggesting there was a prior nerve injury and regeneration.

- Most neuropathies produce a combination of changes in NCV and CMAP size. This combination reflects mixed myelin and axonal pathology.
- Temporal dispersion of the CMAP (it tails off in a series of decreasing undulations) indicates demyelination.

CRITICAL VALUES
None

INTERFERING FACTORS
Drugs That May Alter Results of the Procedure
Neuromuscular blockade, if induced under anesthesia, will prevent a CMAP from being elicited.

Conditions That May Interfere with Performing the Procedure
Other than diseases that contraindicate anesthesia, no conditions interfere with performing nerve conduction studies specifically.

Procedure Techniques or Handling That May Alter Results
- Temperature affects NCV: A 1°C limb temperature reduction decreases NCV by a factor of 1.7–1.8 m/s.
- Severe muscle atrophy can make it difficult to record a CMAP from the interosseous muscles. This does not necessarily indicate abnormal nerve function, and recordings from a larger muscle should be attempted.
- Performing and interpreting nerve conduction studies is specialized and typically performed by a neurologist.

Influence of Signalment on Performing and Interpreting the Procedure
Species
NCV is ≈20–30 m/s faster in cats than dogs.

Breed
NCV decreases with increasing limb, and thus nerve, length.

Age
Nerve conduction matures by 6–12 months of age and starts to decrease after 7 years of age in dogs. In cats, NCV increases for the first 3 months and is then stable.

Gender
None

Pregnancy
None

CLINICAL PERSPECTIVE
- Nerve conduction studies are specialized tests usually performed by a neurologist to evaluate an animal with signs of lower motor neuron dysfunction.
- It is unusual to perform this diagnostic test without concurrently performing electromyography (EMG).
- Although nerve conduction studies do locate pathology and, to a certain extent, differentiate between myelinopathies and axonopathies, further diagnostics tests, ideally nerve biopsy, are needed to establish a definitive diagnosis.

MISCELLANEOUS

ANCILLARY TESTS
- Nerve conduction studies are usually performed after EMG.
- Abnormal results usually need further characterization by a nerve biopsy.
- If NCV is reduced, results of a thyroid panel should be evaluated.
- A nerve conduction study evaluates the nerve distal to the most proximal point of stimulation. Additional electrodiagnostic studies to evaluate the proximal nerve include evaluation of the dorsal and ventral nerve roots and dorsal horn of the spinal cord [evaluation of F and H (*late*) waves and cord dorsum potential].

- Additional electrodiagnostic testing in the form of repetitive stimulations may be performed to evaluate the neuromuscular junction.

SYNONYMS
- Nerve conduction studies
- Nerve conduction velocity (NCV)

SEE ALSO
Blackwell's Five-Minute Veterinary Consult: Canine and Feline Topics
None
Related Topics in This Book
- Electromyography
- Muscle and Nerve Biopsy

ABBREVIATIONS
- CMAP = compound muscle action potential
- EMG = electromyography
- NCV = nerve conduction velocity

Suggested Reading
Kimura J. *Electrodiagnosis in Diseases of Nerve and Muscle: Principles and Practice*. Oxford: Oxford University Press, 2001.
Lorenz MD, Kornegay JN. *Handbook of Veterinary Neurology*. Philadelphia: WB Saunders, 2004.
Poncelet L. Electrophysiology. In: Platt S, Olby N, eds. *BSAVA Manual of Canine and Feline Neurology*, 3rd ed. Ames, IA: Blackwell, 2004: 54–69.

INTERNET RESOURCES
Steiss JE. Electrodiagnostic evaluation. In: Vite CH, ed. Braund's Clinical Neurology in Small Animals: Localization, Diagnosis and Treatment. Veterinary Neurology and Neurosurgery (IVIS), http://www.ivis.org/advances/Vite/toc.asp.

AUTHOR NAME
Natasha Olby

ELECTRORETINOGRAPHY

BASICS

TYPE OF PROCEDURE
Electrodiagnostic

PROCEDURE EXPLANATION AND RELATED PHYSIOLOGY
The electroretinogram (ERG) is a surface recording of electrical changes that occur in the retina in response to light stimulus. The resulting ERG tracing includes an *a wave*, a negative deflection generated from the photoreceptors; a *b wave*, a positive deflection from the inner nuclear layers; and a variably present *c wave*, a positive deflection indicating retinal pigmented epithelium activity. Veterinary ophthalmologists can vary the light stimulus to distinguish between rod and cone function by using colored filters, variable light intensities, and patterns such as flicker fusion. Both the amplitude and the duration (implicit time) of each wave provide valuable information about retinal function.

The ERG is useful to determine whether a patient's blindness is caused by retinal disease (e.g., progressive retinal atrophy (PRA), sudden acquired retinal degeneration syndrome (SARDS), retinal degeneration, or retinal detachment), or central disease (i.e., pathology of the optic nerve, chiasm, or cerebral cortex). A decreased or flat waveform supports a diagnosis of blindness caused by retinal disease. Alternatively, a normal waveform in the absence of other ocular pathology, such as a cataract, suggests that further workup should be pursued for causes of central blindness. The ERG is also an invaluable tool to ensure adequate retinal function prior to cataract surgery, since the retina cannot be visualized through the opaque lens.

INDICATIONS
• Determine whether clinical blindness is retinal as opposed to central in origin.
• Confirm adequate retinal function prior to cataract surgery.
• Identify specific defects (i.e., rods vs cones) in retinal dystrophy or degeneration.
• Identify the presence of suspected inherited retinal disease in breeding stock or young litters before the onset of clinical signs.

CONTRAINDICATIONS
The ERG should not be used to assess retinal function in cases of full-thickness corneal perforation. In such cases, the dazzle reflex and consensual pupillary light reflex (PLR) obtained with a bright light source should be used to for a crude prognostic assessment of retinal function.

POTENTIAL COMPLICATIONS
Superficial corneal ulceration may occur with inadequate lubrication between the cornea and the contact-lens electrode.

CLIENT EDUCATION
Restrict food prior to the test if anesthesia is necessary.

BODY SYSTEMS ASSESSED
Ophthalmic

PROCEDURE

PATIENT PREPARATION
Preprocedure Medication or Preparation
• The eyes must be dilated with topical tropicamide or atropine.
• Topical anesthesia is achieved with proparacaine administration.

Anesthesia or Sedation
The ERG can be performed on awake animals although sedation or general anesthesia may be needed to eliminate a patient's movement artifact.

Patient Positioning
Sternal or seated

Patient Monitoring
As needed if anesthetized

Equipment or Supplies
• An electroretinograph with a computer to amplify the retinal potential and average the generated signals
• A light stimulator and electrodes
• Tropicamide
• Topical proparacaine
• A viscous coupling tear replacement

TECHNIQUE
• The eyes are dilated.
• Dark adaptation: The patient acclimates to a dark room for 5–30 min so that rod (scotopic) function can be assessed.
• The reference electrode is placed SC 1 cm temporal to the lateral canthus.
• The ground electrode is placed SC over the occipital protuberance.
• Topical proparacaine is applied for anesthesia.
• A gold-plated contact lens is placed on the cornea by using a viscous coupling tear replacement.
• The light source is flashed (≈20 cm) from the open eye and the resulting waveform is recorded.

SAMPLE HANDLING
N/A

APPROPRIATE AFTERCARE
Postprocedure Patient Monitoring
As needed if anesthesia was required

Nursing Care
None

Dietary Modification
None

Medication Requirements
None

Restrictions on Activity
None

Anticipated Recovery Time
None

INTERPRETATION

NORMAL FINDINGS OR RANGE
• Normal values are difficult to standardize because of wide variation in technique.
• While results may vary substantially between diagnostic centers, mean a-wave and b-wave implicit times are generally approximately 15 ms and 40 ms, respectively. Mean a-wave amplitudes may vary from 60 to 140 μV, whereas b-wave amplitudes may vary from 140 to 240 μV. The amplitude values will increase with longer dark adaptation and increased light intensity.
• Rod and cone function can be separated by taking advantage of differences between their photoreceptor responses to light intensities. At a certain light intensity of a single flash or rapid series of flashes, the rods will not be able to recover and the ERG will be able to isolate cone function. Alternatively, after dark adaptation, the rod response will be so great that it will mask smaller waveforms generated by the cones.

ABNORMAL VALUES
• Any diminished amplitude of an a or b wave.
• Increased implicit time of an a or b wave.

CRITICAL VALUES
Animals with severely diminished or flat waveforms should not be considered good breeding stock or good candidates for cataract surgery.

INTERFERING FACTORS
Drugs That May Alter Results of the Procedure
• Several drugs, such as isoflurane, can affect the waveform, so their use should be avoided.

Conditions That May Interfere with Performing the Procedure
• Fractious or anxious animals may require sedation or general anesthesia.
• Hypoxia or decreased temperature during anesthesia can decrease the ERG amplitude.

Procedure Techniques or Handling That May Alter Results
Any 60-cycle electrical interference from external currents. An ERG must be performed in an electrically shielded room.

Influence of Signalment on Performing and Interpreting the Procedure
Species
None

Breed
Several breeds are predisposed to retinal degeneration or dystrophy, and the ERG can be used to identify affected individuals before the onset of clinical signs.

Age
Retinal function may decrease with age.

Gender
None

Pregnancy
None

CLINICAL PERSPECTIVE
• An ERG should be performed in any dog or cat with clinical blindness in which another ocular pathology, such as cataracts, cannot be identified. The ERG is particularly helpful in blind animals in which the retina appears normal (such as SARDS) to help rule out central blindness.

• The ERG should be used as preoperative cataract surgery screening to ensure adequate retinal function. Animals with minimally diminished ERG waveforms can benefit from surgery, but owners should be warned that vision may decrease in the future because of suspected retinal degeneration. Animals with severe to absent ERG waveforms are not good candidates for cataract surgery.
• Inherited retinal diseases can be identified and qualified with specific ERG techniques.

MISCELLANEOUS
ANCILLARY TESTS
Ocular ultrasound can be performed in conjunction with the ERG, particularly if the eye is opaque (i.e., hyphema, hypopyon, cataract), to rule out retinal detachment, masses, or infiltrate.

SYNONYMS
ERG

SEE ALSO
Blackwell's Five-Minute Veterinary Consult: Canine and Feline Topics
• Cataract
• Blind Quiet Eye
• Retinal Degeneration
• Retinal Detachment

Related Topics in This Book
Ocular Ultrasonography

ABBREVIATIONS
ERG = electroretinogram

Suggested Reading
Gelatt KN, ed. *Veterinary Ophthalmology,* 3rd ed. Philadelphia: Lippincott Williams & Wilkins, 1990.

INTERNET RESOURCES
None

AUTHOR NAME
A. Brady Beale

BASICS

TYPE OF PROCEDURE
Radiographic

PROCEDURE EXPLANATION AND RELATED PHYSIOLOGY
Epidurography is a radiographic procedure in which iodinated contrast material is injected into the epidural space to delineate mass lesions that are compressing cauda equina structures. Neutral, flexed, and extended lateral radiographs are taken toward the end of the contrast injection; some operators take DV projection radiographs, as well. Mass lesions in the epidural space (especially those located ventrally in the vertebral canal) may be identified by lack of contrast filling in the region of the mass. However, because the epidural space has irregular contours and contains normal structures (e.g., nerve roots, epidural fat) that cause filling defects within the contrast, epidurography can be difficult to interpret.

Epidurography is generally used to evaluate the lumbosacral region of large-breed dogs suspected of having lumbosacral degenerative stenosis. Diagnostic myelography is often not possible in these cases, as the subarachnoid space of large-breed dogs generally does not extend caudally into this region. In cats and small dogs, myelography may be diagnostic in the lumbosacral region because the dural sac commonly extends past the lumbosacral disk space in these patients. Myelography may be attempted in these patients when a lumbosacral lesion is suspected.

Epidurography does not directly image the cauda equina itself.

INDICATIONS
To assess suspected compressive cauda equina lesions, especially those located ventrally within the vertebral canal. Lumbosacral degenerative stenosis is the most common disease syndrome evaluated by epidurography.

CONTRAINDICATIONS
• Conditions that preclude general anesthesia
• Known allergy to iodinated contrast agents

POTENTIAL COMPLICATIONS
• The procedure is generally low risk.
• Rarely, injury to the nerve roots of cauda equina can cause incontinence or motor deficits to the tail.
• Death is rare but may result from an anesthetic accident or an anaphylactic reaction to the contrast agent.

CLIENT EDUCATION
• Fast the patient overnight for general anesthesia.
• Informed consent, which addresses risks of the procedure

BODY SYSTEMS ASSESSED
• Musculoskeletal
• Nervous

PROCEDURE

PATIENT PREPARATION
Preprocedure Medication or Preparation
Fast the patient overnight for general anesthesia.

Anesthesia or Sedation
General anesthesia

Patient Positioning
Lateral recumbency

Patient Monitoring
• Standard anesthetic monitoring

• Maintain an adequate depth of anesthesia prior to and during contrast injection.

Equipment or Supplies
• A 22-gauge spinal needle, $1^1/_2$ inches (38.1 mm) long
• An extension tube
• Iohexol (240 or 300 mg/mL) or iopamidol (200, 250, or 300 mg/mL) contrast agent, drawn into a syringe and warmed to body temperature, if possible. Dose for the first injection is 0.15 mL/kg and is 0.1 mL/kg for subsequent injections. Draw up sufficient contrast for the series of injections planned, usually 4–5. Add additional volume of contrast to account for dead space in the extension tube.
• An empty tube to collect cerebrospinal fluid (CSF)
• Supplies to prepare the injection site aseptically
• Sterile gloves
• Radiographic equipment, preferably with fluoroscopic capabilities
• Sandbags and sponges for patient positioning

TECHNIQUE
• Make survey radiographs of the spine.
• Place patients in lateral recumbency. Clip and prep the skin on dorsal midline from the level of the wings of the ileum to the fifth caudal vertebra.
• Prop the patient's abdomen with sponges as necessary to ensure that the lumbar spine is positioned in perfect lateral recumbency.
• The contrast agent is injected at the sacrocaudal junction or between the first 2 caudal veterbrae (Cd1-Cd2).
• Don sterile gloves. Insert the needle with stylet in place to the floor of the vertebral canal at the sacrocaudal junction. Fluoroscopic guidance is helpful. The bevel of the needle should be directed cranially.
• The first injection is made with the patient in a neutral lateral position. Make the radiograph as the injection is completed.
• Additional injections are made with the lumbosacral joint flexed and extended. In each instance, make the radiograph as the injection is completed.
• If DV projection views are to be made, roll the patient into a frog-leg sternal position with the spinal needle in place, taking care to avoid movement of the spinal needle. Inject the contrast and make DV projection radiograph as the injection is completed.

SAMPLE HANDLING
N/A

APPROPRIATE AFTERCARE
Postprocedure Patient Monitoring
• Standard postanesthetic monitoring
• Assess anal tone, urinary and fecal continence, and tail movements upon the patient's full recovery from anesthesia.

Nursing Care
None

Dietary Modification
None

Medication Requirements
None

Restrictions on Activity
None

Anticipated Recovery Time
Anesthesia recovery time is 1–12 h, depending on the anesthetic regimen and general health of the patient.

INTERPRETATION

NORMAL FINDINGS OR RANGE
Irregular filling of the epidural space from S3 to L5 with contrast is normal. Normal nerve roots may be seen as linear filling defects, and

normal epidural fat may cause amorphous filling defects and pooling of contrast. Contrast may also pool in the dependent intervertebral foramina. Contrast commonly is more prominent in the ventral aspect of the vertebral canal but should cross the lumbosacral disk space without attenuation.

ABNORMAL VALUES

Attenuation or deviation of the contrast is abnormal. Dorsal deviation of the contrast, or contrast that fills the sacral region but abruptly stops at the level of the lumbosacral junction, is indicative of a ventrally located compressive lesion such as a disk protrusion. Contrast that is elevated by ≥50% of the height of the vertebral canal is considered most clinically significant, but lesser degrees of contrast deviation may be clinically significant, particularly when clinical signs and ancillary diagnostics (e.g., electrodiagnostic studies, myelography) are supportive. Abnormal findings are usually most apparent on the lateral, neutral and extended views. Flexed views may be normal or show a lesser degree of elevation of the contrast; such a finding particularly supports the diagnosis of lumbosacral degenerative stenosis. DV views are occasionally helpful in the diagnosis of lateralized lumbosacral lesions.

CRITICAL VALUES

None

INTERFERING FACTORS

Drugs That May Alter Results of the Procedure

None

Conditions That May Interfere with Performing the Procedure

- Anatomic anomalies in the region of the sacrocaudal junction could preclude needle placement.
- Severe lumbar spinal stenosis could cause the results of the study to be nondiagnostic because of extravasation of contrast along the nerve roots, into soft tissues, and into the vertebral venous sinus.

Procedure Techniques or Handling That May Alter Results

- An inadequate volume of contrast material may result in poor filling of the epidural space, causing the results of the study to be nondiagnostic.
- Contrast injection into the vertebral venous sinus may result in poor filling of the epidural space and the false impression of severe lumbar spinal stenosis.

Influence of Signalment on Performing and Interpreting the Procedure

Species
None

Breed
None

Age
None

Gender
None

Pregnancy
The use of epidurography and other radiographic procedures are generally avoided in pregnant patients because of the risk to the fetuses.

CLINICAL PERSPECTIVE

- The presence of contrast material within the epidural space usually renders myelography nondiagnostic. Therefore, if both the spinal cord and cauda equina are to be evaluated, myelography should be performed prior to epidurography.
- MRI and computed tomographic scanning are generally considered superior in the diagnosis of disease affecting the cauda equina. MRI

especially should be considered the diagnostic modality of first choice in the evaluation of cauda equina disease.

MISCELLANEOUS

ANCILLARY TESTS

- Electrodiagnostic studies are useful in the evaluation of cauda equina disease.
- Meningitis or myelitis may be differential diagnoses for lumbar pain or lower motor neuron signs to the tail, bladder, anus, and hind limbs, or a combination of these signs. CSF analysis is necessary to diagnose these conditions. CSF analysis is occasionally helpful in diagnosing nerve-root disorders. CSF may be collected either before or after an epidurogram is performed.
- Because lower motor neuron signs of the tail, bladder, anus, and hind limbs may be caused by spinal cord disease involving lumbosacral intumescence, as well as the cauda equina, myelography is commonly performed prior to epidurography. Alternatively, MRI of the lumbar and lumbosacral spine could be performed.

SYNONYMS

None

SEE ALSO

Blackwell's Five-Minute Veterinary Consult: Canine and Feline Topics

- Ataxia
- Diskospondylitis
- Hip Dysplasia
- Incontinence, Fecal
- Incontinence, Urinary
- Intervertebral Disc Disease, Thoracolumbar
- Lumbosacral Stenosis and Cauda Equina Syndrome
- Neck and Back Pain
- Paralysis
- Spondylosis Deformans

Related Topics in This Book

- General Principles of Radiography
- Cerebrospinal Fluid Tap
- Computed Tomography
- Electromyography
- Fluoroscopy
- Magnetic Resonance Imaging

ABBREVIATIONS

- CSF = cerebrospinal fluid
- DV = dorsoventral
- MRI = magnetic resonance imaging

Suggested Reading
Park RD. Diagnostic imaging of the spine. *Prog Vet Neurol* 1990; 1: 371–386.
Ramirez O, Thrall DE. A review of imaging techniques for canine cauda equina syndrome. *Vet Radiol Ultrasound* 1998; 39: 283–296.
Roberts RE, Selcer BA. Myelography and epidurography. *Vet Clin North Am Small Anim Pract* 1993; 23: 307–329.

INTERNET RESOURCES

None

AUTHOR NAME

Stacey A. Sullivan

ERYTHROPOIETIN

BASICS

TYPE OF SPECIMEN
Blood

TEST EXPLANATION AND RELATED PHYSIOLOGY
Epo is a glycoprotein hormone that is primarily produced by the kidneys and acts on bone marrow to stimulate erythropoiesis. Whereas peritubular interstitial cells (fibroblasts) of the renal cortex are the major source of Epo, liver and bone marrow macrophages have been identified as extrarenal sources. Epo causes erythroid progenitor cells to express specific cell surface receptors, inhibits their apoptosis, and promotes their viability, proliferation, and differentiation. Epo production is stimulated by tissue hypoxia and, accordingly, increases in response to hypoxemia and anemia. The anemia accompanying chronic renal disease is a significant exception in that Epo does not increase in response to the anemia. Serum Epo concentration appears to be regulated by both the rate of renal production and the rate of use by erythroid cells. Epo concentration is likely to be highest in disorders with low marrow erythroid activity (e.g., erythroid aplasia).

Epo is most frequently measured to differentiate the cause of erythrocytosis as primary or secondary. With primary erythrocytosis (polycythemia vera), Epo concentrations will be normal or decreased, whereas secondary erythrocytosis is caused by increased Epo concentrations. In an animal with secondary erythrocytosis, measurement of PaO_2 can help determine whether the Epo concentration is appropriate. Epo is expected to be increased in instances of decreased PaO_2. However, an increase in Epo in the face of a normal PaO_2 and concurrent erythrocytosis would be inappropriate. Physiologically inappropriate increases in Epo, and subsequent erythrocytosis, can be seen in patients with renal lesions (usually tumors that induce localized renal hypoxia). There are also rare reports of increased production of Epo or of an Epo-like substance by nonrenal tumors, including embryonal nephroma, renal carcinoma, nasal fibrosarcoma, uterine leiomyoma, cerebellar hemangioma, hepatoma, and other endocrine neoplasms. The considerable overlap in values among patients with primary and secondary erythrocytosis limits the diagnostic value of the Epo assay. Epo may also be measured to rule out a deficiency (e.g., chronic renal failure) as a cause of anemia.

INDICATIONS
- Unexplained erythrocytosis
- Suspected anemia caused by chronic renal disease

CONTRAINDICATIONS
None

POTENTIAL COMPLICATIONS
None

CLIENT EDUCATION
12-h fast to avoid lipemic serum

BODY SYSTEMS ASSESSED
- Endocrine and metabolic
- Hemic, lymphatic, and immune
- Renal and urologic

SAMPLE

COLLECTION
1–2 mL of venous blood

HANDLING
- Plain red-top tube
- Centrifuge the sample soon as possible and transfer the serum to plastic tube; freeze immediately.
- Ship the frozen sample with 1–2 ice packs via next-day delivery in a Styrofoam container.

STORAGE
- Avoid the use of polymer gel tubes.
- Store the sample frozen.

STABILITY
- Hormone labile at room temperature
- Frozen ($-20°C$): weeks to months if repeated freezing and thawing is avoided

PROTOCOL
None

INTERPRETATION

NORMAL FINDINGS OR RANGE
- Dogs: 8.4–28.0 mIU/mL
- Cats: 10–30 mIU/mL
- Reference ranges were established by the Diagnostic Endocrinology Laboratory at the University of Tennessee College of Veterinary Medicine. Values may vary depending on the laboratory and assay.

ABNORMAL VALUES
Values above or below the reference range

CRITICAL VALUES
None

INTERFERING FACTORS
Drugs That May Alter Results or Interpretation
Drugs That Interfere with Test Methodology
None

Drugs That Alter Physiology
- Androgens increase Epo release.
- Estrogens and corticosteroids decrease Epo release.

Disorders That May Alter Results
None

Collection Techniques or Handling That May Alter Results
Avoid the use of gross hemolysis, icterus, or lipemia.
Influence of Signalment
Species
None

Breed
None

Age
- Epo reportedly is twice as high in dogs 1–2 months old than in dogs 1–7 years old.
- Epo reportedly is 40% lower in dogs >8 years old than in dogs 1–7 years old.

Gender
None

Pregnancy
None

LIMITATIONS OF THE TEST
Sensitivity, Specificity, and Positive and Negative Predictive Values
N/A

Valid If Run in a Human Lab?
Commercial tests developed for human assays may not cross-react sufficiently for use in other species; individual radioimmunoassay must be

validated for each species to be tested prior to clinical use. Therefore, use of a veterinary diagnostic laboratory is recommended.

Causes of Abnormal Findings

High values	Low values
Erythrocytosis	Erythrocytosis
Secondary erythrocytosis with hypoxemia	Primary erythrocytosis (polycythemia vera)
High altitude	Normal PaO$_2$ with normal or decreased Epo
Chronic pulmonary disease	
Cardiovascular anomalies with right-to-left shunting of blood	
Secondary erythrocytosis with inappropriate Epo production (normal PaO$_2$)	Anemia
Renal lesions	Chronic kidney disease
Neoplasia	
Hereditary methemoglobinemia	
Anemia	
Hemolysis	
Hemorrhage	
Marrow abnormalities	
Aplasia	
Myelofibrosis	
Myelodysplasia	
Neoplasia	
Anemia of inflammatory/chronic disease	
Epo normal or increased but not as much as expected	

CLINICAL PERSPECTIVE

• Epo will increase with any anemia (other than anemia caused by chronic renal disease or inflammatory disease). The elevated value represents an appropriate, physiologic response to the anemia.
• Measurements of plasma Epo must be interpreted in light of CBC and blood-gas analysis.

MISCELLANEOUS

ANCILLARY TESTS
• Blood-gas analysis
• Clinical chemistry tests for renal function
• Diagnostic imaging, particularly of the kidneys
• Renal aspiration cytology or biopsy

SYNONYMS
Epo

SEE ALSO
Blackwell's Five-Minute Veterinary Consult: Canine and Feline Topics
• Hypoxemia
• Polycythemia
• Polycythemia Vera
• Renal Failure, Chronic

Related Topics in This Book
• Blood Gases
• Hematocrit
• Red Blood Cell Count
• Red Blood Cell Morphology
• Renal Ultrasonography

ABBREVIATIONS
• Epo = erythropoietin
• PaO$_2$ = arterial blood oxygen tension

Suggested Reading
Brockus CW, Andreasen CB. Erythrocytes. In: Latimer KS, Mahaffey EA, Prasse KW, eds. *Duncan and Prasse's Veterinary Laboratory Medicine*, 4th ed. Ames: Iowa State Press, 2003: 3–45.
Coles EH. *Veterinary Clinical Pathology*, 4th ed. Philadelphia: WB Saunders, 1986.

INTERNET RESOURCES
None

AUTHOR NAMES
Rebekah Gray Gunn-Christie and John W. Harvey

ESOPHAGOGASTRODUODENOSCOPY

BASICS

TYPE OF PROCEDURE
Endoscopic

PROCEDURE EXPLANATION AND RELATED PHYSIOLOGY
Esophagogastroduodenoscopy is a minimally invasive technique whose goal is to obtain tissue, examine the mucosa, and hopefully remove foreign objects without having to resort to invasive surgery.

INDICATIONS
- Biopsy the gastric and intestinal mucosa.
- Remove esophageal, gastric, or high duodenal foreign bodies.
- Detect the site of bleeding or stop bleeding with electrocautery or injection.
- Search for infiltrative or erosive disease.
- Remove gastric polyps.
- Identify benign and malignant strictures, and hopefully dilate benign strictures.

CONTRAINDICATIONS
- Known alimentary tract perforation (a relative contraindication)
- Severe coagulopathy (a relative contraindication)
- High anesthetic risk (a relative contraindication)

POTENTIAL COMPLICATIONS
- Excessive bleeding (rare)
- Perforation (rare)

CLIENT EDUCATION
- Do not feed the patient for at least 24 h (preferably 36 h) prior to the procedure (except when feeding small, high-fat meals 6–8 h prior to endoscopy of patients with protein-losing enteropathy).
- The morning of the procedure, administer only those medications approved by your veterinarian.
- Sometimes surgery will be necessary if (1) there are complications with the procedure or (2) the endoscopy is not successful.

BODY SYSTEMS ASSESSED
Gastrointestinal

PROCEDURE

PATIENT PREPARATION
Preprocedure Medication or Preparation
- Fast the patient for 24 h, making its last meal a soft one as opposed to dry kibble. If the patient has a protein-losing enteropathy, it is sometimes advantageous to feed a small, soft, high-fat meal 8–10 h prior to the procedure to make lymphangiectasia more obvious during endoscopy.
- Do not administer sucralfate (Carafate) or barium sulfate within 24–36 h of the procedure.
- Avoid the use of prokinetic drugs and opioids (e.g., fentanyl, hydromorphone).
- It is usually a good idea to evaluate the abdomen via ultrasound before performing a biopsy (to ensure that the lesion is not out of reach of the endoscope) and to radiograph the patient immediately before removing a foreign body (to ensure the foreign body has not moved).

Anesthesia or Sedation
- In all but the rarest of procedures, the patient will be fully anesthetized.
- Preanesthetic medications in dogs: acepromazine or butorphanol, glycopyrrolate
- Preanesthetic medications in cats: ketamine, glycopyrrolate
- Induction: propofol

- Maintenance: isoflurane (for brief procedures, administer intermittent propofol boluses to effect)

Patient Positioning
- Left lateral recumbency for most procedures; right lateral recumbency when placing a gastrostomy tube with endoscopic assistance
- Rarely, dorsal recumbency when having difficulty directing tip of scope into the gastric antrum of larger dogs

Patient Monitoring
- Standard anesthetic monitoring
- Watch out for stomach overinflation, which puts excessive pressure on the diaphragm, making it difficult to breath.
- Watch out for tension pneumothorax caused by unsuspected esophageal perforation (primarily seen with foreign bodies).

Equipment or Supplies
- For fiberoptic scopes: a standard flexible scope (4-way deflection, aspiration/biopsy channel, air/water insufflation channel), a light source, and a vacuum source
- For video endoscopes: a standard flexible scope (see the preceding paragraph), a light source, a vacuum source, a monitor, and a video processor
- Many different-sized scopes are available: Optimal flexible scopes have an external diameter of ≤9.0 mm plus an aspiration/biopsy channel that is at least 2.8 mm in diameter.
- Biopsy forceps that are elongated (i.e., ellipsoidal) as opposed to round—the largest that will fit through the biopsy channel
- Long, flexible tubing may facilitate obtaining washes of the duodenum or stomach for select parasites.
- Protected cytology brushes may be used, especially for focal lesions.
- Foreign body retrieval devices: Many are available, but a 4-wire basket, a W-type coin-retrieval device, and either a shark's tooth or an alligator jaw forceps are typically the most useful and important devices.
- Balloon catheters are available for dilating esophageal strictures.
- Electrocautery devices (e.g., snares, knives, probes) are available; however, special training is recommended before using them lest damage to the patient, endoscopic equipment, or both occurs.

TECHNIQUE
- The endoscope is passed down the esophagus, into the stomach, through the pylorus, and as far into the duodenum (and even proximal jejunum) as possible. All mucosal surfaces are methodically examined as the scope is advanced. Multiple biopsy samples (≥8) are taken of the duodenal and gastric mucosa in almost all cases (except for some patients with foreign bodies) regardless of how normal the mucosa appears.
- If appropriate, brush cytology may be performed or the gastric or duodenal lumen may be washed.

SAMPLE HANDLING
- Mucosal tissue samples fixed in neutral buffered formalin are submitted to the lab.
- Gastric tissue is relatively tough, but duodenal tissue is very delicate and needs careful handling.
- The endoscopist should work with the histopathology laboratory to ensure proper handling, orientation, and sectioning of tissue samples (see Mansell and Willard 2003).
- Cytology and washings are handled routinely.

APPROPRIATE AFTERCARE
Postprocedure Patient Monitoring
Standard postanesthesia monitoring

Nursing Care
None

Dietary Modification
Start feeding the patient small amounts late in the afternoon of the procedure. The diet should be normal by the morning after procedure.

Medication Requirements
None

Restrictions on Activity
None

Anticipated Recovery Time
Recovery should be complete when the patient awakes from anesthesia.

 INTERPRETATION

NORMAL FINDINGS OR RANGE
• No masses, foreign objects, obvious lymphangiectasia, or protozoal organisms
• No abnormal mucosal infiltrates
• No obvious architectural changes (e.g., villous atrophy, crypt lesions, epithelial necrosis)

ABNORMAL VALUES
• Grossly: The presence of ulcers, erosions, and masses is abnormal, but not all foreign bodies cause problems.
• The presence of large white dots (i.e., dilated lacteals) that are erratically placed and of varying sizes is very suggestive of lymphangiectasia, even if not seen histologically.
• Histology: This topic is controversial and extensive. Intestinal mucosa is expected to have lymphocytes and plasma cells. Diagnosis of inflammatory bowel disease (IBD) requires more than just finding such cells. As of this writing, there is no standardization in nomenclature for histopathology of gastric or intestinal histopathology.
• Cytology: The presence of neoplastic cells, substantial numbers of inflammatory cells (especially neutrophils or eosinophils), or protozoal parasites (e.g., *Giardia*) is abnormal.

CRITICAL VALUES
• Vigorous bleeding
• Apparent perforation

INTERFERING FACTORS
Drugs That May Alter Results of the Procedure
• Administration of NSAIDs or high-dose dexamethasone often causes erosions or ulcers (especially when administered concurrently).
• Barium and sucralfate may obscure lesions.
• Prokinetics, and some narcotics, make it difficult to enter the duodenum, and lesions may be missed.

Conditions That May Interfere with Performing the Procedure
Excessive food in the stomach may obscure lesions and foreign objects.

Procedure Techniques or Handling That May Alter Results
If the tissue samples (especially the duodenal samples) are handled roughly or allowed to dry out, there may be so much artifact that histopathology is misleading.

Influence of Signalment on Performing and Interpreting the Procedure
Species
• It can be harder to enter the feline duodenum, and ketamine as a preanesthetic sometimes helps.
• It is easy to run out of insertion tube length when entering the duodenum of larger dogs (i.e., weighing >30–40 kg). Sometimes it is best to enter the duodenum before distending and examining the stomach in such patients.

Breed
• It is sometimes difficult to enter the duodenum of greyhounds.
• It is sometimes difficult to enter the duodenum of smaller dogs and of cats (i.e., weighing <3 kg).

Age
None

Gender
None

Pregnancy
None

CLINICAL PERSPECTIVE
• Biopsy of the stomach and intestine is typically the most important endoscopic procedure and the principal means of paying for the equipment. Removing foreign objects is important but will rarely pay for the equipment. Therefore, it is critical to be able to take excellent tissue samples.
• It is not always appropriate to automatically biopsy the GI tract of dogs or cats with chronic vomiting, diarrhea, or both. Although IBD (a major reason for endoscopic biopsy) is an important disease, many patients with chronic vomiting, diarrhea or both are responsive to *appropriate* dietary and/or antibacterial therapeutic trials. The number of endoscopic procedures performed by the author over the last 10 years has diminished as more attention has been paid to conducting excellent therapeutic trials.
• A major concern has been whether endoscopic biopsies are sensitive in distinguishing IBD from lymphoma. In many (not all, but possibly most) cases in which there is diagnostic confusion, much of the fault lies in the quality of the biopsy sample that was taken or the maturity of the lymphocytes (i.e., well-differentiated lymphoma is typically more difficult to diagnose), not in the capability of endoscopy to provide diagnostic samples. It is imperative that the endoscopist be able to obtain excellent tissue samples, which is something that is often not stressed during training.
• Rigid endoscopes are often superior to flexible endoscopes in removing esophageal foreign objects.
• It is often advisable to perform endoscopy before surgery to remove bleeding gastric lesions because gastric lesions that are obvious during endoscopy may be impossible to see from the serosal surface. Sometimes, intraoperative endoscopy is needed to find and remove bleeding gastric lesions.
• Rarely, duodenal washes may find *Giardia* when other techniques fail.
• Cytology of masses and mucosal lesions sometimes facilitates a rapid, presumptive diagnosis of malignant or eosinophilic disease.

 MISCELLANEOUS

ANCILLARY TESTS
Abdominal ultrasound is very important in deciding which cases are good candidates for endoscopy. If obvious lesions are beyond the range of the endoscope or if lesions can be aspirated percutaneously, endoscopy may be inappropriate.

SYNONYMS
Gastroduodenoscopy

SEE ALSO
Blackwell's Five-Minute Veterinary Consult: Canine and Feline Topics
• Inflammatory Bowel Disease
• Lymphoma

Related Topics in This Book
• General Principles of Endoscopy
• Colonoscopy

ESOPHAGOGASTRODUODENOSCOPY

ABBREVIATIONS
IBD = inflammatory bowel disease

Suggested Reading
Jergens AE, Andreasen CB, Hagemoser WA, *et al.* Cytological examination of exfoliative specimens obtained during endoscopy for diagnosis of gastrointestinal tract disease in dogs and cats. *J Am Vet Med Assoc* 1998; 213: 1755–1759.
Leib MS, Dalton MN, King SE, Zajac AM. Endoscopic aspiration of intestinal contents in dogs and cats: 394 cases. *J Vet Intern Med* 1999; 13: 191–193.
Mansell J, Willard MD. Biopsy of the gastrointestinal tract. *Vet Clin North Am* 2003; 33: 1099–1116.
Weinstein WM. Mucosal biopsy techniques and interaction with the pathologist. *Gastrointest Endosc Clin North Am* 2000; 10: 555–572.
Willard MD, Mansell J, Fosgate GT, *et al.* Effect of sample quality upon the sensitivity of endoscopic biopsy for detecting gastric and duodenal lesions in dogs and cats. *J Am Vet Intern Med* 2008; 22: 1084–1089.

INTERNET RESOURCES
None

AUTHOR NAME
Michael D. Willard

BASICS

TYPE OF PROCEDURE
Radiographic

PROCEDURE EXPLANATION AND RELATED PHYSIOLOGY
A variety of different positive contrast media may be administered orally in an attempt to better identify the esophagus and, in some instances, to evaluate esophageal function. Images are obtained via standard radiography, or preferably with fluoroscopy. Standard radiography provides a snapshot image, which can be useful for evaluation of esophageal anatomy but can provide little information on esophageal function. Fluoroscopy provides continuous real-time imaging of the examination of the esophagus and is ideal for evaluating esophageal anatomy, as well as function. Contrast-medium selection is extremely important and should be tailored to the patient's suspected clinical problem and risk of complications. Barium paste adheres well to the esophageal mucosa and is the best choice for evaluating esophageal anatomy and location. Barium mixed with food is ideal for evaluating dysphagia, strictures, and functional abnormalities of the esophagus because it closely mimics normal feeding.

INDICATIONS
- Bronchoesophageal fistulas
- Dysphagia
- Esophageal identification
- Esophageal or periesophageal neoplasia
- Esophageal perforation
- Esophageal reflux
- Esophagitis
- Foreign bodies
- Gastroesophageal intussusception
- Hiatal hernias
- Motility disorders
- Regurgitation
- Strictures or diverticuli
- Vascular ring anomalies

CONTRAINDICATIONS
- Barium should not be administered to patients that have underlying pneumonia. Aspiration of barium by a patient with normal lungs usually does not cause significant problems. Even though barium is inert, if aspirated, it may exacerbate underlying pneumonia.
- Barium should not be administered to patients with suspected esophageal perforation. Barium leakage into the mediastinum can lead to a secondary granulomatous reaction. Nonionic iodinated contrast agents that have an osmolarity similar to blood may be used instead. If aspirated, they are usually rapidly absorbed with no complications.
- Ionic iodinated contrast agents should never be administered orally. Because of their high osmolarity, aspiration of these agents may cause severe acute pulmonary edema and death.

POTENTIAL COMPLICATIONS
- Development or exacerbation of aspiration pneumonia, particularly in animals with dysphagia
- Aspiration of barium
- Acute pulmonary edema (seen with aspiration of hyperosmolar ionic iodinated contrast media)
- Mediastinitis in cases of esophageal perforation

CLIENT EDUCATION
- Esophagography is a useful procedure to better identify the esophagus, which is normally invisible on radiographs. The images obtained via radiography represent a snapshot of the esophagus, but facilitate the diagnosis of many common esophageal abnormalities. Fluoroscopy may be needed in some cases to evaluate the esophagus in real time for functional abnormalities or more complicated cases. Endoscopy may also be useful in many cases to better evaluate the esophageal mucosa.

BODY SYSTEMS ASSESSED
- Endocrine and metabolic
- Gastrointestinal
- Musculoskeletal
- Nervous
- Neuromuscular

PROCEDURE

PATIENT PREPARATION
Preprocedure Medication or Preparation
If clinically stable, the patient should ideally be fasted for 6–8 h before the procedure. Survey radiographs of the thorax should be made prior to the esophagram, including both right and left lateral and ventrodorsal or dorsoventral projections. A lateral projection of the cervical region should also be obtained.

Anesthesia or Sedation
- Preferably none
- Motility may be altered and patients predisposed to aspiration.
- For noncompliant patients, acepromazine may be administered SC or IM at a dose of 0.05–0.1 mg/kg.

Patient Positioning
- Right lateral recumbency is usually sufficient. For select cases (e.g., midline caudal thoracic mass), dorsoventral and oblique projections may provide additional information.
- The patient should be adequately restrained with tape and sandbags to minimize manual restraint and personnel radiation exposure.
- The X-ray beam should be centered on the thorax and cervical region and tightly collimated.

Patient Monitoring
Monitor the patient closely during the procedure for possible aspiration or difficulty breathing.

ESOPHAGOGRAPHY

Equipment or Supplies
• Positive contrast agent (barium sulfate suspension, 45%–85% wt/wt; barium paste; nonionic iodinated contrast diluted to a 1:1 ratio of contrast to water). Barium sulfate paste provides good mucosal coating but may not disperse around intraluminal lesions. Barium sulfate suspension is a satisfactory general-purpose contrast agent, but provides inferior mucosal coating compared to paste.
• A 35- or 60-mL syringe
• Palatable dry dog or cat food
• Absorbable pads to place beneath the patient's head

TECHNIQUE
• Choose the appropriate contrast agent.
• For evaluation of motility disorders, barium sulfate suspension should be administered alone first, followed by a food and barium suspension mixture.
• Barium sulfate in any form should not be administered to patients with underlying aspiration pneumonia or suspected esophageal perforation or to patients that soon may undergo esophagoscopy.
• Despite poor mucosal coating and higher expense, nonionic iodinated contrast agents should be used for the specific instances described in the previous paragraph. The agent should be diluted at a 1:1 ratio with water before administration. Ionic iodinated contrast agents should not be used for oral administration.
• Place absorbable pads beneath the patient's head to avoid contamination of the X-ray table with contrast.
• After appropriate positioning and restraint, orally administer a 10- to 30-mL bolus of the contrast agent. Immediately or shortly after the patient has swallowed, the radiograph should be exposed. Several boluses may have to be administered and multiple radiographic exposures made to obtain a diagnosis.

SAMPLE HANDLING
N/A

APPROPRIATE AFTERCARE
Postprocedure Patient Monitoring
Watch closely for persistent coughing or dyspnea.
If the patient has megaesophagus, then removal of food or fluid from esophagus after the procedure is indicated to help prevent aspiration pneumonia.

Nursing Care
Not normally required

Dietary Modification
None

Medication Requirements
None. Any complication that develops should be treated appropriately.

Restrictions on Activity
None

Anticipated Recovery Time
None

INTERPRETATION

NORMAL FINDINGS OR RANGE
Barium paste, barium sulfate suspension, and nonionic contrast medium should result in minimum dilation of the esophagus and should be cleared relatively quickly. Functional abnormalities may affect different phases of swallowing, which are divided into the oral, oropharyngeal, and esophageal phases. The *oral phase* consists of prehension, mastication, and stripping of a food bolus to the base of the tongue. The *oropharyngeal phase* consists of transferring the bolus from the base of the tongue into the cranial esophagus in a coordinated movement. The *esophageal phase* is controlled by primary, secondary, and tertiary peristaltic contractions of the esophagus, based on impulses obtained from neuromuscular fibers within the esophagus when they become distended. Small boluses within the esophagus may appear static; adequate distention stimulates neuromuscular fiber activity, which causes secondary and tertiary peristaltic contractions to move the bolus into the stomach.

ABNORMAL VALUES
• Esophageal dilation, abnormal motility, obstruction, intraluminal lesions, mucosal irregularity, contrast leakage, and changes to esophageal shape or position are considered abnormal.
• Anatomic abnormalities of the esophagus are classified as intraluminal, intramural, or periesophageal.
• Functional abnormalities are classified as affecting the oral, oropharyngeal, or esophageal phases of swallowing.
• Appropriate differentials depend on generalized or segmental involvement of the esophagus and the specific type of anatomic or functional abnormality as classified in the 2 preceding paragraphs.

CRITICAL VALUES
N/A

INTERFERING FACTORS
Drugs That May Alter Results of the Procedure
Any drug that depresses the central nervous system may alter esophageal motility.

Conditions That May Interfere with Performing the Procedure
Diagnostic esophagography cannot be performed on heavily sedated or anesthetized patients because of the effects of sedation or anesthesia on normal esophageal motility.

Procedure Techniques or Handling That May Alter Results
None

Influence of Signalment on Performing and Interpreting the Procedure
Species
Normal dogs have a linear mucosal esophageal pattern, and the esophagus is composed entirely of skeletal muscle. The caudal one-third of a cat's esophagus has a herringbone type of appearance because of the presence of smooth muscle in this portion.

Breed
None

Age
None

Gender
None

Pregnancy
None

CLINICAL PERSPECTIVE

While radiographic esophagography may be sufficient for lower esophageal disorders, real-time fluoroscopy is usually needed to diagnose upper esophageal and pharyngeal disorders such as cricopharyngeal achalasia.

 MISCELLANEOUS

ANCILLARY TESTS

- Endoscopy
- Fluoroscopy

SYNONYMS

Barium swallow

SEE ALSO

Blackwell's Five-Minute Veterinary Consult: Canine and Feline Topics

- Dysphagia
- Esophageal Diverticula

- Esophageal Foreign Bodies
- Esophageal Stricture
- Esophagitis
- Gastroesophageal Reflux
- Hiatal Hernia
- Laryngeal Disease
- Mediastinitis
- Megaesophagus
- Peripheral Neuropathies (Polyneuropathies)
- Pneumonia, Bacterial
- Vascular Ring Anomalies

Related Topics in This Book

- Esophagogastroduodenoscopy
- Fluoroscopy
- General Principles of Radiography

ABBREVIATIONS

None

Suggested Reading
Ettinger SJ, Feldman EC, eds. *Textbook of Veterinary Internal Medicine,* 6th ed. St Louis: Saunders Elsevier.
Thrall DE, ed. *Textbook of Veterinary Diagnostic Radiology,* 4th ed. Philadelphia: WB Saunders, 2002.
Wallack ST. *The Handbook of Veterinary Contrast Radiography.* Solano Beach, CA: San Diego Veterinary Imaging, 2003.

INTERNET RESOURCES

None

AUTHOR NAMES

Paul M. Rist and Reid Tyson

ESTRADIOL

BASICS

TYPE OF SPECIMEN
Blood

TEST EXPLANATION AND RELATED PHYSIOLOGY
Estradiol-17β is the main estrogen in circulation. The primary source of estradiol in sexually intact females is the ovarian follicle, whereas in sexually intact males the testes produce a small amount of estradiol. In both genders, estradiol in peripheral tissue is derived by the aromatization of circulating androgens, testosterone, and androstenedione. This process is responsible for the majority of circulating estradiol in male dogs. Androstenedione is of adrenal origin.

In bitches, serum [estradiol] typically increases to >25 pg/mL during proestrus. It peaks at >60 pg/mL shortly before the onset of estrus and declines through estrus. Serum [estradiol] is <15 pg/mL during diestrus and anestrus. During estrus in queens, estradiol is also typically >25–50 pg/mL. It returns to basal levels of <15 pg/mL between cycles and during the seasonal anestrus.

Deficiencies in circulating concentrations of estradiol are rare. Pathologic amounts of estradiol are produced occasionally by testicular tumors in dogs. Hyperestrogenism in male dogs can cause alopecia, gynecomastia, and pendulous prepuce and suppress bone marrow hematopoiesis. In bitches and queens, cystic ovarian follicles, or rarely granulosa cell tumors, may produce estradiol continuously and cause persistent signs of heat and, much less commonly, alopecia.

[Estradiol] is determined by radioimmunoassay and chemiluminescent immunoassay made for human specimens, and assays are relatively imprecise in measuring the low hormone levels found in dogs and cats. Differentiating pathologic findings from normal physiologic variations in [estradiol], especially in intact females, is often quite difficult.

INDICATIONS
• Evaluate male dogs that are suspected to have an estrogen-producing testicular tumor.
• Assess the aspects of ovarian function:
  • Ovarian remnant
  • Ovarian follicular cysts
  • Primary anestrus

CONTRAINDICATIONS
None

POTENTIAL COMPLICATIONS
None

CLIENT EDUCATION
None

BODY SYSTEMS ASSESSED
• Dermatologic
• Endocrine and metabolic
• Reproductive

SAMPLE

COLLECTION
1–2 mL of venous blood

HANDLING
• Use a plain red-top tube. Avoid the use of a serum-separator gel.
• Centrifuge and harvest the serum within 1 h.

STORAGE
Refrigerate or freeze the serum.

STABILITY
• Room temperature: 2 h
• Refrigerated (2°–8°C): ≈2 days
• Frozen (−20°C): ≈6 months

PROTOCOL
GnRH response test
• Measure estradiol at 0, 60, and 90 min after IV administration of GnRH, 0.02–0.03 μg/kg.
• If responsive ovarian tissue is present, serum estradiol should exceed 15–20 pg/mL.

INTERPRETATION

NORMAL FINDINGS OR RANGE
• <15 pg/mL in bitches and queens during diestrus and anestrus
• 25 to >50–60 pg/mL in bitches and queens during proestrus and estrus
• Reference intervals vary among labs and assays.

ABNORMAL VALUES
• Estradiol >15 pg/mL in a supposedly spayed queen or bitch displaying characteristic physical or behavioral signs of heat is consistent with an ovarian remnant. The gonad is a more likely source of elevated estrogen than the adrenal in those species.
• High [estradiol] in an animal displaying signs of estrogen-induced paraneoplastic syndrome justifies a search for an estrogen-producing tumor or exogenous source of estrogen.

CRITICAL VALUES
None

INTERFERING FACTORS
Drugs That May Alter Results or Interpretation
Drugs That Interfere with Test Methodology
Estrogenic compounds may cross-react with assays.

Drugs That Alter Physiology
Estrogen, progesterone, and testosterone suppress GnRH and/or luteinizing hormone (LH) and therefore gonadal function.

Disorders That May Alter Results
None

Collection Techniques or Handling That May Alter Results
• Prolonged storage with RBCs
• Use of serum-separator tubes; estradiol values may be decreased by exposure to the separator gel.

Influence of Signalment
Species
Estrogen-producing ovarian and testicular tumors have not been reported in cats.

Breed
None

Age
Testicular and ovarian tumors are seen in older dogs (8–10 years of age).

Gender
Male dogs: testicular tumors
Female dogs: granulosa cell tumors; primary anestrus
Female dogs and cats: ovarian remnants and ovarian follicular cyst

Pregnancy
None

LIMITATIONS OF THE TEST
Single, random samples may not yield results sufficiently different from normal reference ranges to be of diagnostic significance.

Sensitivity, Specificity, and Positive and Negative Predictive Values
N/A

Valid If Run in a Human Lab?
Yes—if the lab has established reference intervals for the veterinary species.

Causes of Abnormal Findings

High values	Low values
Estrus	Ovariohysterectomy
Ovarian cystic follicle or remnant	Ovarian failure or aplasia
Ovarian neoplasm (granulosa cell tumor)	Secondary anestrus
Testicular tumor (Sertoli cell tumor)	Glucocorticoid or progestin therapy
Atypical hyperadrenocorticism	

CLINICAL PERSPECTIVE

• Estradiol causes maturation and cornification of vaginal and preputial epithelia. Evaluation of epithelial morphology is easy to perform and far more convenient than measuring serum estradiol.
  • In bitches and queens suspected of having ovarian remnant, a preponderance of cornified superficial epithelial cells in a vaginal cytology smear indicates estrogenic stimulation and suggests that estrogen is the likely cause of clinical signs.
  • In dogs with classic clinical signs of the estrogen paraneoplastic syndrome, cornified vaginal or preputial epithelial cells help confirm that excessive estrogen is present.
  • Given the low assay sensitivity, finding a normal [estradiol] does not necessarily exclude ovarian remnant. However, finding non-cornified vaginal epithelium during supposed signs of heat would.
• When the clinical signs are cyclic in nature, testing should be done when signs of heat are present.

MISCELLANEOUS

ANCILLARY TESTS
• Vaginal or preputial cytology
• Some females with ovarian remnants do ovulate. If signs of heat have passed, consider measuring serum progesterone.

SYNONYMS
• Estradiol-17β
• Estrogen

SEE ALSO
Blackwell's Five-Minute Veterinary Consult: Canine and Feline Topics
• Ovarian Remnant Syndrome
• Ovarian Tumors

Related Topics in This Book
Progesterone

ABBREVIATIONS
• [estradiol] = estradiol concentration
• GnRH = gonadotropin-releasing hormone

Suggested Reading
Feldman EC, Nelson RW. *Canine and Feline Endocrinology and Reproduction,* 3rd ed. St Louis: Saunders Elsevier, 2004.
Johnston SD, Root Kustritz MV, Olson PN. *Canine and Feline Theriogenology.* Philadelphia: WB Saunders, 2001.

INTERNET RESOURCES
None

AUTHOR NAME
Cheri A. Johnson

ETHYLENE GLYCOL

BASICS

TYPE OF SPECIMEN
Bait
Blood
Tissue (stomach content and/or vomitus)
Urine

TEST EXPLANATION AND RELATED PHYSIOLOGY
Ethylene glycol (EG) is an ingredient in many radiator antifreeze products and other automotive and industrial solvents. It is both commonly used and well known for its toxic potential. EG is known to cause central nervous system depression, polyuria/polydipsia, and GI irritation, but EG is metabolized to more toxic products, thus severe clinical signs and death are usually delayed. EG is slowly converted to glycoaldehyde by alcohol dehydrogenase, which in turn is rapidly converted to glycolic acid. Glycolic acid causes metabolic acidosis and some renal tubular epithelial damage. Glycolic acid is slowly converted to glyoxylic acid, which is then converted to oxalic acid. Oxalic acid can bind to calcium, producing hypocalcemia and oxalate crystal formation in renal tubules and other tissues. The presence of unmeasured osmotically active particles in the serum (e.g., EG and its metabolites) increases osmolarity early in the course of toxicosis. With access to an osmometer, the difference between measured and calculated osmolality (the *osmolal gap*) can be used diagnostically.

Methods frequently used to test for EG include a commercially available test kit [EGT (ethylene glycol test) kit; PRN Pharmacal, Pensacola, FL], gas chromatography/mass spectroscopy (GC/MS), and enzymatic assays. The EGT kit provides results within 30 min. False-positive results may occur with this kit because of the presence of propylene glycol or glycerol, common ingredients in pharmaceuticals and some foods. GC/MS and enzymatic tests are more specific for EG and may be more sensitive, but these tests must be performed by a reference laboratory and therefore will take more time. EG may not be detectable in serum after >1–3 days. Some antifreeze preparations contain fluorescein, which appears bright yellow-green when viewed under a Wood's lamp. In human patients, urine fluorescence can serve as an adjunctive test in suspected EG ingestion. However, certain commonly administered medications, such as antibiotics or vitamins, can induce fluorescence. In addition, both glass and plastic specimen containers have a high native fluorescence. Samples for testing should be deposited on filter paper.

INDICATIONS
- A history consistent with EG exposure
- A vomiting patient with central nervous system signs (e.g., depression, stupor, ataxia)
- Oxalate crystals in urine
- Increased osmolal and anion gaps

CONTRAINDICATIONS
None

POTENTIAL COMPLICATIONS
None

CLIENT EDUCATION
EG toxicosis is frequently lethal, and early diagnosis is absolutely essential for successful treatment. Prognosis is excellent in animals treated within 3–6 h of EG ingestion but grave after onset of renal failure, which may occur within 24 h.

BODY SYSTEMS ASSESSED
Renal and urologic

SAMPLE

COLLECTION
- 10 mL of heparinized or EDTA whole blood
- 10 mL of urine
- Bait or stomach content

HANDLING
Ship on ice.

STORAGE
- Refrigerate the blood sample.
- Freeze the urine or stomach content and the bait.

STABILITY
N/A

PROTOCOL
None

INTERPRETATION

NORMAL FINDINGS OR RANGE
Negative for EG

ABNORMAL VALUES
Positive for EG

CRITICAL VALUES
The presence of EG in the sample is diagnostic for exposure.

INTERFERING FACTORS
Drugs That May Alter Results or Interpretation
Drugs That Interfere with Test Methodology
Compounds in drug formulations that may interfere with test kit results:
- Glycerol
- Propylene glycol

Drugs That Alter Physiology
None

Disorders That May Alter Results
None

Collection Techniques or Handling That May Alter Results
False negative if biologic samples collected >1–3 days after exposure
Influence of Signalment
Species
False negatives may be more likely in cats, a highly sensitive species.

Breed
None

Age
None

Gender
None

Pregnancy
None

LIMITATIONS OF THE TEST
- The EGT kit yields rapid results but is less specific than GC/MS or enzymatic tests.
- The EGT kit may cross-react with propylene glycol and glycerol found in foods and some pharmaceuticals.
- Samples taken >1–3 days after exposure may be negative.

Sensitivity, Specificity, and Positive and Negative Predictive Values
N/A

Valid If Run in a Human Lab?
Yes.

Causes of Abnormal Findings

High values	Low values
Ingestion of EG containing antifreeze	Usually insignificant
Commercial kit cross-reacts with these compounds:	May occur with metabolism of EG into by-products not detected by assay
Propylene glycol	
Glycerol	
Enzymatic assay value can be increased by increased lactate or by lactate dehydrogenase	

CLINICAL PERSPECTIVE

- EG concentrations in serum and urine are detectable by 1–2 h after ingestion.
- Calcium oxalate crystalluria in cats and dogs can occur as early as 3 and 6 h, respectively, after ingestion in cats and dogs.
  - Monohydrate calcium oxalate crystals (clear, elongated, flat picket-fence shaped) are more common than dihydrate calcium oxalate crystals (shaped like a Maltese cross or envelope).
  - The dihydrate crystals can be seen in normal animals; the monohydrate crystals are more clinically significant.
- Serum osmolality can be increased as much as 100 mOsm/kg above normal (280–310 mOsm/kg) within 3 h of EG ingestion and is significantly higher than the calculated value (increased osmolal gap). An increased osmolal gap suggests the presence of unmeasured osmotically active molecules such as EG. However, an increased osmolal gap is a relatively nonspecific finding that can also be associated with alcohol toxicity, lactic acidosis, chronic renal failure, and diabetic ketoacidosis.
- By the time patients show signs of renal failure, test results for EG may be negative.

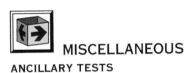

MISCELLANEOUS

ANCILLARY TESTS
- Urinalysis
- Serum chemistries
- Anion gap
- Serum osmolarity and calculated osmolal gap
- Renal impression smears
- Renal histopathology
- Fluorescent marker in urine (not definitive)

SYNONYMS
None

SEE ALSO
Blackwell's Five-Minute Veterinary Consult: Canine and Feline Topics
- Ethylene Glycol Poisoning
- Renal Failure, Acute Uremia

Related Topics in This Book
- Anion Gap
- Osmolality
- Urine Sediment
- Urine Specific Gravity

ABBREVIATIONS
- EG = ethylene glycol
- GC/MS = gas chromatography/mass spectroscopy

Suggested Reading
Dalefield R. Ethylene glycol. In: Plumlee KH, ed. *Clinical Veterinary Toxicology,* 1st ed. St Louis: CV Mosby, 2003: 444–446.
Hull W. Ethylene glycol testing. *Vet Tech* 2001; **22**: 201–202, 216.
Thrall MA, Connally HE, Grauer GF, Hamar D. Ethylene glycol test. In: Peterson ME, Talcott PA, eds. *Small Animal Toxicology,* 2nd ed. Philadelphia: WB Saunders, 2005: 702–726.

INTERNET RESOURCES
Beasley V. Toxicants that cause acidosis. In: Beasley V, ed. Veterinary Toxicology. Ithaca, NY: International Veterinary Information Service (IVIS), 1999, http://www.ivis.org/advances/Beasley/Cpt4/ivis.pdf.
Braund KG. Neurotoxic disorders. In: Braund KG, ed. Clinical Neurology in Small Animals: Localization, Diagnosis, and Treatment. Ithaca, NY: International Veterinary Information Service (IVIS), 2003, http://www.ivis.org/advances/Vite/braund22/ivis.pdf.
PRN Pharmacal EGT Kit: Ethylene glycol test kit, http://prnpharmacal.com/egtkit/index.php.

AUTHOR NAME
Karyn Bischoff

EXCRETORY UROGRAPHY

BASICS

TYPE OF PROCEDURE
Radiographic

PROCEDURE EXPLANATION AND RELATED PHYSIOLOGY
An excretory urogram is the bolus IV administration of sterile, io-dinated (ionic or nonionic) contrast medium to define the renal parenchyma, the renal collecting system, and the ureters. as well as to fill the urinary bladder physiologically (without catheterization). The basis of the procedure is the glomerular filtration of the iodinated contrast medium administered IV with subsequent tubular concentration of the iodine to foster radiographic visibility of the renal parenchyma (nephrogram) and the ureteropelvic collecting system (pyelogram).

INDICATIONS
- Locate and, as necessary, measure the kidneys, renal pelves, and ureters.
- Qualitatively assess renal function (i.e., nephrographic and pyelographic opacity) both as a comparison between the kidneys and as a general assessment of the functional state of the glomerular filtration and tubular concentrating capacity of the kidneys.
- Compare the relative sizes of the renal pelvis, the pelvic recesses, and the ureter to facilitate differentiation of pyelonephritis from hydronephrosis.
- Assess the relationship among the kidneys, the ureters, and the bladder (e.g., ectopic ureter, ureteral duplication, ectopic kidney, retroflexed bladder, herniated bladder).
- Assess bladder sphincter competence by using IV urography as a physiologic means to fill the urinary bladder and determine whether there is urethral or vaginal staining with the iodinated contrast medium, indicating incontinence as the bladder fills.
- Assess for vaginal pooling of urine mimicking incontinence, perform IV urography, allow the bladder to fill, and then look for vaginal staining by radiographing again after voluntary voiding.
- Assess the renal collecting system for leaks, particularly in the presence of retroperitoneal fluid.
- Assess for bladder leaks when retrograde catheterization is impossible or contraindicated.
- Assess the relevance of focal retroperitoneal opacities (e.g., possible stones) or masses to determine their effect on or location relative to the renal parenchyma and collecting system.
- Investigate suspected renal-origin hematuria.
- Assess the ureteral effects of a bladder trigone mass.

CONTRAINDICATIONS
- A dehydrated patient
- An oliguric or anuric patient
- A patient with a medical history of contrast-media reactions (e.g., life-threatening hypotension, collapse, anaphylaxis)
- *Note*: Azotemia in the presence of adequate urine flow and reasonable hydration is not a contraindication to IV urography, but the contrast dose must be increased to increase the probability of a diagnostic study.

POTENTIAL COMPLICATIONS
In addition to the peracute contrast medium–related reactions, contrast medium–induced renal failure is an unlikely possibility. Contrast medium–induced renal failure is usually reversible with fluid therapy alone, but several days of hemodialysis or peritoneal dialysis may be required before renal function returns to preprocedure levels. As a precaution, it is best to use nonionic, iodinated contrast medium in high-risk and geriatric patients.

CLIENT EDUCATION
- The animal should not have any food for at least 18 h prior to the procedure unless it is an emergency.
- The animal should have a cleansing, tepid water enema at least 2 h before the procedure except in an emergency.
- There is a limited, although not insignificant, risk of a life-threatening contrast-medium reaction.

BODY SYSTEMS ASSESSED
Renal and urologic

PROCEDURE

PATIENT PREPARATION

Preprocedure Medication or Preparation
- Ensure adequate urine production and reasonable hydration.
- Verify that the animal has not experienced previous contrast-medium hypersensitivity reactions. If it has, consider an alternative procedure or premedicate it for 24 h with at least 2 doses of corticosteroids.
- Withhold food for at least 18 h prior to the procedure unless it is an emergency.
- Administer a cleansing, tepid water enema at least 2 h before the procedure unless it is an emergency.

Anesthesia or Sedation
In general, IV urography is best performed without sedation or anesthesia unless patient compliance precludes adequate positioning.

Patient Positioning
Right recumbent and dorsally recumbent views are indicated before the contrast-medium administration and at the specified intervals after the administration. Where applicable, oblique views may facilitate ureter or trigone assessment.

Patient Monitoring
Generally observe the patient's well-being, specifically including capillary refill rate (or blood pressure, if available) and heart rate during the 45-min period after the contrast administration.

Equipment or Supplies
- A sodium-based, ionic (e.g., diatrizoate or iothalamate) or nonionic (e.g., iopamidol or iohexol) iodinated contrast medium approved for IV use
- An IV catheter that can remain in place during dosing and for at least 30 min after dosing with contrast medium (in case fluids or drugs are needed)
- Radiographic facilities capable of creating adequate abdominal views
- An emergency or crash cart: IV fluids (including an appropriate administration set), 1:10,000 epinephrine, atropine, rapid-acting corticosteroids, an appropriate-size endotracheal tube, oxygen, a ventilation apparatus (e.g., Ambu bag or anesthesia machine), and parenteral antihistamines

TECHNIQUE
- Expose survey radiographs to ensure that the patient has been adequately prepared and that radiographic techniques are adequate.
- Administer 180 mg of iodine (as sterile sodium diatrizoate or sterile sodium iothalamate or iopamidol or iohexol in high-risk patients) per kilogram of body weight (400 mg/lb) as a rapid IV (bolus) injection through a preplaced cephalic, jugular, or saphenous vein catheter. The catheter should remain usable for at least 30 min for fluid or drug administration in case of a reaction to the contrast medium.
- Expose a VD view at 15–20 s after bolus injection (the best time to see kidneys).
- Expose lateral and VD views at 5, 20, and 40 min after injection.

- Expose VD oblique views (15°–30° off VD in both directions) at 5 min after injection (only in patients suspected of having an ectopic ureter).
- To ensure progressive bladder filling, prevent the patient from urinating during the procedure.

SAMPLE HANDLING
None

APPROPRIATE AFTERCARE
Postprocedure Patient Monitoring
- Monitor the capillary refill rate (or blood pressure, if available) and heart rate for ≈45 min after the contrast administration to be sure there is no evidence of shock or hypotension.
- Watch for any difficulty breathing that might suggest airway problems (e.g., laryngeal edema or bronchial spasm) for the same time frame.
- Be sure the patient continues to produce urine over the next 24 h. If urine production declines, IV fluids should be administered immediately.
- Administer parenteral antihistamines to manage erythematous or hivelike cutaneous reactions, if they occur.
- Manage hypotensive or shock reactions with appropriate fluids, steroids, airway assurance, and epinephrine as prescribed for general resuscitation protocols in the unlikely event of a severe contrast-medium reaction.
- Administer atropine to manage contrast-induced bradycardia, if observed.

Nursing Care
None

Dietary Modification
None

Medication Requirements
None

Restrictions on Activity
None

Anticipated Recovery Time
None

 ## INTERPRETATION

NORMAL FINDINGS OR RANGE
After completion of IV contrast-medium administration, normal findings include a peak symmetrical renal parenchymal opacification (nephrogram) within 15–20 s that progressively fades toward that seen on the survey radiographs during the 40-min sequence of postinjection radiographs. Renal length measurements (from the VD view) for dogs should be between 2.5 and 3.5 times the length of the second lumbar vertebral body, and for cats they should be between 1.9 and 3.2 times the length of the second vertebral body. Peak symmetrical renal pelvic and ureter opacification (pyelogram) should be between 5 and 20 min after contrast-medium administration (Figure 1). Renal pelvic (lateral to medial at the ureteropelvic junction) width and ureteral (maximum diameter of the proximal ureter) measurements (from the VD view) should be <3–4 mm regardless of patient size.

Note: The opacity of the pyelogram should be much greater than that of the nephrogram because the pyelogram represents contrast medium acted upon by both the GFR and the tubular concentration.

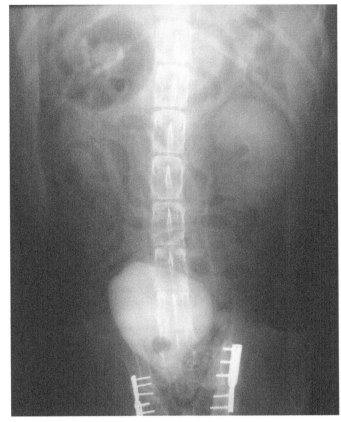

(a)

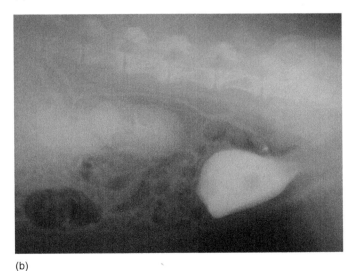

(b)

Figure 1

VD view (a) and right lateral view (b) of a normal canine IV urogram at 5 min after administration of contrast medium.

EXCRETORY UROGRAPHY

ABNORMAL VALUES

- *Nephrogram*: poor opacification (hypotension, outflow obstruction, ischemia, poor GFR); focal or multifocal areas of poor opacification (tumor, cyst, abscess, granuloma, hydronephrosis); apparent renal silhouette larger than nephrogram (perinephric pseudocyst or abscess)
- *Pyelogram*: renal pelvic, ureteral, *and* pelvic recess dilation (hydronephrosis); pelvic and ureteral dilation *with* short, blunted pelvic recesses (pyelonephritis); filling defects in any pyelographic structure (urolith, blood clot, polyp, tumor, parasite); failure of distal ureter(s) to terminate in the bladder trigone with any evidence of contrast medium in vagina, urethra, or rectum (ectopic ureter); poor to nonexistent pyelogram opacity (poor GFR or tubular concentration capacity, renal outflow obstruction); ureteral leakage
- *Bladder*: displaced bladder (pelvic or retroflexed); leakage of urine from bladder into proximal urethra (suspicious for sphincter incontinence); ureteropelvic dilation (if found, check for trigone masses); bladder leakage

CRITICAL VALUES

Patient collapse from a contrast-medium reaction

INTERFERING FACTORS

Drugs That May Alter Results of the Procedure

Aggressive fluid administration may physiologically decrease the opacity of pyelogram.

Conditions That May Interfere with Performing the Procedure

- Severe azotemia (e.g., BUN >100 mg/dL) may result in poor nephrographic and pyelographic opacification. If the risk of the procedure is deemed appropriate, the contrast-medium dose should be doubled [e.g., 1760 mg of iodine/kg of body weight (800 mg/lb)], preferably with nonionic contrast medium, if available.
- Poor patient compliance might require sedation.

Procedure Techniques or Handling That May Alter Results

- Perivascular injection, or inadequate dosing, of the contrast medium
- Poor positioning of patient during image exposure
- *Beware* of contrast-medium effects on urinalysis results probably for at least 24 h, including specifically false increases in urine specific gravity and some interference with culturing success of some organisms.

Influence of Signalment on Performing and Interpreting the Procedure

Species

Dog and cat normal renal measurements differ as discussed in the Normal Findings or Range section.

Breed

None other than to be aware of breed predispositions to hereditary renal diseases.

Age

In general, as cats age, their kidneys progress toward the low end of the specified range for normal length. (This is more prominent in neutered than intact cats.)

Gender

None

Pregnancy

None for the patient, but the risk of contrast medium to the fetuses has not been fully explored, and the radiation effects on first trimester fetuses can be problematic. This procedure is, therefore, a risk/benefit judgment when dealing with pregnant patients.

CLINICAL PERSPECTIVE

IV urography provides morphologic (e.g., size, shape, location) information on both the kidneys and urinary bladder that is similar to that provided by ultrasound. However, the physiologic information provided (e.g., how serious the ureteral stone effect is, whether the differences in function between the kidneys are significant, whether the urethral sphincter is competent in awake dogs) is rarely matched by other procedures. In addition, other than computed tomography, IV urography is about the only procedure that provides primary information on both ureteral morphology and function. IV urography can better characterize the status of ectopic ureters than ultrasound, but is less exacting (and less expensive) than computed tomography for that purpose.

MISCELLANEOUS

ANCILLARY TESTS

- Abdominal ultrasound
- Renal ultrasound

SYNONYMS

- Intravenous pyelogram (IVP)
- Intravenous urogram

SEE ALSO

Blackwell's Five-Minute Veterinary Consult: Canine and Feline Topics

Many

Related Topics in This Book

- General Principles of Radiography
- Cystourethrography
- Renal Biopsy and Aspiration
- Renal Ultrasonography

ABBREVIATIONS

- GFR = glomerular filtration rate
- VD = ventrodorsal

Suggested Reading

Burk RL, Feeney DA. The abdomen In:. *Small Animal Radiology and Ultrasonography*, 3rd ed. Philadelphia: WB Saunders, 2003: 355–399.

Feeney DA, Johnston GR. Kidneys and ureters. In: Thrall DE, ed. *Textbook of Veterinary Diagnostic Radiology*, 4th ed. Philadelphia: WB Saunders, 2002: 556–571.

Johnston GR, Walter PA, Feeney DA. Diagnostic imaging of the urinary tract. In: Osborne CA, Finco DR, eds. *Canine and Feline Nephrology/Urology*. Baltimore: Williams & Wilkins, 1995: 230–276.

INTERNET RESOURCES

http://www.cvm.umn.edu/vetrad/

AUTHOR NAME

Daniel A. Feeney

BASICS

TYPE OF SPECIMEN
Feces

TEST EXPLANATION AND RELATED PHYSIOLOGY
Direct fecal smear cytology is performed to examine the fecal bacterial flora and any nucleated cells that are present (epithelial, inflammatory) and to detect other pathogens that may be present (i.e., bacterial, fungal, protozoal, algal, oomycetal). Although evaluation of fecal cytology may enable one to diagnose the primary cause of GI signs in some cases, abnormalities detected by using fecal cytology are often nonspecific, representing an incidental finding associated with other underlying diseases or processes that may or may not be contributing to the patient's ongoing GI signs (e.g., diarrhea). Direct fecal smear cytology is not synonymous with a *rectal scrape*, which is a somewhat more invasive method of sampling the rectal mucosa by direct scraping of its surface with a swab or blunt spatula. Rectal scraping is typically required to identify some deeper infections (e.g., histoplasmosis, protothecosis).

INDICATIONS
- Diarrhea (the most common indication)
- Less commonly, other GI signs (e.g., vomition)

CONTRAINDICATIONS
None

POTENTIAL COMPLICATIONS
None

CLIENT EDUCATION
- This test may not reveal the primary cause of a patient's GI signs. Instead, abnormalities secondary to other underlying primary or secondary GI disease may be detected.
- Normal direct fecal smear cytology does not definitively exclude the possibility of GI disease, including underlying infection or inflammation.

BODY SYSTEMS ASSESSED
Gastrointestinal

SAMPLE

COLLECTION
Collect feces from the rectum by using a slightly moistened cotton-tipped applicator or use the feces present on one's gloved finger after a digital rectal exam.

HANDLING
- Smear the feces onto a clean, glass microscope slide to form a thin film.
- Prepare a wet preparation by adding a few drops of saline and a coverslip. Do not make the wet preparation too thick; one should be able read newsprint through the wet prep. Adding a drop of iodine to the preparation may improve visualization of protozoa.
- Air-dry the thin film of feces.
  - Stain with a Romanovsky stain (e.g., Diff-Quik; Dade Behring, Newark, DE) for cytologic examination.
  - Use acid-fast stain in looking for *Cryptosporidia* sp.
  - Heat-fix prior to Gram staining.

STORAGE
- Wet preparations should be prepared and immediately examined.
- For other preparations, the sample should be processed within 2 h or feces should be refrigerated.

- Store air-dried fecal smears at room temperature and protected from light.
- Fecal smear slides should not be refrigerated or frozen.
- Wet preparations should be read immediately and cannot be stored.

STABILITY
- Feces at room temperature: 2 h
- Refrigerated feces: variable stability, depending on abnormality of interest. Parasite ova are stable, but cellular deterioration and changes in bacteria flora occur over time.
- Wet preparations cannot be stored.
- Fixed-stain smears are stable indefinitely if protected from light and humidity.

PROTOCOL
- Examine the wet preparation for motile parasites or parasite ova.
- Examine the Romanovsky-stained smear for the following:
  1. Background bacterial flora
  2. Noninflammatory cells (e.g., epithelial cells, neoplastic cells)
  3. Inflammatory cells
  4. The number of spore-forming bacteria per 1,000× high-power field
  5. The presence of pathogens, such as the following (depending on geographic location):
  - Short spiral or gull wing–shaped bacteria (e.g., *Campylobacter, Helicobacter, Anaerobiospirillum*, treponeme-like bacteria, *Serpulina* spp.)
  - Protozoa (e.g., *Giardia, Trichomonas, Entamoeba*)
  - Dimorphic fungi (e.g., *Histoplasma*)
  - Other fungi (e.g., *Cryptococcus, Candida, Aspergillus*)
  - Algae (e.g., *Prototheca*)
  - Oomycetes (e.g., *Pythium*)

INTERPRETATION

NORMAL FINDINGS OR RANGE
- A polymorphic bacterial population of bacilli. Cocci should be absent or very rarely observed.
- A low number of well-differentiated epithelial cells
- Amorphous material, representing digesta
- A small amount of plant material
- A small amount of extracellular yeast (e.g., *Cyniclomyces*; formerly known as *Saccharomycopsis*) may be observed occasionally.

ABNORMAL VALUES
- Monomorphic bacterial flora
- An increased number of cocci
- The presence of inflammatory cells
- The presence of abnormal noninflammatory cells (e.g., reactive epithelial cells, neoplastic cells)
- The presence of potential pathogens (e.g., protozoa, fungi, algae, oomycetes, gull wing–shaped bacteria)
- The presence of >10 spore-forming bacteria per 1,000× high-power field
  - Specifically, sporulated *Clostridium* has a safety-pin or tennis-racket appearance because the spore produces a swollen, colorless area.

CRITICAL VALUES
None

INTERFERING FACTORS
Drugs That May Alter Results or Interpretation
Drugs That Interfere with Test Methodology
None

FECAL DIRECT SMEAR AND CYTOLOGY

Drugs That Alter Physiology
Prior antimicrobial administration may alter the GI flora, resulting in abnormal direct fecal smear cytologic results.

Disorders That May Alter Results
Prior GI procedures (e.g., surgery, enema) may alter GI flora, resulting in abnormal direct fecal smear cytologic results.

Collection Techniques or Handling that May Alter Results
Deeper scraping of the rectal mucosa will increase the number of epithelial cells observed in direct fecal smear cytology. Deeper scraping may be helpful when certain infections (e.g., histoplasmosis, protothecosis) are suspected.

Influence of Signalment
Species
None

Breed
None

Age
None

Gender
None

Pregnancy
None

LIMITATIONS OF THE TEST
Sensitivity, Specificity, and Positive and Negative Predictive Values
None

Valid If Run in a Human Lab?
Yes, if the observer (i.e., pathologist or technician) is acquainted with veterinary species.

Causes of Abnormal Findings

CLINICAL PERSPECTIVE
• Abnormal background bacterial flora is often an incidental finding associated with other primary or secondary GI diseases, with GI procedures, or with prior antimicrobial administration. In some cases, though, abnormal flora may be a factor contributing to ongoing diarrhea in some patients.
• Observation of inflammatory cells suggests the presence of transmural colonic or rectal inflammation. Fecal culture may be useful to exclude underlying infection by invasive bacteria (e.g., salmonellosis).
• Identification of atypical noninflammatory cells, such as abnormal epithelial cells, may indicate the presence of underlying neoplasia or hyperplasia.
• The primary cause of diarrhea may be determined when pathogens (e.g., bacterial, protozoal, fungal, algal, oomycetal) or an increased number of spore-forming bacteria are observed.

MISCELLANEOUS
ANCILLARY TESTS
• Fecal culture and determination of antibiotic sensitivities are useful when inflammatory cells or pathogens are observed.
• Gram stain of the direct fecal smear is useful in evaluating the background flora and potential bacterial pathogens.
• Warthin-Starry silver stain of the direct fecal smear is useful in evaluating potential bacterial pathogens (e.g., *Lawsonia*).
• Submission of direct fecal smear to a referral laboratory for cytologic evaluation is useful when abnormal noninflammatory cells (e.g., atypical epithelial cells) or when potential pathogens are observed.
• Other tests employed as part of routine GI diagnostic evaluation may include serum biochemistry, fecal flotation, and radiography.

Preparation	Abnormal finding	Possible causes
Wet preparation	Motile protozoa	*Giardia, Balantidium, Entamoeba, Trichomonas trophozoites*
	Parasitic larvae	*Strongyloides, Aelurostrongylus, Filaroides, saprophytic larvae caused by environmental* contamination
	Parasite ova	*Coccidia sp., Toxocara, Trichuris, Ancylostoma, Uncinaria*
Romanovsky stain	Monomorphic population of bacteria	Bacterial overgrowth caused by 1° or 2° GI disease or antibiotic treatment
	Sporulated bacteria	Clostridium overgrowth
	Short spiral or gull wing–shaped bacteria	*Campylobacter, Helicobacter, Anaerobiospirillum*
	White (colorless) rods in macrophages and free in background	*Mycobacterium sp.*
	Neutrophils	Nonspecific sign of GI inflammation or suggests the presence of transmural colonic or rectal inflammation
	Eosinophils	Allergic hypersensitivity or parasitic infection
	Small lymphocytes, plasma cells	Lymphocytic, plasmacytic enteritis
	Monomorphic large lymphocytes	Lymphoma
	Teardrop-shaped protozoan organisms with 2 nuclei that "appear to be looking back at you"	*Giardia sp.*
	Spindle-shaped protozoa with whiplike flagella and an undulating or wavy membrane	*Trichomonas sp.*
	Ciliated protozoan with a large sausage-shaped macronucleus that surrounds a small micronucleus	*Balantidium*
	Round intracellular yeast (within macrophages), 3- to 5-μm diameter	*Histoplasma*
	Septate branching hyphae	*Aspergillus, other fungus, or Pythium*
	Round or oval algae with basophilic granular cytoplasm (3 × 16 μm)	*Prototheca*
Acid-fast stain	4- to 5-μm round magenta structures	*Cryptosporidia sp.*
	Intracellular magenta linear inclusions	*Mycobacterium*

SYNONYMS
Fecal cytology

SEE ALSO
Blackwell's Five-Minute Veterinary Consult: Canine and Feline Topics
- Diarrhea, Acute
- Diarrhea, Chronic—Cats
- Diarrhea, Chronic—Dogs

Related Topics in This Book
- Fecal Flotation
- Fecal Sedimentation and Baermann Exam

ABBREVIATIONS
None

Suggested Reading

Andreason CB, Jergens AE, Meyer DJ. Oral cavity, gastrointestinal tract, and associated structures. In: Raskin RE, Meyer DJ, eds. *Atlas of Canine and Feline Cytology*. Philadelphia: WB Saunders, 2001: 207–229.

Broussard J. Optimal fecal assessment. *Clin Tech Small Anim Pract* 2003; 18: 218–230.

Lassen ED. Laboratory evaluation of digestion and intestinal absorption. In: Thrall MA, ed. *Veterinary Hematology and Clinical Chemistry*. Philadelphia: Lippincott Williams & Wilkins, 2004: 387–399.

INTERNET RESOURCES
None

AUTHOR NAME
Heather L. Wamsley

FECAL ELASTASE

 BASICS

TYPE OF SPECIMEN
Feces

TEST EXPLANATION AND RELATED PHYSIOLOGY
Loss of >90% of exocrine pancreatic secretory function results in clinical EPI. Elastase is a protease formed as a zymogen in the pancreas. Upon entering the intestinal lumen, this enzyme is activated and used to digest elastin in the ingesta. Canine elastase is not appreciably degraded within the GI tract and may be measured in the feces by using a commercially available ELISA. Patients with EPI will have low or negligible fecal elastase.

The commercial ELISA demonstrates no appreciable cross-reactivity with human, bovine, or porcine elastase. Therefore, specimens may be analyzed without disruption of therapeutic enzyme supplementation. Additionally, because the canine elastase ELISA quantifies elastase rather than measuring function, this assay may be more sensitive than methods measuring activity of enzymes which may be degraded by the digestive process.

The cTLI assay is the most robust indicator of decreased exocrine pancreatic function and is considered the gold standard among the tests. A recent report on a study in which cTLI was used as the standard suggests that decreased fecal elastase levels may be seen in a significant number of dogs with small-intestinal disease but no evidence of pancreatic insufficiency (TLI within or above the reference range) (Steiner & Pantchev 2006). The low fecal elastase levels may be caused, in part, by decreased cholecystokinin stimulation of pancreatic acini.

INDICATIONS
- Chronic small-intestinal diarrhea
- Chronic weight loss

CONTRAINDICATIONS
None

POTENTIAL COMPLICATIONS
None

CLIENT EDUCATION
None

BODY SYSTEMS ASSESSED
Gastrointestinal

 SAMPLE

COLLECTION
Fresh feces: at least 100 mg

HANDLING
Use a clean, laboratory-approved container.

STORAGE
Refrigerate the sample for short-term storage.

STABILITY
The sample is stable for up to 3 weeks at 4°C.

PROTOCOL
None

 INTERPRETATION

NORMAL FINDINGS OR RANGE
>40 μg elastase/g feces

ABNORMAL VALUES
<10 μg elastase/g feces

CRITICAL VALUES
None

INTERFERING FACTORS
Drugs That May Alter Results or Interpretation
Drugs That Interfere with Test Methodology
None

Drugs That Alter Physiology
None

Disorders That May Alter Results
None

Collection Techniques or Handling That May Alter Results
Concurrent intestinal inflammation causes no appreciable increase in fecal elastase.

Influence of Signalment
Species
The use of fecal elastase for diagnosis of EPI has been validated only for dogs.

Breed
None

Age
None

Gender
None

Pregnancy
None

LIMITATIONS OF THE TEST
It may be associated with a high rate of false-positive results.
Sensitivity, Specificity, and Positive and Negative Predictive Values
When a cutoff of 10 μg elastase/g feces is used:
- Sensitivity, 95.3%
- Specificity is more controversial:
  - 92% (Spillman et al. 2001)
  - 76.9% (Steiner et al. 2006)

Valid If Run in a Human Lab?
No—species-specific assays are required.

Causes of Abnormal Findings

High values	Low values
None known	EPI
	Pancreatic duct obstruction

CLINICAL PERSPECTIVE
- Fecal elastase is a rapid and sensitive method for assessing exocrine pancreatic function in dogs but may suffer from a high rate of false-positive results in dogs with small-intestinal disease.

- Serum cTLI is still considered the gold standard for diagnosing EPI, and, in dogs with low fecal elastase levels, confirmation by serum cTLI measurement is recommended

MISCELLANEOUS

ANCILLARY TESTS
- Cobalamin
- cTLI
- Fecal flotation
- Folate

SEE ALSO

Blackwell's Five-Minute Veterinary Consult: Canine and Feline Topics
- Exocrine Pancreatic Insufficiency
- Gastroenteritis, Eosinophilic
- Gastroenteritis, Lymphocytic-Plasmacytic
- Pancreatitis
- Small Intestinal Bacterial Overgrowth

Related Topics in This Book
- Alpha-1 Protease Inhibitor
- Cobalamin
- Fecal Fat
- Folate
- Trypsin-like Immunoreactivity

ABBREVIATIONS
- cTLI = canine trypsin-like immunoreactivity
- EPI = exocrine pancreatic insufficiency
- TLI = trypsin-like immunoreactivity

Suggested Reading

Battersby IA, Peters IR, Day MJ, *et al.* Effect of intestinal inflammation on fecal elastase concentration in dogs. *Vet Clin Pathol* 2005; 34: 49–51.

Ettinger SJ, Feldman EC, eds. *Textbook of Veterinary Internal Medicine,* 5th ed. Philadelphia: WB Saunders, 2000: 1355–1361.

Spillman T, Wittker A, Tiegelkamp S, *et al.* An immunoassay for canine pancreatic elastase 1 as an indicator for exocrine pancreatic insufficiency in dogs. *J Vet Diagn Invest* 2001; 13: 468–474.

Steiner JM, Pantchev N. False positive results of measurement of fecal elastase concentration for the diagnosis of exocrine pancreatic insufficiency in dogs [Abstract]. *J Vet Intern Med* 2006: 20: 751.

Steiner JM, Rehfeld JF, Pantchev N. Serum CCK concentrations in dogs with severely decreased fecal elastase concentrations [Abstract]. *J Vet Intern Med* 2006; 20: 1520.

INTERNET RESOURCES
ScheBo Biotech, Veterinary Diagnostic, ScheBo elastase 1, canine, http://www.schebo.co.uk/vet/en/index.html.

Texas A&M University, College of Veterinary Medicine, Gastrointestinal Laboratory: New: updated assay reference ranges, http://www.cvm.tamu.edu/gilab.

AUTHOR NAME
Michael Logan

FECAL FAT

BASICS

TYPE OF SPECIMEN

Feces

TEST EXPLANATION AND RELATED PHYSIOLOGY

The disorders affecting assimilation of dietary fat can be separated into 2 broad categories: The *malabsorptive processes* include alterations in micelle formation, absorption from the bowel, and transport, whereas *maldigestive disease* involves pancreatic insufficiency and brush border disease. Any of these disorders of fat assimilation may significantly elevate fecal fat output over that expected in normal animals.

Fecal fat can be analyzed by semiqualitative means or by quantitative analysis. *Semiqualitative* analysis involves Sudan III stain placed upon a thin fecal smear. Orange-stained globules are then enumerated and measured according to a scoring system (Drummey et al. 1961). Semiqualitative analysis is subjective and may underestimate the fat content because acidification of the sample is required to enable Sudan stain to mark fatty acids in addition to triglycerides. The addition of acetic acid and boiling to reveal digested lipids is sometimes referred to as the *indirect fecal fat test*.

Quantitative measurement is a more accurate assessment of the degree of steatorrhea than is the gross exam (Burrows et al. 1979). Titrational methods, though more labor intensive, are more frequently discussed in veterinary literature and involve precise chemical measurement of lipid in the stool.

INDICATIONS

• Chronic small-intestinal diarrhea
• Weight loss

CONTRAINDICATIONS

None

POTENTIAL COMPLICATIONS

None

CLIENT EDUCATION

• Patients must be fed a high-fat diet prior to semiqualitative analysis and should be acclimated to the diet before testing.
• For best sensitivity, patients must be fed a controlled diet and all feces must be collected over a 3-day period.

BODY SYSTEMS ASSESSED

Gastrointestinal

SAMPLE

COLLECTION

• Semiqualitative testing requires 1 drop of fresh feces.
• Quantitative analysis requires all feces produced over 3 days.

HANDLING

• Semiqualitative testing is done on fresh feces only.
• Quantitative testing requires the sample be placed in a laboratory-approved container and transported on ice or frozen.

STORAGE

• Semiqualitative testing is done on fresh feces only.
• Quantitative testing allows for feces to be refrigerated at 4° C or frozen at −20°C.

STABILITY

• Refrigerated (4°C): up to 3 days
• Frozen (−20°C): up to 1 week

PROTOCOL

None

INTERPRETATION

NORMAL FINDINGS OR RANGE

• Quantitative
  • Dogs: <1 g fat/kg body weight/24 h
  • Cats: < 0.8 g of fat/kg body weight/24 h
• Semiqualitative: up to 100 small (1–4 μm) globules of orange Sudan–positive material per high-power field

ABNORMAL VALUES

• Quantitative
  • Dogs: >1 g fat/kg body weight/24 h
  • Cats: >0.8 g fat/kg body weight/24 h
• Semiqualitative: >100 large (6–75 μm) globules of orange Sudan–positive material per high-power field

CRITICAL VALUES

None

INTERFERING FACTORS

Drugs That May Alter Results or Interpretation

Drugs That Interfere with Test Methodology

Administration of castor oil may falsely elevate fecal fat.

Drugs That Alter Physiology

• Administration of cholystyramine or azathioprine may falsely elevate fecal fat.
• Orally administered aminoglycosides may prevent fat absorption, thereby elevating fecal fat.
• Administration of medium-chain triglycerides may decrease fecal fat.

Disorders That May Alter Results

None

Collection Techniques or Handling That May Alter Results

Incomplete collection of feces for the full 3-day period

Influence of Signalment

Species

None

Breed

Clinically, normal small dogs have significantly lower fecal fat measurement than clinically normal large dogs.

Age

None

Gender

None

Pregnancy

None

LIMITATIONS OF THE TEST

Fecal fat measurement cannot definitively characterize a steatorrheic process as malabsorptive or maldigestive, and does not indicate a specific underlying etiology.

Sensitivity, Specificity, and Positive and Negative Predictive Values

- Specificity is poor for any method.
- Quantitative determination of fecal fat excretion is a more sensitive screen for malabsorptive or maldigestive conditions than is the semiqualitative method, but sensitivity values are not available.

Valid If Run in a Human Lab?
Yes.

Causes of Abnormal Findings

High values	Low values
Malabsorption	Improper diet acclimation
Enteritis (infectious, allergic, villous atrophy)	
Neoplasia (e.g., lymphoma)	
Lymphangiectasia	
Rapid intestinal transit (e.g., hyperthyroidism)	
Maldigestion	
Exocrine pancreatic insufficiency	
Abnormal micelle formation	
Hepatic dysfunction	
Biliary obstruction	

CLINICAL PERSPECTIVE
- Semiqualitative determination of fecal fat is a relatively fast and inexpensive method for screening appropriate patients for malabsorptive or maldigestive conditions.
- Trypsin-like immunoreactivity has largely replaced fecal fat excretion for diagnosing pancreatic insufficiency.
- Normal amounts of fecal fat do not exclude a diagnosis of maldigestion or malabsorption.

MISCELLANEOUS

ANCILLARY TESTS
- Trypsin-like immunoreactivity
- Cobalamin, folate, and xylose absorption tests for intestinal malabsorption and/or small-intestinal bacterial overgrowth
- Intestinal biopsy

SYNONYMS
None

SEE ALSO

Blackwell's Five-Minute Veterinary Consult: Canine and Feline Topics
- Exocrine Pancreatic Insufficiency
- Inflammatory Bowel Disease
- Pancreatitis
- Small Intestinal Bacterial Overgrowth

Related Topics in This Book
- Alpha-1 Protease Inhibitor
- Cobalamin
- Fecal Elastase
- Folate
- Trypsin-like Immunoreactivity

ABBREVIATIONS
None

Suggested Reading

Burrows CF, Merritt AM, Chiapella AM. Determination of fecal fat and trypsin output in the evaluation of chronic canine diarrhea. *J Am Vet Med Assoc* 1979; **174**: 62–66.

Drummey GD, Benson JR, Jones CM. Microscopic examination of the stool for steatorrhea. *N Engl J Med* 1961; **264**: 85–87.

Lassen ED. Laboratory evaluation of digestion and intestinal absorption. In: Thrall MA, ed. *Veterinary Hematology and Clinical Chemistry*. Philadelphia: Lippincott Williams & Wilkins, 2004: 387–399.

Lewis LD, Boulay JP, Chow FH. Fat excretion and assimilation by the cat. *Feline Pract* 1979; **9**: 46–49.

Simpson JW, Doxey DL. Evaluation of faecal analysis as an aid to the detection of exocrine pancreatic insufficiency. *Br Vet J* 1988; **144**: 174–178.

INTERNET RESOURCES
Merck Veterinary Manual: Malabsorption syndromes, http://www.merckvetmanual.com/mvm/index.jsp?cfile = htm/bc/23313.htm&word = fecal%2cfat.

AUTHOR NAME
Michael Logan

FECAL FLOTATION

BASICS

TYPE OF SPECIMEN
Feces

TEST EXPLANATION AND RELATED PHYSIOLOGY
Fecal flotation, which is designed to recover parasitic eggs, oocysts, and cysts, is based on the physical property of specific gravity (SG). Eggs, oocysts, and cysts will float in solutions of a higher SG than the parasitic life stage. The importance of proper SG of flotation solutions cannot be overemphasized. The SG of most parasite eggs is between 1.05 and 1.23. For parasite eggs to float, the SG of the flotation solution must be greater than that of the eggs.

    Flotation solutions are made by adding a measured amount of salt or sugar to a specific amount of water to produce a solution with the desired SG. Solutions may be made from scratch or bought premixed from veterinary supply houses. Common flotation solutions include sugar (Sheather's solution; SG, 1.27–1.33), sodium nitrate (NaNO$_3$; SG, 1.18–1.2), and zinc sulfate (ZnSO$_4$; SG, 1.2). Most parasitology laboratories routinely use Sheather's solution, which will float most common parasite eggs. Many commercially available kits supply sodium nitrate with an SG of 1.18. Zinc sulfate is considered the gold standard for flotation of *Giardia* cysts. The SG of a flotation solution should be verified with a hydrometer and then checked on a routine basis (e.g., monthly) to detect SG changes caused by evaporation. Too high an SG can rupture eggs, oocytes, or cysts.

INDICATIONS
- Routine health screening
- Digestive upsets; vomiting and/or diarrhea

CONTRAINDICATIONS
None, other than insufficient fecal output

POTENTIAL COMPLICATIONS
None

CLIENT EDUCATION
- Because pets can have normal stools and still be infected with intestinal parasites, it is good medicine to perform routine fecal exams on all pets. The absence of diarrhea or visible worms in dog feces does not mean that the animal is not infected.
- Negative fecal flotation does not completely exclude the possibility of intestinal parasites. For example, tapeworm segments may be seen in the feces, and the flotation may be negative for several reasons: eggs were not released from the segment, the SG of the solution used was not high enough to float the heavy eggs of *Taenia*, or perhaps owners mistook grains of rice for tapeworm segments.

BODY SYSTEMS ASSESSED
- Gastrointestinal
- Respiratory

SAMPLE

COLLECTION
Minimum of 2–5 g of fresh feces

HANDLING
- Place the sample in an airtight container (e.g., screw-top jar, ziplock bag).
- The sample is best analyzed on the day of collection.

STORAGE
Refrigeration

STABILITY
The stability of organisms and life stages varies; e.g., *Giardia* cysts are very fragile and delicate, whereas ascarid eggs are very hardy.

PROTOCOL
- Fecal flotation with centrifugation has been shown to be the most accurate way to recover parasite life stages and consistently recovers more eggs than standing flotation methods.
  1. Weigh out 2–5 g of feces.
  2. Mix feces with ≈10 mL of flotation solution and pour the mixture through a tea strainer into a beaker or fecal cup.
  3. Pour the strained solution into a 15-mL centrifuge tube.
  4. Fill the tube with flotation solution until a slight positive meniscus forms. Do not overfill tube. Doing so will cause some floating eggs to be forced down the side of tube when the coverslip is placed.
  5. Place a coverslip on the tube and put the tube in the centrifuge.
  6. Centrifuge at 1,200 RPM (280 g) for 5 min.
  7. Remove the tube and let it stand for 10 min.
  8. Remove the coverslip and place on a glass slide.
- Systematically examine the entire area under the coverslip by using the 10× objective lens (100× magnification). The 40× objective lens can be used to confirm the diagnosis and make measurements; however, with practice, most identification can be made at 100× magnification.
- Note that steps 5 and 6 are done only if the centrifuge has a swinging-bucket rotor (swing head). If the centrifuge has a fixed-angle head (fixed head), the tube is spun without being filled completely. After centrifuging, the tube is moved to a test-tube rack and filled with flotation solution until a slight positive meniscus forms. A coverslip is then placed on the tube, and the tube is allowed to stand for an additional 10 min before the coverslip is removed and examined.

Causes of Abnormal Findings

Common parasites of dogs with stage of life cycle found in feces

Parasite	Life stage	Location of mature life stage	How infected
Toxocara canis	Large egg	Small intestine	In utero or ingestion of infected paratenic hosts or infective larvated eggs
Toxascaris leonina	Large egg	Small intestine	In utero or ingestion of infected paratenic hosts or infective larvated eggs
Physaloptera spp.	Thick-shelled, larvated egg	Stomach	Ingestion of infected intermediate hosts (e.g., insects, arthropods) or paratenic hosts (e.g., frogs, mice)
Taenia spp.	Egg	Small intestine	Ingestion of metacestode stage in intermediate hosts (e.g., rabbits)
Dipylidium spp.	Egg packet	Small intestine	Ingestion of metacestode stage in intermediate hosts (fleas)
Ancylostoma caninum	Strongyle-type egg	Small intestine	Ingestion of L_3 from environment, bitches milk, or skin penetration by L_3
Uncinaria caninum	Strongyle-type egg	Small intestine	Ingestion of L_3 from environment or rarely skin penetration by L_3
Eucoleus boehmi	Bipolar egg	Nasal passages	Ingestion of larvated egg or infected paratenic host
Trichuris vulpis	Bipolar egg	Cecum, large intestine	Ingestion of larvated egg
Pearsonema plica (formerly known as Capillaria plica)	Bipolar egg	Bladder	Ingestion of larvated egg
Strongyloides stercovalis	Larvae	Small intestine	Ingestion or skin penetration by L_3
Cystoisospora spp. (formerly known as Isospora sp.)	Oocyst	Small intestine	Ingestion of sporulated oocysts, tachyzoites, or bradyzoites in mice
Giardia spp.	Cyst	Small intestine	Ingestion of cysts
Alaria canis	Egg	Stomach, small intestine	Ingestion of mesocercaria in fish, frogs, or rodents

Common parasites of cats with stage of life cycle found in feces

Parasite	Life stage	Location of mature life stage	How infected
Toxocara cati	Large egg	Small intestine	Ingestion of infected paratenic hosts or infective larvated eggs or larvae in milk
Toxascaris leonina	Large egg	Small intestine	Ingestion of infected paratenic hosts or infective larvated eggs
Physaloptera spp.	Thick-shelled, larvated egg	Stomach	Ingestion of infected intermediate hosts (e.g., insects, arthropods) or paratenic hosts (e.g., frogs, mice)
Taenia spp.	Egg	Small intestine	Ingestion of metacestode stage in intermediate hosts (e.g., rabbits)
Dipylidium spp.	Egg packet	Small intestine	Ingestion of metacestode stage in intermediate hosts (fleas)
Ancylostoma tubaeformae	Strongyle-type egg	Small intestine	Ingestion of L_3 from environment, queen's milk, or skin penetration
Capillaria sp.	Bipolar egg	Bladder or lungs	Ingestion of infective larvated eggs
Cystoisospora sp. (formerly known as Isospora sp.)	Oocyst	Small intestine	Ingestion of sporulated oocysts, tachyzoites, or bradyzoites in mice
Toxoplasma gondii	Oocyst	Small intestine	Ingestion of sporulated oocysts, tachyzoites, or bradyzoites in mice or other meat
Giardia spp.	Cyst	Small intestine	Ingestion of cysts
Aelurostrongylus abstrusus	Larvae	Lungs	Ingestion of intermediate hosts (snails or slugs) or paratenic hosts (mice and birds)
Alaria	Egg	Stomach, small intestine	Ingestion of mesocercaria in fish, frogs, or rodents

Demodex, Cheyletiella, and Otodectes sp. mites may be seen in fecal flotations. Echinococcus eggs are similar to Taenia.

FECAL FLOTATION

INTERPRETATION

NORMAL FINDINGS OR RANGE
No parasitic ova, oocysts, or cysts seen

ABNORMAL VALUES
Parasitic ova, oocysts, or cysts seen

CRITICAL VALUES
None

INTERFERING FACTORS
Drugs That May Alter Results or Interpretation
Drugs That Interfere with Test Methodology
None

Drugs That Alter Physiology
None

Disorders That May Alter Results
None

Collection Techniques or Handling That May Alter Results
• Insufficient sample size
• Old samples: the presence of free-living nematodes and protozoa

Influence of Signalment
Species
None

Breed
None

Age
Most puppies and kittens should be checked for internal parasites and medicated according to the recommendations of the American Association of Veterinary Parasitologists, American Animal Hospital Association, and the Companion Animal Parasite Council.

Gender
None

Pregnancy
None

LIMITATIONS OF THE TEST
• Sample size can be an issue in anorexic or very small animals with minimal fecal output.
• Some eggs (*Trichuris vulpis*) and cysts (*Giardia* sp.) are shed in low numbers or intermittently. If suspicion is high, fecal flotation should be run on samples from 3 consecutive days.

Sensitivity, Specificity, and Positive and Negative Predictive Values
N/A

Valid If Run in a Human Lab?
No. Few technicians are trained in the identification of animal parasite life stages.

CLINICAL PERSPECTIVE
• A good-quality microscope with a micrometer is required. A micrometer makes it possible to measure objects seen under the microscope, thus ensuring the accurate diagnosis of parasites.
• *Giardia* cysts are often mistaken for yeast, but *Giardia* cysts are all about the same size, whereas yeasts vary greatly in size and shape.
• "Proper techniques are imperative for the accurate diagnosis of intestinal parasites. Veterinarians and their staff should reevaluate their attitude of 'it's only a fecal' and better utilize these important techniques in their routine diagnostic plan" (Dryden et al. 2005:27).
• Due to coprophagy, strongyle-type eggs from horses or cows, or coccidia oocysts from ruminants, rabbits, or birds, may be found in canine feces. To determine whether these eggs are just passing through, confine the dog away from these animals for 24–48 h and recheck.

MISCELLANEOUS

ANCILLARY TESTS
• Fecal sedimentation techniques to look for larvae and/or large trematode ova
• In animals with diarrhea, consider evaluating fecal cytology, cobalamin, folate, and trypsin-like immunoreactivity.

SYNONYMS
Fecal float

SEE ALSO
Blackwell's Five-Minute Veterinary Consult: Canine and Feline Topics
• Coccidiosis
• Diarrhea, Chronic—Cats
• Diarrhea, Chronic—Dogs
• Giardiasis
• Hookworms (Ancylostomiasis)
• Roundworms (Ascariasis)
• Strongyloidiasis
• Tapeworms (Cestodiasis)
• Whipworms (Trichuriasis)

Related Topics in This Book
• Fecal Direct Smear and Cytology
• Fecal Sedimentation and Baermann Exam
• *Giardia* Fecal Antigen

ABBREVIATIONS
• L_3 = third-stage larva(e)
• SG = specific gravity

Suggested Reading
Dryden MW, Payne PA, Ridley R, Smith V. Comparison of common fecal flotation techniques for the recovery of parasite eggs and oocysts. *Vet Ther* 2005; 6: 15–28.
Foreyt W, ed. *Veterinary Parasitology Reference Manual*, 5th ed. Ames: Iowa State Press, 2001.

INTERNET RESOURCES
Penn Veterinary Medicine, Veterinary Parasitology CAL Program, http://cal.vet.upenn.edu/projects/parasit06/website/index.htm.
University of Wisconsin–Madison, School of Veterinary Medicine: Veterinary parasitology, http://www.vetmed.wisc.edu/pbs/vetpara/gallery.html.

AUTHOR NAME
Patricia A. Payne

FECAL OCCULT BLOOD

BASICS

TYPE OF SPECIMEN
Feces

TEST EXPLANATION AND RELATED PHYSIOLOGY
In normal veterinary patients, only minimal amounts of blood are passed into the GI tract. Benign and malignant GI tumors can cause GI hemorrhage. As a tumor grows into the intestinal lumen, any friable tissue, subjected to repeated trauma from the fecal stream, can ulcerate and bleed. Other causes of GI hemorrhage include ulcers, inflammatory bowel disease, and the presence of foreign bodies. Blood in the lower GI tract is often grossly visible, but blood can be lost into the proximal GI tract without being grossly visible in feces because the blood is digested. In addition, occult blood in the stool can originate from oral or nasopharyngeal lesions if the blood is swallowed and presented to the GI tract.

Chemical assays are available to detect the fecal occult blood (FOB) by use of either a paper strip or a tablet. The Hemoccult test (Beckman Coulter, Fullerton, CA) uses guaiac-impregnated paper; Hgb catalyzes the oxidation of guaiac to form a blue compound. Blood in feces can also be detected by use of the orthotolodine tablet method (Hematest; Siemens Healthcare Diagnostics, Tarrytown NY).

A positive result obtained on multiple samples collected on successive days warrants further evaluation of the GI tract. However, it is important to remember that ingestion of red meat, which contains Hgb, can cause a false-positive FOB test result.

INDICATIONS
- Microcytic, hypochromic anemia
- Anemia with low total protein and no obvious sign of blood loss
- Workup for suspected GI ulceration or neoplasia

CONTRAINDICATIONS
None

POTENTIAL COMPLICATIONS
None

CLIENT EDUCATION
- Feed the patient rice and cottage cheese for 3 days prior to the test.
- Avoid the use of nonsteroidal anti-inflammatory medications for 1 week prior to the test.
- Avoid feeding the patient vitamin C supplements or vitamin C–enriched foods 3 days prior to the test.
- If the test is performed at home, slides must be returned within 2 weeks after the first sample is obtained.

BODY SYSTEMS ASSESSED
- Gastrointestinal
- Hemic, lymphatic, and immune

SAMPLE

COLLECTION
- Feces can be obtained by gentle digital rectal examination. Traumatic digital collection can cause a false-positive result.
- Clients can be given specimen cards, tissue wipes, or test paper to obtain samples at home.
- Do not mix urine with the stool specimen.
- Multiple specimens obtained on separate days can increase test accuracy.

HANDLING
- Protect the slides from heat, light, and volatile chemicals (e.g., ammonia, bleach, iodine, household cleaners).
- Feces can be placed in any clean, dry container.

STORAGE
- Store the feces at room temperature (15°–30°C).
- Do not refrigerate or freeze the sample.

STABILITY
- Feces are stable for up to 2 weeks at room temperature.
- Hgb in liquid stool samples is inherently unstable.
- Hemoccult test cards are best developed *no sooner than 3 days* after sample application. This allows any peroxidases present to degrade.
- If testing immediately, wait 3–5 min before applying the developing solution (see the Protocol section).

PROTOCOL
Hemoccult Slide Test
- Apply a small amount of feces on 1 side of paper (thin smear).
- Place 2 drops of developer on the other side.
- Bluish discoloration indicates FOB.

Hematest Tablet Test
- Apply the feces to the test paper.
- Place 1 tablet on top of the stool specimen.
- Put 2–3 drops of tap water on the tablet and allow the water to flow onto the paper.
- Bluish discoloration indicates FOB.

INTERPRETATION

NORMAL FINDINGS OR RANGE
Negative test result (no color change)

ABNORMAL VALUES
Positive test result (bluish discoloration)

CRITICAL VALUES
None

INTERFERING FACTORS
Drugs That May Alter Results or Interpretation
Drugs That Interfere with Test Methodology
Ascorbic acid (vitamin C) is an antioxidant and can cause a false-negative result.

Drugs That Alter Physiology
Anticoagulants, aspirin, NSAIDs, colchicine, and steroids can all cause GI bleeding and therefore positive test results.

Disorders That May Alter Results
Mucosal bleeding secondary to dental procedures or rhinoscopy may affect results.

Collection Techniques or Handling That May Alter Results
Ingestion of products containing red meat or fish up to 3 days prior to test

Influence of Signalment
Species
None

Breed
None

Age
None

Gender
None

Pregnancy
None

LIMITATIONS OF THE TEST
- Naturally occurring peroxidases and catalases in red meat, fish, and some fruits and vegetables can cause false-positive test results.
- The test can miss very low-grade blood loss. An abnormal (positive) result requires losses of >20 mL/day.

Sensitivity, Specificity, and Positive and Negative Predictive Values
- The Hemoccult test is less sensitive but has fewer false positives with both restricted and unrestricted diets and is highly specific for occult blood in human stool samples.
- The Hematest test is more sensitive but has higher numbers of false positives in both restricted and unrestricted diets in human patients.

Valid If Run in a Human Lab?
Yes.

Causes of Abnormal Findings

High values	Low values
Ulceration within alimentary tract	Normal to see a negative result
Bleeding intestinal and/or colonic neoplasm	
Bloodsucking intestinal parasites	
Inflammatory bowel disease	

CLINICAL PERSPECTIVE
- FOB is not specific for any single disease. It should be used to screen patients suspected of having GI bleeding.
- Microcytic, hypochromic anemia warrants testing for FOB because this combination of abnormal RBC indices suggests iron deficiency, which is often the result of chronic blood loss into GI tract.
- High-fiber diets can increase test accuracy by helping uncover silent lesions, which bleed intermittently.

MISCELLANEOUS

ANCILLARY TESTS
- Barium series
- Endoscopy
- Fecal flotation

SYNONYMS
None

SEE ALSO
Blackwell's Five-Minute Veterinary Consult: Canine and Feline Topics
- Esophagitis
- Gastroduodenal Ulcer disease
- Gastroenteritis, Eosinophilic
- Gastroenteritis, Lymphocytic-Plasmacytic
- Inflammatory Bowel Disease
- Leiomyoma/Sarcoma, Stomach, Small and Large Intestine
- Rectoanal Polyps
- Whipworms (Trichuriasis)

Related Topics in This Book
- General Principles for Performing Fecal Tests
- General Principles of Endoscopy
- Fecal Direct Smear and Cytology
- Fecal Flotation

ABBREVIATIONS
- FOB = fecal occult blood
- Hgb = hemoglobin

Suggested Reading
Lassen ED. Laboratory evaluation of digestion and intestinal absorption. In: Thrall MA, ed. *Veterinary Hematology and Clinical Chemistry.* Philadelphia: Lippincott Williams & Wilkins, 2004: 387–399.
Willard MD, Twedten DC. Gastrointestinal, pancreatic and hepatic disorders. In: Willard MD, Tvedten H, eds. *Small Animal Clinical Diagnosis by Laboratory Methods,* 4th ed. St Louis: Saunders Elsevier, 2004: 217–29.

INTERNET RESOURCES
None

AUTHOR NAME
Jennifer Steinberg

FECAL SEDIMENTATION AND BAERMANN EXAM

 BASICS

TYPE OF SPECIMEN
Feces

TEST EXPLANATION AND RELATED PHYSIOLOGY
Because of very high specific gravity (fluke eggs) or fragility (lungworm larvae), not all diagnostic stages of parasites may be found in routine fecal flotation. The sedimentation technique is useful to concentrate fluke eggs from feces, and the Baermann exam concentrates larvae from fresh feces so they may be identified.

INDICATIONS
Sedimentation: Suspicion of Fluke Infestation
- *Signs of hepatic disease, extrahepatic biliary obstruction, pancreatic insufficiency, or pancreatitis
- Suspected salmon-poisoning disease (transmitted by *Nanophyetus salmincola*): fever, hemorrhagic enteritis, thrombocytopenia, and a history of eating fish from the Pacific Northwest
- *Paragonimus kellicoti*: respiratory signs (e.g., coughing, dyspnea, pneumothorax, bronchiectasis, hemoptysis)
- *Heterobilharzia americana* and *Alaria* spp.: diarrhea, vomiting, and occasional pulmonary hemorrhage (*Alaria*)

Baermann: Suspicion of Lungworm or *Strongyloides* sp. Intestinal Infection
- Lungworm: respiratory signs or tracheal wash with eosinophilic inflammation
- *Angiostrongylus vasorum* (French heartworm): Canada, Europe, South America, Africa; *Aleurostrongylus abstrusus*: worldwide distribution in cats, rarely dogs
- *Crenosoma vulpis*: Europe; rare in the United States
- *Strongyloides* sp.: watery diarrhea with or without respiratory signs, especially in young or immunosuppressed animals

CONTRAINDICATIONS
None

POTENTIAL COMPLICATIONS
None

CLIENT EDUCATION
None

BODY SYSTEMS ASSESSED
- Gastrointestinal
- Hepatobiliary
- Respiratory

 SAMPLE

COLLECTION
At least 5 g of fresh feces (≤1 day old)

HANDLING
- Place the sample in an airtight container.
- Wear gloves and use caution when handling fecal material because *Strongyloides* sp. is zoonotic to humans.

STORAGE
- Sedimentation: Refrigerate the sample.
- Baermann: Do not refrigerate the sample! It must be fresh and at room temperature.

STABILITY
- Sedimentation: 1–2 days
- Baermann: <1 day

PROTOCOL
Sedimentation
- Mix ≈5 g of feces with 15 mL of water in cup or beaker.
- Strain the mixture through a tea strainer into a 50-mL conical tube.
- Let the mixture stand for 10 min.
- Decant 75% of water and refill the tube with fresh water.
- Repeat 3–5 times until the supernatant is clear.
- Decant 95% of the water and pour the sediment into a petri dish.
- Examine the sample under a dissecting scope for large, operculated eggs.
  Hint: The addition of a few drops of new methylene blue to the sediment will color the background blue while most fluke ova remain slightly orange. Sediment in a petri dish can also be examined by using a stereoscope, although the eggs will appear smaller and may require evaluation by microscope for positive identification.

Baermann
- Equipment: a ring stand with funnel, rubber tubing, a clamp, and a centrifuge tube or a disposable plastic champagne glass
- Fill the funnel or champagne glass partially with warm water. Break up 5 g of fresh feces into small pieces and place them in double layers of gauze or loosely woven cloth with its edges folded over the top. Place the wrapped feces in a funnel or champagne glass. Add enough warm water to cover the fecal packet.
- After 3–4 h, discard the fecal packet into biohazard trash. Clamp off the rubber tubing and carefully remove the centrifuge tube.
- Pipette a few drops of solution from the bottom of the centrifuge tube or champagne glass onto a slide, coverslip the slide, and examine it microscopically for live larvae.

 INTERPRETATION

NORMAL FINDINGS OR RANGE
- Sedimentation: no parasitic life stages seen; no fluke eggs
- Baermann: no ova or larvae recovered

ABNORMAL VALUES
- Sedimentation: identification of large operculated eggs
- Baermann: identification of the larvae of *Strongyloides* sp., *Ancylostoma* L_1 (in old samples), *Aelurostrongylus* spp., and *Crenosoma vulpis*; not recommended for *Oslerus* (formerly *Filaroides*) *osleri* (these will float in zinc sulfate)

CRITICAL VALUES
None

INTERFERING FACTORS
Drugs That May Alter Results or Interpretation
None

Drugs That Interfere with Test Methodology
None

Drugs That Alter Physiology
None

Disorders That May Alter Results
None

Collection Techniques or Handling That May Alter Results
- Sedimentation: false negatives from too small a sample size
- Baermann: Failure to use fresh feces may result in finding free-living larvae or other strongyle larvae that have hatched from eggs. Leaving the Baermann test set up longer than recommended may result in dead or distorted larvae.

Influence of Signalment
Species
None

Breed
None

Age
• Sedimentation: Animals must be as old as, or older than, the prepatent period of the various flukes.
• Baermann: Animals must be as old as, or older than, the prepatent period of various lungworms or other parasites that are diagnosed through identification of larvae rather than eggs.

Gender
None

Pregnancy
None

LIMITATIONS OF THE TEST

Infection cannot be ruled out on the basis of a negative test result, because false negatives can be caused by technical errors and/or low numbers of eggs or larvae in the feces.

Sensitivity, Specificity, and Positive and Negative Predictive Values
N/A

Valid If Run in a Human Lab?
No.

Causes of Abnormal Findings

Parasite larva	Distinguishing features
Strongyloides L_1	Large genital rudiment (primordium)
Ancylostoma L_1	Small, barely noticeable genital rudiment
Angiostrongylus vasorum	Cephalic button on anterior end, S-shaped curve in tail, dorsal spine
Aelurostrongylus abstrusus	Tightly coiled; undulating tail with a spine
Crenosoma vulpis	Characteristic C shape; tail has slight deflection but no definite kink or dorsal spine

CLINICAL PERSPECTIVE

• Clinical signs associated with trematode infections depend on the species of trematode involved.
• Repeated tests may be needed to confirm a diagnosis of *Stongyloides* sp. because larvae can be absent in feces or in low numbers even in symptomatic cases.
• Lungworms and migrating *Strongyloides* larvae can sometimes be found in a tracheal wash sample.

MISCELLANEOUS

ANCILLARY TESTS
• Flukes: liver function tests
• Lungworms: chest radiography, bronchoscopy, or tracheal wash

SYNONYMS
None

SEE ALSO
Blackwell's Five-Minute Veterinary Consult: Canine and Feline Topics
• Liver Fluke Infestation
• Salmon Poisoning Disease
• Strongyloidiasis

Related Topics in This Book
• Fecal Direct Smear and Cytology
• Fecal Flotation

ABBREVIATIONS
L_1 = first-stage larva(e)

Suggested Reading
Zajac AM, Conboy GA. *Veterinary Clinical Parasitology*, 7th ed. Ames, IA: Blackwell, 2006.

INTERNET RESOURCES
Nolan TJ. Canine strongyloidiasis. In: Bowman DD, ed.

AUTHOR NAME
Patricia A. Payne

FELINE CORONAVIRUS

 BASICS

TYPE OF SPECIMEN
Blood

TEST EXPLANATION AND RELATED PHYSIOLOGY
Feline enteric coronavirus (FECV) is a pathogen of minor clinical significance, but spontaneous mutation of this virus can result in feline infectious peritonitis (FIP), a disease associated with high mortality. An effusive form of FIP occurs when immune complexes aggregate in the vasculature and attract complement, causing a vasculitis and subsequent effusion. The dry form of disease is characterized by multiple granulomas or pyogranulomas in various organs, including lungs, liver, kidneys, intestines, and central nervous system. This is believed to result from a partially protective cell-mediated immune response that cannot contain the virus. Often, affected cats have a combination of both the effusive and noneffusive forms, with one form predominating over the other. Several testing options are available for these organisms. The three most common are the following:

IFA and ELISA
These are used to detect host antibodies directed against the organism of interest. Assays for anti–feline coronavirus (anti-FCoV) IgG are widely available. IFA techniques are most commonly used in the commercial laboratory setting and have good sensitivity and specificity for coronavirus. In-house ELISA-based testing kits are also available and have shown good correlation with IFA results. Unfortunately, antibody tests cannot distinguish between pathogenic FCoV and the avirulent FECV.

Reverse Transcriptase–Polymerase Chain Reaction (RT-PCR)
This is used to amplify a specific piece of RNA from the organism of interest. Like serology tests, routine RT-PCR assays for viral RNA cannot necessarily distinguish FECV from active FIP. However, a new RT-PCR test, which detects the subgenomic RNA of the highly conserved FCoV virus M gene, may be better able to differentiate FIP from FECV infection. Specifically amplifying only subgenomic forms of the viral RNA means that only actively replicating virus will be detected. FIP virus is believed to replicate in peripheral blood monocytes, whereas it is thought that enteric coronaviruses cannot replicate in peripheral blood. Therefore, detection of actively replicating virus in blood by using this RT-PCR assay may be more specific for FIP.

INDICATIONS
Clinical signs consistent with FIP:
- Lethargy
- Anorexia
- Weight loss or failure to gain weight
- Pyrexia
- Jaundice
- Ascites and/or pleural effusion
- Neurologic signs
- Ocular changes

CONTRAINDICATIONS
Screening of asymptomatic cats is not recommended because test results can be difficult to interpret.

POTENTIAL COMPLICATIONS
None

CLIENT EDUCATION
- The patient is required to fast for 12 h before sampling.
- It is important that owners understand interpretation of test results—in particular that a positive antibody titer does not indicate that a cat has FIP, nor does it indicate whether the cat might develop FIP in the future.

BODY SYSTEMS ASSESSED
- Gastrointestinal
- Hemic, lymphatic, and immune
- Hepatobiliary
- Nervous
- Neuromuscular
- Ophthalmic
- Renal and urologic

 SAMPLE

COLLECTION
- 0.5–1.0 mL of venous blood, effusion, or cerebrospinal fluid
- Aspiration or biopsy of the affected organ

HANDLING
- IFA/ELISA: Collect the sample into a plain tube without anticoagulant or into a serum-separator tube.
- RT-PCR: Collect blood into EDTA. Effusion can be collected into either EDTA or a plain tube. Aspirated or biopsied tissue can be preserved in buffer.

STORAGE
No special requirements

STABILITY
- Refrigerated (2°–8°C): days to weeks
- Frozen (−20° to −80°C): months to years

PROTOCOL
None

 INTERPRETATION

NORMAL FINDINGS OR RANGE
- IFA/ELISA: negative test result—no anti-FCoV present, antibodies present
- RT-PCR: negative test result—no FCoV RNA present

ABNORMAL VALUES
IFA/ELISA
- A positive antibody titer confirms exposure to FCoV, but does not indicate active FIP. Extremely high titers (>1:16,000) may increase the clinical suspicion of FIP in a cat with compatible signalment and clinical signs, but is not confirmatory.
- Cats with FIP can have low titers, and a negative titer does not exclude a diagnosis of FIP.

RT-PCR
- The presence of FCoV RNA in the sample indicates infection with a coronavirus, but virus particles have been detected in the blood of healthy cats with FECV.
- The detection of subgenomic viral RNA suggests actively replicating virus particles in the blood, which is thought to be more specific for FIP.

CRITICAL VALUES
None

INTERFERING FACTORS
Drugs That May Alter Results or Interpretation
Drugs That Interfere with Test Methodology
None

Drugs That Alter Physiology
None

Disorders That May Alter Results
Immunosuppressed cats may have lower IgG titers.

Collection Techniques or Handling That May Alter Results
None

Influence of Signalment
Species
None

Breed
Signalment will not affect the test result. However, FIP disease is more common in purebred cats.

Age
Signalment will not affect the test result. However, FIP disease is more common in young cats.

Gender
None

Pregnancy
None

LIMITATIONS OF THE TEST
• As many as 40% of the general domestic cat population have been exposed to FCoV and will therefore have antibodies against the virus. Exposure rates in multicat households tend to be much higher at 80%–90%.
• Cats with FIP can have low antibody titers, and a negative titer does not exclude a diagnosis of FIP.

Sensitivity, Specificity, and Positive and Negative Predictive Values
• Sensitivity and specificity of the IFA and ELISA tests are both very good for detecting exposure to FCoV, but this does not correlate with development of FIP.
  • Serum serology predictive values for detecting FIP (Hartman et al. 2003)
    • Positive predictive value: 44%
    • Positive predictive value for antibody concentrations at the highest measurable titer: 94%
    • Negative predictive value: 90%
  • Measuring the antibody titer within effusive fluid is a more useful ancillary test for FIP than measuring serum antibody titers (Hartman et al. 2003).
    • Positive predictive value: 90%
    • Negative predictive value: 79%
• RT-PCR (Simons et al. 2005)
  • Specificity: 95%
  • Sensitivity
    • Positive RT-PCR test results in 93% of cats with FIP confirmed by necropsy
    • Positive RT-PCR test results in 46% of cats with suggestive clinical signs, but no confirmatory testing
    • Sensitivity can be increased by using RT-PCR to simultaneously test several nonintestinal samples from a symptomatic cat (e.g., blood, effusion, and biopsy samples or aspirate from the affected organ (e.g., kidney, enlarged lymph node).

Valid If Run in a Human Lab?
No. Species-specific assays are required.

CLINICAL PERSPECTIVE
FCoV serology is a commonly tested method and may be helpful as part of the diagnostic profile. However, antibody titer results can be confusing in the clinical situation and are often misinterpreted. A positive titer simply confirms past exposure to FCoV. It offers no infor-

mation about whether the cat has developed FIP, is not correlated with severity of disease, and does not indicate active infection. A tentative diagnosis of FIP should therefore be made only based on a combination of appropriate signalment, clinical signs and suggestive laboratory results.

MISCELLANEOUS
ANCILLARY TESTS
• CBC: Routine hematologic evaluation classically shows lymphopenia, mature neutrophilia, and mild anemia, but their absence does not exclude a diagnosis of FIP.
• Serum biochemical analysis frequently shows hyperbilirubinemia and hyperglobulinemia. A serum albumin/globulin ratio of <0.4 has been shown to be suggestive of FIP, whereas a ratio of >0.8 is unlikely to support that diagnosis.
• Protein electrophoresis: Polyclonal gammopathy is common. α_2-Globulins usually increase in early disease but switch to a γ-globulin response as clinical signs progress.
• α_1-Acid glycoprotein is an acute phase protein. Serum levels can be elevated in any inflammatory disease, but values of >1.5 g/dL may be helpful in distinguishing FIP from conditions with similar presenting signs.
• Ascitic fluid analysis is one of the most useful tests for FIP but is only possible in cats with effusive disease. The fluid tends to be a clear, yellow, viscous exudate. The protein content is extremely high, and fibrin strands can often be seen with the naked eye. The cell count is usually between 1,600 and 25,000 cells/μL, and bacterial culture is negative.
• In patients with neurologic signs, measuring antibody titers in the cerebrospinal fluid may be helpful.
• Diagnostic imaging may help in identifying effusions or granulomatous lesions.
• For definitive diagnosis of FIP, histopathologic evaluation of affected tissues is required, and this can be combined with immunohistochemical staining to confirm the presence of FCoV antigens within lesions.

SYNONYMS
• FCoV
• Feline infectious peritonitis (FIP)

SEE ALSO
Blackwell's Five-Minute Veterinary Consult: Canine and Feline Topics
• Feline Infectious Peritonitis (FIP)
• Pericardial Effusion
• Peritonitis
• Renal Failure, Chronic
• Renomegaly
• Seizures (Convulsions, Status Epilepticus)—Cats

Related Topics in This Book
• Fluid Analysis
• Globulins
• Protein Electrophoresis
• Toxoplasmosis Serology

ABBREVIATIONS
• FCoV = feline coronavirus
• FECV = feline enteric coronavirus
• RT-PCR = reverse transcriptase–polymerase chain reaction

Suggested Reading

Addie D, Jarrett O. Feline coronavirus infections. In: Greene CE, ed. *Infectious Diseases of the Dog and Cat,* 3rd ed. Philadelphia: WB Saunders, 2006: 88–102.

Foley JE. Feline infectious peritonitis and feline enteric coronavirus. In: Ettinger SJ, Feldman EC, eds. *Textbook of Veterinary Internal Medicine,* 6th ed. Philadelphia: WB Saunders, 2004: 663–666.

Hartman K, Binder C, Hirschberger, *et al.* Comparison of different tests to diagnose feline infectious peritonitis. *J Vet Intern Med* 2003; **17**: 781–790.

Horzinek MC. The bright future of coronavirology [Editorial]. *J Feline Med Surg* 2004; **6**: 49–132.

Simons FA, Vennema H, Rofina JE, *et al.* A mRNA PCR for the diagnosis of feline infectious peritonitis. *J Virol Methods* 2005; **124**: 111–116.

Sturgess K. Feline infectious peritonitis (FIP). In: Sturgess C., ed. *Notes on Feline Internal Medicine.* Oxford: Blackwell, 1996: 262–266.

INTERNET RESOURCES

Auburn University, College of Veterinary Medicine, Molecular Diagnostics: Feline infectious peritonitis virus, http://www.vetmed.auburn.edu/index.pl/feline_infectious_peritonitis_virus.

Feline Advisory Bureau (FAP). Cat Group policy statement 5: Feline infectious peritonitis (FIP), http://www.fabcats.org/cat_group/policy_statements/fip.html.

Feline Advisory Bureau (FAP). Frequently asked questions: Feline infectious peritonitis (FIP), http://www.fabcats.org/cat_group/faq/fipfaq.html.

Horzinek MC, Lutz H. An update on feline infectious peritonitis. Vet Sci Tomorrow 2001(1), http://www.vetscite.org/issue1/reviews/txt_index_0800.htm.

AUTHOR NAME

Charlotte Dye

BASICS

TYPE OF SPECIMEN
Blood

TEST EXPLANATION AND RELATED PHYSIOLOGY
FIV is a retrovirus closely related to the human immunodeficiency virus (HIV). As a lentivirus, it is characterized by a long incubation period. In cats, the virus is shed in saliva, and infections are transmitted through bite wounds. Cats remain infected for life. After a transient period of fever, lymphadenopathy, and neutropenia, cats can be asymptomatic for months to years. The terminal phase of infection is characterized by disruption of normal immune function and chronic secondary and opportunistic infections. FIV-infected cats also have an increased incidence of B-cell lymphoma and myeloproliferative disorders. Neurologic disease has also been reported. Several testing options are available for diagnosis of this infection:

ELISA and Immunochromatographic Assay (ICA)
These detect antibodies against FIV viral proteins, usually the core protein p24 and/or envelope glycoprotein gp40. In addition to commercial laboratory tests, in-practice kits are available. The SNAP FIV/FeLV Test (IDEXX Laboratories, Portland, ME, USA) uses ELISA methodology, whereas the Witness HW (Synbiotics, Kansas City, MO, USA), Speed HW (Bio Veto Test Laboratories, La Seyne sur Mer, France), and Heartworm IC (Agrolabo, Scarmagno, Italy) use ICA methodology.

Western Blotting
This detects antibodies to a variety of FIV proteins, which can be useful because variation in the antibodies produced by infected cats means that some infected cats may be negative for the antibodies detected by ELISA. It is available in commercial laboratories only.

IFA
This uses cultured FIV-infected cells that are bound to a slide to detect antibodies in cat serum. This enables detection of antibodies to numerous FIV viral proteins, as opposed to just 1 or 2 viral proteins present in an ELISA or an ICA test kit. In this way, it is more sensitive. In addition, the detection of antibodies actually bound to the FIV-infected cells adds a level of specificity by limiting nonspecific antibody binding.

   In general, the presence of serum antibodies is directly correlated with the presence of virus in cells and saliva. Antibody tests become positive following seroconversion, which can take up to 3 months after infection. Some infected cats may remain seronegative indefinitely.

Virus Isolation
This detects whole virus, but its availability is limited because the test is time-consuming and technically difficult.

PCR
This detects viral nucleic acids sequences. The commercially available PCR assays usually detect FIV proviral DNA. Real-time FIV PCR is also available, quantifying the amount of FIV DNA present in the blood and thus indirectly assessing viral load. This may be useful to monitor progression of infection in FIV-infected cats, but more work is required to evaluate this potential application.

INDICATIONS
The following are possible indications for FIV testing. A decision to test a patient for FIV will be influenced by the individual circumstances of the cat, financial considerations, and whether any clinical signs are present.

ELISA and ICA
- Cats with stomatitis and/or chronic or recurrent infections of the skin, urinary bladder, and upper respiratory tract
- Cats with slow but progressive weight loss or severe wasting
- Prior to a cat's rehoming
- Prior to a cat's introduction into a multicat household
- Following a cat's potential exposure (test >2 months after exposure)
- If a cat is residing with FIV-infected cats
- The presence of high-risk factors (e.g., an intact male with a history of fighting)
- As part of a general health screen

PCR
- Testing of cats that are vaccinated against FIV and for kittens <6 months old
- Confirmatory testing

IFA, Western Blotting, and Virus Isolation
Alternative confirmatory tests

CONTRAINDICATIONS
Tests that look for antibodies against FIV are unreliable in the following:
- Cats known to have been vaccinated against FIV
- Kittens (<6 months old) of FIV-positive queens. In these cases, a positive result cannot be used to indicate FIV infection (because of the presence of maternally derived antibodies) although a negative result in a kitten means that it is likely to be FIV negative.

POTENTIAL COMPLICATIONS
None

CLIENT EDUCATION
Clients should be aware of the following:
- False-positive and false-negative test results can occur.
- Test findings need to be interpreted in the light of the health status of the cat.
- Use of an alternative test may be required to confirm the FIV status of a cat.

BODY SYSTEMS ASSESSED
- Dermatologic
- Gastrointestinal
- Hemic, lymphatic, and immune
- Hepatobiliary
- Musculoskeletal
- Nervous
- Ophthalmic
- Renal and urologic
- Respiratory

SAMPLE

COLLECTION
0.5 mL of venous blood

HANDLING
- EDTA or a heparin tube (spun down to yield plasma)
- Send the sample at room temperature (no special transport requirements).

STORAGE
No special requirements

FELINE IMMUNODEFICIENCY VIRUS

STABILITY
IFA, ELISA, or Western Blot
- Refrigerated (2°–8°C): stable for days to weeks
- Frozen (−20° to −80°C): stable for months to years

PCR
- Refrigerated (2°–8°C): stable for days to weeks
- Frozen (−20° to −80°C): stable for months to years

PROTOCOL
- Although most manufacturers of in-practice test kits state that whole blood can be used, it has been known that this can lead to false-positive results, so the use of serum or plasma is preferable.
- When in-practice test kits are used, to avoid technical errors that may lead to false results, it is important to follow the manufacturer's protocol accurately.
  - Test kits and samples should be allowed to equilibrate to room temperature before the test is performed if this is specified by the manufacturer's instructions.
  - The test results should be read at the precise time stated by the manufacturer.

INTERPRETATION

NORMAL FINDINGS OR RANGE
- Uninfected cats should be negative on all tests. False-negative results can occur with the ELISA and ICA, but, in a truly uninfected cat, PCR, Western blot, and IFA would be expected to be negative.
- *Note*: Equivocal in-house test results cannot be interpreted and should be repeated.

ABNORMAL VALUES
In cats >6 months old and those not vaccinated against FIV, a positive ELISA result raises a strong suspicion of FIV infection; however, positive ELISA results should always be confirmed with PCR or IFA, especially in healthy cats. Confirmation of positive results indicates lifelong FIV infection.

CRITICAL VALUES
None

INTERFERING FACTORS
Drugs That May Alter Results or Interpretation
Drugs That Interfere with Test Methodology
FIV vaccination will cause false-positive antibody test results.

Drugs That Alter Physiology
None

Disorders That May Alter Results
Hemolyzed or lipemic serum may interfere with ELISAs.

Collection Techniques or Handling That May Alter Results
ELISA in-practice test kit instructions should be followed accurately because a technical error can lead to false results.

Influence of Signalment
Species
Only feline species are susceptible to this viral infection.

Breed
None

Age
Positive antibody test results due to maternal antibody can be seen in kittens <6 months of age born to FIV-infected queens. In this case, a positive test result does not necessarily indicate FIV infection.

Gender
FIV infection is most common in intact male cats because they are more likely to fight with other cats, but infection can occur in both genders, intact or neutered.

Pregnancy
If FIV infection is identified in a pregnant cat, only a proportion of its kittens are likely to become infected. Kittens should be tested with ELISA at >6 months of age or can be tested at any age with a reliable FIV PCR.

LIMITATIONS OF THE TEST
- False-negative ELISA and ICA test results can be seen with acute infections or in cats that fail to produce antibodies as a result of immunosuppression.
- PCR may not detect all FIV subtypes, so false-negative results can occur.

Sensitivity, Specificity, and Positive and Negative Predictive Values
- Estimates of ELISA and ICA sensitivities and specificities are variable, but manufacturers suggest they are >99% sensitive and 97%–99.5% specific. Positive and negative predictive values depend on the health status of the cat and the prevalence on FIV infection in the population being tested.
- PCR sensitivity and specificity vary among laboratories because sensitivity and specificity depend on assay design and validation and on the FIV subtypes (clades) detected by the PCR and those present in the population being tested. Different FIV subtypes have marked variation in DNA sequences, and therefore it is impossible for a single PCR to detect all subtypes, which creates a problem in those geographic areas where several FIV subtypes exist. There is also some variability within clades that can also confound PCR tests. PCR sensitivity can therefore be a problem, but specificity should be high, provided a reliable PCR is used. Reliability data should be obtained from the laboratory performing the test.

Valid If Run in a Human Lab?
No. A species-specific assay is required.

CLINICAL PERSPECTIVE
- ELISA is good for screening for FIV infection in cats, except for kittens <6 months of age and for cats vaccinated against FIV.
- A negative ELISA result is generally regarded as reliable in healthy cats. However, as it may take up to 3 months for seroconversion to occur, the test should be repeated if there has been recent exposure. Occasional false-negative results may also occur in some cats that do not produce detectable antibodies. Therefore, if ELISA is negative in a cat in which there is strong suspicion of FIV infection, another type of test should also be performed.
- A positive antibody result should always be confirmed with another test methodology such as PCR or IFA, particularly in healthy cats.

MISCELLANEOUS

ANCILLARY TESTS
In FIV-infected cats, further investigations to assess for evidence of FIV-related disease and concurrent infectious diseases may be indicated (e.g., routine hematology, biochemistry, urinalysis, fecal analysis, imaging, FeLV testing, PCR testing for hemoplasma species).

SYNONYMS
- Feline T-lymphotropic lentivirus
- FIV

SEE ALSO
Blackwell's Five-Minute Veterinary Consult: Canine and Feline Topics
Feline Immunodeficiency Virus Infection (FIV)

Related Topics in This Book
Feline Leukemia Virus

ABBREVIATIONS
- FIV = feline immunodeficiency virus
- ICA = immunochromatographic assay

Suggested Reading

Bienzle D, Reggeti F, Sello RK, Hartmann K. Feline Immunodeficiency Virus infection. In: Greene CE, ed. *Infectious Diseases of the Dog and Cat,* 3rd ed. Philadelphia: WB Saunders, 2006: 131–141.

Levy JK, Crawford PC, Slater MR. Effect of vaccination against FIV on results of serologic testing in cats. *J Am Vet Med Assoc* 2004; **225**: 1558–1561.

Wen X, Little S, Hobson J, Kruth S. The variability of serological and molecular diagnosis of FIV infection. *Can Vet J* 2004; **45**: 753–757.

INTERNET RESOURCES
American Association of Feline Practitioners (AAFP). Report of the American Association of Feline Practitioners and Academy of Feline Medicine Advisory Panel on Feline Retrovirus Testing and Management. Hillsborough, NJ: AAFP, 2005, http://www.aafponline.org/resources/guidelines/Felv_FIV_Guidelines.pdf.

Feline Advisory Bureau (FAP). Cat Group policy statement 3: Feline immunodeficiency virus (FIV), http://www.fabcats.org/cat_group/policy_statements/fiv.html. IDEXX Laboratories, In-house Tests: SNAP FIV uses ELISA technology, http://www.idexx.com/animalhealth/testkits/fivfelv/technology.jsp.

AUTHOR NAME
Andrea Harvey

FELINE LEUKEMIA VIRUS

BASICS

TYPE OF SPECIMEN
Blood
Tissue

TEST EXPLANATION AND RELATED PHYSIOLOGY
FeLV is a feline retrovirus that causes several diseases of the immune and hematopoietic systems, including immunosuppression, immune dysregulation, and neoplasms. The virus spreads through contact with saliva (and, to a lesser extent, blood) from infected cats and, if unchecked by the immune system, can infect many tissues, including salivary glands and bone marrow. Within host cells, viral RNA is transcribed by reverse transcriptase and the resulting DNA (provirus) is randomly inserted into the host's DNA, potentially leading to lifelong infection.

The viral genome contains some regulatory sequences believed to be involved in oncogenesis. A structural protein, p27, is produced in large amounts and is abundant in the cytoplasm of infected cells, as well as in plasma. The envelope glycoprotein gp70 appears to be responsible for inducing immunity, whereas p15e interferes with host immune responses. Several FeLV testing options are available:
- FeLV ELISAs and immunochromatographic assays (ICAs) detect free soluble FeLV p27 antigen. The results of these tests become positive during the primary viremic phase, within a few weeks of FeLV infection and before bone marrow infection.
- IFA detects cell (neutrophils and platelets)-associated FeLV p27 antigen, and IFA results become positive once FeLV bone marrow infection occurs.
- PCR detects viral nucleic acid sequences. The PCR assays currently commercially available detect FeLV proviral DNA.
- ELISAs and ICAs are good for FeLV screening and their results become positive early in infection. IFA is a confirmatory test since most IFA-positive cats remain persistently viremic, but transient viremia will also yield positive results. PCR test results will be positive during transient and persistent viremia, and can detect latent FeLV infection.

INDICATIONS
The following are possible indications for FeLV testing. A decision to test a patient for FeLV will be influenced by the individual circumstances of the cat, the client's financial considerations, and the clinical signs present.
- Sick cats, especially those with anemia, lymphoma, bone marrow disease, or polyarthritis
- After potential exposure: Test at least 1 month after exposure.
- Before a cat's FeLV vaccination or rehoming
- Part of a general health screen
- PCR may be indicated in ELISA/ICA-negative cats with suspected latent FeLV infection (e. g., bone marrow suppression, lymphoma).

CONTRAINDICATIONS
- None
- *Note*: Antibodies induced by FeLV vaccination do not interfere with FeLV testing, so prior FeLV vaccination is *not* a contraindication for testing.

POTENTIAL COMPLICATIONS
None

CLIENT EDUCATION
- Test findings must be interpreted in light of the health status of the cat being tested, and repeat testing or use of an alternative test may be required to confirm a cat's FeLV status.
- An FeLV-infected cat may be asymptomatic for many years, though 85% die within 3 years. A positive test result should not be the sole criterion for euthanasia.

- Infection is caused by close contact with other cats (oronasal and bite wounds), so outdoor cats and cats in contact with cats of unknown viral status are at the highest risk of infection. A new cat should be isolated from other cats in a household until its FeLV status is known.
- FeLV is fragile, survives only moments outside of its host, and is susceptible to all disinfectants.

BODY SYSTEMS ASSESSED
Hemic, lymphatic, and immune

SAMPLE

COLLECTION
- ELISA/ICA: 1 mL of venous blood
- IFA: 1 mL of venous blood or aspirated bone marrow
- PCR: 1 mL of venous blood or 0.5 mL of aspirated bone marrow cells

HANDLING
- ELISA/ICA: red-top tube; EDTA or heparinized whole blood to yield plasma or serum
- IFA
  - Prepare several smears from blood or freshly aspirated marrow.
  - Use EDTA or heparinized blood for buffy coat preparations.
  - Air-dry smears and ship, unfixed (and unstained), at room temperature.
- PCR: blood, bone marrow, or fine-needle aspirate collected into EDTA

STORAGE
- Refrigeration of blood is recommended.
- Freeze serum or plasma for prolonged storage.
- Store smears at room temperature.

STABILITY
- ELISA/ICA
  - Refrigerated blood (2°–8°C): ≈3 days
  - Frozen serum or plasma (−20° to −80°C): months to years
- IFA: Unstained smears can be stored for several days.

PROTOCOL
In-house ELISAs or ICAs exist, and these should be performed following the manufacturers' protocol, including test kit temperature and timing of results. Even though some kits allow the use of whole blood, false-positive results can occur compared to the results with the use of serum or plasma.

INTERPRETATION

NORMAL FINDINGS OR RANGE
- Cats completely free of FeLV infection should test negative on all tests.
- Recovered immune cats may test PCR positive but will be ELISA/ICA and IFA negative.

ABNORMAL VALUES
- A positive ELISA or ICA result indicates the presence of free FeLV p27 in a cat's blood, indicating the presence of viremia at that stage. However, the cat may be able to overcome the infection so that the viremia is only transient. Transient viremia can last a few weeks (≈3 weeks but up to 4 months has been reported) so repeat ELISA and/or ICA testing up to 4 months later is recommended to confirm persistent viremia. Alternatively another test method can be used to evaluate the cat's FeLV status (e. g., IFA or PCR).

- A positive IFA result indicates the presence of cell-associated FeLV p27, indicating FeLV bone marrow infection. Since bone marrow infection occurs after a few weeks of FeLV infection, most cats that are IFA positive will be persistently viremic, but transient viremia is still possible, so repeat testing may be indicated to confirm the cat's FeLV status.
- A positive proviral PCR indicates the presence of FeLV provirus in the sample, which occurs with viremia (transient or persistent) and latent and recovered infections. With latent and recovered infections, ELISA/ICA and IFA test results will be negative. Large amounts of provirus (measured by quantitative PCR) usually equate with persistent viremia, whereas lower amounts indicate latent or recovered infections. The significance of a positive PCR result, concurrent with negative ELISA/ICA or IFA test results, is currently unknown, but there is a *theoretical* possibility that the presence of provirus could cause disease or reactivate infection or induce neoplasia.
- Discordant results are defined as conflicting results obtained with different FeLV tests. These can arise due to the stage of infection, test technical errors, or the presence of latent or localized FeLV infections. ELISA/ICA-positive but IFA-negative cases are most commonly encountered. Half of these discordant cats remain so on repeat testing (suggesting possible localized infection that releases p27 antigen but not whole virus); most of the rest will become ELISA/ICA negative, whereas a small proportion will become IFA positive.

CRITICAL VALUES
None

INTERFERING FACTORS
Drugs That May Alter Results or Interpretation
Drugs That Interfere with Test Methodology
None

Drugs That Alter Physiology
None

Disorders That May Alter Results
- Hemolysis or lipemia may interfere with ELISAs and ICAs.
- Neutropenia and thrombocytopenia may cause a false-negative IFA result.

Collection Techniques or Handling That May Alter Results
- Hemolyzed plasma or serum may interfere with ELISAs and ICAs.
- Technical errors can occur with in-house ELISAs and ICAs, leading to inaccurate results, especially if the manufacturers' instructions are not followed with regard to temperature for performance of the test and with regard to timings.
- The use of whole blood in some ELISA and/or ICA kits leads to false-positive results.
- An excessively thick blood smear may cause a false-positive IFA result.

Influence of Signalment
Species
Cats only

Breed
None

Age
FeLV infection in kittens may not become detectable until around 3 months after birth.

Gender
Intact males with outdoor access are at greater risk.

Pregnancy
None

LIMITATIONS OF THE TEST
- ELISAs for use on saliva or tears are not as accurate as those using serum or plasma and thus cannot be recommended.
- No test used for FeLV infection is 100% accurate at all times under all conditions.

Sensitivity, Specificity, and Positive and Negative Predictive Values
- The reported sensitivity and specificity of ELISAs and ICAs vary but generally are 90%–98% sensitive and 98%–99% specific. Positive predictive values are poorer (as low as ≈80%) than negative predictive values (≈99%).
- PCR performance relies on the assay being properly designed, validated, and executed, and laboratories offering diagnostic PCR should make validation data available to veterinarians. A recent study (Pinches *et al.* 2007) showed proviral FeLV PCR had a sensitivity of 98% and specificity of 86% compared to virus isolation as a gold standard for FeLV diagnosis. Although the specificity sounds poor, it reflects the ability of PCR to detect provirus in nonviremic cats. Quantitative FeLV PCR enables the provirus load in the blood to be measured, and use of a cutoff level for determining the significance of a positive PCR result is likely to be helpful.

Valid If Run in a Human Lab?
No.

CLINICAL PERSPECTIVE
- Positive ELISA/ICA results can indicate transient or persistent viremia. Therefore, positive results in healthy cats must be confirmed by using alternative or repeat FeLV testing methods.
- For ELISA/ICA tests: In populations with a low prevalence of FeLV infection (particularly healthy cats), a large proportion of positive results obtained will be false positive, so positive test results must be confirmed.
- For ELISA/ICA tests: Negative results are more reliable because most populations are associated with a low prevalence of FeLV infection.
- Positive IFA results usually indicate persistent viremia.
- PCR results usually agree with those of ELISA/ICA and IFA, but PCR-positive cats exist that are negative on all other testing. These most likely represent recovered cats, but the possibility of a subsequent pathogenic effect of latent FeLV infection in these cats has not been ruled out.

MISCELLANEOUS
ANCILLARY TESTS
- Since FIV can cause clinical signs similar to those of FeLV, concurrent FIV testing may be indicated.
- Hematologic and biochemistry investigations to assess for evidence of FeLV-related disease, as well as investigations for concurrent infectious diseases, may be indicated.

SYNONYMS
FeLV

SEE ALSO
Blackwell's Five-Minute Veterinary Consult: Canine and Feline Topics
Feline Leukemia Virus Infection (FeLV)
Related Topics in This Book
- Blood Sample Collection
- Blood Smear Preparation
- Bone Marrow Aspirate Cytology: Microscopic Evaluation
- Feline Immunodeficiency Virus

FELINE LEUKEMIA VIRUS

ABBREVIATIONS
- FeLV = feline leukemia virus
- ICA = immunochromatographic assay

Suggested Reading
Hartmann K. Feline leukemia virus infection. In: Greene CE, ed. *Infectious Diseases of the Dog and Cat*, 3rd ed. St Louis: Saunders Elsevier, 2006: 105–131.
Hofmann-Lehmann R, Tandon R, Boretti FS, et al. Reassessment of feline leukaemia virus (FeLV) vaccines with novel sensitive molecular assays. *Vaccine* 2006; **24:**1087–1094.
Pinches MD, Helps CR, Gruffydd-Jones TJ, et al. Diagnosis of feline leukaemia virus infection by semi-quantitative real-time polymerase chain reaction. *J Feline Med Surg* 2007; **9**: 8–13.

INTERNET RESOURCES
American Association of Feline Practitioners (AAFP). Report of the American Association of Feline Practitioners and Academy of Feline Medicine Advisory Panel on Feline Retrovirus Testing and Management. Hillsborough, NJ: AAFP, http://www.aafponline.org/resources/guidelines/Felv_FIV_Guidelines.pdf.
Feline Advisory Bureau (FAP). Cat Group policy statement 2: Feline leukemia virus (FeLV), http://www.fabcats.org/cat_group/policy_statements/felv.html.

AUTHOR NAME
Séverine Tasker

BASICS

TYPE OF SPECIMEN
Blood

TEST EXPLANATION AND RELATED PHYSIOLOGY
Iron plays an important role in the metabolism of all living organisms. There are several iron compartments in mammalian species, most notable being the oxygen-carrying hemoglobin molecule present in erythrocytes. The tissue iron compartment is made up of other heme-containing (myoglobin, cytochromes, cytochrome oxygenase, and peroxidases) and non–heme-containing enzymes and proteins. Examples of non–heme-containing enzymes include, but are not limited to, aconitase and ribonucleotide reductase, and enzymes involved in ATP synthesis and DNA synthesis, respectively. With such a wide tissue distribution, it is easy to see why iron deficiency is so detrimental to veterinary patients.

Following intestinal absorption and transport to the tissues by transferrin, the iron-transferrin complex is endocytosed, iron is incorporated into proteins, and enzymes and transferrin are recycled. Excess iron is included into ferritin, a water-soluble iron storage protein. Ferritin is present in the cytoplasm of virtually all cells and in tissue fluids. Small amounts of ferritin are present in plasma/serum and usually correlate with total body iron stores. In iron deficiency, concentrations of serum ferritin decrease and, in cases of iron overload, they increase. Ferritin is also an acute phase protein and can increase in response to significant inflammatory reactions.

Serum ferritin is measured using antibody-driven methods such as radioimmunoassay and ELISA. Unfortunately, the antibodies in these methods are usually species specific and therefore do not cross-react across species.

INDICATIONS
- Assess iron metabolism in patients with suspected iron deficiency or overload.
- Monitor iron therapy.
- Assess iron reserves in at-risk patients.
- Differentiate between iron-deficiency anemia and anemia of chronic disease and/or inflammation.

CONTRAINDICATIONS
None

POTENTIAL COMPLICATIONS
None

CLIENT EDUCATION
None

BODY SYSTEMS ASSESSED
Hemic, lymphatic, and immune

SAMPLE

COLLECTION
1–2 mL of venous blood

HANDLING
- Collect blood into a plain red-top tube or serum-separator tube.
- Centrifuge and remove the serum from a Vacutainer with plastic pipette to *plastic* tube within 2h.

STORAGE
- Refrigerate for short-term storage.
- Freezing is recommended for long-term storage. Separate serum from RBCs before freezing.

STABILITY
- Room temperature and refrigerated: 1 week
- Frozen (−20°C): 6 months to 1 year; avoid repeated thawing and freezing.

FERRITIN

PROTOCOL
None

 INTERPRETATION

NORMAL FINDINGS OR RANGE
- Dogs: 80–800 ng/mL
- Cats: 31–146 ng/mL
- Kansas State University College of Veterinary Medicine diagnostic lab reference intervals. Values may vary depending on the laboratory and assay.

ABNORMAL VALUES
Values above or below the reference interval

CRITICAL VALUES
None

INTERFERING FACTORS
Drugs That May Alter Results or Interpretation
Drugs That Interfere with Test Methodology
None

Drugs That Alter Physiology
- Colchicine
- Iron preparations cause increased ferritin synthesis.

Disorders That May Alter Results
- Hemolysis/hemolytic disease may increase serum ferritin.
- Recent transfusions can increase serum ferritin.

Collection Techniques or Handling That May Alter Results
Marked hemolysis can cause false elevations of serum ferritin because of release of intracellular ferritin from lysed cells.

Influence of Signalment
Species
None

Breed
None

Age
None

Gender
None

Pregnancy
None

LIMITATIONS OF THE TEST
In the anemia of chronic and/or inflammatory disease, serum ferritin levels may be normal or increased and therefore may mask underlying iron deficiency or impaired iron metabolism.

Sensitivity, Specificity, and Positive and Negative Predictive Values
N/A

Valid If Run in Human a Lab?
No. Species-specific assays are required.

Causes of Abnormal Findings

High values	Low values
Acute inflammation	Chronic blood loss
Chronic disease	Iron deficiency
Liver disease	Hemodialysis
Hemochromatosis	
Hemosiderosis	
Certain neoplastic diseases	

CLINICAL PERSPECTIVE
- In dogs and cats, serum ferritin concentration correlates well with liver and splenic iron stores.
- Serum ferritin is an acute phase protein and often increased in inflammatory disease. This can mask concurrent iron deficiency or impaired iron metabolism.
- Ferritin can also be increased in some neoplastic diseases.
- Antibodies to serum ferritin are species specific and do not cross-react.

MISCELLANEOUS
ANCILLARY TESTS
- Serum iron and total iron-binding capacity
- Percent saturation of transferrin
- C-reactive protein
- Fecal occult blood
- CBC with RBC and reticulocyte indices

SYNONYMS
None

SEE ALSO
Blackwell's Five-Minute Veterinary Consult: Canine and Feline Topics
- Anemia, Iron-Deficiency
- Anemia, Nonregenerative

Related Topics in This Book
- Fecal Occult Blood
- Iron Level and Total Iron-Binding Capacity
- Red Blood Cell Count
- Red Blood Cell Indices

ABBREVIATIONS
None

Suggested Reading
Harvey JW. Microcytic anemias. In: Feldman BF, Zinkl JG, Jain NC, eds. *Schalm's Veterinary Hematology.* Baltimore: Lippincott Williams & Wilkins, 2000: 200–204.
Smith JE. Iron metabolism and its disorders. In: Kaneko JJ, Harvey JW, Bruss ML, eds. *Clinical Biochemistry of Domestic Animals,* 5th ed. San Diego: Academic, 1997: 223–237.
Stockham SL, Scott MA. *Fundamentals of Veterinary Clinical Pathology.* Ames: Iowa State Press, 2002.

INTERNET RESOURCES
None

AUTHOR NAME
Jennifer Steinberg

FIBRIN DEGRADATION PRODUCTS

BASICS

TYPE OF SPECIMEN
Blood

TEST EXPLANATION AND RELATED PHYSIOLOGY
Fibrin(ogen) degradation products (FDPs) are nonclottable fragments of fibrinogen or fibrin generated by the fibrinolytic system. This system is activated in response to intravascular coagulation (clotting) and consists of the proteolytic enzyme, plasmin. Plasmin is generated from its inactive precursor, plasminogen, by plasminogen activators released from injured endothelial cells. Plasmin binds to and sequentially cleaves fibrinogen and non–cross-linked (soluble) fibrin at identical sites, initially yielding large fragments, X and Y. These are further degraded to fragments consisting of the terminal (D domain) and central (E domain) portions of fibrinogen or fibrin, called fragments D and E, respectively. Thus, identical degradation products (X, Y, D, and E) are generated from plasmin's action on fibrinogen and soluble fibrin; hence the term *fibrin(ogen) degradation products*.

FDPs are constantly produced during normal physiologic hemostasis and are found in low levels (<10 μg/mL) in healthy individuals. However, large amounts of FDPs will be generated when there is excessive plasmin generation or fibrinolysis. This is usually in response to systemic intravascular activation of coagulation, as occurs in the syndrome of DIC. However, high FDP concentrations can also be seen with hyperplasminemia without preexisting coagulation (primary fibrinolysis) or possibly with extravascular coagulation, i.e., hemorrhage into body cavities. Also, proteases, including neutrophil elastase, cathepsin G, and trypsin, other than plasmin can degrade fibrinogen or fibrin.

FDPs are detected by latex agglutination tests, which contain polyclonal or monoclonal antibodies against FDPs. A major disadvantage with polyclonal antibodies is that they cross-react with intact (not degraded) fibrinogen. Thus, assays containing these antibodies must be performed on serum (which lacks intact fibrinogen) and require the use of special FDP-collection tubes. In contrast, assays containing monoclonal antibodies can measure the FDP concentration in plasma because the antibodies react with regions that are exposed or altered by thrombin or fibrin polymerization. These monoclonal antibodies do not cross-react with intact fibrinogen.

INDICATIONS
- A direct indicator of in vivo activation of fibrinolytic system
- An indirect marker of thrombosis: Since thrombi are subject to plasmin degradation, FDPs are released as a sequel to thrombosis (secondary fibrinolysis).
- Most commonly used as an ancillary diagnostic test for DIC, the systemic hypercoagulable and thromboembolic disorder.

CONTRAINDICATIONS
None

POTENTIAL COMPLICATIONS
None

CLIENT EDUCATION
None

BODY SYSTEMS ASSESSED
Hemic, lymphatic, and immune

SAMPLE

COLLECTION
1–3 mL of venous blood

HANDLING
Choice of tube depends on the assay. Check with the lab for its preference.
- Serum must be collected into a special FDP-collection tube. These tubes contain additives that either remove intact fibrinogen by initiating clotting (*Bothrops atrox* venom [Reptilase] or thrombin) or inhibit in vitro fibrinolysis (soybean trypsin inhibitor).
- Plasma should be collected into citrate anticoagulant (blue-top tube).

STORAGE
- Refrigeration is recommended for short-term storage.
- Freeze serum or plasma for long-term storage. Separate serum or plasma from RBCs before freezing it.

STABILITY
- Refrigerated (2°–8°C): serum, 1 week; plasma, 1 day (based on human data)
- Frozen (−20°C): serum, several months; plasma, 1 month (based on human data)

PROTOCOL
None

INTERPRETATION

NORMAL FINDINGS OR RANGE
- Dogs: serum, <10 μg/mL; plasma, <5 μg/mL
- Cats: serum, <10 μg/mL

ABNORMAL VALUES
- Values above the reference interval

CRITICAL VALUES
None

INTERFERING FACTORS
Drugs That May Alter Results or Interpretation
Drugs That Interfere with Test Methodology
Heparin inhibits clotting induced by thrombin-based collection tubes, increasing the FDP concentration. Reptilase-based collection tubes are not affected.

Drugs That Alter Physiology
Fibrinolytic drugs (e.g., streptokinase and tissue plasminogen activator) will increase the FDP concentration by inducing clot lysis.

Disorders That May Alter Results
• Human conditions reported to affect FDP concentration (unknown effect in animals)
  • Rheumatoid arthritis is associated with false-positive serum or plasma FDP results.
  • Inflammation may increase the FDP concentration when neutrophil proteases degrade fibrinogen or fibrin.
  • Monoclonal gammopathy (e.g., multiple myeloma) may cause false-positive serum FDP results because the monoclonal immunoglobulin inhibits fibrin polymerization and removal of intact fibrinogen in the collection tube.
  • Disorders associated with abnormal fibrinogen (dysfibrinogenemia) may cause false-positive serum FDP reactions (fibrinogen is not completely removed during clotting) (e.g., acute myeloid leukemia).
• An increased serum FDP concentration is seen in human patients with acute and chronic renal disease and in dogs with uremia. This could be secondary to renal intravascular coagulation with secondary fibrinolysis or decreased renal catabolism of FDPs.
• Liver disease may increase the FDP concentration because of decreased clearance.
• Extravascular coagulation (e.g., hemorrhage into tissue or body cavities, severe burns) may increase the FDP concentration. The increase in the FDP concentration in some dogs with anticoagulant rodenticide toxicosis has been attributed to this mechanism. However, experimental induction of muscle hematomas or hemoperitoneum did not increase the serum FDP concentration in dogs.

Collection Techniques or Handling That May Alter Results
• Failure to collect blood into FDP collection tube will falsely increase the serum FDP concentration (intact fibrinogen is not removed; in vitro fibrinolysis is not inhibited).
• Poor venipuncture may contaminate the sample with tissue factor, which could initiate clotting in vitro, falsely increasing the FDP concentration.

Influence of Signalment
Species
Plasma FDP assays have not been validated in cats.

Breed
None

Age
None

Gender
None

Pregnancy
None

LIMITATIONS OF THE TEST
• Plasma FDP assays have not been validated in cats.
• Positive FDP results have been observed in healthy dogs and cats by use of plasma and serum assays, respectively. The reason for this is unclear (these may be false-positive reactions).
• Antibodies vary in their ability to detect specific FDP fragments. Serum FDP assays are more sensitive to the terminal fragments, D and E. In contrast, validated plasma FDP assays detect fragments X and Y. Thus, results depend on stage of clot lysis and assay used. False-negative results may occur if fragments detected by the assay are not present.

• False-negative results may occur with serum FDP assays if the fragments (particularly the early fragment X) adsorb to the clot.
• Serum and plasma assays are not directly comparable, yielding discrepant results in individual canine patients. This is likely due to differences in antibody specificities.

Sensitivity, Specificity, and Positive and Negative Predictive Values
N/A

Valid If Run in a Human Lab?
Yes, for serum FDPs. Specific plasma FDP assays should be used in dogs (not all commercially available kits cross-react with canine FDPs).

Causes of Abnormal Findings

High values	Low (normal) values
Primary fibrinogenolysis	Not clinically
Parvovirus (mechanism unknown)	significant
Secondary fibrinolysis (disorders associated with	
coagulation or thrombosis)	
DIC (e.g., sepsis, heatstroke)	
Protein-losing nephropathy and/or enteropathy	
Hyperadrenocorticism, corticosteroid therapy	
Hemorrhage	
Trauma	
Extravascular fibrinolysis	
Hemorrhage into body cavities or tissues; e.g.,	
secondary to anticoagulant rodenticide	
toxicosis	
Fibrinolytic therapy	
Streptokinase	
Tissue plasminogen activator	
Decreased clearance	
Liver disease	
Renal failure	

CLINICAL PERSPECTIVE
• Determination of FDP level is mostly used as an ancillary diagnostic test for DIC in animals. Serum FDP concentrations are increased in 38%–95% of dogs with DIC, whereas high plasma FDP concentrations occur in 74%–90% of dogs with DIC. Fewer data are available for cats.
• Determination of FDP concentration should not be the sole diagnostic test for DIC; values should be interpreted concurrently with results of coagulation and platelet testing.
  • A high FDP concentration is not specific for DIC. The plasma FDP level may be increased, but the serum FDP concentration may be normal in dogs with thrombosis not associated with DIC (e.g., amyloidosis, hyperadrenocorticism).
  • A negative test result does not exclude a diagnosis of DIC, particularly if other clinical and laboratory data support this diagnosis.
• The FDP value does not correlate with severity or prognosis of DIC or thrombosis, and the degree of FDP increase does not appear to be diagnostically useful; i.e., any increase in FDP is considered abnormal.
• Serum FDP assays are less sensitive than plasma assays for detection of FDPs in dogs with DIC or thrombosis. For this reason, plasma FDP assays are preferred.

FIBRIN DEGRADATION PRODUCTS

• The plasma FDP concentration may be increased, with a normal D-dimer, with primary fibrin(ogen)olysis. This is due to systemic release of tissue plasminogen activator and occurs secondary to hypotension, heatstroke, surgical trauma, and certain neoplasms (e.g., prostatic carcinoma) in human patients. Fortunately, primary fibrinogenolysis is a rare (or poorly recognized) entity in animals; therefore, increases in the FDP concentration are considered indicative of secondary fibrin(ogen)olysis (i.e., in response to coagulation).

• FDPs may interfere with hemostasis by interfering with platelet function and inhibiting fibrin polymerization. This may affect interpretation of diagnostic tests, such as the thrombin clot time, which is prolonged in the presence of a markedly increased FDP concentration. This is also important clinically because the FDPs may worsen hemorrhagic symptoms in patients with DIC.

MISCELLANEOUS

ANCILLARY TESTS
• Platelet count
• Hemostasis testing (i.e., evaluation of prothrombin time, activated partial thromboplastin time, and antithrombin)
• D-dimer

SYNONYMS
• FDPs
• Fibrinogen degradation products

SEE ALSO
Blackwell's Five-Minute Veterinary Consult: Canine and Feline Topics
• Disseminated Intravascular Coagulation

• Protein-Losing Enteropathy
• Proteinuria
• Sepsis and Bacteremia

Related Topics in This Book
• Anticoagulant Proteins
• D-Dimer
• Partial Thromboplastin Time, Activated
• Prothrombin Time

ABBREVIATIONS
• DIC = disseminated intravascular coagulation
• FDP = fibrin(ogen) degradation product

Suggested Reading

Bateman SW, Mathews KA, Abrams-Ogg ACG, *et al.* Diagnosis of disseminated intravascular coagulation in dogs admitted to an intensive care unit. *J Am Vet Med Assoc* **999**; 215: 798–804.

Boisvert AM, Swenson CL, Haines CJ. Serum and plasma latex agglutination tests for detection of fibrin(ogen) degradation products in clinically ill dogs. *Vet Clin Pathol* 2001; **30**: 133–136.

Stokol T, Brooks M, Erb H, Mauldin GE. Evaluation of kits for the detection of fibrin(ogen) degradation products in dogs. *J Vet Intern Med* 1999; **13**: 478–484.

INTERNET RESOURCES
Cornell University, College of Medicine, Animal Health Diagnostic Center, Clinical Pathology Laboratory—Hemostasis, http://www.diaglab.vet.cornell.edu/clinpath/modules/coags/coag.htm.

AUTHOR
Tracy Stokol

BASICS

TYPE OF SPECIMEN
Blood

TEST EXPLANATION AND RELATED PHYSIOLOGY
Fibrinogen is a plasma protein synthesized by the liver with roles in both the coagulation system and the acute phase of the inflammatory response. It is a component of the coagulation system (factor I) and is activated by thrombin to form fibrin, the end stage of the coagulation cascade.

Fibrinogen levels can be reduced by decreased production (e.g., liver disease and congenital afibrinogenemia), abnormal function (congenital dysfibrinogenemia), or increased consumption. Fibrinogen can be consumed in hypercoagulable states, such as DIC, resulting in hypofibrinogenemia. There are rare reported cases of inherited coagulopathies caused by dysfibrinogenemia and afibrinogenemia. Hyperfibrinogenemia is commonly seen in animals with inflammatory disease of any cause.

At reference laboratories, fibrinogen is quantified by a modified thrombin clot test, which measures how much time it takes for a thrombin reagent to convert fibrinogen to fibrin, forming a clot. This test determines the level of functional fibrinogen. Immunoassays for fibrinogen antigen are available in specialized laboratories and differentiate between lack of fibrinogen and abnormal fibrinogen function (congenital dysfibrinogenemia). Fibrinogen levels can be estimated in-house by a heat-precipitation method.

INDICATIONS
- Assessment of clotting disorders
- Identification of the presence of inflammation

CONTRAINDICATIONS
Clotted sample or traumatic venipuncture

POTENTIAL COMPLICATIONS
Hemorrhage from the collection site

CLIENT EDUCATION
None

BODY SYSTEMS ASSESSED
- Hemic, lymphatic, and immune
- Hepatobiliary

SAMPLE

COLLECTION
1–2 mL of venous blood

HANDLING
- Clean venipuncture is essential; clotted samples are not acceptable
- For quantitative fibrinogen, collect blood into sodium citrate (blue-top tube) or in a syringe and mix it with sodium citrate.
  - An exact ratio of blood: citrate (9 parts:1 part) is critical.
  - Centrifuge citrated blood immediately and remove the plasma.
- For a heat-precipitation estimate, collection of blood into EDTA is also acceptable.
- Do not draw samples from a heparinized catheter.

STORAGE
- Refrigerate the plasma if it will be analyzed in <1 day after collection.
- Freeze the plasma if analysis will be delayed >1 day after collection.

STABILITY
- Room temperature: 4 h
- Refrigerated (2°–8°C): 1 day
- Frozen (−20°C): at least 1 week

PROTOCOL
Heat-precipitation method:
- Fill 2 microhematocrit tubes with anticoagulated blood and centrifuge as usual.
- Determine the total protein of 1 tube with a refractometer.
- Incubate a second microhematocrit tube for 3 min in a 56°C water bath. Heating denatures fibrinogen, causing its precipitation.
- The sample is again centrifuged, pushing denatured fibrinogen into the buffy coat layer.
- Determine the total protein of the heat-treated plasma.
- Estimated fibrinogen is the difference between heat-treated and untreated plasma proteins.

INTERPRETATION

NORMAL FINDINGS OR RANGE
- Dogs: 200–400 mg/dL
- Cats: 50–300 mg/dL
- Reference intervals may vary depending on the laboratory and assay.

ABNORMAL VALUES
Values above and below the reference interval

CRITICAL VALUES
None

INTERFERING FACTORS
Drugs That May Alter Results or Interpretation
Drugs That Interfere with Test Methodology
Heparin can reduce measured fibrinogen, particularly at the dose present in a heparinized catheter or in a heparinized tube.

Drugs That Alter Physiology
Drugs that may decrease fibrinogen include phenobarbital, asparaginase, and fibrinolytic agents (e.g., streptokinase, urokinase).

Disorders That May Alter Results
• Hemolysis
• Lipemia

Collection Techniques or Handling That May Alter Results
• Traumatic venipuncture or a clotted sample
• Drawing a sample from a heparinized catheter

Influence of Signalment
Species
None

Breed
None

Age
None

Gender
None

Pregnancy
In dogs, fibrinogen levels and other acute phase reactants increase during days 30–50 of pregnancy.

LIMITATIONS OF THE TEST
Heat precipitation is not sensitive enough to detect hypofibrinogenemia.

Sensitivity, Specificity, and Positive and Negative Predictive Values
N/A
Valid If Run in Human Lab?
Yes.
Causes of Abnormal Findings

High values	Low values
Inflammation	Disseminated intravascular coagulation
Tissue necrosis	Severe liver disease
	Severe malnutrition
	Congenital afibrinogenemia (rare)
	Acquired afibrinogenemia secondary to:
	Fibrinogen antibody formation after transfusion
	Rattlesnake envenomation
	Sodium valproate administration (rare)

CLINICAL PERSPECTIVE
• In dogs and cats, leukogram changes are relatively sensitive for the detection of inflammation. Fibrinogen is rarely used to assess inflammation. Increased fibrinogen cannot differentiate between causes of inflammation.
• The increased consumption seen in DIC can be masked by concurrent inflammation, which often increases fibrinogen production greater than the level of consumption. Because of this, normal or increased fibrinogen values can be seen in patients with DIC.
• If decreased fibrinogen is caused by severe liver disease, other indicators of impaired liver function are expected, such as increased bile acids and decreased albumin, BUN, and other coagulation factors.
• Dysfibrinogenemia is very rare and results in an abnormal thrombin clot time but normal amounts of fibrinogen antigen as determined by immunoassay.

MISCELLANEOUS

ANCILLARY TESTS
- WBC count and differential
- Prothrombin time and activated partial thromboplastin time
- Platelet count
- Fibrin degradation products
- D-dimers

SYNONYMS
None

SEE ALSO
Blackwell's Five-Minute Veterinary Consult: Canine and Feline Topics
- Cirrhosis and Fibrosis of the Liver
- Disseminated Intravascular Coagulation
- Hepatic Failure, Acute
- Hepatitis, Chronic Active

Related Topics in This Book
- D-Dimer
- Fibrin Degradation Products

- Partial Thromboplastin Time, Activated
- Platelet Count and Volume
- Prothrombin Time
- White Blood Cell Count and Differential
- White Blood Cells: Neutrophils

ABBREVIATIONS
DIC = disseminated intravascular coagulation

Suggested Reading
Latimer KS, Mahaffey EA, Prasse KW, eds. *Duncan and Prasse's Veterinary Laboratory Medicine: Clinical Pathology*. Ames: Iowa State Press, 2003.
Stockham SL, Scott MA eds. *Fundamentals of Veterinary Clinical Pathology*, 2nd ed. Ames: Iowa State Press, 2008.

INTERNET RESOURCES
Cornell University, College of Medicine, Animal Health Diagnostic Center, Clinical Pathology Laboratory—Hemostasis, http://www.diaglab.vet.cornell.edu/clinpath/modules/coags/coag.htm.

AUTHOR NAME
Stephanie Corn

FINE-NEEDLE ASPIRATION

BASICS

TYPE OF PROCEDURE
Diagnostic sample collection

PROCEDURE EXPLANATION AND RELATED PHYSIOLOGY
Cytologic examination of samples collected via fine-needle aspiration (FNA) is an integral first step in assessing masses, lymphadenopathy, and other organ changes. When examined by a trained clinical pathologist, properly collected and processed samples can aid in identification of inflammatory and infectious processes and in distinguishing between neoplastic and nonneoplastic conditions. In many cases, cytologic examination of masses may enable the broad categorization of neoplastic processes as round cell, epithelial, or mesenchymal neoplasia. In the case of lymphadenopathy, cytologic evaluation may help classify changes as inflammatory, hyperplastic, reactive, or neoplastic.

Poorly prepared smears can make interpretation difficult. Extremely thick smears, for example, can cloud assessment by limiting the evaluation of individual cell characteristics.

INDICATIONS
• Evaluation of cutaneous and subcutaneous masses
• Evaluation of lymphadenopathy
• Evaluation of nodules or masses or other identified changes within organs

CONTRAINDICATIONS
• FNA is difficult to perform on very small masses.
• FNA entails a risk of hemorrhage when used to assess cavitary masses.
• Patients with a condition that includes severe bleeding tendencies, as with marked thrombocytopenia or coagulopathies

POTENTIAL COMPLICATIONS
• Bleeding, bruising
• Release of bioactive substances (e.g., mast cell tumor)
• Potential spread of malignant neoplasia (rare)

CLIENT EDUCATION
While risks are minimal when FNA cytology of internal organs or masses is performed, clients should be advised of the potential for hemorrhage or pneumothorax in the case of lung aspiration.

BODY SYSTEMS ASSESSED
All

PROCEDURE

PATIENT PREPARATION
Preprocedure Medication or Preparation
• None needed for external palpable masses
• The use of an aseptic skin preparation is indicated prior to FNA of internal masses.

Anesthesia or Sedation
• Generally, none is needed for external palpable masses or lymph nodes.
• Mild to heavy sedation is beneficial for obtaining diagnostic ultrasound-guided or bone FNA.

Patient Positioning
Any that enables optimal access to the site being aspirated

Patient Monitoring
For minor bruising or bleeding at the FNA site

Equipment or Supplies
• A needle of appropriate gauge: A 22-gauge, 1-inch (25.4 mm) needle is appropriate for most masses.
• A 6- or 12-mL syringe
• Glass microscopic slides

TECHNIQUE
Sample Collection
Needle Only
The mass or tissue is stabilized as much as possible while the needle is inserted into it and vigorously moved in and out of it in several directions. The needle is then withdrawn, a syringe filled with air is attached to the needle hub, and pressure is applied to the plunger to empty the needle's contents onto a glass slide.

Needle and Syringe with Continuous Negative Pressure
The mass or tissue is stabilized as well as possible, and the needle with attached empty syringe is inserted into the mass or tissue. Negative pressure is then applied to the syringe and maintained while the needle is redirected several times within the mass or tissue. Negative pressure is then released, and the needle with attached syringe is withdrawn. The syringe is detached from the needle, filled with air, reattached to the hub of the needle, and pressure is applied to the plunger to empty the needle's contents onto a glass slide.

Needle and Syringe with Repeated Negative Pressure
The mass or tissue is stabilized as well as possible while the needle with attached empty syringe is inserted into the mass or tissue. Negative pressure is applied to the syringe and released several times. The needle can be redirected and negative pressure again applied and released several times. This can be repeated in several directions within the mass or tissue. Once the sample has been collected for evaluation, negative pressure is released, and the needle with attached syringe is withdrawn. The syringe is detached from the needle, filled with air, reattached, and pressure is applied to the plunger to empty the needle's contents onto a glass slide.

Slide Preparation
Flat Spreader Slide Technique
A second slide is laid gently atop and perpendicular to the slide containing the sample and gently drawn down the length of the sample slide to achieve an even, thin layer of cells.

Angled Spreader Slide Technique
A second slide is positioned over the slide containing the sample and angled at 45° with the sample located in the small angle created between the 2 slides. The spreader slide is then drawn along the sample slide so that the cells are spread in an even layer down the latter slide's length.

SAMPLE HANDLING
• Air-dried samples can be stored at room temperature.
• Samples should be fixed and stained as soon after collection as possible (ideally within 3–7 days) for optimal assessment of cellular morphology.
• Once fixed and stained, FNA smears are stable for months to years, depending on storage conditions.

APPROPRIATE AFTERCARE
Postprocedure Patient Monitoring
Generally, no postprocedure monitoring is required, although if FNA is performed on highly vascular internal masses or tissues, monitoring for evidence of hemorrhage (i.e., mucous membrane color, attitude, with or without PCV and total solids) may be performed in the hours after the procedure.

Nursing Care
None

Dietary Modification
None

Medication Requirements
None

Restrictions on Activity
None

Anticipated Recovery Time
Immediate

 INTERPRETATION

NORMAL FINDINGS OR RANGE
• A bullet-shaped tissue smear that extends approximately one-half to two-thirds the length of the slide

ABNORMAL VALUES
• Abnormal cell ratios, numbers, or types
• The presence of infectious agents
• The presence of neoplastic cells

CRITICAL VALUES
None

INTERFERING FACTORS
Drugs That May Alter Results of the Procedure
None

Conditions That May Interfere with Performing the Procedure
None

Procedure Techniques or Handling That May Alter Results
• Hemorrhage with numerous RBCs evident cytologically may limit interpretation.
• Failure to fix and stain slides within 1–2 weeks may alter cellular characteristics and limit value of interpretation.

Influence of Signalment on Performing and Interpreting the Procedure

Species
None

Breed
None

Age
None

Gender
None

Pregnancy
None

CLINICAL PERSPECTIVE
Cytologic examination of FNA samples is a useful first step in assessing masses, lymphadenopathy, and other organ changes. Examination of prepared slides can provide information on potential pathology affecting the tissue sampled, including hyperplastic, reactive, inflammatory, and neoplastic changes. Although an important first step, a follow-up biopsy may be indicated, in some instances, for definitive diagnosis.

 MISCELLANEOUS

ANCILLARY TESTS
A biopsy with a histopathologic diagnosis to confirm the FNA results if they are equivocal or if the biopsy is indicated for definitive diagnosis and grading

SYNONYMS
Fine-needle aspiration biopsy

SEE ALSO
Blackwell's Five-Minute Veterinary Consult: Canine and Feline Topics
Numerous

Related Topics in This Book
• Blood Smear Preparation
• Impression Smear
• Ultrasound-Guided Mass or Organ Aspiration

ABBREVIATIONS
FNA = fine-needle aspiration

Suggested Reading
Cowell RL, Tyler RD, Meinkoth JH, eds. *Diagnostic Cytology and Hematology of the Dog and Cat.* St Louis: CV Mosby, 1999.
Raskin RE, Meyer DJ, eds. *Atlas of Canine and Feline Cytology*, 2nd ed. Philadelphia: WB Saunders, 2001.

INTERNET RESOURCES
None

AUTHOR NAME
Laurel E. Williams

FLUID ANALYSIS

BASICS

TYPE OF SPECIMEN
Tissue

TEST EXPLANATION AND RELATED PHYSIOLOGY
The abdominal and thoracic cavities of dogs and cats normally contain a small amount of fluid that is an ultrafiltrate of blood and whose purpose is to provide lubrication that enables frictionless movement of adjacent organ surfaces and the body cavity walls. An increased amount of fluid in any body cavity lined by mesothelial cells is termed an *effusion*. An effusion is not a disease itself but, rather, the result of a pathologic alteration in the process of fluid production and/or the removal system or an accumulation from an ectopic source.

Fluid analysis, including protein concentration, total and differential cell counts, and other biochemical analyses, is a rapid, simple, inexpensive, and reasonably safe way of gaining useful information regarding disease processes that cause effusions. Classification schemes are designed to help clinicians generate a short list of differential diagnoses and generally attempt to characterize an effusion based on the primary underlying pathophysiologic mechanism. Effusions are usually classified as a pure transudate, modified transudate, exudate, hemorrhagic effusion, or neoplastic effusion. Exudates are further divided into subcategories of septic or nonseptic exudates. The classification of these fluids is based on 3 parameters: total protein, nucleated cell counts (NCCs), and cytologic appearance.

Pure transudates usually form via a passive process resulting from decreased colloidal osmotic pressure rather than an alteration in capillary permeability. Pure transudates most frequently form as a result of hypoproteinemia from either increased loss or decreased production of albumin, the primary contributor to plasma colloidal osmotic pressure. Infrequently, transudates precede modified transudates before developing an increased NCC and/or protein concentration. A modified transudate occurs when vascular fluids leak from normal, noninflamed vessels (e.g., via increased capillary hydrostatic pressure or lymphatic obstruction). This fluid is modified by the addition of protein and/or cells as compared to that of a pure transudate. A chylous effusion is a type of modified transudate that results from leakage of noninflamed lymphatics into the thoracic and/or abdominal cavity. Exudates are the result of increased vascular permeability and inflammation and are further classified as septic or nonseptic depending on whether infectious agents are identified in the fluid. Nonseptic exudates may result from conditions that cause long-standing modified transudates, as well as from other, more inflammatory disease conditions. Hemorrhagic effusions can be caused by ruptured vessels or alterations in vascular endothelial integrity that is normally maintained by the interaction of platelets and various clotting factors. Neoplasia is a common cause of effusions in dogs and cats although neoplastic cells are often not identified on cytologic preparations. Furthermore, neoplasia may cause various effusions, including modified transudates, exudates, and hemorrhagic effusions. The term *neoplastic effusion* is reserved for fluids in which a neoplastic cell population is definitively identified. However, this determination is frequently difficult because neoplastic cells are absent or are present in low numbers and reactive mesothelial cells often have cytologic criteria that mimic malignancy.

INDICATIONS
- Accumulation of fluid because of an unknown cause
- Suspicion of neoplasia or sepsis

CONTRAINDICATIONS
None

POTENTIAL COMPLICATIONS
- Hemorrhage
- Infection
- Trauma to surrounding viscera (i.e., perforation, laceration)

CLIENT EDUCATION
None

BODY SYSTEMS ASSESSED
- Cardiovascular
- Gastrointestinal
- Hemic, lymphatic, and immune
- Hepatobiliary
- Renal and urologic

SAMPLE

COLLECTION
2–6 mL of fluid

HANDLING
- Collect the sample into EDTA-containing tube to prevent clotting.
- Place the aliquot into a sterile tube without EDTA if culture is needed (EDTA is bacteriostatic) or if biochemical testing is anticipated.
- Prepare smears immediately if the sample will be processed within >1–2 h after collection.
- Transport the sample chilled.

STORAGE
- Refrigerate fluid.
- Stores slides away from light or humidity.

STABILITY
- Fluid
  - Room temperature: 2–4 h
  - Refrigerated (4°C): 24–36 h
- Unstained smears of fluid can be stored for days. Stained slides can be stored for years.

PROTOCOL
In-house fluid analysis:
- Note the gross appearance of fluid.
- Prepare smears of fluid by using the same technique used to make blood smears. Smears should be thin enough to dry quickly. Be sure that the smear has a stainable feathered edge.
- Air-dry smears and stain with a Romanovsky-type stain (e.g., Wright stain, Hema III).
- Perform an NCC via hematology analyzer or hemocytometer.
- Centrifuge an aliquot of fluid and note the appearance of the supernatant.
- Determine the total protein of supernatant via refractometer.
- If the NCC is <3,000/μL, prepare additional smears of sedimented cellular material.

INTERPRETATION

NORMAL FINDINGS OR RANGE
No free fluid should be found in the pleural cavity, peritoneal cavity, and pericardium.

ABNORMAL VALUES
The presence of an abnormal, increased amount of fluid within a body cavity

CRITICAL VALUES
Evidence of septic peritonitis, uroabdomen, or bile peritonitis may require immediate surgical intervention.

Classification	Gross appearance	Protein g/dL	Cells/μL	Cell types present
Pure transudate	Colorless; clear	<2.5	<1,500	Mixed (macrophages, nondegenerate neutrophils, mesothelial cells)
Modified transudate	White to red; variable turbidity	2.5–5.0	1,000–7,000	Mixed (nondegenerate neutrophils, macrophages, mesothelial cells, small lymphocytes)
Chylous effusion[a]	Milky white, tan, or pink	2.5–5.0	1,000–7,000	Predominantly small lymphocytes
Exudate[b]	Amber, white, or red; turbid or cloudy	>3.0	>7,000	Predominantly neutrophils
Hemorrhagic effusion[c]	Pink or red; cloudy or opaque	Variable	Variable	Similar to peripheral blood but lacks platelets and may have erythrophagia
Neoplastic effusion	Variable	Variable	Variable	Overtly neoplastic cells present

[a]Chylous effusions have a triglyceride concentration of >100 mg/dL and a fluid cholesterol/triglyceride ratio of <1.0.
[b]Further classification of exudates depends on whether microorganisms are present (i.e., septic versus nonseptic).
[c]The PCV of fluid is ≥10%–25% of the PCV of peripheral blood.

INTERFERING FACTORS
Drugs That May Alter Results or Interpretation
Drugs That Interfere with Test Methodology
None

Drugs That Alter Physiology
• Corticosteroids may artifactually decrease the percentage and total number of neutrophils.
• Antibiotic administration greatly hinders the cytologic identification of bacteria.

Disorders That May Alter Results
• High triglyceride concentration in chylous effusions, or other causes of turbidity, may artificially increase protein determination by refractometry. If possible, clear such samples prior to determining protein concentration by refractometer.
• The dilutional effect of urine in uroperitoneum may decrease the protein concentration and NCC.
• Peracute hemorrhagic effusions may not have detectable erythrophagocytosis.
• The protein concentration in an effusion can be affected by serum protein concentration (e.g., mildly increased with dehydration; decreased with protein-losing enteropathies or nephropathies) regardless of the effusion mechanism.

Collection Techniques or Handling That May Alter Results
• Excessive pressure when preparing cytologic preparations (e.g., direct or sediment smears) may lyse cells.
• Delayed processing may lead to in vitro artifacts such as erythrophagocytosis, lysed cells, and/or poor cellular preservation. Bacterial overgrowth may occur if a preservative is not used or the specimen is not refrigerated.

Influence of Signalment
Species
None

Breed
None

Age
None

Gender
None

Pregnancy
None

LIMITATIONS OF THE TEST
Sensitivity, Specificity, and Positive and Negative Predictive Values
N/A

Valid If Run in Human Lab?
Yes.
Causes of Abnormal Values

Type of effusion and mechanisms	Possible causes

Pure transudate
  Decreased plasma colloidal osmotic pressure (i.e., hypoalbuminemia)—more common
  Early cardiac disease or portal hypertension—infrequent
	Decreased production of albumin
	  Liver failure
	  Maldigestion/malabsorption
	  Starvation
	Increased loss of albumin
	  Protein-losing nephropathy
	  Protein-losing enteropathy
	Other
	  Iatrogenic overhydration

Modified transudate
  Increased capillary hydrostatic pressure
  Lymphatic obstruction
	Cardiac disease
	Portal hypertension
	Neoplasia
	Acute organ torsion

Chylous effusion Leakage of lymphatics from noninflamed vessels	Cardiac disease (cats) Hernia Neoplasia Trauma Idiopathic Lung torsion Intestinal lymphangiectasia (dogs) Mediastinal granuloma
Exudate Increased vascular permeability and inflammation caused by septic and nonseptic etiologies	Uroperitoneum Bile peritonitis Feline infectious peritonitis Inflammation and/or infection of internal organs Foreign bodies Neoplasia

Eosinophilic effusion
  Eosinophils >10% of the NCC
  Secretion of interleukin 5 by sensitized T lymphocytes, mast cells, or neoplastic cells
	Neoplasia (e.g., mast cell tumor, lymphoma, carcinoma)
	Infection (e.g., fungus, parasite, protozoa)

Hemorrhagic effusion
  Ruptured vessels
  Coagulopathies
	Traumatic injury
	Rodenticide toxicity
	Neoplasia

Neoplastic effusion Exfoliation of identifiable neoplastic cells into fluid	Carcinomas Round cell tumors (e.g., lymphoma) Mesotheliomas Sarcomas

FLUID ANALYSIS

CLINICAL PERSPECTIVE

• Turbidity caused by lipids (e.g., chylous effusion) will not clear with centrifugation, unlike the turbidity caused by an increased NCC.

• Inadvertent venipuncture or aspiration of the spleen is possible at time of collection; therefore, fluid should be watched as it is collected. True hemorrhagic effusions should have the same color and turbidity throughout the draw, whereas with accidental venipuncture and splenic aspirate samples usually change color and turbidity during collection.

• Because lipid can be irritating, chronic chylous effusions may have a mixed inflammatory cell population, including neutrophils and macrophages, in addition to lymphocytes.

• If infectious agents are identified cytologically, the effusion is a septic one, regardless of its protein concentration and NCC.

• If fluid collected by abdominocentesis has low cellularity, abundant mixed bacteria, ingesta, and/or intestinal parasite ova, consider accidental enterocentesis or acute intestinal perforation.

MISCELLANEOUS

ANCILLARY TESTS

• Albumin

• Creatinine (fluid): A value of ≥2-fold serum creatinine is diagnostic for uroperitoneum.

• Total bilirubin (fluid): A value of ≥2-fold serum bilirubin is diagnostic for bile peritonitis.

• Triglycerides (fluid; for diagnosis of chylothorax)

• Glucose (fluid): A value of 20 mg/dL less than that for blood glucose has been suggested to be specific for sepsis, but low glucose may simply reflect the concurrent elevated NCC.

• Microbial culture and sensitivity

SYNONYMS

Body cavity effusion (BCE)

SEE ALSO

Blackwell's Five-Minute Veterinary Consult: Canine and Feline Topics

• Chapters on cardiac disease
• Chapters on hepatic disease
• Ascites
• Bile Peritonitis
• Feline Infectious Peritonitis (FIP)
• Hemothorax
• Lymphangiectasia

Related Topics in This Book

• Abdominocentesis and Fluid Analysis
• Thoracocentesis and Fluid Analysis

ABBREVIATIONS

NCC = nucleated cell count

Suggested Reading

Rakich PM, Latimer KS. Cytology. In: Latimer KS, Mahaffey EA, Prasse KW, eds. *Duncan and Prasse's Veterinary Laboratory Medicine: Clinical Pathology*, 4th ed. Ames: Iowa State Press, 2003: 315–318.

INTERNET RESOURCES

None

AUTHOR NAMES

Rebekah Gray Gunn-Christie and J. Roger Easley

BASICS

TYPE OF PROCEDURE
Miscellaneous

PROCEDURE EXPLANATION AND RELATED PHYSIOLOGY
The fluorescein dye test is a diagnostic procedure to assess the structural integrity of the cornea. Externally to internally, the cornea consists of epithelium, stroma, Descemet's membrane, and endothelium. The epithelium is composed of stratified, squamous, nonkeratinized epithelial cells with a basement membrane and comprises ≈10% of the overall corneal thickness. One of its functions, maintaining an optically clear ocular surface by limiting fluid uptake into the stroma, is achieved in part because of its hydrophobic nature. The underlying stroma is hydrophilic, composed of a lamellar arrangement of collagen fibrils in an extracellular matrix, and comprises ≈90% of the corneal thickness. Descemet's membrane, which is the basement membrane for the endothelium, and the endothelial cells themselves are hydrophobic and also inhibit water uptake by the stroma.

Sodium fluorescein is a weak dibasic acid that is water soluble and can be applied topically to the cornea to detect breaks in the hydrophobic epithelial barrier. When this barrier is absent (as in an ulcer), fluorescein dye gains access to the hydrophilic stroma and stains the intercellular spaces. Blue light (490 nm) is absorbed by the dye and causes fluorescence at 520 nm, which is visually detected as green dye uptake corresponding to the epithelial defect, or corneal ulcer. In addition to dye uptake in the presence of superficial ulcers (where only epithelium is absent), deeper stromal defects will also take up dye through their entire depth. In the presence of a *descemetocele* (a full-thickness stromal defect with intact Descemet's membrane and endothelium), fluorescein dye will be visible in the surrounding stroma, but Descemet's membrane itself will not retain stain, which leaves a clear spot at the deepest portion of the defect.

In addition to identifying the presence or absence of an intact epithelium, fluorescein dye can indicate patency of the nasolacrimal system by appearance of dye at both nostrils (the Jones test). Subtle leakage of aqueous humor from deep corneal wounds or defects may be detected when fluorescein swirls on the corneal surface near the point of leakage (the Siedel test). Qualitative abnormalities in the mucin layer of the tear film, responsible for adherence of the tear film to the corneal surface, may be detected with the tear-film breakup time, which is evaluated by monitoring the appearance of dye on the corneal surface over time.

INDICATIONS
- Corneal vascularization
- Epiphora
- Decreased tear production
- History of trauma
- Ocular pain (e.g., blepharospasm, rubbing)
- Ocular redness
- Visible corneal surface irregularities

CONTRAINDICATIONS
Use caution in the presence of deep corneal ulcer because the eye may rupture with excessive manipulation of the patient.

POTENTIAL COMPLICATIONS
- Eye rupture in the case of a deep corneal ulcer with excessive manipulation
- Ocular irritation (unlikely)
- Staining of the periocular hairs (which can be cleaned with eyewash)

CLIENT EDUCATION
None

BODY SYSTEMS ASSESSED
Ophthalmic

PROCEDURE

PATIENT PREPARATION
Preprocedure Medication or Preparation
- Perform a Schirmer tear test prior to instilling anything onto the ocular surface.
- Some patients may be more easily handled after the administration of topical anesthetic, but this is generally not necessary.

Anesthesia or Sedation
None

Patient Positioning
Sternal recumbency, sitting, or standing

Patient Monitoring
None

Equipment or Supplies
- Fluorescein dye strips
- Eyewash
- Cotton balls or gentle tissue

FLUORESCEIN DYE TEST

- Topical anesthetic for select patients
- A focal light source, with or without a blue light

TECHNIQUE

- Fluorescein dye inactivates commonly used ophthalmic preservatives, and solutions may become contaminated with bacteria, so the use of freshly opened fluorescein dye strips is safest.
- Flush the eye gently with eyewash to remove discharge or debris prior to performing the test.
- Moisten the strip with a few drops of eyewash, leaving a drop on the edge of the strip.
- Alternatively, place the dye-impregnated end of the strip in a 3-mL syringe, to which eyewash may be added to a volume of 1–2 mL.
- Place a drop of diluted dye (either from end of the strip or from the syringe tip) on the conjunctiva over the dorsal sclera, taking care not to touch the cornea and leave a defect.
- The eye should be blinked and then rinsed with eyewash to remove excess dye.
- The use of cotton balls or gentle tissue around the eye is recommended because gauze sponges may traumatize the cornea or conjunctiva.
- Use a focal light source (blue light will help if ulceration is difficult to visualize, but white light is often sufficient).
- If attempting to assess patency of nasolacrimal ducts (NLDs), fill the conjunctival sac with dilute dye solution and tip the nose toward the floor, watching for appearance of dye at each nares.

SAMPLE HANDLING

N/A

APPROPRIATE AFTERCARE

Postprocedure Patient Monitoring

None

Nursing Care

None

Dietary Modification

None

Medication Requirements

Appropriate topical therapy when an ulceration is present

Restrictions on Activity

None

Anticipated Recovery Time

Immediate

INTERPRETATION

NORMAL FINDINGS OR RANGE

- A normal cornea with an intact epithelial barrier will demonstrate no fluorescein dye uptake.
- Mucoid discharge or roughened cornea [e.g., chronic keratoconjunctivitis sicca (KCS) or other surface disorders] may demonstrate false retention of stain.

ABNORMAL VALUES

- Retention of fluorescein dye on the cornea indicates loss of the epithelial barrier (ulceration).
- A rim of dye retention with a clear, dark area in the deepest portion indicates a descemetocele.
- Absence of dye at either nares may indicate congenital or acquired blockage of the NLD.

CRITICAL VALUES

Dye retention indicates ulceration.

INTERFERING FACTORS

Drugs That May Alter Results of the Procedure

None

Conditions That May Interfere with Performing the Procedure

Deep corneal ulcer, which may rupture with excessive manipulation

Procedure Techniques or Handling That May Alter Results

- Excessive dilution of the stain may produce variable staining.
- Ocular discharge should be removed prior to testing to reduce false positives.

Influence of Signalment on Performing and Interpreting the Procedure

Species

Equally applicable to dogs and cats

Breed
Equally applicable to all dog and cat breeds

Age
Equally applicable to patients of all ages

Gender
Equally applicable to all genders

Pregnancy
Can be safely performed on pregnant animals

CLINICAL PERSPECTIVE
- The fluorescein dye test should be a routine part of an ophthalmologic examination.
- It should be performed on all patients with ocular pain, redness, tearing, or low Schirmer tear test values.
- It should be performed on all patients receiving topical medications, especially topical steroids.
- The entire ocular surface should be examined after fluorescein instillation, and blue light should be used, if necessary, to detect smaller lesions.
- Conjunctival ulcerations and abrasions will also retain fluorescein dye.
- If the NLD is not patent, further evaluation is indicated.

MISCELLANEOUS

ANCILLARY TESTS
- Schirmer tear test
- Jones test

- Siedel test
- Tear-film breakup time
- Rose Bengal dye test
- Evaluation of cytology
- Microbial culture and sensitivity

SYNONYMS
None

SEE ALSO
Blackwell's Five-Minute Veterinary Consult: Canine and Feline Topics
- Corneal and Scleral Lacerations
- Corneal Sequestrum—Cats
- Keratitis, Nonulcerative
- Keratitis, Ulcerative
- Keratoconjunctivitis Sicca

Related Topics in This Book
- Conjunctival Scraping and Cytology
- Schirmer Tear Test

ABBREVIATIONS
NLD = nasolacrimal duct

Suggested Reading
Gelatt KN, ed. *Veterinary Ophthalmology*, 3rd ed. Baltimore: Lippincott Williams & Wilkins, 1999.

INTERNET RESOURCES
None

AUTHOR NAME
Alison Clode

BASICS

TYPE OF PROCEDURE
Radiographic

PROCEDURE EXPLANATION AND RELATED PHYSIOLOGY
This modality uses the differential attenuation of X-rays to produce images of patients as in radiography. Whereas radiographs depict a snapshot of the patient's internal structure, fluoroscopy depicts the patient's internal structure dynamically over a short period.

INDICATIONS
Fluoroscopy is used to examine internal body parts where abnormal motion is a major feature of the disease (e.g., dysphagia, tracheal collapse, diaphragmatic paralysis). Observing motion also is important during certain procedures when guiding instruments into position—such as catheter placement during angiography, needle placement during biopsy or myelography, or repairing a bone fracture. Although image quality generally is inferior to most other imaging modalities, fluoroscopy may be used to evaluate structural abnormalities when custom positioning of a patient is desired to show the lesion better (e.g., ureteral ectopia) and cross-sectional imaging is not selected because of general anesthesia or cost.

CONTRAINDICATIONS
None

POTENTIAL COMPLICATIONS
• Some examinations will be inconclusive when a patient is non-compliant, not allowing the examination to proceed, and sedation is contraindicated or will alter motility (and assessing altered motility is the reason for the examination).
• Administering contrast medium per os could result in aspiration of the contrast medium when it is administered too quickly or the patient has a dysphagia.
• Severe adverse reactions are always a potential risk when contrast medium is administered IV.
• Although rare, patients may be exposed to sufficiently high radiation doses to produce deterministic harmful effects (e.g., skin burn) during extremely long (i.e., hours) interventional procedures.

CLIENT EDUCATION
N/A

BODY SYSTEMS ASSESSED
• Cardiovascular
• Digestive
• Nervous
• Respiratory

 PROCEDURE

PATIENT PREPARATION
Preprocedure Medication or Preparation
None

Anesthesia or Sedation
Variable from awake anesthesia (e.g., for barium swallow or tracheal examination) to general anesthesia (e.g., for angiocardiography or myelography)

Patient Positioning
Variable

Patient Monitoring
None or as for general anesthesia

Equipment or Supplies
Iodinated contrast agent or barium-sulfate suspension

TECHNIQUE
• Patients generally are awake except during procedures that require placement of a needle or catheter.
• During tracheal fluoroscopy, patients stand or are in lateral recumbency and the entire trachea is observed for several seconds during normal (unstressed) respiration and during cough or after exercise. The image detector is oriented such that a lateral projection of the neck and thorax is obtained.
• During fluoroscopy of swallowing, dogs are placed in lateral recumbency and lateral projections are obtained. Movement of a bolus of barium-sulfate paste from the pharynx into the esophagus should be observed at least 3 times, and at least 1 bolus should be followed caudally until it enters the stomach. This observation then should be repeated with barium-coated kibble.
• During evaluation of diaphragm movement, patients are often examined in multiple recumbent positions (e.g., dorsal, ventral, left lateral, and right lateral) and multiple projections are obtained. The X-ray beam is centered on the diaphragm, and the image is collimated such that simultaneous evaluation of movement of the thoracic body wall and diaphragm is possible.
• During needle or catheter placement, advancement of the needle or catheter is observed directly during fluoroscopy. Orthogonal imaging might be helpful when a patient can be repositioned safely or the imaging detector can be rotated.

SAMPLE HANDLING
Captured images currently may be printed and/or stored digitally or on videotape.

APPROPRIATE AFTERCARE
Postprocedure Patient Monitoring
None

Nursing Care
None

Dietary Modification
None

Medication Requirements
N/A

Restrictions on Activity
None

Anticipated Recovery Time
Immediate

 INTERPRETATION

NORMAL FINDINGS OR RANGE
Tracheal Motion
The trachea has a roughly uniform dorsoventral height during both inhalation and exhalation. Mild motion of the dorsally located tracheal muscle into and out of the tracheal lumen may be seen with respiration.

Swallowing
Normal swallowing is divided into 3 phases: oropharyngeal, esophageal and gastroesophageal. The oropharyngeal phase is further divided into 3 stages: oral, pharyngeal, and cricopharyngeal. The oral stage, when dogs grasp the food, chew it, and move it caudally with the tongue to the pharynx, generally may be observed directly, so fluoroscopy is not needed except for tongue motion. The pharyngeal and cricopharyngeal stages are tightly coordinated. When a sufficiently large bolus is present in the pharynx, the pharyngeal muscles contract, the cranial-esophageal sphincter mechanism relaxes, and the bolus

is moved caudally into the esophagus. Immediately thereafter, the cranial-esophageal sphincter mechanism contracts, and the pharyngeal muscles relax. Once a sufficiently large bolus is present in the cranial esophagus, a primary peristaltic wave is initiated that brings the bolus to the stomach. The bolus has a blunt leading (caudal) edge and a tapering trailing (cranial) edge. It is common for a small amount of the bolus to break off and remain in the caudal cervical region. Secondary peristaltic waves then strip the esophagus of any remaining contents. The bolus pauses briefly at the caudal-esophageal sphincter mechanism before entering the stomach. It is normal to see thin linear streaks of contrast medium in the esophagus after the bolus has entered the stomach.

Diaphragmatic Motion
During inhalation, the thoracic body wall expands outwardly and the diaphragm moves caudally. During exhalation, the thoracic body wall moves inwardly and the diaphragm moves cranially.

ABNORMAL VALUES
Collapsing Trachea
The dorsoventral height of the tracheal lumen may be reduced statically or dynamically. During dynamic collapse, the height of the cervical part of the trachea is reduced during inhalation and the height of the thoracic part is reduced during exhalation. In severe cases, collapse of the principal bronchi may be detected and folding of the trachea with cranial displacement through the thoracic inlet may be detected during coughing. The disease severity might be underrepresented compared to that found via tracheoscopy or necropsy.

Dysphagia
Dysphagias may be classified as structural or functional. Some structural abnormalities include detection of a foreign body, neoplasm, or vascular ring anomaly. The functional dysphagias may be further classified by the stage or phase of swallowing where the abnormality is detected (e.g., esophageal phase dysphagia), which helps to define the differential diagnosis and select the appropriate treatment (e.g., cricopharyngeal myotomy). Mixed-stage and mixed-phase dysphagias also occur. Some functional abnormalities include absent, weak, or ineffectual pharyngeal or cranial-esophageal sphincter mechanism contractions; asynchronous contraction and relaxation of the pharynx and cranial-esophageal sphincter mechanism; reflux into the nasopharynx; aspiration; absent, weak, or ineffectual primary or secondary peristaltic waves; and reflux into the esophagus from the stomach.

Diaphragmatic Paralysis
There is paradoxical movement of the diaphragm relative to the body wall during both inhalation and exhalation. For example, during inhalation, the thoracic body wall expands outwardly and the diaphragm moves *cranially*. The entire diaphragm may be involved or only the left or right half.

CRITICAL VALUES
N/A

INTERFERING FACTORS
Drugs That May Alter Results of the Procedure
Many sedatives alter normal esophageal motility or may make the esophagus appear enlarged. The use of antitussive drugs (e.g., butorphanol) should be avoided when patients with suspected tracheal collapse are being examined.

Conditions That May Interfere with Performing the Procedure
For tracheal and swallowing studies, undesirable patient behavior (e.g., aggression) is the major issue that interferes with performing the examination satisfactorily.

Procedure Techniques or Handling That May Alter Results
None

Influence of Signalment on Performing and Interpreting the Procedure
Species
None

Breed
None

Age
None

Gender
None

Pregnancy
One might want to consider the necessity of exposing fetuses to ionizing radiation.

CLINICAL PERSPECTIVE
Fluoroscopy allows one to view both normal and abnormal motion during a radiographic procedure. Therefore, fluoroscopy becomes a necessary procedure when one is evaluating an animal for a disease in which abnormal motion is suspected. For example fluoroscopy is an important component of esophagography in the evaluation of an animal with dysphagia. Fluoroscopy is also helpful in the evaluation of certain structural abnormalities. For example, fluoroscopy is an essential component of excretory urography in the evaluation of animals suspected to have ectopic ureters.

MISCELLANEOUS
ANCILLARY TESTS
N/A

SYNONYMS
None

SEE ALSO
Blackwell's Five-Minute Veterinary Consult: Canine and Feline Topics
- Dysphagia
- Tracheal Collapse

Related Topics in This Book
- General Principles of Radiography
- Angiography and Angiocardiography
- Cystourethrography
- Epidurography
- Esophagography
- Excretory Urography
- Myelography
- Thoracic Radiography

ABBREVIATIONS
None

Suggested Reading
None

INTERNET RESOURCES
http://rpop.iaea.org/RPOP/RPoP/Content/InformationFor/
    HealthProfessionals/1_Radiology/Fluoroscopy.htm
http://www.fda.gov/cdrh/radhealth/products/fluoroscopy.html

AUTHOR NAME
Peter V. Scrivani

FOLATE

BASICS

TYPE OF SPECIMEN
Blood

TEST EXPLANATION AND RELATED PHYSIOLOGY
Folate is a water-soluble vitamin that is abundant in commercial canine and feline diets, making nutritional deficiency unlikely. Dietary folate is usually present in a poorly absorbable polyglutamate form. Folate deconjugase, a brush border enzyme secreted in the jejunum, removes all but 1 glutamate residue from the molecule. Specific carriers for folate monoglutamate in the proximal small intestine are responsible for folate uptake. Proximal or diffuse small intestinal disease (e.g., inflammatory bowel disease) can reduce folate absorption either by interfering with folate polyglutamate deconjugation or by reducing the presence of folate carrier proteins, thus decreasing serum folate concentrations.

Bacteria present in the distal small intestine and the large intestine produce large quantities of folate, which is normally excreted in feces. Folate carriers responsible for folate uptake are located exclusively in the proximal small intestine, and thus folate produced in distal sections of the intestine will not be absorbed. If folate-producing bacteria migrate upward into the proximal small intestine, folate of bacterial origin can be absorbed by the host, thus elevating serum folate concentrations. Dogs with EPI have a decreased secretion of antibacterial products, with subsequent small intestinal bacterial overgrowth (SIBO). As a consequence, dogs with EPI often have increased serum folate concentrations. The clinical significance of increased serum folate concentrations in cats remains unknown.

Most laboratories measure serum folate via a competitive chemiluminescence assay (Immulite; DPC, Los Angeles, CA). However, radioimmunoassays that have been validated for use in dogs and cats are also available.

INDICATIONS
• Assessment of GI function (proximal small intestine) in dogs and cats
• SIBO in dogs

CONTRAINDICATIONS
None

POTENTIAL COMPLICATIONS
None

CLIENT EDUCATION
Patients should be fasted—ideally, at least 12 h—prior to testing.

BODY SYSTEMS ASSESSED
Gastrointestinal

SAMPLE

COLLECTION
1–2 mL of venous blood

HANDLING
• Collect the sample into a red-top or serum-separator tube.
• Take steps to avoid hemolysis.

• Separate the serum from the blood clot and transfer the serum into a new tube. Do *not* submit unseparated serum to the laboratory.
• Ship the sample, with an ice pack, to laboratory.

STORAGE
Although short-term storage at room temperature will not affect test results, storing serum frozen at −20 °C is recommended.

STABILITY
• Room temperature: a few days
• Frozen (−20°C): at least 6–8 weeks

PROTOCOL
None

INTERPRETATION

NORMAL FINDINGS OR RANGE
• Dogs: 7.7–24.4 μg/L
• Cats: 9.7–21.6 μg/L
• References ranges are from the GI Laboratory at Texas A&M University. Values may vary depending on the laboratory and assay.

ABNORMAL VALUES
Values above or below the reference range

CRITICAL VALUES
None

INTERFERING FACTORS
Drugs That May Alter Results or Interpretation
Drugs That Interfere with Test Methodology
Folic acid

Drugs That Alter Physiology
None

Disorders That May Alter Results
None

Collection Techniques or Handling That May Alter Results
RBCs contain large quantities of folate, and hemolysis will falsely increase serum folate concentrations.

Influence of Signalment
Species
None

Breed
None

Age
None

Gender
None

Pregnancy
None

LIMITATIONS OF THE TEST
Sensitivity, Specificity, and Positive and Negative Predictive Values
• The sensitivity and the specificity for proximal small intestinal disease are unknown.
• The sensitivity for SIBO is 50%–66%.

Valid If Run in a Human Lab?
Yes, if the laboratory has validated the assay for dogs and cats and has established species-specific reference ranges.

Causes of Abnormal Findings

High values	Low values
Dogs: SIBO Increased dietary intake of folic acid Cats: clinical significance unknown	Mucosal disease in the upper small intestine or diffuse small intestinal disease (e.g., inflammatory bowel disease, lymphoma, fungal disease)

CLINICAL PERSPECTIVE

- In dogs and cats with increased serum folate concentrations, assess trypsin-like immunoreactivity to rule out EPI.
- Dietary deficiency of folate is unlikely. Subnormal serum folate concentrations reflect a state of chronic folate malabsorption, and patients with severely decreased serum folate concentrations may benefit from folate supplementation.
- Not all proximal intestinal diseases causing malabsorption are sufficiently severe or long-standing to deplete the body stores of folate and to cause abnormal test results.
- In contrast to dogs, the clinical significance of increased serum folate concentrations remains unknown in cats.
- Serum folate concentrations are not useful for monitoring therapeutic success in patients with SIBO.

MISCELLANEOUS

ANCILLARY TESTS

- Cobalamin for assessing distal small intestinal disease (i.e., ileum)
- Trypsin-like immunoreactivity to rule out EPI
- Pancreatic lipase immunoreactivity to rule out pancreatitis.

SYNONYMS
Folic acid

SEE ALSO
Blackwell's Five-Minute Veterinary Consult: Canine and Feline Topics
- Exocrine Pancreatic Insufficiency
- Protein-Losing Enteropathy
- Small Intestinal Bacterial Overgrowth

Related Topics in This Book
- Cobalamin
- Gastrointestinal Ultrasonography
- Pancreatic Lipase Immunoreactivity
- Pancreatic Ultrasonography
- Trypsin-like Immunoreactivity

ABBREVIATIONS
- EPI = exocrine pancreatic insufficiency
- SIBO = small intestinal bacterial overgrowth

Suggested Reading
German AJ, Day MJ, Ruaux CG, *et al*. Comparison of direct and indirect tests for small intestinal bacterial overgrowth and antibiotic-responsive diarrhea in dogs. *J Vet Intern Med* 2003; **17**: 33–43.
Johnston KL. Small intestinal bacterial overgrowth. *Vet Clin North Am Small Anim Pract* 1999; **29**: 5235–5250.

INTERNET RESOURCES
Texas A&M University, College of Veterinary Medicine, Gastrointestinal Laboratory: Serum cobalamin (vitamin B_{12}) and folate, http://www.cvm.tamu.edu/gilab/assays/b12folate.shtml.

AUTHOR NAMES
Jan S. Suchodolski and Jörg M. Steiner

FOOD TRIAL

BASICS

TYPE OF PROCEDURE
Allergy testing

PROCEDURE EXPLANATION AND RELATED PHYSIOLOGY
A significant number of dogs with chronic diarrhea, vomiting, and weight loss, or nonseasonal pruritus, or a combination of these signs, respond favorably to treatment with elimination diet and are therefore suspected of having food allergy. In true *food allergy*, an immunologic reaction in the intestinal mucosa causes the associated clinical signs. To the contrary, *food intolerance* is defined as a repeatable reaction toward food ingredients that is not immune mediated (i.e., idiosyncrasy or poisoning). Food intolerance and food allergy cannot be differentiated clinically. The current gold standard for the diagnosis of food allergy or food intolerance is the oral food challenge test during which dogs or cats are fed an elimination diet for 6–14 weeks, leading to resolution of clinical signs if the diagnosis is confirmed. Thereafter, challenges with the diet that previously elicited clinical symptoms or single proteins from the original diet are performed until the clinical signs recur.

An elimination dietary trial should be conducted before the provocative dietary trial is commenced. To find a suitable elimination diet, the client is asked about the diets that the dog or cat have been given over its lifetime. Any protein source that has never been fed to the animal is suitable for an elimination dietary trial. Dogs and cats can be allergic to a food ingredient that has been fed for only a few days. The allergy can start at any age but is most often seen in young animals. Most allergens from nutrients that have been identified in cats and dogs are proteins or polypeptides. The most frequently encountered food allergens in dogs are beef, chicken, cow milk, gluten (in wheat), and lamb. In cats, food allergens frequently eliciting reactions are fish, cow's milk, and beef.

INDICATIONS
• Clinical signs of chronic diarrhea, vomiting, weight loss, or nonseasonal pruritus, especially in a young animal (<3 years of age)
• Suspected food allergy or food intolerance
• Dermatologic signs similar to atopy in dogs, but with nonseasonal pruritus
• Dermatologic signs in cats of nonseasonal pruritus, with lesions mostly on face, head, and back

CONTRAINDICATIONS
None

POTENTIAL COMPLICATIONS
Since this procedure may provoke an allergic reaction, dogs may react with signs of general anaphylaxis, such as elevated heart rate, decreased blood pressure, and hives. Minor signs of a reaction are diarrhea, vomiting, and pruritus.

CLIENT EDUCATION
The goal of the provocative food trial is to provoke clinical signs such as vomiting, diarrhea, bloating, abdominal cramps, or pruritus. A combination of these signs may develop. Clients need to be aware that these are signs of a positive reaction and should stop feeding the offending food as soon as such a reaction is noticed.

BODY SYSTEMS ASSESSED
• Dermatologic
• Gastrointestinal
• Hemic, lymphatic, and immune

PROCEDURE

PATIENT PREPARATION
Preprocedure Medication or Preparation
Before the provocative dietary trial is commenced, a strict elimination dietary trial should be conducted for 6–8 weeks or until all clinical

Table 1 Example of a daily formulation for healthy adult dogs, weighing 18 kg

Ingredient	Grams	%
Carbohydrate, cooked (e.g., rice, potato, pasta, oatmeal)	240	58
Meat, cooked (all typical meats, poultry, fish, and liver)	120	29
Fat (chicken fat, beef fat, vegetable oil, fish oil)	10	2
Fiber (prepared high-fiber cereals)	30	7
Bone meal or dicalcium phosphate	4	
Potassium chloride	1	

symptoms subside. Commercially available diets are preferable because they are complete and there is no need to cook or add vitamins and calcium. Especially for growing dogs, pregnant bitches, and large-breed dogs, it is preferable to use commercial diets. It is very difficult to supply a complete home-cooked diet for cats because of their special need for amino acids like taurine and arginine. In cats, it is advisable to always use a commercial diet for either elimination or provocation diets.

Anesthesia or Sedation
None

Patient Positioning
None

Patient Monitoring
None

Equipment or Supplies
• For the provocative dietary trial, either a commercial elimination diet containing a single protein source with the offending allergen in question or a homemade diet containing the protein in question is fed for 6–8 weeks or until the clinical signs recur. In Table 1 is a recipe for a homemade provocative dietary trial. This recipe will yield 820 kcal (as fed) with the nutrient content listed in Table 2.
• If the homemade provocative diet is fed, 1 human adult vitamin-mineral tablet is given (9 g/tablet; give 1 tablet/day).

TECHNIQUE
Dogs and cats are fed the provocative diet solely and are observed for newly occurring—or an increase in frequency of—vomiting, diarrhea, and pruritus during the trial. The trial is conducted for 6–8 weeks or until clinical signs recur. GI symptoms such as vomiting and diarrhea tend to recur more quickly than dermatologic signs such as pruritus (e.g., a few days to 2 weeks for GI signs as opposed to several weeks to months for dermatologic signs).

SAMPLE HANDLING
N/A

APPROPRIATE AFTERCARE
Postprocedure Patient Monitoring
In case of excessive provocation of clinical signs during the trial, symptomatic therapy for vomiting, diarrhea, or pruritus may be indicated.

Table 2 Nutrient content of the recipe shown in Table 1

Nutrient	% DM
Protein	21
Fat	20
Crude Fiber	6.5
Calcium	0.66
Phosphorus	0.59
Magnesium	0.1
Sodium	0.2
Potassium	0.6

Nursing Care
None

Dietary Modification
After the provocative dietary trial, the animals can be fed either a diet containing only protein sources that have not elicited any clinical signs or their specific elimination diet.

Medication Requirements
None

Restrictions on Activity
None

Anticipated Recovery Time
None

INTERPRETATION

NORMAL FINDINGS OR RANGE
Negative reaction: no evidence of vomiting, diarrhea, or pruritus during the trial

ABNORMAL VALUES
• Positive reaction: newly occurring or increased frequency of vomiting, diarrhea, or pruritus during the trial
• False-negative results: False-negative reactions may occur if the allergenic food was not given long enough or if subtle reactions such as bloating or mild pruritus are overlooked.
• False-positive results: During testing for a specific true food allergy, false-positive reactions will probably be frequent because nonimmunologic reactions, such as food intolerance, will also elicit clinical signs.

CRITICAL VALUES
A sudden increase in heart rate, tachypnea, or a drop in mean arterial blood pressure after the provocation diet is fed may indicate anaphylactic shock and must be treated immediately by IV shock doses of fluids and epinephrine.

INTERFERING FACTORS
Drugs That May Alter Results of the Procedure
Any drugs that relieve the symptoms of a possible positive reaction, such as symptomatic or other treatment for vomiting, diarrhea, and pruritus, should be withheld during the trial (e.g., antihistamines, corticosteroids).

Conditions That May Interfere with Performing the Procedure
Very young, pregnant, or growing dogs of large breeds may not tolerate a homemade diet because it is difficult to supplement the diet with the correct amount of vitamins and minerals. In these cases, it may be better to conduct the trial with a commercially available elimination diet or postpone the trial.

Procedure Techniques or Handling That May Alter Results
It is important to educate clients about the strict feeding regimen that their dog or cat undergoes while either an elimination or provocative dietary trial is conducted. No food should be given other than the one chosen for the trial.

Influence of Signalment on Performing and Interpreting the Procedure
Species
Provocative dietary trials can be conducted in both cats and dogs.

Breed
None

Age
None

Gender
None

Pregnancy
It may be advisable to postpone the trial until after delivery.

CLINICAL PERSPECTIVE
• The provocative dietary trial is the gold standard for diagnosis of food allergy. It is the best clinically available test to diagnose food allergy and food intolerance in small animals.
• The food trial is a time-consuming test, and dog owners need to be thoroughly informed about the benefit for their animal.
• It does not differentiate between food allergy and food intolerance.
• If conducted accurately, the trial will enable a specific diet to be found that can be fed to the animal without risk of adverse reactions.
• There is a risk that an animal may be sensitized to the new diets over time.

MISCELLANEOUS

ANCILLARY TESTS
• A mucosal allergy test, either gastroscopic or colonoscopic, may help identify which allergens should be tested in the provocative dietary trial.
• Serum tests for allergen-specific IgE and IgG are not helpful in identifying dogs with food allergy.
• Fecal IgE testing may help identify possible allergens, particularly when performed on several fecal samples during the provocative dietary trial. Unfortunately, a commercial assay is not available at this time.

SYNONYMS
• Oral challenge test
• Provocative dietary trial

SEE ALSO
Blackwell's Five-Minute Veterinary Consult: Canine and Feline Topics
• Atopic Dermatitis
• Food Reactions (Dermatologic)
Related Topics in This Book
Gastroscopic and Colonoscopic Food-Sensitivity Testing

ABBREVIATIONS
None

Suggested Reading
August JR. Dietary hypersensitivity in dogs: Cutaneous manifestations, diagnosis, and management. *Compend Contin Educ Pract Vet* 1985; 7: 469–477.
Guilford WG. Adverse reactions to food: A gastrointestinal perspective. *Compend Contin Educ Pract Vet* 1994; **16**: 957–968.
Guilford WG, Jones BR, Markwell PJ, *et al.* Food sensitivity in cats with chronic idiopathic gastrointestinal problems. *J Vet Intern Med* 2001; **15**: 7–13.
Hall EJ. Gastrointestinal aspects of food allergy: A review. *J Small Anim Pract* 1994; **35**: 145–152.
Vaden SL, Sellon RK, Melgarejo LT, *et al.* Evaluation of intestinal permeability and gluten sensitivity in soft-coated Wheaten terriers with familial protein-losing enteropathy, protein-losing nephropathy, or both. *Am J Vet Res* 2000; **61**: 518–524.
White SD. Food allergy in dogs. *Compend Contin Educ Pract Vet* 1998; **20**: 261–268.

INTERNET RESOURCES
None

AUTHOR NAME
Karin Allenspach

BASICS

TYPE OF SPECIMEN
Blood

TEST EXPLANATION AND RELATED PHYSIOLOGY
Glucose covalently binds to the free amino groups of many types of proteins by a nonenzymatic reaction. When this glycation reaction occurs with albumin, the result is known as fructosamine (aka glycoalbumin). Because plasma proteins have a longer circulating half-life than the glucose molecule, fructosamine is thought to provide information about the average glucose status over the preceding 2 weeks.

Elevated fructosamine levels can be seen with any condition that causes persistent hyperglycemia. Acute hyperglycemia associated with the stress of sample collection does not affect fructosamine, making this assay useful for confirming a diagnosis of diabetes mellitus and for monitoring therapeutic control of blood glucose. Hyperadrenocorticism may also be associated with increased fructosamine concentrations. Disorders that cause prolonged hypoglycemia may lower fructosamine concentrations in patients. These disorders include starvation, hepatic insufficiency, or neoplasms such as insulinomas. Patients with hypoalbuminemia or hypoproteinemia may also have lowered fructosamine concentrations in their serum. Hyperthyroid cats may have decreased fructosamine levels, independent of their blood glucose level and despite having normal serum protein levels, because of an increased protein turnover rate.

A reagent system using a reducing reaction to form a color change is readily available.

INDICATIONS
- Hyperglycemia of uncertain cause
- Monitoring of a diabetic patient under therapy

CONTRAINDICATIONS
None

POTENTIAL COMPLICATIONS
None

CLIENT EDUCATION
- Because fructosamine is not affected by the stress of sample collection, this assay is useful for confirming a diagnosis of diabetes mellitus, especially in cats.
- The patient should undergo a fast to prevent lipemia.

BODY SYSTEMS ASSESSED
Endocrine and metabolic

SAMPLE

COLLECTION
2–3 mL of venous blood

HANDLING
- A plain red-top tube or serum-separator tube
- Sodium heparin, lithium heparin, or EDTA anticoagulant is acceptable.
- Prompt separation of cells from serum or plasma is recommended to prevent hemolysis.

STORAGE
Refrigerate for short-term storage; freeze for longer storage.

STABILITY
- Room temperature: 3 days
- Refrigerated (2°–8°C): 2 weeks
- Frozen (−20°C): 2 months

PROTOCOL
None

INTERPRETATION

NORMAL FINDINGS OR RANGE
- Dogs: 259–344 μmol/L
- Cats: 219–347 μmol/L
- Reference intervals may vary depending on the laboratory and assay.

ABNORMAL VALUES
Values above or below the reference range

CRITICAL VALUES
None

INTERFERING FACTORS
Drugs That May Alter Results or Interpretation
Drugs That Interfere with Test Methodology
None

Drugs That Alter Physiology
- Insulin therapy will affect the carbohydrate status of an animal and alter results.
- The administration of drugs with long-term effects on glucose metabolism will affect results and include corticosteroids, progestins, estrogens, and megestrol acetate.
- *Note*: Alteration of glucose metabolism by drug therapy must occur over several days to affect test results. Transient or short-term alteration of glucose metabolism will not be reflected in fructosamine results.

Disorders That May Alter Results
- Low fructosamine levels are seen with disorders that cause prolonged hypoglycemia.
- Low fructosamine levels can be caused by hypoalbuminemia or hypoproteinemia.
- Diabetes mellitus is the most common disorder causing increased concentrations of fructosamine.
- Hyperadrenocorticism may also be associated with increased fructosamine concentrations.

Collection Techniques or Handling That May Alter Results
- Hemolysis may cause falsely elevated results.
- Although lipemia does not directly affect results, it will often cause hemolysis. Therefore, patients should be undergo a fast to avoid lipemia.

Influence of Signalment
Species
None

Breed
None

Age
None

Gender
None

Pregnancy
None

LIMITATIONS OF THE TEST
- This test may miss short-term or transient abnormalities in blood glucose values (e.g., daily episodes of hypoglycemia or hyperglycemia). Therefore, serial measurements of blood and/or urine glucose are necessary for detecting these short-term alterations and establishing an initial protocol for feeding and medication of diabetic patients.
- False low fructosamine results may be seen with decreased protein levels or increased protein loss.

Sensitivity, Specificity, and Positive and Negative Predictive Values

For diagnosis of diabetes mellitus when using 343.8 μmol/L as upper limit of reference interval:
- Sensitivity: 88%
- Specificity: 99%
- Positive predictive value: 82%
- Negative predictive value: 99%

Valid If Run in a Human Lab?

Yes.

Causes of Abnormal Findings

High values	Low values
Prolonged hyperglycemia	Prolonged hypoglycemia
Diabetes mellitus, especially	Starvation
with poor glycemic control	Hepatic insufficiency
Hyperadrenocorticism	Insulinomas or other neoplasms
Drugs	Inappropriate insulin therapy
Corticosteroids	Hypoproteinemia
Progestins	Starvation
Megestrol acetate	Hepatic insufficiency
	Protein-losing nephropathy
	Protein-losing enteropathy
	Hyperthyroidism

CLINICAL PERSPECTIVE
- When monitoring glycemic control in diabetic patients:
  - Diabetic dogs
    - Excellent control: <400 μmol/L
    - Good control: 400–475 μmol/L
    - Fair control: 475–550 μmol/L
    - Poor control: >550 μmol/L
  - Diabetic cats
    - Excellent control: <400 μmol/L
    - Good control: 400–475 μmol/L
    - Fair control: 475–550 μmol/L
    - Poor control: >550 μmol/L

- Consider the Somogyi effect if clinical signs suggest poor glycemic control [e.g., polyuria-polydipsia, weight loss], but the fructosamine level is <400 μmol/L.

MISCELLANEOUS

ANCILLARY TESTS
- Glucose curve to rule out transient episodes of hypoglycemia
- Glycosylated hemoglobin
- Serum protein or albumin

SYNONYMS
Glycoalbumin

SEE ALSO
Blackwell's Five-Minute Veterinary Consult: Canine and Feline Topics
- Diabetes Mellitus Without Complication—Cats
- Diabetes Mellitus Without Complication—Dogs
- Hyperadrenocorticism (Cushing's Disease)—Cats
- Hyperadrenocorticism (Cushing's Disease)—Dogs

Related Topics in This Book
- Glucose
- Glucose Curve
- Glycosylated Hemoglobin

ABBREVIATIONS
None

Suggested Reading
Kaneko JJ. Carbohydrate metabolism and its diseases. In: Kaneko JJ, Harvey JW, Bruss ML, eds. *Clinical Biochemistry of Domestic Animals,* 5th ed. New York: Academic, 1997: 45–81.

INTERNET RESOURCES
Cornell University, College of Medicine, Clinical Pathology Modules, Veterinary Clinical Chemistry: Fructosamine, http://www.diaglab.vet.cornell.edu/clinpath/modules/chem/fructose.htm.

AUTHOR NAME
Denise Wunn

GAMMA-GLUTAMYLTRANSFERASE

BASICS

TYPE OF SPECIMEN
Blood

TEST EXPLANATION AND RELATED PHYSIOLOGY
Gamma-Glutamyltransferase (GGT) is a cell membrane–bound enzyme thought to be involved in glutathione metabolism. GGT is present in most cell types (excluding myocytes), but bile duct and renal tubular epithelial (brush border) cells have high GGT activity. Although GGT is present in many tissues (with particularly high levels in pancreas, kidney, and intestinal mucosa), increases in serum GGT are primarily considered a marker of hepatic disease. Increased levels may occur with either cholestasis or biliary necrosis. The precise mechanism of increased serum GGT activity in these disorders is not completely understood, but may be due to induction of GGT (increased GGT production) and/or release of GGT from cell membranes (solubilization).

INDICATIONS
Suspected hepatic disease

CONTRAINDICATIONS
None

POTENTIAL COMPLICATIONS
None

CLIENT EDUCATION
None

BODY SYSTEMS ASSESSED
Hepatobiliary

SAMPLE

COLLECTION
0.5–2.0 mL of venous blood

HANDLING
• A plain red-top tube or serum-separator tube, though EDTA or heparin anticoagulant is acceptable
• Separate serum and/or plasma from cells within 48 h at 2°–8°C (refrigerated).

STORAGE
Refrigerate serum for the short-term; freeze serum for long-term storage.

STABILITY
• Refrigerated (4°C): at least 3 days
• Frozen (−20°C): at least 8 months

PROTOCOL
None

INTERPRETATION

NORMAL FINDINGS OR RANGE
• Dogs: 2–10 IU/L
• Cats: <3 IU/L
• Reference intervals may vary depending on the laboratory and assay.

ABNORMAL VALUES
Values above the reference interval

CRITICAL VALUES
None

INTERFERING FACTORS
Drugs That May Alter Results or Interpretation
Drugs That Interfere with Test Methodology
None

Drugs That Alter Physiology
• Corticosteroids: They cause increased GGT (in dogs) due to enzyme induction and/or cholestasis.
• Phenobarbital: It is typically associated with normal GGT, but mild increases may be observed.
• Halothane: It may increase GGT activity 2–7 days after anesthesia.

Disorders That May Alter Results
None

Collection Techniques or Handling That May Alter Results
Extended storage or heating of sample may decrease GGT activity.

Influence of Signalment
Species
In cats, GGT is a more sensitive indicator of cholestatic disease than is ALP. (ALP is generally considered more sensitive in dogs.) GGT may not increase, or may be only mildly increased, in cats with hepatic lipidosis, however, despite increases in other indicators of cholestatic disease (i.e., ALP, bilirubin).

Breed
None

Age
Serum GGT levels in 1- to 3-day-old puppies may be >100-fold higher than normal adult values because of a large amount of GGT in colostrum. These decrease to adult levels after ≈10 days.

Gender
None

Pregnancy
None

LIMITATIONS OF THE TEST
Sensitivity, Specificity, and Positive and Negative Predictive Values
The sensitivity and predictive values of GGT for liver disease depend on the type of disorder present.

Dogs
For steroid hepatopathy
• Sensitivity: 81%
• PPV: 62%
• NPV: 95%
For cholestasis
• Sensitivity: 68%
• PPV: 81%
• NPV: 78%
For hepatic necrosis
• Sensitivity: 59%
• PPV: 56%
• NPV: 88%
For chronic hepatitis
• Sensitivity: 50%
• PPV: 47%
• NPV: 89%

Cats
For hepatobiliary disease in general (excluding portal vascular anomalies)
• Sensitivity: 86%
• Specificity: 67%
• PPV: 90%
• NPV: 59%

Valid If Run in a Human Lab?
Yes.

Causes of Abnormal Findings

High values	Low values
Cirrhosis	No significance
Hepatitis/cholangiohepatitis	
Cholelithiasis/cholecystitis	
Hepatic or biliary neoplasia	
Corticosteroid treatment or increased endogenous corticosteroids (dogs)	
Corticosteroid hepatopathy	
Biliary hyperplasia	

CLINICAL PERSPECTIVE

- Cholestatic diseases are most likely to have increased GGT, whereas hepatocellular injury (carbon tetrachloride toxicity) and portal vascular anomalies typically do not increase GGT activity.
- Cats with hepatic lipidosis often exhibit an increased ALP level with a normal or mildly increased GGT level.
- GGT is not considered more sensitive than ALP in dogs, but is less affected by noncholestatic factors (e.g., not increased by bone lesions, less influenced by anticonvulsant therapy).
- Renal tubular disease or nephrotoxicity may increase levels of urinary (rather than serum) GGT.
- Acute hepatocellular injury alone will not increase serum GGT unless there is also an element of cholestasis.

MISCELLANEOUS

ANCILLARY TESTS

- ALP, serum bile acids, or bilirubin to confirm cholestatic disease
- Serum bile acids or plasma ammonia levels to assess hepatic function
- ALT and/or AST may be tested concurrently to assess potential hepatocellular injury.

SYNONYMS

- γ-GT
- Gamma GT
- GGT

SEE ALSO

Blackwell's Five-Minute Veterinary Consult: Canine and Feline Topics

- Bile Duct Obstruction
- Bile Peritonitis
- Cholangitis/Cholangiohepatitis Syndrome
- Cholecystitis and Choledochitis
- Hepatitis, Chronic Active
- Hepatitis, Infectious Canine

Related Topics in This Book

- Alkaline Phosphatase
- Bile Acids
- Bilirubin
- Liver and Gallbladder Ultrasonography
- Urine Gamma-Glutamyltransferase/Creatinine Ratio

ABBREVIATIONS

- ALP = alkaline phosphatase
- NPV = negative predictive value
- PPV = positive predictive value

Suggested Reading

Bain PJ. Liver. In: Latimer KS, ed. *Duncan and Prasse's Veterinary Laboratory Medicine: Clinical Pathology,* 4th ed. Ames: Iowa State Press, 2003: 193–214.

Center SA. Diagnostic procedures for evaluation of hepatic disease. In: Guilford WG, Center SA, Strombeck DR, *et al.,* eds. *Strombeck's Small Animal Gastroenterology.* Philadelphia: WB Saunders, 1996: 130–188.

Center SA, Slater MR, Manwarren T, Prymak K. Diagnostic efficacy of serum alkaline phosphatase and gamma-glutamyltransferase in dogs with histologically confirmed hepatobiliary disease: 270 cases (1980–1990). *J Am Vet Med Assoc* 1992; **201**: 1258–1264.

Willard MD, Twedten DC. Gastrointestinal, pancreatic, and hepatic disorders. In: Willard MD, Tvedten H, eds. *Small Animal Clinical Diagnosis by Laboratory Methods,* 4th ed. St Louis: Saunders Elsevier, 2004: 208–246.

INTERNET RESOURCES

Maddison J. Diagnosing liver disease in dogs: What do the tests really mean? In: Scherk M, ed. 26th Congress of the World Small Animal Veterinary Association (WSAVA), Vancouver, 2001, http://www.vin.com/VINDBPub/SearchPB/Proceedings/PR05000/PR00128.htm.

Maddison J. The diagnostic and therapeutic challenges of hepatobiliary disease in the cat. In: Scherk M, ed. 26th Congress of the World Small Animal Veterinary Association (WSAVA), Vancouver, 2001, http://www.vin.com/VINDBPub/SearchPB/Proceedings/PR05000/PR00113.htm.

University of Georgia, College of Veterinary Medicine, Veterinary Clinical Pathology Clerkship Program: Turner B, LeRoy BE, Tarpley HL, et al. Feline hepatic lipidosis, http://www.vet.uga.edu/vpp/clerk/turner/index.php.

AUTHOR NAME

Perry J. Bain

GASTRIN

BASICS

TYPE OF SPECIMEN
Blood

TEST EXPLANATION AND RELATED PHYSIOLOGY
Gastrin is a 34-amino acid (big gastrin), 17-amino acid (little gastrin) or 14-amino acid (minigastrin) peptide hormone produced by G cells of the gastric antrum and duodenal mucosa. Gastrin is secreted in response to dietary protein, antral distention, vagal stimulation, and increased gastric pH. Gastrin stimulates histamine production, and both gastrin and histamine stimulate gastric acid production. Pancreatic tumors called *gastrinomas* have been reported in dogs and cats. Although gastrinomas in people occur in the duodenum, duodenal gastrinomas are rarely reported in dogs. Tumor cells produce an excess of gastrin, which results in hypersecretion of gastric acid, GI ulceration, and hypertrophic gastropathy (which may be referred to as Zollinger-Ellison syndrome). Hypergastrinemia is also seen in other disorders, so caution should be practiced in using fasting serum gastrin concentrations as the sole diagnostic criterion. Provocative testing for assessing gastrin secretion in response to secretin administration, may help confirm a gastrinoma if gastrin concentration after fasting is normal or only mildly increased.

INDICATIONS
• Suspected gastrinoma: chronic vomiting, intermittent diarrhea, and/or progressive weight loss, especially with melena, hematemesis, and abdominal pain
• A gastric or duodenal ulcer of unknown cause

CONTRAINDICATIONS
None

POTENTIAL COMPLICATIONS
None

CLIENT EDUCATION
Animals should be fasted 24 h before testing.

BODY SYSTEMS ASSESSED
• Endocrine and metabolic
• Gastrointestinal

SAMPLE

COLLECTION
1–2 mL of venous blood

HANDLING
• Collect the sample into a red-top or serum-separator tube.
• Separate the serum from cells within 1 h of collection.
• Perform the assay within 4 h or freeze the sample (−20°C); ship frozen.

STORAGE
Keep the sample frozen (−20°C). Avoid repeated freezing and thawing.

STABILITY
• Gastrin will gradually degrade if kept at 2°–8°C for >4 h.
• Frozen (−20°C): at least 2 weeks

PROTOCOL
• Provocative testing is useful if the gastrin concentration after fasting is equivocal (100–1,000 pg/mL).

• Gastrin levels are evaluated at 0, 2, 5, 10, 15, and 20 min after IV injection of secretin (2–4 IU/kg).

INTERPRETATION

NORMAL FINDINGS OR RANGE
Values may vary depending on the laboratory and assay.
• Dogs: Studies suggest a fasting basal level of <100 pg/mL.
  • Up to a 2-fold increase after feeding
  • Decreased levels after secretin administration
• Cats: Data suggest a reference interval of <18 pg/mL.

ABNORMAL VALUES
• A fasting basal level of >100 pg/mL
• With gastrinoma
  • Fasting gastrin concentrations in dogs and cats range from 100 to >10,000 pg/mL.
  • Gastrin concentrations of >200 pg/mL over basal levels within 15 min of secretin administration have been reported in dogs with gastrinoma (Simpson and Dykes 1997).
• Dogs with chronic lymphocytic-plasmacytic enteritis have mean serum gastrin concentrations of 40.62 pg/mL.

CRITICAL VALUES
An increase of ≥10-fold in basal serum gastrin

INTERFERING FACTORS
Drugs That May Alter Results or Interpretation
Drugs That Interfere with Test Methodology
None

Drugs That Alter Physiology
• Proton-pump inhibitors (e.g., omeprazole) and histamine type-2 receptor antagonists (e.g., cimetidine, ranitidine) reduce acid gastric secretion and therefore increase gastrin secretion.
• Insulin can stimulate gastrin secretion.

Disorders That May Alter Results
Lipemia, hemolysis, and icterus

Collection Techniques or Handling That May Alter Results
• Failure to freeze the sample within 4 h after collection
• Repeated freezing and thawing

Influence of Signalment
Species
Gastrinoma has been reported in both dogs and cats.

Breed
None

Age
• The mean age of dogs with gastrinoma is 9 years.
• Gastrinoma has been reported in cats 10–12 years of age.

Gender
None

Pregnancy
None

LIMITATIONS OF THE TEST
Sensitivity, Specificity, and Positive and Negative Predictive Values
N/A

Valid If Run in a Human Lab?
Yes.

Causes of Abnormal Findings

High values	Low values
Gastrinoma	Not significant
Renal failure	
Chronic lymphocytic-plasmacytic enteritis (in dogs)	
Immunoproliferative enteropathy of basenjis	
Achlorhydria (primary or secondary to antisecretory drugs)	
Hypercalcemia	
A nonfasted sample	
Potential causes	
Antral G-cell hyperplasia	
Atrophic gastritis	
Gastric dilatation-volvulus	
Gastric cancer	
Gastric outlet obstruction	
Helicobacter pylori infection	
Hyperparathyroidism	
Liver disease	

CLINICAL PERSPECTIVE

- Gastrinomas are rare and typically are associated with vomiting, hematemesis, anorexia, progressive weight loss, intermittent diarrhea, and melena.
- Other laboratory abnormalities associated with gastrinoma may include these:
  - Hypokalemia, hypochloremia, and metabolic alkalosis, suggestive of upper GI obstruction
  - Hypoproteinemia, hypoalbuminemia, and anemia due to chronic blood loss
  - Increased alkaline phosphatase and ALT activities because of metastasis to the liver
- Endoscopic findings associated with gastrinoma in dogs include esophagitis, ulceration of the gastric or duodenal mucosa, and hypertrophy of the gastric mucosa. In cats with gastrinoma, there is duodenal ulceration without hypertrophic gastropathy and gastric ulceration.

- Values of $\geq$10-fold the normal range are relatively diagnostic for gastrinoma. With lesser, unclear results, gastrin measurement after exogenous secretin administration may be diagnostic.

MISCELLANEOUS

ANCILLARY TESTS
- Endoscopy
- Measure the gastric pH, which should be decreased because of increased gastric acid secretion.
- Radiolabeled somatostatin analogs bind to receptors on gastrinomas to facilitate nonsurgical localization of the tumor.
- Immunocytochemical confirmation of gastrinoma is available.

SYNONYMS
None

SEE ALSO
Blackwell's Five-Minute Veterinary Consult: Canine and Feline Topics
Gastroduodenal Ulcer Disease
Related Topics in This Book
- Fecal Occult Blood
- Gastrointestinal Ultrasonography

ABBREVIATIONS
None

Suggested Reading
Fukushima R, Ichikawa K, Hirabayashi M, *et al.* A case of canine gastrinoma. *J Vet Med Sci* 2004; **66**: 993–995.
Garcia-Sancho M, Rodriguez-Franco F, Sainz A, *et al.* Serum gastrin in canine chronic lymphocytic-plasmacytic enteritis. *Can Vet J* 2005; **46**: 630–634.
Simpson KW, Dykes NL. Diagnosis and treatment of gastrinoma. *Semin Vet Med Surg (Small Anim)* 1997; **12**: 274–281.
Ward CR, Washabau RJ. Gastrointestinal endocrine disease. In: Ettinger SJ, Feldman EC, eds. *Textbook of Veterinary Internal Medicine*, 6th ed . Philadelphia: WB Saunders, 2005: 1622–1632.

INTERNET RESOURCES
None

AUTHOR NAMES
Cecilia Parrula and Maxey L. Wellman

GASTROINTESTINAL ULTRASONOGRAPHY

BASICS

TYPE OF PROCEDURE
Ultrasonographic

PROCEDURE EXPLANATION AND RELATED PHYSIOLOGY
Transabdominal ultrasound of the GI tract provides different and complementary information to that provided by radiography and barium studies. To prevent gas and food content from interfering with examination of the GI tract and surrounding structures, patients should be fasted for 12 h prior to examination. If the stomach is empty and contracted, the patient may be allowed to drink or water may be administered per os. Fluid in the stomach will appear anechoic and facilitate good visualization of the gastric wall. The ventral and lateral abdomen of the patient must be clipped and acoustic gel applied to the skin to obtain good contact and to reduce artifacts. Animals can be scanned in either dorsal or lateral recumbency. Barium should not be administered prior to an ultrasound examination because barium can produce artifacts that obscure the intestinal wall as well as the surrounding organs. Enemas should not be administered immediately prior to the sonographic examination because air artifacts in the colon may prevent visualization of abdominal structures.

INDICATIONS
- Vomiting and weight loss
- Chronic diarrhea
- Fresh blood in the feces
- Melena
- Clinically thickened intestinal segments
- A palpable abdominal mass

CONTRAINDICATIONS
None

POTENTIAL COMPLICATIONS
None

CLIENT EDUCATION
Ultrasound is a safe, noninvasive imaging procedure. Patients should be fasted 12 h prior to the examination. Water may be given a few hours prior to the procedure. The hair on the ventral abdomen will need to be clipped to perform the ultrasound examination.

BODY SYSTEMS ASSESSED
Gastrointestinal

PROCEDURE

PATIENT PREPARATION
Preprocedure Medication or Preparation
The patient should be fasted 12 h prior to examination.

Anesthesia or Sedation
Anesthesia or sedation may be required in noncompliant patients or those with a painful abdomen. If fine-needle tissue aspiration or biopsy of the gastric or intestinal wall is required, then sedation or anesthesia is usually required.

Patient Positioning
The ultrasound examination may be performed in either dorsal or lateral recumbency according to the sonographer's preference. Both left and right lateral recumbency may be required for examination of different areas of the GI tract. Fluid will accumulate in dependent regions of the stomach, providing an acoustic window for better visualization of the gastric wall layering. Luminal gas rising to nondependent regions will cause artifacts that may prevent visualization of those re-

gions. Therefore, alternating between ventral and lateral recumbency will enable better assessment of the entire GI tract.

Patient Monitoring
None

Equipment or Supplies
An ultrasound machine equipped with high-frequency transducers is needed. Both curved and linear 7.5- to 14-MHz, high-frequency transducers are required for optimal resolution of the GI wall. Linear probes are best for examination of the small intestines, and curved-array probes enable examination of the entire GI tract. Low-frequency sector probes may be required for examination of the stomach in large dogs. Documentation with video recordings, black-and-white printers, or digital acquisition of still images or clips is required.

TECHNIQUE
- The hair of the ventral abdomen is clipped, and acoustic gel is applied to the skin to ensure good contact with the ultrasound probe.
- Scanning may be carried out with the patient in either dorsal or lateral recumbency, and the position can be changed multiple times during the examination, if necessary. The use of both right and left lateral recumbency may be advantageous because fluid in the stomach will be displaced to the dependent region, providing an optimal acoustic window for examining the gastric wall.
- The stomach and small intestinal segments should be scanned in both the transverse and the longitudinal sections to assess completely each region's wall thickness, layering, and echogenicity. The lumen is used to orient the transducer in either the transverse or the longitudinal plane.
- The examination of the GI tract is part of a complete abdominal ultrasound examination. Changes in the liver, hepatobiliary system, and pancreas may cause GI signs and should be examined along with the GI tract.

SAMPLE HANDLING
N/A

APPROPRIATE AFTERCARE
Postprocedure Patient Monitoring
None

Nursing Care
None

Dietary Modification
None

Medication Requirements
None

Restrictions on Activity
None

Anticipated Recovery Time
Immediate

INTERPRETATION

NORMAL FINDINGS OR RANGE
Stomach
- The stomach is located directly behind the liver and is easily recognized. Its size will vary from small and contracted to large and fluid or food filled. After a 12-h fast, the stomach should mostly be empty. If large amounts of food are present, then either a delayed gastric emptying or obstruction may be present. The fundus can be identified in the left lateral abdomen, and the splenic head will be adjacent to it. The body of the stomach can be followed across the midline to which it lies perpendicularly. Depending on thoracic conformation in dogs, the antrum and pylorus may be difficult to identify. The portal vein

entering the liver hilus is a good landmark for identifying the antrum and pylorus.

- The normal wall is made up of 4 layers that can be well differentiated with ultrasound. The wall appears as alternating hyperechoic and hypoechoic bands starting from the outer serosa, which is hyperechoic. The prominent anechoic muscularis makes a dark outer rim and is followed by the hyperechoic submucosa and hypoechoic mucosa. A more irregular hyperechoic zone of variable thickness representing the junction between the mucosa and the lumen can be identified. Rugae are easily recognized as invaginations of the wall at regular intervals in the transverse section. In the longitudinal section, the rugal folds appear as linear layered structures aligned parallel to one another.
- The gastric wall is 3–5 mm thick in dogs and 2–4 mm thick in cats.
- Peristaltic contractions can be identified and occur at ≈5/min.

Small Intestine
- The duodenum can be identified from the pylorus and cranial flexure to the caudal flexure in most dogs and cats. The pylorus may be difficult to identify in deep-chested dogs or those with excessive abdominal pressing as a result of a lack of cooperation or pain. In cats, the pylorus and proximal duodenum can be identified at the midline of the abdomen in the region of the porta hepatis. The duodenum in both dogs and cats can be seen as a linear segment lying superficially to and parallel with the right body wall. The duodenal papilla can often be identified in both cats and dogs. Outpouchings of the mucosa at regular intervals along the antimesenteric border of the duodenum are normal structures and should not be confused with ulcerations. The jejunal segments are distributed uniformly throughout the abdomen. The ileum is short and has a prominent, hyperechoic submucosal layer differentiating it from duodenal segments. In fasted animals, the jejunum should be empty and the lumen contracted.
- Beginning from the outer surface, the serosa can be identified as a thin hyperechoic band. Moving toward the lumen, the next layer is the thin, hypoechoic muscular layer, followed by the thin hyperechoic submucosa and then the thick hypoechoic mucosa. Between the lumen and the mucosa, a hyperechoic band representing the transition to the lumen can be identified.
- Duodenal wall thickness is 3–6 mm in dogs, depending on their body size.
- Jejunal wall thickness is 2–4 mm in dogs, depending on their body size, and ≈2 mm in cats.
- Peristaltic contractions occur at 1–3/min in the small intestine.
- The ileum can be identified as a short segment of small intestine entering the cecocolic junction. The ileum can be differentiated from the jejunum by the ileum's prominent hyperechoic submucosa and association with the cecum.

Colon
The ileum, ileocecal junction, cecum, and ascending, transverse, and descending colon can be identified. The descending colon can be easily identified in the caudal abdomen at the left lateral aspect of the urinary bladder in cats and dogs. From there, it can be followed cranially to the transverse and ascending portions. The cecum is generally gas filled and therefore difficult to assess. The ileocolic junction can often be identified in the right midabdomen. The colon wall appears thin, with 3 layers visible. The thickness is generally 1–2 mm. The presence of feces and air creates shadowing artifacts and reverberations that enable only the near wall to be examined. The empty colon contracts down, and the walls have a more irregular or wavy appearance compared to the small intestines. This should not be confused with corrugated walls or neoplasia. The bony pelvis also limits examination of the colon; however, the rectum, perirectal, and perineal regions can be easily examined from a perineal approach.

ABNORMAL FINDINGS
The most common abnormalities are wall thickening and altered wall layering. Others include motility disturbances, abnormal contents and multiorgan or systemic involvement of disease. Ultrasonography can

be used to inspect the stomach, small intestine and colon for altered wall layering, thickening, dilation, peristalsis as well as for intraluminal, intramural and extraluminal causes of obstruction.

Stomach
Wall Thickening
Focal, diffuse, concentric, or asymmetrical wall thickening may be detected in dogs that experience chronic vomiting. Oblique scanning of the gastric wall may lead to the appearance of wall thickening in normal animals. Scanning in multiple planes should avoid misinterpretation. Criteria include the following:
- >5 mm in dogs; >3 mm in cats
- Focal thickening with disrupted wall layering can represent the following:
  - Neoplasia
  - Granulomatous, fungal infiltration
  - Ulcer
- Generalized thickening with intact wall layering can represent the following:
  - Chronic inflammatory disease, gastritis
  - Gastric wall edema
  - Mild uremic gastropathy
  - Eosinophilic gastritis
- To differentiate neoplastic from inflammatory disease, evaluation of histolopathology or cytology is required.

Foreign Bodies
Hyperechoic structures of different shapes and sizes may be identified in the stomach. Foreign material such as bone, wood, fruit pits, rubber, and plastic all create shadowing. Food particles from dry or canned food will have the same appearance. Fluid and gas interfaces can also create hyperechoic structures with shadowing. Reexamining the patient while it is in different positions can be used to observe air and fluid movement. If a dog has recently eaten and a foreign body is suspected, radiographs and ultrasound should be repeated later.

Pyloric Obstruction
Congenital hypertrophic pyloric stenosis and chronic hypertrophic gastropathy appear similar sonographically. Circumferential thickening (>3 mm) of the outer muscular layer can be recognized as a hypoechoic layer forming a ring in cross section.

Gastric Ulcers
- Focal wall thickening with mucosal defects causing an irregular surface may be recognized under optimal conditions. Free air in the lumen may prevent their visualization. The adherence of gas bubbles, which appear hyperechoic with reverberation artifacts, suggests the presence of an ulcer.
- Benign and malignant ulcers can appear similarly in ultrasound.
- Biopsy is required to rule out an underlying neoplastic infiltration. Ulcers are commonly seen with gastric carcinomas.

Gastric Neoplasia
- Diffuse and localized wall infiltrations can be detected with ultrasound. The thickened portion will show a loss or disruption of the wall layering. Pseudolayering may be present and appears as alternating hyperechoic and hypoechoic thick concentric layers. Peristaltic activity is usually decreased.
- Adenocarcinomas are the most common gastric neoplasia in dogs and are often located in the antrum and lesser curvature. Enlarged regional lymph nodes may be detected in addition to the thickened wall.
- Leiomyoma and leiomyosarcoma may also cause focal wall thickening and masses.
- Lymphoma and malignant histiocytosis generally cause diffuse wall thickening. Gastric lymphoma occurs in both dogs and cats and causes a generalized, hypoechoic thickening of the stomach wall, with loss of wall layering and regional lymphadenomegaly.

GASTROINTESTINAL ULTRASONOGRAPHY

• Chronic inflammation may appear as nodular infiltration or masses that resemble tumors. Tissue aspiration or biopsy is required for a definitive diagnosis.

• Ultrasound-guided percutaneous fine-needle aspiration (with a 20-gauge needle) or biopsy (with an 18-gauge, spring-loaded Tru-cut device) of the gastric wall may be performed to differentiate neoplastic from inflammatory infiltrates. Gastroscopy can be used to obtain mucosal biopsy samples.

Small Intestine

Wall Thickening

• Inflammation, fungal disease, and neoplasia can cause wall thickening. Fungal and neoplastic infiltrations may cause strictures, and patients may have signs of obstructions, both clinically and radiographically. The presence or absence of normal wall layering will help in differentiating inflammatory from neoplastic disease. Lymphadenomegaly can occur in both cases.

• Evaluation of histopathology is required in order to differentiate inflammatory, fungal, and neoplastic diseases.

Wall Layering

• Disrupted wall layering is most commonly seen with neoplasia.
  • Most common neoplasias include adenocarcinoma, lymphoma, leiomyoma, and leiomyosarcoma.
  • Lymphoma leads to either symmetrical or asymmetrical transmural or circumferential thickening. The wall usually appears diffusely hypoechoic. Lesions may be solitary, multifocal, or diffuse. Regional lymph node enlargement is common.
  • Granulomatous lesions caused by fungal infiltration result in loss of wall layering and are difficult to distinguish from neoplastic disease. Histoplasmosis and pythiosis are common in dogs and cats in endemic regions. Lymphadenomegaly is often present.
  • Carcinoma usually appears as a focal, irregular, annular thickening of the small intestinal wall and causes stenosis of the lumen. Carcinomas usually have a mixed echogenicity but are variable in appearance.
  • Leiomyomas are smaller in size and appear as echogenic nodules.
  • Leiomyosarcomas are much larger masses of mixed echogenicity growing out of the intestinal wall.
• Maintained layering is more common in inflammatory disease.
  • Lymphocytic, plasmacytic, and eosinophilic inflammatory infiltrations may lead to wall thickening with preservation of wall layering.
  • Muscular hypertrophy can create thickening localized to the muscular layer, which will appear thicker than the neighboring submucosa or equal in thickness to the mucosa. It may be associated with chronic enteritis, proximal foreign bodies, or lymphoma.

Solitary GI Mass

Intestinal carcinoma, leiomyoma, leiomyosarcoma, and polyps are common and will appear as solitary masses of the intestinal wall. Less common are mast cell tumors, hemangiosarcomas, and histiocytic sarcomas.

Peristaltic Abnormalities

• Lack of peristalsis and generalized mild to moderate intestinal dilation are commonly found with functional ileus. All of the intestines and possibly the stomach and colon will be fluid filled and show to-and-fro movements of the luminal contents. Causes include the following:
  • Viral infection (parvovirus)
  • Gastroenteritis or hemorrhagic gastroenteritis
  • Distal jejunal obstructions
  • Sedation or anesthesia
• Segmental or multifocal decreased peristalsis can be seen with intestinal wall infiltrations caused by either inflammatory or neoplastic disease.

Obstructions

• The finding of severe dilation of 1 or more segments of jejunum in combination with empty, contracted bowel segments distally should raise the suspicion of a complete or partial obstruction.

• Both radiopaque and radiolucent foreign bodies may be detected with ultrasound. A hyperechoic interface casting an acoustic shadow from the intestinal lumen can be seen with rubber balls, fruit pits, bones, plastic, and wood.

• Linear foreign bodies are often difficult to see, but their presence can be recognized by the observation of plicated jejunal segments that gather together.

Intussusceptions

• Multilayered, concentric rings of small intestine can be easily identified in most cases. The inner segments of small intestine often appear normal but are surrounded by hyperechoic mesentery and vessels.

• The jejunal segments involved in the intussusception should be examined carefully for the presence of focal masses or wall infiltrations, which may be the cause.

• Jejunal-jejunal, ileocolic, or gastrogastric intussusceptions may also occur.

Colon

Colitis

In dogs with signs of colitis, the colon may appear normal, irregular in form, or air or fluid filled. Colonoscopy for mucosal biopsies is the diagnostic method of choice in both dogs and cats with suspicion of colitis.

Focal Wall Infiltrations and Masses

Sonographically, focal infiltrations or intramural masses of the colon wall may be detected and are associated with either neoplasms or granulomas. Adenocarcinomas are the most frequently diagnosed colonic neoplasms in dogs and cats. Lymphoma has been described in cats.

CRITICAL VALUES

N/A

INTERFERING FACTORS

Drugs That May Alter Results of the Procedure

Sedation or anesthesia may affect peristaltic activity of the stomach and small intestines.

Conditions That May Interfere with Performing the Procedure

• Abdominal pain
• A food-filled GI tract
• Aerophagia
• Barium in the GI tract
• Postoperative free abdominal air

Procedure Techniques or Handling That May Alter Results

Sedation in animals that are noncompliant or have a painful abdomen will greatly improve the ability to examine the abdomen.

Influence of Signalment on Performing and Interpreting the Procedure

Species
None

Breed
None

Age
None

Gender
None

Pregnancy
None

CLINICAL PERSPECTIVE

• Abdominal ultrasound has become extremely useful in the assessment of intestinal disease in dogs and cats. As with all forms of

ultrasound, the quality of the results depends on the quality of the equipment and the training and experience of the operator.
• Ultrasound and endoscopy are complementary imaging modalities that together enable a complete assessment of the GI tract.

MISCELLANEOUS

ANCILLARY TESTS
• Vomiting patients should undergo radiography and those results should be compared with the sonographic findings.
• If a foreign body is suspected but not detected sonographically, radiography and a barium study may be required.
• If the GI tract appears normal in patients with GI signs, gastroduodenoscopy or colonoscopy, which includes mucosal biopsy samples for histologic analysis, is generally required.

SYNONYMS
Abdominal sonography

SEE ALSO
Blackwell's Five-Minute Veterinary Consult: Canine and Feline Topics
• Adenocarcinoma, Stomach, Small and Large Intestine, Rectal
• Colitis and Proctitis
• Colitis, Histiocytic
• Gastroenteritis, Eosinophilic
• Gastroenteritis, Hemorrhagic
• Gastroenteritis, Lymphocytic-Plasmacytic
• Histoplasmosis
• Ileus
• Inflammatory Bowel Disease
• Intussusception
• Lymphoma—Cats
• Lymphoma—Dogs
• Lymphoma, Epidermotropic
• Protein-Losing Enteropathy
• Pythiosis
• Vomiting, Chronic

Related Topics in This Book
• General Principles of Ultrasonography
• Abdominal Ultrasonography
• Esophagogastroduodenoscopy
• Lower Gastrointestinal Radiographic Contrast Studies
• Upper Gastrointestinal Radiographic Contrast Studies

ABBREVIATIONS
None

Suggested Reading
Graham JP, Newell SM, Roberts GD, Lester NV. Ultrasonographic features of canine gastrointestinal pythiosis. *Vet Radiol Ultrasound* 2000; **41**: 273–277.
Hoffmann KL. Sonographic signs of gastroduodenal linear foreign body in 3 dogs. *Vet Radiol Ultrasound* 2003; **44**: 466–469.
Newell SM, Graham JP, Roberts GD, *et al.* Sonography of the normal feline gastrointestinal tract. *Vet Radiol Ultrasound* 1999; **40**: 40–43.
Penninck D. Gastrointestinal tract. In: Nyland TG, Mattoon JS, eds. *Textbook of Small Animal Diagnostic Ultrasound,* 2nd ed. Philadelphia: WB Saunders, 2002: 206–229.
Penninck D, Smyers B, Webster CR, *et al.* Diagnostic value of ultrasonography in differentiating enteritis from intestinal neoplasia in dogs. *Vet Radiol Ultrasound* 2003; **44**: 570–575.

INTERNET RESOURCES
None

AUTHOR NAME
Lorrie Gaschen

GASTROSCOPIC AND COLONOSCOPIC FOOD-SENSITIVITY TESTING

BASICS

TYPE OF PROCEDURE
Allergy testing

PROCEDURE EXPLANATION AND RELATED PHYSIOLOGY
• During gastroscopy or colonoscopy, suspected food allergens are injected into the mucosa, and a mucosal wheal-and-flare reaction is evaluated to assess the possibility of an immediate type I hypersensitivity reaction.
• A significant number of dogs with chronic diarrhea, vomiting and weight loss, or nonseasonal pruritus, or a combination of these signs, respond favorably to treatment with an elimination diet and are therefore suspected of having food allergy. In animals with true food allergy, an immunologic reaction in the intestinal mucosa causes the associated clinical signs.
• The food trial (i.e., oral provocation test) is the gold standard of diagnosis for food allergy. The 2 tests available for a direct mucosal allergen test in dogs are the gastric food-sensitivity test (GFST) and the colonoscopic allergen test (COLAP). Both tests rely on the hypothesis that some of the clinical signs in food allergic dogs are caused by an immediate type I hypersensitivity reaction, which can be assessed directly on the stomach or colonic mucosa. If the test is performed after an animal has been fed an elimination diet for several weeks, in which the clinical signs should completely subside, GFST or COLAP could be helpful in identifying candidates for a subsequent oral food challenge.

INDICATIONS
• Suspected food allergy or food intolerance in dogs
• Signs of chronic diarrhea, vomiting, weight loss, or nonseasonal pruritus, especially in a young animal (<3 years of age)
• Dermatologic signs similar to inhalant allergy in a dog, but with nonseasonal pruritus
• The tests can be performed before or after an oral food challenge test to confirm the findings of the food challenge.

CONTRAINDICATIONS
• If general anesthesia cannot be performed
• If gastroscopy or colonoscopy are contraindicated

POTENTIAL COMPLICATIONS
Since this procedure provokes a type I hypersensitivity reaction, dogs may react with signs of general anaphylaxis (increased heart rate, tachypnea, decreased blood pressure) or local hypersensitivity reactions (excessive swelling of the area where the allergen has been applied, excessive stomach or colonic contractions). In case of an anaphylactic reaction, the allergen injection should be stopped and epinephrine (0.01–0.02 mg/kg IV) should be administered.

CLIENT EDUCATION
• Risks are associated with general anesthesia.
• It is advisable to take mucosal biopsy samples for histologic evaluation of the stomach and duodenum or colon after performing the allergy test.
• Performing the GFST or COLAP procedure takes ≈30 min.
• There is a low risk of anaphylaxis or local allergic reactions. Only 1 case has been reported of a possible anaphylaxis during a GFST.

BODY SYSTEMS ASSESSED
• Gastrointestinal
• Hemic, lymphatic, and immune

PROCEDURE

PATIENT PREPARATION
Preprocedure Medication or Preparation
• Ideally, an elimination dietary trial is conducted before the procedure. (Feed a protein and carbohydrate source that has never been fed to the animal before for 6–8 weeks or until all clinical symptoms subside.)
• Alternatively, a liquid elemental diet can be fed for several days prior to the procedure.
• The dog is fasted for 12 h before gastroscopy or 48 h before colonoscopy.
• For colonoscopy, an electrolyte solution (i.e., Golytely, 30 mL/kg; Braintree Laboratories, Braintree, MA) should be given to the dog by stomach tube the day before anesthesia to cleanse the colon.

Anesthesia or Sedation
The anesthetic procedure should avoid the use of any medications, such as acepromazine, benzodiazepines, propofol, or antihistamines, that may interfere with histamine release during the test. One possibility is using atropine (0.02 mg/kg SC) and oxymorphone (0.05 mg/kg IV) as premedication and isoflurane for induction and maintenance. Oxymorphone (0.05 mg/kg IV) as analgesic medication can be administered during recovery from anesthesia as needed.

Patient Positioning
Left lateral recumbency is favorable for gastroenteroscopy and colonoscopy.

Patient Monitoring
• Monitoring of anesthesia
• Monitoring for possible allergic reactions during application of the allergens

Equipment or Supplies
• Gastroscope or colonoscope, if possible attached to a video camera that enables easy identification of the injection sites
• Sclerotherapy needle for human esophageal varices, with a length appropriate for the gastroscope or colonoscope
• Allergen solutions for intracutaneous applications are used at a concentration of 1 mg/mL; 0.3 mL per injection and allergen is administered.
• Negative control: 0.9% saline
• Positive control: histamine for intracutaneous application

TECHNIQUE
• For both GFST and COLAP, 1 mL of the allergen solution, negative control, or histamine is drawn up into a syringe that fills the channel of the sclerotherapy needle. When the needle is visualized via endoscopy at the correct injection site, 0.3 mL of the allergen solution or control is injected into the needle and in or on the application site.
• GFST: Allergen solutions are dropped around the rugal folds in the most ventral portion of the stomach during gastroscopy. During several minutes after the application of the allergen, the site is watched for a wheal-and-flare reaction as a sign of a positive reaction.
• COLAP: Injection sites for the allergens are selected in a clockwise fashion around the ileocolic valve. Allergens are injected into the colonic mucosa by using a human sclerotherapy needle. The needle is washed between each injection with 5 mL of 0.9% saline and subsequently injected with 10 mL of air. All injection sites are observed for 15 min after application of the allergen. The reactions are interpreted as positive when clearly demarcated swelling, edema, and hyperemia are observed (Figure 1). It may help interpretation to videotape the procedure and review the tape at a later time.

GASTROSCOPIC AND COLONOSCOPIC FOOD-SENSITIVITY TESTING

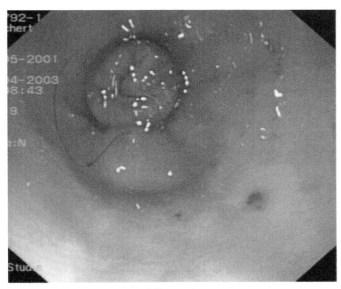

Figure 1

Example of a positive test result as seen during the COLAP procedure immediately after injection of the allergen solution. There is a clearly demarcated swelling visible below the ileocolic valve.

• If bleeding occurs during the injection in the COLAP procedure, a new injection site should be chosen for that allergen, because the blood may interfere with interpretation of the test.
• Injection or application of the negative control should be used as a guideline for interpretation. During the COLAP procedure, care must be taken to interpret the negative control (0.9% saline), because a small swelling will be visible at the injection site and should not be mistaken for a positive reaction.

SAMPLE HANDLING
N/A

APPROPRIATE AFTERCARE
Postprocedure Patient Monitoring
Oxymorphone (0.05 mg/kg IV) can be administered to reduce pain. Usually, dogs can be sent home the same day.

Nursing Care
None

Dietary Modification
It is not necessary to modify the diet after the procedure, unless an elimination or provocative dietary trial is planned for the dog.

Medication Requirements
Since this test may provoke an allergic reaction, dogs may react with signs of general anaphylaxis, such as elevated heart rate, tachypnea, or decreased blood pressure. In case of an anaphylactic reaction, the allergen injection should be stopped and epinephrine (0.01–0.02 mg/kg IV) should be administered.

Restrictions on Activity
None

Anticipated Recovery Time
Dogs can be discharged from the hospital 1–2 h after recovery from anesthesia.

INTERPRETATION
NORMAL FINDINGS OR RANGE
Negative reaction: The injection or application site can be visualized but no swelling, hyperemia, or edema is seen.

ABNORMAL VALUES
• Positive reaction: A clearly demarcated swelling, edema, and hyperemia at the injection or application site 1–2 min after application of the allergen (Figure 1).
• In the GFST, the allergen solution can run off the application site, which could account for false-negative results
• Catheter injuries to the mucosa or the gastric rugal folds, or marking the injection site by taking a biopsy sample, may be misread as mucosal swelling, producing false-positive results.
• False-negative reactions as compared to the oral challenge test may occur during both GFST and COLAP because only part of the GI mucosa is naturally exposed to the allergen during digestion.

CRITICAL VALUES
In case of an anaphylactic reaction, the allergen injection should be stopped and epinephrine (0.01–0.02 mg/kg IV) should be administered.

INTERFERING FACTORS
Drugs That May Alter Results of the Procedure
The anesthetic procedure should avoid the use of any medications, such as acepromazine, benzodiazepines, propofol and antihistamines, that may interfere with histamine release during the test.

Conditions That May Interfere with Performing the Procedure
If severe inflammation of the gastric or colonic mucosa is present, the tests will be difficult to interpret and should be delayed until the inflammation has subsided

Procedure Techniques or Handling That May Alter Results
Lyophilized allergen solutions should be freshly dissolved before the test and stored at 4°C until use. Otherwise, freshly dissolved allergen solutions can be aliquoted and frozen at −80°C until use. Improperly handled allergen solutions may lead to false-negative results.

Influence of Signalment on Performing and Interpreting the Procedure
Species
GFST and COLAP have both been performed only in dogs.

Breed
COLAP is difficult to perform in small-breed dogs.

Age
None

Gender
None

Pregnancy
It may be advisable to postpone the test until after whelping.

CLINICAL PERSPECTIVE
• GFST or COLAP may help in identifying which allergens should be tested in the provocative dietary trial.
• Both GFST and COLAP assess only immediate-type hypersensitivity reactions that can be appreciated during the time endoscopy is performed. Some dogs may clinically show protracted signs after having been fed a provocation diet, which implies type II or type IV hypersensitivity reactions that will not be assessed by either technique.

GASTROSCOPIC AND COLONOSCOPIC FOOD-SENSITIVITY TESTING

• The COLAP probably has a higher sensitivity and specificity than GFST when compared to oral food challenge testing. In the GFST, stomach contractions are frequently encountered and may hamper interpretation of the test. In the COLAP test, the injection is administered directly into the colonic mucosa, which helps to relocate the specific injection sites after a contraction.

MISCELLANEOUS

ANCILLARY TESTS
• The provocative dietary trial is the gold standard test for diagnosis of food allergy.
• Serum tests for allergen-specific IgE and IgG cannot identify dogs with food allergy.
• Fecal IgE testing may help identify possible allergens, particularly when performed on several fecal samples during the provocative dietary trial, but are not routinely available.

SYNONYMS
• Colonoscopic allergy provocation
• Gastroscopic allergy provocation
• Mucosal allergy testing

SEE ALSO
Blackwell's Five-Minute Veterinary Consult: Canine and Feline Topics
• Atopic Dermatitis
• Food Reactions, Dermatologic
• Food Reactions (Gastrointestinal)

Related Topics in This Book
• General Principles of Endoscopy
• Allergen-Specific Serology
• Colonoscopy
• Esophagogastroduodenoscopy
• Food Trial
• Intradermal Testing

ABBREVIATIONS
• COLAP = colonoscopic allergy provocation
• GFST = gastroscopic food-sensitivity test

Suggested Reading

Allenspach K, Vaden S, Harris T, *et al.* Validation of colonoscopic allergen provocation (COLAP) in dogs with proven food hypersensitivity reactions. *J Small Anim Pract* 2006; 47: 21–26.

Elwood CM. Gastroscopic food sensitivity testing in 17 dogs. *J Small Anim Pract* 1994; 35: 199–203.

Guilford WG, Strombeck DR, Rogers Q, *et al.* Development of gastroscopic food sensitivity testing in dogs. *J Vet Intern Med* 1994; 8: 414–422.

Vaden SL, Hammerberg B, Davenport DJ, *et al.* Food hypersensitivity reactions in soft-coated Wheaten terriers with protein-losing enteropathy or protein-losing nephropathy or both: Gastroscopic food sensitivity testing, dietary provocation, and fecal immunoglobulin E. *J Vet Intern Med* 2000; 14: 60–67.

INTERNET RESOURCES
None

AUTHOR NAME
Karin Allenspach

BASICS

TYPE OF SPECIMEN
Blood
Tissue

TEST EXPLANATION AND RELATED PHYSIOLOGY
Genetic tests, looking at an animal's DNA, are most often used to diagnose genotypes associated with specific familial disease. These tests rely on PCR testing.

Direct mutation tests identify specific nucleotide sequence mutations in a tested gene. These tests are usually breed specific unless the mutation occurred in an ancestor that predated the separation of breeds. For example, the ancestrally old mutation for the prcd form of progressive retinal atrophy is shared by over 17 diverse breeds, including American cocker spaniels, Chinese cresteds, Entlebucher mountain dogs, Labrador retrievers, and toy poodles. The mutation-based test can be used in all of these breeds. Direct mutation tests for susceptibility genes may not reflect the observed phenotype, which may be influenced by other factors.

Linked marker tests identify the presence of a nucleotide sequence that is located on a chromosome close to the defective gene. The genetic mutation in the breed has not been identified. The problem with linked marker tests is if a genetic crossover occurs between the marker and the defective gene during meiotic formation of egg or sperm, the marker will no longer be linked to the defective gene. This results in false-positive or false-negative test results. Such tests of all offspring and descendents of such an individual that inherit the false marker will have inaccurate results. For example, because of ancestral crossovers, entire families of Bedlington terriers had false results in their linked marker genetic tests for copper toxicosis. Knowledge of pedigrees, previous family test results, and clinical history were required to evaluate the accuracy of the test results. The genetic mutation was eventually identified, and a direct genetic test for copper toxicosis is now available for the breed.

Recently, genetic testing has been offered to determine the breed composition of mixed-breed dogs.

INDICATIONS
- Diagnosis of familial disease
- Screening for genetic disease

CONTRAINDICATIONS
None

POTENTIAL COMPLICATIONS
None

CLIENT EDUCATION
Genetic counseling on the use of genetic test results is of the utmost importance with purebreds. Dog and cat breeds have finite genetic diversity and gene pool resources. If all carriers of a defective gene were eliminated from a gene pool, it would reduce the genetic diversity of the breed. The emotional response to a carrier test result is not to use the animal for breeding. The proper use of genetic tests is to breed quality carrier-positive animals with normal testing animals and thus replace the carrier parent with a quality, normal-testing offspring for breeding in the next generation. No affected offspring will be produced. This eliminates the single defective gene, but maintains the tens of thousands of other genes in the genetic line without reducing genetic diversity. Many breeds have been devastated by having all carriers of defective genes discarded from their gene pool.

BODY SYSTEMS ASSESSED
Depends on the genetic disorder being tested

SAMPLE

COLLECTION
- 2–3 mL of venous blood
- Cheek swabs: The animal should not have eaten or nursed recently.

HANDLING
- Collect blood into an EDTA tube, ensure blood is not clotted, and ship with ice packs.
- Cheek swabs
  - A cytology brush should be applied to the buccal cheek and pinched between 2 fingers on the outer cheek. Rotate the swab several times to collect buccal epithelial cells.
  - Return the swab to the original container and ship it by regular mail.

STORAGE
- Refrigerate the blood.
- Maintain the cheek swabs at room temperature.

GENETIC TESTING

STABILITY
- DNA-based PCR tests on EDTA-anticoagulated blood
  - Refrigerated ($2°-8°C$): days to weeks
  - Frozen ($-20°$ to $-80°C$): months to years; if cold centrifuged into a WBC pellet.
- Cheek swabs are stable indefinitely at room temperature.

PROTOCOL
None

 INTERPRETATION

NORMAL FINDINGS OR RANGE
Homozygous normal (2 normal copies of the tested gene)

ABNORMAL VALUES
The presence of a specific genetic mutation:
- Heterozygous
  - If testing for a recessive gene, the animal will be an asymptomatic carrier.
  - If testing for a dominant gene, the animal will be affected (i.e., symptomatic).
- Homozygous mutant: Note that a homozygous mutation will result in an affected (i.e., symptomatic) animal regardless of whether the genetic mutation is dominant or recessive.
- The presence of susceptibility genes provide increased risk, but not necessarily disease occurance.

CRITICAL VALUES
None

INTERFERING FACTORS
Drugs That May Alter Results or Interpretation
Drugs That Interfere with Test Methodology
None

Drugs That Alter Physiology
None

Disorders That May Alter Results
None

Collection Techniques or Handling That May Alter Results
- DNA from a recent meal, from nursing (breast epithelial cells), or from licking another animal can be captured with a cheek swab. Wiping the inner cheek prior to sampling can reduce DNA contamination.
- Clotting of EDTA-anticoagulated blood

Influence of Signalment
Species
Direct genetic tests are usually species specific.

Breed
Direct genetic tests are usually breed specific.

Age
Direct genetic tests can be conducted on animals of any age.

Gender
While certain traits may be carried on the X-chromosome, gender does not directly affect the specific genetic test.

Pregnancy
N/A

LIMITATIONS OF THE TEST
Sensitivity, Specificity, and Positive and Negative Predictive Values
- PCR-based direct genetic tests are highly sensitive and specific.
- Linkage-based genetic tests can have false-positive and false-negative predictive values if a genetic crossover occurs between the linked marker and the defective gene.

Valid If Run in a Human Lab?
No.

CLINICAL PERSPECTIVE
Genetic counseling recommendations will vary based on the mode of inheritance and the availability of tests for the disorder.

 MISCELLANEOUS

ANCILLARY TESTS
Phenotype testing depends on the trait and might include radiography, biopsy, blood chemistry analysis, etc.

SYNONYMS
None

SEE ALSO
Blackwell's Five-Minute Veterinary Consult: Canine and Feline Topics
None

Related Topics in This Book
- Red Blood Cell Enzyme Activity
- Von Willebrand Factor

ABBREVIATIONS
None

Suggested Reading
None

INTERNET RESOURCES
Proceedings of the Tufts Breeding and Genetics Conference, Sturbridge, MA, 2007, http://www.vin.com/TUFTS/2007.

Testing Centers
Alfort School of Veterinary Medicine, France: Centronuclear Myopathy (CNM), http://www.labradorcnm.com/.

Animal Health Trust (AHT) (UK), http://www.aht.org.uk.

Auburn University, College of Veterinary Medicine, M.K. Boudreaux Lab, http://www.vetmed.auburn.edu/index.pl/mary_k._boudreaux. Characterization of congenital platelet disorders.

Cornell University, College of Veterinary Medicine, Goldstein Laboratory: Canine primary hyperparathyroidism, http://www.vet.cornell.edu/labs/goldstein/.

GenMARK, DNA Services: Canine—Merle gene, http://www.genmarkag.com/home_companion.php.

HealthGene, http://www.healthgene.com. Veterinary DNA diagnostic services.

MARS Veterinary, Wisdom Panel: Mixed breed analysis, http://www.wisdompanel.com/.

Michigan State University, Microbiology and Molecular Genetics, Laboratory of Comparative Medical Genetics, http://mmg.msu.edu/92.html.

Optigen, http://www.optigen.com. Veterinary genetic services.

University of Pennsylvania, Penn Veterinary Medicine, PennGen, http://www.vet.upenn.edu/penngen.

VetGen, http://www.vetgen.com. Veterinary genetic services.

University of California–Davis, Veterinary Genetic Services, http://www.vgl.ucdavis.edu/.

University of Missouri–Columbia, College of Veterinary Medicine: Canine genetic diseases network, http://www.caninegeneticdiseases.net.

Washington State University, College of Veterinary Medicine, Veterinary Cardiac Genetics Laboratory (VCGL), http://www.vetmed.wsu.edu/deptsVCGL/.

Washington State University, College of Veterinary Medicine, Veterinary Clinical Pharmacology Lab: Multidrug sensitivity, http://www.vetmed.wsu.edu/depts-VCPL/.

AUTHOR NAME
Jerold S. Bell

GIARDIA FECAL ANTIGEN

BASICS

TYPE OF SPECIMEN
Feces

TEST EXPLANATION AND RELATED PHYSIOLOGY
Giardia is a flagellated protozoan parasite that can cause chronic intestinal infections in dogs, cats, and many other mammals. Transmission occurs through ingestion of cysts in contaminated water, food, or fomites, or through self-grooming. Infections may be subclinical and asymptomatic or may produce weight loss due to chronic malabsorption, with continual or intermittent, chronic diarrhea. It appears that some *Giardia* spp. are species specific whereas others can infect a variety of mammals. Wild animals may be reservoirs for infection of domestic animals. There is a zoonotic concern with *Giardia* infections in family pets. The zoonotic potential of this parasite is currently under discussion. With new molecular techniques, this important issue should be resolved in the next few years.

The accurate diagnosis of this parasite is often a challenge because of intermittent shedding and difficulty identifying cysts and trophozoites. Yeasts may be mistaken for *Giardia* spp. cysts because of their similar size and shape. The IDEXX SNAP *Giardia* Antigen Test (IDEXX Laboratories, Portland, ME) may be a useful tool for small-animal practices when used in conjunction with fecal flotation in zinc sulfate with centrifugation. This rapid enzyme immunoassay test will indicate the presence of a cyst protein found on *Giardia* organisms in canine and feline feces.

INDICATIONS
• Dogs and cats with diarrhea

CONTRAINDICATIONS
None

POTENTIAL COMPLICATIONS
None

CLIENT EDUCATION
• *Giardia* spp. in family pets have potential zoonotic implications.
• All susceptible pets must be treated in the home.
• Cysts in feces are infective and can survive several months in the environment, especially in cool water. They are a source of infection and reinfection, particularly for animals in crowded conditions (e.g., kennels and catteries). Environmental contamination can be limited by prompt removal of feces from runs and yards.

BODY SYSTEMS ASSESSED
Gastrointestinal

SAMPLE

COLLECTION
A small amount of fresh feces

HANDLING
• Wear gloves when handling feces.
• Sample and test kits must both be at room temperature before the test is performed.

STORAGE
Refrigerate the sample for short-term storage; freeze it for long-term storage.

STABILITY
• Refrigerated (2°–7°C): stable for up to 1 week
• Frozen (−20°C): stable indefinitely

PROTOCOL
See the kit directions for the SNAP test.

INTERPRETATION

NORMAL FINDINGS OR RANGE
Negative (blue only in the positive control spot and no color in the negative control spot)

ABNORMAL VALUES
• Positive (blue in both the positive control spot and the sample spot). Even a slight bluish tinge is considered to be positive.
• Invalid result: no color in the positive control spot

CRITICAL VALUES
None

INTERFERING FACTORS
Drugs That May Alter Results or Interpretation
Drugs That Interfere with Test Methodology
Barium in the feces may adversely affect the accuracy of this test. The fecal sample should be obtained before barium is administered for intestinal contrast studies.

Drugs That Alter Physiology
None

Disorders That May Alter Results
None

Collection Techniques or Handling That May Alter Results
• The sample and/or the kit not at room temperature
• An old sample
• An outdated test kit

Influence of Signalment
Species
None

Breed
None

Age
Giardia infections in young animals may be severe and can be life threatening especially in puppies or kittens that are in stressful situations.

Gender
None

Pregnancy
None

LIMITATIONS OF THE TEST
False positives and false negatives do occur:
• Occasionally, with centrifugation, *Giardia* cysts are found in fecal flotation with zinc sulfate and the *Giardia* Antigen Test will be negative and vice versa.
• For unknown reasons, results for some clinically normal animals will remain positive on the *Giardia* Antigen Test after treatment.

Sensitivity, Specificity, and Positive and Negative Predictive Values
Compared with direct immunofluorescence microscopy:
• 95% sensitive for the protein
• 99% specific for the protein

Valid If Run in a Human Lab?
No, unless the IDEXX Giardia Fecal Antigen Test is used

CLINICAL PERSPECTIVE
Use the test only on symptomatic dogs and cats for the most accurate results.

MISCELLANEOUS

ANCILLARY TESTS
• Fecal flotation in zinc sulfate with centrifugation is highly recommended in symptomatic animals.
• Motile trophozoites can sometimes be seen in saline smears of loose feces.

SYNONYMS
None

SEE ALSO
Blackwell's Five-Minute Veterinary Consult: Canine and Feline Topics
• Coccidiosis
• Cryptosporidiosis
• Diarrhea, Chronic—Cats
• Diarrhea, Chronic—Dogs
• Giardiasis

Related Topics in This Book
• Fecal Direct Smear and Cytology
• Fecal Flotation
• Fecal Sedimentation and Baermann Exam

ABBREVIATIONS
None

Suggested Reading
Hill SL, Cheney JM, Taton-Allen GF, *et al.* Prevalence of enteric zoonotic organisms in cats. *J Am Vet Med Assoc* 2000; 216: 687–692.
Lieb MS, Zajac AM. Giardiasis in dogs and cats. *Vet Med* 1999; 793–802.
Payne PA, Ridley RK, Dryden MW, *et al.* Efficacy of a combination febantel-praziquantel-pyrantel product, with or without vaccination with a commercial *Giardia* vaccine, for treatment of dogs with naturally occurring giardiasis. *J Am Vet Med Assoc* 2002; 220: 330–333.

INTERNET RESOURCES
Companion Animal Parasite Council (CAPC), Protozoa: Giardiasis guidelines, http://www.capcvet.org/?p = Guidelines_giardiasis&h = 0&s = 0.
IDEXX Laboratories, In-house Tests: SNAP *Giardia* Test, http://www.idexx.com/animalhealth/testkits/giardia_canine/giardiavideo.jsp. *Giardia* life-cycle animation.

AUTHOR NAME
Patricia A. Payne

BASICS

TYPE OF PROCEDURE
Miscellaneous

PROCEDURE EXPLANATION AND RELATED PHYSIOLOGY
Periodontal disease is a common bacterial infection of the tissues surrounding the teeth: attached gingiva, periodontal ligament, cementum, and alveolar bone. At a healthy site, the normal space between the free gingival margin and the tooth is called the *gingival sulcus*. When infection destroys these tissues, a *periodontal pocket*, or defect deeper than the normal gingival sulcus depth, may form in between the tooth and remaining periodontal tissues. The presence of a pocket indicates a need for subgingival cleaning or root planing. The extent of periodontal attachment loss is assessed initially with a periodontal probe, measuring both the depth of a pocket as well as the extent of gingival and bone recession that can result in root exposure, or a combination of the 2.

INDICATIONS
• Every patient that is anesthetized for any dental procedure should undergo a complete dental examination, including periodontal probing of every tooth surface.
• Specific conditions that necessitate accurate probing may include the following:
  • Inflamed gingiva indicates potential tissue involvement.
  • Areas of gingival recession (bone recession may also be present)
  • Loose teeth

CONTRAINDICATIONS
None

POTENTIAL COMPLICATIONS
Because a complete oral examination that includes periodontal probing necessitates general anesthesia, appropriate measures should be taken.

CLIENT EDUCATION
• Appropriate preanesthetic considerations should be discussed with the owner.
• A complete oral examination, including periodontal probing, will often reveal lesions not previously anticipated during the procedure. The owner must be available for contact during the procedure to discuss appropriate therapeutic choices.

BODY SYSTEMS ASSESSED
Gastrointestinal

 PROCEDURE

PATIENT PREPARATION
Preprocedure Medication or Preparation
The preanesthetic regimen includes appropriate antimicrobial and pain medication as indicated.
Anesthesia or Sedation
General anesthesia, with a cuffed endotracheal tube, is required.
Patient Positioning
N/A
Patient Monitoring
Appropriate monitoring, as for any general anesthetic procedure
Equipment or Supplies
Periodontal Probe
• Round or flat
• Marked in millimeters; varied formats (Figure 1)
  • Some are marked with millimeter indentations.

• Some are marked in alternating 3-mm bands of black and silver.
• Become familiar with the measurements marked on the instruments you use.

Pressure Sensitive Probe
This a plastic probe with additional indicator that is depressed when too much pressure is applied.

Periodontal Explorer
The other end of many probes (Figure 2).
• Shepherd's hook: A sharp, slender tip used as a tactile instrument to detect soft enamel (pre-carious), open canals, and enamel defects, especially feline tooth resorption.
• The periodontal explorer can be gently used subgingivally to detect calculus deposits.

TECHNIQUE
• To identify specific areas of concern, some individuals prefer to initially probe before dental therapy.
• Complete probing and charting must be performed after plaque and calculus are removed because areas may be occluded with the debris.
• After cleaning each half-mouth, examine and probe the buccal or facial surfaces of the up side and the lingual or palatal surfaces of the down side.
• Gently insert the probe into the gingival sulcus, advancing to the depth of the sulcus or pocket until touching the base (Figure 3).
  • *Note*: With inflamed pockets, the probe can easily be pushed past the base attachment because the tissue is delicate. Use great care!
• Probing the *6 points*, refers to placing the probe gently at the 6 line angles of the tooth (mesiolingual, mesiobuccal, etc.) In human dentistry with interproximal contact points, the probe cannot be advanced circumferentially around the tooth, so these areas are evaluated.
• Areas of note: Although every tooth surface should be probed and examined, specific areas demand special attention or can often be accompanied by minimal outward abnormalities.
  • Palatal surface of maxillary canines: Often a deep pocket may be present when unanticipated, and, if advanced, the bone loss can form a communication into the nasal cavity, which would then necessitate extraction of the canine tooth and special closure of the oronasal fistula. Early intervention with root planing and pocket therapy is necessary to prevent fistulation.
  • Rostral or mesial surface of mandibular canines: A significant pocket beside the lower third incisor can significantly compromise the lower canine. Advanced procedures may be used to save the incisor or more thoroughly treat the lower canine once the incisor is extracted.
  • Lower first molar—mesial and distal surfaces: Deep pockets at either aspect of this tooth can lead to further compromise of the mandible itself, especially in small-breed dogs. The gingival margins may look relatively normal, so careful probing is essential.
• Periodontal explorer: Its sharp tip is very tactile.
  • Evaluate areas of tooth wear or fracture to determine whether the canal is exposed (Figure 4).
  • In cats, evaluate areas of potential tooth resorption.

SAMPLE HANDLING
N/A

APPROPRIATE AFTERCARE
Postprocedure Patient Monitoring
Appropriate for general anesthesia
Nursing Care
None
Dietary Modification
None
Medication Requirements
None

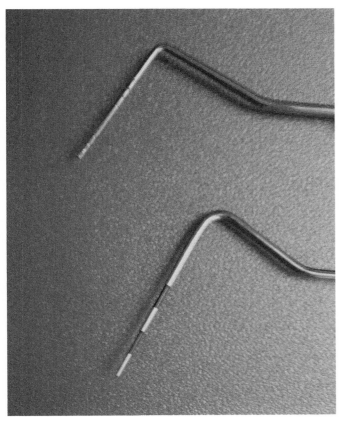

Figure 1

Two periodontal probes: the **top** one with marked indentations at 1–3, 5, and 7–10 mm, and the **bottom** one with alternating black and silver bands of 3 mm each.

Restrictions on Activity
None

Anticipated Recovery Time
As expected for anesthesia

 INTERPRETATION

NORMAL FINDINGS OR RANGE
- Normal sulcus depth
  - Dogs: 2–3 mm
  - Cats: <0.5 mm
- No root or furcation exposure

ABNORMAL VALUES
Measure and record any abnormalities encountered.

Periodontal Pocket
- Its pathologic depth is greater than that of the normal sulcus. These are the pocket (abnormal) depths:
  - >2–3 mm in dogs (take the patient's size into account)
  - >0.5 mm in cats
- Mark "PP" (periodontal pocket) and millimeter depth on the chart: Several measurements may be recorded around an individual tooth.

Root Exposure
- The exposed root area is now visible because of gingival and alveolar bone loss.

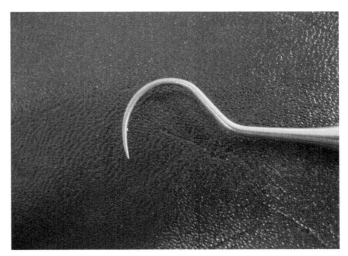

Figure 2

Explorer tip (Shepherd's hook).

- Mark "RE" (root exposure) and millimeter depth on the chart.
- If there is additional pocket formation, mark that, as well.

Attachment Loss
- A combination of root exposure and periodontal pocket
- Total attachment loss is the measurement from the neck of the tooth (cementoenamel junction) to the depth of the pocket.

Furcation Exposure
Space between roots of multirooted teeth is exposed because of gingiva and bone loss.
- F1: depression at the furcation area into soft tissue and some bone
- F2: extension into bone, past halfway
- F3: through and through

CRITICAL VALUES
None

INTERFERING FACTORS
Drugs That May Alter Results of the Procedure
None

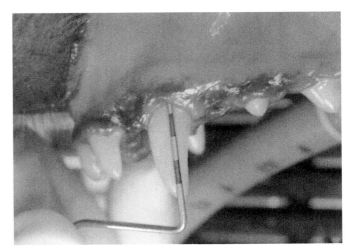

Figure 3

The tip of a periodontal probe is inserted gently into the gingival sulcus or pocket and advanced carefully to the base, without penetrating tissue further.

GINGIVAL SULCUS MEASUREMENT

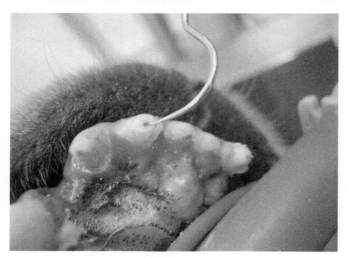

Figure 4

The explorer should be used on a worn tooth surface to determine whether a canal is exposed or, as in this case, whether the surface glides along the very smooth surface of the worn tooth with reparative dentin (brown appearance). Gradual wear may protect the pulp.

Conditions That May Interfere with Performing the Procedure
• Gingival hyperplasia may result in a thicker or taller gingival margin that may present the appearance of a deeper pocket but without attachment loss present—a pseudopocket.
• Excessive calculus deposition may hinder initial probing.

Procedure Techniques or Handling That May Alter Results
Using an aggressive probing technique may advance the probe tip deeper into inflamed tissues, past the original depth of the pocket.

Influence of Signalment on Performing and Interpreting the Procedure
Species
None

Breed
None

Age
None

Gender
None

Pregnancy
None

CLINICAL PERSPECTIVE
• The initial oral examination can only estimate the level of periodontal attachment loss, and extensive lesions may be inapparent until full examination under general anesthesia.
• Probing should be performed in every patient.
• Intraoral radiographs are essential to continue the evaluation of the bone.

MISCELLANEOUS

ANCILLARY TESTS
A complete oral examination, including intraoral radiology

SYNONYMS
Periodontal probing

SEE ALSO
Blackwell's Five-Minute Veterinary Consult: Canine and Feline Topics
• Gingivitis
• Periodontitis

Related Topics in This Book
Dental Radiography

ABBREVIATIONS
None

Suggested Reading
Holmstrom SE, Frost Fitch P, Eisner ER. *Veterinary Dental Techniques for the Small Animal Practitioner*, 3rd ed. Philadelphia: WB Saunders, 2004.
Wiggs RB, Lobprise HB. *Veterinary Dentistry: Principles and Practice*. Philadelphia: Lippincott-Raven (Blackwell), 1997.

INTERNET RESOURCES
None

AUTHOR NAME
Heidi B. Lobprise

BASICS

TYPE OF SPECIMEN
Blood

TEST EXPLANATION AND RELATED PHYSIOLOGY
Globulins are a heterogeneous group of >1,000 proteins that perform a variety of different physiologic functions. The major site of globulin synthesis is the liver, although the immune system also contributes significantly. In routine serum chemistry profiles, the globulin value is calculated by subtracting the albumin concentration from the total protein concentration. Individual globulins can also be measured and quantified by specialized immunochemical and radioimmunologic methods (see the "Immunoglobulin Assays" chapter). Globulins are divided into 3 main classes or fractions (alpha, beta, and gamma) based on their electrophoretic mobility (see the "Protein Electrophoresis" chapter). Variations in 1 or more of the fractions can occur in response to several physiologic and pathologic processes. If abnormal globulin values are present, knowing which fraction(s) is abnormal can help refine the differential diagnosis. Examples of globulins include proteins that are components of the immune system (i.e., immunoglobulins or antibody molecules, complement), proteins involved with coagulation (i.e., fibrinogen and other clotting factors), acute phase proteins, lipoproteins, several enzymes (e.g., α_1-antitrypsin), and proteins that act as transport molecules for a variety of substances (e.g., hormones, vitamins, certain metal ions).

INDICATIONS
- To evaluate unexplained dysproteinemias
- To screen for antibody-producing neoplasia (multiple myeloma)
- To screen for failure of passive transfer (neonates) or inherited or acquired immune deficiency (puppies)

CONTRAINDICATIONS
None

POTENTIAL COMPLICATIONS
None

CLIENT EDUCATION
None

BODY SYSTEMS ASSESSED
- Hemic, lymphatic, and immune
- Hepatobiliary

SAMPLE

COLLECTION
0.5–2.0 mL of venous blood

HANDLING
- Plain red-top tube or serum-separator tube
- Sodium heparin or lithium heparin anticoagulant also acceptable

STORAGE
- Store at room temperature for short-term use.
- Refrigerate for up to 1 month.
- Freeze for the long term.

STABILITY
- Room temperature: 1 week
- Refrigerated (2°–8°C): 1 month
- Frozen (−18°C): >1 month

PROTOCOL
None

INTERPRETATION

NORMAL FINDINGS OR RANGE
- Dogs: 2.7–4.4 g/dL (27–44 g/L)
- Cats: 2.6–5.1 g/dL (26–51 g/L)
- Reference intervals may vary depending on the laboratory and assays used for total protein and albumin determinations.

ABNORMAL VALUES
Values above or below the reference range

CRITICAL VALUES
None

GLOBULINS

INTERFERING FACTORS

Drugs That May Alter Results or Interpretation

Drugs That Interfere with Test Methodology
None

Drugs That Alter Physiology
None

Disorders That May Alter Results
None

Collection Techniques or Handling That May Alter Results
None

Influence of Signalment

Species
None

Breed
None

Age
• A minimal immunoglobulin level is present at birth. The immunoglobulin concentration rises rapidly in newborns because of absorption of maternal immunoglobulins after ingestion of colostrum.
• Newborns begin to synthesize immunoglobulins as maternally derived immunoglobulins are metabolized and decline (within 1–5 weeks). Adult levels of immunoglobulins are attained upon reaching young adulthood (6 months to 1 year).
• There is a general increase in globulins with advancing age.

Gender
None

Pregnancy
The globulin concentration may decrease during the third trimester of pregnancy and whelping (in association with colostrum production).

LIMITATIONS OF THE TEST

Sensitivity, Specificity, and Positive and Negative Predictive Values
N/A

Valid If Run In a Human Lab?
Yes.

Causes of Abnormal Findings

High values	Low values
Inflammation (increased acute phase proteins)	Loss
Immunoglobulins—polyclonal gammopathies from chronic antigenic stimulation	Hemorrhage
	Exudative skin disease
	Exudative effusion
	Vasculitis
Infectious processes	Protein-losing enteropathy
Bacterial, rickettsial	Deficient protein synthesis or increased protein catabolism
Viral	
Fungal	Severe malnutrition or cachexia
Protozoal	Maldigestion/malabsorption
Immune-mediated diseases	Hepatic insufficiency
Liver disease (hepatitis)	Failure of passive transfer
Immunoglobulins—monoclonal gammopathies caused by production of homogeneous immunoglobulin molecule	Severe combined immunodeficiency (dogs)
	Selective IgM, IgA, and IgG deficiencies (in dogs)
Lymphoid neoplasia—B cell	Transient hypogammaglobulinemia (dogs)
Plasma cell myeloma, plasmacytoma	
Lymphoma	
Lymphocytic leukemia	
Macroglobulinemia	
Nonneoplastic (infrequent)	
Canine ehrlichiosis*	
Canine amyloidosis	
Visceral leishmaniasis*	
Feline infectious peritonitis*	
Immunoglobulin light chains (Bence-Jones proteins)	
Idiopathic	
Nephrotic syndrome	

*May actually be oligoclonal, but usually polyclonal.

CLINICAL PERSPECTIVE
• If both the albumin and the globulin levels are decreased, consider loss of proteins through hemorrhage (low PCV), vasculitis, exudative skin disease, exudative effusion, severe malnutrition, or protein-losing enteropathy.
• If the globulin level is low, but the albumin level is normal, consider immunodeficiency.
• If both the albumin and the globulin levels are elevated, consider hemoconcentration (dehydration), perhaps with concurrent antigenic stimulation.
• Marked increases are usually caused by increased immunoglobulin production either because of neoplasia (e.g., multiple myeloma) or chronic antigenic stimulation (e.g., FIP, ehrlichiosis, leishmaniasis).

MISCELLANEOUS
ANCILLARY TESTS
• Albumin
• Total protein
• Serum protein electrophoresis to look for monoclonal gammopathy or immunodeficiency
• Bence-Jones proteins
• Quantification of immunoglobulins through radial immunodiffusion

SYNONYMS
None

SEE ALSO
Blackwell's Five-Minute Veterinary Consult: Canine and Feline Topics
• Ehrlichiosis
• Feline Infectious Peritonitis (FIP)
• Immunodeficiency Disorders, Primary
• Leishmaniasis
• Multiple Myeloma
Related Topics in This Book
• Albumin
• Immunoglobulin Assays
• Protein Electrophoresis
• Total Protein

ABBREVIATIONS
None

Suggested Reading
Evans EW, Duncan JR. Proteins, lipids and carbohydrates. In: Latimer KS, Mahaffey EA, Prasse KW, eds. *Duncan and Prasse's Veterinary Laboratory Medicine Clinical Pathology,* 4th ed. Ames: Iowa State Press, 2003: 162–192.
Lassen ED. Laboratory evaluation of plasma and serum proteins. In: Thrall MA, ed. *Veterinary Hematology and Clinical Chemistry.* Philadelphia: Lippincott Williams & Wilkins, 2004: 401–412.

INTERNET RESOURCES
None

AUTHOR NAME
Rob Simoni

GLOMERULAR FILTRATION RATE

BASICS

TYPE OF PROCEDURE
Function tests

PROCEDURE EXPLANATION AND RELATED PHYSIOLOGY
Chronic kidney disease (CKD) is a common problem in dogs and cats: In some surveys, as many as 1 in 3 elderly animals have CKD. Early diagnosis of CKD enables a veterinarian to avoid treatments that may damage a compromised kidney and enables early institution of renoprotective therapy that will slow the progression of CKD. Early diagnosis is problematic because of the tremendous functional reserve of the kidneys and because routine laboratory tests enable identification of CKD only when a majority of renal tissue has already been destroyed. For example, a loss of urinary concentrating ability is generally not seen until at least two-thirds of renal tissue is destroyed. Furthermore, dilute urine may be observed in many nonrenal conditions. The central and most critical renal function is glomerular filtration rate (GFR). In patients with CKD, elevations of plasma concentrations of urea and creatinine (Cr) are used as clinical markers for estimating GFR. Unfortunately, BUN is affected by several nonrenal factors, making it inferior to Cr for estimation of GFR. Further, the relation between GFR and both Cr and BUN is nonlinear, and the reference ranges for both indices reflect a wide interanimal variability in normal values. Thus, neither BUN nor Cr can be expected to exceed the normal reference range until ≈75% of nephrons have been destroyed. Serial determinations of Cr over time in the same animal (using the same laboratory) are more useful than a single determination. Serial increases in Cr, even within the reference range, are usually indicative of either declining GFR or changing body condition. Nonetheless, patients with early to moderate CKD often have normal Cr and BUN. In nonazotemic patients suspected to have early CKD, and in conditions in which a precise measure of renal function is important, GFR measurement is indicated.

Classically, measurement of GFR relies upon timed urine collections and the use of either inulin or Cr as a marker. Although urinary clearance procedures are more accurate, they are time and labor intensive and largely have been replaced in clinical practice by quantitative imaging modalities such as nuclear scintigraphy or measurements of plasma clearance of marker substances following a single IV injection. Appropriate markers for plasma clearances that have been studied in dogs and cats include radionuclides, inulin, Cr, and iohexol. Radionuclides and nuclear imaging require specialized equipment and are technically difficult to master, making them impractical for routine use in clinical patients. Assays for inulin are not routinely available, and injectable preparations for inulin and Cr are not commercially available in many countries, including the United States. Iohexol is readily available as an injectable product (Omnipaque: a nonionic, iodinated radiographic contrast agent), and a reliable assay for iohexol is commercially available. Measurement of the rate of disappearance (clearance) from plasma after a single iohexol injection provides a useful estimate of GFR in dogs and cats. Although urinary clearance of exogenously administered Cr remains an option for measurement of GFR, the most commonly used method for GFR estimation is plasma clearance of iohexol.

INDICATIONS
- Early diagnosis of CKD: The usual purpose here is to determine whether clinical findings, such as polyuria, in a patient are due to CKD. Early diagnosis will enable the adoption of an appropriate diagnostic regimen and therapeutic interventions and enable a veterinarian to avoid potentially nephrotoxic situations in animals with preexisting renal compromise.
- Monitoring changes in renal function (GFR) during patient management

- Adjusting drug therapy for agents that are eliminated by the kidneys, particularly those with a narrow therapeutic index, narrow therapeutic range, or with known potential for nephrotoxicity
- Screening for the presence of familial renal disease where there is an index of suspicion in a dog or cat. Such suspicion may arise as a result of knowledge of family members affected with kidney disease or in animals of a potentially affected breed (e.g., Abyssinian cats).

CONTRAINDICATIONS
- A history of an adverse reaction to iohexol: Adverse reactions are rare but may include allergic manifestations.
- The presence of renal azotemia is not a true contraindication, although it obviates the use of the test for early identification of CKD. The iohexol and exogenous Cr clearance tests may be used in azotemic patients when an accurate measure of GFR is important for the management of the animal.

POTENTIAL COMPLICATIONS
- Adverse reactions to iohexol are rare but can occur. These include anaphylaxis, hypotension, arrhythmias, nausea, vomiting, renal vasoconstriction, and acute renal failure. The low dosage used for this test makes acute nephrotoxicity extremely unlikely, and plasma clearance of iohexol is generally accepted as safe in normal dogs and cats and in those with CKD.
- Cr is a normal, endogenous molecule, and true adverse reactions to Cr will not occur. However, the solution as described in the Equipment or Supplies section is mildly hypertonic and may induce postprocedure discomfort.
- If principles of sterility and asepsis are not followed, introduction of bacteria may lead to complications at injection sites or systemically with either the plasma clearance of iohexol or exogenous Cr clearance procedure.
- Urethral catheterization during an exogenous Cr clearance test may cause a urinary tract infection through introduction of bacteria into the urinary bladder.

CLIENT EDUCATION
- Do not feed the animal the morning of the procedure. There is a small risk of adverse reactions. Shaving of an extremity may be necessary for injections and blood sample procurement. Plan to leave the animal at the clinic for an entire day.
- Report any posttest changes in an animal's behavior, such as an alteration in eating, drinking, or urination, to the veterinarian immediately.
- For exogenous Cr clearance, the patient should be returned for urine culture in 3–7 days.

BODY SYSTEMS ASSESSED
Renal and urologic

PROCEDURE

PATIENT PREPARATION
Preprocedure Medication or Preparation
- Either procedure: Patients should be well hydrated and fasted for 12 h prior to the clearance study and during the study.
- Iohexol clearance: Water should be provided ad libitum throughout the fasting period and clearance study.
- Cr clearance: After the water gavage (see the Technique section), additional water is not provided during the urinary clearance procedure.

Anesthesia or Sedation
Contraindicated because general anesthesia and most sedatives will alter GFR

Patient Positioning
N/A

Patient Monitoring

Routine physical observation with assessment of temperature, pulse, respiration, and pulse character for 15 min after iohexol administration or for 30 min after Cr administration

Equipment or Supplies

Iohexol Clearance
- Iohexol (Omnipaque)
- An IV catheter, syringes, and needles

Cr Clearance
- Cr (Sigma, St. Louis, MO) solution containing 50 mg of Cr/mL water. The solution should be autoclaved or filtered to ensure the absence of bacteria.
- A urinary catheter, syringes, and needles
- A stomach tube and oral speculum
- Sterile water

TECHNIQUE

Iohexol Clearance

- Determine and record the animal's body weight (kilograms). As this weight is used in the calculation of the GFR, accuracy of this measurement is important.
- Place an IV catheter. It is critical that the catheter is patent and that there is no perivascular leakage of injected material. Test the catheter patency with sterile isotonic solution prior to injection of iohexol.
- Determine the dose of iohexol:
  - The standard dosage is 300 mg iodine/kg of body weight.
  - For moderate to severe azotemia (serum Cr, >3 mg/dL or >250 μmol/L), a dosage of either 300 mg iodine/kg or 150 mg iodine/kg may be used.
  - The actual dose is used in calculating the GFR, so accuracy is critical.
- Administer the iohexol dose as a single, rapid IV bolus through the injection catheter, followed immediately by flushing with an isotonic solution. The dose may be administered by syringe and needle, but there is a greater risk of perivascular extravasation with this approach. Record the exact time of injection to the nearest minute. Use only a single clock or timing device for all time determinations.
- Remove the catheter ≈15 min after the injection. This interval allows venous access until certain an immediate adverse reaction will not occur. Do not use the injection catheter to procure blood because the catheter is contaminated with significant amounts of iohexol, even after flushing.
- Collect ≈3 mL of whole blood (in a clot tube for serum) by venipuncture at 2, 3, and 4 h after the injection. It is important to be as close to these hourly intervals as possible but more important to record the exact time (to the nearest minute) that blood samples were collected.

Creatinine Clearance

- Determine and record the animal's body weight (kilograms). As this weight is used in the calculation of GFR, accuracy of this measurement is important.
- Inject the Cr solution at a dosage of 2.0 mL/kg of body weight SC. Accuracy of this dosage is less critical than with iohexol clearance. Do not inject >10 mL/site. This becomes time = 0 min.
- Immediately pass a stomach tube and administer a volume of tap water equal to 3% of body weight. For example, a 15-kg dog should receive 450 mL of water orally.
- Place an indwelling urinary catheter so that it is in place at time = 60 min.
- At 60 min, remove and discard all urine from the bladder. Flush the bladder with 10 mL (for cats) to 50 mL (for dogs) of sterile water, remove all flush, and discard this as well. Record the exact time of bladder emptying as T1.
- Obtain a 1.5- to 2.5-mL blood sample (B1) by venipuncture or via an indwelling venous catheter and place the blood in a clot tube.

- Collect and save all urine ≈20 min later. After the urine is collected, flush the bladder with sterile water as described previously and collect all flush carefully. Note the exact time flush is complete as T2. Thoroughly mix the urine and flush, and label it U1. Measure the total volume of mixed flush and urine as V1 and save an aliquot of this urine. Immediately obtain a 1.5- to 2.5-mL blood sample as B2 in a clot tube.
- Collect and save all urine ≈20 min later. Flush the bladder with sterile water as described previously and collect all flush. Note the exact time the flush is complete as T3. Thoroughly mix the urine and flush, and label it U2. Measure the total volume of mixed flush and urine as V2 and save an aliquot of this urine. Immediately obtain a 1.5- to 2.5-mL blood sample as B3 in a clot tube.
- Remove the urinary catheter.

SAMPLE HANDLING

Iohexol Clearance

- Allow the blood to clot and transfer at least 1.2 mL of serum to a labeled plastic vial. Samples may be refrigerated or frozen.
- Ship the chilled or frozen serum samples to the appropriate laboratory, being certain to include the exact dose of iohexol administered (milligrams of iodine per kilograms of body weight), the exact time of iohexol administration, and the exact time that the blood samples were collected. The Animal Health Diagnostic Laboratory at Michigan State University (B629 West Fee Hall, East Lansing, MI 48824) provides this assay commercially.

Creatinine Clearance

- Allow the blood to clot and transfer the serum samples (B1–B3; at least 0.5 mL) and the urine and urine-flush mixture (U1 and U2) to labeled plastic vials. Samples should be refrigerated but not frozen.
- Submit the samples to any clinical pathology laboratory. Notify the laboratory as to which of the samples contain urine, because the lab may need to perform appropriate dilutions.

APPROPRIATE AFTERCARE

Postprocedure Patient Monitoring

- Observe the injection site for bleeding or infection.
- Cr clearance: Perform follow-up bacterial urine culture within 3–7 days after the procedure.

Nursing Care

None

Dietary Modification

None

Medication Requirements

None

Restrictions on Activity

None

Anticipated Recovery Time

Immediate

INTERPRETATION

NORMAL FINDINGS OR RANGE

- Individual laboratories will provide reference (normal) values specifically determined for their assay and GFR determination methodology. Substantial variation may occur in reference ranges for plasma clearance procedures because these techniques rely on specifics of sample timing and kinetic modeling to calculate GFR.
- A value for GFR that lies within the normal range for that species is considered normal.
- A value for GFR that is below the normal range is diagnostic of kidney disease if prerenal and postrenal factors have been eliminated as considerations. The percent reduction in GFR is determined by

GLOMERULAR FILTRATION RATE

comparison of the patient's value with the mean normal value for that species.

- A high value for GFR is generally not considered to be of significance, though certain disease states, such as poorly regulated diabetes mellitus, may lead to the undesirable condition of chronically sustained hyperfiltration.
- For the iohexol clearance procedure performed in accordance with the protocol outlined by the Michigan State University Animal Health Diagnostic Laboratory, the GFR will be calculated by the laboratory. The mean normal GFR by this method for dogs is 5.48 mL/min/kg of body weight (normal range, 2.89–8.07) and for cats is 1.94 mL/min/kg (normal range, 1.15–2.73).
- For the exogenous urinary Cr clearance procedure (as outlined here), GFR should be taken as the average of the two 20-min clearance periods. The clearance formula is as follows:
  - GFR = (urine volume × urine Cr concentration)/(mean plasma concentration × duration of collection × body weight). Body weight is measured in kilograms, Cr concentrations in milligrams per deciliter, and time in minutes.
- For the first collection period, GFR = [V1 × [creatinine] in U1]/[(0.5) × (B1 + B2) × (T2 − T1) × body weight].
- For the second collection period, GFR = [V2 × [creatinine] in U2]/[(0.5) × (B2 + B3) × (T3 − T2) × body weight].
- For the exogenous Cr clearance, the mean normal GFR in dogs is 3.8 mL/min/kg of body weight (normal range, 2.8–4.8) and in cats is 2.8 mL/min/kg (normal range, 2.1–3.5).

CRITICAL VALUES
N/A

INTERFERING FACTORS
Drugs That May Alter Results of the Procedure
For iohexol clearance, iodine-containing compounds, such as radiographic contrast agents

Conditions That May Interfere with Performing the Procedure
Any prerenal or postrenal cause of azotemia

Procedure Techniques or Handling That May Alter Results
For Either Procedure
Failure to note body weight or times accurately

For Iohexol Clearance
- Use of an injection catheter to procure blood samples will contaminate the sample significantly
- Inaccurate dose administration: Perivascular extravasation of iohexol invalidates the test result. If repeated, the intertest interval should be at least 48 h.

For Urinary Clearance of Cr
- Failure to empty the urinary bladder completely
- Failure to mix the flush and urine thoroughly and to measure urine volume accurately
- Failure to administer the water gavage will lower urine volumes and artifactually reduce the measured value for GFR.

Influence of Signalment on Performing and Interpreting the Procedure
Species
There are species-specific normal values for GFR.

Breed
Interbreed differences in normal values for GFR exist but have not been well studied. Historically, these differences have been presumed to be small. Unfortunately, this is almost certainly an inaccurate presumption. Until further studies are published, the only viable approach is to accept a single reference range for GFR for each species.

Age
Normal values are for adult animals only. Although the prevalence of

CKD rises with advancing age, normal dogs and cats experience only a small decline in GFR with advancing age.

Gender
Differences in normal values for GFR among genders have not been well studied but are generally presumed to be small.

Pregnancy
Differences in values for GFR during pregnancy have not been well studied, although a substantial increase in GFR should be expected during pregnancy.

CLINICAL PERSPECTIVE
- GFR estimation is the best way to assess the severity of kidney dysfunction, particularly in preazotemic stages.
- Plasma clearance of iohexol is a readily available method for GFR estimation that avoids the labor-intensive and time-intensive aspects of urinary clearances.

MISCELLANEOUS

ANCILLARY TESTS
- A complete urinalysis, including sediment examination and quantification of proteinuria with the urinary protein/Cr ratio or albumin-specific assays, or both, along with determination of plasma concentrations of BUN and Cr should always accompany this procedure.
- Renal imaging studies (survey or contrast radiography and ultrasonography) to evaluate the urinary tract for structural abnormalities
- Renal biopsy, particularly if the kidneys are normal sized or enlarged or if marked proteinuria is present

SYNONYMS
None

SEE ALSO
Blackwell's Five-Minute Veterinary Consult: Canine and Feline Topics
- Azotemia and Uremia
- Polyuria and Polydipsia

Related Topics in This Book
- Creatinine
- Urea Nitrogen
- Urethral Catheterization

ABBREVIATIONS
- CKD = chronic kidney disease
- Cr = creatinine
- GFR = glomerular filtration rate

Suggested Reading
Brown SA, Finco DR, Boudinot D. Evaluation of a single injection method, using iohexol, for estimating glomerular filtration rate in dogs and cats. *Am J Vet Res* 1996; 57: 105–110.
Finco DR, Coulter DB, Barsanti JA. Procedure for a simple method of measuring glomerular filtration rate in the dog. *J Am Anim Hosp Assoc* 1982; 18: 804–806.
Heiene R, Moe L. Pharmacokinetic aspects of measurement of glomerular filtration rate in the dog: A review. *J Vet Intern Med* 1998; 12: 401–414.

INTERNET RESOURCES
None

AUTHOR NAME
Scott A. Brown

BASICS

TYPE OF SPECIMEN
Blood

TEST EXPLANATION AND RELATED PHYSIOLOGY
Glucose analysis is one of the most important laboratory procedures because glucose provides the cellular energy for nearly all tissues in the body. Glucose is regulated by many hormones, the most important of which is insulin. Insulin lowers plasma glucose by promoting entry of glucose into myocytes and adipocytes. Several hormones, including glucagon, catecholamines, glucocorticoids, and growth hormone (GH), counter the effects of insulin. Glucagon increases plasma glucose by stimulating glycogenolysis and gluconeogenesis. Cortisol also increases gluconeogenesis but also creates a state of insulin resistance by decreasing the number of glucose membrane transporters in target cells. GH also causes a peripheral insulin resistance and reduces glucose uptake by myocytes and adipocytes. Catecholamines alter blood glucose through a variety of mechanisms, including increased gluconeogenesis and decreased insulin secretion.

Diabetes mellitus (DM), caused by either insulin deficiency or defects in insulin action (i.e., insulin resistance), is an important cause of hyperglycemia. DM is often caused by pancreatic disease (e.g., immune-mediated destruction of pancreatic β cells or damage following pancreatitis). In addition, a variety of endocrine diseases can cause secondary DM, including hyperadrenocorticism (excess cortisol), acromegaly (excess GH), pheochromocytomas (excess catecholamines), and glucagonomas. Hepatocutaneous syndrome, seen in some dogs with cirrhosis or other hepatic lesions, includes a multifactorial hyperglycemia. In addition, DM must be distinguished from the hyperglycemia produced by acute or chronic stress and the subsequent effect of catecholamines and cortisol.

Hypoglycemia can be caused by increased tissue use of glucose (e.g., endotoxemia, marked exertion), decreased glucose production (e.g., hepatic insufficiency, starvation), or both (hypoadrenocorticism). Neoplasia is an occasional cause of hypoglycemia. Excessive insulin from β-cell neoplasms is occasionally seen in dogs and causes persistent hypoglycemia because of excessive tissue use of glucose. Other neoplasms such as leiomyomas or leiomyosarcomas have been associated with hypoglycemia caused by either secretion of an insulin-like substance or excessive use of glucose by the neoplastic cells. Hepatic neoplasia may also cause hypoglycemia by decreasing the functional hepatic mass.

Most reference laboratories use enzymatic analytical methods that incorporate the reaction of hexokinase or glucose oxidase on glucose, and subsequent color changes are detected photometrically. A wide variety of benchtop instruments and handheld instruments (glucometers) are available for in-hospital office testing. Many of these rely on strips or slides coated with chemicals (i.e., glucose oxidase, dehydrogenase, or hexokinase) that interact with blood glucose and then measure the amount of light reflected from the strip after the chemical reaction has occurred (i.e., a reflectance meter). Other meters quantify glucose by measuring the amount of electricity that can pass through the sample. These methods have variable correlation, particularly when significantly increased glucose concentrations are involved. Point-of-care meters tend to display values lower than those determined by reference laboratories because plasma glucose levels tend to be $\approx$10%–15% higher than whole blood glucose levels.

INDICATIONS
- Weakness
- Seizures, altered mentation, or coma
- Sepsis
- Polyuria-polydipsia
- Suspected hepatic or endocrine disease

CONTRAINDICATIONS
None

POTENTIAL COMPLICATIONS
None

CLIENT EDUCATION
- Glucose is the first line of tests in diagnosing DM, but additional tests such as fructosamine or glycosylated hemoglobin may be needed to confirm the diagnosis.
- Patients should undergo a fast.

BODY SYSTEMS ASSESSED
- Endocrine and metabolic
- Gastrointestinal
- Hepatobiliary
- Nervous
- Renal and urologic

SAMPLE

COLLECTION
- 2–3 mL of venous blood
- Minimize patient struggling as much as possible.

HANDLING
- Collect the sample into a plain red-top tube, serum-separator tube, heparin, or EDTA.
- To prevent the use of the glucose, separate the serum or plasma from the cellular portion of the blood soon after sample collection.
  - A decreased glucose level can be seen within 30 min if serum is not separated from cells with up to a 10% decrease per hour.
  - The administration of sodium fluoride (NaF) anticoagulant can prevent cellular consumption of glucose. However, NaF interferes with the glucose oxidase method of glucose determination used in some glucometers.

STORAGE
Refrigeration is recommended.

STABILITY
- Room temperature: at least 2 days (if the serum or plasma is separated from the cells)
- Refrigerated (4°C): at least 3 days (if the serum or plasma is separated from the cells)
- Frozen (−20°C): at least 1 week

PROTOCOL
None

INTERPRETATION

NORMAL FINDINGS OR RANGE
- Dogs: 70–120 mg/dL (3.89–6.66 mmol/L)
- Cats: 70–130 mg/dL (3.89–7.22 mmol/L)
- Reference intervals may vary depending on the laboratory and assay.

ABNORMAL VALUES
Results above or below the reference range

CRITICAL VALUES
- Mentation may be altered or coma caused if the glucose level is ≤40 mg/dL, so this requires immediate treatment.
- A glucose level of >1,000 mg/dL may also alter mentation or cause coma because of a hyperosmotic state.

GLUCOSE

INTERFERING FACTORS

Drugs That May Alter Results or Interpretation

Drugs That Interfere with Test Methodology
None

Drugs That Alter Physiology
- β-Adrenergic blockers, antihistamines, ethanol, sulfonylureas, salicylates, and anabolic steroids may decrease blood glucose.
- In diabetic patients, recent insulin treatment or the administration of sulfonylurea compounds such as glipizide may cause hypoglycemia.
- Hyperglycemia can be seen with L-asparaginase, β-adrenergic blockers, corticosteroids, α_2-agonist sedatives (e.g., xylazine, detomidine), ketamine, diazoxide, furosemide and thiazide diuretics, acetazolamide, phenothiazines, morphines, megestrol acetate, and heparin.
- Patients receiving parenteral nutrition may also develop hyperglycemia.

Disorders That May Alter Results
- Hormones such as glucagon, thyroxin, progestins, and estrogens in cats are associated with hyperglycemia.
- The hematocrit will affect assays that use whole blood. An elevated hematocrit will lower glucose values and vice versa.

Collection Techniques or Handling That May Alter Results
- Delay in separation of cells from the serum or plasma may falsely lower the glucose level. The rate of glucose consumption varies with glucose concentration, temperature, WBC count, and other factors. Extreme leukocytosis or bacterial contamination of the sample accelerates glucose consumption.
- Patients, particularly cats, that struggle or are very fearful during sample collection may have transient hyperglycemia due to stimulation of gluconeogenesis from catecholamine secretion.
- Postprandial sampling may elevate glucose concentrations.

Influence of Signalment

Species
- Dogs: DM is usually caused by insulin deficiency as a result of pancreatic β-cell destruction.
- Cats: DM is often produced by a combination of defective insulin secretion and insulin receptor defects.

Breed
- Hunting breeds of dogs may develop hypoglycemia after time in the field, perhaps due to increased glucose use.
- Glycogen storage diseases are a rare cause of hypoglycemia. Type III glycogen storage disease has been reported in German shepherds.
- Some families of keeshonds have a predilection for DM.

Age
Neonates or juvenile animals, particularly toy-breed dogs, can be prone to develop hypoglycemia, perhaps due to insufficient gluconeogenesis relative to metabolic rate.

Gender
Diestrus in bitches has been associated with hyperglycemia as caused by progesterone-stimulated mammary gland secretion of GH.

Pregnancy
Dogs in late pregnancy may develop a ketogenic hypoglycemia, although the causal mechanism has not been clearly established.

LIMITATIONS OF THE TEST
- Temperature and humidity can have unpredictable effects on glucometer results.
- Although glucometers may have a broad working range (e.g., 0–600 mg/dL), their results are not necessarily linear over this entire range. Therefore, extremely high or low values should be verified with another method.

Sensitivity, Specificity, and Positive and Negative Predictive Values
N/A

Valid If Run in a Human Lab?
Yes.

Causes of Abnormal Findings

High values	Low values
DM	Delayed separation of cells from
Insulin deficiency	serum or plasma
Immune-mediated β-cell	Sepsis
destruction	Paraneoplastic syndrome
Pancreatitis	Insulinoma
Insulin resistance	Leiomyosarcoma
Hyperadrenocorticism	Hepatic insufficiency
Acromegaly	Hypoadrenocorticism
Pheochromocytoma	Exertional—hunting dogs
Glucagonoma	Juvenile dogs (especially
Excitement or fear	toy breeds)
Hyperthyroidism	Late pregnancy
Drug therapy	
Hepatocutaneous syndrome	

CLINICAL PERSPECTIVE
- Serum or plasma glucose level constantly changes throughout the day in response to activity, meals, and other factors. Since a single glucose determination is therefore a "snapshot in time," follow-up testing is usually needed in patients with disorders of carbohydrate metabolism.
- In hypoglycemic patients, neutropenia or an inflammatory leukogram with toxic neutrophils suggests sepsis.
- When working up hyperglycemic patients, it is important to rule out the excitement induced by patient handling or drug therapy. Documenting the persistence of hyperglycemia may be an important first part of the diagnostic plan, particularly if the hyperglycemia is mild.

MISCELLANEOUS

ANCILLARY TESTS

In Hypoglycemic Patients
- CBC and evaluation of WBCs
- Analysis of serum bile acids to evaluate hepatic function
- Determination of the insulin/glucose ratio in patients suspected of having an insulinoma
- A possible ACTH stimulation test to look for hypoadrenocorticism

In Hyperglycemic Patients
- Evaluation of urine glucose, fructosamine, or glycated hemoglobin to rule out hyperglycemia induced by transient stress or excitement
- An ACTH stimulation or low-dose dexamethasone suppression test to look for hyperadrenocorticism

SYNONYMS
None

SEE ALSO
Blackwell's Five-Minute Veterinary Consult: Canine and Feline Topics
- Cirrhosis and Fibrosis of the liver
- Diabetes mellitus without complication–Cats

- Diabetes mellitus without complication–Dogs
- Diabetes with hyperosmolar Coma
- Diabetes with Ketoacidosis
- Hyperadrenocorticism (Cushing's Disease)—Cats
- Hyperadrenocorticism (Cushing's Disease)—Dogs
- Hyperglycemia
- Hypoglycemia
- Sepsis and Bacteremia

Related Topics in This Book
- Fructosamine
- Glucose Curve
- Glycosylated Hemoglobin
- Insulin and Insulin/Glucose Ratio

ABBREVIATIONS
- ACTH = adrenocorticotropic hormone
- DM = diabetes mellitus
- GH = growth hormone

Suggested Reading

Kaneko JJ. Carbohydrate metabolism and its diseases. In: Kaneko JJ, Harvey JW, Bruss ML, eds. *Clinical Biochemistry of Domestic Animals,* 5th ed. San Diego: Academic, 1997: 45–81.

Stockham SL, Scott MA. Glucose and related regulatory hormones. In: *Fundamentals of Veterinary Clinical Pathology.* Ames: Iowa State Press, 2002: 487–506.

INTERNET RESOURCES
Cornell University, College of Medicine, Clinical Pathology Modules, Veterinary Clinical Chemistry: Blood glucose, http://www.diaglab.vet.cornell.edu/clinpath/modules/chem/glucose.htm.

AUTHOR NAME
Denise Wunn

GLUCOSE CURVE

BASICS

TYPE OF SPECIMEN
Blood

TEST EXPLANATION AND RELATED PHYSIOLOGY
Determination of a blood glucose (BG) curve is a method of evaluating glucose control in diabetic dogs or cats. Serial BG measurement enables assessment of the effect of food and medication (insulin or oral hypoglycemic drugs) on glucose control. The dose, and if necessary the type, of medication (e.g., intermediate-acting vs long-acting insulin) can be altered, depending on results.

The lowest (nadir) and highest BG concentrations should be noted, as well as the duration of action of insulin (the number of hours the glucose is in a desired range, provided the nadir is acceptable). Hypoglycemia (a BG concentration of <65 mg/dL) or a rapid drop in glucose concentration (e.g., from 500 to 200 mg/dL in 2 h) can result in the Somogyi phenomenon, whereby counterregulatory hormones, notably glucagon and epinephrine, cause a variable period of hyperglycemia (up to 3 days) after hypoglycemia occurs.

INDICATIONS
- To regulate a new diabetic patient
- To investigate a poorly controlled diabetic patient
- To diagnose transient diabetes mellitus, a temporary or permanent resolution of diabetes in cats

CONTRAINDICATIONS
- Inappetence or illness on the day of the test
- Hypoglycemia (a BG concentration of <60) on admission: In this case, cancel the BG curve analysis and recommend a 10%–25% insulin-dose reduction.
- Stress hyperglycemia: If a patient, especially a cat, is very anxious, the curve may be meaningless. If glucose readings in an extremely stressed patient are normal, insulin overdosage may be suspected.

POTENTIAL COMPLICATIONS
None

CLIENT EDUCATION
- The goal is to have all BG concentrations between 80 and 200 mg/dL in diabetic dogs and between 100 and 300 mg/dL in cats. Measurements outside that range may require a dose adjustment, an alternative insulin type, or further investigation and/or monitoring.
- Owners can be taught to monitor glucose at home by using lancets to obtain a small drop of blood from the marginal ear vein, ventral medial pinna, buccal mucosa of a lip (dogs), or elbow calluses (dogs). Warming the site first with a moist hot cloth will improve sample size. Glucose should be measured by using portable glucometers that use the least amount of blood, such as Ascensia Elite and Ascensia Contour (Bayer, Tarrytown, NY), One Touch Ultra (Lifescan, Milpitas, CA), and the veterinary product AlphaTrak (Abbott Laboratories, Abbott Park, IL).
- Owners need to be instructed carefully in the home use of glucometers and informed about calibration and coding of the devices according to the manufacturer's directions.

BODY SYSTEMS ASSESSED
Endocrine and metabolic

SAMPLE

COLLECTION
- Generally, a very small amount of blood (<0.2 mL) is drawn using an insulin or tuberculin syringe.
- The goal is to be minimally invasive while enabling multiple sequential sample collections.
- For home glucose monitoring, the glucometer with test strip inserted is held to the drop of blood, which is then drawn up by capillary action.

HANDLING
The sample should be analyzed immediately by using a portable glucometer.

STORAGE
Immediate analysis is recommended.

STABILITY
- Room temperature: at least 2 days (if serum or plasma is separated from cells)
- Refrigerated (4°C): at least 3 days (if serum or plasma is separated from cells)
- Frozen (−20°C): at least 1 week

PROTOCOL
- The patient is admitted to the hospital shortly after being *fed* and given *insulin* at home.
- The owner's feeding schedule should be followed for the remainder of the day.
- Appetite and stress level are noted during the day.
- BG concentration is measured every 2 h for 12 h. Collect blood from any easily accessible peripheral vein by using minimal restraint to avoid stress hyperglycemia.
- Measure glucose by using a portable glucose meter or a point-of-care analyzer.
- Note the nadir, duration of effect, and highest BG concentration. Bear in mind that BG concentrations obtained with glucometers using whole blood are ≈10%–15% lower than BG concentrations obtained through methods using plasma or serum.

INTERPRETATION

NORMAL FINDINGS OR RANGE
- Dogs: The ideal BG concentration range for diabetic dogs is 80–200 mg/dL.
- Cats: The ideal BG concentration range for diabetic cats is 100–300 mg/dL. Higher BG concentrations are tolerated because cats are more prone to life-threatening episodes of hypoglycemia.
- Normal or below-normal BG concentration readings in cats with diabetes mellitus suggest transient diabetes, especially if normal findings are repeatable with dose reduction or discontinuation of insulin administration.
- See Figure 1A.

ABNORMAL VALUES
BG concentrations above or below ideal range require evaluation.

CRITICAL VALUES
- A BG concentration of <60 requires monitoring, dose adjustment, and treatment to avoid subsequent hypoglycemic attacks.
- A BG concentration persistently at >500 may be associated with hyperosmolar syndrome.

INTERFERING FACTORS
Drugs That May Alter Results or Interpretation
Drugs That Interfere with Test Methodology
None

Drugs That Alter Physiology
The administration of drugs such as corticosteroids and megestrol acetate cause insulin resistance that predisposes patients to diabetes or worsening glucose control.

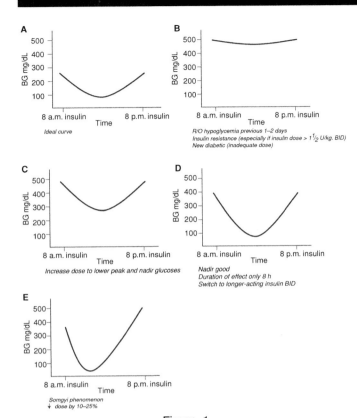

Figure 1

Examples of possible blood glucose curves and suggested treatment adjustments.

Disorders That May Alter Results
Any underlying disease can make diabetes more difficult to regulate: especially Cushing's disease, infection, pancreatitis, acromegaly, or thyroid disease, as well as diestrus.

Collection Techniques or Handling That May Alter Results
• Stress hyperglycemia in cats and, to a lesser degree, in dogs may falsely increase the BG concentration.
• Failure to separate serum promptly may falsely lower the BG concentration when the assay relies on serum sample.

Influence of Signalment
Species
None

Breed
None

Age
None

Gender
Intact females with diabetes are very difficult to regulate and should be spayed.

Pregnancy
The same as for gender

LIMITATIONS OF THE TEST
Handheld portable glucometers may overestimate or underestimate glucose levels when compared to reference methods. Generally, they tend to underestimate the higher readings, which needs to be considered when interpreting a blood-sugar curve.

Sensitivity, Specificity, and Positive and Negative Predictive Values
N/A

Valid If Run in a Human Lab?
Yes.

Causes of Abnormal Findings

Abnormal finding	Suggested response
Nadir and peak BG concentration are greater than the ideal (Figure 1B and C).	Increase the dose of insulin.
The nadir is acceptable, but the effect of insulin was of insufficient duration (Figure 1D).	Switch to a longer-acting insulin: Dogs: Switch from NPH (neutral protamine Hagedorn) insulin to lente insulin. Cats: Switch from NPH or lente to PZI (protamine zinc insulin) or insulin glargine, a long-acting synthetic version of human insulin.
Hypoglycemia followed by hyperglycemia is diagnostic for the Somogyi phenomenon (Figure 1E).	Decrease the dose by 10%–25% and, in cats, consider transient diabetes mellitus. Switch to a less potent insulin such as PZI or insulin glargine in cats and lente in dogs.
Persistent hyperglycemia (Figure 1B) may be caused by insulin overdose (Somogyi), insulin underdose, or insulin resistance.	After ruling out Somogyi and underdose, and if the insulin dose is >1.5 U/kg, evaluate for causes of the insulin resistance.

CLINICAL PERSPECTIVE
• BG curves are only 1 indicator of diabetic control, and results can vary from day to day, even when there is little change in the patient's status. Therefore, the results should be interpreted along with how the animal is doing clinically (e.g., presence of PU/PD, polyphagia, weight loss, cataracts). If the patient appears well (no PU/PD, stable weight, active), then changes made may be small or the curve might be repeated.
• Other reasons for persistent hyperglycemia [BG concentrations of >300 mg/dL (Figure 1B)] are mishandling of insulin, poor injection technique, inadequate absorption, and insulin resistance (e.g., infection, drugs, Cushing's disease, diestrus, acromegaly, hypothyroidism, hyperthyroidism, Somogyi due to insulin overdose, severe obesity).
• Hyperglycemia may persist for up to 3 days following hypoglycemia, making the Somogyi effect sometimes difficult to detect.
• It is important that portable glucometers be calibrated regularly and readings compared to gold standard methods.

MISCELLANEOUS
ANCILLARY TESTS
• Serial urine glucose testing can enable veterinarians to make some dose increases in new diabetic patients before fine-tuning with a BG curve.
• Fructosamine and glycosylated hemoglobin can be used in addition to analysis of BG curves and, in fractious animals, may replace the analysis of a BG curve.
• Continuous glucose monitoring using SC sensors (e.g., CGMS System Gold; Medtronic MiniMed, Minneapolis, MN) enables continuous interstitial fluid glucose concentration to be measured for up to 3 days.

GLUCOSE CURVE

SYNONYMS
None

SEE ALSO
Blackwell's Five-Minute Veterinary Consult: Canine and Feline Topics
- Diabetes Mellitus with Hyperosmolar Coma
- Diabetes Mellitus with Ketoacidosis
- Diabetes Mellitus without Complication—Cats
- Diabetes Mellitus without Complication—Dogs
- Hyperglycemia

Related Topics in This Book
- Fructosamine
- Glucose
- Glycosylated Hemoglobin

ABBREVIATIONS
- BG = blood glucose
- PU/PD = polyuria-polydipsia

Suggested Reading

Freeman L, Rank J. Evaluation of day to day variability of serial blood glucose concentration curves in diabetic dogs. *J Am Vet Med Assoc* 2003; 22: 317–321.

Kley S, Casella M, Reusch C. Evaluation of long-term home monitoring of blood glucose concentrations in cats with diabetes mellitus: 26 cases (1999–2002). *J Am Vet Med Assoc* 2004; 225: 261–266.

Rand J, Kinnaird E, Baglioni A, *et al.* Acute stress hyperglycemia in cats is associated with struggling and increased concentrations of lactate and norepinephrine. *J Vet Intern Med* 2004; 16: 123–132.

Reusch C, Kley S, Casella M. Home monitoring of the diabetic cat. *J Feline Med Surg* 2005; 8: 119–127.

Wess G, Reusch C. Assessment of five portable blood glucose meters for use in cats. *Am J Vet Res* 2000; 61: 1587–1592.

Whitley N, Drobatz K, Panciera D. Insulin overdose in dogs and cats: 28 cases (1986–1993). *J Am Vet Med Assoc* 1997; 211: 326–330.

Wiedmeyer CE, Johnson PJ, Cohn LA, Meadows RL. Evaluation of a continuous glucose monitoring system for use in dogs, cats and horses. *J Am Vet Med Assoc* 2003; 223: 987–992.

INTERNET RESOURCES
Canine Diabetes, http://www.caninediabetes.org.
Feline Diabetes, http://www.felinediabetes.com.
Harry's Home BG Testing Website, http://sugarcats.net/sites/harry/.
Pet Diabetes Easy Reference List, http://www.petdiabetes.com. Pet diabetes support site.

AUTHOR NAME
Orla Mahony

BASICS

TYPE OF SPECIMEN
Blood

TEST EXPLANATION AND RELATED PHYSIOLOGY
Glucose covalently binds to free amino groups of many types of proteins in biologic systems by a nonenzymatic reaction. In addition to glycation of albumin (see the "Fructosamine" chapter), glycation can occur on hemoglobin. The product is also known as hemoglobin A1 (HbA1). Because canine RBCs circulate 100 days, with a half-life of 60 days, glycosylated hemoglobin (Ghb) reflects canine glucose control over the previous 2 months. Feline erythrocytes circulate 70 days with a half-life of 40 days. Hence, feline Ghb reflects glucose control over the previous 40 days.

Unlike the ready availability of fructosamine assays, Ghb has more limited availability because of more complex and difficult analysis. High-performance liquid chromatography, the reference method in human patients, does not adequately distinguish glycated hemoglobin from normal hemoglobin in dogs. However, affinity chromatography, ion-exchange chromatography, and colorimetric methods have been validated and are available in some specialized laboratories.

INDICATIONS
- Hyperglycemia of uncertain cause
- Monitoring diabetic patients under therapy

CONTRAINDICATIONS
None

POTENTIAL COMPLICATIONS
None

CLIENT EDUCATION
- Ghb is most often used to obtain further information about the duration of hyperglycemia and may be used to confirm a diagnosis of diabetes mellitus.
- Ghb may also be used either alone or in conjunction with other procedures such as the glucose curve or fructosamine to monitor therapy for diabetes.
- The patient should be fasted prior to testing.

BODY SYSTEMS ASSESSED
Endocrine and metabolic

SAMPLE

COLLECTION
1–2 mL of venous blood

HANDLING
- Collect the sample into EDTA anticoagulant (purple-top tube).
- Do not centrifuge or separate the cells.

STORAGE
Refrigerate the sample.

STABILITY
- Room temperature: 3 days
- Refrigerated: 1 week

PROTOCOL
None

INTERPRETATION

NORMAL FINDINGS OR RANGE
- Dogs, <4%
- Cats, <2.6%
- Reference intervals may vary depending on the laboratory and assay.

ABNORMAL VALUES
Above the upper limit of the reference range

CRITICAL VALUES
None

INTERFERING FACTORS
Drugs That May Alter Results or Interpretation
Drugs That Interfere with Test Methodology
None

Drugs That Alter Physiology
- Insulin therapy of diabetic patients is the most common treatment that will affect the carbohydrate status of an animal and alter results.
- Any drugs that affect glucose metabolism over more than several days will affect the results of this test. However, a transient or short-term alteration in glucose metabolism will not be reflected in Ghb results. Drugs that may have long-term effects on glucose metabolism may include corticosteroids, progestins, estrogens, and megestrol acetate.

Disorders That May Alter Results

• Diabetes mellitus, due to either insulin deficiency or insulin resistance, is the most common disorder causing increased concentrations of Ghb.

• Hyperadrenocorticism may also be associated with increased Ghb concentrations.

• Changes in RBC mass can affect the Ghb concentration:
  • Decreased by anemia, especially due to hemolysis
  • Increased by polycythemia

• Insulinomas can be associated with decreased Ghb levels.

Collection Techniques or Handling That May Alter Results

• Lipemia and hemolysis

• Because Ghb represents long-term evaluation of glucose metabolism, struggling or excitement at the time of sample collection does not affect results, unlike as with glucose.

Influence of Signalment

Species

The cat RBC membrane is less permeable to glucose compared to that of the dog, and this results in lower Ghb levels.

Breed

None

Age

None

Gender

None

Pregnancy

None

LIMITATIONS OF THE TEST

Although an elevated Ghb in animals being treated for diabetes mellitus can suggest poor glycemic control, it does not provide information about the underlying problem and possible insulin adjustments. For example, it cannot distinguish between a dog receiving an insufficient dose of insulin and one that has a rebound hyperglycemia following an insulin overdose (Somogyi effect).

Sensitivity, Specificity, and Positive and Negative Predictive Values

Sensitivity, specificity, and predictive values are not established in the literature, but Ghb is considered to be a sensitive and specific procedure for the diagnosis of diabetes mellitus.

Valid If Run in a Human Lab?

Yes—if the laboratory uses an assay validated in animals.

Causes of Abnormal Findings

High values	Low values
Persistent hyperglycemia	Not usually clinically significant
Diabetes mellitus with poor	Insulinoma
glycemic control	Anemia
Hyperadrenocorticism	
Polycythemia	

CLINICAL PERSPECTIVE

• Because Ghb is not affected by struggling at the time of sample collection and does not require strict separation of cells from the serum, elevated Ghb may provide confirmation of the diagnosis of diabetes mellitus.

• An elevated Ghb concentration does not distinguish between type I (insulin dependent) and type II (insulin resistant) diabetes mellitus.

• Ghb provides information about the average blood glucose concentration over a longer period of a pet's past life (8–12 weeks) as compared to the fructosamine concentration (7–10 days).

Guidelines for Monitoring Diabetic Dogs

• Excellent control, <5%
• Good control, 5%–6%
• Fair control, 6%–7%
• Poor control, >7%

Guidelines for Monitoring Diabetic Cats

• Excellent control, <2%
• Good control, 2.0%–2.5%

- Fair control, 2.5%–3.0%
- Poor control, >3%

MISCELLANEOUS

ANCILLARY TESTS
- Fructosamine
- Glucose
- Glucose curve

SYNONYMS
- Glycated hemoglobin
- Hemoglobin A1 (HbA1)

SEE ALSO
Blackwell's Five-Minute Veterinary Consult: Canine and Feline Topics
- Diabetes Mellitus with Hyperosmolar Coma
- Diabetes Mellitus with Ketoacidosis
- Diabetes Mellitus without Complication—Cats
- Diabetes Mellitus without Complication—Dogs

- Hyperadrenocorticism (Cushing's Disease)—Cats
- Hyperadrenocorticism (Cushing's Disease)—Dogs

Related Topics in This Book
- Fructosamine
- Glucose
- Glucose Curve

ABBREVIATIONS
Ghb = glycosylated hemoglobin

Suggested Reading
Kaneko JJ. Carbohydrate metabolism and its diseases. In: Kaneko JJ, Harvey JW, Bruss ML, eds. *Clinical Biochemistry of Domestic Animals,* 5th ed. New York: Academic, 1997: 45–81.

INTERNET RESOURCES
Cornell University, College of Veterinary Medicine, Clinical Pathology Modules, Specialized Chemistry Tests: Glycosylated hemoglobin, http://www.diaglab.vet.cornell.edu/clinpath/modules/chem/glycos.htm.

AUTHOR NAME
Denise Wunn

HEARTWORM SEROLOGY

 BASICS

TYPE OF SPECIMEN
Blood

TEST EXPLANATION AND RELATED PHYSIOLOGY
Heartworm antigen tests detect antibodies against the adult female heartworm, *Dirofilaria immitis*. Serologic testing is the recommended screening for heartworm disease in dogs. Approximately 25% of dogs with adult heartworms do not have circulating microfilariae. This can occur in cases where the worms are too young to produce microfilariae, in a unisex or single-sex infection, in cases where microfilariae are produced but removed by the host's immune response, or because of infection in which the microfilariae are killed by a drug but the adults are not affected. In cats, serologic testing is required because cats with heartworm disease are usually infected with low numbers of adult worms and typically remain amicrofilaremic. Antibody testing is recommended in cats because the low worm burden may result in insufficient amounts of circulating antigen to detect.

INDICATIONS
Dogs
• Part of annual physical exam in animals that are >7 months of age, to detect infection occurring during the preceding transmission season
• Animals that have changed chemoprophylaxis products
• Dogs with clinical signs (e.g., cough, exercise intolerance), radiographic changes, or other laboratory abnormalities suggestive for heartworm disease
• To evaluate the efficacy of adulticide treatment

Cats
Showing clinical signs (e.g., coughing, syncope, unexplained vomiting), radiographic changes, or other laboratory abnormalities consistent with heartworm disease

CONTRAINDICATIONS
• Animals that are <7 months of age, because of the *prepatent period* (the interval between the first infection and the appearance of microfilariae)
• Indiscriminate testing of dogs at any time in the year may result in false negatives if the date of the test is within the predetection period.

POTENTIAL COMPLICATIONS
None

CLIENT EDUCATION
• Dogs: The antigen test result is usually positive 6–7 months after infection. False negatives can occur during the prepatent period, in infections by male worms only, and in animals with low worm burdens.
• Cats: Antibody testing is recommended. A negative antibody test result suggests there is no heartworm disease or a low worm burden. A positive test result should be followed by further diagnostic testing to confirm the diagnosis.

BODY SYSTEMS ASSESSED
• Cardiovascular
• Respiratory

 SAMPLE

COLLECTION
1 mL of venous blood

HANDLING
• Collect into EDTA, a red-top tube, or a serum-separator tube (this varies with the test kit). Check the package insert or contact the reference laboratory for recommendations.
• Test anticoagulated whole blood samples within 24 h of collection.
• If analysis is delayed, separate the plasma or serum from the cells before storing the sample.

STORAGE
• Refrigerate the sample for short-term storage.
• For longer storage, freeze the serum or plasma in vials with airtight seals.

STABILITY
Refrigerated (2°–8°C): 4 days

PROTOCOL
None

 INTERPRETATION

NORMAL FINDINGS OR RANGE
Negative

ABNORMAL VALUES
Positive

CRITICAL VALUES
None

INTERFERING FACTORS
Drugs That May Alter Results or Interpretation
Drugs That Interfere with Test Methodology
None

Drugs That Alter Physiology
None. Preventatives (e.g., diethylcarbamazine, ivermectin, milbemycin) will not affect test results.

Disorders That May Alter Results
Marked hemolysis or lipemia

Collection Techniques or Handling That May Alter Results
Failure to separate serum may result in hemolysis (which can affect the test results).

Influence of Signalment
Species
• Dogs: antigen test recommended
• Cats: antibody test recommended

Breed
None

Age
Because of the prepatent period, it is not necessary to test dogs that are <7 months old.

Gender
None

Pregnancy
None

LIMITATIONS OF THE TEST
• Feline antigen tests are specific but have low sensitivity. Antigen testing cannot rule out heartworm disease in cats.
• Feline antibody tests indicate exposure but are not specific for active infection.

Sensitivity, Specificity, and Positive and Negative Predictive Values
In dogs, these statistical measures of assay performance vary with specific test kit used:

- Specificity: ≈97%
- Sensitivity: 78%–84% (sensitivity increases with higher numbers of female worms)
- Positive predictive value varies depending on prevalence of *Dirofilaria*: The false-positive rate is higher in areas with low disease prevalence.

Valid If Run in Human a Lab?

No. The test requires specific ELISA or immunochromatographic test systems.

CLINICAL PERSPECTIVE

- Dogs
  - Occult (amicrofilaremic) infections are relatively common, whereas only 1% of infections are patent but not antigenemic.
  - Antigen assays are the only appropriate tests for dogs receiving a monthly preventative (ivermectin or milbemycin), because these preventatives can result in sterile adult female worms and amicrofilaremia.
  - In areas with a low prevalence of *Dirofilaria*, positive test results should be confirmed through additional workup (radiographs, etc.).
- Diagnosis of heartworm disease in cats is challenging because they often have nonspecific clinical signs. The antibody test is recommended, but positive cats should be antigen tested.
- Microfilarial testing (modified Knott's test) is recommended in dogs receiving diethylcarbamazine as a preventative.

 MISCELLANEOUS

ANCILLARY TESTS

- Dogs: Antigen positive dogs should also be screened for microfilariae.
- Other testing (e.g., CBC, thoracic radiography, echocardiography) as clinically indicated

SYNONYMS

Dirofilaria test

SEE ALSO

Blackwell's Five-Minute Veterinary Consult: Canine and Feline Topics

- Heartworm Disease—Cats
- Heartworm Disease—Dogs

Related Topics in This Book

- Electrocardiography
- Knott's Test
- Thoracic Radiography

ABBREVIATIONS

None

Suggested Reading

Atkins C. Canine heartworm disease. In: Ettinger SJ, Feldman EC, eds. *Textbook of Veterinary Internal Medicine,* 6th ed. St Louis: Saunders Elsevier, 2006: 1118–1128.

Atkins C. Feline heartworm disease. In: Ettinger SJ, Feldman EC, eds. *Textbook of Veterinary Internal Medicine,* 6th ed. St Louis: Saunders Elsevier, 2006: 1137–1144.

Nelson CT, McCall JW, Rubin SB, *et al.* 2005 Guidelines for the diagnosis, prevention and management of heartworm (*Dirofilaria immitis*) in dogs. *Vet Parasitol* 2005; 133: 255–266.

Nelson CT, McCall JW, Rubin SB, *et al.* 2005 Guidelines for the diagnosis, prevention and management of heartworm (*Dirofilaria immitis*) in cats. *Vet Parasitol* 2005; 133: 267–275.

INTERNET RESOURCES

American Heartworm Society: Canine heartworm disease, http://www.heartwormsociety.org/article.asp?id = 11. Canine heartworm information.

American Heartworm Society: Feline heartworm disease, http://www.heartwormsociety.org/article.asp?id = 16. Feline heartworm information.

Michigan State University, Some Sites, Health Concerns: Canine heartworm disease, http://www.msu.edu/~silvar/heartworm.htm.

AUTHOR NAME

Deborah Groppe Davis

HEINZ BODIES

BASICS

TYPE OF SPECIMEN
Blood

TEST EXPLANATION AND RELATED PHYSIOLOGY
Heinz bodies are aggregates of denatured hemoglobin that form as a result of oxidative damage to hemoglobin. The denatured hemoglobin binds to erythrocyte membrane proteins, causing these erythrocytes to become more susceptible to autoantibodies and also decreasing the deformability of these cells. This can lead to erythrocyte removal from the circulation or lysis and anemia.

On a blood film stained with a Romanovsky-type stain (e.g., Wright's stain, Diff-Quick), Heinz bodies appear as small, pale, eccentrically located structures seen in or protruding from erythrocytes. Although Heinz bodies can be detected in routine smears, they are more easily identified when blood is incubated with a vital stain such as new methylene blue or brilliant cresyl blue prior to the smear preparation. With vital stains, Heinz bodies are dark blue to turquoise, round structures associated with the erythrocyte membrane.

INDICATIONS
• An anemic animal, especially with a history of exposure to oxidizing agents
• Staining with a vital dye should be performed to confirm suspected Heinz bodies seen in a Romanovsky-stained smear.

CONTRAINDICATIONS
None

POTENTIAL COMPLICATIONS
None

CLIENT EDUCATION
• Onions and garlic (raw, cooked, dehydrated, or powdered), or foods containing these substances, can cause hemolytic anemia in dogs and cats because these species are more susceptible to the oxidative effects of these substances than are people.
• Ingestion of zinc-containing ointments (e.g., zinc oxide, creams with sun-blocking action) or pennies produced after 1982 can cause oxidative RBC damage and anemia.
• Acetaminophen administration can cause severe hemolytic anemia, especially in cats.

BODY SYSTEMS ASSESSED
Hemic, lymphatic, and immune

SAMPLE

COLLECTION
0.5–1.0 mL of venous blood

HANDLING
Collect blood into an anticoagulant such as EDTA or heparin.

STORAGE
• Refrigeration is recommended for short-term storage of blood.
• Stained smears should be protected from light.

STABILITY
• Morphologic features of erythrocytes are generally stable for several hours at 25°C and for up to 24 h at 4°C.
• Stained smears are stable for many years if protected from light.

PROTOCOL
Vital stains:
• New methylene blue or other vital stains can be purchased as liquid stain or in individual test tubes containing dehydrated stain.
• Whole blood is mixed with an equivalent volume of stain.
• The suspension should be mixed thoroughly and then incubated for 10 min at 37°C.
• Slides should be prepared as a normal blood film.

INTERPRETATION

NORMAL FINDINGS OR RANGE
• Dogs: no Heinz bodies seen
• Cats: small Heinz bodies in up to 1%–2% of healthy cat RBCs

ABNORMAL VALUES
• Heinz bodies are abnormal findings in dogs and indicate oxidative damage to erythrocytes.
• Cats with increased numbers of Heinz bodies should be evaluated for exposure to oxidants and for diabetes mellitus, hyperthyroidism, or lymphoma.

CRITICAL VALUES
None

INTERFERING FACTORS
Drugs That May Alter Results or Interpretation
Drugs That Interfere with Test Methodology
None

Drugs That Alter Physiology
Drugs that can cause oxidative injury to hemoglobin include acetaminophen, phenazopyridine, benzocaine, propofol, phenylhydrazine, and vitamin K.

Disorders That May Alter Results
Increased numbers of large Heinz bodies can be seen in cats with diabetes mellitus, hyperthyroidism, and lymphoma.

Collection Techniques or Handling That May Alter Results
• Morphology of erythrocytes is best preserved on smears made from fresh blood.
• Proper technique for blood film preparation is needed to ensure an adequate monolayer for erythrocyte evaluation.

Influence of Signalment
Species
Healthy cats may have low numbers of small Heinz bodies.

Breed
None

Age
None

Gender
None

Pregnancy
None

LIMITATIONS OF THE TEST
Sensitivity, Specificity, and Positive and Negative Predictive Values
N/A

Valid If Run in a Human Lab?
Yes.

Causes of Abnormal Findings

High values	Low values
Plants and food additives	Not significant
Allium sp., including onions, chives, leeks, and garlic	
Brassica sp., including cabbages, collards, cauliflower, broccoli, brussel sprouts, and kale	
Propylene glycol	
Drugs	
Acetaminophen	
Benzocaine	
Phenazopyridine	
Propofol	
Phenylhydrazine	
Vitamin K	
Zinc	
Copper	
Naphthalene	
Metabolic disease (in cats)	
Diabetes mellitus	
Hyperthyroidism	
Lymphoma	

CLINICAL PERSPECTIVE
• Formation of Heinz bodies typically leads to extravascular hemolysis. However, oxidants can also cause formation of eccentrocytes and methemoglobin. Oxidation of membrane lipids can cause intravascular hemolysis.
• Identification of Heinz bodies on a canine blood film should initiate a search for exposure of the patient to potentially oxidative substances.
• The toxicity of onions and garlic is dose dependent.
• Heinz bodies are less likely to cause significant anemia in cats, as compared to dogs, although finding large numbers of Heinz bodies in an anemic cat should initiate a search for exposure to potentially oxidative substances.
• In cats, increased numbers of large Heinz bodies have also been associated with diabetes mellitus, hyperthyroidism, and lymphoma.
• In cats, increased numbers of Heinz bodies have been associated with semimoist cat foods containing propylene glycol.

MISCELLANEOUS
ANCILLARY TESTS
• A complete CBC with evaluation of RBC morphology
• A reticulocyte count if anemia is present
• A chemistry profile and urinalysis
• Other testing (e.g., of zinc or copper levels) depends on the cause of the Heinz body formation.

SYNONYMS
None

SEE ALSO
Blackwell's Five-Minute Veterinary Consult: Canine and Feline Topics
• Acetaminophen Toxicity
• Anemia, Heinz Body
• Zinc Toxicity
Related Topics in This Book
• Red Blood Cell Count
• Red Blood Cell Morphology
• Zinc

ABBREVIATIONS
None

Suggested Reading
Desnoyers M. Anemias associated with Heinz bodies. In: Feldman BF, Zinkl JG, Jain NC, eds. *Schalm's Veterinary Hematology,* 5th ed. Baltimore: Lippincott Williams & Wilkins, 2000: 178–183.
Stockham SL, Scott MA. Basic hematologic assays. In: *Essentials of Veterinary Clinical Pathology.* Ames: Iowa State Press, 2002: 31–48.
Stockham SL, Scott MA. Erythrocytes. In: *Essentials of Veterinary Clinical Pathology.* Ames: Iowa State Press, 2002: 85–154.
Thrall MA. Regenerative anemia. In: Thrall MA, ed. *Veterinary Hematology and Clinical Chemistry.* Baltimore: Lippincott Williams & Wilkins, 2004: 95–119.

INTERNET RESOURCES
Cope RB. *Allium* species poisoning in dogs and cats [Toxicology brief]. Vet Med 2005 (August), http://www.aspca.org/site/DocServer/vetm0805_562–566.pdf?docID = 5602&AddInterest = 1101.
University of Georgia, College of Veterinary Medicine, Veterinary Clinical Pathology Clerkship Program: Tarigo-Martinie J, Krimer P. Heinz body anemia in cats, 2002, http://www.vet.uga.edu/vpp/CLERK/Tarigo.

AUTHOR NAME
Karen Zaks

HEMATOCRIT

BASICS

TYPE OF SPECIMEN
Blood

TEST EXPLANATION AND RELATED PHYSIOLOGY
The terms packed cell volume (PCV) and hematocrit (Hct) are used synonymously, although their values actually are enumerated differently. A *PCV* is a *measured* number that represents the percentage of RBCs in whole blood. A microcapillary tube full of blood is centrifuged, and the height of the RBC column is measured relative to the top of the plasma column. An *Hct* is a *calculated* number generated by automated hematology analyzers. *Hematology analyzers* measure the number of erythrocytes and their mean cell volume, and then use an equation to calculate the Hct [Hct % = RBCs × $10^6/\mu$L × MCV (fL)/10].

A centrifuged microcapillary tube will display 3 distinct layers: packed RBCs at the bottom; a thin, middle band composed of WBCs and platelets (the *buffy coat*); and the plasma on top. The plasma may be evaluated for evidence of lipemia, hemolysis, and icterus, and may be used for total plasma protein determination by refractometry. The PCV provides a rapid determination of RBC mass when hematology analyzers are unavailable. A decreased PCV is termed *anemia*, and an increased PCV is termed *polycythemia* or, more appropriately, *erythrocytosis*. Measurement of PCV determines the presence or absence of abnormalities in erythrocyte mass but does not determine the underlying cause for the abnormality. Concurrent evaluation of the erythrocyte indices (MCV, MCHC) and a peripheral blood smear evaluation often help to identify the cause of the alteration.

Measurement of PCV and its comparison to automated analyzer–generated Hct can be used as quality control for the analyzer. PCV determined by the centrifugation method and Hct determined by an automated analyzer will vary slightly. However, if the variation exceeds 3%–5%, a technical problem may exist in 1 of the 2 methods.

INDICATIONS
• Estimation of erythroid mass
• Gross examination of the plasma for evidence of hemolysis, lipemia, or icterus

CONTRAINDICATIONS
None

POTENTIAL COMPLICATIONS
None

CLIENT EDUCATION
None

BODY SYSTEMS ASSESSED
Hemic, lymphatic, and immune

SAMPLE

COLLECTION
Venous blood: Only fractions of 1 mL of blood are required to fill a microcapillary tube, but 1–3 mL of blood is usually collected so that a CBC may concurrently be performed.

HANDLING
• EDTA is preferred, but heparin may also be used.
• Evacuated tubes must be filled appropriately to prevent dilutional effects of the anticoagulant.
• Transport the sample on ice to the laboratory.

STORAGE
• Anticoagulated blood samples should be refrigerated if not processed within 2–4 h.
• Spun samples in microcapillary tubes will desiccate and thus should be read soon after centrifugation.

STABILITY
• Room temperature: 2–4 h
• Refrigerated (2°–8°C): RBCs are generally stable for up to 48 h.

PROTOCOL
PCV determination:
• Equipment needed: microcapillary tubes, tube sealant (putty), a microcapillary centrifuge, and a device to read the tube
• Place the open end of a microcapillary tube into a well-mixed EDTA blood sample and allow capillary action to fill tube. Holding the tube horizontally or tipping it downward slightly will facilitate filling.
• Fill the tube approximately two-thirds to three-quarters full and seal 1 end with the sealant putty by pressing the tube into the putty.
• Place the tube into the microcapillary centrifuge, putty facing out, and centrifuge it at high speed for ≈5 min. The exact speed and centrifugation time depend on the centrifuge manufacturer recommendations.
• Use a tube-reading device to measure the PCV.

INTERPRETATION

NORMAL FINDINGS OR RANGE
Reference intervals vary depending on geographic location, the laboratory performing the analysis, and the age, gender, and breed of the patient. The following intervals are only general guidelines:
• Dogs: 40%–60%. Note: Hct may be reported in SI units as 0.4–0.6 L/L.
• Cats: 30%–45%. Note: Hct may be reported in SI units as 0.30–0.45 L/L.

ABNORMAL VALUES
Any value 5% above or below the reference interval is interpreted to be an abnormal finding.

CRITICAL VALUES
• Dogs: <20%
• Cats: <15%

INTERFERING FACTORS
Drugs That May Alter Results or Interpretation
Drugs That Interfere with Test Methodology
Use of Oxyglobin [hemoglobin glutamer-200 (bovine)] discolors the plasma, which makes it difficult to distinguish the RBC layer from the buffy coat and plasma layers.

Drugs That Alter Physiology
None

Disorders That May Alter Results
• Centrifugal packing of RBCs may be less than complete if the PCV is >50%, causing overestimation of the PCV.
• A PCV of <25% results in tighter packing of RBCs, which underestimates the PCV.
• Changes in plasma volume will affect PCV.
• Calculated Hct may be erroneous if there is artifactual alteration in the MCV or absolute RBC count.
• RBC agglutination can result in spuriously decreased calculated Hct.
• Cats naturally have large platelets and small RBCs, which may be difficult for automated analyzers to discern from one another. Enumeration of platelets as small RBCs may falsely increase RBC counts and thus calculated Hct.

Collection Techniques or Handling That May Alter Results

- If microcapillary tubes are filled to more than two-thirds to three-quarters full, cell packing is incomplete and the PCV may be overestimated.
- Spinning too briefly or too slowly will lead to an overestimation of PCV, and poor centrifuge maintenance may result in insufficient *g* forces.
- Failure to align the microcapillary tube properly on the tube-reading device or card can result in erroneous measurements.
- Underfilling evacuated tubes causes artifactual dilution of the sample by excess EDTA.

Influence of Signalment

Species
Cats have lower PCV as compared to dogs.

Breed
The PCV of some breeds (e.g., greyhounds and dachshunds) may be higher than average.

Age
Neonatal animals (<6 months of age) typically have mildly decreased PCV as compared to adults.

Gender
Gender differences do occur, but reference intervals are generated from both genders, so gender differences will be masked.

Pregnancy
PCV may decrease to 29%–35% in pregnant dogs because of increased plasma volume.

LIMITATIONS OF THE TEST

Sensitivity, Specificity, and Positive and Negative Predictive Values
Properly performed, centrifugal determination of PCV is an accurate measurement with little inherent error (+/−1%).

Valid If Run in Human Lab?
- Spun PCV: Yes, but interpretation should be based on veterinary reference intervals.
- Calculated Hct from an automated analyzer: No, unless the automated hematology analyzer has been calibrated for veterinary species. Hematology analyzers calibrated for human patients may not correctly categorize small feline erythrocytes or large feline platelets, which could interfere with RBC count, MCV, and subsequently Hct (since it is calculated from measured RBCs and MCV).

Causes of Abnormal Findings

High values	Low values
Relative	Anemia of chronic disease/inflammation
Hemoconcentration	Lack of erythropoietin caused by chronic kidney disease
Splenic contraction	
Absolute	Blood loss
Hypoxia (heart or lung disease)	GI ulceration
High altitude	Hemostasis defects
Erythropoietin producing tumors or cysts	Neoplasia
	Parasitism
Renal neoplasia (e.g., lymphoma)	Surgery
	Trauma
Primary erythrocytosis (aka polycythemia vera)	Hemolysis
	Immune-mediated (primary or secondary)
	RBC parasites
	Oxidants (e.g., acetaminophen, onions)
	Zinc toxicity or copper toxicity
	Fragmentation (e.g., disseminated intravascular coagulation, neoplasia, heartworm)
	Snake envenomation
	Iron deficiency
	Endocrine disorders (e.g., hypothyroidism)
	Bone marrow disease (decreased production)
	Infections (*Ehrlichia canis*, FeLV, FIV, panleukopenia, parvovirus)
	Myelophthisis
	Toxic bone marrow damage
	Pure RBC aplasia
	Erythroid myeloproliferative or myelodysplastic diseases
	Nutritional deficiencies (rare)

HEMATOCRIT

CLINICAL PERSPECTIVE

- Decreased Hct (PCV) is often arbitrarily categorized as mild, moderate, or severe.
  - Dogs: mild, 30%–37%; moderate, 20%–29%; severe, 13%–19%
  - Cats: mild, 20%–26%; moderate, 14%–19%; severe, 10%–13%
- Changes in plasma volume will affect PCV and therefore interpretation should be made with knowledge of the patient's hydration status.
- It can be useful to interpret Hct and TP together.
  - Decreases in both Hct and TP suggest blood loss, although, in stressed dogs, splenic contraction may temporarily mask the decreased Hct.
  - Increases in both Hct and TP suggest hemoconcentration (dehydration).
- PCV should always be interpreted with the erythrocyte indices (MCV and MCHC) and a peripheral blood smear evaluation.
  - Decreases in both MCV and MCHC suggest iron deficiency.
  - An increased MCV and decreased MCHC suggest a regenerative response to anemia.

MISCELLANEOUS

ANCILLARY TESTS

- Total protein
- Complete CBC, including evaluation of RBC morphologic features
- Bone marrow aspiration and biopsy may be warranted in animals with chronic nonregenerative anemias.

SYNONYMS

Packed cell volume (PCV)

SEE ALSO

Blackwell's Five-Minute Veterinary Consult: Canine and Feline Topics

- Anemia, Aplastic
- Anemia, Heinz Body
- Anemia, Iron-Deficiency
- Anemia, Metabolic (Anemias with Spiculated Red Cells)
- Anemia, Nonregenerative
- Anemia, Regenerative
- Polycythemia
- Polycythemia Vera

Related Topics in This Book

- Blood Smear Microscopic Examination
- Hemoglobin
- Red Blood Cell Count
- Red Blood Cell Indices
- Red Blood Cell Morphology
- Reticulocyte Count

ABBREVIATIONS

None

Suggested Reading

Lassen ED, Weiser G. Laboratory technology for veterinary medicine. In: Thrall MA, ed. *Veterinary Hematology and Clinical Chemistry*. Philadelphia: Lippincott Williams & Wilkins, 2004: 3–37.

INTERNET RESOURCES

Rebar AH, MacWilliams PS, Feldman BF, *et al*. Laboratory methods in hematology. In: Rebar A, MacWilliams P, Feldman BF, *et al*., eds. A Guide to Hematology in Dogs and Cats. Jackson, WY: Teton NewMedia, 2001; Ithaca, NY: International Veterinary Information Service (IVIS), 2004, http://www.ivis.org/docarchive/A3303.1204.pdf.

AUTHOR NAME

Jennifer L. Brazzell

BASICS

TYPE OF SPECIMEN
Blood

TEST EXPLANATION AND RELATED PHYSIOLOGY
Hemoglobin concentration, RBC count, and PCV are all measures of RBC mass and generally increase and decrease together. Hemoglobin concentration is the most direct measure of the oxygen-carrying capacity of blood, but its measurement does not provide significantly more information than measurement of PCV or absolute RBC count. Hemoglobin concentration may provide a more reliable measurement of RBC mass if artifactual cell swelling, cell shrinkage, or increased cell fragility have occurred. If RBC size is within normal limits, the hemoglobin concentration should be roughly one-third of the calculated Hct or measured PCV. Hemoglobin is measured spectrophotometrically by hematology analyzers after dilution and chemical lysis of the RBCs in the blood sample. (*Spectrophotometry* measures the absorbance of light passed through the sample.) Increased hemoglobin concentrations result in increased light absorbance and vice versa. Unlike other analyzers, the IDEXX QBC VetAutoread (IDEXX Laboratories, Portland, ME) reports a calculated hemoglobin concentration.

INDICATIONS
- To estimate the erythroid mass (usually to document anemia)
- Enables calculation of the MCHC

CONTRAINDICATIONS
None

POTENTIAL COMPLICATIONS
None

CLIENT EDUCATION
Lipemia interferes with plasma light transmission and may cause hemolysis. Consider withholding food for 12 h prior to sampling.

BODY SYSTEMS ASSESSED
Hemic, lymphatic, and immune

SAMPLE

COLLECTION
1–3 mL of venous blood

HANDLING
- EDTA is the preferred anticoagulant, but heparin may also be used.
- Refrigerate.
- If it is being sent to a diagnostic laboratory, transport the sample on ice.

STORAGE
- Anticoagulated blood samples should be refrigerated if not processed within 2–4 h.

STABILITY
- Room temperature: 2–4 h
- Refrigerated (2°–8°C): Erythrocytes are generally stable for up to 24–48 h.

PROTOCOL
None

INTERPRETATION

NORMAL FINDINGS OR RANGE
Reference intervals depend on geographic location; the laboratory performing the analysis; and the age, gender, and breed of the patient. The following intervals are only general guidelines:
- Dogs: 13–20 g/dL (SI units, 130–200 g/L)
- Cats: 10–15 g/dL (SI units, 100–150 g/L)

ABNORMAL VALUES
Values above or below the normal reference interval

CRITICAL VALUES
- Dogs: <7 g/dL (SI units, <70 g/L)
- Cats: <5 g/dL (SI units, <50 g/L)

INTERFERING FACTORS
Drugs That May Alter Results or Interpretation
Drugs That Interfere with Test Methodology
With most hematology instruments, Oxyglobin (chemically modified bovine hemoglobin) is measured along with patient hemoglobin. Although the measurement does not reflect RBC numbers, it does indicate oxygen-carrying capacity.

Drugs That Alter Physiology
None

Disorders That May Alter Results
• Lipemia increases sample opacity and may cause in vitro hemolysis resulting in falsely increased concentrations.
• Iatrogenic or pathologic hemolysis of a sample results in falsely increased concentrations.
• Increased numbers of Heinz bodies result in falsely increased concentrations.

Collection Techniques or Handling That May Alter Results
• Traumatic venipuncture or inappropriate sample handling may result in hemolysis that artifactually increases the measured hemoglobin concentration.

Influence of Signalment
Species
Cats have lower hemoglobin concentrations than dogs.

Breed
Hemoglobin concentrations of some breeds (e.g., greyhounds and dachshunds) may be higher than average.

Age
Neonatal animals (<6 months of age) typically have more mildly decreased hemoglobin concentrations than adults.

Gender
Gender differences do occur, but because reference intervals are generally generated from both genders, any differences are masked.

Pregnancy
Hemoglobin concentration may decrease in pregnant dogs because of increased plasma volume and hemodilution.

LIMITATIONS OF THE TEST
Sensitivity, Specificity, and Positive and Negative Predictive Values
N/A

Valid If Run in a Human Lab?
Yes—but interpretation should be based on veterinary reference intervals.

Causes of Abnormal Findings

High values	Low values
Relative	Anemia of chronic disorders
Hemoconcentration	Erythropoietin lack because
Splenic contraction	of chronic kidney disease
Absolute	Blood loss
Hypoxia (e.g., heart or	Trauma
lung disease)	Neoplasia
High altitude	Surgery
Erythropoietin-producing tumors	GI ulceration
Primary erythrocytosis	Parasitism
(aka polycythemia vera)	Hemostasis defects
	Hemolysis
	Immune mediated
	(primary or secondary)
	RBC parasites
	Oxidants (e.g.,
	acetaminophen,
	onions)
	Zinc or copper toxicity
	Fragmentation (e.g.,
	disseminated intravascular
	coagulation, neoplasia,
	heartworm)
	Snake envenomation
	Iron deficiency
	Endocrine disorders
	(e.g., hypothyroidism)
	Bone marrow disease
	(decreased production)
	Infections (e.g., FeLV, FIV,
	panleukopenia, parvovirus,
	Ehrlichia canis)
	Myelophthisis
	Toxic bone marrow damage
	Pure red cell aplasia
	Erythroid myeloproliferative
	and myelodysplastic
	diseases
	Nutritional deficiencies (rare)

CLINICAL PERSPECTIVE

- Changes is plasma volume will affect PCV and hemoglobin concentrations, so their interpretation should be made with knowledge of the patient's hydration status.
- Hemoglobin determinations are useful for calculating MCHC.
  - Elevated MCHC suggests an artifact in hemoglobin measurement (e.g., lipemia).
  - Decreased MCHC could be due to a regenerative response to anemia, iron or copper deficiency, or a portosystemic shunt.
- Measurement of hemoglobin concentration in patients that have received Oxyglobin likely provides a truer estimate of oxygen-carrying capacity than do absolute RBC counts or PCV.

 MISCELLANEOUS

ANCILLARY TESTS

Bone marrow aspiration and biopsy may be warranted in cases of chronic nonregenerative anemias.

SYNONYMS

None

SEE ALSO

Blackwell's Five-Minute Veterinary Consult: Canine and Feline Topics

- Anemia, Aplastic
- Anemia, Heinz Body
- Anemia, Iron-Deficiency
- Anemia, Metabolic (Anemias with Spiculated Red Cells)
- Anemia, Nonregenerative
- Anemia, Regenerative

Related Topics in This Book

- Blood Smear Microscopic Examination
- Hematocrit
- Red Blood Cell Count
- Red Blood Cell Indices
- Red Blood Cell Morphology

ABBREVIATIONS

None

Suggested Reading

Thrall MA, ed. *Veterinary Hematology and Clinical Chemistry*. Philadelphia: Lippincott Williams & Wilkins, 2004.

INTERNET RESOURCES

Cornell University, College of Veterinary Medicine, Clinical Pathology Modules, Hemogram Basics: Hemoglobin, http://www.diaglab.vet.cornell.edu/clinpath/modules/hemogram/hb.htm.

AUTHOR NAME

Jennifer L. Brazzell

BASICS

TYPE OF SPECIMEN
Blood

TEST EXPLANATION AND RELATED PHYSIOLOGY
Hemotrophic mycoplasmas are Gram-negative erythrocyte parasites. Previously classified as rickettsia in the genera *Haemobartonella* and *Eperythrozoon*, these organisms are now classified as mycoplasmas. The exact means of transmission has not been definitively determined. In cats, bloodsucking arthropods such as fleas are thought to be the primary means of transmission. In dogs, the brown dog tick (*Rhipicephalus sanguineus*) has been shown experimentally to transmit the disease. Iatrogenic transmission via blood transfusions has also been documented.

There are 2 hemotrophic mycoplasmas in cats: *Mycoplasma haemofelis* (formerly *Haemobartonella felis* large variant) and *Mycoplasma haemominutum* (formerly *Haemobartonella felis* small variant). The 2 species in cats have different pathogenicities. *Mycoplasma haemofelis* is the cause of feline infectious anemia. Acute infection with *M. haemofelis* is associated with high numbers of organisms in the peripheral blood with a severe (and possibly fatal) hemolytic anemia. Commonly, cats will present with lethargy, anorexia, fever, and anemia. The anemia is typically regenerative. Cats infected with *M. haemominutum* are often subclinical or have only mild clinical signs. The hematocrit usually remains within the normal range for cats.

Mycoplasma haemocanis (formerly *Haemobartonella canis*) is the organism found in dogs. The acute form of the disease is found in splenectomized or immunocompromised animals. There is a rapidly developing anemia with numerous parasites seen in the peripheral blood. It can also be found in animals with intact spleens and concurrent infections (e.g., babesiosis, ehrlichiosis, and/or septicemia). Clinical signs include anorexia, lethargy, weight loss, and fever. The anemia is typically regenerative.

Organisms can often be seen on a air-dried Romanovsky stained (Wright's stain or Diff-Quick; Dade Behring, Deerfield, IL). Organisms are rod-shaped, spherical, or ring-shaped structures individually and in chains (especially *M. haemocanis*) across the RBC surface. The organisms range in size from 0.3 to 0.8 μm. Low numbers of organisms can be difficult to see with Diff-Quick. Differentiation of organisms from artifacts such as stain precipitate, drying artifacts, basophilic stippling, siderotic inclusion, and Howell-Jolly bodies can be challenging. PCR is a more sensitive molecular technique that amplifies a specific fragment of the organism's DNA and can be used to either confirm infection or identify asymptomatic carriers.

INDICATIONS
- A cat with regenerative anemia, especially if associated with fever
- A splenectomized dog
- An immunocompromised dog, especially if anemic
- A potential blood donor

CONTRAINDICATIONS
None

POTENTIAL COMPLICATIONS
None

CLIENT EDUCATION
- Hemotrophic mycoplasmas can be found in ≈25% of anemic cats in the United States. Without therapy, approximately one-third of cats infected with *M. haemofelis* will die of severe anemia.
- Of cats with hemotrophic mycoplasmosis, 40%–50% are FeLV positive and should be tested for this disease.

- Long-term feline infection with *M. haemominutum* can be associated with concurrent FIV and FeLV infections, as well as with other debilitating diseases.

BODY SYSTEMS ASSESSED
Hemic, lymphatic, and immune

SAMPLE

COLLECTION
0.5–1.0 mL of venous blood

HANDLING
Collect into EDTA anticoagulant and make a blood smear immediately after sample collection.

STORAGE
- Refrigerate whole blood (2°–8°C).
- Store slides at room temperature, protected from light and humidity.

STABILITY
- Refrigerated blood (2°–8°C): 2 days
- Slides can be stored for months or years.

PROTOCOL
None

INTERPRETATION

NORMAL FINDINGS OR RANGE
No parasites detected on the peripheral blood or by PCR analysis

ABNORMAL VALUES
The presence of organisms in the peripheral blood and/or PCR positive

CRITICAL VALUES
None

INTERFERING FACTORS
Drugs That May Alter Results or Interpretation
Drugs That Interfere with Test Methodology
None

Drugs That Alter Physiology
Antibiotic therapy can mask infection.

Disorders That May Alter Results
None

Collection Techniques or Handling That May Alter Results
Storage of EDTA tube for >6–8 h can cause organisms to fall off RBC membranes, making their identification much more challenging. Preparation of a blood film at the time of sample collection can avoid this artifact.

Influence of Signalment
Species
Dogs: clinical disease is usually only seen in splenectomized or immunocompromised animals.

Breed
None

Age
None

Gender
None

Pregnancy
None

LIMITATIONS OF THE TEST
Sensitivity, Specificity, and Positive and Negative Predictive Values
N/A

Valid If Run in a Human Lab?
Yes and no. Blood smears can be evaluated by properly trained personnel, but the PCR assay requires specific primers unique to the organism that are currently available only in veterinary laboratories.

CLINICAL PERSPECTIVE
• *Mycoplasma haemofelis* parasitemia is often cyclical, with the lowest hematocrit associated with the highest numbers of organisms. Hematocrit increases rapidly as organisms disappear from peripheral blood.
• PCR for hemotrophic mycoplasmas is highly sensitive. Blood-donor cats and dogs should be tested regularly.
• Animals that are treated and recover are often chronic carriers.

MISCELLANEOUS
ANCILLARY TESTS
• Serial CBC to monitor the anemia
• PCR after therapy is completed to check for a possible chronic carrier
• FIV and FeLV tests in cats
• In nonsplenectomized dogs, consider testing for concurrent *Ehrlichia, Babesia,* bacterial, or viral infections.

SYNONYMS
• Feline infectious anemia
• *Haemobartonella*
• *Mycoplasma haemocanis*
• *Mycoplasma haemofelis*
• *Mycoplasma haemominutum*

SEE ALSO
Blackwell's Five-Minute Veterinary Consult: Canine and Feline Topics
• Anemia, Regenerative
• Hemotrophic Mycoplasmosis (Haemobartonellosis)
Related Topics in This Book
• Hematocrit
• Red Blood Cell Count
• Red Blood Cell Morphology

ABBREVIATIONS
None

Suggested Reading
Messick JB. Hemotrophic mycoplasmas (hemoplasmas): A review and new insights into pathogenic potential. *Vet Clin Pathol* 2004; 33: 2–13.
Messick JB. New perspectives about hemotrophic mycoplasma (formerly *Haemobartonella* and *Eperythrozoon* species) infections in dogs and cats. *Vet Clin Small Anim* 2003; 33: 1453–1465.

INTERNET RESOURCES
None

AUTHOR NAME
Deborah Groppe Davis

HIGH-DOSE DEXAMETHASONE SUPPRESSION TEST

 BASICS

TYPE OF SPECIMEN
Blood

TEST EXPLANATION AND RELATED PHYSIOLOGY
Cortisol is the major glucocorticoid secreted by the adrenal cortex. Synthesis and secretion of cortisol are stimulated by ACTH from the pituitary gland. ACTH secretion is regulated by corticotropin-releasing hormone (CRH) from the hypothalamus. In turn, rising levels of cortisol suppress secretion of both CRH and ACTH though negative feedback.

The high-dose dexamethasone suppression test (HDDST) works on the principle that, in normal patients, administration of exogenous glucocorticoid (dexamethasone) inhibits secretion of CRH and ACTH, thus suppressing endogenous cortisol secretion. Animals with hyperadrenocorticism are abnormally resistant to physiologic levels of negative feedback. However, administration of large doses of dexamethasone should eventually suppress ACTH (and therefore cortisol) in dogs with pituitary-dependent hyperadrenocorticism (PDH). Cortisol remains unchanged in patients with a functional adrenal tumor (AT) because ACTH levels are already maximally suppressed by chronic excess cortisol levels.

INDICATIONS
Used to differentiate PDH from an AT after a positive screening test result for hyperadrenocorticism is obtained

CONTRAINDICATIONS
• Do not use as a screening test for hyperadrenocorticism.
• Its use is inappropriate as a screen for iatrogenic hyperadrenocorticism.
• Do not use to monitor treatment of hyperadrenocorticism.
• Its use may not be necessary in dogs with hyperadrenocorticism if the low-dose dexamethasone suppression test (LDDST) shows adequate suppression at 4 h (<1.4 μg/dL).

POTENTIAL COMPLICATIONS
None

CLIENT EDUCATION
• Fasting samples are preferred.
• Basal levels of cortisol alone provide limited information about adrenocortical function.
• Ancillary tests may be required if the results are inconclusive.

BODY SYSTEMS ASSESSED
• Endocrine and metabolic

 SAMPLE

COLLECTION
1–2 mL of venous blood

HANDLING
• Choice of the collection tube depends on the assay: Some labs use serum (red-top tube), whereas others use plasma (EDTA), so check with the laboratory before submitting the sample.
• Centrifuge and transfer the serum or plasma into a transport tube. Do not store the sample in a serum-separator tube.
• Label the tubes with the time of collection.
• Refrigerate or freeze and ship the sample with cold packs in an insulated container.

STORAGE
Refrigerate for short-term storage and freeze for long-term storage.

STABILITY
• Refrigerated (2°–8°C): 1 week
• Frozen (−20°C): up to 3 months

PROTOCOL
1. Collect a baseline serum sample.
2. Administer dexamethasone sodium phosphate or dexamethasone in polyethylene glycol (e.g., Azium):
   • Dogs: 0.1 mg/kg IV
   • Cats: 1.0 mg/kg IV
3. Collect samples at 4 and 8 h after dexamethasone injection.
4. Submit all 3 samples for cortisol assay.

 INTERPRETATION

NORMAL FINDINGS OR RANGE
• Normal values are established for each laboratory, but ranges are usually very similar.
• Typical basal cortisol levels:
   • Dogs: 0.6–6.0 μg/dL (17–170 nmol/L)
   • Cats: 0.6–5.0 μg/dL (17–140 nmol/L)
• Cortisol <1.4 μg/dL (40 nmol/L) at 4 and 8 h

ABNORMAL VALUES
• PDH, <1.4 μg/dL at 4 and/or 8 h; or cortisol level, $<50\%$ of baseline at 4 and/or 8 h
• PDH or AT, >1.4 μg/dL at 4 and 8 h; or cortisol level, $>50\%$ of baseline at 4 and 8 h

CRITICAL VALUES
None

INTERFERING FACTORS
Drugs That May Alter Results or Interpretation
Drugs That Interfere with Test Methodology
• Prednisone and prednisolone (or structurally related steroids) cross-react in the cortisol assay, falsely elevating results. Discontinue steroid therapy for 2 days prior to performing test.
• Dexamethasone does not interfere with the cortisol assay.

Drugs That Alter Physiology
Anticonvulsant therapy

Disorders That May Alter Results
• Nonadrenal illness and stress can elevate cortisol concentrations.
• Severe hyperbilirubinemia (>20 mg/dL) can falsely elevate cortisol levels measured by a chemiluminescent enzyme immunoassay.

Collection Techniques or Handling That May Alter Results
• Storage of serum in a serum-separator tube may alter results. Cortisol levels, as measured by a chemiluminescent enzyme immunoassay, can be increased when blood is collected into Becton Dickinson SST vacutainer tubes (BD Diagnostics, Franklin Lakes, NJ). However, the effects on cortisol measurements vary depending on the type of assay, as well as the type of blood collection tube used, since the latter can contain different additives (e.g., physical barriers or clot activators).
• Nonfasting samples with excessive lipemia may affect some assays.
• Inappropriate use of anticoagulant can produce an assay dependent effect:
   • Use of heparinized plasma can decrease cortisol levels measured by a chemiluminescent enzyme immunoassay.
   • Use of EDTA plasma can increase cortisol levels by as much as 30% when measured by radioimmunoassay.

Influence of Signalment

Species
Cats are more resistant than dogs to the suppressive effects of dexamethasone.

Breed
None

Age
None

Gender
None

Pregnancy
None

LIMITATIONS OF THE TEST
Sensitivity, Specificity, and Positive and Negative Predictive Values
- ≈75% of dogs with PDH will meet 1 of the criteria for suppression.
- ≈25% of dogs with PDH will demonstrate no suppression at 4 or 8 h.
- ≈40%–55% of cats with PDH will meet 1 of the criteria for suppression at the 4 h and/or 8 h time points.

Valid If Run in a Human Lab?
Yes—if a cortisol assay validated for dogs and cats is used.

Causes of Abnormal Findings

High values (lack of suppression)	Low values (suppression at 4 or 8 h)
AT	PDH
≈25% of dogs with PDH	Improper handling or storage (see Collection Techniques or Handling That May Alter Results)
Chronic stress	
Nonadrenal illness	
Drugs (prednisone, prednisolone, or other related steroids)	
Improper handling or storage (see Collection Techniques or Handling That May Alter Results)	

CLINICAL PERSPECTIVE
- The HDDST should not be used as a screening test for hyperadrenocorticism because the results for normal dogs and those with PDH can be similar.
- Since some pituitary tumors are resistant to suppression, an abnormal HDDST result requires additional tests to confirm (or rule out) an AT.
- Tumors in the pars intermedia and large pars distalis tumors are more likely to be resistant to dexamethasone.
- The 0.1-mg/kg dexamethasone dose used in dogs suppresses cortisol levels adequately in only ≈20% of PDH cats. The use of this dose is therefore not recommended for discriminating PDH from AT in cats.

MISCELLANEOUS
ANCILLARY TESTS
- Endogenous ACTH can be used to differentiate AT from PDH, especially if the results of the HDDST show lack of suppression or appear inconclusive.
- Ultrasonographic examination of the adrenal glands:
  - PDH: bilaterally symmetrical adrenal glands
  - AT: The affected gland often is irregularly round with mixed echogenicity; sometimes with a homogeneous nodule.

SYNONYMS
None

SEE ALSO
Blackwell's Five-Minute Veterinary Consult: Canine and Feline Topics
- Hyperadrenocorticism (Cushing's Disease)—Cats
- Hyperadrenocorticism (Cushing's Disease)—Dogs

Related Topics in This Book
- ACTH Assay
- ACTH Stimulation Test
- Adrenal Ultrasonography
- Cortisol
- Cortisol/Creatinine Ratio
- Low-Dose Dexamethasone Suppression Test

ABBREVIATIONS
- ACTH = adrenocorticotropic hormone
- AT = adrenal tumor
- CRH = corticotropin-releasing hormone
- HDDST = high-dose dexamethasone suppression test
- LDDST = low-dose dexamethasone suppression test
- PDH = pituitary-dependent hyperadrenocorticism

Suggested Reading
Feldman EC, Nelson RW. *Canine and Feline Endocrinology and Reproduction.* St Louis: Saunders Elsevier, 2004: 252–393.
Ferguson DC, Hoenig M. Endocrine system. In: Lattimer KS, Mahaffey EA, Prasse KW, eds. *Duncan and Prasse's Veterinary Laboratory Medicine: Clinical Pathology*, 4th ed. Ames: Iowa State Press, 2003: 270–303.
Reusch CE. Hyperadrenocorticism. In: Ettinger SJ, Feldman EC, eds. *Textbook of Veterinary Internal Medicine*, 6th ed. Philadelphia: WB Saunders, 2004: 1592–1612.

INTERNET RESOURCES
None

AUTHOR NAME
Janice M. Andrews

HORIZONTAL BEAM RADIOGRAPHY

 BASICS

TYPE OF PROCEDURE
Radiographic

PROCEDURE EXPLANATION AND RELATED PHYSIOLOGY
The X-ray tube head and cassette are rotated 90° from the typical vertical orientation. During exposure, X-rays are emitted parallel to the floor. The patient positioning depends on the goal of the study.

INDICATIONS
Abdomen
Determine or confirm the presence of free peritoneal gas (pneumoperitoneum).

Skeletal System
• An alternate method for making craniocaudal or dorsopalmar (plantar) extremity radiographs
• Obtain a VD projection of animals with suspected spinal fractures.

Thorax
• Improve the visualization of structures (cardiac silhouette, lungs, mediastinum) obscured by the pleural effusion by moving the pleural effusion via gravity.
• Distinguish among lung, pleural, and extrapleural masses.
• Determine whether a lung mass is cavitated.

CONTRAINDICATIONS
• None
• Use caution when positioning an animal with suspected spinal fracture.

POTENTIAL COMPLICATIONS
None

CLIENT EDUCATION
None

BODY SYSTEMS ASSESSED
• Cardiovascular
• Gastrointestinal
• Hepatobiliary
• Musculoskeletal
• Neuromuscular
• Respiratory

 PROCEDURE

PATIENT PREPARATION
Preprocedure Medication or Preparation
None

Anesthesia or Sedation
As needed

Patient Positioning
Abdomen
The animal is in left lateral recumbency (Figure 1). With the animal in this position, any fluid in the stomach will move into the fundus and any gas in the stomach will move to the pylorus. It is easier to distinguish free gas in the peritoneum from gas in the pylorus than from gas in the fundus.

Musculoskeletal System
The animal is in lateral recumbency with the joint or bone being radiographed away from the X-ray table (e.g., to image the right stifle, place the animal in left lateral recumbency) (Figure 2). Aligning the X-ray tube with the cassette is easier when the limb is not directly against the X-ray table. To radiograph the right stifle, place the animal in left lateral recumbency. Lateral projections of the joint or bone also can be made from this position—just remember to adjust the X-ray tube to film distance.

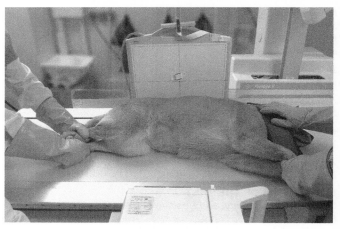

Figure 1

Horizontal beam, VD projection with a dog in left lateral recumbency. The dog is on its left side with its legs toward the front of the X-ray table. The X-ray tube head is oriented parallel to the floor (*bottom* of the figure), and the X-ray cassette is against the dog's spine, perpendicular to the X-ray cassette.

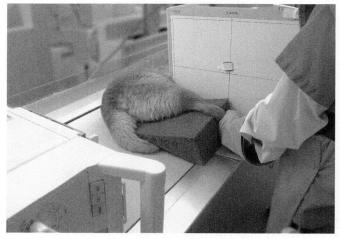

Figure 2

Horizontal beam, caudocranial projection of a dog's right stifle. The dog is on its left side with its legs toward the front of the X-ray table. The X-ray tube head is oriented parallel to the floor (*bottom left* of figure), and the X-ray cassette is cranial the dog's right stifle, perpendicular to the X-ray cassette.

Spine
The animal is positioned in either right or left lateral recumbency (Figure 1).

Thorax
Pleural effusion
The goal is to move pleural fluid away from site of interest.
• Left lungs: The animal is in right lateral recumbency, which moves fluid to the right hemithorax.
• Right lungs: The animal is in left lateral recumbency, which moves fluid to the left hemithorax.
• Cranial mediastinum: Stand the animal erect on its hind limbs; this moves the fluid toward the diaphragm.
• Dorsal lung: Position the animal in sternal recumbency (Figure 3).

Cavitated lung mass
• The animal is in sternal recumbency (see Figure 3).

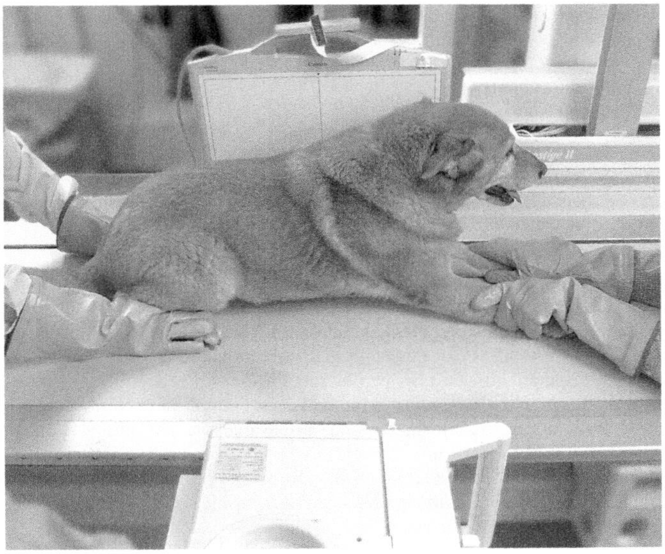

Figure 3

Horizontal beam, right-to-left lateral projection of the thorax of a dog in ventral (sternal) recumbency. The dog is on its sternum. The X-ray tube head is oriented parallel to the floor (*bottom* of figure), and the X-ray cassette is against the dog's left side, perpendicular to the X-ray cassette.

Patient Monitoring
As needed

Equipment or Supplies
• An X-ray machine that allows tube head to be positioned to emit X-rays horizontally (parallel to the floor). One cannot perform horizontal beam radiography if their X-ray tube head does not rotate.
• An X-ray cassette loaded with film or digital x-ray detector.
• A grid is optional. It would be helpful for larger animals, but it may be difficult to align X-ray tube head and cassette with grid.
• An X-ray cassette holder helps to minimize radiation exposure to personnel.
• Patient-restraint devices: Tape and sandbags help to minimize radiation exposure to personnel.

TECHNIQUE
Abdomen
• Horizontal beam radiography of the abdomen is usually used to confirm the presence of free peritoneal gas (pneumoperitoneum). Two views of the abdomen are made beforehand: right or left lateral and a VD projection.
• With the animal in left lateral recumbency, with its legs toward the front of the X-ray table (Figure 1), any fluid in the stomach will move into the fundus and any gas in the stomach will move to the pylorus. It is easier to distinguish free gas in the peritoneum from gas in the pylorus than from gas in the fundus.
• Place the cassette against the animal's dorsum (spine).
• Make the radiographic exposure.

Musculoskeletal System
• Horizontal beam radiography of a bone or joint is an alternative to traditional, vertical beam radiography. Patient positioning may be easier using horizontal beam radiography, especially if one is using passive restraint (tape and sandbags).
• Use sponges or other relatively radiolucent devices to position the limb while the animal is in lateral recumbency with the affected joint away from the table (Figure 2).
• Make a lateral projection by using traditional, vertical beam radiography. Make sure that the distance from the X-ray tube head and cassette is 40 inches (1.016 m).

• For the craniocaudal or dorsopalmar (plantar) projection, do not move the animal, but rather rotate the X-ray tube head 90° so that the X-rays are emitted horizontally, parallel to the floor.
• Place the cassette directly against the limb. You want the bone or joint to be as close to the cassette as possible. For some regions (e.g., stifle and femur), a caudocranial projection is more appropriate.
• Make the radiographic exposure.

Spine
• With the animal in left or right lateral recumbency, with its legs toward the front of the X-ray table (Figure 1), make a lateral projection by using traditional, vertical beam radiography.
• Rotate the X-ray tube head 90° so that the X-rays are emitted horizontally, parallel to the floor.
• Place the cassette against the animal's dorsum (spine).
• Make the radiographic exposure.

Thorax
Pleural Effusion
• Two views of the thorax are made to confirm the presence of pleural effusion. A right or left lateral projection and a VD are recommended.
• Determine whether a suspected cause of pleural effusion is a lesion in the cranial mediastinum, left hemithorax, or right hemithorax.
• Rotate the X-ray tube head 90° so that the X-rays are emitted horizontally, parallel to the floor.

Suspected cranial mediastinal lesion
• Set the kilovoltage peak (kVp) and milliampere exposure time (mAs) based on the VD projection. If a grid is used (taped to the cassette), use the same radiographic technique as that in the VD projection. Without a grid, decrease the mAs by a factor of 4 (e.g., 12 mAs → 3 mAs).
• Estimate how far above the X-ray table the animal's thorax will be with the animal standing erect on its hind limbs or sitting on its bottom.
• Align the X-ray tube and cassette.
• Place the animal's dorsum (spine) against the cassette (Figure 1).
• On full inspiration, make the radiographic exposure.

Suspected left pulmonary or body wall lesion
• With the animal in right lateral recumbency with its legs towards the front of the X-ray table, place the cassette against the animal's dorsum (spine).
• On full inspiration, make the radiographic exposure.

Suspected right pulmonary or body wall lesion
• With the animal in left lateral recumbency with its legs toward the front of the X-ray table, place the cassette against the animal's dorsum (spine).
• On full inspiration, make the radiographic exposure.

Cavitated Lung Lesion
• At least 2 views (right or left lateral and dorsoventral or VD) of the thorax are made first. A possible cavitated lung lesion is noted.
• Rotate the X-ray tube head 90° so that the X-rays are emitted horizontally, parallel to the floor.
• The animal should be in ventral (sternal) recumbency (Figure 3), with the side of the thorax that has the suspected lesion placed toward the back of the X-ray table so that it is closest to the cassette.
• Place the cassette against the animal's side.
• Make the radiographic exposure.

SAMPLE HANDLING
None

APPROPRIATE AFTERCARE
Postprocedure Patient Monitoring
None

Nursing Care
None

Dietary Modification
None

Medication Requirements
None

Restrictions on Activity
None

Anticipated Recovery Time
None

 INTERPRETATION

NORMAL FINDINGS OR RANGE
Abdomen
No gas accumulation between the pylorus and the right body wall

Musculoskeletal System
The appearance of the joint or bone as imaged by horizontal beam radiography is not different from images obtained by vertical beam radiography.

Spine
The spine is often not parallel to the X-ray table.

Thorax
• Horizontal beam VD of the left or right thorax: Aerated lung lobes extend to the body wall. The pleural effusion gravitates toward the recumbent side of the animal. A fluid line, oriented parallel to the X-ray table, will be present.
• Horizontal beam erect VD: Aerated lung lobes extend to the thoracic inlet. The thin cranial mediastinum is seen between the cranial lung lobes. The pleural effusion gravitates toward the diaphragm. A fluid line, oriented parallel to the X-ray table, will be present.

ABNORMAL VALUES
Abdomen
Gas accumulation between the pylorus and the right body wall

Musculoskeletal System
The appearance of abnormal joints or bones as imaged by horizontal beam radiography is not different from images obtained by vertical beam radiography.

Spine
Malalignment or spinal fractures, or both, are noted.

Thorax
• Horizontal beam VD of the left or right thorax: Soft tissue present in the lung lobe may be a pulmonary nodule or mass, interstitial or alveolar disease, a pleural abnormality, or a body wall abnormality (e.g., rib lesion). This radiographic projection is meant to move the pleural effusion away from the lesion, thus enabling better visualization of the pathology.
• Horizontal beam erect VD: The cranial mediastinum contains a soft tissue mass. This radiographic projection is meant to move the pleural effusion away from the lesion, thus enabling better visualization of the pathology.
• Cavitated lung mass: The center of a soft tissue mass contains fluid and gas. Gravity pulls the fluid ventrally, and the gas rises dorsally; this creates a sharp, fluid-gas interface within the soft tissue mass.

CRITICAL VALUES
Pneumoperitoneum (not caused by recent abdominal surgery) is usually caused by a rupture in the GI tract and is a surgical emergency.

INTERFERING FACTORS
Drugs That May Alter Results of the Procedure
None

Conditions That May Interfere with Performing the Procedure
Animals that had recent abdominal surgery will have a pneumoperitoneum for a few days.

Procedure Techniques or Handling That May Alter Results
None

Influence of Signalment on Performing and Interpreting the Procedure
Species
None

Breed
None

Age
None

Gender
None

Pregnancy
None

CLINICAL PERSPECTIVE
• Horizontal beam radiography usually supplements thoracic or abdominal radiography.
• For animals with pleural effusion, a horizontal beam projection of the thorax provides additional, noninvasive information about the underlying structures that are obscured by the pleural effusion. Once identified, pleural effusion should be removed to make the animal more comfortable and provide diagnostic information via sample analysis. The animal should be reradiographed after fluid removal.
• For animals with pulmonary masses, a horizontal beam projection of the thorax noninvasively provides additional radiographic signs that may be the key for achieving a specific radiographic diagnosis.
• For animals with suspected pneumoperitoneum, a horizontal beam projection of the abdomen is often the 1 view that confirms the presence or absence of free gas in the abdomen and helps the clinician decide whether surgery is indicated.

 MISCELLANEOUS

ANCILLARY TESTS
• Thoracocentesis to determine the cause of pleural effusion more definitively
• Abdominocentesis helps support a diagnosis of a rupture in the GI tract and sepsis.

SYNONYMS
Postural radiography

SEE ALSO
Blackwell's Five-Minute Veterinary Consult: Canine and Feline Topics
Pleural Effusion

Related Topics in This Book
• Abdominal Radiography
• Abdominocentesis and Fluid Analysis
• Computed Tomography
• General Principles of Radiography
• Thoracic Radiography
• Thoracic Ultrasonography
• Thoracocentesis and Fluid Analysis

ABBREVIATIONS
• mAs = mA (milliampere) + s (exposure time in seconds)
• VD = ventrodorsal

Suggested Reading
Farrow C. Postural radiography in dogs. *J Am Vet Med Assoc* 1994; 205: 878–887.
Ticer JW, ed. *Radiographic Technique in Small Animal Practice.* Philadelphia: WB Saunders, 1975.

INTERNET RESOURCES
None

AUTHOR NAME
Wm Tod Drost

BASICS

TYPE OF SPECIMEN
Blood
Urine

TEST EXPLANATION AND RELATED PHYSIOLOGY
Radial Immunodiffusion (RID)
RID assays are a type of immunoprecipitation assay used to quantify the immunoglobulin (Ig) isotypes (especially IgG, IgM, and IgA) in a patient's serum and can be helpful in identifying immunodeficiencies. In general, immunoprecipitation tests rely on the fact that, at optimal concentrations, antigens and antibodies will form large immune complexes that precipitate out of solution. In the RID assay, gel is impregnated with antibody against the constant region (Fc, crystallizable fragment) of 1 of the Ig isotypes. Patient serum is added to a well cut into the gel, and standard solutions, with known antibody concentrations, are placed in adjacent wells. Igs in the serum will diffuse out from the well, interact with the antibody in the gel, and form a visible precipitate when the 2 substances reach optimal concentrations (zone of equivalence). The diameter of the precipitin ring is proportional to the concentration of the specific Ig isotype and can be calculated by generating a standard curve using the standards. A slightly different immunoprecipitation assay known as Ouchterlony agar gel immunodiffusion (AGID) uses similar principles to detect antibodies against a variety of infectious agents.

Immunoelectrophoresis (IEP)
IEP is an immunoprecipitation assay that uses diffusion and precipitation in conjunction with an electric current. Basically, this test is used to identify relative concentrations of monoclonal proteins, primarily Igs, including κ and λ light chains. It can be performed on serum, urine and, occasionally, cerebral spinal fluid. Test and control fluids are placed in wells that are equidistant from a trough containing antiserum to the target Ig. The proteins are allowed to diffuse through the gel while an electric current is applied. The test substance forms an arc at the zone of equivalence between the antigen and specific antisera. The test arc is compared to the control arc to determine relative increases or decreases in Ig concentration. This test is most frequently used to identify the class of Igs present when a monoclonal hyperglobulinemia is seen with serum electrophoresis. It can help confirm the presence of a monoclonal hyperglobulinemia versus a restricted polyclonal gammopathy, such as sometimes seen with *Ehrlichia* and FIP infections. This test can also be helpful in identifying relative immunodeficiencies, but a test that quantifies Ig, such as RID, may provide more information. Immunofixation is a slightly different technique that can be used to estimate Ig levels. IEP and immunofixation are both specialty tests that are performed in only a few select laboratories. Antisera containing species-specific monoclonal reagents (e.g., anti–λ antibody) are not often available.

INDICATIONS
RID
• Quantification of Igs or complement protein concentrations
• Identification of specific inherited or acquired Ig deficiencies (IgG, IgM, and IgA)
• Identification and quantification of a specific Ig isotype (IgG, IgM, or IgA) produced by neoplastic plasma cells (myeloma)
AGID
• Identification of antibodies against a variety of infectious agents (e.g., fungi, viruses)
• Determination of the efficacy of vaccination
IEP
• IEP is most often used to confirm a monoclonal gammopathy and identify the isotype present, including κ and λ light chains.

• IEP for κ and λ light chains can also be performed on urine to confirm Bence-Jones proteinuria. With a monoclonal gammopathy, only 1 type of light chain (κ or λ) will be present, not both.
• This test may also be helpful in determining the relative immunodeficiency of a specific class of Ig.

CONTRAINDICATIONS
None

POTENTIAL COMPLICATIONS
None

CLIENT EDUCATION
None

SYSTEMS ASSESSED
Hemic, lymphatic, and immune

SAMPLE

COLLECTION
• 1–2 mL of venous blood
• 5–10 mL of urine for IEP
  • Cystocentesis is preferred, but a clean free-catch sample or a catheterized sample is acceptable.
  • Early morning urine collection is preferred.

HANDLING
• Serum: Collect into a serum-separator tube or plain tube without anticoagulant.
• Urine: Collect into clean urine-specimen container. Transfer the sample to sterile, plastic, leakproof container or to a red-top tube. Do not submit urine in a syringe.
• Ship the sample on ice packs.

STORAGE
Refrigerate or freeze.

STABILITY
• Room temperature: ≈2 h
• Refrigerated (2°–8°C): 1 week
• Frozen (−18°C): 1 month

PROTOCOL
None

INTERPRETATION

NORMAL FINDINGS OR RANGE
RID
• Canine IgA: 35–270 mg/dL
• Canine IgG: 670–1,650 mg/dL
• Canine IgM: 100–400 mg/dL
• Feline values unavailable
• Reference intervals may vary depending on the laboratory and assay.
IEP
The sample needs to be compared with control serum from a healthy patient of the same species.

ABNORMAL VALUES
• RID: a value above or below the reference interval
• IEP: a increased or decreased amount of Ig compared with the control

CRITICAL VALUES
None

INTERFERING FACTORS
Drugs That May Alter Results or Interpretation
Drugs That Interfere with Test Methodology
None

Drugs That Alter Physiology
None

Disorders That May Alter Results
• Monoclonal gammopathies have been reported with multiple myeloma, Waldenstrom's macroglobulinemia (IgM), lymphoma, chronic lymphocytic leukemia, *Ehrlichia* infection, FIP, amyloidosis, heartworm infection, leishmaniasis, and, rarely, they are of undetermined cause.
• In dogs, neoplasm-associated monoclonal gammopathies are usually IgG or IgA, with approximately equal incidence. In cats, most Ig-secreting neoplasms secrete IgG.
• Immunodeficiency diseases can decrease the concentrations of certain Igs. Primary immunodeficiencies are considered rare, but secondary immunodeficiencies are fairly common. RID may be helpful in identifying failure of passive transfer in neonates (i.e., low IgG concentration).

Collection Techniques or Handling That May Alter Results
Samples should be kept refrigerated to help ensure stability.

Influence of Signalment
Species
None

Breed
• Combined immunodeficiency has been reported in the bassett hounds, Cardigan Welsh corgis, and Jack Russell terriers. These dogs may have decreased Ig levels.
• German shepherds, beagles, Irish wolfhounds, rottweilers, Weimaraners, miniature dachshunds, and English bull terriers have been reported to have IgA deficiencies associated with different clinical syndromes.
• Sharpei immunodeficiency can be associated with low serum concentrations of 1 or more of IgG, IgM, and IgA.
• IgG deficiency has been reported in Cavalier King Charles spaniels, Weimaraners, rottweilers, and miniature dachshunds.

Age
• Igs are low at birth with a rapid rise because of absorption of maternal Igs through ingestion of colostrum.
• Occasionally, puppies have transient hypogammaglobulinemia caused by delayed onset of IgG and IgM production. These puppies are susceptible to infections once maternal antibodies are gone but spontaneously recover between 5 and 7 months of age.
• IgA levels do not reach adult values until 12–18 months of age. Submission of a sample from an aged matched normal dog may be necessary when testing for possible IgA deficiency.

Gender
None

Pregnancy
None

LIMITATIONS OF THE TEST
Sensitivity, Specificity, and Positive and Negative Predictive Values
N/A

Valid If Run in a Human Lab?
No—species-specific antibodies to the Ig being measured are needed.

Causes of Abnormal Findings

High values	Low values
Multiple myeloma	Inherited Ig deficiency
Waldenstrom's macroglobulinemia (IgM)	Acquired immunodeficiency
	Viral infection
Lymphoma	FIV
Chronic lymphocytic leukemia	Canine distemper
Amyloidosis	Canine parvovirus
Chronic infection or	Feline panleukopenia virus
inflammation	Feline leukemia virus
Ehrlichia	Drugs
FIP	Chemotherapeutic drugs
Heartworm	Glucocorticoids
Leishmania	Severe protein malnutrition

CLINICAL PERSPECTIVE
• RID and IEP are most useful in determining absolute and relative concentrations of Igs and other serum proteins. IEP can also be performed on urine and occasionally on cerebrospinal fluid. When one is confronted with a monoclonal gammopathy, these tests are helpful in classifying the class of Ig secreted. This may help narrow differential diagnoses. For example, *Ehrlichia*-induced monoclonal gammopathies are usually IgG. An IgM hypergammopathy would be more indicative of Waldenstrom's macroglobulinemia.
• Some authors suggest that the monoclonal peaks associated with infectious etiologies may represent oligoclonal or restricted polyclonal bands (i.e., multiple Igs that fail to spread and form a compact band with routine protein electrophoresis). IEP and RID may be helpful in determining whether the band is truly monoclonal.
• These tests can also be used to help classify immunodeficiency syndromes, including failure of passive transfer and specific breed-associated immunodeficiencies.

MISCELLANEOUS
ANCILLARY TESTS
• If an immune deficiency is suspected, ancillary testing, including leukocyte function tests and subpopulation counts, may be helpful.
• If myeloma is suspected, additional workup should include serum protein electrophoresis, bone marrow aspiration, serum calcium determination, and radiography to look for lytic bone lesions.

SYNONYMS
• Agar gel immunodiffusion (AGID)
• Immunoelectrophoresis
• Quantitative immunoglobulins
• Radial immunodiffusion (RID)

SEE ALSO
Blackwell's Five-Minute Veterinary Consult: Canine and Feline Topics
• Immunodeficiency Disorders, Primary
• Multiple Myeloma
Related Topics in This Book
• Bence-Jones Proteins
• Globulins
• Protein Electrophoresis

ABBREVIATIONS

- AGID = agar gel immunodiffusion
- FIP = feline infectious peritonitis
- IEP = immunoelectrophoresis
- Ig = immunoglobulin
- RID = radial immunodiffusion

Suggested Reading

Fike DJ. Precipitation. In: Sheehan C, ed. *Clinical Immunology: Principles and Laboratory Diagnosis*. Philadelphia: Lippincott Williams & Wilkins, 1990: 123–134.

Modiano JF, Ritt MG. Immunoassays. In: Feldman BF, Zinkl JG, Jain NC, eds. *Schalm's Veterinary Hematology*. Philadelphia: Lippincott Williams & Wilkins, 2000: 910–916.

Stockham SL, Scott MA. Proteins. In: *Essentials of Veterinary Clinical Pathology*. Ames: Iowa State Press, 2002: 251–275.

INTERNET RESOURCES

Day MJ. Immunodeficiency disease in the dog. In: 29th World Congress of the World Small Animal Veterinary Association. Rhodes, Greece, October 2004, http://www.vin.com/proceedings/Proceedings.plx?CID = WSAVA2004&PID = 8598&O = Generic.

AUTHOR NAME

Karen Zaks

IMPRESSION SMEAR

BASICS

TYPE OF PROCEDURE
Diagnostic sample collection

PROCEDURE EXPLANATION AND RELATED PHYSIOLOGY
Impression smears obtained from superficial lesions or from tissue biopsy samples may reveal cellular details not visible after collection and processing for histologic evaluation. Individual cell types, including infectious organisms and neoplastic cells, may be more readily apparent when impression smears are evaluated cytologically, and this technique may therefore serve as a valuable adjunct to histologic examination.

CONTRAINDICATIONS
None

POTENTIAL COMPLICATIONS
None

CLIENT EDUCATION
None

BODY SYSTEMS ASSESSED
All

PROCEDURE

PATIENT PREPARATION
Preprocedure Medication or Preparation
None

Anesthesia or Sedation
None

Patient Positioning
None

Patient Monitoring
None

Equipment or Supplies
- A paper towel for blotting
- A scalpel blade
- Glass slides

TECHNIQUE
Impression smears may be made directly from superficial ulcerated lesions or from harvested biopsy tissue.
- Directly from a lesion: An imprint is made by touching the center of a clean glass slide to the uncleaned lesion. After an initial impression smear, the lesion can be gently blotted and cleaned with saline solution and gauze and a second impression made.
- For a harvested biopsy tissue: A freshly cut surface is exposed by sectioning the tissue biopsy sample with a scalpel blade (this is not required if the sample being evaluated is freshly removed via needle or punch biopsy). An important aspect of obtaining diagnostic impression smears is blotting the tissue on a clean absorbent material, such as a paper towel, to remove excess blood, moisture, and tissue fluid prior to imprinting the tissue on a slide. The blotted tissue can be gently touched onto the middle of a clean glass slide and lifted off. Multiple impression smears may be made onto separate glass slides.

SAMPLE HANDLING
- Air-dried samples can be stored at room temperature.
- Samples should be fixed and stained as soon after collection as

possible (ideally within 3–7 days) for optimal assessment of cellular morphology.

APPROPRIATE AFTERCARE
Postprocedure Patient Monitoring
N/A

Nursing Care
N/A

Dietary Modification
N/A

Medication Requirements
N/A

Restrictions on Activity
N/A

Anticipated Recovery Time
N/A

INTERPRETATION

NORMAL FINDINGS OR RANGE
- A blot of tissue centered on the glass slide
- Identification of cells normally seen in sampled tissue

ABNORMAL FINDINGS
- Abnormal ratios, numbers, or types of cells present
- Infectious agents
- Neoplastic cells

CRITICAL VALUES
None

INTERFERING FACTORS
Drugs That May Alter Results of the Procedure
None

Conditions That May Interfere with Performing the Procedure
None

Procedure Techniques or Handling That May Alter Results
- Failure to blot the sample adequately prior to making an impression smear may obscure evaluation.
- Failure to fix and stain slides within 3–7 days may alter cellular characteristics and limit the value of the interpretation.

Influence of Signalment on Performing and Interpreting the Procedure

Species
None

Breed
None

Age
None

Gender
None

Pregnancy
None

CLINICAL PERSPECTIVE
Impression smears are simple to make and, when obtained from superficial lesions or from tissue biopsy samples, these smears may reveal cellular details not visible following collection and processing for histologic evaluation. Individual cell types, including infectious organisms and neoplastic cells, may be more readily apparent when impression smears are evaluated cytologically and, when combined with histologic examination, this technique may enhance diagnostic accuracy.

MISCELLANEOUS

ANCILLARY TESTS
- Fine-needle aspiration and cytology
- Biopsy with histopathologic evaluation

SYNONYMS
- Touch prep
- Touch prep cytology

SEE ALSO
Blackwell's Five-Minute Veterinary Consult: Canine and Feline Topics
Many
Related Topics in This Book
- Fine-Needle Aspiration

- Tissue Biopsy: Needle and Punch
- Ultrasound-Guided Mass or Organ Aspiration

ABBREVIATIONS
None

Suggested Reading
Cowell RL, Tyler RD, Meinkoth JH, eds. *Diagnostic Cytology and Hematology of the Dog and Cat.* St Louis: CV Mosby, 1999.
Raskin RE, Meyer DJ, eds. *Atlas of Canine and Feline Cytology*, 2nd ed. Philadelphia: WB Saunders, 2001.

INTERNET RESOURCES
None

AUTHOR NAME
Laurel E. Williams

INSULIN AND INSULIN/GLUCOSE RATIO

BASICS

TYPE OF SPECIMEN
Blood

TEST EXPLANATION AND RELATED PHYSIOLOGY
Insulin is a polypeptide hormone secreted by pancreatic β cells in response to increased concentrations of glucose, amino acids, fatty acids, ketones, and the neurotransmitter acetylcholine, as well as some hormones (i.e., glucagon, gastrin, secretin, pancreozymin, GI polypeptide, growth hormone, β-adrenergic hormones), and drugs (e.g., sulfonylureas, isoproterenol). Conversely, insulin release is inhibited by hypoglycemia and some other hormones (i.e., somatostatin, α_2-adrenergic agonists, β-adrenergic antagonists) and drugs (e.g., dilantin, phenothiazines, epinephrine, norepinephrine).

Glucose is used by all cells of the body, either as an energy source or to produce another product, such as glycogen, triglycerides, or amino acids. A substantial part of the body mass (e.g., skeletal, muscle, heart, and adipose tissue) requires insulin for transmembrane transport of glucose; insulin is also required for multiple enzymatic reactions in the liver, which is the primary organ for regulating glucose homeostasis. Insulin has other actions, as well, such as the cellular uptake and utilization of amino acids. The immediate effect of insulin is decreased blood glucose concentration because of increased cellular glucose uptake and conversion to glycogen, protein, and fat. Because of the close relationship between insulin and glucose concentrations in physiologic and pathologic states, the reader is referred to the chapter on glucose for a more comprehensive understanding of both tests.

Serum insulin concentration is more frequently measured in cases of hypoglycemia in order to establish a diagnosis of a pancreatic β-cell tumor (insulinoma). With an insulinoma, hypoglycemia does not exert the same suppressive effect on insulin secretion, because of hyporesponsiveness of the neoplastic cells. The concentration of insulin is normal to increased in light of a concurrent hypoglycemia. However, many variables can affect serum insulin concentration, necessitating that the concentration must be interpreted in conjunction with corresponding blood glucose concentration measured from the same blood sample. Insulin is infrequently measured in hyperglycemic animals (i.e., DM cases).

The *insulin/glucose ratio*, which is a mathematical equation that describes the physiologic relationship between insulin and glucose, can be useful to calculate in animals with persistent hypoglycemia. In the physiologic state, hypoglycemia should produce negative feedback on insulin secretion. In the case of an insulinoma, this negative feedback does not work, resulting in an insulin concentration that is inappropriately high for the concurrent hypoglycemia. Therefore, determination of the ratio should indicate whether the concentration of insulin is appropriate for the degree of glucose stimulation. However, the insulin/glucose ratio is not specific, and substances other than glucose influence insulin release from β cells. Hepatic tumors, sepsis, and other conditions may produce a detectable serum insulin concentration (although it is generally low normal) despite a concurrent hypoglycemia; the end result would be an abnormal (increased) insulin/glucose ratio. Furthermore, much of the released insulin is removed from portal blood by hepatocytes and thus does not appear in peripheral blood. The clinician is encouraged to evaluate absolute serum insulin concentration during hypoglycemia in conjunction with clinical history, physical exam findings, and results of other diagnostic tests rather than relying on the insulin/glucose ratio in making a diagnosis.

The amended insulin/glucose ratio was first proposed by Turner and associates in 1971, who theorized that amending the measured concentration of insulin prior to determining the ratio would establish a direct relationship between insulin and glucose. To amend the ratio, they proposed subtracting 30 mg/dL from the measured glucose concentration. However, subsequent clinical application and research have not validated the amended insulin/glucose ratio, so it should not be used.

INDICATIONS
- Diagnosis of an insulin-secreting β-cell tumor of the pancreas
- To assess β-cell function in animals with DM
- To increase the clinician's index of suspicion for circulating insulin-binding antibodies in animals with DM and insulin resistance

CONTRAINDICATIONS
None

POTENTIAL COMPLICATIONS
Complications associated with marked hypoglycemia

CLIENT EDUCATION
- If the animal does not experience clinical signs attributable to states of hypoglycemia, a 12-h fast is recommended.
- If the animal experiences clinical signs attributable to states of hypoglycemia, the animal should be fed as usual and the glucose should be measured by the clinic. If the glucose is not <60 mg/dL at this time, an in-house fast with careful monitoring may be conducted.

BODY SYSTEMS ASSESSED
Metabolic and endocrine

SAMPLE

COLLECTION
1 mL of venous blood

HANDLING
- Collect blood into a plain red-top tube or serum-separator tube.
- Harvest the serum from clotted blood within 1 h and then immediately assay or freeze it.
- Ship the frozen samples in a Styrofoam container with ice packs.

STORAGE
Refrigerate or freeze samples.

STABILITY
- Room temperature: at least 5 h
- Refrigerated (2°–8°C): 1 week
- Frozen (−20°C): several months
- Avoid thawing and refreezing of samples.

PROTOCOL
- If a dog is sporadically hypoglycemic, serum should be measured when the animal is hypoglycemic. Fast the dog until its serum glucose concentration is <60 mg/dL and then collect a sample for blood glucose and insulin determination. Freeze the serum immediately after harvesting it from clotted blood.
- Most dogs with insulin-secreting tumors develop hypoglycemia 8–10 h after a meal, although >24 h of fasting may be required in some patients.
- After sample collection, feed the animal several small meals before returning to the previous feeding schedule.

INTERPRETATION

NORMAL FINDINGS OR RANGE
These reference intervals were established by the Endocrine Section of the Diagnostic Center for Population and Animal Health at Michigan State University. Reference intervals may vary depending on the laboratory and assay used.

INSULIN AND INSULIN/GLUCOSE RATIO

Dogs (Fasting Values)
- Insulin: 58–229 pmol/L (8.1–32.0 μIU/mL)
- Glucose: 4.2–6.6 mmol/L (76–120 mg/dL)
- Insulin/glucose ratio (SI units): 14–43

Cats (Fasting Values)
- Insulin: 72–583 pmol/L (10.0–81.3 μIU/mL)
- Glucose: 3.1–7.2 mmol/L (56–131 mg/dL)
- Insulin/glucose ratio (SI units): not established

ABNORMAL VALUES
Values above or below the reference interval and/or ratio

CRITICAL VALUES
None, unless accompanied by marked hypoglycemia

INTERFERING FACTORS
Drugs That May Alter Results or Interpretation
Drugs That Interfere with Test Methodology
- Insulin from an insulin injection may be measured for up to 24 h after the injection.
- Chronic exogenous insulin therapy in diabetes may cause insulin antibody formation, which may interfere with single antibody radioimmunoassay systems, resulting in artifactually increased values.

Drugs That Alter Physiology
- Insulin release is stimulated by certain drugs: e.g., sulfonylureas or isoproterenol.
- Insulin release is inhibited by certain drugs: e.g., dilantin, phenothiazines, epinephrine, or norepinephrine.

Disorders That May Alter Results
The presence of anti-insulin antibodies may increase or decrease measured insulin concentrations.

Collection Techniques or Handling That May Alter Results
Avoid the use of specimens that are grossly hemolyzed, icteric, or lipemic.

Influence of Signalment
Species
- Cats tend to have higher insulin concentrations than dogs.
- Some radioimmunoassays for measuring insulin reportedly do not work in cats.

Breed
None

Age
None

Gender
None

Pregnancy
None

LIMITATIONS OF THE TEST
Sensitivity, Specificity, and Positive and Negative Predictive Values
N/A

Valid If Run in a Human Lab?
There is sufficient cross-immunoreactivity that commercial human assays have been validated for canine insulin. However, commercial assays may not be valid for feline insulin.

Causes of Abnormal Findings

High insulin values	Low insulin values
Increased insulin production and release	Pathologic hypoinsulinemia
Functional pancreatic β-cell neoplasia (insulinoma)	Decreased insulin production because of destruction of pancreatic β cells (type I DM)
Appropriate response to physiologic hyperglycemia	Advanced stages of pancreatic amyloidosis involve β-cell damage and thus decreased insulin production
Presence of anti-insulin antibodies	Physiologic hypoinsulinemia Hypoglycemic states should be accompanied by hypoinsulinemia if the response is appropriate
	Presence of anti-insulin antibodies

CLINICAL PERSPECTIVE
- Serum insulin and glucose concentrations must be evaluated from the same blood sample for appropriate interpretation.
- Any serum insulin concentration that falls below the normal range is consistent with insulinopenia and does not indicate the presence of an insulin-secreting tumor.
- If an insulinoma is suspected, a sample obtained while the animal is hypoglycemic is of more benefit than one obtained during normoglycemia. Confidence in identifying inappropriate hyperinsulinemia depends on the severity of the hypoglycemia. The lower the blood glucose concentration is, the more confident the clinician can be in identifying inappropriate hyperinsulinemia.
- The insulin/glucose ratio is not specific and can be affected by several disorders other than an insulinoma. Therefore, absolute serum insulin concentration during hypoglycemia should be interpreted in conjunction with the history, physical findings, drug administration, and results of other diagnostic tests.

MISCELLANEOUS
ANCILLARY TESTS
Glucose evaluation

SYNONYMS
None

SEE ALSO
Blackwell's Five-Minute Veterinary Consult: Canine and Feline Topics
- Diabetes mellitus without complication–Cats
- Diabetes mellitus without complication – Dogs
- Diabetes with Hyperosmolar Coma
- Diabetes with ketoacidosis
- Hyperglycemia
- Hypoglycemia
- Insulinoma

Related Topics in This Book
- Glucose
- Glucose Curve

INSULIN AND INSULIN/GLUCOSE RATIO

ABBREVIATIONS
DM = diabetes mellitus

Suggested Reading
Feldman EC, Nelson RW. Beta-cell neoplasia: Insulinoma. In: Feldman EC, Nelson RW, eds. *Canine and Feline Endocrinology and Reproduction*, 3rd ed. St Louis: Saunders Elsevier, 2004: 616–644.
Stockham SL, Scott MA. Glucose, ketoamines, and related regulatory hormones. In: *Fundamentals of Veterinary Clinical Pathology*, 2nd ed. Ames: Iowa State Press, 2008: 707–738.
Turner RC, Oakley NW, Nabarro JDN. Control of basal insulin secretion with special reference to the diagnosis of insulinomas. *Br Med J* 1971; 2: 132–135.

INTERNET RESOURCES
Michigan State University, Diagnostic Center for Population and Animal Health, http://animalhealth.msu.edu/.

AUTHOR NAMES
Rebekah Gray Gunn-Christie and J. Roger Easley

BASICS

TYPE OF PROCEDURE
Allergy testing

PROCEDURE EXPLANATION AND RELATED PHYSIOLOGY
Sterile dilutions of allergen are introduced by injection into the dermis. At a cellular level, allergen is then captured by 2 adjacent allergen-specific IgE molecules bound to dermal mast cells, stimulating subsequent mast cell degranulation. The release of preformed inflammatory mediators, in particular histamine, produces local edema and erythema at the site of injection, which can be observed clinically. Positive (histamine) and negative (saline) controls are also injected. In theory, animals with atopic disease should have more allergen-specific IgE bound to dermal mast cells, and the mast cells themselves may be more labile in these individuals, resulting in visible positive reactions.

INDICATIONS
Intradermal testing (IDT) is indicated only when a diagnosis of atopic dermatitis (AD) is suspected on clinical grounds and other pruritic skin diseases have been ruled out. IDT is not a diagnostic test for AD. Positive reactions support the diagnosis and are generally used to formulate allergen-specific immunotherapy used in the management of AD.

CONTRAINDICATIONS
• IDT should not be performed unless other pruritic skin diseases have been ruled out.
• IDT with food allergens does not facilitate a reliable diagnosis of food allergy.
• Certain drugs, as listed in the Interfering Factors section, will interfere with IDT.
• IDT should not be performed when there is evidence of pyoderma at the site of testing.

POTENTIAL COMPLICATIONS
• Generalized reactions such as urticaria, angioedema, or anaphylaxis are possible but rare.
• Pruritus at the site of injection can commonly occur.

CLIENT EDUCATION
• The patient should be fasted overnight because sedation is generally required.
• A large area of the hair coat will be clipped on the lateral thorax to perform the procedure.
• False-positive and false-negative results can occur with IDT.
• The potential exists for more generalized reactions, such as urticaria, angioedema, or anaphylaxis.

BODY SYSTEMS ASSESSED
Dermatologic

PROCEDURE

PATIENT PREPARATION
Preprocedure Medication or Preparation
None

Anesthesia or Sedation
For the majority of cases, light sedation is required. Sedatives and anesthetics that do not affect skin reactivity and are acceptable for IDT include xylazine hydrochloride, medetomidine, thiamylal, halothane, isoflurane, methoxyflurane, and tiletamine-zolazepam combination.

Patient Positioning
The patient should be positioned in lateral recumbency.

Patient Monitoring
Monitoring should be appropriate for the sedation or anesthesia used.

Equipment or Supplies
• Tuberculin or 1.0-mL syringes with a 26- to 27-gauge needle containing diluted allergen
• Clippers with a no. 40 blade
• An indelible marker
• A scoring sheet
• A timer
• A flashlight or other handheld light source

TECHNIQUE
• Preparation of the allergen solutions: Allergens to be used in veterinary IDT should be selected according to the regional location in which the testing is performed. Aqueous allergen extracts used as glycerin-preserved extracts may cause irritation. Allergen extracts are not standardized in veterinary medicine, and therefore allergen content may vary. The use of allergen mixtures should be avoided. Optimal concentrations of allergen for use in IDT in companion animals have not been determined. Pollens and molds are usually tested at 1,000 protein nitrogen units (PNU)/mL; house dust mites at 1:50,000 wt/vol; fibers, hair, and feathers at 250–500 PNU/mL; and insects at 1,000 PNU/mL. Allergens kept in aqueous solution lose potency with time. Once diluted, they can be stored for 2 months in glass or 2 weeks in plastic syringes.
• Positive and negative controls are usually employed. Histamine phosphate 1:100,000 and 0.9% buffered solution, respectively, are commonly used.
• By convention, the IDT is performed on the lateral thorax. The site is lightly clipped with a no. 40 blade and should not be scrubbed. Test

INTRADERMAL TESTING

sites are marked with an indelible marker and should be at least 3 cm apart. By convention, a volume of 0.05 mL of each solution is injected intradermally. Air bubbles should be expelled from the syringe prior to injection because these can confuse interpretation. Reactions are read at 15–20 min after injection. A positive reaction is characterized by local edema and erythema. There are no standardized criteria for evaluating IDT. Many clinicians record reactions on a scale of 0–4 where 0 is equal to the negative control and 4 is equal to the positive control. Reactions scored as 2+ or greater are considered clinically significant. The diameter of each reaction may also be measured, and those greater or equal to the difference between the histamine and saline reactions are considered positive. Darkening the room and viewing the reactions with incidental light with a handheld light source might enhance visualization.

APPROPRIATE AFTERCARE
• Patients should be monitored for sedation or anesthetic recovery, if indicated.
• The intradermal injection of allergens may induce significant pruritus in some individuals. If this is noted, an IM injection of 0.2 mg/kg of dexamethasone can be administered.

 INTERPRETATION

NORMAL FINDINGS OR RANGE
It is well documented that apparently clinically normal dogs can have positive reactions to the intradermal injection of allergen. Therefore, it is imperative that IDT be carried out only in dogs in which other pruritic skin diseases have been ruled out and AD is suspected. Positive reactions should correlate with recent environmental exposure.

ABNORMAL VALUES
• False-positive reactions can arise if the allergen concentration is too high or contains irritants.
• False-negative reactions may arise if the allergen concentration is too low, there is drug interference, poor injection technique is used, or the selection of allergens is incorrect. The timing of the test may also be important. Many dermatologists prefer to perform IDT during or immediately after a period of overt clinical disease.
• A subpopulation of dogs with clinical signs consistent with AD has negative skin-test reactivity to allergen. The reason for this is currently undetermined.

INTERFERING FACTORS
Drugs That May Alter Results of the Procedure
A number of drugs can adversely affect the results of IDT. The following table lists the class of drug and recommended withdrawal time. This should be used as a guide because there may be some variation among individuals and with the dose and duration of previous drug administration.

Drug	Withdrawal time
Oral antihistamines	10 days
Topical glucocorticoids	3 weeks
Oral glucocorticoids	3 weeks, minimum
Injectable glucocorticoids	8 weeks, minimum

• Other drugs can interfere with IDT but have specific withdrawal times that have not been determined, including progestational compounds, β_2-adrenergic agonists, bronchodilators, and theophylline.

Conditions That May Interfere with Performing the Procedure
• Endogenous hyperadrenocorticism
• The effect of previously administered allergen-specific immunotherapy on IDT is unknown.
• Performing the test during a period of partial or complete remission of clinical signs

Procedure Techniques or Handling That May Alter Results
• Surgical scrubbing
• Poor injection technique
• Improper allergen concentration or storage

Influence of Signalment on Performing and Interpreting the Procedure
Species
The technical performance of IDT in cats may be more difficult for inexperienced operators. Reactions in cats can develop more quickly (10–15 min) and be more transient than those seen in dogs.

Breed
None

Age
In young dogs with clinical AD, the results of IDT may be negative. The test should be repeated at a later date.

Gender
None

Pregnancy
None

CLINICAL PERSPECTIVE
At the time of writing, IDT as commonly used in veterinary medicine is considered a valuable procedure used to indicate allergen-specific hypersensitivity in individuals with atopic disease. However, many aspects of this test could be improved. Many dermatologists perform allergen-specific serologic testing in conjunction with IDT.

MISCELLANEOUS

ANCILLARY TESTS
Serum allergy testing

SYNONYMS
Intradermal skin testing

SEE ALSO
Blackwell's Five-Minute Veterinary Consult: Canine and Feline Topics
Atopic Dermatitis
Related Topics in This Book
None

ABBREVIATIONS
- AD = atopic dermatitis
- IDT = intradermal testing
- PNU = protein-nitrogen units

Suggested Reading
Hillier A, DeBoer DJ. The ACVD task force on canine atopic dermatitis (XVII): Intradermal testing. *Vet Immunol Immunopathol* 2001; **81**: 289–304.

INTERNET RESOURCES
None

AUTHOR NAME
Hilary A. Jackson

IRON LEVEL AND TOTAL IRON-BINDING CAPACITY

BASICS

TYPE OF SPECIMEN
Blood

TEST EXPLANATION AND RELATED PHYSIOLOGY
Iron (Fe) plays an important role in the metabolism of all living organisms. There are several Fe compartments in mammalian species, most notable being the oxygen-carrying hemoglobin molecule present in RBCs. The tissue Fe compartment is made up of other heme-containing (e.g., myoglobin, cytochromes, peroxidases) and non–heme-containing enzymes and proteins, including some involved in ATP synthesis (aconitase) and DNA synthesis (ribonucleotide reductase). With such a wide tissue distribution, it is easy to see why Fe deficiency is so detrimental to veterinary patients.

Intestinal absorption of dietary Fe depends on the amount of dietary Fe and its bioavailability, as well as previous exposure to dietary Fe, the amount of storage Fe, and erythropoietic activity. Once absorbed by enterocytes, Fe is released into the circulation, where it binds to transferrin, which transports 2 Fe molecules to other cells. Once internalized, Fe dissociates from transferrin to be incorporated into Fe-containing proteins. Excess Fe is stored either as water-soluble ferritin or water-insoluble hemosiderin. Transferrin is a negative acute phase protein produced by the liver. With acute inflammatory reactions and some chronic illnesses, transferrin levels decrease.

Serum Fe can be determined by colorimetry, coulometry, and atomic absorption (uncommon). Colorimetric determinations are most common and involve liberation of ferric (oxidized) Fe from transferrin in an acidic environment, followed by reduction with ascorbic acid. Ferrous (reduced) Fe can then be detected photometrically after it interacts with a reagent to form a colored complex. Coulometry can also be used to measure serum Fe and requires smaller sample volumes.

TIBC is a measure of all proteins available for binding Fe. Because transferrin represents the largest quantity of Fe-binding proteins, TIBC is an indirect measure of this protein. Typically, excess Fe is added to the serum sample to saturate all the Fe-binding sites. Excess (free) Fe is removed, and bound Fe is measured colorimetrically. Additional information can be obtained by dividing serum Fe concentration by TIBC to calculate the percent transferrin saturation (%sat), another useful indicator of Fe status.

INDICATIONS
Assess the Fe metabolism in patients with suspected Fe deficiency or overload.

CONTRAINDICATIONS
Patients with hemolytic disease, because they may have artificially elevated Fe

POTENTIAL COMPLICATIONS
None

CLIENT EDUCATION
None

BODY SYSTEMS ASSESSED
• Gastrointestinal
• Hemic, lymphatic, and immune
• Hepatobiliary

SAMPLE

COLLECTION
1–2 mL of venous blood

HANDLING
Plain red-top tube or serum-separator tube

STORAGE
Refrigerate or freeze the serum for long-term storage.

STABILITY
• Room temperature: 1 week
• Refrigerated (4°– 8°C): 3 weeks
• Frozen (−20°C): 1 year

PROTOCOL
None

INTERPRETATION

NORMAL FINDINGS OR RANGE
Iron
Values are from the Kansas State University College of Veterinary Medicine Diagnostic Lab. Reference intervals may vary depending on the laboratory and assay.
• Dogs: 33–147 μg/dL
• Cats: 33–134 μg/dL

TIBC
• Dogs: 282–386 μg/dL
• Cats: 169–325 μg/dL

ABNORMAL VALUES
Values above or below the reference intervals

CRITICAL VALUES
None

INTERFERING FACTORS
Drugs That May Alter Results or Interpretation
Drugs That Interfere with Test Methodology
None

Drugs That Alter Physiology
Corticosteroids increase serum Fe in dogs.

Disorders That May Alter Results
• Marked hemolysis can falsely increase Fe levels because of Fe contained within RBCs.
• Marked icterus can falsely increase Fe levels.

Collection Techniques or Handling That May Alter Results
Marked hemolysis

Influence of Signalment
Species
None

Breed
None

Age
• Kittens <5 weeks old can be transiently Fe deficient because of rapid growth.
• Puppies and kittens are prone to Fe deficiency because of limited tissue Fe stores.

Gender
None

Pregnancy
Late pregnancy can decrease serum Fe and increase TIBC.

LIMITATIONS OF THE TEST
Sensitivity, Specificity, and Positive and Negative Predictive Values
N/A

IRON LEVEL AND TOTAL IRON-BINDING CAPACITY

Valid If Run in a Human Lab?
Yes.

Causes of Abnormal Findings

High values	Low values
Serum Fe	Serum Fe
Recent transfusion	Chronic blood loss
Increased glucocorticoids	Shift of Fe to tissue stores
Fe injections	Acute inflammation
Release of Fe from tissue	Chronic inflammation
Hemolytic anemia	Portosystemic shunt (in dogs)
Hepatocyte damage	Decreased dietary absorption
Hemosiderosis	Severe intestinal mucosal disease
	Severe dietary deficiency
	Hypothyroidism
	Renal disease
	Hemodialysis
	Overuse of blood donors
TIBC	TIBC
Fe deficiency	Acute phase inflammation
Polycythemia vera	Hepatic insufficiency
Late pregnancy	Hypoproteinemia (transferrin loss)
	Hemolytic anemia

CLINICAL PERSPECTIVE
• A low serum Fe concentration, normal to elevated TIBC, and low transferrin %sat are characteristic findings with Fe deficiency.
• Chronic illness and/or inflammation are characterized by a low serum Fe concentration, decreased TIBC, and normal transferrin %sat.
• In young animals, severe parasitemia—fleas in kittens and puppies, and hookworms and whipworms in dogs—causes external blood loss and subsequent Fe deficiency.
• In adults, chronic blood loss, usually from the intestinal tract and less commonly the urinary tract, can cause Fe deficiency.

 MISCELLANEOUS

ANCILLARY TESTS
• Serum ferritin evaluation
• Fecal occult blood test
• MCHC and MCV: Microcytosis and hypochromasia suggest Fe deficiency or a defect in Fe metabolism.

SYNONYMS
• TIBC
• Transferrin

SEE ALSO
Blackwell's Five-Minute Veterinary Consult: Canine and Feline Topics
• Anemia, Iron-Deficiency
• Anemia, Nonregenerative
Related Topics in This Book
• Fecal Occult Blood
• Ferritin
• Red Blood Cell Indices

ABBREVIATIONS
• Fe = iron
• %sat = percent saturation
• TIBC = total iron-binding capacity

Suggested Reading
Harvey JW. Microcytic anemias. In: Feldman BF, Zinkl JG, Jain NC, eds. *Schalm's Veterinary Hematology*. Baltimore: Lippincott Williams & Wilkins, 2000: 200–204.
Smith JE. Iron metabolism and its disorders. In: Kaneko JJ, Harvey JW, Bruss ML, eds. *Clinical Biochemistry of Domestic Animals*, 5th ed. San Diego: Academic, 1997: 223–237.
Stockham SL, Scott MA. *Fundamentals of Veterinary Clinical Pathology*. Ames: Iowa State Press, 2002: 144–154.

INTERNET RESOURCES
None

AUTHOR NAME
Jennifer Steinberg

BASICS

TYPE OF SPECIMEN
Blood

TEST EXPLANATION AND RELATED PHYSIOLOGY
Although microfilariae can often be found in a blood smear examined as part of a routine CBC, since only a single drop of blood is examined low numbers of circulating microfilariae can be easily missed with this technique. The Knott's test improves the odds of finding microfilariae by concentrating them from a larger volume of blood. This test is typically performed in dogs that test positive on serologic heartworm testing to confirm the diagnosis. Additionally, this test enables differentiation between the pathogenic *Dirofilaria immitis* and the nonpathogenic *Dipetalonema reconditum* (now called *Acanthocheilonema reconditum*).

INDICATIONS
• Dogs with clinical signs of heartworm disease
• Dogs about to undergo prophylactic therapy, especially those that are administered diethylcarbamazine as a preventive
• Dogs with a CBC positive for microfilariae

CONTRAINDICATIONS
Cats rarely have circulating microfilariae. Serologic testing is more reliable in this species.

POTENTIAL COMPLICATIONS
None

CLIENT EDUCATION
• This test is highly recommended prior to initiation of diethylcarbamazine therapy because that drug can cause fatal reactions in animals with circulating microfilariae.
• False negatives (a negative Knott's test result when adult organisms are present) can occur.

BODY SYSTEMS ASSESSED
• Cardiovascular
• Respiratory

 SAMPLE

COLLECTION
1 mL of venous blood

HANDLING
Collect the sample into either EDTA or heparin anticoagulant.

STORAGE
Store the sample at room temperature.

STABILITY
Room temperature: whole blood is stable for 24 h.

PROTOCOL
• Mix 1 mL of whole blood with 9 mL of 2% formalin.
• Centrifuge at 1,500 RPM for 5 min and then pour off the supernatant.
• Mix the sediment with methylene blue and transfer the mixture to a slide for microscopic evaluation.

 INTERPRETATION

NORMAL FINDINGS OR RANGE
No microfilariae

ABNORMAL VALUES
• The presence of microfilariae in any amount
• Differentiation between the 2 species seen in North America is important (see the table).
   • In animals >6 months old, any number of circulating *Dirofilaria immitis* microfilariae is diagnostic for heartworm disease. The quantity of microfilariae is not indicative of the adult burden.
   • *Dipetalonema reconditum* (now called *Acanthocheilonema reconditum*) is nonpathogenic and does not require therapy.

CRITICAL VALUES
None

INTERFERING FACTORS
Drugs That May Alter Results or Interpretation
Drugs That Interfere with Test Methodology
None

Drugs That Alter Physiology
Infected dogs on a heartworm preventive (such as ivermectin or milbemycin) often do not have circulating microfilariae.

Disorders That May Alter Results
None

Collection Techniques or Handling That May Alter Results
Blood should be mixed well prior to the addition of formalin solution.

Influence of Signalment
Species
Cats are usually amicrofilaremic or have very low numbers of circulating microfilariae.

Breed
None

Age
Animals that are <4–5 months of age can have circulating microfilariae because of transplacental transfer.

Gender
None

Pregnancy
None

LIMITATIONS OF THE TEST
• False negatives (a negative Knott's test result when adult organisms are present) can occur because of immune-mediated destruction of microfilariae, unisex or sterile adult infection, or cyclic variation in the numbers of circulating microfilariae.
• Cytologic methods for detection of microfilariae (such as the Knott's test) are not recommended in cats because the methods have poor sensitivity.

Sensitivity, Specificity, and Positive and Negative Predictive Values
• The Knott's test is highly specific but is less sensitive. Up to 40% of dogs can have occult heartworm disease without any circulating microfilariae.
• Up to 1% of infected dogs are microfilaria positive and antigen negative.

Valid If Run in a Human Lab?
Yes, if personnel are trained in the distinction between pathogenic and nonpathogenic microfilarial species.

Causes of Abnormal Findings

Dipetalonema reconditum	Dirofilaria immitis
Usually present in low numbers	Usually present in high numbers
Progressive motion	Stationary
Curved body, blunt head, button-hook tail	Straight body and tail, tapered head
Length, 250–288 µm	Length, 295–325 µm

CLINICAL PERSPECTIVE
• Microfilaria testing should be done as a confirmatory test after a positive antigen test result. Certain heartworm treatments and preventives are contraindicated in microfilaremic dogs.
• Knott's testing can be used to differentiate between pathogenic and nonpathogenic circulating microfilariae.
• Occult heartworm infections are common, and a negative Knott's test result does not exclude heartworm infection.

MISCELLANEOUS
ANCILLARY TESTS
• The Difil-Test (EVSCO Pharmaceuticals, Beuna, NJ), which uses Millipore filtration, is another method of microfilaria detection. The protocol is slightly different from the Knott's test, but both tests use whole, anticoagulated blood with subsequent concentration and microscopic evaluation for microfilariae. The Difil-Test kit contains complete instructions.
• Heartworm antigen serology
• Thoracic radiography or echocardiography as clinically indicated

SYNONYMS
None

SEE ALSO
Blackwell's Five-Minute Veterinary Consult: Canine and Feline Topics
• Heartworm Disease—Cats
• Heartworm Disease—Dogs

Related Topics in This Book
• Electrocardiography
• Heartworm Serology
• Thoracic Radiography

ABBREVIATIONS
None

Suggested Reading
Atkins C. Canine heartworm disease. In: Ettinger SJ, Feldman EC, eds. *Textbook of Veterinary Internal Medicine*, 6th ed. St Louis: Saunders Elsevier, 2006: 1118–1128.
Atkins C. Feline heartworm disease. In: Ettinger SJ, Feldman EC, eds. *Textbook of Veterinary Internal Medicine*, 6th ed. St Louis: Saunders Elsevier, 2006: 1137–1144.
Bowman DD. *Georgi's Parasitology for Veterinarians*. Philadelphia: WB Saunders, 1999: 207–212 and 309–311.
Nelson CT, McCall JW, Rubin SB, *et al*. 2005 Guidelines for the diagnosis, prevention and management of heartworm (*Dirofilaria immitis*) in cats. *Vet Parasitol* 2005; **133**: 267–275.
Nelson CT, McCall JW, Rubin SB, *et al*. 2005 Guidelines for the diagnosis, prevention and management of heartworm (*Dirofilaria immitis*) in dogs. *Vet Parasitol* 2005; **133**: 255–266.

INTERNET RESOURCES
American Heartworm Society, Canine heartworm disease, http://www.heartwormsociety.org/article.asp?id = 11. Canine heartworm information.
American Heartworm Society, Feline heartworm disease, http://www.heartwormsociety.org/article.asp?id = 16. Feline heartworm information.
Michigan State University, Health Concerns: Canine heartworm disease, http://www.msu.edu/~silvar/heartworm.htm.
Western Medical Supply, http://www.westernmedicalsupply.com. Difil-Test kits.

AUTHOR NAME
Deborah Groppe Davis

LACTATE

BASIC

TYPE OF SPECIMEN
Blood

TEST EXPLANATION AND RELATED PHYSIOLOGY
Lactic acid is the end product of anaerobic glucose metabolism and is produced daily (e.g., by exercise) but also during pathologic processes (e.g., shock). At physiologic pH, lactic acid immediately dissociates to lactate and hydrogen ion, with lactate cleared by the liver and kidney. Clinically significant lactate accumulation is due to tissue hypoperfusion and subsequent tissue hypoxia, with the shift to anaerobic glycolysis. Inadequate perfusion, severe hypoxemia, increased oxygen demands, decreased hemoglobin concentration, or combinations of these factors cause tissue hypoxia. *Hyperlactatemia* is a mild increase in blood lactate concentration without the presence of acidosis. *Lactic acidosis* is an elevated blood lactate concentration associated with metabolic acidosis (pH, <7.35). *Type A* lactic acidosis is caused by tissue hypoperfusion, either because of inadequate delivery or increased oxygen utilization. *Type B* lactic acidosis is caused by mechanisms other than tissue hypoperfusion (e.g., abnormal utilization of oxygen, errors of metabolism).

INDICATIONS
• To assess the presence and severity of tissue hypoperfusion and/or hypoxia (the higher the lactate level, the worse the problem)
• To predict the outcome (the higher the lactate level, the higher the mortality)
• To assess the response to therapy (lactate clearance is correlated with survival; inability to normalize is correlated with death)

CONTRAINDICATIONS
None

POTENTIAL COMPLICATIONS
None

CLIENT EDUCATION
None

BODY SYSTEMS ASSESSED
• Cardiovascular
• Endocrine and metabolic
• Gastrointestinal
• Musculoskeletal

SAMPLE

COLLECTION
• 0.5–1.0 mL of blood (peripheral venous, central venous, or arterial). Use the same source for repeated measurements.
• Avoid prolonged restraint and venous stasis during sample collection.

HANDLING
• Lithium heparin, sodium fluoride, or indoacetate are the preferred anticoagulants.
• Centrifuge and harvest plasma, which is preferred to whole blood.
• Keep the sample on ice or refrigerate it if it is not measured immediately.

STORAGE
Freeze the plasma if measurement is delayed for >30 min (heparin) or >2 h (fluoride or indoacetate).

STABILITY
• Room temperature

• 30 min (heparin)
• 2 h (indoacetate or fluoride tubes)
• Refrigerated (4°C) or on ice: 2 h
• Frozen (−20°C): stable indefinitely

PROTOCOL
None

INTERPRETATION

NORMAL FINDINGS OR RANGE
• Adult dogs and puppies >70 days of age: 1.6 mmol/L
• Puppies <4 days of age: 3.8 mmol/L; and 4–28 days of age: 2.7 mmol/L
• Adult cats: 1.8 mmol/L
• Reference intervals may vary depending on the lab and analyzer. Generally, findings are considered clinically normal if the concentration is ≤2.5 mmol/L.

ABNORMAL VALUES
A lactate concentration of >1.6 mmol/L for dogs or >1.8 mmol/L for cats, especially if acidemia also present

CRITICAL VALUES
A lactate concentration of >6.0–6.5 mmol/L suggests severe global tissue hypoperfusion (e.g., shock) or severe local ischemia (e.g., gastric necrosis in patients with gastric dilatation and volvulus syndrome).

INTERFERING FACTORS
Drugs That May Alter Results or Interpretation
Drugs That Interfere with Test Methodology
None

Drugs That Alter Physiology
• Acetaminophen
• Activated charcoal
• Bicarbonate
• Catecholamines
• Halothane
• Nitroprusside
• Propylene glycol
• Salicylates
• Terbutaline

Disorders That May Alter Results
Seizures or extreme muscular exertion can increase the lactate concentration (≈4–10 mmol/L), which generally returns to normal in 2 h or less.

Collection Techniques or Handling That May Alter Results
• Stress, trembling, resisting restraint, excitement, venous stasis, and exercise increase the lactate concentration (≈2.5–5.0 mmol/L), which generally returns to normal in 2 h or less.
• Failure to separate plasma from RBCs falsely increases the result.

Influence of Signalment
Species
Cats have slightly higher normal lactate levels than dogs.

Breed
None

Age
Lactate levels are higher in neonatal puppies <70 days of age.

Gender
None

Pregnancy
None

LIMITATIONS OF THE TEST
- Significant regional hypoperfusion (e.g., splanchnic ischemia) may be present with a normal blood lactate concentration. Thus, a normal lactate concentration does not rule out tissue hypoperfusion or tissue hypoxia.
- Hyperlactatemia can be due to causes other than hypoperfusion.

Sensitivity, Specificity, and Positive and Negative Predictive Values
N/A

Valid If Run in a Human Lab?
Yes.

Causes of Abnormal Findings

High values	Low values
Type A lactic acidosis	Sodium citrate anticoagulant
Systemic hypoperfusion (e.g., shock, heart failure)	
Regional hypoperfusion (e.g., gastric/splanchnic ischemia, thromboembolism)	
Severe hypoxemia	
Severe anemia	
Increased anaerobic activity (e.g., seizures, exercise, trembling)	
Type B_1 lactic acidosis	
Neoplasia	
Sepsis	
Renal failure	
Liver failure	
Type B_2 lactic acidosis	
Drugs (see the Drugs that Alter Physiology section)	
Toxins (e.g., ethylene glycol, ethanol, sorbitol, xylitol, propylene glycol, carbon monoxide)	
Type B_3 lactic acidosis due to inborn errors of metabolism (e.g., metabolic myopathy of Labrador retrievers)	

CLINICAL PERSPECTIVE
- Lactate is a global marker of tissue hypoperfusion or regional ischemia.
- The severity of increase in lactate concentration is roughly equal to severity of the underlying disorder and can be used to predict outcome.
- Lactate clearance over time is useful in assessing response to therapy, in guiding therapy changes, and in predicting outcome.
- Clearance suggests improvement, whereas failure to normalize implies clinical deterioration and should prompt a change in therapy.

MISCELLANEOUS

ANCILLARY TESTS
Arterial blood-gas analysis and specific tests (e.g., anion gap, ethylene glycol, serum and urine glucose, serum and urine ketones) may define the type of acid-base disorder present and its etiology.

SYNONYMS
Lactic acid

SEE ALSO
Blackwell's Five-Minute Veterinary Consult: Canine and Feline Topics
- Acidosis, Metabolic
- Lactic Acidosis

Related Topics in This Book
- Anion Gap
- Bicarbonate
- Blood gases

ABBREVIATIONS
None

Suggested Reading

Boag A, Hughes D. Assessment and treatment of perfusion abnormalities in the emergency patient. *Vet Clin North Am Small Anim Pract* 2005; 35: 319–342.

Karagiannis M, Reniker A, Kerl M, Mann FA. Lactate measurement as an indicator of perfusion. *Comp Contin Educ Pract Vet* 2006; 28: 287–300.

McMichael M, Lees G, Hennessey J, *et al.* Serial plasma lactate concentrations in 68 puppies aged 4 to 80 days. *J Vet Emerg Crit Care* 2005; 15: 17–21.

Pang DS, Boysen S. Lactate in veterinary critical care: Pathophysiology and management. *J Am Anim Hosp Assoc* 2007; 43: 270–279.

INTERNET RESOURCES
None

AUTHOR NAME
Michael S. Lagutchik

BASICS

TYPE OF PROCEDURE
Endoscopic

PROCEDURE EXPLANATION AND RELATED PHYSIOLOGY
This is a sterile procedure in which a rigid endoscope (telescope) is introduced into the abdomen to view abdominal structures and obtain biopsy samples (Figure 1). Surgical procedures may also be performed. The technique enables exploration of and surgery within the abdomen without the need for a full abdominal wall incision. The procedure is less painful and stressful than open surgery.

To view structures within the abdomen, a pneumoperitoneum must be created. Carbon dioxide (CO_2) is passed through tubing into a needle or a trochar than enters the abdomen. CO_2 is used because it carries the least risk of causing an air embolism. The intra-abdominal pressure must be controlled during insufflation to avoid causing cardiovascular and respiratory compromise.

INDICATIONS
- Evaluation of abdominal organs and abdominal surfaces
- Liver, kidney, intestinal, or pancreatic biopsies
- Gallbladder aspiration
- Visualization and biopsy of abdominal masses
- Exploration for causes of abdominal effusion
- Splenoportography

CONTRAINDICATIONS
Absolute
- Diaphragmatic hernia
- Septic peritonitis
- Obvious need for open surgery

Relative
- Small body size
- Obesity
- Coagulopathy

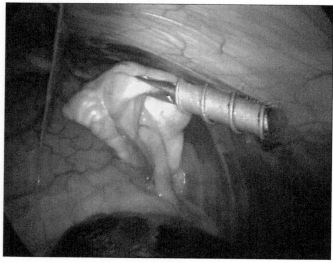

Figure 1

Laparoscopic view of the abdomen. The endoscopic grasper is holding the vas deferens.

POTENTIAL COMPLICATIONS
- SC emphysema
- Cardiorespiratory compromise
- Internal organ damage
- Bleeding
- A need to convert to an open procedure
- Wound-healing complications
- Infection

CLIENT EDUCATION
- This procedure requires heavy sedation or anesthesia. The animal must not be fed for 12 h before surgery.
- This is a sterile surgical procedure. The animal will be clipped for a full abdominal exploratory surgery because there may be a need to convert from a minimally invasive procedure to an open surgery.

BODY SYSTEMS ASSESSED
- Endocrine and metabolic
- Gastrointestinal
- Hemic, lymphatic, and immune
- Hepatobiliary
- Renal and urologic
- Reproductive

PROCEDURE

PATIENT PREPARATION
Preprocedure Medication or Preparation
- The animal must be fasted for 12 h before the procedure.
- The bladder should be as empty as possible.
- Routine preanesthetic drugs are administered.

Anesthesia or Sedation
- The procedure is almost always performed using inhalant general anesthesia.
- In rare cases, total IV anesthesia or heavy sedation may be used in conjunction with local anesthetic blocks.

Patient Positioning
- It depends on the procedure, but usually dorsal recumbency.
- If the patient is sedated, rather than anesthetized, lateral recumbency may minimize patient movement.

Patient Monitoring
- Blood pressure measurement, pulse oximetry, ECG monitoring, and respiratory rate monitoring are used.
- Intra-abdominal pressure is monitored using a pressure gauge that is part of the gas-insufflation device.

Equipment or Supplies
Basic
- Hair clippers
- Sterile preparation supplies
- 0° 5-mm or 10-mm rigid telescope
- A video camera and monitor
- A light source and cable
- An insufflator-gas and CO_2 source
- A Veress needle (if this technique is being used)
- A trocar-cannula
- Laparoscopic probe and retractors
- Laparoscopic grasping forceps
- Laparoscopic biopsy instruments

- Biopsy and aspiration needles
- Surgical instruments
- Suture material
- A scalpel blade

Additional
- A table that enables the animal to be easily tipped sideways, head down, or head up.
- Other telescopes: those with angled viewing ports or that are smaller; an operating telescope
- Specific instruments used to perform various laparoscopic surgeries
- A suction device
- Devices to control hemorrhage (i.e., bipolar electrocautery, stainless-steel clips, harmonic scalpel)

TECHNIQUE

- Performing laparoscopy requires special training. See the Internet Resources for basic equipment, videos, and training courses.
- The patient is anesthetized and placed in dorsal recumbency. The bladder is expressed. The abdomen is clipped for full abdominal exploratory surgery. The clipped area is surgically prepared. The patient is draped.
- *Veress needle technique*: The Veress needle has a spring-loaded blunt obturator that prevents damage to viscera. The skin behind the umbilicus is nicked with a scalpel. The needle is passed through the abdominal wall. A hanging-drop technique is used to ensure correct placement of the needle into the peritoneal cavity. Once placement is assured, tubing is attached to the needle and the peritoneal cavity is filled with CO_2 to a pressure of 5–15 mmHg. A skin incision is made to the diameter of the trocar-cannula, and the tissues are dissected to the level of the body wall. A sharp trocar-cannula combination is used. The trocar is advanced through the body wall. Once the wall is penetrated, the trocar is withdrawn and the cannula is advanced. The CO_2 tubing is moved to the stopcock on the cannula, and the Veress needle is withdrawn. The major complication associated with the Veress needle technique is SC emphysema caused by insufflation without confirmation of placement into the peritoneal cavity (wherein the needle slides off the external rectus fascia and lateral to midline). This complication is more likely to occur in obese or large animals and with inexperienced operators. Once emphysema is present, it may be very difficult to enter the peritoneal cavity accurately. Thus, some clinicians prefer to use an open technique, particularly if an animal is large or obese.
- *Open technique*: A 2-cm ventral midline incision is made caudal to the umbilicus. The tissues are dissected to the level of the body wall.

A short stab incision is made through the body wall. A mattress or purse-string suture is placed around the incision. A towel clamp (or large suture) is used to grasp the body wall and elevate it away from the viscera. A blunt trocar-cannula combination is used. The trocar is advanced into the abdomen, the cannula is advanced, and then the trocar is withdrawn. The suture is tightened around the cannula to prevent gas from escaping. The CO_2 tubing is attached to a stopcock on the side of the cannula, and the peritoneal cavity is filled with CO_2 to a pressure of 10–15 mmHg.
- The telescope tip is placed in warm saline (to prevent fogging), and the light cable and camera are attached. The camera is color balanced, the orientation of the camera is selected, and the telescope is then introduced into the cannula. If an operating telescope (which has a channel for instruments) is used, this will be the only cannula placed. If a regular telescope is used, at least 1 additional cannula will be placed to introduce an instrument. The telescope is used to observe the peritoneal cavity during additional cannula placement to ensure that no organs are harmed during penetration of the sharp trocar. If separate instrument cannulas are used, instruments are always introduced into the abdominal cavity under direct visualization to ensure that no organs are damaged. The CO_2 tubing is attached to the instrument cannula to help prevent fogging.
- Once the camera and instrument cannulas are in place, exploration of the abdomen may begin. It is critical that the operator know the orientation of the camera, and care must be taken to ensure that the orientation does not change during exploration. Camera fogging or obscured vision is controlled by keeping the telescope warm, by wiping the tip on the peritoneal surface, or by removing the telescope and wiping the tip with warm saline in a gauze sponge. Blunt probes, fan retractors, and grasping instruments may be used to manipulate viscera during exploration. Exploration is greatly eased if the animal is on a table that enables the body to be tipped head down, head up, or side to side.
- *Liver biopsy*: This is the most basic technique and is usually performed with the patient positioned in left lateral recumbency or tipped left 45° from dorsal midline, with the cannula port(s) in the right flank. If ascites is present, enough fluid is removed to enable visualization of the liver. The biopsy sample is obtained by using 5-mm oval cup (clamshell) biopsy forceps. The forceps are opened, closed over the selected site, held for 30 s, and then pulled away with a twisting motion. Usually 3–4 samples are obtained. The sites are observed for hemorrhage. The blunt probe may be used to provide compression, or saline-soaked Gelfoam may be placed on the biopsy site, if needed.

LAPAROSCOPY

• For other techniques, see the references listed in Suggested Reading. Once the procedure is finished, the gas is expelled from the abdomen by opening the stopcocks on the cannulas, and the cannulas are removed. The body wall, subcutaneous tissue, and skin defects are closed routinely. Each surgery site is injected with bupivacaine.

SAMPLE HANDLING
• Biopsy samples are placed in formalin and submitted for histopathologic examination.
• Fluid samples are submitted for cytologic evaluation and culture, as indicated.

APPROPRIATE AFTERCARE
Postprocedure Patient Monitoring
• Body temperature
• Heart and respiratory rate
• Blood pressure, if indicated
• Sedation score
• Pain score
• Observation of incision sites

Nursing Care
Provide a warm, quiet environment for recovery from anesthetic.

Dietary Modification
Feed the animal once it awakes from anesthesia.

Medication Requirements
Analgesics

Restrictions on Activity
Leash walk the patient until the incisions are healed and any sutures or staples are removed.

Anticipated Recovery Time
• Patients recover rapidly, usually within 12–24 h, from minimally invasive surgery.
• Sutures or staples are removed 7–10 days after the procedure.

 INTERPRETATION

NORMAL FINDINGS OR RANGE
Normal size and shape of abdominal organs and abdominal surfaces

ABNORMAL VALUES
• Abnormal size, shape, or color of abdominal organ
• An abdominal mass or masses
• Diffuse neoplastic disease
• Rupture of or leakage from an organ

CRITICAL VALUES
Any condition requiring immediate open surgery, such as peritonitis, severe hemoabdomen, or vascular compromise of the bowel

INTERFERING FACTORS
Drugs That May Alter Results of the Procedure
None

Conditions That May Interfere with Performing the Procedure
• Obesity
• Abdominal fluid
• Hemorrhage
• Clinician inexperience

Procedure Techniques or Handling That May Alter Results
None

Influence of Signalment on Performing and Interpreting the Procedure
Species
Because their bodies are usually smaller, cats are more difficult than dogs.

Breed
Small breeds are more difficult than large breeds.

Age
None

Gender
None

Pregnancy
It may make visualization difficult.

CLINICAL PERSPECTIVE
• This technique is used to explore the abdomen and obtain biopsy samples with minimal pain and stress for the animal. It is an ideal technique for use in medically compromised patients and provides a faster return to function in all patients.

- Results of the exploration and biopsies will enable a treatment plan to be developed or realistic expectations to be provided in the event of a terminal illness.

 MISCELLANEOUS

ANCILLARY TESTS
- Abdominal ultrasonography
- Abdominal radiography

SYNONYMS
Minimally invasive surgery

SEE ALSO
Blackwell's Five-Minute Veterinary Consult: Canine and Feline Topics
Many
Related Topics in This Book
- General Principles of Endoscopy
- Liver Biopsy
- Renal Biopsy and Aspiration
- Thoracoscopy

ABBREVIATIONS
None

Suggested Reading
Richter K. Laparoscopy in dogs and cats. *Vet Clin North Am Small Anim Pract* 2001; **31**: 707–727.
Twedt DC, Monnet E. Laparoscopy: Technique and clinical experience. In: McCarthy TC, ed. *Veterinary Endoscopy for the Small Animal Practitioner*. St Louis: Saunders Elsevier, 2005: 357–386.

INTERNET RESOURCES
BioVision Technologies, Resources: Enabling better medical visualization, http://biovisiontech.com/resources/. Operating-telescope equipment, videos, and training courses.
Storz: Laparoscopy/thoracoscopy, http://www.ksvea.com/small_laparoscopy.html. Equipment and videos.
University of Georgia, College of Veterinary Medicine: Minimally invasive surgery/endoscopic surgery: http://www.vet.uga.edu/mis/index.php. Examples of minimally invasive surgery and training courses.

AUTHOR NAME
Elizabeth M. Hardie

LEAD

 BASICS

TYPE OF SPECIMEN
Blood
Urine

TEST EXPLANATION AND RELATED PHYSIOLOGY
Lead (Pb) poisoning, or plumbism, is of great contemporary and historical significance. Sources of Pb for small animals include old paint (before 1977), artist paints, Pb pipes, caulking, some shot, sinkers, weights for toys and draperies, foil from wine bottles, improperly glazed ceramics, newsprint ink, and industrial contamination of soil.

Most circulating Pb is bound to erythrocytes; thus, blood Pb concentrations are commonly measured as an estimate of body burden. Blood Pb levels do not correlate well with clinical signs. Ca-EDTA–chelated Pb is eliminated in the urine. When blood Pb concentrations are equivocal, urine Pb levels have been used to determine the change in Pb excretion with chelation therapy.

The concentration of Pb in blood or urine is measured by graphite furnace atomic absorption spectrometry or anodic stripping voltammetry. While graphite furnace atomic absorption is considered to be the gold standard, results obtained through anodic stripping voltammetry correlate well with those obtained by atomic absorption spectroscopy.

INDICATIONS
- Blood Pb: screening test for exposure to Pb or Pb poisoning
  - GI signs, such as diarrhea and vomiting
  - Neurologic signs, such as blindness, seizures, difficulty walking, tremors, or unusual behavior
  - Anemia, if present, is usually mild and may be accompanied by an unusually high number of nucleated RBCs, ± basophilic stippling.
- Urine Pb: confirmation of Pb poisoning by determination of the degree of Pb excretion during chelation therapy

CONTRAINDICATIONS
None

POTENTIAL COMPLICATIONS
None

CLIENT EDUCATION
- Low blood Pb concentrations do not rule out Pb poisoning.
- Urinary Pb concentrations, before and after chelation therapy, may be used to confirm the diagnosis of Pb poisoning.
- The diagnosis of Pb poisoning must be based on clinical signs, history of exposure, and other clinical findings in addition to blood or urine Pb concentrations.

BODY SYSTEMS ASSESSED
- Gastrointestinal
- Hemic, lymphatic, and immune
- Nervous
- Renal and urologic

 SAMPLE

COLLECTION
- 1 mL of whole blood
- 5 mL of urine; paired samples:
  - An initial urine sample collected before chelation therapy with either Ca-EDTA, penicillamine, or succimer (DMSA)
  - A second urine sample collected 24-h after chelation
  - Samples may be collected individually or over a 24-h period.

HANDLING
- Heparinized blood collection tubes
- A sterile container for urine
- Ship the sample on ice.

STORAGE
Keep the sample refrigerated.

STABILITY
- Up to 10 weeks at 2°–8°C (refrigerated)
- Stable indefinitely if the blood is sonicated and frozen in plastic tubes

PROTOCOL
When confirming toxicity or monitoring therapy, a baseline urine sample is collected before therapy and another sample is collected after 24 h of chelation therapy.

 INTERPRETATION

NORMAL FINDINGS OR RANGE
- Canine blood should contain <10 µg/dL (0.10 ppm) of Pb.
- Feline blood should contain <14 µg/dL (0.14 ppm) of Pb.

ABNORMAL VALUES
- A concentration of >30–35 µg/dL (0.30–0.35 ppm) of Pb may be associated with clinical signs.
- A >10-fold increase in urinary Pb between prechelation and postchelation therapy samples supports the diagnosis of Pb toxicosis. A <10-fold increase does not support the diagnosis of Pb toxicosis.

CRITICAL VALUES
A concentration of >60 µg/dL in blood (0.60 ppm) is considered diagnostic for Pb poisoning.

INTERFERING FACTORS
Drugs That May Alter Results or Interpretation
Drugs That Interfere with Test Methodology
None

Drugs That Alter Physiology
Chelation therapy may alter blood Pb concentrations.

Disorders That May Alter Results
None

Collection Techniques or Handling That May Alter Results
- Serum and plasma are inappropriate samples.
- Some labs prefer heparin and citrate over EDTA blood tubes.

Influence of Signalment
Species
Cats may be more susceptible to Pb poisoning.

Breed
None

Age
Young animals may be more susceptible Pb poisoning.

Gender
None

Pregnancy
None

LIMITATIONS OF THE TEST
Blood Pb concentrations do not correlate directly with clinical signs.
Sensitivity, Specificity, and Positive and Negative Predictive Values
N/A

Valid If Run in a Human Lab?
Yes.

CLINICAL PERSPECTIVE

- Blood Pb concentrations of >30–35 μg/dL in dogs or cats are consistent with exposure to Pb.
  - Blood Pb concentrations may not represent the total body burden.
  - Blood Pb concentrations may not correlate with clinical signs.
  - Most laboratories have established reference ranges for blood Pb.
- Diagnosis of Pb poisoning is based on a combination of clinical and analytical findings, which may include blood Pb concentrations, prechelation and postchelation therapy urine Pb concentrations, clinical signs, evidence of exposure, and ancillary testing.
- Pb poisoning may cause inappropriate rubricytosis (circulating nucleated RBCs without polychromatophils or in the absence of anemia) as a result of damage to marrow sinuses.
- Pb poisoning may cause basophilic stippling of RBCs by inhibiting the enzyme that helps degrade RNA.
- The absence of nucleated RBCs or basophilic stippling does not rule out Pb toxicosis.

MISCELLANEOUS

ANCILLARY TESTS

- CBC
- Radiography
- Blood aminolevulinic acid dehydratase (δ-ALAD) levels have been recommended but are not available at most veterinary laboratories.
- Zinc protoporphyrin levels have been recommended but are not available at most veterinary laboratories.
- Liver and kidney Pb concentrations

SYNONYMS

- Blood lead
- Pb

SEE ALSO

Blackwell's Five-Minute Veterinary Consult: Canine and Feline Topics
Lead Poisoning
Related Topics in This Book
None

ABBREVIATIONS

- Ca-EDTA = calcium ethylenediaminetetraacetic acid
- DMSA = 2,3-dimercaptosuccinic acid
- Pb = lead

Suggested Reading
Casteel SW. Lead. In: Peterson ME, Talcott PA, eds. *Small Animal Toxicology,* 2nd ed. Philadelphia: WB Saunders, 2005: 795–805.
Gwaltney-Brant S. Lead. In: Plumlee KH, ed. *Clinical Veterinary Toxicology,* 1st ed. St Louis: CV Mosby, 2003: 204–209.
Knight TE, Kumar MSA. Lead toxicosis in cats: A review. *J Feline Med Surg* 2003; 6: 249–255.
Mount ME. Toxicology. In: Ettinger SJ, ed. *Textbook of Veterinary Internal Medicine: Diseases of the Dog and Cat,* 3rd ed. Philadelphia: WB Saunders, 1989: 469–470.
Puls R. *Mineral Levels in Animal Health,* 2nd ed. Aldergrove, Canada: Sherpa, 1994: 146–151.

INTERNET RESOURCES

Beasley V. Toxicants with mixed effects on the central nervous system. In: Beasley V, ed. Veterinary Toxicology. Ithaca, NY: International Veterinary Information Service (IVIS), 1999, http://www.ivis.org/advances/Beasley/Cpt2D/ivis.pdf.

AUTHOR NAME

Karyn Bischoff

LEPTOSPIRA

BASICS

TYPE OF SPECIMEN
Blood
Tissue
Urine

TEST EXPLANATION AND RELATED PHYSIOLOGY

Leptospirosis is a significant zoonotic disease that has been traditionally thought of as important in wild animals, livestock, and hunting dogs. However, in recent years, the incidence of leptospirosis has increased in suburban, as well urban, areas and is now being diagnosed in small to toy breeds of dogs. Dogs become infected with leptospires by directly contacting or ingesting them in stagnant water, by venereal and placental transfer, through bite wounds, or by ingesting contaminated meat. Leptospires penetrate the mucous membranes and migrate to the blood vascular space. The organism then replicates in many organs, including the kidney, liver, central nervous system, eyes, and genital tract. Neutralizing antibodies clear the organisms from most tissues except the renal tubular epithelial cells, where the organisms often persist. Subclinical infections are common, but severe, sometimes fatal, disease also occurs.

Although there are >200 known *Leptospira* serovars, only a handful have been shown to cause disease in animals: *L. canicola*, *L. icterohaemorrhagiae*, *L. bratislava*, *L. grippotyphosa*, *L. pomona*, *L. hardjo*, *L. autumnalis*, *L. ballum*, *L. tarassovi*, and *L. australis* are among the most commonly tested. Clinical signs are similar regardless of the serovar, with renal and liver failure being 2 of the most common manifestations. Renal failure results from interstitial swelling and decreased renal perfusion, leading to decreased glomerular filtration. Liver dysfunction can occur through subcellular damage or hepatic necrosis. In addition, endothelial damage can result in disseminated intravascular coagulation. Several types of diagnostic tests are available.

Serologic Tests
Microscopic Agglutination Test (MAT)

This is a test for *Leptospira*-agglutinating antibodies and is currently the 1 most widely used for diagnosing the disease in dogs. Cultured spirochetes are exposed to serial dilutions of patient serum, and the highest serum dilution to cause agglutination of 50% of the organisms is reported. Agglutinating antibodies usually appear 1–2 weeks after infection and then generally decline over several months to moderate levels that may persist for years. Laboratories test for several serovars, and the highest titer is interpreted as the likely cause of infection. However, in human patients, when compared to culture the highest serovar on the MAT was comparable in only ≈50% of the cases. Lowered titers represent cross-reactivity between serovars and/or vaccination titers.

IgM/IgG ELISA

This assay is used to detect IgM or IgG antibodies to leptospires. IgM antibodies are detectable within 1 week after infection, peak around 2 weeks after infection, and then decline. IgG antibodies begin to develop 2–3 weeks after infection and reach a peak level at 1 month after infection. The IgM ELISA is more sensitive at detecting leptospirosis in the early stages than is the MAT and is better than the MAT at distinguishing naturally infected dogs from vaccinated dogs. However, this test does not distinguish between serovars and is not widely available.

Direct Identification of Organisms
PCR

This test relies on amplification of a specific piece of leptospiral DNA. Some studies suggest that PCR may be more sensitive than the MAT, with an ability to detect subclinical carriers. However, negative results can occur because organisms may not be shed in urine until 4–10

days after the onset of clinical signs and thereafter can be shed intermittently. This test does not distinguish between serovars and is available only through laboratories that specialize in PCR testing.

Visualization of Organisms

Leptospires cannot be seen in a routine urinalysis but can be visualized through the use of a special dark-field microscope condenser. This is not recommended as a screening test. The sensitivity and the specificity of this assay are poor because leptospires are only transiently shed in urine and false-positive results occur if cell debris, fibrin strands, or other types of bacteria are mistaken for leptospires.

Spirochetes can be seen in a biopsy stained with a silver stain. Direct immunofluorescence assays (dIFAs) can be used to visualize leptospires in smears of urine sediment or imprints of liver and/or kidney. These tests do not distinguish between serovars.

Culture

Culture of organisms from urine is difficult. Multiple samples may be required because of intermittent shedding. In addition, leptospires are difficult to culture and require special culture media. They may take weeks to months to grow.

INDICATIONS

These include dogs with any of the following:
- Acute renal failure
- Acute hepatitis
- Anterior uveitis
- Meningitis
- Multisystemic disease
- Polyarthritis
- Vasculitis

CONTRAINDICATIONS

None

POTENTIAL COMPLICATIONS

None

CLIENT EDUCATION

- Urine from infected dogs can cause disease in people if it contacts their mucosal surfaces.
- Leptospires persist in the kidney despite an effective immune response, and infected dogs can shed organisms in urine for months to years. Doxycycline is the treatment of choice to eliminate the carrier state and chronic shedding.
- Urine-contaminated areas should be cleaned with detergent and iodophor disinfectants.

BODY SYSTEMS ASSESSED

- Hepatobiliary
- Nervous
- Ophthalmic
- Renal and urologic
- Reproductive

SAMPLE

COLLECTION

- 2 mL of venous blood for serologic tests
- 5–10 mL of urine for PCR, dIFA, or culture
- 1 mL of cerebrospinal fluid or aqueous humor for PCR, IFA, or culture
- Renal biopsy

HANDLING

- Serologic tests: Collect the sample into a plain red-top tube or serum-separator tube.

- PCR, dIFA, or culture: Collect the sample into a sterile container. Special transport medium is recommended for culture (contact the laboratory).
- Biopsied tissue should be fixed in formalin.

STORAGE
- Refrigeration is recommended for short-term storage.
- Serum or plasma (not urine) should be frozen for long-term storage.
- Samples for culture should be processed as soon as possible.

STABILITY
- Serologic tests
  - Room temperature: 1 day
  - Refrigerated (2°–8°C): 1 week
  - Frozen (−20°C): months to years
- PCR: Samples can be stored for days to weeks at 2°–8°C or months to years at −20° to −80°C.
- Culture: Process the samples as soon as possible.

INTERPRETATION

NORMAL FINDINGS OR RANGE
- Negative for all tested serovars, in the absence of a history of vaccination
- 1:100, 1:200, and 1:400 are considered normal vaccinal titers. The 4 serovars currently available in canine leptospirosis vaccines include *L. canicola*, *L. icterohaemorrhagiae*, *L. grippotyphosa*, and *L. pomona*.

ABNORMAL VALUES
- Any serovar ≥1:800 is considered positive for leptospirosis.
- Any nonvaccinated dog with clinical signs and a negative titer or a 1:100, 1:200, or ≥1:400 titer may have an early infection.
- A 4-fold increase in titer in paired samples is positive for infection.
- A cross-reaction between serovars is possible.
- Coinfection with more than 1 serovar is possible.
- Collection of convalescent samples 10–14 days apart are recommended to look for an increase in titer.

CRITICAL VALUES
None

INTERFERING FACTORS
Drugs That May Alter Results or Interpretation
Drugs That Interfere with Test Methodology
None

Drugs That Alter Physiology
Antibiotic therapy can decrease or prevent rising MAT titers in acutely infected animals.

Disorders That May Alter Results
None

Collection Techniques or Handling That May Alter Results
None

Influence of Signalment
Species
Cats are less susceptible than dogs to clinical illness, although they may have leptospiral antibodies.

Breed
None

Age
Dogs <6 months old are more severely affected and more likely to have signs of hepatic dysfunction.

Gender
None

Pregnancy
Abortion and infertility have been reported with some serovars.

LIMITATIONS OF THE TEST
Dogs acutely infected with leptospirosis may have a negative or low MAT result despite clinical signs. Dogs still suspected of having leptospirosis should be treated appropriately. Samples to determine convalescent titers should be submitted in 2–3 weeks to confirm the diagnosis.

Sensitivity, Specificity, and Positive and Negative Predictive Values
N/A

Valid If Run in Human a Lab?
No.

Causes of Abnormal Findings

High values (positive test)	Low values (negative test)
MAT/ELISA	MAT/ELISA
Infection	Healthy
Vaccination	Early infection
Cross-reaction with	Urine dIFA
nonleptospiral	Healthy
spirochetes (low titer)	Early infection
Urine dIFA	Organisms not currently
Infection (cannot	being shed
distinguish dead vs live	Urine PCR
spirochetes)	Healthy
Urine PCR	Early infection
Infection (cannot	Organisms not currently
distinguish dead vs	being shed
live spirochetes)	

CLINICAL PERSPECTIVE
- Most dogs infected with leptospirosis present with acute renal failure. However, some infected dogs present with acute liver failure and are icteric.
- Dogs acutely infected with leptospirosis may have a titer of ≤1:400. PCR or dIFA may facilitate the diagnosis of these cases. Alternatively, these dogs should be treated presumptively and retested in 2–3 weeks to confirm infection.
- A titer of ≥1:800 generally indicates active infection or a subclinical carrier state.

MISCELLANEOUS

ANCILLARY TESTS
- Chemistry profile and urinalysis to look for evidence of renal failure and liver disease
- CBC
- Renal biopsy

SYNONYMS
- *Leptospira australis*
- *L. autumnalis*
- *L. ballum*
- *L. bratislava*
- *L. canicola*
- *L. grippotyphosa*
- *L. hardjo*
- *L. icterohaemorrhagiae*
- *L. pomona*
- *L. tarassovi*

SEE ALSO
Blackwell's Five-Minute Veterinary Consult: Canine and Feline Topics
- Hepatitis, Infectious Canine
- Leptospirosis
- Renal Failure, Acute Uremia
- Renal Failure, Chronic

Related Topics in This Book
- Chapters on urine tests
- Creatinine
- Urea Nitrogen

ABBREVIATIONS
- dIFA = direct immunofluorescent assay
- MAT = microscopic agglutination test

Suggested Readings
Greene CE, Sykes JE, Brown CA, Hartmann K. Leptospirosis. In: Greene CE, ed. *Infectious Diseases of the Dog and Cat,* 3rd ed. St Louis: Saunders Elsevier, 2005: 402–417.
Hartmann K, Greene CE. Diseases caused by systemic bacterial infections. In: Ettinger SJ, Feldman EC, eds. *Textbook of Veterinary Internal Medicine,* 6th ed. Philadelphia: WB Saunders, 2005: 616–618.
Moore, GE, Guptill LF, Glickman NW, *et al.* Canine leptospirosis, United States, 2002–2004. *Emerg Infect Dis* 2006; 12: 501–503.

INTERNET RESOURCES
None

AUTHOR NAME
Terri Wheeler

BASICS

TYPE OF SPECIMEN
Blood

TEST EXPLANATION AND RELATED PHYSIOLOGY
Lipase is an enzyme that hydrolyzes triglycerides to fatty acids and glycerol. Similar to amylase, the major source of lipase is the pancreas, with other organs, such as the stomach, liver, intestine, and other locations also producing lipase. Lipase is removed from the circulation by the kidney. In the intestine, bile salts and the enzyme colipase enhance the activity of lipase.

Elevations of this enzyme in dogs are often associated with pancreatitis. Like amylase, lipase levels rise and peak within ≈12–48 h and return to normal within 8–14 days after experimental induction of pancreatic inflammation. However, elevated lipase can also be caused by decreased GFR or with diseases of other lipase-producing nonpancreatic tissues. Extremely high lipase levels have also been reported with some pancreatic and hepatocellular carcinomas. Lipase is an unreliable indicator of pancreatitis in cats.

A kinetic procedure has been developed for automated methods of determining lipase. Methods that add colipase to the reaction mixture were found to increase analytical sensitivity and specificity of lipase. An immunoassay is available that measures only the lipase of pancreatic origin. This pancreas-specific lipase assay is of higher sensitivity and specificity in the diagnosis of pancreatitis (see the "Pancreatic Lipase Immunoreactivity" chapter).

INDICATIONS
• Clinical signs suggestive of canine pancreatitis (e.g., vomiting, anorexia, abdominal pain, icterus)
• Nonseptic, inflammatory abdominal exudate

CONTRAINDICATIONS
None

POTENTIAL COMPLICATIONS
None

CONTRAINDICATIONS
None

CLIENT EDUCATION
• Dogs should be fasted for the most accurate results.
• Clients should be made aware that lipase is a nonspecific test and can be associated with pancreatitis, as well as disease in other organs such as kidney or intestine.

BODY SYSTEMS ASSESSED
• Gastrointestinal
• Hepatobiliary
• Renal and urologic

 SAMPLE

COLLECTION
• 1–2 mL of venous blood
• Abdominal fluid

HANDLING
• A red-top tube or serum-separator tube is preferred.
• A lithium-heparinized tube (green top) is acceptable but not preferred.

STORAGE
Refrigerate or freeze the serum for long-term storage.

STABILITY
• Room temperature: 1 week
• Refrigerated (2°–8°C): at least 1 month
• Frozen (−20°C): at least 8 months

PROTOCOL
None

 INTERPRETATION

NORMAL FINDINGS OR RANGE
• Dogs: 90–527 IU/L
• Cats: 0–83 IU/L
• Reference intervals may vary depending on the laboratory and assay.

ABNORMAL VALUES
Values above the reference range

CRITICAL VALUES
None

INTERFERING FACTORS
Drugs That May Alter Results or Interpretation
Drugs That Interfere with Test Methodology
None

Drugs That Alter Physiology
• Corticosteroids may increase serum lipase levels up to 5 times the upper limit of the reference interval without histologic evidence of pancreatitis.
• Some drugs have been associated with pancreatitis:
  • Antibiotics, such as metronidazole, sulfonamides, tetracycline
  • Diuretics, including furosemide and thiazides
  • Other drugs, such as asparaginase and azathioprine

Disorders That May Alter Results
None

LIPASE

Collection Techniques or Handling That May Alter Results
None

Influence of Signalment

Species
Lipase is less reliable as a marker of pancreatitis in cats than in dogs.

Breed
None

Age
None

Gender
None

Pregnancy
None

LIMITATIONS OF THE TEST
• Lipase is considered moderately sensitive and specific for the diagnosis of pancreatitis but is still affected by other diseases, such as renal disease, or intestinal disorders.
• The level of lipase activity is not proportional to the severity of pancreatitis, and normal levels can be seen in some patients with severe acute pancreatitis.
• Some of the highest lipase levels can be seen with pancreatic and liver neoplasms.

Sensitivity, Specificity, and Positive and Negative Predictive Values
Not available

Valid If Run in a Human Lab?
Yes.

Causes of Abnormal Findings

High values	Low values
Decreased GFR	Not significant
Severe dehydration	
Renal disease	
Urinary tract obstruction	
Pancreatitis	
GI disease	
Liver disease, including	
hepatocellular	
carcinoma	
Pancreatic carcinoma	
Glucocorticoids	
(endogenous or	
exogenous)	

CLINICAL PERSPECTIVE
• If a patient has high lipase values, additional workup is needed to rule out liver disease, GI disease, or causes of decreased GFR.
• Nonpancreatic diseases usually raise lipase no more than 2–3 times normal, although renal disease and glucocorticoids will occasionally increase levels as much as 4 or 5 times normal, respectively.
• Pancreatic masses should be biopsied because both chronic pancreatitis and pancreatic neoplasms can cause elevated lipase levels.
• Newer tests such as canine pancreatic lipase immunoreactivity (PLI) offer greater sensitivity and specificity than amylase for the diagnosis of this disorder.
• Abdominal fluid lipase levels of >2-fold the serum lipase levels suggest pancreatitis, although bowel rupture is also possible.

MISCELLANEOUS

ANCILLARY TESTS

- Amylase, pancreatic lipase immunoreactivity, or trypsin-like immunoreactivity (TLI) to confirm pancreatic disease
- BUN, creatinine, and urinalysis for evaluation of renal function
- Biopsy of the liver or pancreatic masses
- Liver enzymes
- Ultrasound of the liver and pancreas

SYNONYMS

None

SEE ALSO

Blackwell's Five-Minute Veterinary Consult: Canine and Feline Topics

Pancreatitis

Related Topics in This Book

- Amylase
- Pancreatic Lipase Immunoreactivity
- Pancreatic Ultrasonography
- Trypsin-like Immunoreactivity

ABBREVIATIONS

GFR = glomerular filtration rate

Suggested Reading

Brobst DF. Pancreatic function. In: Kaneko JJ, Harvey JW, Bruss ML, eds. *Clinical Biochemistry of Domestic Animals,* 5th ed. San Diego: Academic, 1997: 353–366.

Quigley KA, Jackson ML, Haines DM. Hyperlipasemia in 6 dogs with pancreatic or hepatic neoplasia: Evidence for tumor lipase production. *Vet Clin Pathol* 2001; **30**: 114–120.

Steiner JM. Diagnosis of pancreatitis. *Vet Clin North Am Small Anim Pract* 2003; **33**: 1181–1195.

INTERNET RESOURCES

Cornell University, College of Veterinary Medicine, Clinical Pathology Modules, Specialized Chemistry Tests: Lipase, http://www.diaglab.vet.cornell.edu/clinpath/modules/chem/lipase.htm.

Texas A&M University, College of Veterinary Medicine, Gastrointestinal Laboratory: Pancreatic lipase immunoreactivity (PLI), http://www.cvm.tamu.edu/gilab/cPLI.shtml.

AUTHOR NAME

Denise Wunn

LIVER AND GALLBLADDER ULTRASONOGRAPHY

BASICS

TYPE OF PROCEDURE
Ultrasonographic

PROCEDURE EXPLANATION AND RELATED PHYSIOLOGY
Hepatic ultrasonography is a valuable tool for differentiating focal from multifocal disease and solid versus fluid-filled lesions. Ultrasonography is sensitive for identifying liver nodules and masses but less sensitive for detecting diffuse liver disease. Although diffuse disease may be present, the liver may still appear normal sonographically. Differentiating benign from malignant nodules can be difficult with ultrasound and generally requires tissue sampling. In icteric patients, ultrasonography is very helpful for differentiating obstructive from nonobstructive lesions. The pancreas can be ruled out with ultrasound as the source at the same time. In obstructive disease, dilation of the intra- and extrahepatic bile ducts can be detected. Gallbladder distention, wall thickening, and abnormal content can be examined with ultrasound. Ultrasound can also be used for screening for portosystemic shunts, both congenital and acquired. Lastly, ultrasound-guided tissue aspiration, as well as cholecystocentesis, can be performed.

INDICATIONS
- Liver parenchyma, biliary tract, and vascular system abnormalities
- Increased liver enzyme activities
- Focal, multifocal, and diffuse liver disease differentiation
- Icterus
- A space-occupying lesion of the cranial abdomen
- Hepatomegaly
- Chronic vomiting
- Detect portosystemic shunts
- Ascites

CONTRAINDICATIONS
None

POTENTIAL COMPLICATIONS
None

CLIENT EDUCATION
- Ultrasound is a safe, noninvasive imaging procedure.
- The animal should be fasted 12 h prior to the examination. Water may be given up to a few hours prior to the procedure.
- The hair on the ventral and lateral abdomen will need to be clipped in order to perform the ultrasound examination.

BODY SYSTEMS ASSESSED
Hepatobiliary

PROCEDURE

PATIENT PREPARATION
Preprocedure Medication or Preparation
- Patients should be fasted 12 h prior to examination. Water may be given up to a few hours prior to the procedure.
- Hair should be clipped from the abdomen and from the costal arch both ventrally and bilaterally.

Anesthesia or Sedation
- Anesthesia or sedation may be required in noncompliant patients or those with a painful abdomen.
- If fine-needle tissue aspiration or biopsy of the gastric or intestinal wall is required, then sedation or anesthesia is usually required.

Patient Positioning
The ultrasound examination may be carried out with patients in either dorsal or lateral recumbency according to the sonographer's preference. Both left and right lateral recumbency may be required.

Patient Monitoring
None

Equipment or Supplies
- An ultrasound machine equipped with high-frequency transducers. Curved array transducers between 7.5 and 14 MHz may be used, depending on the region being examined and the size of the patient. A 5.0-MHz sector or curved linear transducer is necessary to examine the liver in mid-sized to large dogs. A ≥7.5-MHz transducer will improve resolution in cats and small-breed dogs. A ≤3-MHz transducer may be necessary in obese or giant-breed dogs.
- Documentation with video recordings, black-and-white printers, or digital acquisition of still images or clips is required.
- Clippers
- Acoustic coupling gel

TECHNIQUE
- The hair of the ventral abdomen is clipped, and acoustic gel is applied to the skin to ensure good contact with the ultrasound probe.
- The position of the animal can be changed during the examination, if necessary.
- Intercostal imaging from the left and right through the 10th to 13th intercostal spaces should also be used to ensure complete assessment of the liver.
- The entire abdomen, including the pancreas, should be examined because many diseases affecting the liver may involve multiple organ systems.
- Scanning should start at the xyphoid with the transducer angled craniodorsally toward the dog's head. Both the sagittal and transverse planes should be used to examine the liver. The beam should be swept from cranial to caudal and left to right in both the transverse and sagittal planes.
- When examining patients with suspected hepatic disease, the liver, gallbladder, biliary tract, duodenal papilla, and pancreas should be examined with high-frequency transducers. Generally, curved array transducers with a small footprint are advantageous for examining these structures because of their location just behind and underneath the costal arch. Larger transducers make it more difficult to access these regions, especially in cats.
- The internal architecture, including its portal, venous, arterial, and biliary vasculature, in addition to its echogenicity and echotexture, should be evaluated. The gallbladder wall, size, and contents, as well as the size of the cystic and bile ducts, can be determined. In addition, the proximal duodenal papilla can be assessed for signs of obstruction. The hepatic hilar region and cranial duodenum can be challenging regions to examine with ultrasound.

SAMPLE HANDLING
N/A

APPROPRIATE AFTERCARE
Postprocedure Patient Monitoring
None

Nursing Care
None

Dietary Modification
None

Medication Requirements
None

Restrictions on Activity
None

Anticipated Recovery Time
None

INTERPRETATION

NORMAL FINDINGS OR RANGE
- Dogs: The liver has a uniform echogenicity and is hypoechoic in comparison with the spleen and either hyperechoic or isoechoic to the renal cortex (Figure 1). The echotexture is coarse compared to the spleen.
- Cats: The liver has uniform echogenicity and is hypoechoic to the adjacent falciform fat. It may become hyperechoic to the surrounding fat in obese but otherwise healthy cats.
- A mirror-image artifact is often present on the thoracic side of the diaphragm.
- The portal and hepatic venous systems are clearly identifiable and make the echotexture appear coarse. Portal veins have a branching pattern with hyperechoic walls. Hepatic veins appear as anechoic branching structures that can be traced to the vena cava at the liver hilus.
- Intrahepatic arteries and bile ducts are not visible in normal animals.
- The gallbladder is round to oval with a thin wall of <2 mm and visible to the right of midline in most dogs and cats (Figure 2). The gallbladder is larger in fasted animals. The contents are generally anechoic, but it is common to observe hyperechoic, mobile sediment in most dogs, though less so in cats. Sludge balls may appear as small round hyperechoic mobile structures within the gallbladder.
- Acoustic enhancement and edge-shadowing artifacts are usually present distal to the gallbladder.
- If the common bile duct is visible, it should be <5 mm in diameter and located ventral to the portal vein at the liver hilus. It can be more easily visualized in cats.
- The assessment of liver size is subjective and should be determined by using ultrasound in combination with radiography.

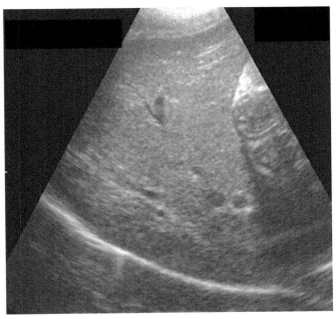

Figure 1

Sagittal section of a normal liver in a dog. The liver has a homogeneous echotexture of middle echogenicity. The portal veins are identified by their thin hyperechoic wall.

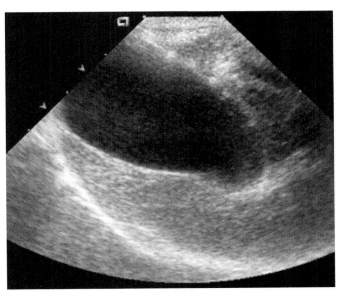

Figure 2

Sagittal section of a normal canine gallbladder. The wall is thin and hyperechoic. The content in this instance is anechoic.

ABNORMAL VALUES
Hepatic Parenchymal Disease
Sonographic changes in hepatic parenchymal disorders are generally focal, multifocal, or diffuse. Although ultrasound is sensitive in detecting focal or multifocal changes, diffuse processes are more difficult to recognize. In diffuse disease, the liver may appear normal or have an increased, decreased, or mixed echogenicity. Because the evaluation of liver echogenicity is rather subjective and the findings nonspecific, changes should also be correlated with the clinical findings. In acute liver disease, the liver may appear normal or enlarged. In chronic disease, the liver may be small to normal. Because of the wide variations in the sonographic appearance of different inflammatory and neoplastic diseases, either fine-needle aspiration for cytologic evaluation or Tru-cut biopsy for histopathologic evaluation is required for a more definitive diagnosis.

Hepatomegaly
- Because only extreme alterations in liver size are readily recognizable with ultrasound, the size should be determined in combination with radiography.
- Hepatomegaly can be suspected when the distance between the diaphragm and stomach is increased, the liver lobes are extended caudally, and the liver margins are rounded.
- Common causes include hyperadrenocorticism, diabetes mellitus, acute hepatitis, hepatic venous congestion, and neoplasia.

Microhepatica
- Suspected when there is poor visualization of the liver or close approximation of the stomach to the diaphragm. Potential causes are these:
  - Cirrhosis and chronic hepatitis are the most common. Fibrosis is usually present.
  - Portosystemic shunt
  - Displacement caused by diaphragmatic hernia
- Difficult to diagnose based on ultrasound appearance alone
- The hepatic echotexture may appear coarse, and hyperplastic nodules may be present. Ascites may be present.

LIVER AND GALLBLADDER ULTRASONOGRAPHY

Diffuse Liver Changes: Hyperechogenicity

Hyperechogenicity can be detected in a number of conditions, including fatty infiltration, steroid therapy, hyperadrenocorticism, chronic liver disease, diabetes, histiocytic sarcoma, and lymphoma. Sonographically, the liver will appear homogeneous and isoechoic to the spleen. This can be difficult to observe unless a high-frequency transducer is used. In most cases, the liver will also be enlarged unless the disease is chronic. The liver may be so hyperechoic that attenuation of the beam occurs and the dorsal regions of the liver appear hypoechoic. If this occurs, gain should be increased in the far field, or a lower-frequency transducer should be used. Chronic hepatitis and cirrhosis may also result in a diffusely hyperechoic liver, and the liver will be small to normal sized, with or without ascites.

Feline hepatic lipidosis

The liver in affected cats is enlarged, rounded, and shows an increased echogenicity equal to or greater than that of the spleen. It may appear isoechoic or hyperechoic compared to omental and falciform fat. Beam attenuation may occur, and the dorsal region of the liver in the far field may be difficult to visualize. The appearance of vascular structures is diminished. Fatty infiltration of the liver (from obesity or diabetes mellitus) will appear similar to hepatic lipidosis sonographically. Fine-needle aspiration is usually adequate for a cytologic diagnosis and to rule out neoplastic disease.

Diffuse Liver Changes: Hypoechogenicity

When hypoechogenicity is present, the portal veins will appear more echogenic and the liver will appear to have a high contrast between the vessels and the parenchyma. Differentials include hepatitis and cholangiohepatitis, toxic injury, metabolic disease, trauma, vascular compromise, amyloidosis, lymphoma, and passive congestion. If the hepatic veins are dilated, right heart disease should be ruled out.

Diffuse Liver Changes: Mixed Echogenicity

Mixed echogenicity is most often due to neoplasia, with the hepatic parenchyma appearing diffusely complex or disrupted with poorly circumscribed areas of both increased and decreased echogenicities. Other causes of a complex echostructure in the liver are inflammation, toxicity, necrosis, and canine superficial necrolytic dermatitis (hepatocutaneous syndrome).

Focal or multifocal disease

- Abscesses and granulomas
  - Generally produce focal lesions of mixed echogenicity but are variable depending on age. The content of an abscess may be anechoic, hypoechoic, or isoechoic with the surrounding parenchyma.
  - A distinct wall may or may not be present, and the margins may even be irregular.
  - Hyperechoic foci with reverberation artifacts represent gas content.
  - Suspected abscesses can be safely aspirated for cytologic and bacteriologic examination using a small-gauge needle (22–25 gauge).
- Neoplasia
  - A wide range of appearances is possible for different tumor types, and no specific pattern enables differentiation of primary from metastatic neoplasia.
  - Neoplasia may present as solitary or multifocal nodules or masses with well defined borders.
  - Target lesions may be present showing a hyperechoic center and hypoechoic outer rim.
  - Focal or multifocal hypoechoic or mixed lesions are most common in most primary or metastatic disease.
  - Lymphoma can cause hepatomegaly with either a normal appearing parenchyma or focal or multifocal changes. Lymphadenomegaly is not always present.
  - Liver nodules are often discovered on examination of older animals. Benign hyperplastic nodules in older dogs cannot be differen-

tiated from metastases by using 2-dimensional gray-scale ultrasound. Therefore, aspiration or biopsy is required to determine their cause.
- Hematoma
  - Appearance varies with age.
  - Acute bleeding appears hyperechoic.
  - As the hematoma ages, it will become hypoechoic to anechoic and hyperechoic coaguli may also be identified.
  - Irregular or poorly defined margins are often present.
  - Hematomas cannot be differentiated form abscesses, necrosis, or neoplasia.
- Cysts
  - Thin-walled structures of varying size with an anechoic center
  - Congenital or acquired
  - Solitary or multiple
  - Can be within the parenchyma or biliary tract
  - Can be seen together with polycystic kidney disease
  - Usually of little clinical importance if enough normal appearing liver parenchyma is present
- Nodular hyperplasia
  - Variable appearance
  - Common in older dogs
  - Usually present as well marginated, hypoechoic nodules but other patterns are possible
  - Requires a fine-needle aspiration or biopsy to differentiate it from hematomas, abscesses, necrosis. and primary or metastatic liver disease
- Mineralization
  - Hyperechoic structures within the hepatic parenchyma may be caused by mineralization of the parenchyma due to fibrosis, dystrophic mineralization of old hematomas, or granulomas, as well as foreign bodies or gas.

Vascular Abnormalities

Congenital and acquired abnormalities of the portal, venous, and arterial hepatic vasculature may occur in both dogs and cats. Experience with color and spectral Doppler ultrasound and knowledge of normal blood flow are necessary in order to detect vascular diseases.

Portosystemic Shunts

- Common 2-dimensional gray-scale findings:
  - Microhepatica
  - A decreased number of intrahepatic portal veins
  - Bilateral renomegaly
  - Urolithiasis
  - Ascites
- Shunts are best identified by examining the vena cava and portal vein from the right craniolateral abdomen with the dog in left lateral recumbency. The hilus of the liver should be scanned between the right 11th and 13th ribs.
- The vena cava and portal vein should be examined with color Doppler to identify regions of turbulence. The search for shunting vessels should then be focused to that region.
- If a shunt is not identified with ultrasound, then scintigraphic detection or positive contrast portograms are additional diagnostic methods that can be pursued.

Intrahepatic shunts

- Occur mainly in young large-breed dogs
- Appear as large anechoic dilations within the liver parenchyma near the hilus of the liver and vena cava
- Are generally easier to identify than extrahepatic shunts

Extrahepatic shunts

- They occur most commonly in young, small-breed dogs and young cats.
- They can be difficult to detect and require experience with Doppler ultrasound and a good understanding of ultrasound vascular anatomy.

- The type of shunt is highly variable, and communications may occur between the portal vein and the vena cava, renal, azygous, splenic, and left gastric veins.
- Because of either their small size or poor visualization because of overlying GI structures and air artifacts, a normal study does not rule out an extrahepatic shunt.
- The vena cava is examined from the hilus of the liver to its bifurcation in the caudal abdomen. Color Doppler is used to search for areas of turbulence in the vena cava so that the examination can be focused on that region.
- Small tortuous shunt vessels showing turbulent flow may be identified from the hilus of the liver to the midabdomen in the region of the vena cava.

Secondary, acquired shunts
- Occur in older dogs and cats
- Most commonly due to hepatic disease causing portal hypertension
- Identified as numerous tortuous dilated vessels in the region of the kidneys and caudal vena cava
- Ascites and microhepatica are generally present. Sonographic evidence of cirrhosis or fibrosis may also be detected.

Other Vascular Abnormalities
Passive venous congestion
- The liver appears enlarged and hypoechoic, and ascites is usually present.
- Dilated vessels that converge with the vena cava at the hilus can be identified.
- High-frequency and highly pulsatile waveforms can be detected with pulsed-wave Doppler examination of the caudal vena cava and hepatic veins.
- Causes include pericardial effusion, right heart failure, restrictive pericardial disease, or severe tricuspid insufficiency.

Portal vein thrombosis
- Not common
- If it is anechoic, the thrombus may or may not be directly visualized with 2-dimensional gray-scale ultrasound. It can sometimes be visualized as an intraluminal hyperechoic structure at the liver hilus.
- Use of Doppler ultrasound is necessary for showing reduced or absent flow in the portal vein.
- Extraluminal compression by a mass or lymphadenomegaly may also occur but is less common.

Arteriovenous fistulas
- Not common
- The clinical signs are similar to those in a patient with a portosystemic shunt.
- Tortuous vessels can be identified within the liver.
- Use of Doppler ultrasound is required to show high-velocity arterial signals, which differentiates them from portosystemic venous shunts.

Biliary Tract Disease
Ultrasound is useful for differentiating hepatic parenchymal disease from biliary obstruction in patients with icterus.

Nonobstructive Biliary Tract Disease
Cholecystitis
- The main sonographic finding is wall thickening. The disease may be seen together with hepatitis, cholangitis, and cholangiohepatitis. Edema of the wall may occur in inflammatory diseases, causing it to appear thickened and hypoechoic.
- The wall will appear hyperechoic, often with an irregular mucosal surface.
- Varying amounts of gallbladder sediment may be identified and is a nonspecific finding.

Double gallbladder wall
A double-rimmed wall with a hypoechoic space between an outer and inner hyperechoic wall may be detected in animals with ascites, hypoalbuminemia, sepsis, inflammation, or neoplasia.

Gallbladder mucoceles
In general, the gallbladder wall is thickened, and the contents show a complex echostructure and echogenicity. Hyperechoic membranes, irregular sludge, or stellate patterns that are not mobile can be demonstrated. The gallbladder may be obstructed, and wall necrosis can cause bile peritonitis. Exploratory surgery is generally indicated when this disease is detected in conjunction with hepatic disease. The presence of ascites can indicate the presence of rupture and bile peritonitis.

Emphysematous cholecystitis
This can be identified by the presence of reverberation echoes creating "dirty" shadowing coming from the gallbladder wall or lumen.

Choleliths
- These can be identified as hyperechoic structures with acoustic shadowing in the gallbladder. The surface of the structures may be smooth and curvilinear or irregular.
- They may or may not be associated with clinical signs.
- The common bile duct should be examined in its entirety for the presence of choleliths potentially causing obstruction.

Polyps
These are focal or multifocal wall infiltrations or nodules that may appear as hyperechoic rounded structures attached by a stalk to the gallbladder wall. Sessile or polypoid lesions are rarely tumors.

Neoplasia
Rare. It is difficult to differentiate it from neoplasia of the hepatic parenchyma.

Obstructive Biliary Tract Disease
Pancreatitis, biliary calculi and neoplasia, lymphadenomegaly, abscesses, and granulomas may be causes of obstructive disease. A normal finding does not exclude the presence of an obstruction.

Extrahepatic cholestasis
- The pancreas and duodenal papilla can be sources of obstruction and should be evaluated sonographically.
- Biliary calculi, pancreatitis, neoplasia, granulomas, abscesses, and liver flukes are possible causes of obstruction.
- Lymphoma in cats, bile duct carcinoma, and pancreatic carcinoma are neoplastic causes.
- The gallbladder may or may not be enlarged.
- The common bile duct may be dilated to >5 mm.

Intrahepatic cholestasis
- Intrahepatic bile ducts may take days to weeks to dilate following common bile duct obstruction.
- Long-standing obstructions may lead to a "gunshot" appearance of the liver, with numerous, tortuous anechoic tubular structures in the liver parenchyma. Color Doppler ultrasound will show an absence of flow, indicating that they are biliary vessels. Differentials for this finding include the following:
  - Long-standing obstruction
  - Biliary cysts
  - Pseudocysts
  - Biliary cystadenomas
  - Bile duct carcinoma

CRITICAL VALUES
None

LIVER AND GALLBLADDER ULTRASONOGRAPHY

INTERFERING FACTORS

Drugs That May Alter Results of the Procedure
The use of medetomidine to sedate animals will slow blood flow significantly and make color Doppler investigations for portosystemic shunts difficult.

Conditions That May Interfere with Performing the Procedure
None

Procedure Techniques or Handling That May Alter Results
The hilus of the liver and regional vasculature will be difficult to examine in patients with large amounts of ingesta in the stomach.

Influence of Signalment on Performing and Interpreting the Procedure

Species
None

Breed
None

Age
None

Gender
None

Pregnancy
None

CLINICAL PERSPECTIVE

• Although ultrasound is sensitive for the detection of focal or multifocal liver abnormalities, it is much less sensitive for detecting diffuse disease.
• A sonographically normal appearing liver may still be abnormal.
• Liver diseases are often involved in multiorgan or systemic disease. The entire abdomen should be examined with ultrasound when hepatic disease is suspected.
• Because of wide variation in the sonographic appearance of many liver diseases, the use of fine-needle aspiration or biopsy or both is usually required to differentiate inflammatory, neoplastic, and hyperplastic diseases.
• Ruling out obstructive biliary tract disease in patients with icterus requires excellent understanding of the regional anatomy of the porta hepatis and advanced sonography experience.
• Detecting portosystemic shunts with ultrasound requires advanced knowledge of Doppler ultrasound techniques and vascular anatomy.

MISCELLANEOUS

ANCILLARY TESTS

• If a suspected portosystemic shunt cannot be detected with ultrasound, per-rectal portal scintigraphy, transsplenic portal scintigraphy, positive contrast portograms, or computed tomographic examination may be required to confirm the diagnosis.
• Fine-needle aspiration or biopsy is indicated if the findings on examination of the liver are normal.

SYNONYMS

• Hepatic ultrasound
• Hepatobiliary ultrasonography

SEE ALSO

Blackwell's Five-Minute Veterinary Consult: Canine and Feline Topics
• Arteriovenous Malformation of the Liver
• Cirrhosis and Fibrosis of the Liver
• Hemangiosarcoma, Spleen and Liver
• Hepatic Amyloid
• Hepatic Failure, Acute
• Hepatic Lipidosis
• Hepatic Nodular Hyperplasia
• Hepatitis, Chronic Active
• Hepatitis, Granulomatous
• Hepatitis, Infectious Canine
• Hepatitis, Suppurative and Hepatic Abscess
• Hepatocellular Adenoma
• Hepatocellular Carcinoma
• Hepatomegaly
• Hepatoportal Microvascular Dysplasia
• Juvenile Fibrosing Liver Disease
• Liver Fluke Infestation
• Portosystemic Shunting, Acquired
• Portosystemic Vascular Anomaly, Congenital

Related Topics in This Book
• General Principles of Ultrasonography
• Abdominal Radiography
• Abdominal Ultrasonography
• Computed Tomography
• Liver Biopsy
• Transsplenic Portal Scintigraphy
• Ultrasound-Guided Mass or Organ Aspiration

ABBREVIATIONS
None

Suggested Reading
Biller DS, Kantrowitz B, Miyabayashi T. Ultrasonography of diffuse liver disease: A review. *J Vet Intern Med* 1992; 6: 71–76.
Bromel C, Leveille R, Scrivani PV, *et al.* Gallbladder perforation associated with cholelithiasis and cholecystitis in a dog. *J Small Anim Pract* 1998; 39: 541–544.
Daniel GB, Berry CR. Scintigraphic detection of portosystemic shunts. In: Daniel GB, Berry CR, eds. *Textbook of Veterinary Nuclear Medicine,* 2nd ed. Harrisburg, PA: American College of Veterinary Radiology, 2006: 231–255.
Fahie MA, Martin RA. Extrahepatic biliary tract obstruction: A retrospective study of 45 cases (1983–1993). *J Am Anim Hosp Assoc* 1995; 31: 478–482.
Nyland TG, Mattoon JS, Hergesell EJ, Wisner ER. Liver. In: Nyland TG, Mattoon JS, eds. *Small Animal Diagnostic Ultrasound,* 2nd ed. Philadelphia: WB Saunders, 2002: 93–127.

INTERNET RESOURCES
None

AUTHOR NAME
Lorrie Gaschen

BASICS

TYPE OF PROCEDURE
Biopsy

PROCEDURE EXPLANATION AND RELATED PHYSIOLOGY
Liver biopsy enables sampling of the hepatic parenchyma and intra-hepatic vascular and biliary structures. Three general methods are used depending on clinician skill with the procedure, patient status, and considered differential diagnoses. Percutaneous liver biopsy samples are collected under ultrasonographic guidance; spring-loaded automated cutting needles are most commonly used. Laparosocpic liver biopsy samples are collected using a cup biopsy forceps. Laparoscopic procedures are desirable because they provide gross visualization of the liver and peritoneal cavity, and enable detection of acquired portosystemic shunts (caused by portal hypertension), assessment of extrahepatic biliary structures, and safe biopsy of any liver lobe or specific lesions. Similar benefits are achieved by laparotomy, where liver biopsy is generally collected using a wedge biopsy method or a Baker's skin biopsy punch. Patients recover from laparoscopy much faster than from exploratory laparotomy. Jaundiced patients with suspected extrahepatic bile duct occlusion should undergo exploratory laparotomy rather than needle or laparoscopic procedures for liver assessment.

INDICATIONS
• Essential for definitive diagnosis of most forms of hepatobiliary disease
• Differentiates acquired from congenital or inherited hepatobiliary disorders
• Distinguishes anatomic distribution (acinar zonal involvement) of hepatobiliary injury, enabling subjective appraisal of the extent of hepatic fibrosis; type, extent, and location of hepatobiliary inflammation; and presence and location of transition metal (copper, iron) accumulation, hepatocellular necrosis or apoptosis, biliary hyperplasia, cholestasis (bile canalicular plugs), biliary epithelial hyperplasia, and hepatocellular vacuolar transformation
• Detection, differentiation, and staging of primary hepatobiliary and metastatic hepatic neoplasia
• Characterization of hepatic disorders causing ascites
• Assessment of treatment efficacy
• Detection of bacterial infections of the hepatobiliary system

CONTRAINDICATIONS
• Symptomatic coagulopathy
• Needle biopsies are ill-advised in patients with ascites or suspected extrahepatic bile duct occlusion or that weigh ≤2 kg.
• Tru-cut biopsy procedures should not be performed with only local anesthesia or sedation.
• Needle biopsy procedures are contraindicated in patients with nonsolid lesions (cystic lesions, vascular malformations, abscess) and patients with ascites.
• Septic peritonitis
• Laparoscopy is difficult in patients weighing <2 kg.
• Liver biopsy is not recommended as a first-line diagnostic maneuver in cats with suspected hepatic lipidosis (HL), owing to their bleeding tendencies, severe metabolic and electrolyte aberrations, and frequent inability to recover from general anesthesia. Liver aspiration cytology combined with signalment and classic clinicopathologic features is used to initiate supportive care in the treatment of HL.

POTENTIAL COMPLICATIONS
• Life-endangering iatrogenic postbiopsy hemorrhage. However, correlation between coagulation test results and hemorrhage complications is poor. Bleeding may develop acutely or within 24 h.

• Hemobilia: bleeding into the biliary tree from an inadvertent laceration of large biliary structures after Tru-cut type biopsy sampling of the liver
• Bile peritonitis caused by puncture of large biliary structures during Tru-cut biopsy sampling
• Severe hypotension due to vasovagal reaction: secondary to pressure on the gallbladder or to liver biopsy
• Patients demonstrating signs of hepatic encephalopathy are at high risk of anesthetic complications.
• Cats with systemic amyloidosis involving the liver may develop catastrophic hepatic hemorrhage after liver biopsy.
• Systemic sepsis resulting from biopsy of septic hepatobiliary lesions
• Pneumoperitoneum can rarely develop subsequent to laceration of the diaphragm and lung after Tru-cut automated needle biopsy.
• See the Laparoscopy chapter for additional complications.

CLIENT EDUCATION
• Owners must be fully informed of risks and benefits of liver biopsy before the procedure.
• Owners must be informed of the need for postbiopsy surveillance for bleeding or other complications.
• Owners must be informed of the need for general anesthesia and its attendant risks in patients with advanced liver disease.
• Owners must be informed that animals with ascites may have postbiopsy complications because of fluid leaking into the subcutaneous tissues.

BODY SYSTEMS ASSESSED
Hepatobiliary

PROCEDURE

PATIENT PREPARATION
Preprocedure Medication or Preparation
Patients should undergo a 12-h fast because of the need for general anesthesia.

Anesthesia or Sedation
All procedures are performed with patients under general anesthesia.

Patient Positioning
• Percutaneous needle biopsy technique: dorsal recumbency, individually modified according to the ultrasonographic image and best assessed path for needle biopsy to avoid nonhepatic viscera or vasculature
• Laparoscopic biopsy procedure: dorsal or left lateral recumbency
• Open liver biopsy during laparotomy: generally dorsal recumbency

Patient Monitoring
• Coagulation assessments: routine tests (PT, APTT, fibrinogen), protein C activity, and BMBT should be evaluated before the procedure.
• Although prolonged coagulation times indicate increased risk of bleeding, there is poor correlation between routine coagulation tests and provoked bleeding. The clinician should be prepared to intervene with fresh frozen plasma, packed RBCs, or whole fresh blood should a hemorrhage complication be encountered.
• Low protein C activity (<70%) indicates either the presence of substantial portosystemic shunting or severe liver dysfunction or failure.
• In pure-breed dogs with a risk of von Willebrand factor deficiency (e.g., Doberman pinschers), a von Willebrand disease test should be conducted to anticipate the need for cryoprecipitate.
• Patients with prolonged PT, APTT, or fibrinogen should be treated with fresh frozen plasma, initiated before and continued during the procedure.

• Dogs with prolonged BMBT should be treated with DDAVP ≈30 min before the procedure (repeat dosing is not known to provide benefit): DDAVP, 0.5–1.0 μg/kg IV in saline increases coagulation factors, shortens bleeding times, and reduces bleeding tendencies (mechanism unclear).

Equipment or Supplies
All Procedures
• Clippers
• Sterile scrub supplies
• Neutral buffered formalin (ph 7.0)
• Transport media for aerobic and anaerobic culture of biopsy samples
• Vacutainer clot (red top) tube for transport for metal quantification. Place a plastic wrap over the rubber cap to protect against biopsy sample contact.
• Microscopic slides with which to make imprint cytology

Percutaneous Needle Biopsy Procedure
• Needles used for percutaneous liver biopsy are categorized as suction needles, cutting needles, and spring-loaded or automated cutting needles (which have a triggering mechanism). Manual cutting needles require a longer time in the liver tissue and their use is not advised because it increases the chance for iatrogenic hemorrhage. An 18-gauge needle is preferred. A greater incidence of bleeding after biopsy has been variably reported with large-diameter needles. If hepatic fibrosis is suspected, a cutting needle is preferred over a suction needle because fibrotic tissue tends to fragment with suction needles.
• Ultrasound equipment, including a needle guide, if available

Laparoscopic Biopsy Procedure
• Laparoscopic instruments, including a Veress needle, trocar and trocar-cannula, telescope, second cannula, biopsy instrument, Kelly forceps, blunt visceral probe, cautery unit, suction devise, and digital photographic equipment
• A source of CO_2
• Sterile saline
• Gelfoam

Open Liver Biopsy During Laparotomy
• Surgical instruments
• Absorbable suture
• Gelfoam
• Circular skin biopsy punch (Baker's punch), optional

TECHNIQUE
Biopsy of the caudate lobe should be avoided in dogs with suspected vascular anomalies because this lobe often has the most normal vasculature (receives the first branch off the portal vein).

Percutaneous Needle Biopsy Procedure
• Needle biopsy sampling has a greater risk of iatrogenic injury in cats in which other tissues are inadvertently sampled because of small patient size or the depth of the device's cutting notch.
• Ultrasound guidance is essential to verify the location of the most accessible left liver lobes and to avoid large vascular structures, the gallbladder, and large bile ducts.
• A needle guide on the ultrasound probe assists in sampling accuracy.
• The ventral and lateral abdominal and thoracic regions are aseptically prepared, and the pet is positioned in dorsal recumbency to optimize liver sampling. Leaning the patient slightly to the right often is helpful but there is wide individual variation.
• Since a minimum of 8 portal triads and an optimum of 15 portal triads are needed to ascertain acinar distribution of lesions, use of an 18-gauge biopsy needle requires collection of at least 3–4 samples. Risk of iatrogenic injury increases with each sample.
• The biopsy site should be investigated with ultrasound immediately after sample acquisition and again in 30 min to detect serious iatrogenic hemorrhage.

• If possible, the patient should be maintained with the biopsy site on the down side to augment pressure hemostasis.

Laparoscopic Biopsy Procedure
• Gross visualization of the liver and peritoneal cavity increases the quality of disease severity assessment when combined with histologic findings.
• The ventral thoracoabdominal area from an area 2 inches (5.08 cm) cranial to the costochondral junction to 2 inches caudal to the umbilicus is aseptically prepared.
• The urinary bladder is fully emptied to avoid puncture during Veress needle and trocar-cannula insertions.
• Patients are positioned either in dorsal recumbency, tilted slightly to the left, or in left lateral recumbency. Some clinicians prefer a right lateral approach because it provides good visualization of the pancreas, gallbladder and extrahepatic biliary structures, and a large area of liver. The left lobes of liver are difficult to evaluate with patients in this position. An approach with the initial cannula placed to the right of midline, at the level of the umbilicus, halfway lateral and midline works well. A second trocar is usually placed in a similar position in the left abdominal wall. Such positioning allows patient repositioning to either the right or left side to facilitate full liver inspection and sampling of all gross lesions and all liver lobes. If the falciform ligament is obtrusive to visualization and instrumentation, a third cannula can be placed in the lateral quadrant.
• The site of Veress needle penetration (the Veress needle provides initial CO_2 abdominal insufflation) is used for initial trocar-cannula insertion. After considering liver size (ultrasound and radiographic imaging), an appropriate location for Veress needle insertion is estimated [at least 4 inches (10.16 cm) from the liver margin]. Before needle insertion, the abdomen is palpated to ascertain the location of the spleen so that it will not be lacerated.
• Before CO_2 insufflation via the Veress needle, sterile saline is injected into the needle with a syringe, the needle is aspirated, and a "hanging drop" assessment made. These steps verify safe, correct needle placement (i.e., not in muscle planes, which will result in SC emphysema on insufflation, or the needle not penetrating the spleen, large vessels, or other visceral structures, thereby reducing the risk of gas embolization).
• The abdomen is insufflated to tense distention (≤15 mmHg, tympanic on percussion) to protect the viscera during the initial trocar-cannula insertion. The trocar is removed and the telescope (with a fiberoptic extension attached to a digital camera) inserted for inspection of the abdominal cavity. A lower abdominal pressure (≈10 mmHg) is maintained during the procedure. The peritoneal cavity is inspected carefully for iatrogenic hemorrhage, acquired portosystemic shunts, unexpected lesions, and appropriate cannula position relative to the liver. A second cannula is strategically inserted, providing a port for instrumentation (biopsy instrument, Kelly forceps, blunt visceral probe, cautery unit, or suction device).
• Digital photographs document the gross appearance of the liver and extrahepatic biliary structures.
• If present, ascites is removed by using an appropriate aspirator and vacuum system enabling visualization of biopsy sites, subsequent verification of postbiopsy hemostasis, or hemostasis assistance. Ascites removal reduces postoperative complications associated with fluid draining through the trocar insertion sites.
• Gelfoam is preplaced (Kelly forceps) on the liver capsule or other visceral surfaces in the visual field to provide immediate postbiopsy accessibility.
• A 5-mm oval cupped clamshell biopsy instrument is used for biopsy collection. The liver tissue is collected into the clamshell instrument and held tightly 90 s to promote vascular associated primary hemostasis responses. The cannula is gently advanced along the shaft of the biopsy instrument toward the liver such that the biopsy sample may be gently extracted from the liver while it is stabilized by the cannula

orifice. This avoids capsular tearing and other traumatic injuries to the liver or vascular structures. Gelfoam is packed into the biopsy site with Kelly forceps.
- The response to the first biopsy acquisition is used to ascertain the propriety of collecting a series of samples from several liver lobes. Generally, 4 tissue samples are collected from different liver lobes or areas with gross lesions.

Open Liver Biopsy During Laparotomy
- Prepare the abdomen aseptically for laparotomy.
- Express the urinary bladder.
- The liver and biliary structures are grossly examined, and the peritoneal cavity is inspected for acquired portosystemic shunts secondary to portal hypertension and unexpected lesions.
- Three methods of tissue collection and hemostasis control are commonly used employing absorbable suture and Gelfoam:
  - A marginal wedge biopsy with closure by using preplaced mattress suture(s) deep within the adjacent liver tissue (surgeon's knot applied to the suture). Gelfoam can be incorporated into the tissue defect if hemostasis is problematic.
  - Modified guillotine method: A loop of suture is used to encircle a naturally protruding margin of a liver lobe. Before the ligature is tied, it is tightened to crush through hepatic parenchyma. A sharp blade is used to sever liver tissue 5 mm distal to the ligature. Iatrogenic vascular stasis and vascular dilation are routinely observed upon histologic evaluation of such biopsies.
  - Circular skin biopsy punch (Baker's punch): Lesional areas are sampled by using a sterile disposable Baker's punch. Tissue is lifted gently with forceps and severed with fine Metzenbaum scissors or a scalpel blade (no. 15 or ll). The created tissue defect is packed with Gelfoam to promote hemostasis and closed with a simple interrupted or cruciate mattress suture pattern.

SAMPLE HANDLING
The biopsy specimen should be divided to enable the following:
1. Fixation of representative samples in neutral buffered formalin (pH 7.0) for histopathologic evaluations: The use of routine hematoxylin-eosin, and special stains for connective tissue, reticulin, iron, copper, fat, or glycogen, may be appropriate. In some cases, the use of immunohistochemical stains may be necessary to characterize cell infiltrates, infectious agents, or abnormal storage debris.
2. Aerobic and anaerobic tissue culture for infectious organisms
3. Transition metal quantification (copper, iron, zinc) expressed on a dry-weight basis
4. Imprint cytology may disclose the presence of bacterial organisms in septic disorders (histopathologic evaluation infrequently discloses bacteria) or the presence of neoplasia.

APPROPRIATE AFTERCARE
Postprocedure Patient Monitoring
- Postprocedure patient monitoring is essential for any type of liver biopsy to detect iatrogenic hemorrhage, sepsis, or other complications.
- Patients that have undergone needle biopsy should be observed closely for at least 2 h in the hospital.
- Patients that have undergone laparoscopic biopsy are monitored in the hospital overnight.
- Patients that have undergone laparotomy will require several days of hospitalization.
- Monitor vital signs (heart rate, respiratory rate, mucous membrane color, pulse quality, and blood pressure) every 15 min for 2 h. Unexpected tachycardia, rapid bounding pulses, pallor, and rapid respiration may indicate substantial blood loss or unusual pain. On the basis of such changes, clinicians should initiate ultrasonographic evaluation of the abdominal cavity, initiate blood component therapy if hemorrhage is suspected, and possibly perform abdominocentesis to confirm bleeding in patients with ascites.

Nursing Care
- Monitor the surgical wound for heat, pain, swelling, discharge, or redness.
- Leakage of ascitic fluid into the surgical plane may necessitate application of an abdominal bandage to locally compress surgical site. (*Note*: Taut abdominal wraps can increase portal pressure and should not be applied to animals with advanced liver disease or abdominal hemorrhage.)
- Remove the sutures in 10 days.

Dietary Modification
None for the procedure. However, dietary modifications may be required for specific disease entities.

Medication Requirements
- Analgesics should be provided to all patients. In most patients undergoing needle or laparoscopic liver biopsy, analgesia with butorphanol is satisfactory.
- Laparotomy requires postoperative hospitalization for several days and a judicious use of analgesia during that interval.
- If an infectious disorder is possible, broad-spectrum antimicrobial drugs targeting enteric opportunistic bacteria can be administered until microbial culture and histopathology results are available.

Restrictions on Activity
- Needle biopsies: Activity is restricted throughout the next day, with owner observational vigilance necessary.
- Laparoscopic biopsies: Activity is restricted for the next 3 days, with owner observational vigilance necessary.
- Laparotomy acquired biopsies: These require several days of restricted activity afterward.

Anticipated Recovery Time
Within several hours for needle and laparoscopic procedures, longer for recovery from laparotomy, depending on disease severity, anesthesia used, and analgesics provided

INTERPRETATION
NORMAL FINDINGS OR RANGE
- A normal liver should have a normal histologic appearance.
- Histologic evaluation of liver tissue should clarify acinar zonal involvement, presence or absence and severity of inflammation, hepatocellular necrosis, biliary epithelial hyperplasia, bile stasis, and fibrosis; variation from normal in vascular structures; qualitative estimates of iron and copper storage; and increased hepatocellular cytosolic stores of glycogen or lipid if a vacuolar change is described. For necroinflammatory disorders, the type of cellular infiltrate must be clearly characterized.

ABNORMAL VALUES
- Histologic findings should be reconciled with clinical pathologic features, including hepatic function test results. Sequential demonstration of high liver enzyme activities (for several weeks) may be the sole indication for a need for liver biopsy in animals with chronic hepatitis before liver function is compromised. High bile acid values may indicate the need for liver biopsy in animals with chronic asymptomatic liver disease.
- Necroinflammatory active inflammation
- Hepatic fibrosis with or without associated necroinflammatory liver injury
- Biliary epithelial hyperplasia is a common response to zone 1 (portal) inflammation or disease, directly involving biliary structures or recovery from panlobular necrosis.
- Hepatocellular vacuolation with glycogen in canine vacuolar hepatopathy syndrome and with neutral fat (triglyceride) in cats with the HL syndrome

• Increased arteriolar cross sections (so-called portal arterialization) reflect portal hypoperfusion and are observed with compromised portal venous perfusion of any cause. Liver biopsy cannot be used to diagnose portal hypoplasia or atresia. Portal vascular anomalies are difficult to clarify with needle biopsy specimens.
• Lobular atrophy versus parenchymal collapse helps differentiate portal hypoperfusion from acquired degenerative disorders.
• Hepatic amyloid verification requires special stains (e.g., Congo red) and examination with a polarizing lens.

CRITICAL VALUES
Panlobular hepatic necrosis portends a grave prognosis.

INTERFERING FACTORS
Drugs That May Alter Results of the Procedure
Glucocorticoid medications may induce a severe vacuolar change in dogs (glycogen) or facilitate development of HL in inappetent cats and may reduce the intensity of inflammation in patients with necroinflammatory liver disease.

Conditions That May Interfere with Performing the Procedure
• Antecedent treatment with aspirin may increase bleeding tendencies.
• Morbid obesity
• Symptomatic von Willebrand disease or an other symptomatic coagulopathy
• Severe liver dysfunction causing hepatic encephalopathy increases the risk of adverse drug responses and complicates general anesthesia.
• Ascites

Procedure Techniques or Handling That May Alter Results
• Needle biopsy samples may be too small to achieve accurate diagnoses without collection of multiple samples, especially in congenital vascular malformations, cats with cholangiohepatitis, and dogs with chronic hepatitis.
• Needle biopsies may lead to an erroneous diagnosis of liver disease in patients without liver disease.
• Tissue damage during specimen acquisition (e.g., removal from the cutting notch of the biopsy needle) or specimen preparation may compromise the pathologic interpretation.
• Imprint cytologic evaluation may not accurately represent histopathologic lesions. Specifically, a diagnosis of hepatic fibrosis, chronic hepatitis, cholangiohepatitis, or copper storage disease cannot be substantiated on the basis of cytopathologic features.
• Tissue contamination can lead to false-positive culture results.
• Delay in tissue formalin fixation or inappropriately buffered formalin can cause cellular artifacts (e.g., ballooning degeneration, acid hematin).

Influence of Signalment on Performing and Interpreting the Procedure
Species
Small cats and dogs (weighing <2 kg) should not undergo needle biopsy or laparoscopic procedures.

Breed
• Small cats and dogs (weighing <2 kg) should not undergo needle biopsy or laparoscopic procedures.
• With established genetic defects for which there is a reliable genetic test (e.g., copper transport abnormality in Bedlington terriers or polycystic disease in certain breeds of cats), individuals should undergo genetic testing rather than liver biopsy as a first diagnostic step.

Age
Animals with suspected congenital portosystemic vascular abnormalities should not undergo needle biopsy sampling, owing to ambiguous findings with slender tissue samples.

Gender
None

Pregnancy
Avoid the use of percutaneous needle biopsy and laparoscopy in pregnant animals.

CLINICAL PERSPECTIVE
• Liver biopsy is the only method of ascertaining a definitive diagnosis in most forms of liver disease.
• The value of liver biopsy depends on the quality of the sample secured, tissue stains applied, cultures for infectious agents, transition metal quantification, and, in some cases, immunohistochemical investigations.
• The value of liver biopsy is substantially influenced by the examining pathologist's expertise in hepatic histopathology and the use of specific stains that increase the accuracy of morphologic characterizations.
• Quantitative metal measurements must be used to assess the role of iron and copper objectively in tissue lesions. Metals must be expressed on a dry-weight basis (parts per million/gram of dry tissue). Metal measurements should be reconciled with subjective interpretation of tissue staining.
• Liver biopsy should not be coupled with dentistry procedures, owing to risk of systemic bacteremia and seeding of biopsy sites.

MISCELLANEOUS
ANCILLARY TESTS
• Coagulation profile
• Aerobic and anaerobic bacterial culture and sensitivity testing
• Histopathology
• Routine hematologic and biochemical assessment; serum or urine bile acid measurements
• Routine coagulation assessments; special coagulation tests (e.g., protein C activity)

SYNONYMS
• Core Tru-cut liver biopsy
• Guillotine liver biopsy
• Laparoscopic liver biopsy
• Surgical wedge liver biopsy

SEE ALSO
Blackwell's Five-Minute Veterinary Consult: Canine and Feline Topics
• Chapters on specific hepatobiliary disorders
• Coagulopathy of Liver Disease
Related Topics in This Book
• Bacterial Culture and Sensitivity
• Impression Smear
• Laparoscopy
• Liver and Gallbladder Ultrasonography
• Tissue Biopsy: Needle and Punch

ABBREVIATIONS
• APTT = partial thromboplastin time
• BMBT = buccal mucosal bleeding time
• DDAVP = desmopressin acetate
• HL = hepatic lipidosis
• PT = prothrombin time

Suggested Reading
Cole TL, Center SA, Flood SN, *et al.* Diagnostic comparison of needle and wedge biopsy specimens of the liver in dogs and cats. *J Am Vet Med Assoc* 2002; 220: 1483–1490.

Monnet E, Twedt DC. Laparoscopy. *Vet Clin North Am Small Anim Pract* 2003; 33: 1147–1163.

Wang KY, Panciera DL, Al-Rukibat RK, *et al.* Accuracy of ultrasound-guided fine-needle aspiration of the liver and cytologic findings in dogs and cats: 97 cases (1990–2000). *J Am Vet Med Assoc* 2004; 224: 75–78.

INTERNET RESOURCES

Storz (Karl Storz Veterinary Endoscopy): Laparoscopy in a dog [movie], http://www.karlstorzvet.com/movie_lap_small.html.

AUTHOR NAME

Sharon A. Center

LOW-DOSE DEXAMETHASONE SUPPRESSION TEST

BASICS

TYPE OF SPECIMEN
Blood

TEST EXPLANATION AND RELATED PHYSIOLOGY
Cortisol is the major glucocorticoid secreted by the adrenal cortex. The synthesis and secretion of cortisol are stimulated by ACTH released from the pituitary gland. ACTH is regulated by CRH from the hypothalamus. In turn, rising levels of cortisol suppress secretion of both CRH and ACTH though negative feedback.

The LDDST works on the principle that, in normal patients, the administration of exogenous glucocorticoid (i.e., dexamethasone) inhibits secretion of CRH and ACTH, thus suppressing endogenous cortisol secretion. Animals with hyperadrenocorticism are abnormally resistant to negative feedback.

INDICATIONS
- Screening test for hyperadrenocorticism (Cushing's disease)
- Potential discrimination test for an ACTH-secreting pituitary adenoma (PDH) and a functional adrenal tumor

CONTRAINDICATIONS
- Inappropriate as a screen for iatrogenic hyperadrenocorticism
- Should not be used to monitor the treatment of hyperadrenocorticism

POTENTIAL COMPLICATIONS
None

CLIENT EDUCATION
- Basal cortisol levels alone provide limited information regarding adrenocortical function.
- Normal results do not exclude a diagnosis of spontaneous hyperadrenocorticism and may necessitate an ACTH stimulation test.
- A false-positive test result can occur in patients with nonadrenal illness or stress.

BODY SYSTEMS ASSESSED
Endocrine and metabolic

SAMPLE

COLLECTION
1–2 mL of venous blood

HANDLING
- The choice of collection tube depends on the assay: some labs use serum (red top), whereas others use plasma (EDTA or heparin). Check with the lab before submitting the sample.
- Centrifuge and transfer the serum or plasma into a transport tube. Do not store the sample in a serum-separator tube.
- Label the tubes with the time of collection.
- Refrigerate or freeze the sample and ship it with cold packs in an insulated container.

STORAGE
Refrigerate or freeze the sample.

STABILITY
- Refrigerated (2°–8°C): 7 days
- Frozen (−20°C): up to 3 months

PROTOCOL
1. Collect a baseline serum sample.

2. Administer dexamethasone sodium phosphate or dexamethasone in polyethylene glycol (e.g., Azium; Schering-Plough Animal Health, Union, NJ).
- Dogs: 0.01 mg/kg IV
- Cats: 0.1 mg/kg IV
3. Collect the samples at 4 and 8 h after dexamethasone injection.
4. Submit all 3 samples for cortisol assay.

INTERPRETATION

NORMAL FINDINGS OR RANGE
- Normal values are established by each laboratory, but the ranges are usually very similar.
- Typical cortisol basal levels:
  - Dogs: 0.6–6.0 μg/dL (17–170 nmol/L)
  - Cats: 0.6–5.0 μg/dL (17–140 nmol/L)
- Cortisol concentration of <1.4 μg/dL (40 nmol/L) at 4 and 8 h

ABNORMAL VALUES
Dogs
- Hyperadrenocorticism: at 8 h, a cortisol level of >1.4 μg/dL
- Inconclusive: at 8 h, a cortisol level of 1.0–1.4 μg/dL
- LDDST can differentiate PDH (in ≈60% of dogs with PDH). Criteria for PDH:
  - Cortisol concentration of <1.4 μg/dL at 4 h after dexamethasone administration
  - Cortisol concentration of <50% of the baseline at 4 and/or 8 h

Cats
- Hyperadrenocorticism: at 4 and 8 h, a cortisol concentration of >1.4 μg/dL
- Inconclusive: at 4 and 8 h, a cortisol concentration of 1.0–1.4 μg/dL

CRITICAL VALUES
None

INTERFERING FACTORS
Drugs That May Alter Results or Interpretation
Drugs That Interfere with Test Methodology
- Prednisone or prednisolone (or structurally related steroids) cross-react with the cortisol assay and falsely elevate results. Discontinue steroid therapy for 48 h prior to the test.
- Dexamethasone does not interfere with the cortisol assay.

Drugs That Alter Physiology
Anticonvulsant therapy

Disorders That May Alter Results
- Any cause of chronic stress or a nonadrenal illness can lead to elevated cortisol levels and false-positive results.
- Severe hyperbilirubinemia (>20 mg/dL) can falsely elevate cortisol levels measured by a chemiluminescent enzyme immunoassay.

Collection Techniques or Handling That May Alter Results
- Storage of serum in a serum-separator tube may alter results. Cortisol levels, as measured by a chemiluminescent enzyme immunoassay, can be increased when blood is collected into Becton Dickinson SST vacutainer tubes (BD Diagnostics, Franklin Lakes, NJ). However, the effects on cortisol measurements vary depending on the type of assay as well as the type of blood collection tube used, since the latter can contain different additives (e.g., physical barriers or clot activators).
- Nonfasting samples with excessive lipemia may affect some assays.
- Inappropriate use of an anticoagulant can produce an assay-dependent effect:
  - Use of heparin can decrease cortisol levels measured by a chemiluminescent enzyme immunoassay.

- Use of EDTA plasma can increase cortisol levels by as much as 30% when measured by radioimmunoassay.

Influence of Signalment
Species
Cats are more resistant than dogs to the suppressive effects of dexamethasone.

Breed
None

Age
None

Gender
None

Pregnancy
None

LIMITATIONS OF THE TEST
- This test is not useful for diagnosing iatrogenic hyperadrenocorticism.
- Any significant chronic disease can result in a positive test (failure to sufficiently suppress cortisol levels).
- In cats, this test is not sensitive for discriminating PDH from AT, although a >50% suppression of cortisol levels from the baseline value at either 4 or 8 h may indicate PDH.

Sensitivity, Specificity, and Positive and Negative Predictive Values
Dogs
- Overall sensitivity: ≈95%
- Specificity: ≈50%

Cats
- Overall sensitivity: >80%
- Specificity: unknown

Valid If Run in a Human Lab?
Yes—if the cortisol assay in use has been validated for dogs and cats.

Causes of Abnormal Findings

High values (failure to suppress)	Low values
Hyperadrenocorticism	Improper handling and/or storage (see Collection Techniques or Handling That May Alter Results)
Stress	
Nonadrenal illness	
Drugs (prednisone, prednisolone, or related steroids)	
Improper handling and/or storage (see Collection Techniques or Handling That May Alter Results)	

CLINICAL PERSPECTIVE
- A definitive diagnosis of hyperadrenocorticism should not be based solely on the results of abnormal LDDST results. A final interpretation must be made in context with medical history, clinical signs, and other laboratory findings supportive of hyperadrenal cortical function. False positives occur in animals with nonadrenal illness or stress.

- In cats, the 0.01-mg/kg dexamethasone dose used in dogs is not recommended because as many as 15%–50% of healthy cats will fail to demonstrate adequate suppression of cortisol levels after receiving this dose of dexamethasone.
- In cats, the 0.1-mg/kg LDDST is more sensitive for the diagnosis of hyperadrenocorticism than either the urine cortisol/creatinine ratio or the ACTH stimulation test.

 MISCELLANEOUS

ANCILLARY TESTS
- The high-dose dexamethasone suppression test can be used to differentiate PDH from adrenal tumor if the LDDST is inconclusive.
- Endogenous ACTH can be used to differentiate PDH from adrenal tumor.

SYNONYMS
None

SEE ALSO
Blackwell's Five-Minute Veterinary Consult: Canine and Feline Topics
- Hyperadrenocorticism (Cushing's Disease)—Cats
- Hyperadrenocorticism (Cushing's Disease)—Dogs

Related Topics in This Book
- ACTH Assay
- ACTH Stimulation
- Adrenal Ultrasonography
- Cortisol
- Cortisol/Creatinine Ratio
- High-Dose Dexamethasone Suppression Test

ABBREVIATIONS
- ACTH = adrenocorticotropic hormone
- CRH = corticotropin-releasing hormone
- LDDST = low-dose dexamethasone suppression test
- PDH = pituitary-dependent hyperadrenocorticism

Suggested Reading
Ferguson DC, Hoenig M. Endocrine system. In: Lattimer KS, Mahaffey EA, Prasse KW, eds. *Duncan and Prasse's Veterinary Laboratory Medicine: Clinical Pathology,* 4th ed. Ames: Iowa State Press, 2003: 270–303.
Feldman EC, Nelson RW. *Canine and Feline Endocrinology and Reproduction,* 3rd ed. St Louis: Saunders Elsevier, 2004: 252–393.
Reusch CE. Hyperadrenocorticism. In: Ettinger SJ, Feldman EC, eds. *Textbook of Veterinary Internal Medicine,* 6th ed. Philadelphia: WB Saunders, 2004: 1592–1612.

INTERNET RESOURCES
Kintzer P. Beware of false positives, negatives in canine hyperadrenocorticism testing. DVM Newsmagazine, September 3, 2003, http://www.dvmnewsmagazine.com/dvm/article/articleDetail.jsp?id = 70245.

AUTHOR NAME
Janice M. Andrews

LOWER GASTROINTESTINAL RADIOGRAPHIC CONTRAST STUDIES

BASICS

TYPE OF PROCEDURE
Radiographic

PROCEDURE EXPLANATION AND RELATED PHYSIOLOGY
The lower GI radiographic contrast study is a radiographic study that uses negative contrast, positive contrast, or both (double contrast) for a morphologic assessment of the cecum and large intestine. This study enables assessment of the size, shape, and position of the colon, and radiographic visualization of the mucosal lining of the colon and assessment of colonic wall thickness.

INDICATIONS
• To aid in the evaluation of colonic disease such as colitis, ileocolic intussusception, cecal inversion, and mass lesions involving the colonic wall (e.g., tumor, granuloma)
• To determine the location and position of the large bowel relative to the small bowel and other abdominal organs (e.g., uterus, ovary, prostate gland)

CONTRAINDICATIONS
Positive contrast studies should not be performed in animals with suspected perforation of the large intestine or cecum.

POTENTIAL COMPLICATIONS
Complications are rare, but can include rupture of the large bowel related to either disease of the bowel wall or to faulty contrast technique.

CLIENT EDUCATION
The client should be informed as to the value of the contrast study and that a definitive diagnosis may or may not be obtained.

BODY SYSTEMS ASSESSED
Gastrointestinal

PROCEDURE

PATIENT PREPARATION
Either oral laxatives [e.g., Golytely (PEG-3350 plus electrolytes)] 24 h before the procedure or a cleansing enema 4–6 h prior to the procedure is optimum.

Preprocedure Medication or Preparation
None

Anesthesia or Sedation
For a pneumocolon examination, sedation is not usually required. For a barium enema or double contrast barium study, general anesthesia is highly recommended.

Patient Positioning
For most studies, a left lateral and ventrodorsal projection following the instillation of contrast media is sufficient. A right lateral projection may be helpful as an additional projection.

Patient Monitoring
None required

Equipment or Supplies
• Barium sulfate mixtures with suspending agents are diluted to a percent of 10% wt/vol. A balloon-type catheter (Foley or Bardex) is advantageous for most large-bowel studies to occlude the rectum.
• Recommended barium sulfate preparations: liquid Barosperse (Lafayette Pharmaceuticals, Lafayette, IN); Novapaque (Picker International, Cleveland, OH); and E-Z Paque (E-Z-EM, Westbury, NY)

TECHNIQUE
• Obtain survey recumbent lateral and ventrodorsal abdominal radiographs immediately prior to the study.
• For a single-contrast colonic examination (air or barium), place the balloon catheter in the rectum and inflate the balloon with air or saline. Insufflate the large bowel with a volume sufficient to fill the large bowel and cecum completely. The usual dose is 5-mL/lb of body weight. If available, fluoroscopic observation is recommended. Obtain left lateral and ventrodorsal projections. Develop and evaluate the radiographs. If incomplete distention of the bowel is observed, continue additional insufflation and make additional radiographs. If satisfied with the results, aspirate the contrast out of the colon and then deflate the balloon and withdraw the catheter from the rectum.
• For a double contrast study, insufflate the large bowel with barium as outlined in the previous paragraph. Once satisfied with the radiographs, remove as much barium as possible by aspirating it via the catheter. Then, instill an adequate amount of air to reinflate the large bowel. Obtain radiographs to ensure that all regions of the large bowel and cecum are visualized. Once satisfied with the radiographs, remove all air by aspiration from the catheter, deflate the balloon catheter, and withdraw the catheter from the rectum.

SAMPLE HANDLING
N/A

APPROPRIATE AFTERCARE
Postprocedure Patient Monitoring
None

Nursing Care
None

Dietary Modification
None

Medication Requirements
None

Restrictions on Activity
None

Anticipated Recovery Time
30 min to 2 h, depending on type of anesthesia used

INTERPRETATION

NORMAL FINDINGS OR RANGE
The entire large bowel, including the cecum, should be visualized adequately. If the distal ileum also contains contrast, the ileocolic valve can also be seen. The colon should have a uniform diameter and a smooth mucosal border. Filling defects, associated with the clumping of barium and mucus or residual fecal material, have to be differentiated from mucosal lesions such as ulcers, granulomas, or tumors.

ABNORMAL VALUES
• Abnormal position of the colon (e.g., in abdominal hernia)
• Filling defects affecting the colonic wall (e.g., tumor, stricture)
• Filling defects affecting the colonic lumen (e.g., cecal inversion, ileocolic or colic intussusception)
• Incomplete distention of the colon can result from faulty technique (e.g., poor preparation, insufficient contrast) or from mass lesions, such as focal areas of colonic wall thickening from stricture or tumor, or intraluminal masses (e.g., tumor, granuloma, foreign body, intussusception).
• With diffuse colitis, mucosal irregularities consisting of ulcers, spasticity, rigidity, and shortening of the colon may result.
• An abnormal tortuous colon may be seen with colonic volvulus, internal hernia or abdominal wall hernia.

LOWER GASTROINTESTINAL RADIOGRAPHIC CONTRAST STUDIES

CRITICAL VALUES
Leakage of contrast into the abdominal cavity, although rare, indicates a perforated bowel that would require immediate surgical intervention.

INTERFERING FACTORS
Drugs That May Alter Results of the Procedure
None

Conditions That May Interfere with Performing the Procedure
None

Procedure Techniques or Handling That May Alter Results
• Poor patient preparation with residual fecal matter in the large bowel will cause artifactual filling defects.
• If the balloon dislodges from the rectum, incomplete colonic distention will result.
• Spilled contrast on the tabletop may adhere to the patient's hair and be an artifact on subsequent radiographic exposures.

Influence of Signalment on Performing and Interpreting the Procedure

Species
None

Breed
None

Age
None

Gender
None

Pregnancy
None

CLINICAL PERSPECTIVE
With the availability of flexible endoscopy and ultrasonography, the need for contrast studies of the large bowel is greatly diminished. The size and extent of a colonic wall mass can be more accurately estimated with contrast studies and distention of the large bowel, which may be helpful in preoperative staging assessment.

 MISCELLANEOUS

ANCILLARY TESTS
For most colonic diseases, abdominal ultrasound and colonoscopy used individually or in combination have replaced the need for most contrast studies of the large intestine. Ultrasound can readily identify mass lesions involving the cecum and large bowel and assess for adjacent lymphadenopathy. Colonoscopy enables direct visualization of erosive or ulcerative lesions, polyps, and tumors and the acquisition of biopsy specimens.

SYNONYMS
None

SEE ALSO
Blackwell's Five-Minute Veterinary Consult: Canine and Feline Topics
• Colitis and Proctitis
• Colitis, Histiocytic Ulcerative

Related Topics in This Book
• General Principles of Radiography
• Abdominal Ultrasonography
• Colonoscopy

ABBREVIATIONS
None

Suggested Reading
Biery DN. The large bowel. In: Thrall DE, ed. *Veterinary Diagnostic Radiology,* 4th ed. Philadelphia: WB Saunders, 2002: 660–673.
Kealy JK, McAllister H. *Diagnostic Radiology and Ultrasonography of the Dog and Cat,* 4th ed. St Louis: Elsevier Saunders, 2005.
Mahaffey MB, Barber DL. The stomach. In: Thrall DE, ed. *Veterinary Diagnostic Radiology,* 4th ed. Philadelphia: WB Saunders, 2002: 615–638.
Owens JM, Biery DN. *Radiographic Interpretation for the Small Animal Clinician,* 2nd ed. Baltimore: Williams & Wilkins, 1999.
Riedesel EA. The small bowel. In: Thrall DE, ed. *Veterinary Diagnostic Radiology,* 4th ed. Philadelphia: WB Saunders, 2002: 639–659.

INTERNET RESOURCES
None

AUTHOR
Jerry M. Owens

LOWER URINARY TRACT ULTRASONOGRAPHY

 BASICS

TYPE OF PROCEDURE
Ultrasonographic

PROCEDURE EXPLANATION AND RELATED PHYSIOLOGY
The abdominal ultrasound examination includes complete examination of the lower urinary tract. This portion of the total examination includes the bladder, urethra, and prostate gland (if present). Ultrasound is an ideal modality to examine these structures. These organs are of soft tissue radiographic opacity. Without a contrast examination, the wall and luminal contents appear similar in opacity. Ultrasound is useful in interrogating the wall, as well as the luminal contents. It is also useful in identifying all types of calculi, which may be radiopaque or radiolucent. Anesthesia or urinary catheterization is not necessary for the examination. Vascularization of a mass can be seen with Doppler interrogation, and a blood clot can be discriminated from a bladder tumor.

INDICATIONS
• Hematuria
• Dysuria
• Pyuria
• Mass palpated or suspected via abdominal radiographs
• Recent pelvic trauma
• Azotemia
• Peritoneal effusion and suspected bladder rupture
• Bladder not found
• Assistance in cystocentesis

CONTRAINDICATIONS
None

POTENTIAL COMPLICATIONS
• If a cystocentesis is performed, some urine could leak.
• Aspiration of a bladder that contains a mass consistent with a transitional cell carcinoma should be avoided because that might disseminate cancerous cells along the needle tract.

CLIENT EDUCATION
The hair will be removed in order to image the abdomen.

BODY SYSTEMS ASSESSED
• Renal and urologic
• Reproductive

 PROCEDURE

PATIENT PREPARATION
Preprocedure Medication or Preparation
• Recent voiding should be avoided because it is best to have partial distention of the bladder.
• For complete evaluation, it is best to avoid having a catheter in place.
• Cystocentesis should be delayed until after the procedure.
• Prior catheterization or cystoscopy prior to the procedure should be avoided because it may introduce air into the bladder, creating an artifact that may mimic disease or hide disease.

Anesthesia or Sedation
It usually is not required. However, if the patient is unruly or very anxious, sedation may be administered.

Patient Positioning
Right and left lateral recumbency and possibly dorsal recumbency as needed to check the influence of gravity on a structure

Patient Monitoring
Routine monitoring if the patient is in critical condition

Equipment or Supplies
• An ultrasound unit with a high-resolution transducer (7.5–13.0 MHz)
• Ultrasound gel is needed for acoustic coupling.
• Clippers
• Alcohol for cleaning the skin

TECHNIQUE
• Clip the hair as needed.
• Apply acoustic gel as needed.
• Place the patient in lateral recumbency with the pelvic limbs positioned caudally for the bladder and cranially for the male urethra. This is especially helpful if the bladder is in a pelvic location and to evaluate the prostate gland and urethra.
• The positional markers should indicate that the longitudinal images have the head to the left and the transverse images have the left side of the image representing the dorsal aspect of the organ. If oblique images are made, the appropriate positional identifiers need to be placed on them.
• With the animal in lateral recumbency, the entire bladder is swept with the transducer from dorsal to ventral, from right to left, and from cranial to caudal.
• As much of the urethra as possible is imaged.
• Particular areas of interest include the dependent part of the bladder (Figure 1A), the entrance of the ureters, and the trigone of the bladder (Figure 1B), the prostate gland, and the urethra (Figure 1C). Luminal content, wall thickness, or irregularity is of particular interest. If a mass is identified, the vascular flow is demonstrated to ensure that the mass is not a blood clot and to determine the site from where the mass arises. The use of gravity is often helpful in determining whether a mass is free or attached.
• Regional lymph nodes should be imaged for possible regional metastasis.
• Ureteral or urethral obstruction should be evaluated and documented.
• A cause of peritoneal effusion or evidence of leakage of urine should be determined.
• A cystocentesis should be performed following the procedure because cystocentesis may cause a bladder wall defect or a blood clot.

SAMPLE HANDLING
NA

APPROPRIATE AFTERCARE
Postprocedure Patient Monitoring
None

Nursing Care
None

Dietary Modification
None

Medication Requirements
None

Restrictions on Activity
None

Anticipated Recovery Time
Immediate

 INTERPRETATION

NORMAL FINDINGS OR RANGE
• The bladder size varies, dependent upon fluid intake, when voiding occurred and if the patient is reluctant or unable to void.

LOWER URINARY TRACT ULTRASONOGRAPHY

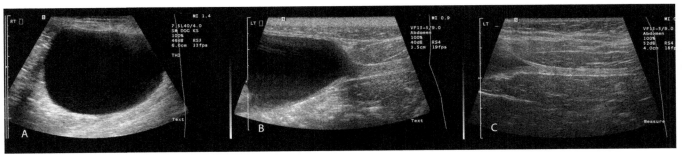

Figure 1

A: The bladder contains anechoic contents. The entire bladder is carefully and completely scanned, including its dependent part. Its wall and the luminal contents are scrutinized. **B:** This is the trigone of the bladder. The wall, the luminal contents, and the entrance of the ureters are imaged and evaluated. **C:** The trigone to the urethra is imaged. The urethra is a linear parallel structure that is usually collapsed and uniformly echogenic. Its serosal surface is smooth.

- The internal contents should be anechoic.
- The wall thickness should be uniform, ≈2.0–2.3 mm, and is normally thicker if the animal recently voided.
- The urethra in the female can be imaged from both the abdominal and the perineal approaches. Its thickness should be uniform. The female urethra should be empty of luminal contents and have a uniform echogenic appearance with smooth margins. Imaging of the male urethra should include the prostate gland.
- The prostate gland in an intact male is ≈3 cm in width, height, and length, depending on the age and size of the patient. In a neutered dog, the size will depend on when the animal was neutered; it should be only slightly larger than the urethra if the animal was neutered when sexually immature. If the dog is intact, the testicles should be included in the exam.
- Ducts within the prostate gland may be seen to communicate with the urethra. The parenchyma of the gland should be uniform and mildly hypoechoic to surrounding fat but more echogenic than the spleen and without mineral or cystic areas. The urethra will course through the center of the gland. The muscle around the urethra is often mildly hypoechoic.

ABNORMAL VALUES
- Focally or diffusely thickened bladder wall or urethra
- A mass in the lumen
- A mass in the wall, with extension into the lumen
- Mineralized mass(es) free in the lumen or attached to the wall
- Obstruction of the ureters or urethra
- Leakage from the bladder into the peritoneal cavity
- Regional metastasis to the lymph nodes
- Ureteroceles
- Ectopic ureters
- An enlarged prostate gland with small cystic areas
- Cystic areas with echogenic contents within the prostate lobes
- Mineralized foci within the prostate gland
- Periprostatic cystic masses

CRITICAL VALUES
- Evidence for a ruptured bladder
- Prostatic abscess that is suspected to have ruptured
- Obstruction of the urethra or ureter(s)

INTERFERING FACTORS
Drugs That May Alter Results of the Procedure
None

Conditions That May Interfere with Performing the Procedure
- Recent trauma and severe pain
- A pelvic bladder
- Recent bladder emptying

- Artifacts from the wall of an emphysematous bladder may interfere with complete examination.

Procedure Techniques or Handling That May Alter Results
- Not systematically imaging the complete bladder, especially its dependent part
- Recent negative or double-contrast cystogram where air in the lumen will cause artifacts
- Recent cystocentesis may result in cellular contents in the lumen and a thickening or mass effect in the wall from a hematoma that may mimic disease.
- Recent introduction of air into the bladder via catheterization, cystoscopy, or surgery

Influence of Signalment on Performing and Interpreting the Procedure
Species
The position and length of the urethra and the appearance of the prostate gland vary with the species. The cat prostate gland is not usually imaged.

Breed
None

Age
The prostate gland is small in a sexually immature male. As the male matures, there is an increase in the gland's size and the incidence of prostatic hyperplasia.

Gender
The urethra in the male will require imaging of its entire length. The section in the pelvic canal is harder to image in both the male and the female because of the overlying bone surrounding the pelvic canal. The prostate gland size is directly influenced by the male sex hormones.

Pregnancy
The bladder may be displaced in late-term pregnancy.

CLINICAL PERSPECTIVE
- This exam is easy to perform and has reduced the need for other radiographic contrast procedures.
- Bladder and urethral tumors, cystitis, blood clots, calculi, bladder rupture, ectopic ureters, and ureteroceles are abnormalities frequently identified.
- Prostatic neoplasia, abscesses, cysts, and periprostatic cysts are prostatic abnormalities frequently identified.
- If a mass identified in the bladder is consistent with a transitional cell carcinoma, an aspiration should not be performed because that might disseminate cancerous cells along the needle tract.

MISCELLANEOUS

ANCILLARY TESTS
- Abdominal radiography
- Cystocentesis
- Computed tomography or magnetic resonance imaging
- Cystoscopy
- Fine-needle aspirations of lymph nodes and prostate gland
- Urinary radiographic contrast examinations

SYNONYMS
- Bladder sonography
- Urethral sonography

SEE ALSO
Blackwell's Five-Minute Veterinary Consult: Canine and Feline Topics
- Ectopic Ureter
- Hematuria
- Incontinence, Urinary
- Lower Urinary Tract Infection, Bacterial
- Lower Urinary Tract Infection, Fungal
- Pelvic Bladder
- Prostate Disease in the Breeding Male Dog
- Prostatic Cysts
- Prostatitis and Prostatic Abscess
- Prostatomegaly
- Rhabdomyosarcoma, Urinary Bladder
- Transitional Cell Carcinoma, Renal, Bladder, Urethra
- Ureterolithiasis
- Urinary Retention, Functional
- Urinary Tract Obstruction
- Urolithiasis, Calcium Oxalate
- Urolithiasis, Calcium Phosphate
- Urolithiasis, Cystine
- Urolithiasis, Struvite—Cats
- Urolithiasis, Struvite—Dogs
- Urolithiasis, Urate
- Urolithiasis, Xanthine

Related Topics in This Book
- General Principles of Ultrasonography
- Abdominal Radiography
- Abdominal Ultrasonography

ABBREVIATIONS
None

Suggested Reading
Nyland TG, Mattoon JS, eds. *Small Animal Diagnostic Ultrasound.* Philadelphia: WB Saunders, 2002.

INTERNET RESOURCES
None

AUTHOR NAME
Kathy Spaulding

LUPUS ERTHEMATOSUS CELL PREPARATION

BASICS

TYPE OF SPECIMEN
Blood

TEST EXPLANATION AND RELATED PHYSIOLOGY
The lupus erythematosus (LE) cell test (or LE cell preparation) is most commonly performed in patients with an elevated ANA titer and strong clinical suspicion of systemic lupus erythematosus (SLE). The test is used to diagnose, or confirm a diagnosis, of SLE. LE cells are neutrophils that have phagocytosed nuclear material from another cell after it has been complexed with ANAs. In rare circumstances, naturally occurring LE cells may be found in smears of bone marrow, buffy coat preparations, or joint fluid from animals with SLE. The LE cell test manipulates patient's blood in an attempt to promote formation of these cells in vitro. Blood is either vortexed or filtered to rupture WBCs and liberate free nuclei. Once nuclear contents are exposed, they are opsonized by any ANAs present, which attach to different components in DNA (e.g., histones, ribosomal proteins). The opsonized nuclear material is then phagocytosed by neutrophils (those that are intact and still viable). A smear of buffy coat from this sample is prepared and examined for neutrophils containing the intracytoplasmic nuclear material that is round and has a smooth, homogeneously pink to purple appearance (LE cells). Detection of 3–4 LE cells or more per slide is necessary for a positive test result. If LE cells are not detected on the first attempt, the test is usually repeated 2–3 times to verify a negative test result. A certain level of skill and experience is necessary to interpret the test properly. For example, it may be difficult to differentiate LE cells from leukocytes that have phagocytosed generic intact nuclei (aka tart cells).

The LE cell test is labor intensive and time consuming. It has good specificity but it is far less sensitive a test than the ANA test. False positives and false negatives may occur (see the table). Because of the limitations of this preparation, the LE cell test has fallen out of favor among veterinary internists, but while the use of this test to screen patients for SLE is discouraged, it is still used occasionally for confirmation purposes in canine and feline patients. In human medicine, the development of more advanced diagnostics for patients with suspected SLE has rendered the LE cell test obsolete.

INDICATIONS
Clinical suspicion of SLE

CONTRAINDICATIONS
Conditions in which false-negative results may occur (see the chart)

POTENTIAL COMPLICATIONS
None

CLIENT EDUCATION
None

BODY SYSTEMS ASSESSED
Hemic, lymphatic, and immune

SAMPLE

COLLECTION
10 mL of venous blood

HANDLING
• Collect the blood sample in a red-top tube and allow the sample to clot.

- Some laboratories will accept samples in a lithium or sodium heparin tube (green-top tube).
- Freshly collected blood should be processed as soon as possible.

STORAGE
Refrigeration is recommended for very short-term storage (1–2 days).

STABILITY
The test should not be run on stored or aged blood samples, because test requires viable neutrophils.

PROTOCOL
None

 INTERPRETATION

NORMAL FINDINGS OR RANGE
A negative test (i.e., no LE cells seen)

ABNORMAL VALUES
A positive test (i.e., LE cells found)

CRITICAL VALUES
None

INTERFERING FACTORS
Drugs That May Alter Results or Interpretation
Drugs That Interfere with Test Methodology
Blood samples containing excessive heparin may produce false-negative test results.

Drugs That Alter Physiology
A previous or concurrent administration of corticosteroids may cause false-negative results.

Disorders That May Alter Results
Serum containing low levels of complement because of concurrent disorders may produce false-negative test results.

Collection Techniques or Handling That May Alter Results
Aged blood samples or blood samples containing excessive heparin are associated with false-negative test results.

Influence of Signalment
Species
None

Breed
None

Age
None

Gender
None

Pregnancy
None

LIMITATIONS OF THE TEST
Sensitivity, Specificity, and Positive and Negative Predictive Values
Very low sensitivity. Even dogs with SLE rarely have a positive test.

Valid If Run in a Human Lab?
Yes.

Causes of Abnormal Findings

Positive result	Negative (normal) result
SLE: good specificity (low sensitivity)	Corticosteroid therapy
Osteochondritis dissecans	Serum containing low levels of complement
Non–immune-mediated joint disease	Sample containing excessive heparin
Disseminated intravascular coagulation	An old sample
Neoplasia	
Rheumatoid arthritis	

CLINICAL PERSPECTIVE

- Because of its high specificity, the LE cell test may be used to confirm SLE in patients with elevated ANA titers and clinical signs compatible with SLE.
- The use of the LE cell prep has declined due to poor sensitivity (i.e., limited usefulness for disease screening) and technical challenges involved in running the test.

MISCELLANEOUS

ANCILLARY TESTS
ANA test

SYNONYMS
- LE cell preparation
- LE prep

SEE ALSO
Blackwell's Five-Minute Veterinary Consult: Canine and Feline Topics
Lupus Erythematosus, Systemic (SLE)
Related Topics in This Book
- Antinuclear Antibody
- Rheumatoid Factor

ABBREVIATIONS
- ANA = antinuclear antibody
- LE = lupus erythematosus
- SLE = systemic lupus erythematosus

Suggested Reading
Day MJ. Systemic lupus erythematosus. In: Feldman BF, Zinkl JG, Jain NC, eds. *Schalm's Veterinary Hematology,* 5th ed. Ames, IA: Blackwell, 2006: 824–825.
Medleau L, Miller WH. Immunodiagnostic tests for small animal practice. *Vet Clin North Am Small Anim Pract* 1983; 5: 707–711.
Tizard IR. The systemic immunological diseases. In: Tizard IR, ed. *Veterinary Immunology: An Introduction,* 6th ed. Philadelphia: WB Saunders, 2000: 386–390.
Werner LL, Turnwald GH, Willard MD. Immunologic and plasma protein disorders. In: Willard MD, Tvedten H, eds. *Small Animal Clinical Diagnosis by Laboratory Methods,* 4th ed. Philadelphia: WB Saunders, 2004: 301–303.

INTERNET RESOURCES
None

AUTHOR NAME
Maria Vandis

LUTEINIZING HORMONE

BASICS

TYPE OF SPECIMEN
Blood

TEST EXPLANATION AND RELATED PHYSIOLOGY
Luteinizing hormone (LH) is produced by the pituitary, under the control of hypothalamic GnRH. It is secreted in pulses in ever increasing magnitude until a so-called surge occurs. The surge causes mature ovarian follicles, which were producing estrogen, to ovulate, luteinize, and produce progesterone. The LH surge is relatively brief, usually occurring within a 24-h window, although it may remain elevated for somewhat longer.

In bitches, ovulation occurs 2–3 days after the LH surge. Primary oocytes are released, which must undergo a meiotic division to become secondary oocytes before they can be fertilized. This happens 2–3 days after ovulation. The fertile life of mature oocytes is ≈2–3 days. Therefore, the optimal time for insemination, the so-called fertile period, is ≈4–6 days after the LH surge.

In cats, a neuroendocrine reflex initiated by coital stimulation of the vagina causes the LH surge. Multiple breedings are usually necessary to reach the threshold that causes a single LH surge during the cycle. Although domestic cats are generally considered to be induced ovulators, LH is also released, and ovulation occurs, in the absence of coital stimulation.

In male dogs and cats, LH stimulates testosterone secretion by the Leydig cells. Gonadal hormones, in turn, feed back to the hypothalamus and pituitary. Following gonadectomy, this negative feedback control of LH is lost, and serum concentrations of LH are persistently elevated. A semiquantitative immunochromogenic assay is commercially available for in-house use (ICG Status-LH; Synbiotics, San Diego, CA). Concentrations of >1 ng/mL are reported as positive or high. Concentrations of <1 ng/mL are reported as negative or low. At this time, none of the veterinary diagnostic laboratories in the United States offer a quantitative LH assay for clinical use, although several can provide it for research.

INDICATIONS
• Determine the presence or absence of gonads.
  • Confirm the reproductive status (intact vs spayed) of newly acquired animals.
  • Confirm the presence of an ovarian remnant.
• Ovulation timing in a bitch

CONTRAINDICATIONS
None

POTENTIAL COMPLICATIONS
None

CLIENT EDUCATION
• Newly acquired animals may have an unknown reproductive status. When there are no testes in the scrotum, it is usually presumed that the male has been castrated rather than the less likely possibility of bilateral cryptorchidism. In females, there are no such obvious physical findings, other than a scar, to suggest previous spaying. To avoid unnecessary laparotomy, serum concentrations of LH can be measured to determine the presence or absence of gonads.
• LH measurements can be used to determine the optimal time for insemination. Knowing this is especially important when frozen semen is going to be used, because the life of the frozen-thawed spermatozoa is brief, ≈1 day.

BODY SYSTEMS ASSESSED
Reproductive

SAMPLE

COLLECTION
0.5–1.0 mL of venous blood

HANDLING
• Collect the sample into a plain red-top tube. Avoid the use of serum-separator tubes.
• After complete clot formation, separate the serum by centrifugation.
• Ideally, the test should be run on the day of collection.

STORAGE
Refrigerate for short-term storage, and freeze for long-term storage.

STABILITY
• Refrigerated (2°–4°C): 1 day
• Freeze at −20°C for prolonged storage, although the duration of stability has not been documented.

PROTOCOL
None

INTERPRETATION

NORMAL FINDINGS OR RANGE
• Low concentrations of LH (>1.0 ng/mL) indicate the presence of gonads in males and females.
• High concentrations of LH (>1.0 ng/mL) occur in pulses, particularly the LH surge during heat, but also at other times of the cycle in intact females.
• High concentrations of LH (>1.0 ng/mL) are consistently found by 5 days, to as long as 5 years, after ovariectomy in bitches.
• *Note*: the reference intervals provided are simply a guideline; values may vary depending on the laboratory and assay used.

ABNORMAL VALUES
Elevated values in an animal believed to be neutered

CRITICAL VALUES
None

INTERFERING FACTORS
Drugs That May Alter Results or Interpretation
Drugs That Interfere with Test Methodology
None

Drugs That Alter Physiology
Estrogen, progesterone, testosterone, and drugs that alter GnRH or prolactin

Disorders That May Alter Results
• Gonadal disorders, such as ovarian dysgenesis, affecting sex-hormone production (rare)
• Hypothalamic disorders affecting GnRH secretion (rare)
• Pituitary disorders affecting LH secretion (rare)

Collection Techniques or Handling That May Alter Results
The sample must not be hemolyzed or lipemic. These conditions interfere with the flow of the sample into the device and can create a background color that will complicate the interpretation of results.

Influence of Signalment
Species
Dogs and cats

Breed
None

Age
The assay may be performed in animals at, or older than, the expected age of puberty.

Gender
Values vary depending on the presence or absence of gonads.

Pregnancy
None

LIMITATIONS OF THE TEST
Sensitivity, Specificity, and Positive and Negative Predictive Values
- The finding of greatest diagnostic importance is a low LH concentration, because, with rare exceptions, it confirms that a female *has not* been spayed (or *does* have an ovarian remnant). Finding high serum LH concentrations is sensitive for detecting animals that have been spayed. However, it is not as specific, especially in bitches, because a high LH concentration is also normally found in cycling females.
  - Sensitivity: 100% (queens); 98% (bitches)
  - Specificity: 92% in (queens); 78% (bitches)
- The probability that a high LH concentration correctly predicts a spayed animal is fairly high but not perfect, again because intact females also have a high LH concentration at some times during the estrus cycle. However, the probably that a low LH concentration accurately predicts an *intact* animal is very high. Finding a low LH concentration indicates that the female has *not* been spayed.
  - Positive predictive value: 92% (queens); 90% (bitches)
  - Negative predictive value: 100% (queens); 96% (bitches)

Valid If Run in a Human Lab?
No.

Causes of Abnormal Findings

High values	Low values
LH surge just prior to ovulation	Intact female or male
LH pulses during estrous cycle	Female not spayed
Successful ovariectomy	Ovarian remnant in ovariectomized female
	Cryptorchid male if no scrotal testes

CLINICAL PERSPECTIVE
For Use in Predicting Ovulation in Bitches
- Recall that the LH surge may be over in 24 h. Before and after that, the concentrations of LH will be lower but possibly still detectable by the assay. Therefore, to ensure that the LH surge is not missed, it is recommended that samples be obtained every day, at approximately the same time of day.
- Because pulses of LH other than the surge may be of such magnitude to be detected by the assay, it is recommended that serum concentrations of progesterone be measured several days after the surge. Progesterone concentrations of >2 ng/mL (>6 nmol/L) differentiate the actual preovulatory LH surge from the normal proestrus pulses of LH.
- For ovulation timing in bitches, the optimal time to inseminate is ≈4–6 days after the LH surge.

For Determining the Reproductive Status (Intact versus No Gonads)
- Low concentrations of LH indicate the presence of gonads. The female has not been spayed. If no scrotal testes are found, the male is likely cryptorchid.
- High concentrations of LH indicate either impending ovulation in females or the absence of gonads in males and females.

- Examine the female for other signs of heat.
  - If there are no signs of heat rechecking the LH concentration in 2 h is recommended. However, because of its pulsatile secretion at various stages of the cycle, and because the LH surge itself may last 1–4 days, it might be possible, albeit very unlikely, that a sample 2 h later would again be high in an intact animal. Unless there is urgency in deciding on laparotomy that same day, one might wait several days before rechecking the LH concentration.
  - If the second determination is high, and there are still no signs of heat, she has been spayed.
  - An alternative approach for a female with a high LH concentration to differentiate a spayed female from an intact female with a preovulatory surge is to measure progesterone at the same time. Concentrations of >2 ng/mL (>6 nmol/L) indicate the presence of an ovary.

MISCELLANEOUS
ANCILLARY TESTS
- To determine reproductive status: Physical examination for the presence of testes in dogs or cats and of penile spines in cats. Physical examination for signs of heat, or the presence of a scar typical of previous spaying
- For ovulation timing in bitches: Determination of serum concentrations of progesterone and vaginal cytology

SYNONYMS
None

SEE ALSO
Blackwell's Five-Minute Veterinary Consult: Canine and Feline Topics
- Infertility, Female
- Ovarian Remnant Syndrome

Related Topics in This Book
- Progesterone
- Relaxin

ABBREVIATIONS
- GnRH = gonadotropin-releasing hormone
- LH = luteinizing hormone

Suggested Reading
Johnston SD, Root Kustritz MV, Olson PN, eds. *Canine and Feline Theriogenology*. Philadelphia: WB Saunders, 2001.
Löfstedt RM, VanLeeuwen JA. Evaluation of a commercially available luteinizing hormone test for its ability to distinguish between ovariectomized and sexually intact bitches. *J Am Vet Med Assoc* 2002; 220: 1331–1335.
Olson PN, Mulnix JA, Nett TM. Concentrations of luteinizing hormone and follicle-stimulating hormone in the serum of sexually intact and neutered dogs. *Am J Vet Res* 1992; 53: 662–766.
Scebra LR, Griffin B. Evaluation of a commercially available luteinizing hormone test to distinguish between ovariectomized and sexually intact queens [Abstract 214]. In: Proceedings of the 21st Annual Medical Forum of the American College of Veterinary Internal Medicine (ACVIM), 2003.

INTERNET RESOURCES
None

AUTHOR NAME
Cheri A. Johnson

LYME DISEASE SEROLOGY

BASICS

TYPE OF SPECIMEN
Blood

TEST EXPLANATION AND RELATED PHYSIOLOGY
Lyme disease is caused by the spirochete *Borrelia burgdorferi*, which is transmitted by the *Ixodes* sp. tick. Once the tick transmits the spirochetes, they proliferate locally in the skin and then migrate throughout the body. Genetic recombinations in certain variable regions of the VLsE section of the spirochete's genome produce antigenically distinct surface lipoproteins that help ensure the survival of the organism and the potential for chronic, subclinical infections. Although the spirochetes seem to have a tropism for joints, they can be found anywhere. In experimentally infected animals, it can take up to 30 days after the tick transmits the spirochetes before dogs become symptomatic for Lyme disease. Most dogs with clinical Lyme disease have an acute onset of fever, anorexia, and lameness. The joints become swollen and painful, particularly those of the carpus and tarsus. Rarely, some dogs can develop acute renal failure. However, most dogs infected with Lyme disease show no clinical signs at all.

These are some of the several serologic tests available for Lyme disease:

IFA and ELISA
These assays traditionally use whole spirochetes and measure antibodies to many different proteins, some shared by other bacteria, including *Leptospira*. Cross-reacting antibodies have also been reported in people with inflammatory conditions, such as autoimmune diseases, rheumatoid arthritis, and periodontal disease. Lyme vaccines can also cause antibody titers with these assays. The immune response to *Borrelia* develops relatively slowly, and it takes ≈4–6 weeks after infection for a dog to develop antibodies (IgG).

Western Blot
This is a useful confirmatory test in dogs that are IFA or ELISA positive. This test detects antibodies against a variety of *Borrelia* protein and can distinguish cross-reacting antibodies from Lyme-specific ones. The types of antibodies can be used to differentiate exposure or infection from vaccination.

Assays for Antibodies Against C6 Peptide
• A peptide produced in the 6th nonvariable (constant) area of the VLsE site is diagnostically useful. This is a unique, highly immunogenic surface protein that is rapidly turned over and is highly specific for *Borrelia*. This protein is not present in vaccines, which target membrane proteins expressed while the spirochete is in the tick.
• IDEXX Laboratories (Portland, ME) offers 3 antibody assays that use a synthetic C6 peptide. Two in-office assays (SNAP 3Dx and SNAP 4Dx) provide a rapid screen for *Borrelia* exposure and/or infection. Results are reported as positive or negative. They also test for *Dirofilaria immitis* antigen, *Ehrlichia canis* antibody, and *Anaplasma phagocytophilum* antibody (4Dx).
• The Lyme Quantitative C6 Antibody Test is reported in optical density units, which can be interpreted as would an antibody titer. Serial testing can be used to document a rising titer suggestive of active infection (vs exposure). In addition, since C6 titers seems to wane more quickly after treatment than antibodies measured by IFA/ELISA, this test can also be used to monitor response to treatment.

INDICATIONS
• Test dogs in *Ixodes*-endemic areas.
• Test dogs with acute onset of lameness especially if accompanied by fever, anorexia, and swollen carpal and/or tarsal joints.
• Test dogs in acute renal failure.

CONTRAINDICATIONS
None

POTENTIAL COMPLICATIONS
None

CLIENT EDUCATION
Clients might become infected if bitten by an infected *Ixodes* tick.

BODY SYSTEMS ASSESSED
• Cardiovascular
• Dermatologic
• Musculoskeletal
• Renal and urologic

SAMPLE

COLLECTION
2 mL of venous blood

HANDLING
Collect the sample into a plain red-top tube or serum-separator tube.

STORAGE
• Refrigeration is recommended for short-term storage.
• Serum or plasma should be frozen for long-term storage.

STABILITY
• Room temperature: 1 day
• Refrigerated (2°–8°C): 1 week
• Frozen (−18°C): at least 1 month

PROTOCOL
None

INTERPRETATION

NORMAL FINDINGS OR RANGE
• IFA/ELISA: a negative assay for *Borrelia* antibodies
• Western blot: <5 bands, with no Lyme-specific bands
• 3Dx and 4Dx: a negative C6 test
• Quantitative C6: a concentration of <30 U/mL

ABNORMAL VALUES
• IFA/ELISA: A positive assay for *Borrelia* antibodies; positive titers ranges can vary from lab to lab. Most positive Lyme IFA titers begin at around 1:100. Active Lyme disease is suggested by convalescent titer ≥4 times higher than the acute titer.
• Western blot: The presence of 3–6 Lyme-specific bands suggests exposure or infection. Antibodies against several specific proteins are more typical of natural infection instead of vaccination.
• 3Dx and 4Dx: A positive C6 test (a blue spot) suggests exposure or infection.
• Quantitative C6: A concentration of >30 U/mL suggests exposure or infection. Active Lyme disease is suggested by a convalescent titer ≥50% higher than the acute titer.

CRITICAL VALUES
None

INTERFERING FACTORS
Drugs That May Alter Results or Interpretation
Drugs That Interfere with Test Methodology
None

Drugs That Alter Physiology
None

Disorders That May Alter Results
None

Collection Techniques or Handling That May Alter Results
None

Influence of Signalment

Species
- Lyme disease is primarily a problem in dogs.
- Cats can be seropositive, and experimental infection has been described, but clinical disease due to natural infection has not been reported.
- The C6 assay is currently unavailable for cats.

Breed
None

Age
None

Gender
None

Pregnancy
None

LIMITATIONS OF THE TEST
- Spirochetes can sequester in connective tissue and muscle such that infected dogs can have positive test results for years even after antibiotic therapy. No available assay can distinguish dogs with a previous self-limited or subclinical infection from those with active disease.
- IFA/ELISAs are associated with a large number of false positives because of cross-reacting antibodies.
- Vaccination causes positive results by IFA/ELISA that will sometimes persist for years.
- Negative results are possible if a patient had tick exposure in the last month and is still in the process of seroconversion.
- The 3Dx and 4Dx assays are sensitive screening tests, but provide only a positive or negative result. These assays cannot be used to look for a rising titer as evidence of active infection. They also tend to remain positive even in the face of effective therapy.

Sensitivity, Specificity, and Positive and Negative Predictive Values
SNAP 3Dx and 4Dx C6 assays
- Sensitivity: 92%
- Specificity: 100%

Valid If Run in a Human Lab?
No.

Causes of Abnormal Values

Test	High values	Low values
IFA/ELISA	Exposure to *Borrelia* sp., but self-limiting infection	Not clinically significant
	Lyme disease (active infection)	
	Asymptomatic subclinical infection	
	Lyme vaccination	
	Other cross-reacting bacteria (e.g., leptospirosis)	
	Inflammatory disease (e.g., periodontal disease)	
	Immune-mediated disease (e.g., rheumatoid arthritis in people)	
Western blot	Exposure to *Borrelia* sp., but self-limiting infection	
	Lyme disease (active infection)	
	Asymptomatic subclinical infection	
	Lyme vaccination	
3DX/4DX	Exposure to *Borrelia* sp., but self-limiting infection	
	Lyme disease (active infection)	
	Asymptomatic subclinical infection	
Quantitative C6	Exposure to *Borrelia* sp., but self-limiting infection	
	Lyme disease (active infection)	
	Asymptomatic subclinical infection	

CLINICAL PERSPECTIVE
- A positive test result for *Borrelia burgdorferi* does not prove that a dog has a clinical infection or that any clinical signs present were caused by the organism. Diagnosis of Lyme disease should be based on a combination of (1) seropositivity, (2) tick exposure, (3) compatible clinical signs, and (4) rapid response to antimicrobial therapy.
- The new C6 assays are more specific for *Borrelia burgdorferi* and are not affected by vaccination status. These assays provide a powerful new tool that has largely replaced Western blot in dogs.
  - In a dog with lameness, consider treatment for Lyme disease if the Quantitative C6 is >30 U/mL.
  - In an asymptomatic dog, the significance of a Quantitative C6 is >30 U/mL and benefit of treatment remains unclear.

LYME DISEASE SEROLOGY

- Although a positive C6 test in a dog with joint swelling suggests Lyme disease, coinfection with another tickborne agent (e.g., *Anaplasma phagocytophilum*) should also be considered.
- The Quantitative C6 assay enables clinicians to compare acute and convalescent results.
- A convalescent titer ≥50% higher than acute titer suggests active infection.
- Retesting 6 months after treatment is recommended to monitor its efficacy.
  - If the convalescent C6 level drops ≥50% of that in the acute sample, treatment was probably successful.
  - If the convalescent C6 level fails to decrease or decreases <50% of that in the acute sample, there are several possibilities:
  1. Treatment failure or treatment noncompliance by the owner
  2. Reinfection: A tick-control program should be assessed.
  3. Chronic infection: Long-standing infection and chronic immune stimulation may result in formation of memory cells (lymphocytes). In these cases, antibodies levels are less likely to decline despite effective therapy.

MISCELLANEOUS

ANCILLARY TESTS

- Determination of the urine/protein creatinine ratio to look for protein-losing glomerulonephropathy
- Arthrocentesis and synovial fluid analysis: Lyme disease causes suppurative inflammation (WBCs, 5,000–100,000/μL).
- PCR can detect *Borrelia burgdorferi* nucleic acid in tissue such as skin or synovium. Assay of blood has a much lower sensitivity because of the paucity of circulating organisms. A negative result does not definitively rule out infection.
- Culture of connective tissue (e.g., skin biopsy) is a definitive test but impractical for routine use and not provided by most diagnostic laboratories. Results can take 2–3 weeks and may be negative because of low numbers of organisms.

SYNONYMS

- *Borrelia burgdorferi*
- Borreliosis

SEE ALSO

Blackwell's Five-Minute Veterinary Consult: Canine and Feline Topics

- Lyme Disease
- Polyarthritis, Nonerosive, Immune-Mediated
- Renal Failure, Acute Uremia

Related Topics in This Book

- Arthrocentesis with Synovial Fluid Analysis
- Creatinine
- Urine Albumin
- Urine Protein/Creatinine Ratio
- Urine Specific Gravity

ABBREVIATIONS

None

Suggested Reading

Greene CE, Straubinger RE. Borreliosis. In: Greene CE, ed. *Infectious Diseases of the Dog and Cat,* 3rd ed. St Louis: Saunders Elsevier, 2006: 417–435.

Levy S, O'Connor TP, Hanscom JL, Shields P. Utility of an in-office C6 ELISA test kit for determination of infection status of dogs naturally exposed to *Borrelia burgdorferi*. *Vet Ther* 2002; 3: 308–315.

Philipp MT, Bowers LC, Fawcett PT, *et al.* Antibody response to IR6, a conserved immunodominant region of the VLsE lipoprotein, wanes rapidly after antibiotic treatment of *Borrelia burgdorferi* infection in experimental animals and in humans. *J Infect Dis* 2001; 184: 870–878.

INTERNET RESOURCES

IDEXX Laboratories, Lyme Quant C6 Test, http://www. idexx.com/animalhealth/laboratory/c6

AUTHOR NAME

Terri Wheeler

BASICS

TYPE OF PROCEDURE
Radiographic

PROCEDURE EXPLANATION AND RELATED PHYSIOLOGY
Lymphangiography is an examination of the lymph nodes and lymphatic vessels after the injection of a radiopaque substance. This technique is primarily used to identify the thoracic duct (TD) during surgery in dogs and cats with chylothorax and to verify its complete occlusion. Surgical intervention is warranted in animals with chylothorax that do not have underlying disease and in whom medical management becomes impractical. Medical management becomes impractical when thoracocentesis is required more frequently than once a week or when repeat thoracocentesis fails to relieve the dyspnea. Surgical options include mesenteric lymphangiography and TD ligation, subtotal pericardiectomy, omentalization, passive pleuroperitoneal shunting, active pleuroperitoneal or pleurovenous shunting, and pleurodesis. Of these, only the first 2 (TD ligation and pericardiectomy) are recommended by the author as first-line therapies.

The mechanism by which TD ligation is purported to work is through the formation of abdominal lymphaticovenous anastomoses that develop when the duct has been occluded. Chyle, therefore, bypasses the TD, and the effusion resolves. Advantages of TD ligation are that, if successful, it resolves pleural fluid completely (as compared to palliative procedures) and may prevent fibrosing pleuritis from developing. The disadvantages include that operative time is long (which is problematic in debilitated animals), continued or recurrent chylous or nonchylous (from pulmonary lymphatics) effusion may occur in some animals, and mesenteric lymphangiography is often difficult to perform (particularly in cats). Without mesenteric lymphangiography, complete ligation of the TD cannot be assured; however, this technique might not be uniformly successful in verifying complete ligation of the TD. Additionally, some animals may form collateral lymphatics past the site of the ligature and thus reestablish TD flow. If chyle flow is directed into the diaphragmatic lymphatics, chylothorax may continue or recur.

INDICATIONS
• Lymphangiography is used to help identify the number and location of branches of the TD, which need to be ligated during surgery. It is critical that all branches be ligated or continued effusion can be expected.
• This technique can also help evaluate the extent of lymphangiectasia present in the cranial thorax.
• After ligation of the TD, repeat lymphangiography can be performed to help ensure that no identifiable flow into TD branches might have been missed during the ligation.

CONTRAINDICATIONS
Nonsurgical causes of chylothorax (e.g., heart failure, neoplasia, fungal infections)

POTENTIAL COMPLICATIONS
Serious complications have not been reported; however, mesenteric tears could result in intestinal strangulation and should be repaired.

CLIENT EDUCATION
• Small branches of the TD may not fill with contrast and thus may be difficult to locate and ligate. Failure to locate and ligate these small branches can contribute to continued chylothorax.
• Not all animals respond to TD ligation with resolution of pleural fluid; however, success rates of >80% should be expected when experienced surgeons perform the procedure.

BODY SYSTEMS ASSESSED
Hemic, lymphatic, and immune

PROCEDURE

PATIENT PREPARATION

Preprocedure Medication or Preparation
• Food is withheld 12 h prior to surgery.
• Beginning 3 h prior to surgery, administer corn oil or cream, or a mixture of the 2 (≈2 mL/kg), every hour until anesthetic induction (3 doses), to ensure visualization of lymphatics. If the patient does not absorb the cream or corn oil, the lymphatics will be clear, making catheterization and ligation of them difficult.

Anesthesia or Sedation
General anesthesia is required for this procedure.

Patient Positioning
Dogs are positioned in left lateral recumbency, and cats in right.

Patient Monitoring
Because these animals may have trouble ventilating, close monitoring of respiratory and cardiac parameters is essential.

Equipment or Supplies
• A 22- or 20-gauge over-the-needle catheter
• An extension set
• A 3-way stopcock
• Methylene blue
• 4-0 silk suture material
• A water-soluble contrast agent
• Supplies needed for abdominal surgery
• Radiographic equipment

TECHNIQUE
• The right side of the thorax and abdomen in dogs (left side in cats) is prepared for aseptic surgery.
• Make a right (dogs) or left (cats) paracostal incision and exteriorize the cecum.
• Once the cecum has been exteriorized, locate a lymph node adjacent to it. If necessary, inject a small volume (0.1–1.0 mL) of methylene blue (USP 1%; American Quinine, Shirley, NY) into the lymph node to increase visualization of the lymphatics. Administration of repeated doses of methylene blue should be avoided because of the risk or inducing a Heinz body anemia or renal failure.
• Carefully dissect the mesentery near this node to visualize large lymphatic vessels that can be cannulated. *Note*: Be careful to not tear or cut a lymphatic during this process because then the lymphatic system will decompress, making cannulation very difficult.
• Once the lymphatic has been cleared of surrounding tissue, cannulate it with a 20-gauge (dogs) or 22-gauge (cats) over-the-needle catheter. *Note*: Cannulation of this lymphatic is more difficult in cats than in dogs because cats have more fat in their mesentery and their lymphatics are significantly smaller.
• Place a suture (4-0 silk) in the mesentery and use the suture to secure the catheter and an attached piece of extension tubing in place. (The ends of the suture can be looped over the hub of the extension tubing.) An additional suture may be placed around the extension tubing and through a segment of intestine to prevent dislodgment of the catheter.
• Attach a 3-way stopcock to the end of the extension tubing and inject a water-soluble contrast agent at a dosage of 1 mL/kg diluted with 0.5 mL/kg of saline. Alternatively, a volume of diluted methylene blue (1 part methylene blue to 3 parts sterile saline) sufficient to fill the extension set and catheter plus 1–2 mL may be injected. Repeating the

injection of a similar volume of dye after ligation may help identify any branches bypassing the ligature(s).
• If a radiographic contrast agent is being used, take a lateral thoracic radiograph while the last millimeter is being injected or use a C-arm to observe flow of the contrast into the TD and subsequently into the venous system.
• Repeat the procedure after ligation of the TD.

SAMPLE HANDLING
None

APPROPRIATE AFTERCARE
Postprocedure Patient Monitoring
Observe the patient for evidence of respiratory distress after the procedure. If a thoracotomy has been done to ligate the duct, ensure that all air and fluid have been removed prior to the patient's recovery.

Nursing Care
None

Dietary Modification
Animals with chylothorax are typically fed a low-fat diet. This diet may be continued until the effusion has resolved (generally 1–2 weeks postoperatively).

Medication Requirements
None

Restrictions on Activity
Recovery should be restricted to leash walks for 7–10 days following the procedure. Do not allow patients to run or jump.

Anticipated Recovery Time
7–10 days

INTERPRETATION

NORMAL FINDINGS OR RANGE
A normal lymphangiogram (Figure 1A) will show the TD emptying cleanly into the venous system.

ABNORMAL VALUES
In animals with lymphangiectasia, numerous lymphatics can be visualized in the cranial mediastinum (Figure 1B). A tear or rupture of the TD is extremely rare.

CRITICAL VALUES
None

INTERFERING FACTORS
Drugs That May Alter Results of the Procedure
It can be very difficult to locate and ligate lymphatics in animals that have been fasted and have not been fed cream or corn oil, as described in the Patient Preparation section.

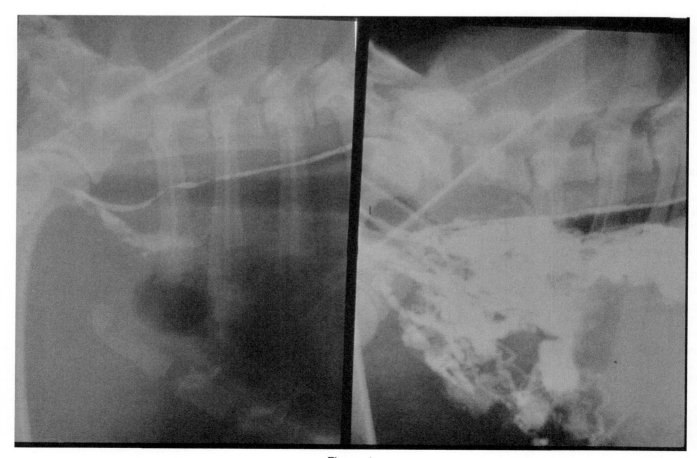

Figure 1

A: A normal lymphangiogram showing the thoracic duct emptying cleanly into the venous system. **B:** A lymphangiogram from a dog with lymphangiectasia and chylothorax. Numerous lymphatics can be seen in the cranial mediastinum.

Conditions That May Interfere with Performing the Procedure
Diffuse lymphangiectasia may make localization of a mesenteric lymphatic very difficult.

Procedure Techniques or Handling That May Alter Results
Use extreme care when dissecting a mesenteric lymphatic for cannulation: A small laceration or tear will cause chyle to leak into the site and the collapse of all lymphatics, making catheterization difficult or impossible.

Influence of Signalment on Performing and Interpreting the Procedure

Species
Lymphangiography is much harder to perform in small cats and dogs than in larger-breed dogs.

Breed
None

Age
None

Gender
None

Pregnancy
None

CLINICAL PERSPECTIVE
• Injection of methylene blue into the catheter to aid in visualization of the duct is of more value than a contrast lymphangiogram.
• Computed tomographic lymphangiography may also be performed in dogs to help discern the course and number of lymphatics in the thoracic cavity.

MISCELLANEOUS

ANCILLARY TESTS
Computed tomographic lymphangiography

SYNONYMS
Lymphography

SEE ALSO
Blackwell's Five-Minute Veterinary Consult: Canine and Feline Topics
Chylothorax
Related Topics in This Book
• General Principles of Radiography
• Computed Tomography
• Thoracic Radiography

ABBREVIATIONS
TD = thoracic duct

Suggested Reading
Fossum TW, Mertens MM, Miller MW, *et al*. Thoracic duct ligation and pericardectomy for treatment of idiopathic chylothorax. *J Vet Intern Med* 2004; 18: 307–310.

INTERNET RESOURCES
None

AUTHOR NAME
Theresa W. Fossum

BASICS

TYPE OF SPECIMEN
Blood

TEST EXPLANATION AND RELATED PHYSIOLOGY
Magnesium (Mg) is the second most abundant intracellular cation behind potassium and is an essential cofactor in hundreds of enzymatic reactions, as well as being associated with ATP production, ion transport, and establishment of transmembrane electrical gradients. Whole-body Mg is found within the bone ($\approx$67%), soft tissues ($\approx$32%), and extracellular fluid/plasma ($\approx$1%). The latter is further divided into an ionized or free fraction ($\approx$55%), a protein-bound fraction ($\approx$30%), and a portion chelated or complexed to various anions and acids ($\approx$15%). Mg homeostasis is largely regulated by the kidneys through glomerular filtration and tubular reabsorption. Intestinal absorption at the distal jejunum and ileum depends on dietary concentrations and is modulated by vitamin D and parathyroid hormone.

Total magnesium (tMg) is most often measured spectrophotometrically. Ionized magnesium (iMg), measured with an ion-specific electrode, is in dynamic equilibrium with intracellular Mg, and is therefore a much more reliable indicator of whole-body Mg levels. Unfortunately, availability of this assay is limited.

INDICATIONS
- Component of a routine biochemical profile (tMg)
- Monitoring in critically ill patients (tMg and iMg)

CONTRAINDICATIONS
None

POTENTIAL COMPLICATIONS
None

CLIENT EDUCATION
Serum total Mg levels may be normal despite an underlying deficiency.

BODY SYSTEMS ASSESSED
- Cardiovascular
- Endocrine and metabolic
- Gastrointestinal
- Neuromuscular
- Renal and urologic

SAMPLE

COLLECTION
1–3 mL of venous blood

HANDLING
- tMg: Collect samples into plain red-top tube, serum-separator tube, or heparin anticoagulant. Anticoagulants that chelate Mg (e.g., EDTA, citrate) are not acceptable.
- iMg: Collect samples anaerobically into heparin or a plain red-top tube, place them on ice, and analyze them immediately or store separated serum or plasma in a tightly sealed container to maintain anaerobic conditions.

STORAGE
- tMg: Refrigerate samples for short-term storage. Freeze serum or plasma for long-term storage.
- iMg: If necessary, serum or plasma can be refrigerated or frozen in an airtight container.

STABILITY
- tMg

- Room temperature: 1 week
- Refrigerated (2°–8°C): 1 week
- Frozen (−20°C): $\approx$1 year
- iMg
  - Room temperature: 1 day
  - Refrigerated (2°–8°C): 3 days
  - Frozen (−20°C): 1 month

INTERPRETATION

NORMAL FINDINGS OR RANGE
Dogs
- tMg: 1.6–2.4 mg/dL (0.66–0.99 mmol/L)
- iMg: 0.92–1.26 mg/dL (0.38–0.52 mmol/L)

Cats
- tMg: 1.7–2.6 mg/dL (0.70–1.07 mmol/L)
- iMg: 1.14–1.53 mg/dL (0.47–0.63 mmol/L)
- Reference intervals may vary among instruments and laboratories.

ABNORMAL VALUES
Values above or below reference interval

CRITICAL VALUES
Not established. Other electrolyte and mineral abnormalities contribute to complications.

INTERFERING FACTORS
Drugs That May Alter Results or Interpretation
Drugs That Interfere with Test Methodology
- Artifactual decreases caused by citrates, Ca gluconate, glucuronic acid, and cefotaxime (if tobramycin is present)
- Artifactual increases caused by cefotaxime, trichloroacetic acid, and Ca

Drugs That Alter Physiology

Physiologic increases
Caused by prolonged aspirin therapy, lithium, Mg salts, medroxyprogesterone, and progesterone

Physiologic decreases
- Nephrotoxicity: aminoglycosides, amphotericin B, cisplatin, cyclosporine, ticarcillin
- Citrates may chelate Mg (blood transfusions).
- Decreased intestinal absorption: neomycin, Ca salts, laxatives
- Enhanced renal loss: digoxin, furosemide, thiazides, mannitol, saline diuresis
- Intracellular shifts with the administration of insulin, glucose, or amino acids

Disorders That May Alter Results
- tMg falsely increased by in vivo hemolysis, hypercalcemia, or hyperproteinemia
- tMg falsely decreased by hyperbilirubinemia, lipemia, or hypoproteinemia
- Acid-base disorders may result in shifts between iMg and protein-bound Mg similar to those observed with Ca.

Collection Techniques or Handling That May Alter Results
- Mg falsely decreased by the use of inappropriate anticoagulants such as citrate, EDTA, lithium heparin, sodium fluoride, or oxalates or by the use of siliconized blood tubes
- Elevated by in vitro hemolysis with Mg release from erythrocytes
- iMg decreased by increased pH from delayed sample processing or exposure to air

Influence of Signalment
Species
None

Breed
None

Age
None

Gender
None

Pregnancy
Maternal Mg may affect the fetus.

LIMITATIONS OF THE TEST
Sensitivity, Specificity, and Positive and Negative Predictive Values
N/A

Valid If Run in a Human Lab?
Yes.

Causes of Abnormal Findings

High values	Low values
Intestinal hypomotility disorders	GI/inadequate intake
	Chronic diarrhea
Renal failure	Malabsorptive syndromes (e.g.,
Postrenal obstruction	exocrine pancreatic insufficiency,
Hypothyroidism	cholestatic disorders,
Hypoadrenocorticism	inflammatory bowel disease)
(reported in human	Gastroenteritis
patients)	Neoplasia
Iatrogenic administration	Intestinal resection
Cathartics	Acute pancreatitis
Laxatives	Inadequate nutrition or parenteral
IV fluids	nutrition with inadequate Mg
	supplementation
	Renal
	Renal tubular disorders (e.g., acute
	tubular necrosis, nephrotoxicity)
	Postobstructive diuresis
	Extrarenal factors
	Diuretics
	Digitalis
	Hypercalcemia, hypokalemia, or
	phosphate depletion
	Endocrine
	Diabetic ketoacidosis (more
	common in cats than dogs)
	Hyperthyroidism
	Primary hyperparathyroidism
	Translocation/chelation
	Elevated catecholamine states:
	sepsis, trauma, or hypothermia
	Rapid insulin or glucose
	administration

CLINICAL PERSPECTIVE
Hypomagnesemia is often undetected, especially in critically ill patients, and may produce clinical signs affecting multiple organ systems. Hypermagnesemia is less common.

MISCELLANEOUS
ANCILLARY TESTS
- Chemistry profile including Ca and electrolytes
- Urinary Mg levels to look for renal loss

SYNONYMS
None

SEE ALSO
Blackwell's Five-Minute Veterinary Consult: Canine and Feline Topics
- Hypermagnesemia
- Hypomagnesemia

Related Topics in This Book
Calcium

ABBREVIATIONS
- Ca = calcium
- iMg = ionized magnesium
- Mg = magnesium
- tMg = total magnesium

Suggested Reading
Gilroy CV, Burton SA, Horney BS, MacKenzie AL. Validation of the NOVA CRT8 for the measurement of ionized magnesium in feline serum. *Vet Clin Pathol* 2005; 34: 124–131.
Martin LG, Van Pelt DR, Wingfield WE. Magnesium and the critically ill patient. In: Bonagura JD, Kirk RW, eds. *Current Veterinary Therapy XII*. Philadelphia: WB Saunders, 1995: 128–131.

INTERNET RESOURCES
None

AUTHOR NAMES
Seth E. Chapman and Karen E. Russell

BASICS

TYPE OF PROCEDURE
Diagnostic imaging

PROCEDURE EXPLANATION AND RELATED PHYSIOLOGY
Many morphologic abnormalities, involving many organ systems, can be detected by using magnetic resonance imaging (MRI). For MRI, an anesthetized patient is placed in a homogeneous high-field magnet. The high-field magnet causes hydrogen protons to align with the magnetic field; hydrogen protons themselves act like small magnets because they have both charge and motion. This process is not limited to hydrogen protons, but this is what is imaged clinically. Any atom with an unbalanced number of protons and neutrons could potentially be imaged. A radiofrequency (RF) pulse is broadcast into the patient, and this energy deposition causes a small but measurable number of hydrogen protons to become excited and align in a higher energy level against the main magnetic field. When the RF pulse is turned off, the protons release the absorbed energy in the form of an RF pulse. The character of the emitted RF pulse is influenced by the local environment with which the hydrogen protons are associated. Hydrogen protons in complex carbon chains, like fat, release the absorbed energy differently from hydrogen protons that are bound to oxygen in a water molecule. The differences in energy-release characteristics are used to generate an image.

Many different pulse sequences are acquired to accentuate the various relaxation properties of hydrogen protons in the region of interest. Each sequence generates a data set of sectional images in a particular plane or volume and may take a few seconds to many minutes to acquire. A standard examination may involve 7 or more sequences, and a completed study comprises >400 images. As with computed tomography, contrast medium is usually administered to accentuate regions of inflammation, infiltration, or vascular disruption. Magnetic resonance (MR) contrast agents are considered safer than iodinated agents used in radiographic imaging.

MRI provides superior soft tissue contrast resolution when compared to any other imaging modality currently available. In addition, despite popular belief, MR provides significant information about bone structure and physiology. Inflammatory and infiltrative conditions of bone are detected earlier on MR images than on radiographs and often earlier than with nuclear medicine.

Magnet field strength has a major impact on image quality and the types of studies that can be performed. Generally speaking, it takes longer to acquire a selection of images on low-field magnets (e.g., 0.3-T field strength) compared to high-field magnets (e.g., 1.5-T field strength). In addition, it is easier to acquire higher-resolution images by using a high-field magnet than a low-field magnet. There is significant variation in the quality of MRI services available to the veterinary profession.

INDICATIONS
- Focal or multifocal intracranial disease
- Seizures (rule out a morphologic cause)
- Cranial nerve disorders
- Chronic nasal discharge
- Nasal deformation
- Cervical or thoracolumbar disk disease
- Focal spinal cord dysfunction from any disorder
- Lumbosacral disorders
- Peripheral nerve tumors
- Suspected spinal tumors or infiltrative disorders
- Orthopedic disorders particularly associated with soft tissue injuries
- Preoperative assessment of cruciate and meniscus integrity
- Chronic shoulder or elbow lameness
- Mediastinal and cardiac masses (requires a high-field system)
- Abdominal masses
- Confirm and map portosystemic shunt vessels
- Pelvic cavity masses
- Radiation therapy planning
- Surgical planning for treatment of soft tissue sarcomas
- Tumor staging

CONTRAINDICATIONS
- Cardiac pacemaker
- Nontitanium metallic implants, gold beads, or ferromagnetic projectiles in close proximity to region of interest
- Within 1 month of surgery where non-MRI-compatible surgical staples were used

POTENTIAL COMPLICATIONS
- Unauthorized entry of personnel with metallic instruments into the scan room poses a severe safety hazard. Metallic objects are attracted to the magnet and will be pulled from pockets or hands at great speed toward its center. This could injure personnel or the patient.
- Those associated with general anesthesia can occur.
- Some metallic implants can move in soft tissue.
- Patients with spinal instability should be handled with extreme care.
- Excessive imaging very rarely elevates the temperature of small patients.
- Pregnant patients should be imaged with caution.
- Although extremely rare, an adverse reaction to gadolinium, a common MR contrast agent, might occur.

CLIENT EDUCATION
- MRI is well accepted in human patients as a high-yield, reliable diagnostic imaging test. The same is true in animal patients.
- Because animals require general anesthesia, the concerns many people have about claustrophobia in bore magnets are not relevant.
- Clients should be made aware that their pet will be anesthetized and that risk is associated with this procedure, particularly in patients with intracranial disease.

BODY SYSTEMS ASSESSED
- Cardiovascular
- Gastrointestinal
- Hepatobiliary
- Musculoskeletal
- Nervous
- Neuromuscular
- Ophthalmic
- Renal and urologic
- Reproductive
- Respiratory

 PROCEDURE

PATIENT PREPARATION
Preprocedure Medication or Preparation
- MRI services are available at many veterinary teaching hospitals and some larger, privately owned, veterinary referral centers. A small number of independent MRI services are available. Different imaging centers will have different patient preparation protocols, so specific requirements should be obtained directly from the center one plans to use. Most centers require referral from a veterinarian.
- Generally, preanesthetic blood tests are required, and any information about the cardiovascular status of the patient with respect to anesthesia should be made available. Food but not water should be withheld for 12 h.
- There cannot be any ferromagnetic material in the patient in close proximity to the region of interest because this produces a susceptibility artifact and the distorted image is usually nondiagnostic. Radiography should be used to rule out ferromagnetic material if there is any doubt. Identification microchips do not usually cause a large enough artifact to prevent a diagnostic spinal study from being made. A total hip prosthesis can sometimes prevent a diagnostic study of the lumbosacral region. Field strengths of ≤1.5 T do not damage identification microchips. Gold beads can interfere with imaging, as can metallic projectiles. Lead and titanium cause less artifact than ferrous materials.
- An accurate and complete record of the patient's medical history will enable the interpreting radiologist to generate a more accurate differential diagnosis for the MR findings.

Anesthesia or Sedation
- General anesthesia is required because patients must be completely immobilized for the duration of the scan. The procedure is not painful, although it is noisy because of gradient switching within the bore of the magnet.

- Fentanyl premedication followed by propofol induction and isoflurane maintenance is a popular anesthetic regimen because patients awake quickly after the procedure and the regimen is considered relatively safe.
- If gaseous anesthesia is used, provision must be made for an MR-compatible anesthetic system.
- Many patients undergoing brain studies have increased intracranial pressure, so it is important that these patients be ventilated adequately. Ventilator equipment must also be MR compatible.

Patient Positioning
- Patient positioning depends on the region of interest.
- Brain studies are usually conducted with patients in sternal recumbency.
- Spine imaging is done with patients in dorsal recumbency, which entails minimal spinal movement.
- As with all cross-sectional imaging, accurate patient positioning results in superior image quality.

Patient Monitoring
Anesthetic monitoring is difficult without dedicated MR-compatible equipment. Standard ECG machines, pulse oximeters, blood pressure monitors, and capnographs usually contain ferromagnetic components and may be attracted to the magnet. In addition, many perform inaccurately when close to the magnetic field. In the absence of dedicated monitoring equipment, continuous monitoring at the magnet via a plastic esophageal stethoscope is the most practical alternative.

Equipment or Supplies
- All diagnostic MR magnets need to be shielded from extraneous electromagnetic radiation. Essentially, the magnet and patient must be isolated from RFs from the environment because RF signals from other sources (e.g., radio stations, cell phones) disrupt the very weak RF signal generated by the patient when the RF pulse is turned off. Shielding is achieved by creating an electrically isolated and contiguous enclosure within which the magnet is placed. This is usually made of copper or copper mesh and is known as a Faraday cage. Smaller magnets are often shielded in a portable cage; with high-field magnets, the shielding is built into the walls, windows, and door.
- If MR examinations are conducted in a local human facility, anesthetic and monitoring equipment will need to be supplied. As stated earlier, gas anesthesia requires MR-compatible equipment. Some clinicians use a high-flow plastic to-and-fro system with the anesthetic machine outside the magnet room. Anesthetic tubes can sometimes be passed through a shielded port in the Faraday cage, negating the need to leave the door ajar and breach the RF seal.

TECHNIQUE
- Dedicated veterinary imaging suites providing an outpatient service usually have a turnaround time of ≈2 h. During this time, the patient is evaluated for anesthesia and anesthetized, the scan is performed, and the patient recovers. Scanning usually takes ≈30–45 min, depending on the region and complexity of the case. Some centers provide an

imaging report. The images are digital and thus easily transferred to a server for remote viewing. A CD is often provided with embedded viewing software that enables the referring veterinarian to review the images.

SAMPLE HANDLING
Images of the study are usually given to, or made available on request by, the referring veterinarian.

APPROPRIATE AFTERCARE
Postprocedure Patient Monitoring
As with all patients undergoing general anesthesia, patients undergoing MRI should be closely monitored for 24 h after the procedure. Outpatient monitoring can usually be done by owners at home.

Nursing Care
• It is uncommon for patients to be clinically worse after MRI.
• It is unlikely patients will be discharged from an imaging center until any complications associated with anesthesia are resolved.

Dietary Modification
Food should be withheld for 12 h prior to the study as a precaution against vomiting secondary to anesthesia.

Medication Requirements
No special medication is required.

Restrictions on Activity
After patients have recovered from anesthesia, normal activity can be resumed.

Anticipated Recovery Time
Recovery time pertains to anesthesia. An MR study has no known side effects.

INTERPRETATION

NORMAL FINDINGS OR RANGE
• The most common pulse sequences in veterinary imaging are conventional and fast T1, T2, and proton density weighted spin echo sequences and combinations thereof. T1 and T2 pertain to the way in which hydrogen protons release the energy absorbed during the RF broadcast. Generally, in conventional and fast T1 weighted spin echo sequences, free fluid [e.g., cerebrospinal fluid (CSF)] is black, tissue with higher fluid content is dark, and fat is bright. In T2 weighted sequences, free fluid is white, and tissue containing an excess of fluid (i.e., edema) is bright. Fat is also bright in fast or turbo spin echo sequences. In a proton density weighted sequence, image contrast is related to the density of protons per volume rather than proton energy dissipation characteristics. In all sequences, cortical bone and normal ligaments and tendons appear dark.
• To better differentiate pathology, modifications of these basic sequences are also acquired. FLAIR (*fl*uid-*a*ttenuated *i*nversion *r*ecovery)

is a T2 weighted sequence, but the signal from true free fluid is removed. This often helps in differentiating tissue edema from true fluid accumulations. Similarly, sometimes bright fat masks the ability to see adjacent tissue edema or infiltration (e.g., edema in fatty marrow cavity) on T2 weighted sequences. STIR (*sh*ort-*t*au *i*nversion *r*ecovery) is a sequence whereby the signal from fat is removed from the image. This enables clinicians to see tissue edema, inflammation, or infiltration easier, without the bright signal from fat masking the pathology.
• Many hundreds of pulse sequences are available to clinicians. The aforementioned are the most basic sequences (and most commonly used) in medical imaging. When specifically investigating blood flow and hemorrhage, 3-D volume and 4-D imaging, angiograms, venograms, and other specialized sequences are commonly used.
• The brain and spinal cord are the most common regions imaged in animals. Normal findings on brain MR study rule out morphologic causes for the clinical signs but they do not rule out toxic, inflammatory, or metabolic causes. Many meningoencephalitides can be detected by MRI, but the absence of meningeal or parenchymal enhancement after contrast medium administration does not rule out an inflammatory or infiltrative process. Normal findings on spinal examination do not rule out degenerative myelopathy. As with intracranial examinations, normal findings on spinal exam do not rule out all inflammatory or infiltrative myelopathies or metabolic causes of the spinal dysfunction. If the results of an MR study are normal, a CSF tap should be performed. Even in the light of abnormal MRI findings, a CSF tap may assist in prioritizing the differential list.

ABNORMAL VALUES
• Many morphologic anomalies can be detected.
• With respect to the brain, congenital and developmental anomalies, intra-axial and extra-axial tumors, some inflammatory conditions, and vascular disruptions (hemorrhagic and nonhemorrhagic) can be detected.
• In the spine, degenerative, prolapsed, and herniated intervertebral disks; parenchymal, dural, epidural, and paraspinal masses; and cord infarcts (fibrocartilaginous embolus) can be detected. Developmental anomalies of the spine and spinal cord can usually be detected. The ability to diagnose the presence of syringohydromyelia, either associated with occipital dysplasia and Chiari-like malformations or secondary to other pathology, has greatly advanced our understanding of spinal disorders in dogs.

CRITICAL VALUES
None

INTERFERING FACTORS
Drugs That May Alter Results of the Procedure
Steroidal and nonsteroidal anti-inflammatory medication may reduce the apparent severity of intracranial edema.

Conditions That May Interfere with Performing the Procedure
• Ferromagnetic implants or projectiles might interfere with the scan, depending on the size of the ferromagnetic material and distance from the region of interest.
• Spinal instability may complicate patient handling.

Procedure Techniques or Handling That May Alter Results
• Many technical factors can influence the quality of an examination. These are mainly associated with selection of the optimum sequences, imaging parameters, and coil. A lot of time can be wasted by inexperienced operators because 1 nondiagnostic sequence could easily waste many minutes. Imaging protocols should be optimized on test patients before being attempted on clinical patients.
• Coil selection is critical in ensuring optimum signal detection. Coils should be as close to the patient as possible to reduce signal loss. Some third-party vendors are generating veterinary specific coils that fit our smaller patients better.

Influence of Signalment on Performing and Interpreting the Procedure

Species
Any species can be imaged that can be chemically restrained adequately, fits in the magnet bore, and does not exceed couch weight limits. Generally, smaller species are much harder to image than larger species because less signal emanates from small volumes and smaller patients require thinner slices.

Breed
It is more difficult to acquire high-resolution, thin-slice images of smaller breeds relative to large breeds. The image generated is the result of the RF broadcast from the region of interest. In many situations, smaller patients require thinner slices than larger patients. The volume of tissue generating the image is less, and therefore the signal is weaker. This results in a low signal-to-noise ratio and a grainy image. This can be overcome by increasing the number of times the data acquisition is repeated. This substantially increases scan time. The most effective way to overcome problems associated with small patients and small body parts is to image patients on a magnet with higher field strength. Higher field strength results in relatively more protons being energized and thus more signal generated per unit volume (*voxel*, or 3-dimensional pixel). This substantially increases signal-to-noise ratio, improving image quality.

Age
The adipose tissue in young patients sometimes appears different relative to that in older patients.

Gender
None

Pregnancy
General anesthesia, the magnetic field, and gadolinium might have negative effects on a pregnancy, although this has not been completely characterized in our patients. Imaging of pregnant patients should be performed only if clinically necessary.

CLINICAL PERSPECTIVE
MRI is the most significant recent advance in veterinary imaging. The technology is expensive, but the benefit with respect to diagnostic sensitivity and specificity is excellent. It is envisioned that MRI will play an increasingly important role in veterinary imaging in the foreseeable future.

 MISCELLANEOUS

ANCILLARY TESTS
A CSF tap is commonly done in conjunction with brain and spinal cord MRI to assist in prioritizing the differential list.

SEE ALSO
Blackwell's Five-Minute Veterinary Consult: Canine and Feline Topics
Many

Related Topics in This Book
None

ABBREVIATIONS
• CSF = cerebrospinal fluid
• FLAIR = fluid-attenuated inversion recovery
• MR = magnetic resonance
• MRI = magnetic resonance imaging
• RF = radiofrequency
• STIR = short-tau inversion recovery
• T = Tesla, the SI unit for magnetic flux density

Suggested Reading
Thrall D. *Textbook of Veterinary Diagnostic Radiology,* 5th ed. Elsevier, 2007 [for veterinary MRI: overview of the physics of MRI and common diagnoses].
Westbrook C, Kaut Roth C, Talbot J. *MRI in Practice,* 3rd ed. Ames, IA: Blackwell, 2005 [for the detailed physics of MRI].

INTERNET RESOURCES
Hesselink JR. Basic principles of MR imaging. University of California–San Diego (UCSD), Center for Functional MRI, UCSD Neuroradiology Teaching File Database, http://spinwarp.ucsd.edu/neuroweb/Text/br-100.htm.
Hornak JP. The Basics of MRI. Rochester, NY: Rochester Institute of Technology (TIT), Chester F. Carlson Center of Imaging Science, http://www.cis.rit.edu/htbooks/mri/.

AUTHOR NAME
Ian Robertson

MASTICATORY MUSCLE MYOSITIS (2M ANTIBODY ASSAY)

BASICS

TYPE OF SPECIMEN
Blood

TEST EXPLANATION AND RELATED PHYSIOLOGY
The muscles of mastication in dogs and cats contain a unique fiber type—type 2M—that is not present in limb muscles. Further, type 2M fibers are biochemically different from limb muscle. Dogs with masticatory muscle myositis (MMM) develop autoantibodies against type 2M fiber proteins that do not cross-react with limb muscle. It has not yet been determined whether these autoantibodies play a role in the pathogenesis of MMM or are just a marker of this disease. Demonstration of autoantibodies by immunohistochemical assay or ELISA provides a reliable diagnosis of canine MMM.

INDICATIONS
- Jaw pain
- Atrophy or swelling of the masticatory muscles
- Trismus
- Exophthalmos or endophthalmos

CONTRAINDICATIONS
- Generalized muscle atrophy
- Weakness and exercise intolerance

POTENTIAL COMPLICATIONS
None

CLIENT EDUCATION
- The animal should undergo a 12-h fast before the test.
- A negative 2M antibody titer does not completely rule out a diagnosis of MMM.

BODY SYSTEMS ASSESSED
- Musculoskeletal
- Neuromuscular

SAMPLE

COLLECTION
1–2 mL of venous blood

HANDLING
- Red-top or serum-separator tube
- Separate the serum from the cells.

STORAGE
Refrigerate the sample.

STABILITY
- Room temperature: 3–5 days
- Refrigerated (2°–8°C): 1–2 weeks
- Frozen (−20°C): years

PROTOCOL
None

INTERPRETATION

NORMAL FINDINGS OR RANGE
- Negative staining of type 2M fibers in normal canine masticatory muscle by immunohistochemistry
- ELISA antibody titers against masticatory muscle proteins of <1:100

ABNORMAL VALUES
- Positive staining of type 2M fibers in normal canine masticatory muscle by immunohistochemistry
- An ELISA serum antibody titer against masticatory muscle type 2M fiber proteins of >1:100
- A serum antibody titer of 1:100 by ELISA is considered borderline.

CRITICAL VALUES
None

INTERFERING FACTORS
Drugs That May Alter Results or Interpretation
Drugs That Interfere with Test Methodology
None

Drugs That Alter Physiology
Corticosteroid therapy at immunosuppressive dosages for >7–10 days will lower autoantibody levels. Effects of other immunosuppressive agents have not been evaluated but likely also lower antibody concentrations.

Disorders That May Alter Results
Severe hemolysis or lipemia

Collection Techniques or Handling That May Alter Results
- Failure to separate serum from cells may be associated with severe hemolysis.
- Serum held at room temperature for longer than advised

Influence of Signalment
Species
- The test is valid for dogs.
- Although cats can rarely have an MMM-like disorder, autoantibodies against type 2M fibers have not been demonstrated in this species.

Breed
- All dog breeds may be affected.
- A severe form of MMM occurs in Cavalier King Charles spaniels, with clinical signs beginning at 3–6 months of age.

Age
Signs usually begin at >6 months of age but can infrequently occur in dogs at 3–4 months of age.

Gender
Both genders are affected.

Pregnancy
May unmask subclinical MMM

LIMITATIONS OF THE TEST
• The 2M antibody titer will be negative in end-stage MMM, where type 2M fibers have been lost and replaced by fibrosis.
• A negative 2M antibody titer does not eliminate a diagnosis of MMM. If the results of the serum assay are normal and clinical signs are consistent with MMM, a muscle biopsy is indicated.

Sensitivity, Specificity, and Positive and Negative Predictive Values
• Sensitivity for MMM is ≈85%.
• The test is specific for MMM, with the exception of rare overlap between syndromes of MMM and polymyositis (PM).

Valid If Run in a Human Lab?
No—the assay is species specific, with no human equivalent.

Causes of Abnormal Findings

High values	Low values
MMM	End-stage MMM
Antibodies rarely	Corticosteroids
increased with PM	Temporomandibular joint
	disease
	Denervation
	Extraocular myositis or PM

CLINICAL PERSPECTIVE
• MMM is a bilateral disease, although 1 side can be more severely affected than the other and present with a unilateral appearance.
• Relapses are common if MMM is not treated appropriately.
• A positive 2M antibody titer is diagnostic of canine MMM.
• Correlation (if any) of the antibody titer and severity of disease has not been determined.
• Vaccination may exacerbate active MMM. It is not known whether vaccination can precipitate the disease.

MISCELLANEOUS

ANCILLARY TESTS
• Oral examination for the presence of retrobulbar abscess
• Radiographic evaluation of the temporomandibular joints
• Evaluation of the serum creatine kinase concentration, which may be mildly elevated or normal

• Masticatory muscle biopsy: A muscle biopsy is recommended, especially if the serum is negative for 2M antibodies. The antibody titer may be low in end-stage MMM or with previous corticosteroid therapy, and the biopsy should confirm this.
• Magnetic resonance imaging (MRI): If the 2M antibody titer is negative, and the muscle biopsy is not confirmatory, MRI could show focal or multifocal areas of increased intensity, supporting inflammation. Hyperintensity of the extraocular muscles could suggest extraocular myositis.
• Testing for hypothyroidism and Cushing's syndrome in older dogs with chronic atrophy of the masticatory muscles

SYNONYMS
2M antibody

SEE ALSO
Blackwell's Five-Minute Veterinary Consult: Canine and Feline Topics
• Myopathy, Focal Inflammatory—Masticatory Muscle Myositis and Extraocular Myositis
• Myopathy, Generalized Inflammatory—Polymyositis and Dermatomyositis
• Myopathy, Noninflammatory—Endocrine

Related Topics in This Book
• ACTH Stimulation Test
• Low-Dose Dexamethasone Suppression Test
• Magnetic Resonance Imaging
• Muscle and Nerve Biopsy
• Thyroxine (T$_4$), Free
• Thyroxine (T$_4$), Total

ABBREVIATIONS
• MMM = masticatory muscle myositis
• MRI = magnetic resonance imaging
• PM = polymyositis

Suggested Reading
Evans J, Levesque D, Shelton GD. Canine inflammatory myopathies: A clinicopathologic review of 200 cases. *J Vet Intern Med* 2004; 18: 679–691.
Melmed C, Shelton GD, Bergman R, Barton C. Masticatory muscle myositis: Pathogenesis, diagnosis, and treatment. *Comp Contin Educ Pract Vet* 2004; 26: 590–605.
Podell M. Inflammatory myopathies. *Vet Clin North Am* 2002; 32: 147–167.

INTERNET RESOURCES
University of California–San Diego, Department of Pathology, School of Medicine, Comparative Neuromuscular Laboratory: Companion animal diagnostics, http://medicine.ucsd.edu/vet_neuromuscular.

AUTHOR NAME
G. Diane Shelton

BASICS

TYPE OF SPECIMEN
Blood

TEST EXPLANATION AND RELATED PHYSIOLOGY
Methemoglobin (metHb) refers to hemoglobin (Hb) in which the iron has been oxidized from the ferrous (+2) to the ferric (+3) state and is therefore unable to bind oxygen. It follows, therefore, that *methemoglobinemia* is the condition that occurs when a significant portion of the Hb is oxidized to metHb and unable to bind to oxygen. Blood from animals with ≥10% of Hb as metHb, when exposed to air, has been described as appearing chocolate brown. Individuals with severe methemoglobinemia may be cyanotic.

A small amount (≈3%) of Hb is oxidized to metHb daily, and, in normal animals, metHb is reduced to Hb by metHb reductase enzymes. Methemoglobinemia occurs when an oxidizing agent overwhelms the animal's natural ability to reduce metHb. Cats are generally more sensitive to metHb-producing agents than are dogs. A few cases of inherited diseases, such as NADH-metHb reductase deficiency, have been reported in people, cats, and dogs.

Methemoglobinemia is usually diagnosed based on clinical signs, physical exam findings, and medical history, which may include cyanosis, chocolate-brown blood, a history of exposure to certain toxicants, and response to treatment. Toxin-induced methemoglobinemia frequently presents as an emergency, requiring immediate treatment. Methemoglobinemia caused by metHb reductase deficiency may present a diagnostic challenge.

Blood metHb can be measured at a few veterinary laboratories using spectrophotometric methods. Hospitals may be willing to run this test, but saponins used routinely to produce hemolysis may affect results of veterinary samples. A control sample should be sent. Contact the laboratory before submitting the sample.

INDICATIONS
- A brown appearance to the blood when exposed to air
  - Test a drop of blood on filter paper.
- Cyanosis of undetermined cause
- Known exposure to certain toxicants that produce oxidative injury:
  - Acetaminophen
  - Chlorates
  - Local anesthetics
  - Naphthalene
  - Nitrites
  - Phenazopyradine
  - Phenols
  - Sulfonamides

CONTRAINDICATIONS
None

POTENTIAL COMPLICATIONS
None

CLIENT EDUCATION
- The metHb test can quantitate the amount of Hb that has been oxidized to metHb but cannot determine the cause.
- A thorough medical history is required.
- Testing for individual toxins may be necessary.
- NADH-metHb reductase activity testing may be required.
- Toxic methemoglobinemia frequently presents as an emergency and may require treatment before test results become available.

BODY SYSTEMS ASSESSED
Hemic, lymphatic, and immune

SAMPLE

COLLECTION
5 mL of venous blood

HANDLING
- Collect the sample into sodium or lithium heparin anticoagulant, and place it on ice immediately.
- Results are most accurate if testing is done soon after collection.
- If necessary, ship the sample with ice packs.
- Determination of metHb levels requires a specialized assay that may not be available through some diagnostic laboratories. Contact the laboratory before submitting the sample.
- If possible, submit a sample from a healthy animal of the same species, breed, gender, and age as a control.

STORAGE
Keep the sample refrigerated.

STABILITY
Refrigerated (2°–8°C): up to 8 h

PROTOCOL
None

INTERPRETATION

NORMAL FINDINGS OR RANGE
Dogs and cats: <1% of Hb exists as metHb.

ABNORMAL VALUES
- Blood may appear brown when ≥10% of Hb has been oxidized to metHb.
- Animals with a metHb concentration of 50% will be moribund.

CRITICAL VALUES
- Organ damage may occur at a metHb concentration of 50% because of hypoxia (centrilobular hepatic necrosis) or hemolysis (hemoglobinuric nephritis).
- Death from toxic methemoglobinemia may occur at metHb concentrations of >60%.

INTERFERING FACTORS
Drugs That May Alter Results or Interpretation
Drugs That Interfere with Test Methodology
None

Drugs That Alter Physiology
Drugs that cause metHb production include acetaminophen, phenazopyradine, some anesthetics, and sulfonamides.

Disorders That May Alter Results
Hemolysis may elevate the metHb concentration.

Collection Techniques or Handling That May Alter Results
- Blood must be cooled immediately and analyzed within 8 h.
- Lysis of red cells with saponins may increase metHb values.

Influence of Signalment
Species
None

Breed
A metHb reductase deficiency has been recognized in chihuahuas, borzois, English setters, terrier mixes, cockapoos, poodles, corgis, pomeranians, toy American Eskimos, cocker–toy American Eskimos, pit bull mixes, and domestic shorthair cats.

Age
None

Gender
None

Pregnancy
None

LIMITATIONS OF THE TEST
Sensitivity, Specificity, and Positive and Negative Predictive Values
N/A

Valid If Run in a Human Lab?
Yes, but use of saponins to hemolyze samples at the laboratory should be avoided.

Causes of Abnormal Findings

High values	Low values
Drugs	Not significant
Acetaminophen	
Phenazopyradine	
Local anesthetics	
Chlorates	
Sulfonamides	
Toxins	
Nitrites	
Naphthalene	
Phenols	
A metHb reductase	
deficiency	

CLINICAL PERSPECTIVE
- Clinical methemoglobinemia may present as an emergency.
- Animals with metHb reductase deficiency may have high blood metHb concentrations but minimal or no clinical signs.
- Chemicals that produce methemoglobinemia (except nitrites) also produce hemolytic anemia.
- RBC oxidation may also produce Heinz bodies and/or eccentrocytes.
- Not all veterinary laboratories run the metHb test. One may need to submit samples to a lab that handles samples from human patients.

MISCELLANEOUS
ANCILLARY TESTS
- Microscopic evaluation of blood smeared after staining with a vital dye such as new methylene blue or brilliant cresyl blue for Heinz body detection
- Toxin analysis for metHb-producing agents
- Analysis of metHb reductase enzyme activity

SYNONYMS
None

SEE ALSO
Blackwell's Five-Minute Veterinary Consult: Canine and Feline Topics
- Acetaminophen Toxicity
- Anemia, Heinz Body
- Methemoglobinemia

Related Topics in This Book
- Complete Blood Count
- Heinz Bodies
- Red Blood Cell Count
- Red Blood Cell Morphology

ABBREVIATIONS
- Hb = hemoglobin
- metHb = methemoglobin

Suggested Reading
Harvey JW. The erythrocyte. In: Kaneko JJ, Harvey JW, Bruss ML, eds. *Clinical Biochemistry of Domestic Animals*, 5th ed. San Diego: Academic, 1997: 184–192.
Harvey JW. Hereditary methemoglobinemia. In: Feldman BF, Zinkl JG, Jain NC, eds. *Schalm's Veterinary Hematology*, 5th ed. Philadelphia: Lippincott Williams & Wilkins, 2000: 1008–1011.
Plumlee K. Hematic system. In: Plumlee KH, ed. *Clinical Veterinary Toxicology*, 1st ed. St Louis: CV Mosby, 2003: 204–209.

INTERNET RESOURCES
Beasley V. Methemoglobin producers. In: Beasley V, ed. Veterinary Toxicology. Ithaca, NY: International Veterinary Information Service (IVIS), 1999, http://www.ivis.org/advances/Beasley/Cpt18b/ivis.pdf.

AUTHOR NAME
Karyn Bischoff

MUSCLE AND NERVE BIOPSY

 BASICS

TYPE OF PROCEDURE
Biopsy

PROCEDURE EXPLANATION AND RELATED PHYSIOLOGY
Muscle and nerve biopsies involve sampling small, but representative, portions of these tissues to submit for histopathologic evaluation. The aim is to establish a definitive diagnosis in neuropathic and myopathic conditions.

INDICATIONS
• Evaluation of muscle atrophy or hypertrophy (muscle and nerve biopsy)
• Evaluation of animals with increased creatine kinase (muscle biopsy)
• Evaluation of animals with lower motor neuron paresis; i.e., weakness characterized by decreased to absent muscle tone and spinal reflexes (muscle and nerve biopsy)
• Evaluation of exercise intolerance or weakness of unknown etiology (muscle biopsy)
• Evaluation of animals with abnormalities on electromyography (muscle biopsy) or nerve conduction studies (nerve biopsy)

CONTRAINDICATIONS
None unless anesthesia is contraindicated

POTENTIAL COMPLICATIONS
• Routine complications of anesthesia or sedation are possible.
• There is an increased risk of aspiration pneumonia during anesthesia if the patient being evaluated has megaesophagus or regurgitation.

Muscle Biopsy
• This is a minor surgical procedure, so complications should be rare.
• Infection if aseptic technique is not used
• Hemorrhage, although it would be extremely unusual to cause significant hemorrhage

Nerve Biopsy
• Infection if aseptic technique is not used
• Hemorrhage
• Motor deficits (which are minimized by the size of the biopsy taken; see Technique section for details)
• Postoperative pain or parasthesias

CLIENT EDUCATION
• Food should be withheld from 10 p.m. the night before the procedure in preparation for anesthesia.
• Clients need to understand that nerve biopsies necessarily sample a very small portion of the peripheral nerve and may not yield a diagnosis.
• Clients should be informed of the possibility of their animals having transient motor deficits and pain following a nerve biopsy.

BODY SYSTEMS ASSESSED
Neuromuscular

 PROCEDURE

PATIENT PREPARATION
Preprocedure Medication or Preparation
The area to be biopsied needs to be clipped and prepared with a routine surgical scrub after the patient has been anesthetized.

Anesthesia or Sedation
These procedures require general anesthesia.

Patient Positioning
The patient is placed in lateral recumbency.

Patient Monitoring
Routine anesthesia monitoring is necessary (heart rate, respiratory rate, blood pressure, pulse oximeter).

Equipment or Supplies
• A surgical drape
• 4 × 4-inch surgical sponges
• A scalpel handle and blades (no. 10 for skin incision; no. 15 for dissection)
• Rat-toothed forceps
• Metzenbaum and suture scissors
• Hemostatic forceps
• Needle holders
• Suture material for closing (absorbable for the muscle and subcutaneous tissues and nonabsorbable for the skin)
• Additional equipment needed for the nerve biopsy:
    • Allis tissue forceps
    • Small rat-toothed forceps
    • 5–0 nylon suture material

TECHNIQUE
Muscle Biopsy
• It is important to select a muscle that is not end stage because the pathology may not be informative of the active disease process. The correct muscle might be selected following electromyographic evaluation or by choosing a muscle that is not severely atrophied. Because muscle pathology can be multifocal, always biopsy more than 1 muscle. If the disease is generalized, sample a muscle from the thoracic and pelvic limbs and consider obtaining a proximal appendicular muscle and a distal appendicular muscle.
• An incision ≈2 cm long is made in the skin overlying the muscle to be biopsied.
• The subcutaneous tissues are dissected to reveal the underlying muscle.
• The fascia overlying the muscle is incised in the direction of the muscle fibers. Using the scalpel blade, 2 cuts, approximately 1 cm long, 5 mm apart, and 5 mm deep, are made in the muscle parallel to the long axis of the myofibers. The cuts are joined at 1 end with a transverse incision made at 90° to the long axis of the myofibers. The cut myofibers are grasped just below the transverse incision with the forceps and peeled down along the long axis cuts by using Metzenbaum scissors, if needed, and then the muscle biopsy is cut at its distal end with scissors. Care is taken to avoid handling the center of the biopsy sample.
• The incision is closed routinely.

Nerve Biopsy
• This is a more specialized surgery. Typically, mixed nerves (motor and sensory) are biopsied, and the histopathologic appearance of the common peroneal nerve has been well described. The nerve selection is usually based on the results of nerve conduction studies.
• A skin incision is made over the nerve to be biopsied and the soft tissues dissected to reveal the nerve. Once the nerve has been identified, ≈2 cm of the nerve is exposed. Using the 5–0 suture material, a suture is placed proximally on the exposed nerve at a distance of approximately one-quarter to one-third of the width of the nerve. The suture is tied, leaving the ends long, and this is used to hold the nerve fibers to be biopsied. A careful incision is made ≈1 mm proximal to the suture and then, using the suture, the nerve fibers are pulled away from the main nerve until there is a piece ≈1.5 cm long. This is cut away from the main nerve, and the incision closed routinely.

SAMPLE HANDLING
Muscle
Ideally, muscle histopathology is examined by using frozen tissue so that enzyme activities can be evaluated. The muscle sample is placed in a gauze sponge that has been moistened in saline and then is shipped overnight on ice packs to a laboratory that evaluates muscle

histopathology. If this is not possible, the muscle sample is pinned at its normal resting length onto a tongue depressor by using 25-gauge needles, placed in 10% formalin, and then submitted for histopathologic evaluation.

Nerve
Nerves can be evaluated histopathologically from frozen, formalin-fixed sections and glutaraldehyde-fixed tissue (the latter for electron microscopy and teased nerve preparations). Histopathologic evaluation of nerve is specialized, so ideally the samples are sent to a suitable laboratory while following the sample-handling and shipping instructions provided by that laboratory. Typically, nerve is placed on a tongue depressor and pinned in place at its normal length with 25-gauge needles and then placed in 10% formalin.

APPROPRIATE AFTERCARE
Postprocedure Patient Monitoring
• The patient's vital parameters should be monitored while it recovers from anesthesia.
• The surgical incisions should be monitored daily for swelling, pain, and discharge (serosanguinous or purulent).

Nursing Care
• If the patient interferes with the surgical incisions, an Elizabethan collar should be placed. A patient is more likely to lick or chew the nerve biopsy site because this procedure may cause parasthesias or pain during recovery.
• To limit swelling, the incisions can be cold packed for 5 min twice daily for 3 days after surgery. This is probably unnecessary for muscle biopsies but is indicated for the nerve biopsies.

Dietary Modification
None

Medication Requirements
• For analgesia, a nonsteroidal anti-inflammatory agent can be administered for 7 days after the biopsy.
• Nerve biopsies may also require an opiate, such as a fentanyl patch, for adequate analgesia.

Restrictions on Activity
Vigorous exercise should be avoided for 2 weeks after surgery.

Anticipated Recovery Time
• Recovery from a muscle biopsy should be complete by the time of suture removal (10–14 days after the procedure).
• Full recovery from a nerve biopsy may take longer but should be complete by 4 weeks after surgery.

INTERPRETATION

NORMAL FINDINGS OR RANGE
There should be no histopathologic abnormalities identified in a normal animal.

ABNORMAL VALUES
• *Muscle*: Histopathologic abnormalities may be classified as infectious or inflammatory myositis, degenerative myopathy, metabolic myopathy, or necrotizing myopathy.
• *Nerve*: Histopathologic abnormalities may be classified as demyelination, axonal loss, infectious or inflammatory process, or degenerative process.

CRITICAL VALUES
None

INTERFERING FACTORS
Drugs That May Alter Results of the Procedure
None

Conditions That May Interfere with Performing the Procedure
Any condition that prevents anesthesia will prevent a muscle or nerve biopsy from being performed.

Procedure Techniques or Handling That May Alter Results
• Handling the center of the muscle or nerve sample is likely to produce artifacts.
• Both nerve and muscle biopsy samples should not be overstretched because this could produce artifacts.
• Incorrect freezing will produce ice-crystal artifact in muscle.

Influence of Signalment on Performing and Interpreting the Procedure
Species
The normal histologic findings vary slightly between species, so it is important that the pathologist is conversant with species differences.

Breed
None

Age
• None for muscle
• In nerves, axonal degeneration and segmental demyelination and remyelination may be incidental findings in patients over 7 years of age.
• The density of axons decreases from birth to ≈1 year of age and then remains stable.

Gender
None

Pregnancy
None

CLINICAL PERSPECTIVE
• A muscle biopsy is straightforward to perform, but the maximum information is obtained by sending the sample to a specialized laboratory.
• A nerve biopsy is a more delicate procedure that is usually performed once electrodiagnostic testing has confirmed the presence of a neuropathy.
• Muscle and nerve biopsies offer the opportunity to establish a definitive diagnosis. However, in many instances, the disorder can be classified through the results of biopsy (e.g., as a metabolic or degenerative process), but further testing is indicated to reach a definitive diagnosis.

MISCELLANEOUS
ANCILLARY TESTS
• Full histopathologic characterization of muscle biopsy samples includes fiber typing by use of adenosine triphosphatase (ATPase) and a variety of histochemical stains to evaluate the oxidative status, glycogen and lipid storage, and structural components. This can be performed only on frozen muscle at an appropriate specialized laboratory.
• If the results of muscle and nerve biopsies indicate infectious or inflammatory disease, serologic testing for infectious diseases (e.g., *Toxoplasma gondii* and *Neospora caninum*) will be needed.
• If the results of muscle biopsy indicate a metabolic or endocrine disorder, additional testing may include evaluation of preexercise and postexercise blood lactate and pyruvate concentrations, evaluation of urine and plasma organic acid concentrations, a thyroid panel, and an ACTH stimulation test.
• If the results of the nerve biopsy indicate a degenerative process, tests evaluating cholinesterase activity (reflects organophosphate toxicity) or blood lead concentrations may be indicated.

MUSCLE AND NERVE BIOPSY

SYNONYMS
None

SEE ALSO
Blackwell's Five-Minute Veterinary Consult: Canine and Feline Topics
- Myopathy
- Paralysis

Related Topics in This Book
- Creatine Kinase
- Electromyography
- Electroneurography

ABBREVIATIONS
None

Suggested Reading
Braund KG. Nerve and muscle biopsy evaluation. In: *Clinical Syndromes in Veterinary Neurology.* St Louis: CV Mosby, 1993: 376–421.
Long S, Anderson TJ. Tissue biopsy. In: *The BSAVA Manual of Canine and Feline Neurology.* Quesgeley, UK: BSAVA, 2004: 84–96.

INTERNET RESOURCES
University of California–San Diego, Department of Pathology, School of Medicine, Comparative Neuromuscular Laboratory: Companion animal diagnostics, http://medicine.ucsd.edu/vet_neuromuscular/.

AUTHOR NAME
Natasha Olby

BASICS

TYPE OF PROCEDURE
Radiographic

PROCEDURE EXPLANATION AND RELATED PHYSIOLOGY
Myelography is a contrast radiographic procedure used to visualize the contours of the spinal cord. Iodinated contrast material is injected into the subarachnoid space to mix with CSF and delineate the surface of the spinal cord. Radiographs (lateral, VD, and oblique views) are then made of the vertebral column to identify lesions that distort the cord's size or shape. Less commonly, myelography may be used to diagnose lesions of the subarachnoid space. Myelography does not directly image the spinal cord parenchyma itself.

INDICATIONS
To assess spinal cord disease

CONTRAINDICATIONS
• Conditions that preclude general anesthesia
• Known allergy to iodinated contrast agents
• Conditions that preclude subarachnoid puncture (increased intracranial pressure or coagulopathy)
• Known encephalitis or meningitis (contrast agents can exacerbate these conditions)
• Cisternal myelography only: Conditions in which flexion of the cervical spine is contraindicated (atlantoaxial subluxation or cervical vertebral fracture or luxation).

POTENTIAL COMPLICATIONS
• Seizures (within the first 12–24 h after the procedure)
• Exacerbation of neurologic signs, which is more commonly seen in patients with chronic spinal cord disease; usually mild and transient, lasting a week or less, but occasionally permanent
• Death is rare but may result from an anesthetic accident, anaphylactic reaction to contrast agent, or penetration of the brain stem or cervical spinal cord by a malpositioned spinal needle.

CLIENT EDUCATION
• Patients should undergo an overnight fast for general anesthesia.
• Animals may need to remain under veterinary care for 24 h or longer should seizures occur.
• Informed consent that addresses the risks of procedure

BODY SYSTEMS ASSESSED
• Musculoskeletal
• Nervous

PROCEDURE

PATIENT PREPARATION
Preprocedure Medication or Preparation
Patients should undergo an overnight fast for general anesthesia, except in emergency situations.

Anesthesia or Sedation
General anesthesia

Patient Positioning
Lateral recumbency. Some prefer patients in sternal recumbency.

Patient Monitoring
• Standard anesthetic monitoring
• Be prepared to ventilate patients if apnea occurs during and after contrast injection.
• Maintain an adequate depth of anesthesia prior to and during contrast injection.

Equipment or Supplies
• A 20- to 22-gauge spinal needle, $1^1/_2$ inches (3.81 cm) (cisternal injection) or $3^1/_2$ inches (8.89 cm) (lumbar injection) long
• Iohexol (240 or 300 mg/mL) or iopamidol (200, 250, or 300 mg/mL) contrast agent, drawn into a syringe and warmed to body temperature, if possible. Dose at either 0.45 mL/kg (entire spine) or 0.3 mL/kg for myelography (single region, either cervical or thoracolumbar). If using a T-piece or extension tube, add an additional volume of contrast to account for dead space in these connectors.
• A T-piece (cisternal injection) or extension tube (lumbar injection) is optional and can be used so that movement of the syringe during contrast injection is not translated to the needle tip. If either is used, connect it to the syringe and fill it with contrast material.
• Empty tube to collect CSF.
• Supplies to prepare the injection site aseptically
• Sterile gloves
• Radiographic equipment, preferably with fluoroscopy
• Sandbags and sponges for patient positioning

TECHNIQUE
Cisternal Injection Myelography
• Make survey radiographs of the spine.
• Place the patient in lateral recumbency. Clip the hair and prepare the skin as for a cisternal CSF tap.
• Have an assistant hold the patient's head in a flexed position at right angles to the body, with nose parallel to the median plane of the body.
• Don sterile gloves and palpate landmarks: the cranial aspect of the wings of C1 and external occipital protuberance.
• Insert the needle through the skin perpendicular to animal's body on the midline at the level of the cranial aspect of the wings of the atlas.
• Advance the needle with the stylet in place and bevel directly caudally until the subarachnoid space is encountered. A pop may be felt as the tip of the spinal needle penetrates the atlanto-occipital membrane and dura mater; however, this is not a consistent indicator of correct needle placement. The only reliable indicator is the presence of CSF in the needle.
• Collect free-flowing CSF into the empty tube for immediate analysis.
• Connect a T-piece or syringe tip to the hub of the spinal needle.
• Inject contrast slowly (over $\approx$1–2 min).
• Remove the spinal needle.
• Repeat the spinal series (lateral and VD projections) with contrast in the subarachnoid space. Make oblique views as necessary to distinguish a left-sided from a right-sided lesion.

Lumbar Injection Myelography
• Make survey radiographs of the spine.
• Place the patient in lateral recumbency. Clip the hair and prepare the skin as for a lumbar CSF tap.
• Prop the patient's abdomen with sponges as necessary to ensure that the lumbar spine is positioned in perfect lateral recumbency.
• Flex the lumbar spine by bringing the animal's hind limbs cranially until they touch the abdomen. Some operators prefer the spine only slightly flexed or in a neutral position.
• Make the injection as far caudally as possible, depending on the location of the caudal extent of the dural sac (in dogs, usually L5–6; in cats and some small dogs, L6–7). Individual variation in anatomy or lesion location may necessitate a myelographic injection 1 intervertebral space cranial or caudal to the planned site of injection.
• Don sterile gloves and palpate landmark: the L6 dorsal spinous process (located on midline just cranial to the cranial aspect of the wings of the ileum; it usually is the most caudal dorsal spinous process that may be readily palpated).
• Insert the needle through the skin with the needle's bevel directed cranially at an angle dependant on the degree of flexion of the animal's lumbar spine. Neutral position: Insert the needle at a 45° angle to the skin. Extremely flexed: Insert the needle at a 60°–80° angle to the skin.

MYELOGRAPHY

• Advance the needle cranially with the stylet in place until the interarcuate ligament is encountered and then further advance the needle to the floor of the vertebral canal. Usually, a twitch of the tail or hind limb indicates correct needle placement.

• Collect free-flowing CSF into the tube for immediate analysis. In some patients, CSF is not obtained despite correct needle placement.

• Make a test injection of 0.2–0.4 mL of contrast by using fluoroscopy or a lateral radiograph to ensure the injection is into the subarachnoid space.

• Inject the remainder of the contrast over 2–5 min, ideally by using fluoroscopy during the injection in order to ensure injection is neither epidural or intraparenchymal.

• Make lateral radiographs with the needle in place, taking care not to move the needle during patient positioning. The needle is left in place in case additional contrast is needed.

• Remove the spinal needle.

• Make VD projection radiographs to complete the study (and oblique views when necessary to distinguish left-sided from right-sided lesions).

SAMPLE HANDLING
None

APPROPRIATE AFTERCARE
Postprocedure Patient Monitoring
Monitor for seizures at least 12 h after the procedure.

Nursing Care
To minimize the risk of seizures, elevate the patient's head 10°–15° during its recovery from anesthesia.

Dietary Modification
None

Medication Requirements
None

Restrictions on Activity
None

Anticipated Recovery Time
Within 12–24 h, or up to 1 week in cases of neurologic deterioration. Some animals may not recover if neurologic deterioration occurs.

INTERPRETATION

NORMAL FINDINGS OR RANGE
Uniform filling of the subarachnoid space without attenuation of contrast columns on any view

ABNORMAL VALUES
• *Extradural lesion*: Attenuation and deviation of 1 contrast column toward the spinal cord, with attenuation of the opposite contrast column. Examples: herniated disk material, tumor (e.g., vertebral tumor, meningioma), abscess, and abnormal bony or ligamentous structures.

• *Intradural lesion*: A filling defect within the affected contrast column, with variable attenuation of the opposite contrast column. Examples: tumor (e.g., meningioma, peripheral nerve sheath tumor). Occasionally, dilation of subarachnoid space. Examples: subarachnoid cyst and meningocele.

• *Intramedullary lesion*: Attenuation of both contrast columns, with deviation of both away from the spinal cord. Examples: tumor (e.g., glioma, metastatic tumor), edema, and myelitis.

CRITICAL VALUES
None

INTERFERING FACTORS
Drugs That May Alter Results of the Procedure
None

Conditions That May Interfere with Performing the Procedure
• Adhesions within the subarachnoid space secondary to previous spinal surgery or meningitis

• Severe articular facet degenerative joint disease may preclude needle placement (lumbar injection).

Procedure Techniques or Handling That May Alter Results
Myelography may be nondiagnostic if epidural or subdural contrast injection is made.

Influence of Signalment on Performing and Interpreting the Procedure
Species

• The spinal cord is longer (relative to the vertebral column length) in cats than dogs. Lumbar injection in cats therefore is usually made at L6–7.

• The spinal cord diameter (relative to the size of the vertebral canal) is greater in cats than dogs, which can make the spinal cord appear falsely enlarged in cats.

Breed

• Spinal cord (relative to vertebral column length) is longer in small dogs than in large dogs; lumbar injection in small dogs therefore is sometimes attempted at L6–7.

• Spinal cord diameter (relative to size of vertebral canal) is greater in small dogs than in large dogs, which can make the spinal cord appear falsely enlarged in small dogs or falsely atrophied in large dogs.

Age
None

Gender
None

Pregnancy
The use of myelography and other radiographic procedures are generally avoided in pregnant patients because of the risk to the fetus.

CLINICAL PERSPECTIVE
• When marked spinal cord edema is present (as is commonly seen with acute disk herniation), it may not be possible to achieve a diagnostic myelogram via cisternal injection, because contrast may travel retrogradely into the cranial vault rather than caudally past the point of spinal cord edema. Many diagnosticians therefore preferentially perform lumbar myelography in cases in which acute disk herniation is suspected. Alternatively, a nondiagnostic cisternal injection myelogram may be followed by a CT scan. CT is more sensitive than conventional radiography at detecting contrast. Postmyelography CT is frequently diagnostic in this scenario.

• There is greater likelihood of a central canal or epidural injection with lumbar myelography. This can worsen neurologic symptoms, result in a nondiagnostic study, or both.

• A diagnosis cannot always be made without transverse imaging. An example is the "pencil point" type II disk protrusion, in which there is a narrow midline disk herniation with spinal cord appearing to be draped over the offending disk. Since there is subarachnoid space to both the left and the right of the disk, lateral and VD projection radiographs may appear normal. Postmyelography CT scan (or, alternatively, foregoing myelography in favor of MRI) may be necessary to make a diagnosis in such a case.

• Because of the increased risk of neurologic deterioration in cases with chronic spinal cord disease, many diagnosticians favor MRI for these patients.

• Because MRI can visualize the spinal cord parenchyma directly, it is a better choice than myelography when such diseases are suspected. Examples: metastatic neoplasia, fibrocartilaginous embolism, and syringomyelia.

• Many cases of acute type I disk disease can be diagnosed noninvasively via either CT or MRI.

- When imaging the spinal cord, it is best to consider the pros and cons of myelography, CT, postmyelography CT, and MRI before recommending a specific procedure.

MISCELLANEOUS

ANCILLARY TESTS
- CSF analysis is recommended prior to myelography because of the possibility of meningitis or myelitis.
- Electrodiagnostic studies may be useful when lower motor neuron disease is present.

SYNONYMS
Myelogram

SEE ALSO
Blackwell's Five-Minute Veterinary Consult: Canine and Feline Topics
- Ataxia
- Atlantoaxial Instability
- Degenerative Myelopathy
- Fibrocartilaginous Embolic Myelopathy
- Incontinence, Fecal
- Incontinence, Urinary
- Intervertebral Disc Disease, Cervical
- Intervertebral Disc Disease, Thoracolumbar
- Lumbosacral Stenosis and Cauda Equina Syndrome
- Myelomalacia and Hematomyelia
- Neck and Back Pain
- Paralysis
- Schiff-Sherrington Phenomenon

- Spondylosis Deformans
- Wobbler Syndrome (Cervical Spondylmyelopathy)

Related Topics in This Book
- General Principles of Radiography
- Cerebrospinal Fluid Tap
- Computed Tomography
- Electromyography
- Fluoroscopy
- Magnetic Resonance Imaging

ABBREVIATIONS
- CSF = cerebrospinal fluid
- CT = computed tomography
- MRI = magnetic resonance imaging
- VD = ventrodorsal

Suggested Reading
Dennis R, Kirkberger RM, Wrigley RH, Barr FJ. Spine. In: *Handbook of Small Animal Radiological Differential Diagnosis*. London: WB Saunders, 2001: 83–102.
Sharp NJH, Wheeler SJ. Diagnostic aids. In: *Small Animal Spinal Disorders Diagnosis and Surgery*, 2nd ed. Edinburgh: Elsevier Mosby, 2005: 41–72.
Widmer WR. Intervertebral disc disease and myelography. In: Thrall DE, ed. *Textbook of Veterinary Diagnostic Radiology*, 3rd ed. Philadelphia: WB Saunders, 1998: 89–104.

INTERNET RESOURCES
VEM 5181: Musculoskeletal Radiology: Radiology of skeletal diseases, http://sacs.vetmed.ufl.edu/Radio/Dr.Taka/main.htm. Note: Click through menu on left of the screen for cases.

AUTHOR NAME
Stacey A. Sullivan

BASICS

TYPE OF PROCEDURE
- Biopsy
- Diagnostic sample collection

PROCEDURE EXPLANATION AND RELATED PHYSIOLOGY

Disease within the nasal cavity and sinuses can be unilateral or bilateral and frequently results in nasal discharge, sneezing, and stertorous breathing. A serous, mucoid, purulent, or hemorrhagic discharge can be seen, and a mixed pattern is often present. The type of discharge can be suggestive of a general disease process, but a specific diagnosis can usually not be made without a cytologic or histopathologic evaluation.

A number of procedures can be performed to obtain a sample when localized nasal disease is present. Cytologic evaluation of a superficial or deep nasal swab can definitively diagnose some fungal diseases (especially *Cryptococcus*). An oropharyngeal examination (with general anesthesia) can reveal significant dental disease, polyps, or foreign bodies. A nasal flush can be performed both to obtain cytologic samples and as temporary therapy to relieve nasal obstruction seen with significant nasal discharge. This procedure is easy to perform and requires no specialized equipment. Biopsy samples are often needed to obtain deeper (and likely more diagnostic) samples. A traumatic nasal flush can be performed to obtain small pieces of nasal tissue for histopathologic evaluation. This procedure is of the most use when diffuse disease is suspected, because the samples are obtained blindly. Again, the equipment necessary to perform this procedure is likely present in most clinics. An otoscope can be used to look for a mass in the nasal cavities. Although only a small area can be visualized by using this method, if a mass effect is seen a core biopsy of that mass can be taken with a stiff catheter or alligator forceps. Multiple blind pinch biopsy samples can also be taken with cup biopsy forceps. All of these procedures can be performed safely in any clinic with minimal specialized equipment.

In all cases of suspected nasal disease, a complete physical examination (including a fundic exam), medical history, CBC, chemistry profile, urinalysis, blood pressure, and thoracic radiographs should be evaluated before proceeding to the more invasive techniques of a nasal flush and biopsy. The information obtained from this initial evaluation may reveal a systemic disease process that could be responsible for the clinical signs or can uncover other clinically significant abnormalities that may need to be addressed before performing a procedure that requires general anesthesia. A coagulation profile should also be evaluated if a nasal biopsy is to be performed. Because epistaxis can be caused by hypertension or platelet abnormalities (i.e., thrombocytopenia or diminished platelet function), it is especially important to evaluate blood pressure, platelet number, and platelet function in these patients. Determination of buccal mucosal bleeding time (BMBT) is an excellent way to evaluate platelet function quickly. Epistaxis can also be caused by vasculitis, hyperviscosity syndromes, and vascular anomalies. Ehrlichial and rickettsial infections can also cause epistaxis, and testing to rule out these diseases should be done prior to performing a complete nasal workup.

INDICATIONS
- Persistent nasal discharge
- Nasal or sinus mass effect
- Nasal or palate deformity
- Persistent sneezing or stertor
- Exophthalmia

CONTRAINDICATIONS
- Thrombocytopenia (platelet count, <50,000/μL)
- Coagulopathy

- Significant hypertension

POTENTIAL COMPLICATIONS
- Hemorrhage
- Aspiration of fluid into the lower airways
- Penetration of the cribriform plate

CLIENT EDUCATION
- Patients should not be fed 12 h prior to the procedure.
- Hemorrhage will always occur and in rare cases can be severe (a transfusion may be required in these cases).
- Even with appropriate diagnostic evaluation, a definitive diagnosis may not be reached.

BODY SYSTEMS ASSESSED
Respiratory

PROCEDURE

PATIENT PREPARATION
Preprocedure Medication or Preparation
None

Anesthesia or Sedation
General anesthesia with tracheal intubation is required. It is important that the endotracheal tube is of the appropriate size and the cuff is adequately inflated.

Patient Positioning
The patient should be in sternal recumbency with the nose pointing slightly downward to facilitate sample collection.

Patient Monitoring
A deep plane of anesthesia is generally required. Continuous patient monitoring is necessary to ensure that the patient remains adequately anesthetized throughout the procedure.

Equipment or Supplies
- 4 × 4-inch gauze squares
- A spay hook
- A dental mirror
- A small Christmas tree adapter (not needed in all cases)
- Cotton-tipped swabs (sterile and nonsterile)
- A 5, 8, or 10 French red rubber catheter (depending on the patient's size)
- A 12- or 20-mL syringe
- Sterile saline
- A polypropylene urinary catheter
- Alligator or Jackson cup biopsy forceps (Figure 1)

TECHNIQUE
- An extensive oropharyngeal examination should be conducted once the patient is anesthetized and prior to sample collection. The hard and soft palates need to be assessed for symmetry, mass effects, or erosive lesions. A dental examination should be performed, including assessment for deep gingival pockets or oronasal fistulas via a dental probe. In cats, a tonsillar swab for viral isolation of both herpesvirus and calicivirus should be considered. A spay hook can be inserted into the mouth, and the curved end used to pull back the soft palate. A dental mirror may then be passed next to the spay hook and be positioned above the soft palate to assess the caudal nasopharynx.
- Fine-needle aspiration should be performed on any masses.
- Prior to sample collection, the caudal pharynx should be packed with 2- × 4-inch gauze squares. A note should be made of how many gauze squares were used.
- To avoid possible penetration of the cribriform plate, sample-collecting devices should never be inserted past the medial canthus of the eye. The distance to the medial canthus should be measured and

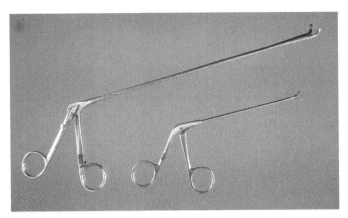

Figure 1

Biopsy cup forceps for nasal biopsy.

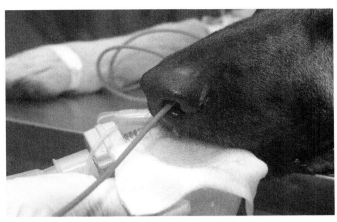

Figure 3

To collect particulate matter, 4 × 4-inch gauze squares are used.

this position marked (with tape or an indelible marker) on the catheter or biopsy instrument.

• Superficial nasal swabs and sterile swabs for culture can be collected by inserting a cotton-tipped swab into the nares and gently rolling it along the nasal mucosa at varying depths to obtain samples for cytologic analysis. This procedure should be performed as carefully as possible to avoid trauma to the nasal cavities and contamination of subsequent samples with blood.

Nasal Flush Technique

• Depending on the size of the patient, a 5, 8, or 10 French catheter is passed from the nares into the caudal nasal cavity. Remember to mark the distance to the medial canthus.

• A 12- or 20-mL syringe filled with sterile saline is attached to the catheter (a Christmas tree adapter may be used to facilitate attachment to some catheters). The saline is then flushed into the nasal cavity (Figure 2).

• The fluid from the nasal cavity is then aspirated back into the syringe, and any fluid draining from the nose is collected in a cup or bowl. A piece of gauze can be placed over the top of collecting cup to catch any particulate matter (Figure 3).

• To obtain adequate samples, each side of the nose should be flushed 3–4 times.

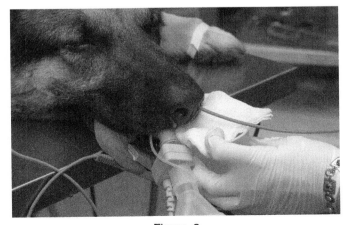

Figure 2

Use of an 8 French red rubber catheter for nasal flush. The catheter is attached to a 35-mL syringe containing 0.9% sodium chloride.

• This procedure may also be performed by passing either the red rubber or a Foley catheter into the mouth and retroflexing the catheter behind and above the palate, through the internal nares, and into the caudal nasal cavity. Sterile saline is again flushed through the catheter, and samples are collected as just described.

Traumatic Nasal Flush

• A 5 or 8 French polypropylene urinary catheter is prepared by cutting the end at a 45° angle, and small "wings" are cut into the sides of the catheter with a scalpel blade.

• A 12-mL syringe filled with sterile saline is attached to the catheter, which is then blindly raked against the nasal mucosa while saline is alternately flushed and aspirated through the catheter.

• Samples are collected into the syringe, and the fluid is allowed to drain into a cup covered with gauze to collect particulate matter.

• Both the particles and fluid can be submitted for analysis.

Biopsy Techniques

• It is important to stress again that care must be taken not to pass any biopsy device past the medial canthus of the eye.

• If a mass is identified with imaging or rhinoscopy, a polypropylene catheter can be used to obtain a direct core biopsy sample. The narrow end of the catheter is cut at a 45° angle, and a 20-mL syringe is attached to the opposite end. The catheter is then advanced to the site of the lesion and moved back and forth into the mass while suction is applied to the syringe. Gentle suction is maintained while the catheter is removed to keep any tissue samples within the catheter itself. Tissue collected can be expelled from the catheter with air or saline and placed in formalin. Collect 3–4 samples.

• If diffuse disease is suspected or a specific mass has not been identified, a cup biopsy instrument can be used to obtain pinch biopsy samples. With the instrument's jaws closed, the forceps are inserted into the nasal cavity. The jaws are then opened, and the forceps are pushed forward into the nasal tissue and closed, and the tissue sample is removed by firmly and quickly pulling the forceps out of the nose. This procedure should be repeated 4–6 times for each side. Excellent quality tissue samples can be obtained with this method.

• After the procedures are finished, the patient's nose should be directed at a more downward angle, and pressure can be applied to the rostral nares to help alleviate excess hemorrhage.

• Excessive bleeding can usually be controlled by 1 of the following methods:
  • Ice packs are applied to the top of the nose.
  • Epinephrine (1:100,000) is instilled into the nares.
  • The nares and caudal nasopharynx are packed with epinephrine-soaked umbilical tape or gauze.

NASAL FLUSH AND BIOPSY

- Once bleeding is under control, the gauze squares are removed, and any particulate matter (excluding blood clots) trapped in the gauze can be submitted for analysis.
- The patient is extubated with the cuff partially inflated to remove any remaining debris.

SAMPLE HANDLING
- Nonsterile nasal swabs should be smeared onto slides and submitted for cytologic evaluation.
- If collected, sterile swabs should be submitted for culture. Aerobic bacterial cultures are usually sufficient.
- Particulate matter can be submitted as touch preparations, smears for cytology, or, if large enough, for histopathologic evaluation.
- Fluid samples can be transferred to EDTA tubes and centrifuged for submission for cytology. Fluid analysis is not necessary.
- Tissue samples should be placed into a biopsy cassette (if small), fixed in formalin, and submitted for histologic evaluation. Prior to placing the samples in formalin, roll preparations may also be made for cytologic analysis.
- Fungal cultures are generally not required.

APPROPRIATE AFTERCARE
Postprocedure Patient Monitoring
- Perform standard monitoring after anesthesia.
- Monitor for excessive bleeding and anemia (i.e., PCV, heart rate, respiratory rate).

Nursing Care
- Clean the muzzle (without dislodging clots initially) and paws.
- Clean the kennel area of hemorrhagic discharge.

Dietary Modification
None

Medication Requirements
- Usually none
- Sedation may be required if the patient is agitated or too active.

Restrictions on Activity
As hemorrhage can be significant in the first 24–48 h after the procedure (if a biopsy was performed), strict cage rest is recommended during this period.

Anticipated Recovery Time
- Patients usually recover from these procedures and general anesthesia within 12 h.
- Increased sneezing and nasal discharge can occur for up to 1 week after biopsy.

INTERPRETATION

NORMAL FINDINGS OR RANGE
- Stratified squamous epithelium, pseudostratified columnar epithelium, and possibly goblet cells
- Some RBCs will usually be seen.

ABNORMAL VALUES
There are numerous general categories of nasal disease. Infectious diseases that are commonly seen include fungal, viral, and parasitic etiologies. Bacterial infections are common but are almost always considered to be secondary in nature. Lymphoplasmacytic inflammation is a frequent but frustrating finding because the underlying cause of this reaction is difficult to determine. Pyogranulomatous inflammation can also be seen and is suspicious for fungal infections or chronic foreign bodies. Numerous forms of neoplasia that can invade the nasal cavity include lymphoma, adenocarcinoma, squamous cell carcinoma, osteosarcoma, fibrosarcoma, and chondrosarcomas. Nasal polyps are common in cats. Foreign bodies and trauma should also be considered on a differential list:

Inflammation
- Neutrophilic (with or without bacteria)
- Eosinophilic
- Lymphoplasmacytic
- Pyogranulomatus

Inflammatory Polyps
Lymphocytes and plasma cells predominate, with neutrophils, monocytes, and rafts of epithelial cells.

Fungal Infection
- *Cryptococcus*
- *Aspergillus*
- *Penicillium*
- *Rhinosporidium*

Neoplasia
- Carcinoma
- Sarcoma
- Lymphoma

Miscellaneous
- Mites
- Foreign bodies

CRITICAL VALUES
None

INTERFERING FACTORS
Drugs That May Alter Results of the Procedure
None

Conditions That May Interfere with Performing the Procedure
- Coagulopathy
- Thrombocytopenia
- Any preexisting condition that precludes general anesthesia

Procedure Techniques or Handling That May Alter Results
- The use of sterile water instead of saline can lyse cells.
- A tissue sample is too small.
- Tissue fixation is inadequate.

Influence of Signalment on Performing and Interpreting the Procedure
Species
- Polyps occur mainly in cats.
- *Cryptococcus* is seen primarily in cats and rarely in dogs.
- *Aspergillus* is seen mainly in dogs.

Breed
Neoplasia and fungal disease are seen more frequently in dolichocephalic dog breeds.

Age
Older patients are more likely to develop neoplasia.

Gender
None

Pregnancy
None

CLINICAL PERSPECTIVE
- Cytologic results may reflect only superficial findings and be misleading. However, some forms of neoplasia and fungal disease (especially *Cryptococcus*) can be diagnosed with cytologic analysis alone.
- Bacterial infections are common but are almost always secondary in nature. Culture results can be confusing to interpret but may be useful to determine appropriate antimicrobial therapy to treat the secondary bacterial component of the nasal disease. As an underlying disease is usually present, the administration of antibiotics will not totally resolve the clinical signs long term.
- Fungal disease is generally diagnosed through cytologic analysis or biopsy. Fungal cultures are not generally necessary.

- Lymphoplasmacytic rhinitis is a nonspecific diagnosis and can have a number of underlying etiologies. The association of this finding with infectious disease is still unknown and currently under investigation.
- Samples may be nondiagnostic, and owners should be warned prior to the procedure that a final diagnosis could be difficult to determine.
- Combining the procedure with nasal computed tomography may increase the likelihood of obtaining a representative biopsy sample of a mass lesion.
- Nasal flushing can be used as a therapeutic technique to alleviate some forms of nasal obstruction.

MISCELLANEOUS

ANCILLARY TESTS
- Skull radiography
- Computed tomographic scan
- Rhinoscopy with retroflexion behind the soft palate
- Fungal serologies
- Von Willebrand disease testing

SYNONYMS
None

SEE ALSO
Blackwell's Five-Minute Veterinary Consult: Canine and Feline Topics
- Adenocarcinoma, Nasal
- Chondrosarcoma, Nasal and Paranasal Sinus
- Epistaxis
- Fibrosarcoma, Nasal and Paranasal Sinus
- Nasal and Nasopharyngeal Polyps

- Nasal Discharge
- Respiratory Parasites
- Rhinitis and Sinusitis
- Rhinosporidiosis
- Squamous Cell Carcinoma, Nasal and Paranasal Sinuses
- Stertor and Stridor

Related Topics in This Book
- Computed Tomography
- Rhinoscopy
- Skull Radiography

ABBREVIATIONS
None

Suggested Reading
King LG, ed. *Respiratory Disease in Dogs and Cats*. St Louis: Saunders Elsevier, 2004: 12–38, 67–69, 100–109.
Nelson RW, Couto CG, eds. *Small Animal Internal Medicine*. St Louis: CV Mosby 2003: 210–240.
Ogilvie GK, LaRue SM. Canine and feline nasal and paranasal sinus tumors. *Vet Clin North Am Small Anim* 1992; 22: 1133–1144.
Rebar AH, Hawkins EC, DeNicola DB. Cytologic evaluation of the respiratory tract. *Vet Clin North Am Small Anim* 1992; 22: 1065–1075.
Windsor RC, Johnson LR, Sykes JE, *et al.* Molecular detection of microbes in nasal tissue of dogs with idiopathic lymphoplasmacytic rhinitis. *J Vet Intern Med* 2006; 20: 250–256.

INTERNET RESOURCES
None

AUTHOR NAME
Karyn Harrell

NASOLACRIMAL IRRIGATION

BASICS

TYPE OF PROCEDURE
Function test

PROCEDURE EXPLANATION AND RELATED PHYSIOLOGY
The preocular tear film that bathes the surface of the eye is removed via the nasolacrimal drainage system. Two oval puncta, 1 in both the upper and lower medial eyelids, are located 1–2 mm from the eyelid margin in the palpebral conjunctiva. A ring of pigment may be present around the puncta and facilitate their detection. Each punctum is an opening to its associated canaliculum. After entering the puncta and canaliculi, the tears enter a poorly developed nasolacrimal sac and then flow into the nasolacrimal duct. The length of the nasolacrimal duct varies with species and breeds. It empties into the floor of the nasal cavity or the nasopharynx.

Prior to irrigation, the nasolacrimal drainage system can be clinically evaluated based on the presence or absence of a lacrimal lake (tear pooling in the ventral conjunctival sac) and passage of fluorescein dye instilled onto the eye. Passage of fluorescein from the eye to the external nares is a reasonable test (i.e., Jones test) for patency of the nasolacrimal system. A fluorescein strip is moistened with sterile eyewash and touched to the upper bulbar conjunctiva. Fluorescein may pass through the puncta and nasolacrimal duct and become apparent at the nares within 1–5 min. The test should be performed in both eyes at the same time to compare passage times. Holding the animal's nose down may facilitate the speed of passage. A positive test means the nasolacrimal system is patent and irrigation is not indicated. A negative test in a brachycephalic dog and most cats is not reliable because the nasolacrimal duct more commonly empties into the nasopharynx. Ultraviolet light can be used to enhance detection of the dye at the nares or inside the mouth.

A negative test, which can occur for several reasons, is an indication to perform nasolacrimal irrigation to evaluate patency. If nasolacrimal irrigation fails, further diagnostic testing is indicated and can involve catheterization of the entire nasolacrimal system and dacryocystorhinography. Nasolacrimal irrigation is a relatively easy test that can be performed and frequently results in clearing of the system. Care must be taken when performing this procedure because trauma to the canaliculi or excessive force used when a blockage is present can inflame and even rupture the system.

INDICATIONS
- Epiphora (i.e., overflow of tears) without an obvious etiology
- Resistant or relapsing conjunctival infection
- Mucopurulent ocular discharge
- Failure of passage of fluorescein dye, combined with ocular signs

CONTRAINDICATIONS
The use of excessive force to irrigate the duct is contraindicated.

POTENTIAL COMPLICATIONS
- Nasolacrimal duct rupture
- Iatrogenic trauma and inflammation causing dacryocystitis
- Iatrogenic trauma and inflammation causing nasolacrimal duct stricture
- Trauma to the cornea with the tip of the irrigating cannula if the animal is not properly restrained

CLIENT EDUCATION
None

BODY SYSTEMS ASSESSED
Ophthalmic

PROCEDURE

PATIENT PREPARATION
Preprocedure Medication or Preparation
None

Anesthesia or Sedation
- Topical anesthesia (e.g., proparacaine hydrochloride) is recommended in all cases.
- Sedation might be necessary in dogs.
- Sedation is usually necessary in cats because of the small size of their nasolacrimal puncta.
- Sedation or general anesthesia may be required if an obstruction is present or the animal is struggling. Heavy sedation or general anesthesia may be required, especially if the force required to unblock the obstruction is uncomfortable for the patient.

Patient Positioning
- Lateral recumbency is easiest.
- The procedure can be performed with patients in the sternal position.

Patient Monitoring
Routine for anesthesia and sedation

Equipment or Supplies
- Topical anesthetic (e.g., proparacaine hydrochloride)
- Human lacrimal cannulas (dogs, 22–23 gauge; cats, 24–27 gauge) or the flexible portion of a 22- to 24-gauge IV catheter
- 3- to 6-mm syringes
- A sterile eyewash or artificial tears as the irrigating solution
- Clean glass microscope slides
- Culturettes

TECHNIQUE
- Identify the upper eyelid and lower eyelid lacrimal puncta.
- The upper eyelid punctum is usually more accessible in dogs and cats.
- Apply topical anesthetic.
- One hand should hold open the patient's eye while the lid is rolled and everted so that the punctum can be visualized.
- The other hand should hold the syringe and cannula so that the irrigating solution can be immediately injected while the cannula is entering the upper punctum.
- Rest the hand holding the syringe against the animal's head (or the hand holding the eyelid) and hold the syringe loosely to minimize traumatizing the duct if the head moves.
- Ensure the eyelid is taut and thread the cannula into the punctum and down the canaliculus.
- Keep the cannula parallel to the canaliculus and lid margin because this will ease the passage of the cannula and prevent obstruction by the wall of the canaliculus.
- Obstruction of the tip of the cannula against the wall commonly gives the false impression that a pathologic obstruction is present. If unsure, move the tip slowly back and forth while irrigating.
- Gently inject fluid and observe it emerging from the lower punctum.
- Now occlude the lower punctum with gentle fingertip pressure and continue to irrigate. Fluid should now exit the distal nares.
- If fluid does not exit the nares, continue to apply gentle pressure until you are convinced there is a blockage.
- Stop immediately if the animal exhibits discomfort or begins to struggle.
- Do not use excessive force to irrigate the duct. If you cannot establish a patent duct, consider medical therapy and repeat irrigation or general anesthesia and further diagnostic testing to pursue the problem.

SAMPLE HANDLING
Mucopurulent discharge that is evacuated from the duct with irrigation should be collected for cytologic analysis, as well as bacterial culture and sensitivity testing.

APPROPRIATE AFTERCARE
Postprocedure Patient Monitoring
As required if sedation or anesthesia was used

Nursing Care
As required if sedation or anesthesia was used

Dietary Modification
None

Medication Requirements
None

Restrictions on Activity
None

Anticipated Recovery Time
Immediate

INTERPRETATION

NORMAL FINDINGS OR RANGE
Fluid should pass easily through both puncta and out the external nares or into the nasopharynx.

ABNORMAL VALUES
• An obstruction is likely present if fluid fails to exit both puncta and the nares or nasopharynx.
• Failure of fluid passage could indicate the presence of dacryocystitis, a foreign body within the nasolacrimal system, stenosis of the nasolacrimal duct, congenital alacrima, or a mass effect obstructing the nasolacrimal duct.

CRITICAL VALUES
None

INTERFERING FACTORS
Drugs That May Alter Results of the Procedure
None

Conditions That May Interfere with Performing the Procedure
• Congenital alacrima
• A foreign body or mass obstruction of the nasolacrimal system
• Dacryocystitis
• Stenosis of the nasolacrimal system

Procedure Techniques or Handling That May Alter Results
Keeping the cannula parallel to the canaliculus and lid margin will ease the passage and prevent obstruction by the wall of the canaliculus. This avoids the false impression of a pathologic obstruction.

Influence of Signalment on Performing and Interpreting the Procedure
Species
• Cats are more difficult to cannulate because of their smaller puncta and possibly the animal's temperament.
• The nasolacrimal drainage system in cats is more likely to empty into their nasopharynx, and dye will not be seen exiting the nares.

Breed
• The puncta in brachycephalic breeds can be located extremely medial in the eyelid and make them more difficult to find.
• The nasolacrimal drainage system in brachycephalic breeds is more likely to empty into their nasopharynx, and dye will not be seen exiting the nares.

Age
Very young animals with epiphora are more likely to have a congenital defect such as alacrima.

Gender
None

Pregnancy
None

CLINICAL PERSPECTIVE
• When the nasolacrimal duct empties into the nasopharynx, patients may choke, sneeze, or swallow as an indication of patency, even if fluid does not exit from the nose.
• If an animal's head is held in an upward position, the fluid may run posteriorly into the pharynx and result in swallowing or a gag reflex.

MISCELLANEOUS

ANCILLARY TESTS
• Catheterization of the nasolacrimal system
• Dacryocystorhinography
• Computed tomography
• Magnetic resonance imaging (MRI)

SYNONYMS
Nasolacrimal flush

SEE ALSO
Blackwell's Five-Minute Veterinary Consult: Canine and Feline Topics
• Conjunctivitis—Cats
• Conjunctivitis—Dogs
• Epiphora

Related Topics in This Book
• Computed Tomography
• Fluorescein Dye Test
• Magnetic Resonance Imaging
• Skull Radiography

ABBREVIATIONS
None

Suggested Reading
Brooks DE. Ocular imaging. In: Gelatt KN, ed. *Veterinary Ophthalmology*, 3rd ed. Philadelphia: Lippincott Williams & Wilkins, 1999: 467–482.
Gelatt KN. Ophthalmic examination and diagnostic procedures. In: Gelatt KN, ed. *Veterinary Ophthalmology*, 3rd ed. Philadelphia: Lippincott Williams & Wilkins, 1999: 427–466.
Martin CL. Anamnesis and the ophthalmic examination. In: Martin CL, ed. *Ophthalmic Disease in Veterinary Medicine*. London: Manson, 2005: 11–38.
Samuelson D. Ophthalmic anatomy. In: Gelatt KN, ed. *Veterinary Ophthalmology*, 3rd ed. Philadelphia: Lippincott Williams & Wilkins, 1999: 31—150.

INTERNET RESOURCES
None

AUTHOR NAME
Tammy Miller Michau

BASICS

TYPE OF SPECIMEN
Blood

TEST EXPLANATION AND RELATED PHYSIOLOGY
Atrial and B-type natriuretic peptides (ANP and BNP) are produced by myocardial tissue in response to increased pressure and wall stress. ANP and BNP elicit vasodilation, diuresis, and natriuresis, and they also counteract activity of the renin-angiotensin-aldosterone system. The clinical utility of ANP and BNP primarily lies in their potential as markers for cardiac dysfunction, differentiation of cardiac from noncardiac causes of dyspnea, prognostication, and as a means to monitor response to therapy. Natriuretic peptide assays are becoming available for companion animals. Because of the short half-life of mature ANP and BNP, clinical assays are likely to target the more stable prohormones: proANP and N-terminal proBNP (NT-proBNP). Commercial canine proANP and NT-proBNP assays are currently available in Europe and the United States. Natriuretic peptide testing, especially with regard to BNP, is relatively new to clinical veterinary medicine, and concrete diagnostic, prognostic, and therapeutic recommendations based on assay results are not yet available.

INDICATIONS
• Canine NT-proANP assay (Vetsign Canine CardioSCREEN; Guildhay, Newton Abbot, UK): differentiation of cardiac versus noncardiac causes of dyspnea
• Canine proBNP assay (Vetsign Canine CardioSCREEN NT-proBNP; Guildhay, Newton Abbot, UK; and Canine Cardiopet proBNP; IDEXX Laboratories, Westbrook, ME) or feline NT-proBNP assay (Feline Cardiopet proBNP, IDEXX Laboratories): differentiation of cardiac versus noncardiac causes of dyspnea
• Future indications may include the following: detection of asymptomatic (occult) cardiac disease in dogs and cats (BNP), quantification of disease severity (ANP, BNP), prognostication (ANP, BNP), and monitoring the efficacy of therapy (ANP, BNP).

CONTRAINDICATIONS
None

POTENTIAL COMPLICATIONS
None

CLIENT EDUCATION
None

BODY SYSTEMS ASSESSED
Cardiovascular

SAMPLE

COLLECTION
0.5 mL of venous blood

HANDLING
• Canine proANP assay is best performed on heparinized plasma, although EDTA plasma and serum can be used. Whether serum or EDTA plasma is used may affect the assay result, with EDTA plasma tending to give higher values. Cutoff values established for each type of sample should therefore be applied.
• NT-proBNP assays in dogs can be performed on serum or plasma. NT-proBNP assays in cats should be performed on EDTA plasma.
• Samples should be centrifuged and plasma or serum separated after collection. For BNP analysis, serum or plasma should be separated from cells within 1 h of collection.
• Ship samples by overnight courier and use cold packs to maintain samples at 4°C during transport.

STORAGE
• ANP samples analyzed the same day as collection should be held at room temperature. If analysis is delayed, freeze the samples. Samples should not be refrigerated.
• Freeze samples (−20°C) until they are shipped.

STABILITY
Frozen (−20°C): 2 days

PROTOCOL
None

INTERPRETATION

NORMAL FINDINGS OR RANGE
• Canine proANP levels of <1,350 fmol/mL (for samples collected into EDTA). When using serum, 1 study suggests that a cutoff of 1,000 fmol/mL can be used to discriminate cardiac from noncardiac causes of dyspnea.
• Canine NT-proBNP levels of ≤210 pmol/L (EDTA plasma or serum)
• Feline NT-proBNP levels of ≤50 pmol/L (EDTA plasma)

ABNORMAL VALUES
• Canine proANP levels of >1,700 fmol/mL (for samples collected into EDTA)
• Canine proANP levels of 1,351–1,700 fmol/mL are suggestive of heart failure, but results are not conclusive (for samples collected into EDTA).
• Canine NT-proBNP levels of ≥300 pmol/L (serum or plasma) are likely to indicate the presence of cardiac disease but not necessarily the presence of congestive heart failure.
• Feline NT-proBNP levels of ≥95 pmol/L (plasma) are likely to indicate the presence of cardiac disease but not necessarily the presence of congestive heart failure.

CRITICAL VALUES
• Canine proANP levels of >1,700 fmol/ml is associated with a 92% probability of congestive heart failure.
• Canine NT-proBNP levels of >1,000 pmol/L accompanied by clinical symptoms are associated with a 95% probability of congestive heart failure.
• Feline NT-proBNP levels of ≥95 pmol/L (plasma) are associated with the presence of cardiac disease.

INTERFERING FACTORS
Drugs That May Alter Results or Interpretation
Drugs That Interfere with Test Methodology
The influence of drugs on test methodology is not known.

Drugs That Alter Physiology
Treatment for heart failure will likely affect the levels of ANP and BNP although this has not been clearly shown for the assays available. Administration of drugs that reduce atrial pressure and left ventricular end diastolic pressure are likely to reduce natriuretic peptide levels.

Disorders That May Alter Results
• Renal failure (reduced glomerular filtration) affects the clearance of natriuretic peptides in human patients, and limited (unpublished) studies suggest that this will also be the case for veterinary patients. Elevated values should therefore be interpreted with caution in patients with known renal disease.
• Rapid fluid administration or treatment with vasoactive agents is also likely to alter circulating natriuretic peptide concentrations.
• Lipemia and hemolysis may cause erroneous results.

Collection Techniques or Handling That May Alter Results
The molecules being measured are small polypeptides. Prolonged periods at room temperature will likely degrade the peptides. Freeze samples at −20°C if overnight shipping at 4°C does not occur immediately after collection.

Influence of Signalment

Species
Species-specific assays are required for NT-proBNP assays because the sequence of these molecules differs significantly between dogs and cats.

Breed
The influence of breed on natriuretic peptide assays has not been evaluated.

Age
There is a relationship between natriuretic peptide concentrations and age in human patients, with higher cutoffs required for older individuals. The influence of age on ANP and BNP concentrations in dogs and cats has not been fully characterized.

Gender
In human patients, gender must be considered when interpreting BNP concentrations. Women tend to have higher values than men, and some of this effect has been attributed to effects of estrogen. This question has not been examined in detail in veterinary patients, but both gender and reproductive status (i.e., intact or neutered) might have some effect.

Pregnancy
The effect of pregnancy on natriuretic peptide levels in veterinary patients is not known.

LIMITATIONS OF THE TEST

Sensitivity, Specificity, and Positive and Negative Predictive Values

Various studies have been conducted with these assays and, as already mentioned, the results have differed slightly according to the study design and whether EDTA plasma or serum has been used.
- When measuring proANP by using EDTA plasma to discriminate dogs with heart failure from normal dogs, a cutoff of 1,350 fmol/mL yields a sensitivity of 93.5% and a specificity of 72.5%. A cutoff of 1,750 fmol/mL yields a sensitivity of 83.9% and a specificity of 97.5%.
- When measuring proANP by using serum to discriminate dogs with dyspnea or cough caused by heart disease from those with respiratory disease, a cutoff of 1,000 fmol/mL yields a sensitivity of 78% and a specificity of 96%.
- Measuring canine NT-proBNP in serum or EDTA plasma using a cutoff of 210 pmol/L yields a sensitivity of 86% and specificity of 83% (EDTA) and a sensitivity of 83% and specificity of 83% (serum) in detecting dogs with heart disease.

Valid If Run in a Human Lab?

No. Species-specific assays are required for NT-proBNP in veterinary patients. Test results are unlikely to be valid if run using assays designed for human patients.

Causes of Abnormal Findings

High values	Low values
Heart disease with elevated filling pressures (with or without heart failure) Renal failure	No pathologic causes

CLINICAL PERSPECTIVE

Increasing numbers of studies demonstrate similarities between the behavior of natriuretic peptides in veterinary patients and human patients with cardiac disease. The assays that are currently available have been clinically validated in a relatively limited number of diagnostic studies, but their use will likely become increasingly widespread. Caution should be exercised when using new diagnostic tests, and further studies must be undertaken to further characterize the utility of these tests for prognostic and therapeutic monitoring purposes.

MISCELLANEOUS

ANCILLARY TESTS
- Thoracic radiographs to determine whether high levels of natriuretic peptides are due to heart failure
- Chemistry profile and urinalysis to rule out renal failure

SYNONYMS
- Atrial natriuretic peptide (ANP)
- B-type natriuretic peptide (BNP)

SEE ALSO
Blackwell's Five-Minute Veterinary Consult: Canine and Feline Topics
Congestive heart failure, left-sided

Related Topics in This Book
- Echocardiography
- Thoracic-Radiography
- Troponin, Cardiac Specific

ABBREVIATIONS
- ANP = atrial natriuretic peptide
- BNP = B-type natriuretic peptide
- NT-proBNP = N-terminal prohormone of BNP

Suggested Reading
Boswood A, Attree S, Page K. Clinical validation of a proANP 31–67 ELISA in the diagnosis of heart failure in the dog. *J Small Anim Pract* 2003; 44: 104–108.
Häggström J, Hansson K, Kvart C, *et al.* Relationship between different natriuretic peptides and severity of naturally acquired mitral regurgitation in dogs with chronic myxomatous valve disease. *J Vet Cardiol* 2000; 2: 7–16.
MacDonald KA, Kittleson MD, Munro C, Kass P. Brain natriuretic peptide concentration in dogs with heart disease and congestive heart failure. *J Vet Intern Med* 2003; 17: 172–177.
Sisson DD. Neuroendocrine evaluation of cardiac disease. *Vet Clin North Am Small Anim Pract* 2004; 34: 1105–1126.

INTERNET RESOURCES
Guildhay Vetsign: Canine CardioSCREEN proANP,
http://www.guildhay.co.uk/veterinary/canine/VC3167.php.
Guildhay Vetsign, Guildhay & AXIOM Veterinary Laboratories: Canine CardioSCREEN proANP,
http://www.axiomvetlab.com/VETSIGN.html.
IDEXX Laboratories: Canine and Feline Cardiopet proBNP,
http://www.idexx.com/animalhealth/laboratory/cardiopetprobnp/.

AUTHOR NAMES
Mark A. Oyama, Adrian Boswood, and David Sisson

OCULAR ULTRASONOGRAPHY

 BASICS

TYPE OF PROCEDURE
Ultrasonographic

PROCEDURE EXPLANATION AND RELATED PHYSIOLOGY
Ocular ultrasonography is an effective and safe method to examine intraocular and retrobulbar structures in awake animals. This technique is most useful whenever direct visualization of intraocular structures is difficult or orbital lesions are suspected.

Ultrasonographic energy is emitted from a transducer. The sound waves strike intraocular structures and are reflected back to the transducer as an echo. In amplitude-mode or *A-scan ultrasonography*, a thin parallel sound beam is emitted that passes through the eye and images 1 small axis of tissue, the echoes of which are represented as spikes arising from a baseline. A-scan ultrasonography is useful for measuring distances between ocular structures. In brightness-mode or *B-scan ultrasonography*, an oscillating sound beam is emitted, and the echoes are represented as a multitude of dots that form a screen image. The stronger the echo is, the brighter the echodensity appears. In veterinary ophthalmology, B-scan ultrasonography provides a 2-dimensional real-time image and is the most common mode of ultrasonography used in a clinical setting.

The transducer probe for ocular ultrasonography is typically smaller than for routine ultrasonography. Direct contact of the transducer with the cornea produces good ocular images. This requires a transducer with a small scan-head diameter (footprint). Ultrasound probes for ophthalmic use are available in a range of frequencies from 5 million cycles per second (5 MHz) up to 50 MHz. The frequency of the sound wave is the number of cycles per second measured in hertz (Hz). The frequency of the transducer is inversely proportional to the wavelength of the sound beam. A direct relationship exists between wavelength and depth of tissue penetration: the higher the frequency is, the shorter is the wavelength, and the more shallow is the tissue penetration. However, as the wavelength shortens, the image resolution actually improves. This is important in ocular ultrasonography where high resolution is more advantageous than deep tissue penetration.

A low-frequency (5 MHz) transducer supplies greater tissue penetration, but poor near-field axial resolution, and is more useful in evaluating deeper structures such as those within the orbit. A higher-frequency (20 MHz) transducer supplies lower tissue penetration, but high near-field axial resolution, and is desirable for evaluating intraocular structures. The optimal ophthalmic transducer is 10–20 MHz. These probes will provide adequate depth of penetration to visualize the retrobulbar structures, enhanced resolution, and the ability to visualize the anterior intraocular structures, such as the iris, ciliary body, anterior and posterior chambers, and cornea. The anterior segment of the globe will be lost in the near-field reverberation artifact of the lower-frequency transducers. The use of a stand-off device, the use of increased sterile coupling gel, or performing the ultrasonographic examination through the animal's closed eyelids may help overcome the near-field loss.

High-frequency ultrasonic biomicroscopy is a relatively new tool that has been used to define, identify, and treat human glaucoma based on numerous iridocorneal and anterior chamber structural changes. The higher-frequency (20–50 MHz) probe enables better resolution of anterior segment structures such as the iridocorneal angle and cornea. These probes penetrate only ≈5–10 mm into the eye but provide incredibly detailed resolution of the anterior segment.

INDICATIONS
- Opacity of the transmitting media of the eye (i.e., cornea, aqueous, lens, vitreous)
- Prior to cataract surgery
- Evaluation of intraocular mass lesions
- Evaluation of the position of the lens (suspected lens luxation)
- Evaluation for suspected retinal detachment
- Assessment of intraocular damage following trauma
- Evaluation of orbital disease
- Differentiation between solid and cystic structures
- Examination for a foreign body
- Determination of globe axial length (determine whether buphthalmia or microphthalmia is present)

CONTRAINDICATIONS
- Full-thickness corneal or scleral ruptures
- Deep corneal ulceration (the structural integrity of the globe is compromised) if a corneal contact probe is being used

POTENTIAL COMPLICATIONS
Rupture of the globe if the structural integrity is compromised

CLIENT EDUCATION
None

BODY SYSTEMS ASSESSED
Ophthalmic

 PROCEDURE

PATIENT PREPARATION
Preprocedure Medication or Preparation
None

Anesthesia or Sedation
Usually only topical anesthesia (e.g., proparacaine hydrochloride) is required.

Patient Positioning
Sitting, or sternal or lateral recumbency

Patient Monitoring
None

Equipment or Supplies
- An ultrasound unit
- Transducers
- An image-recording device to enable freeze-frame evaluation, to obtain measurements, to document the image for record purposes and future reference, and to enable consultation with colleagues
- An offset device, if necessary (available with most transducers or alternately a water-filled balloon can be used)
- Sterile ultrasonographic coupling gel or K-Y Jelly (not cellulose based)
- Topical anesthesia (e.g., proparacaine hydrochloride)
- Sterile eyewash

TECHNIQUE
- Sterile ultrasonographic coupling gel or K-Y Jelly is placed on the transducer tip or on the corneal surface. Avoid the use of cellulose-based coupling gels because they may cause corneal irritation.
- Place the transducer directly on the cornea or perform the scan through the animal's closed eyelids or an offset device.
- Direct corneal contact provides a better image of the posterior segment and orbit. The use of an offset device or closing the animal's eyelids will provide a better image of the anterior aspect of the globe.
- Attempt to keep air bubbles to a minimum when applying the coupling gel or while constructing the water-filled balloon because air bubbles cause substantial reverberation artifact.
- When imaging through eyelids or an offset device, it is sometimes necessary to increase the gain setting.
- The globe should be imaged in both the horizontal and the vertical planes through the visual axis.
- Oblique positioning of the probe should also be used for a complete examination.
- Only gentle contact is required between the probe and the cornea.
- At the completion of the study, the coupling gel should be irrigated from the eye and conjunctiva by using sterile eyewash.

SAMPLE HANDLING
None

APPROPRIATE AFTERCARE
Postprocedure Patient Monitoring
None

Nursing Care
None

Dietary Modification
None

Medication Requirements
None

Restrictions on Activity
None

Anticipated Recovery Time
Immediate

 INTERPRETATION

NORMAL FINDINGS OR RANGE
• The capacity of a structure in the path of an ultrasonographic beam to reflect back sound waves is its *echogenicity*.
• Ultrasonographic images are typically described as hyperechoic, hypoechoic, and anechoic in B-scan ultrasonography.
 • An ultrasonographic image with echoes stronger than normal or than the surrounding structures and are bright on the monitor is termed *hyperechoic*.
 • An ultrasonographic image with weaker echoes than the surrounding structures and are darker on the monitor is termed *hypoechoic*.
• There are 4 major ocular acoustic echoes within a normal eye: anterior cornea; anterior lens capsule; posterior lens capsule; and the retina, choroid, and sclera.
• Additional echodensities may be generated by the iris, corpora nigra, ciliary body, optic nerve, orbital fat, muscles, and other orbital structures.
• The anterior chamber (between the iris and cornea) and posterior chamber (between the iris and lens), lens cortex and nucleus, and vitreous chamber are normally anechoic, appearing dark or black on ultrasonography.
• In a normal eye, the lens appears as 2 distinct echodensities seen at the anterior and posterior axial lens capsules. The anterior echo is slightly convex, whereas the posterior is concave in relationship to the probe. Internally, the lens is anechoic.
• In a normal eye, the retinal echo is indistinguishable from the underlying choroidal and scleral echoes. This echodensity is collectively termed the *posterior eye wall*.
• The optic nerve head, including the lamina cribrosa, appears as a hyperechoic structure. The optic nerve itself is seen as a hypoechoic structure extending posteriorly from the optic nerve head within the orbital cone.
• The orbital muscle cone and fat appear as an area of moderate echodensity extending posteriorly from the equatorial region of the globe and converging toward the orbital apex.
• In normal dogs and cats, the anterior-posterior axial distance of the globe (probe contact on the cornea to the posterior eye wall) is ≈19–21 mm. The axial lens thickness is ≈7 mm. The anterior chamber depth is ≈3–5 mm.

ABNORMAL VALUES
• Abnormalities of globe dimensions include enlargement of the globe (buphthalmia), a decrease in globe size (microphthalmia or phthisis bulbi), increased or decreased lens dimensions, or changes in the relationship of intraocular structures to one another.
• Changes in depth of the anterior chamber or vitreal chamber may result from lens (sub)luxation, corneal rupture, or posterior eye wall rupture. For example, a reduction in the lens–posterior eye wall axial length may indicate a posterior lens luxation, whereas an increase may indicate an anterior lens luxation or a posterior eye wall rupture.
• Metal foreign bodies are highly reflective (hyperechoic) and cause an echodensity with acoustic shadowing behind it because of the absorption of

sound by the object. Glass and organic material tend to be less echodense and more difficult to diagnose by ultrasonography.
• Intraocular mass lesions consist of inflammatory, neoplastic, and cystic structures. During ultrasonography, a cyst will have an echogenic wall but an anechoic, fluid-filled center, whereas a mass appears more homogeneous in its acoustic density.
• In anterior uveitis, fibrin appears as a series of disconnected echodensities throughout the anterior chamber, whereas hypopyon is most often seen ventrally and its echodensity is more uniform.
• Cataracts will result in the typically anechoic area between the hyperechoic anterior and posterior lens capsule becoming hyperechoic, as well. Cataract can also appear with increased visualization of the lens periphery other than the anterior and posterior axial portions. The size and intensity of the echoes will depend on the extent and severity of the cataract.
• Abnormalities of lens size, measured anterior to posterior at the axial position, include both increased and decreased lens dimensions. Lens size increase can be seen in association with a cataract and is the result of imbibition of fluid by the cataract, resulting in lens swelling (i.e., intumescence). An acquired decrease in lens size occurs as a result of resorption of liquefied cortical material as is seen with a hypermature cataract. *Microphakia*, a congenitally small lens, may be seen alone or in association with other congenital intraocular abnormalities.
• Difficulty in obtaining a simultaneous echo of both the anterior and posterior lens capsule and changes in the anterior-posterior axial measurements of the lens or lens-posterior eyeballs may indicate a (sub)luxation of the lens.
• Degeneration or liquefaction of the vitreous results in a decrease in the vitreous gel and an increase in the free water content. As the vitreous gel and water separate, interfaces are created that result in echodensities. These appear as multiple, variable echogenic lines within the vitreous cavity and are best visualized by increasing the far-field gain setting on the ultrasound unit.
• Vitreous hemorrhage appears as discrete to diffuse moderate amplitude echoes that may demonstrate motion when evaluated during a real-time kinetic study.
• Vitreous inflammation appears as multifocal, disconnected, variable echodensities within the vitreous cavity. In addition, fibrin, hypopyon, and retinal detachment may be present if the inflammation extends to involve other structures.
• The presence of calcium-phosphate crystals suspended in the vitreous humor is termed *asteroid hyalosis*. Ultrasonographically, they appear as highly reflective, discrete, freely moving echoes. These echoes will persist even as the gain setting is reduced.
• The retina becomes apparent as a distinct echodensity with a separation of 0.5–1.0 mm. When detached, the retina appears as an echodense linear structure, most often attached at the optic disk posteriorly and the ora ciliaris retinae anteriorly, resulting in the classic funnel-like or gull-wing–like detachment. Initially, retinal detachments will be seen to undulate when viewed in real time, but, with chronicity, the retina will become fixed and less mobile.
• When evaluating a retinal detachment, it is important to evaluate the echo from the subretinal space. An anechoic subretinal space indicates fluid, such as a transudate, that may resorb, whereas the presence of echodense material in the subretinal space may indicate hemorrhage or infiltration of neoplastic or inflammatory cells and should indicate a less favorable prognosis.
• Differentials for a hyperechoic linear structure in the vitreous in addition to retinal detachment include choroidal detachment, vitreous hemorrhage, vitreous detachment, vitreous degeneration, traction bands, and artifacts such as reverberation from the lens.
• Orbital contents include the extraocular muscles, fat, vascular tissues, glands, and the optic nerve. If an orbital mass lesion is present on ultrasonography, an attempt is made to characterize it as cystic or solid and to characterize it with regard to location within the orbit. The normally concave posterior eye wall can be deformed by orbital mass lesions.

CRITICAL VALUES
None

OCULAR ULTRASONOGRAPHY

INTERFERING FACTORS

Drugs That May Alter Results of the Procedure
None

Conditions That May Interfere with Performing the Procedure
• Extreme care should be taken when performing ocular ultrasonography on globes in which the structural integrity is compromised. Corneal contact ultrasonography is contraindicated in the presence of deep corneal ulceration.
• *Absorption artifact* occurs when a dense structure such as a cataract or intraocular foreign body causes an acoustic shadow. This artifact occurs because of the almost complete reflection of sound from the dense structure, with little or no sound passing beyond to image the deeper tissues. The artifact appears as an anechoic area some distance posterior to the hyperechoic structure and can be confused with a mass lesion.
• *Reduplication echoes* result from the echo passing from an intraocular structure to the transducer and back again. As it will take longer for this echo to reach the probe and return into the eye to be imaged, the artifact always appears deeper in the globe than does the tissue of origin. The typical reduplication echo reflects from the lens capsule to the transducer and back again and appears as linear hyperechodensities in the middle to posterior axial vitreous and can be confused with vitreous hemorrhage, inflammatory debris, or degeneration.

Procedure Techniques or Handling That May Alter Results
• Failure to use adequate coupling gel results in a gap between the transducer and the eyelid or cornea and subsequent artifact.
• Substantial air bubbles in the coupling gel will produce artifact.

Influence of Signalment on Performing and Interpreting the Procedure

Species
Dimensions of the globe and intraocular structures, such as the anterior-posterior width of the lens, vary with species

Breed
Dimensions of the globe and intraocular structures, such as the anterior-posterior width of the lens, vary with breeds

Age
Degenerative conditions, such as asteroid hyalosis, are more common in older animals.

Gender
None

Pregnancy
None

CLINICAL PERSPECTIVE
• Ocular ultrasonography is not a replacement for a routine ophthalmic examination that includes assessment of menace, blink and pupillary light response, fluorescein staining, nasolacrimal evaluation, determination of intraocular pressure, and examination of anterior and posterior segments by using a bright focal light source and direct and indirect ophthalmoscopy, respectively.
• Axial vertical sections are the most commonly obtained images with transcorneal probe placement and the probe marker at 12 o'clock.
• Transscleral orientation with the probe placed at the corneal limbus can also be used to bypass the lens and obtain better images of the posterior segment and orbit.
• Care should be taken to avoid traumatizing a globe through excessive pressure exerted on the globe by the ultrasound probe.
• Exposure of intraocular contents to the coupling gel in instances of corneal laceration or uveal prolapse should be avoided because it can cause severe intraocular inflammation.
• Using ultrasonography to evaluate for intraocular foreign bodies is often unrewarding. For a foreign body to be visualized on ultrasonography, it must be of sufficient size (>1.0 mm^3) and have a surface that will reflect enough energy to be visualized among the surrounding tissue.
• Ultrasound-guided fine-needle aspirates or biopsy samples can be obtained to assist in the diagnosis of orbital mass lesions.
• The most common clinical indications for ocular ultrasonography include the following:

• Evaluation for the presence of a retinal detachment in an eye with a cataract
• Assessment of posterior segment damage (retinal detachment, vitreous hemorrhage, etc.) and examination for the presence of a foreign body following trauma
• Evaluation of intraocular structures in eyes with severe corneal opacification
• Evaluation of orbital structures in cases of exophthalmos or orbital trauma

MISCELLANEOUS

ANCILLARY TESTS
• Computed tomography
• Electroretinography
• Fine-needle aspiration
• Magnetic resonance imaging
• Skull radiography

SYNONYMS
None

SEE ALSO
Blackwell's Five-Minute Veterinary Consult: Canine and Feline Topics
• Anterior Uveitis—Cats
• Anterior Uveitis—Dogs
• Cataract
• Glaucoma
• Hyphema
• Hypopyon and Lipid Flare
• Lens Luxation
• Optic Neuritis
• Orbital Diseases (Exophthalmos, Enophthalmos, Strabismus)
• Papilledema
• Retinal Detachment
• Uveal Melanoma—Cats
• Uveal Melanoma—Dogs

Related Topics in This Book
• General Principles of Ultrasonography
• Computed Tomography
• Electroretinography
• Magnetic Resonance Imaging
• Skull Radiography
• Ultrasound-Guided Mass or Organ Aspiration

ABBREVIATIONS
None

Suggested Reading
Bentley E, Miller PE, Diehl K. Use of high-resolution ultrasound as a diagnostic tool in veterinary ophthalmology. *J Am Vet Med Assoc* 2003; 223: 1617–1622.
Brooks .DE Ocular imaging. In: Gelatt KN, ed. *Veterinary Ophthalmology*, 3rd ed. Philadelphia: Lippincott Williams & Wilkins, 1999: 467–482.
Dziezyc J, Hagar DA. Ocular ultrasonography in veterinary medicine. *Semin Vet Med Surg* 1988; 3: 1–9.
Gonzalez EM, Rodriguez A, Garcia I. Review of ocular ultrasonography. *Vet Radiol Ultrasound* 2001; 42: 485–495.
Williams J, Wilkie DA. Ultrasonography of the eye. *Comp Contin Educ Pract Vet* 1996; 18: 667–676.

INTERNET RESOURCES
Waldron RG, Aaberg TM. B-scan ocular ultrasound. eMedicine, http://www.emedicine.com/oph/topic757.htm.

AUTHOR NAME
Tammy Miller Michau

BASICS

TYPE OF SPECIMEN
Blood
Urine

TEST EXPLANATION AND RELATED PHYSIOLOGY
The *osmolality* of a fluid is a measure of the total number of solute particles per kilogram of solvent (mOsm/kg). This is different from *osmolarity*, which is the number of solute particles in a liter of solution. In normal serum, the main contributors (>95%) to osmolality are those present in highest concentrations, with the greatest contribution by Na^+ and Cl^-. This is followed distantly by bicarbonate, K^+, urea, and glucose. Others electrolytes such as magnesium, calcium, and phosphate, and solutes such as protein contribute very little to serum osmolality.

The effective osmolality of blood is due to solute particles that promote water movement across a semipermeable membrane. Effective osmolality is monitored by the hypothalamic osmoreceptors and regulated by ADH produced by the pituitary. With increased plasma osmolality, ADH release increases. ADH then acts on the distal tubules and collecting ducts in the kidney to increase water resorption. The individual also is stimulated to drink. Both result in dilution of solutes and a decrease in plasma osmolality. Alternately, with a decrease in plasma osmolality, ADH production is reduced, resulting in reduced water resorption by the kidney.

Osmolality (Osm_m) is measured by either freezing-point depression or vapor-pressure depression methods. The freezing-point osmometers are preferred and more commonly used because this methodology will detect the presence of volatile solutes. An estimate of serum osmolality can be calculated using various published formulas. One such formula is $Osm_c = 1.86\ ([Na^+] + [K^+]) + [BUN]/2.8 + [glucose]/18$. These calculations take into account the measured values of the major contributing solutes. Osm_c can be used to calculate the serum osmolal gap: $Osm_m - Osm_c$. A large osmolal gap indicates the presence of an unmeasured solute (e.g., ketones) or a foreign solute in the blood (e.g., ethylene glycol, ethyl alcohol, mannitol).

Urine osmolality can be determined and interpreted relative to serum osmolality and urine electrolyte and creatinine measurements. It gives the best estimate of the kidney's ability to concentrate urine because it measures total solute concentration. More commonly, the urine specific gravity, which is a reflection of urine osmolality, is used. The urine specific gravity, however, is not only affected by the number of solutes present but also by the molecular weights of the different solutes. Urine with an osmolality that is similar to that of plasma is considered isosthenuric. Hyposthenuric urine has an osmolality that is less than that of plasma. Hypersthenuric urine has an osmolality greater than that of plasma and is used to describe urine that is very concentrated.

INDICATIONS
- Determine the hydration status (dehydration or overhydration).
- Determine the presence of toxic metabolites in poison ingestion (e.g., ethylene glycol, methanol, ethanol).
- Confirm suspected hyperosmolar syndrome (e.g., hyperglycemia, hypernatremia resulting in seizures, or coma).
- Measure in a water-deprivation test to differentiate between diabetes insipidus and psychogenic polydipsia (comparison of serum and urine osmolality).

CONTRAINDICATIONS
Animals administered mannitol for treatment or IV radiographic contrast agents for diagnostics

POTENTIAL COMPLICATIONS
None

CLIENT EDUCATION
None

BODY SYSTEMS ASSESSED
- Endocrine and metabolic
- Gastrointestinal
- Renal and urologic

SAMPLE

COLLECTION
- 1–2 mL of venous blood
- Urine collection by voiding into a clean receptacle, via catheterization or via cystocentesis

HANDLING
- Collect blood into a red-top tube and centrifuge it as soon as there is clot formation (in <1 h).
- Spin an aliquot of urine to remove cells and other debris. The supernatant is used for measurement of urine osmolality.

STORAGE
- Serum: refrigerated or frozen
- Urine: refrigerated or frozen to prevent bacterial growth

STABILITY
Dependent on the stability of the individual solute:
- Urea: 1 day at room temperature, several days at 4°–6°C, and at least 2–3 months frozen
- Glucose: 8 h at 25°C and up to 3 days at 4°C
- Monovalent electrolytes (i.e., Na^+, K^+, Cl^-: stable for months if dehydration is prevented)

PROTOCOL
None

OSMOLALITY

INTERPRETATION

NORMAL FINDINGS OR RANGE
- Serum osmolality: 290–310 mOsm/kg (dogs and cats)
- Urine osmolality: 500–2400 mOsm/kg (dogs); 1,200–3,200 mOsm/kg (cats)
- Osmolal gap: <10 mOsm/kg (dogs); may be greater in cats

ABNORMAL VALUES
- Serum: greater than or less than the aforementioned reference intervals
- Urine: Osmolality varies depending on serum osmolality and hydration status of the individual.

CRITICAL VALUES
For serum osmolality, the rapidity of change has a greater impact on causing clinical abnormality than does the magnitude of change.
- A concentration of >340–350 mOsm/kg (hyperosmolar syndrome) may result in neurologic and GI abnormalities.
- A concentration of <260–270 mOsm/kg

INTERFERING FACTORS
Drugs That May Alter Results or Interpretation
Drugs That Interfere with Test Methodology
None

Drugs That Alter Physiology
- Diuretics alter electrolytes and fluid balance.
- Insulin alters glucose levels.
- IV fluids increase or decrease osmolality, depending on amount and tonicity of fluid.

Disorders That May Alter Results
- Causes of pseudohyponatremia (increased protein or lipid) will lower Osm_c but not affect Osm_m.
- The use of some drugs for treatment or diagnostics will increase Osm_m:
  - Mannitol
  - IV radiographic contrast medium

Collection Techniques or Handling That May Alter Results
Allowing the serum to sit on the clot for >1 h will cause a falsely decreased glucose through continued glucose utilization by the cells.

Influence of Signalment
Species
None

Breed
A 1° hypodipsia is rarely seen in miniature schnauzers.

Age
None

Gender
None

Pregnancy
None

LIMITATIONS OF THE TEST
Sensitivity, Specificity, and Positive and Negative Predictive Values
N/A

Valid If Run in a Human Lab?
Yes.

Causes of Abnormal Findings

High values	Low values
Increased serum Osm$_m$	**Decreased serum Osm$_m$**
Dehydration (e.g., fever, lack of water)	(Generally causes of hyponatremia with excess free water)
Diabetes mellitus (hyperglycemia, ketoacidosis)	Diarrhea and/or vomiting
Diarrhea and/or vomiting (water loss greater than solute loss)	Congestive heart failure
Renal dysfunction (e.g., postobstruction diuresis, chronic renal failure, nonoliguric renal failure)	Severe renal failure
	Third-space loss (e.g., peritonitis, pancreatitis, uroabdomen)
Hyperadrenocorticism	Hypoadrenocorticism
Presence of toxins or foreign solutes (e.g., ethylene glycol, alcohol)	Drugs (e.g., diuretics, hypotonic fluids)
Diabetes insipidus	Cirrhosis
Third-space loss of hypotonic fluids (e.g., peritonitis, pancreatitis)	Nephrotic syndrome
Other causes for solute gain (e.g., hypertonic fluids, salt poison, hyperaldosteronism)	Psychogenic polydipsia: rare in dogs
Primary hypodipsia	SIADH (syndrome of inappropriate ADH release): rare in dogs
Other (e.g., mannitol, chemical diuretics)	
Hypersthenuric urine	**Hyposthenuric urine**
Useful because it indicates that the kidney is able to concentrate urine. Renal function, therefore, is fine.	Diabetes insipidus (high serum Osm$_m$)
	Primary polydipsia (low serum Osm$_m$)
May be normal or associated with diseases; e.g., congestive heart failure, SIADH	Other causes of free water overload
Isosthenuric urine	
May be normal	
Inappropriate isosthenuria seen with various conditions	
Renal failure	
Chronic hypoadrenocorticism	
Diabetes mellitus	
Hyperadrenocorticism	
Hypercalcemia	
Liver failure	
Post–urinary obstruction diuresis	

CLINICAL PERSPECTIVE
- Measurement of serum osmolality is helpful in a some situations:
  - An increased osmolal gap will indicate the presence of a foreign solute or toxin such as ethylene glycol or paraldehyde, or other unmeasured solutes such as ketones and lactate.
  - Increased Osm_m will help identify a hyperosmolar syndrome responsible for neurologic changes (e.g., depression, stupor, coma, death).
  - Allows monitoring of fluid and electrolyte balance in the body
  - In case of a normal Osm_m, the presence of an increased osmolal gap should cause a suspicion of pseudohyponatremia.
- Urine osmolality is not commonly determined in veterinary medicine. It should be interpreted relative to serum osmolality and along with other measurements of kidney function:
  - It indicates renal concentrating ability.
  - Urine osmolality that is hypersthenuric indicates that renal concentrating ability is good.

- Urine osmolality in the hyposthenuric range has 2 primary differentials:
- Primary polydipsia (low serum and low urine osmolality)
- Diabetes insipidus (high serum and low urine osmolality).

MISCELLANEOUS

ANCILLARY TESTS
- Standard tests (i.e., CBC, serum chemistry panel, urinalysis)
- Subsequent tests depend on the process or disease suspected.

SYNONYMS
None

SEE ALSO
Blackwell's Five-Minute Veterinary Consult: Canine and Feline Topics
- Diabetes Insipidus
- Diabetes Mellitus with Hyperosmolar Coma
- Diabetes Mellitus with Ketoacidosis
- Ethylene Glycol Poisoning
- Hyperosmolarity

Related Topics in This Book
- Chloride
- Ethylene Glycol
- Glucose
- Sodium
- Urea Nitrogen
- Urine Specific Gravity

ABBREVIATIONS
- ADH = antidiuretic hormone (vasopressin)
- Cl^- = chloride
- K^+ = potassium
- Na^+ = sodium
- Osm_c = calculated osmolality
- Osm_m = measured osmolality
- SIADH = syndrome of inappropriate antidiuretic hormone (ADH) secretion

Suggested Reading
DiBartola SP. Disorders of sodium and water: Hypernatremia and hyponatremia. In: DiBartola SP, ed. *Fluid, Electrolyte, and Acid-Base Disorders in Small Animal Practice*, 3rd ed. St Louis: Saunders Elsevier, 2006: 47–79.
Morgan RV, Bright RM, Swartout MS, eds. *Handbook of Small Animal Practice*, 4th ed. Philadelphia: WB Saunders, 2003: 1270.
Stockham SL, Scott MA. Monovalent electrolytes and osmolality. In: *Fundamentals of Veterinary Clinical Pathology*. Ames: Iowa State Press, 2002: 339–372.

INTERNET RESOURCES
Dufour DR. Osmometry: The Rational Basis for Use of an Underappreciated Diagnostic Tool. Presented as an industry workshop at the American Association for Clinical Chemistry Meeting, New York, 1993:1–36. http://www.osmolality.com/pdf/Osmometry.pdf.
Lab Tests Online: Osmolality (osmolarity), http://www.labtestsonline.org.uk/understanding/analytes/osmo/related.html.
Osmolality.com, http://www.osmolality.com/.

AUTHOR NAMES
Brenda Yamamoto and M. Judith Radin

OSMOTIC FRAGILITY

BASICS

TYPE OF SPECIMEN
Blood

TEST EXPLANATION AND RELATED PHYSIOLOGY
The RBC osmotic fragility (OF) test depends primarily on the RBC surface area/volume ratio. During the test, RBCs are suspended in a series of tubes containing serial dilutions of buffered 10% NaCl ranging from 0.9% to 0% in increments of 0.02% or 0.05%; 0.9% represents physiologic saline and 0% is pure water (i.e., distilled water). As cells are exposed to progressively more dilute solutions, water is osmotically drawn into them, causing RBCs to swell and become spherical. The membrane has minimal ability to stretch, so surface area is a limiting factor in determining the volume of water that can be accommodated. Cells initially leak their contents (including Hb) and finally rupture when critical volume is exceeded. OF is partly related to cell size (i.e., erythrocyte volume, MCV): species with smaller RBCs are more osmotically fragile because they have less membrane and a more limited expandability. After incubation, samples are centrifuged and Hb is measured in the supernatant. The Hb concentration at a given NaCl dilution is reported as a percentage of the Hb concentration when all RBCs are lysed (usually 0%; i.e., pure water). Minimum resistance is the dilution at which slight hemolysis above the baseline concentration of Hb (if any) is detectable; maximum resistance is the highest dilution at which all cells are lysed. Mean cell fragility is the NaCl concentration at which 50% hemolysis occurs. RBCs lysing at higher NaCl concentrations have less resistance to hyposmotic solutions and, accordingly, an increased OF.

The OF test is most frequently used to diagnose hereditary RBC disorders. RBCs with decreased membrane area (e.g., hereditary spherocytosis) or a preexisting pathologically increased volume (i.e., hereditary stomatocytosis) such that they can less readily accommodate additional water will have an increased OF. Increased OF can also be seen with conditions that cause membrane damage (e.g., RBC parasites, immune-mediated hemolytic anemia).

INDICATIONS
- Measure OF to provide an index of RBC membrane surface/volume ratio.
- Screen for RBC membrane integrity, decreased membrane, and/or increased volume.
- Screen for hereditary stomatocytosis or spherocytosis.
- Screen for erythrocyte OF of Abyssinian and Somali cats.

CONTRAINDICATIONS
None

POTENTIAL COMPLICATIONS
None

CLIENT EDUCATION
None

BODY SYSTEMS ASSESSED
Hemic, lymphatic, and immune

SAMPLE

COLLECTION
1 mL of venous blood

HANDLING
- EDTA anticoagulant
- Collect blood from a normal animal of same species as a control.

STORAGE
- Refrigerate for short-term storage.
- An increased OF is noted in stored blood for transfusions when it is nearing end of its shelf life (J.W.H., unpublished data).

STABILITY
- Refrigerated (4°C): up to 24 h
- Spontaneous hemolysis is possible with overnight storage, depending on the disorder.
- Do not freeze the sample.

PROTOCOL
None

INTERPRETATION

NORMAL FINDINGS OR RANGE

Species	% Saline minimum resistance	
	Initial hemolysis	Complete hemolysis
Dog	0.45–0.50	0.32–0.36
Cat	0.69–0.72	0.46–0.50

ABNORMAL VALUES
Values above or below the reference range

CRITICAL VALUES
None

INTERFERING FACTORS
Drugs That May Alter Results or Interpretation
Drugs That Interfere with Test Methodology
Oxyglobin [hemoglobin glutamer-200 (bovine); Biopure, Cambridge, MA] therapy will increase the baseline Hb concentration above zero.

Drugs That Alter Physiology
Decreased by drugs with membrane-stabilizing properties, such as synthetic androgens (e.g., danazol)

Disorders That May Alter Results
- Lipemia increases erythrocyte fragility.
- Marked reticulocytosis may mask an underlying increased OF of mature erythrocytes; reticulocytes have more membrane than mature erythrocytes.
- Leptocytes have increased expandability and decreased OF.
- Hemolyzed blood samples will have a preexisting Hb concentration at 0.9% NaCl, potentially affecting test accuracy.
- Hyperbilirubinemia may interfere with spectrophotometric Hb measurement.

Collection Techniques or Handling That May Alter Results
- Hemolysis due to traumatic venipuncture or poor postcollection handling techniques
- Delayed sample processing may cause spontaneous hemolysis of abnormal cells, causing their underrepresentation in the assay; also, baseline Hb content may be increased.

Influence of Signalment
Species
Cats have smaller erythrocytes and increased OF compared to dogs.

Breed
- Hereditary spherocytosis reported in golden retrievers
- Familial stomatocytosis reported in Alaskan malamutes, Drentse patrijshonds (Dutch partridge dogs), miniature schnauzers, standard schnauzers, and Pomeranians
- Erythrocyte OF defect reported in Abyssinian and Somali cats

Age
None

Gender
None

Pregnancy
None

LIMITATIONS OF THE TEST
Sensitivity, Specificity, and Positive and Negative Predictive Values
N/A

Valid If Run in a Human Lab?
Yes.

Causes of Abnormal Values

Decreased OF	Increased OF
Reticulocytosis	Congenital
Leptocytosis	Hereditary spherocytosis
Liver disease	Familial stomatocytosis
Iron deficiency	Erythrocyte OF of Abyssinian and Somali cats
	Hereditary elliptocytosis
	Acquired
	Immune-mediated hemolytic anemia
	Hemotrophic mycoplasmosis (hemobartonellosis)
	Anemia of inflammatory disease
	Chronic azotemia

CLINICAL PERSPECTIVE
The test is best used in predisposed breeds to screen for hereditary erythrocyte disorders resulting in increased erythrocyte fragility.

MISCELLANEOUS
ANCILLARY TESTS
- CBC with erythrocyte indices
- Blood smear evaluation for erythrocyte poikilocytosis (e.g., spherocytes, stomatocytes, Heinz bodies) and/or hemoparasites (e.g., hemotrophic mycoplasmas)
- Coombs' test
- Serology for tick borne pathogens

SYNONYMS
Erythrocyte fragility test

SEE ALSO
Blackwell's Five-Minute Veterinary Consult: Canine and Feline Topics
Anemia, Regenerative

Related Topics in This Book
- Blood Smear Microscopic Examination
- Red Blood Cell Count
- Red Blood Cell Morphology

ABBREVIATIONS
- Hb = hemoglobin
- NaCl = sodium chloride
- OF = osmotic fragility

Suggested Reading
Jain NC. Hematologic techniques: The erythrocyte osmotic fragility test. In: Jain NC, ed. *Schalm's Veterinary Hematology*, 4th ed. Philadelphia: Lea & Febiger, 1986: 69–71.

INTERNET RESOURCES
None

AUTHOR NAMES
Rebekah Gray Gunn-Christie and John W. Harvey

PANCREATIC LIPASE IMMUNOREACTIVITY

BASICS

TYPE OF SPECIMEN
Blood

TEST EXPLANATION AND RELATED PHYSIOLOGY
Lipases are enzymes that hydrolyze water-insoluble substrates, such as triglycerides, into more polar lipolysis products. Many cells are capable of producing lipases, and all lipases of different cellular origin (e.g., pancreatic lipase, gastric lipase) share the same function. However, lipases of different cellular origins differ immunologically from one another, and the clinical usefulness of PLI assays is based on this characteristic. Pancreatic lipase is exclusively synthesized by pancreatic acinar cells and is normally secreted into the pancreatic duct system. Under physiologic conditions, only small amounts of pancreatic lipase enter the circulation. During inflammatory conditions of the pancreas, pancreatic lipase enters the circulation in large quantities and can be detected by the PLI assay.

PLI assays are species-specific immunoassays that are currently available for dogs (i.e., Spec cPL, previously cPLI) and cats (Spec fPL, previously fPLI). In contrast to the traditional catalytic assays for lipase, which indiscriminately measure the activity of lipases regardless of their cellular origin (e.g., pancreatic, duodenal), PLI is specific for the pancreatic lipase and thus specific for pancreatic disease.

Commercial assays for the measurement of serum cPLI concentration (Spec cPL; IDEXX Laboratories, Portland, ME) and fPLI (Spec fPL; IDEXX Laboratories, Portland, ME) have replaced the original cPLI and fPLI assays. The Spec cPL and Spec fPL assays show the same clinical performance as the original PLI assays and are currently available through IDEXX Laboratories and the Gastrointestinal Laboratory at Texas A&M University.

INDICATIONS
- GI signs (e.g., vomiting, diarrhea, abdominal pain)
- Vague clinical signs (e.g., anorexia, depression)
- A history of pancreatitis
- Consider adding a PLI assay to the routine health screen to detect possible subclinical pancreatitis, which could lead to episodes of severe pancreatitis or chronic complications such as exocrine pancreatic insufficiency (EPI) and/or diabetes mellitus.

CONTRAINDICATIONS
None

POTENTIAL COMPLICATIONS
None

CLIENT EDUCATION
- A 12-h fast is recommended.
- Canine and feline patients with subclinical pancreatitis may have increased serum PLI concentrations. These patients should be appropriately managed and monitored to avoid severe pancreatitis and/or chronic complications.

BODY SYSTEMS ASSESSED
Gastrointestinal

SAMPLE

COLLECTION
2 mL of venous blood

HANDLING
- Use a red-top or serum-separator tube.
- Separate the serum from the clot before shipping the sample, preferably on ice.

STORAGE
- Refrigerate the serum for short term storage.
- Freeze the serum for long-term storage (>2 days).

STABILITY
At least 3 weeks at room temperature, in a refrigerator (2°–8°C), or frozen

PROTOCOL
None

INTERPRETATION

NORMAL RANGE
- Spec cPL, 0–200 μg/L
- Spec fPL, 0–3.5 μg/L

ABNORMAL VALUES
Questionable Ranges
- Spec cPL, 201–399 μg/L
- Spec fPL, 3.6–5.3 μg/L
In 2–3 weeks, recheck results that are in a questionable range and evaluate for other conditions.

Diagnostic Ranges for Pancreatitis
- Spec cPL, >400 μg/L
- Spec fPL, ≥5.4 μg/L

CRITICAL VALUES
None

INTERFERING FACTORS
Drugs That May Alter Results or Interpretation
Drugs That Interfere with Test Methodology
None

Drugs That Alter Physiology
Several drugs are considered to be risk factors for pancreatitis in dogs and cats.

Disorders That May Alter Results
None

Collection Techniques or Handling That May Alter Results
None

Influence of Signalment
Species
The PLI assay is species specific and currently available for dogs (Spec cPL) and cats (Spec fPL).

Breed
None

Age
None

Gender
None

Pregnancy
None

LIMITATIONS OF THE TEST
- Single values are not indicative of the severity of pancreatic inflammation.
- Serum PLI concentrations are generally not useful for the diagnosis of EPI because the assay is optimized for the diagnosis of pancreatitis.

Sensitivity, Specificity, and Positive and Negative Predictive Values
Spec cPL
- Sensitivity for clinical pancreatitis, 82%; for mild chronic pancreatitis, 61%

• Specificity, >96%

Spec fPL
• Sensitivity for moderate to severe pancreatitis, 100%; for pancreatitis overall, 67%; for mild pancreatitis, 54%
• Specificity, 91%–100%
• Positive predictive value, 86%–100%
• Negative predictive value, 100% for moderate to severe pancreatitis and 60% for mild pancreatitis

Valid If Run in a Human Lab?
No.

Causes of abnormal findings

High values	Low values
Concentrations of >400 μg/L (dogs) and $\geq$5.4 μg/L (cats) indicate pancreatic inflammation (acute and/or chronic pancreatitis)	Not significant
There are no known causes of falsely increased concentrations.	

CLINICAL PERSPECTIVE
• Current studies suggest that canine and feline PLI assays are more sensitive and specific than any other test currently available, including abdominal ultrasound. In addition, in contrast to abdominal ultrasound, PLI is not dependent on operator skill.
• Sequential measurement of PLI concentrations may help monitor disease progression in individual patients with pancreatitis.
• Increased PLI concentrations in the absence of clinical signs may indicate subclinical pancreatitis.

MISCELLANEOUS

ANCILLARY TESTS
• CBC, serum chemistry profile, and urinalysis to assess the general condition of the patient

• Abdominal radiographs and/or ultrasonography to rule out other conditions or identify complications of pancreatitis (e.g., pancreatic necrosis, presence of abdominal fluid)
• Evaluation of serum cobalamin, folate, and TLI concentrations to look for concurrent intestinal disease and EPI

SYNONYMS
• PLI

SEE ALSO
Blackwell's Five-Minute Veterinary Consult: Canine and Feline Topics
• Acute Abdomen
• Pancreatitis

Related Topics in This Book
• Lipase
• Pancreatic Ultrasonography
• Trypsin-like Immunoreactivity

ABBREVIATIONS
• cPLI = canine PLI
• EPI = exocrine pancreatic insufficiency
• fPLI = feline PLI
• PLI = pancreatic lipase immunoreactivity
• Spec cPL = specific canine pancreatic lipase
• Spec fPL = specific feline pancreatic lipase

Suggested Reading
Forman MA, Marks SL, De Cock HEV, *et al*. Evaluation of serum feline pancreatic lipase immunoreactivity and helical computed tomography versus conventional testing for the diagnosis of feline pancreatitis. *J Vet Intern Med* 2004; **18**: 807–815.
Steiner JM. Diagnosis of pancreatitis. *Vet Clin North Am Small Anim Pract* 2003; **33**: 1181–1195.

INTERNET RESOURCES
Texas A&M University, College of Veterinary Medicine, Gastrointestinal Laboratory: Pancreatic lipase immunoreactivity (PLI), http://www.cvm.tamu.edu/gilab/assays/cPLI.shtml.

AUTHOR NAMES
Panagiotis G. Xenoulis and Jörg M. Steiner

PANCREATIC ULTRASONOGRAPHY

BASICS

TYPE OF PROCEDURE
Ultrasonographic

PROCEDURE EXPLANATION AND RELATED PHYSIOLOGY
Ultrasonography of the pancreas is a noninvasive diagnostic imaging procedure that typically is performed as part of the systematic abdominal ultrasonographic examination. Successful ultrasonographic evaluation of the pancreas in dogs and cats requires operator experience, knowledge of pancreatic anatomy, and an understanding of pancreatic disease. The ultrasonographic examination should focus on the pancreas in patients with anorexia, vomiting, hyperbilirubinemia (suspected pancreatitis), persistent hypoglycemia (insulinoma), or a cranial abdominal mass.

INDICATIONS
- Suspected pancreatitis
- Suspected extrahepatic biliary obstruction caused by pancreatitis
- Suspected insulinoma
- Right cranial quadrant abdominal mass (e.g., pancreatitis, pancreatic neoplasia, abscess, or pseudocyst)

CONTRAINDICATIONS
None

POTENTIAL COMPLICATIONS
Vomiting in patients with abdominal pain and pancreatitis when excessive ultrasound transducer pressure is applied during the ultrasonographic examination

CLIENT EDUCATION
- The patient must not be fed for 12 h prior to the ultrasonographic examination.
- The abdominal hair coat must be clipped to enable a thorough US examination.

BODY SYSTEMS ASSESSED
- Gastrointestinal
- Hepatobiliary

PROCEDURE

PATIENT PREPARATION
Preprocedure Medication or Preparation
A 12-h fast prior to the ultrasonographic examination. The patient may be allowed to drink water and be administered oral medications prior to the procedure.

Anesthesia or Sedation
Sedation may be required for uncooperative patients or those with severe abdominal pain.

Patient Positioning
Determined by operator preference. Typically patients are placed in dorsal, right lateral, or left lateral recumbency. Lateral recumbency is preferred for hemodynamically unstable or vomiting patients.

Patient Monitoring
- Critical patients require monitoring of pulse, respiration, and signs of abdominal pain.
- Transducer pressure may incite vomiting in patients with pancreatitis.

Equipment or Supplies
- A diagnostic ultrasonography machine with higher-frequency (7.5–10 MHz) curvilinear or linear array transducers.

- Pancreatic imaging via an intercostal or paracostal approach is easier using transducers designed with a small skin-contact area.

TECHNIQUE
- The preparation of patients is typical for general abdominal ultrasonography: Clip the hair coat and apply coupling gel.
- The pancreas should be examined as part of a systematic abdominal scan. In addition, the biliary tract and peritoneum should receive attention.
- Patients are positioned as preferred by the operator: dorsal, right, or left lateral recumbency.
- Scanning from the dependent aspect (e.g., right side while in right lateral recumbency) may be used to eliminate artifacts from gastric and intestinal gas.
- The pancreas is difficult to visualize ultrasonographically, and adjacent anatomic landmarks must be used in both dogs and cats: right lobe—descending duodenum; body—pylorus; left lobe—triangle formed by the stomach, spleen and colon in the left cranial quadrant.
- The normal pancreas in dogs is easier to visualize than in cats.
- The right lobe in dogs and the left lobe in cats are the easier portions to identify ultrasonographically.

SAMPLE HANDLING
N/A

APPROPRIATE AFTERCARE
Postprocedure Patient Monitoring
None

Nursing Care
None

Dietary Modification
None

Medication Requirements
None

Restrictions on Activity
None

Anticipated Recovery Time
Immediate

INTERPRETATION

NORMAL FINDINGS OR RANGE
Dogs
A normal right lobe is much easier to identify in dogs. The pancreas is a thin, ribbonlike hypoechoic tissue with sharp borders that is isoechoic to the normal liver, and located immediately dorsomedial to the descending duodenum. Normal right lobe thickness is ≈7–10 mm. The panceaticoduodenal vein will be in the right lobe. The pancreatic body may be followed caudally to the pylorus along the greater curvature, ventral to the portal vein, and between the greater curvature of the stomach and transverse colon. The lateral end of the left lobe is between the stomach and transverse colon and is deep to the spleen. Pancreatic ducts are not typically seen in dogs.

Cats
The left lobe is easier to image in cats. It is a thin (mean width, 5.4 mm) slightly hypoechoic (to surrounding mesentery), sharply demarcated ribbon of tissue seen deep to the spleen in the left cranial quadrant. The left lobe will contain a larger vessel (diameter, ≈2.1 mm) and smaller pancreatic duct (diameter, ≈0.8 mm); color flow Doppler can be used to differentiate the duct from the vessel. The remaining left lobe is followed between the greater curvature of the stomach and transverse colon to the pancreatic body (mean width, 6.6 mm). The right lobe is difficult to image as a slightly hypoechoic

band of tissue (mean width, 4.5 mm) dorsomedial to the descending duodenum.

ABNORMAL FINDINGS
Canine Nonsuppurative, Interstitial Pancreatitis
The pancreas becomes increasingly hypoechoic and slightly thickened. Linear and subcapsular anechoic bands resembling tiger stripes characterize its echotexture. The peripancreatic mesentery becomes hyperechoic with inflammation, and a small volume of peritoneal effusion adjacent to the pancreas is possible.

Canine Acute Necrotizing Pancreatitis
The pancreas resembles a hypoechoic mass, or phlegmon, with hypoechoic and anechoic areas of hemorrhage and necrosis contrasting with hyperechoic peripancreatic mesenteric inflammation. The pancreatic borders are indistinct or irregular. A peritoneal effusion is more likely. An atonic descending duodenum is likely if the right lobe is affected.

Abscess or Pseudocyst
This is a rare sequel to pancreatitis in dogs. It is difficult to differentiate abscess from pseudocyst with ultrasonography, so fluid aspiration and analysis may be required. Both abscess and pseudocyst are characterized by a hypoechoic to anechoic cystic mass in a portion of the pancreas and a hyperechoic peripancreatic mesentery. The amount of cellular debris in the cystic fluid determines the fluid echogenicity and the degree of distal enhancement artifact.

Feline Pancreatitis
This has an extremely variable ultrasonographic appearance. The pancreas can appear normal, mixed echoic (both hypoechoic and hyperechoic), or hypoechoic, with a contrasting hyperechoic peripancreatic mesentery. Further findings include pancreatic enlargement and peritoneal effusion.

Insulinoma
This is a hypoechoic, variably sized nodule in the pancreas or pancreatic region. The ultrasonographic appearance of an enlarged metastatic lymph node will mimic that of an insulinoma. Hepatic metastasis is typically characterized by hypoechoic hepatic nodules.

Pancreatic Adenocarcinoma
This is a hypoechoic or mixed echoic mass or diffuse nodules isolated to the pancreas. Larger mesenteric masses may be attributed to the pancreas by excluding hepatic, splenic, renal, or intestinal origin. Adenocarcinoma is often metastatic at the time of diagnosis as evidenced by carcinomatosis and peritoneal effusion.

CRITICAL VALUES
• A ultrasonographic finding of pancreatitis, insulinoma, or pancreatic carcinoma rarely prompts emergency intervention.
• Surgery may be considered if extremely elevated serum bilirubin levels are combined with US evidence of extrahepatic biliary obstruction (common bile duct, cystic duct, and gallbladder enlargement) because of pancreatitis.
• Ultrasound-guided gallbladder drainage of biliary sludge may be considered in patients with persistent hyperbilirubinemia, pancreatitis, and evidence of biliary obstruction.
• Ultrasound-guided pancreatic cyst aspiration can be used to differentiate pseudocyst from abscess.

INTERFERING FACTORS
Drugs That May Alter Results of the Procedure
None

Conditions That May Interfere with Performing the Procedure
• Excessive GI gas obscuring the pancreas in the ultrasonographic examination
• Extreme abdominal pain because of pancreatitis
• Critical, unstable patients

Procedure Techniques or Handling That May Alter Results
• Poor ultrasound machine image quality or the use of lower-frequency transducers (4–5 MHz)

• Lack of operator experience in finding the normal pancreas and evaluating ultrasonographic pancreatic findings

Influence of Signalment on Performing and Interpreting the Procedure
Species
• *Dogs*: The reported sensitivity for ultrasonographic detection of pancreatitis is 68%. The sensitivity is felt to be higher now because of greater operator experience and improved diagnostic ultrasound equipment.
• *Cats*: The reported sensitivity for ultrasonographic detection of pancreatitis is a poor 24%–35%. Insulinoma is rare in cats.

Breed
• *Dogs*
  • Pancreatitis: terrier breeds, miniature schnauzers, miniature poodles, cocker spaniels, and Labrador retrievers
  • Insulinoma: many breeds, with possibly a higher incidence in Labrador retrievers, German shepherds, Irish setters, and golden retrievers
• *Cats*: Pancreatitis and insulinoma—no breed predilection; mostly domestic shorthairs

Age
• *Dogs*: middle-aged to older for both insulinoma (mean, 10 years) and pancreatitis (mean, 9 years)
• *Cats*: middle-aged to older for both insulinoma (mean, 14 years) and pancreatitis (mean, 6–7 years)

Gender
• *Dogs*: no gender predilection
• *Cats*: no gender predilection

Pregnancy
N/A

CLINICAL PERSPECTIVE
Pancreatitis
This is difficult to diagnose in dogs and particularly in cats based solely on medical history, physical exam findings, and blood chemistry analysis. Radiographic abnormalities are infrequent and nonspecific; ultrasonography is the preferred diagnostic imaging tool. In dogs, ultrasonography has a relatively high sensitivity for detecting pancreatitis and complications (i.e., extrahepatic biliary obstruction, peritonitis). In cats, ultrasonography has a low sensitivity, but other potential complicating diseases can be ruled out. Equivocal ultrasonographic findings in dogs and cats can be followed with the Spec cPL [specific canine pancreatic lipase (IDEXX Laboratories)] (dogs) or fPLI (cats) assays.

Insulinoma
Ultrasonography is performed because clinical suspicion of insulinoma is heightened with persistent hypoglycemia but before insulin/glucose ratio results are available. The ability to identify a pancreatic nodule by ultrasonography depends on the nodule size and location: It is easier to identify a nodule in the right canine pancreatic lobe and the left feline pancreatic lobe. If the pancreas itself is not seen during ultrasonography, an identified nodule in the pancreatic region can represent either an insulinoma or an enlarged metastatic duodenal lymph node. Surgery to remove an identified pancreatic nodule suspected of being an insulinoma may be indicated when normal blood glucose levels cannot be maintained without IV glucose supplementation.

MISCELLANEOUS
ANCILLARY TESTS
• Suspected canine pancreatitis: Spec cPL test
• Suspected feline pancreatitis: fPLI

• Suspected insulinoma: determination of the insulin/glucose ratio or amended insulin/glucose ratio

SYNONYMS
Pancreatic ultrasound

SEE ALSO
Blackwell's Five-Minute Veterinary Consult: Canine and Feline Topics
• Bile Duct Obstruction
• Insulinoma
• Pancreatitis

Related Topics in This Book
• General Principles of Ultrasonography
• Abdominal Ultrasonography

ABBREVIATIONS
• fPLI = feline pancreatic lipase immunoreactivity
• Spec cPL = spec canine pancreatic lipase

Suggested Reading
Etue SM, Penninck DG, Labato MA, *et al.* Ultrasonography of the normal feline pancreas and associated anatomical landmarks:

A prospective study of 20 cats. *Vet Radiol Ultrasound* 2001; 42: 330–336.

Hess RS, Saunders HM, Van Winkle TJ, *et al.* Clinical, clinopathologic, radiographic, ultrasonographic abnormalities in dogs with fatal acute pancreatitis: 70 cases (1986–1995). *J Am Vet Med Assoc* 1998; 213: 665–670.

Lamb CR, Simpson KW, Boswood A, Matthewman LA. Ultrasonography of pancreatic neoplasia in the dog: A retrospective review of 16 cases. *Vet Rec* 1995; 137: 65–68.

Saunders HM, Van Winkle TJ, Kimmel SE, Washabau RJ. Ultrasonographic and radiographic findings in cats with clinical, necropsy, and histologic evidence of pancreatic necrosis: 20 cases (1994–2001). *J Am Vet Med Assoc* 2002; 221: 1724–1730.

INTERNET RESOURCES
None

AUTHOR NAME
H. Mark Saunders

BASICS

TYPE OF SPECIMEN
Blood

TEST EXPLANATION AND RELATED PHYSIOLOGY
Parathyroid hormone (PTH) is a polypeptide hormone that acts to maintain the ionized calcium (iCa) concentration within physiologically normal limits. PTH is secreted by the chief cells in the parathyroid gland in response to decreased concentrations of plasma iCa. PTH is inactivated by Kupffer cells in the liver and, to a lesser extent, in the bone and kidney. iCa levels exert a negative feedback effect on the secretion of PTH. Active vitamin D (calcitriol) also inhibits PTH secretion. High phosphorus (P) levels indirectly promote the release of PTH by decreasing calcitriol levels. PTH exerts its effect after binding to specific receptors in target tissues (i.e., bone, kidneys, intestine). PTH promotes the mobilization of bone Ca and P stores, increases intestinal absorption of Ca (potentiated by calcitriol), and decreases urinary excretion of Ca by increasing Ca resorption in the renal tubules. PTH decreases serum P concentrations by inhibiting P resorption in the renal tubules; thus, the net effect of PTH on P is to reduce plasma P values. PTH promotes the conversion of inactive vitamin D to active vitamin D (calcitriol) by increasing the release of the converting enzyme 1α-hydroxylase from renal tubular cells.

PTH must be interpreted in light of contemporaneous total calcium (tCa) and iCa values, as well as P values. Primary hyperparathyroidism (HPTH) is a disorder characterized by autonomous production of PTH from hyperplastic/adenomatous parathyroid glandular tissue with resultant increases in plasma tCa and iCa values; decreased P levels are expected if there is an adequate glomerular filtration rate. Primary HPTH is found mainly in dogs; however, cats are infrequently affected. Secondary HPTH is characterized by elevated levels of PTH released by normal parathyroid tissue in response to decreased plasma tCa and iCa caused by renal failure or inadequate nutrition. P levels are elevated with renal failure but can be either increased or decreased with nutritional deficiencies. In a small subset of dogs and cats with renal failure, low levels of calcitriol allow excessive PTH secretion, resulting in increases in both tCa and iCa levels. This is sometimes referred to as *tertiary hyperparathyroidism.*

Low levels of PTH can be seen with primary hypoparathyroidism, a condition characterized by inadequate production and secretion of PTH with resultant hypocalcemia and hyperphosphatemia. The few documented cases in dogs and cats are likely due to lymphocytic parathyroiditis or surgical removal of parathyroid tissue following thyroidectomy. Humoral hypercalcemia of malignancy (HHM) is a common disorder associated with overproduction of parathyroid hormone–related protein (PTH-rP) by neoplastic tissue. This causes the same Ca and P disturbances as primary HPTH, but, in this condition, persistent hypercalcemia suppresses secretion of PTH. In dogs, this is most often seen with lymphoma or an anal sac adenocarcinoma. In cats, lymphoma and squamous cell carcinomas are equally likely causes of HHM. Hypervitaminosis D can cause hypercalcemia; however, in contrast to primary HPTH, this disorder also causes hyperphosphatemia. PTH secretion is suppressed. Hypovitaminosis D can also cause hypocalcemia and hypophosphatemia, with a compensatory increase in PTH secretion.

MEASUREMENT OF PARATHYROID HORMONE
• A 2-point immunoradiometric assay (IRMA) for intact PTH is most widely used. Because of structural similarities in PTH from different species, the test designed for humans has also been validated for use with samples from dogs and cats. IRMA kits typically have 2 different antibodies targeting 2 different sites on the intact PTH molecule.

One antibody is specific for the midregion and C terminus of PTH, whereas the other antibody is specific for the N terminus of PTH.
• Another assay targets only 1 site of the PTH molecule: the N-terminal portion of the molecule. The N terminus is found mainly in intact (active) PTH with scant amounts of free (inactive) N-terminal fragments also detected by the assay. In healthy patients, the latter free fragments have a short half-life and are present in insignificant concentrations.
• PTH assays do not detect PTH-rP.

INDICATIONS
To help determine the cause of an abnormal blood Ca concentration

CONTRAINDICATIONS
None

POTENTIAL COMPLICATIONS
None

CLIENT EDUCATION
None

BODY SYSTEMS ASSESSED
Endocrine and metabolic

SAMPLE

COLLECTION
1.0–1.5 mL of venous blood

HANDLING
• Collect the sample into EDTA or a red-top tube; check with the lab about its preference. Protease inhibitors reduce proteolysis of PTH in EDTA plasma, but they are not widely used in practice.
• Centrifuge the sample promptly and separate serum or plasma from RBCs.
• Transfer the sample to plastic and freeze it.

STORAGE
Freeze the serum or plasma for storage.

STABILITY
• Refrigerated (4°C): at least 5 days
• Frozen (−20°C): several weeks

PROTOCOL
None

INTERPRETATION

NORMAL FINDINGS OR RANGE
• Dogs: 2–13 pmol/L
• Cats: 0–4 pmol/L
• Reference intervals may vary depending on the laboratory and the assay used.

ABNORMAL VALUES
• Hypoparathyroidism: PTH low or within the reference interval, with concurrent low iCa
• Hyperthyroidism: PTH >13 pmol/L (dogs) or >4 pmol/L (cats), with concurrent high iCa

CRITICAL VALUES
None

INTERFERING FACTORS
Drugs That May Alter Results or Interpretation
Drugs That Interfere with Test Methodology
None known

PARATHYROID HORMONE

Drugs That Alter Physiology
Substances that cause elevated plasma Ca (IV administration of Ca gluconate or vitamin D) or inhibit osteoclastic resorption of bone (e.g., bisphosphonates) may indirectly affect PTH levels in healthy patients.

Disorders That May Alter Results
• Lipemia or hemolysis
• Renal failure may significantly affect results of assays other than 2-point IRMA or 1-point N-terminal assays.

Collection Techniques or Handling That May Alter Results
Delayed serum or plasma separation, or improper storage allowing proteolysis of PTH

Influence of Signalment
Species
Primary HPTH is much more common in dogs than in cats.

Breed
• There is an increased incidence of canine primary HPTH in Labrador retrievers, German shepherds, keeshonds, shih tzus, golden retrievers, cocker spaniels, Rhodesian ridgebacks, Australian shepherds, Doberman pinschers, poodles, and springer spaniels.
• Primary hypoparathyroidism has been most frequently reported in poodles, miniature schnauzers, retrievers, German shepherds, and terriers.

Age
Primary HPTH is most common in dogs that are >7 years old.

Gender
None

Pregnancy
The exact mechanism of puerperal tetany in small dogs is unclear but may be related to relatively insufficient PTH production or may be due to an inadequate response of PTH receptors.

LIMITATIONS OF THE TEST
• PTH values cannot be fully interpreted without at least knowing the values of concurrent tCa, iCa, and P values.
• Equivocal results are possible. PTH values may be within the reference interval despite a parathyroid disorder and Ca/P homeostasis disturbance.

Sensitivity, Specificity, and Positive and Negative Predictive Values
N/A

Valid If Run in a Human Lab?
Yes.

Causes of Abnormal Findings

	High values			Low values		
		[iCa]	[P]		[iCa]	[P]
Primary HPTH		↑	↓	HMM	↑	↓
Renal 2° HPTH		↓	↑	Primary hypoparathyroidism	↓	↑
Renal 3° HPTH		↑	↑	Excess vitamin D[b]	↑	↑
Nutritional 2° HPTH		↓	↓ or ↑	Canine hypoadrenocorticism[a,b]	↑	↑
Hypomagnesemia[a,b] (impaired PTH receptor)		↓	↑			

2°, secondary; 3°, tertiary; ↓, below the reference interval; and ↑, above the reference interval.
[a] Mechanisms not well documented.
[b] Uncommon cause.
The PTH, Ca, and P concentrations depicted are typical expectations for each disorder, although exceptions and inconclusive results are possible.

CLINICAL PERSPECTIVE
• In conditions associated with abnormal PTH secretion (or secretion of PTH-rP), there may be inverse changes in Ca and P concentrations.
• If the PTH value is low, with concurrent hypercalcemia and hypophosphatemia, PTH-rP values should be evaluated to rule out HHM.
• If the PTH value is above the reference interval, with concurrent hypercalcemia and hypophosphatemia, then consider primary HPTH.
• If the PTH value is above the reference interval, with concurrent hypocalcemia and hyperphosphatemia, then consider renal (or possibly nutritional) secondary HPTH.
• If the PTH value is decreased or low normal, with concurrent hypocalcemia, then consider primary hypoparathyroidism (destruction of the parathyroid glands).
• If the tCa, iCa, and P values are all elevated, rule out renal failure and vitamin D toxicity.

MISCELLANEOUS

ANCILLARY TESTS
• PTH-rP, tCa, iCa, and P should be evaluated concurrently with PTH such that the values are interpreted with respect to one another at a given point in time.
• A vitamin D assay should be performed to rule out toxicosis if PTH is low with increased iCa and P values. Vitamin D values may be secondarily elevated in cases of primary HPTH or HMM; however, in the latter 2 situations, the plasma P levels are expected to be low.
• With hypercalcemia in a dog, a careful rectal exam is recommended to rule out an anal sac adenocarcinoma.
• Cytologic and/or biopsy specimens and bone marrow aspiration are recommended to rule out neoplastic causes of HMM.
• Serum BUN, creatinine, and urine specific gravity should be evaluated to rule out renal failure as a cause of secondary HPTH.
• The nutritional Ca/P ratio should be evaluated to rule out poor nutrition as a cause of secondary HPTH.
• Ultrasonography of the neck is recommended to evaluate parathyroid gland size (nonspecific).
• The parathyroid gland should be evaluated histologically, if indicated.

SYNONYMS
PTH

SEE ALSO
Blackwell's Five-Minute Veterinary Consult: Canine and Feline Topics
• Hypercalcemia
• Hyperparathyroidism
• Hyperparathyroidism, Renal Secondary
• Hyperphosphatemia
• Hypocalcemia
• Hypoparathyroidism

Related Topics in This Book
• Calcium
• Calcitriol
• Magnesium
• Parathyroid-Related Protein
• Phosphorus

ABBREVIATIONS
• Ca = calcium
• HHM = humoral hypercalcemia of malignancy
• HPTH = hyperparathyroidism
• iCa = ionized calcium
• IRMA = immunoradiometric assay
• P = phosphorus
• PTH = parathyroid hormone
• PTH-rP = parathyroid hormone–related protein
• tCa = total calcium

Suggested Reading
Feldman EC, Nelson RW. Hypercalcemia and primary hyperparathyroidism. In: *Canine and Feline Endocrinology and Reproduction*, 3rd ed. St Louis: Saunders Elsevier, 2004: 659–715.
Feldman EC, Nelson RW. Hypocalcemia and primary hypoparathyroidism. In: *Canine and Feline Endocrinology and Reproduction*, 3rd ed. St Louis: Saunders Elsevier, 2004: 716–742.
Rosol TJ, Chew DJ, Nagode LA, Schenck PA. Disorders of calcium: Hypercalcemia and hypocalcemia. In: Dibartola SP, ed. *Fluid Therapy in Small Animal Practice*, 2nd ed. Philadelphia: WB Saunders, 2000: 108–162.
Torrance AG, Nachreiner R. Human-parathormone assay for use in dogs: Validation, sample handling studies, and parathyroid function testing. *Am J Vet Res* 1989; 50: 1123–1127.

INTERNET RESOURCES
Kimball's Biology Pages: The parathyroid glands, http://users.rcn.com/jkimball.ma.ultranet/BiologyPages/T/Thyroid.html#parathyroid.

AUTHOR NAME
Ryan M. Dickinson

BASICS

TYPE OF SPECIMEN
Blood

TEST EXPLANATION AND RELATED PHYSIOLOGY
Parathyroid hormone–related protein (PTH-rP) is a peptide with a similar N-terminal structure and similar function to PTH. Typically, plasma PTH-rP levels are very low or nondetectable in healthy adults. Unlike PTH, PTH-rP is not formed in the parathyroid gland. It is formed, as needed, in various tissues throughout the body. PTH-rP governs fetal calcium homeostasis and, in adults, functions in a paracrine manner (examples: lactation; tooth eruption). An elevated plasma PTH-rP level is an abnormality attributed to inappropriate and excessive production of the molecule by certain tumors such as lymphoma (especially T-cell lymphoma), anal sac apocrine gland carcinoma, mammary carcinoma, and thyroid carcinoma. The PTH-rP molecule activates the PTH receptor and, when PTH-rP levels are increased, the disorder [termed *humoral hypercalcemia of malignancy* (HHM)] can mimic primary hyperparathyroidism (HPTH). Like primary HPTH, HHM is characterized by hypercalcemia via bone resorption and renal resorption of calcium, along with hypophosphatemia via inhibition of phosphorus resorption in renal tubules. The resultant hypercalcemia suppresses PTH release from the parathyroid gland. PTH-rP production by tumor cells is not a consistent finding, and the effect of PTH-rP may be potentiated by cytokines produced by the tumor cells. In any case, HHM associated with such tumors can occur suddenly. Patients with humoral hypercalcemia of malignancy may be intermittently hypercalcemic. Renal failure may be associated with mild elevations in PTH-rP in the absence of a malignancy.

A 2-point immunoradiometric assay used for human patients has been validated for dogs. An N-terminal radioimmunoassay is also available. PTH-rP assays do not detect PTH. Concurrent assays for iCa and PTH are recommended.

INDICATIONS
To aid in determination of the cause of an elevated iCa concentration, especially when a neoplastic etiology is suspected

CONTRAINDICATIONS
None

POTENTIAL COMPLICATIONS
None

CLIENT EDUCATION
Patients should be fasted for 8–12 h prior to sample collection.

BODY SYSTEMS ASSESSED
Endocrine and metabolic

SAMPLE

COLLECTION
1.0–1.5 mL of venous blood

HANDLING
- Collect the sample into an EDTA tube.
- Centrifuge and separate the plasma within 15 min of collection.
- Transfer the sample to a plastic tube and freeze it.
- Ship the frozen plasma with ice packs.

STORAGE
Store the specimen in a freezer.

STABILITY
Frozen (−20°C): several weeks

PROTOCOL
None

INTERPRETATION

NORMAL FINDINGS OR RANGE
- A PTH-rP of <1.0 pmol/L
- Reference intervals may vary depending on the laboratory and assay used.

ABNORMAL VALUES
A PTH-rP of >1.0 pmol/L. This should correlate with hypercalcemia.

CRITICAL VALUES
None

INTERFERING FACTORS
Drugs That May Alter Results or Interpretation
Drugs That Interfere with Test Methodology
None

Drugs That Alter Physiology
None

Disorders That May Alter Results
Lipemia or hemolysis

Collection Techniques or Handling That May Alter Results
- Delayed separation of EDTA plasma from erythrocytes
- Prolonged or improper storage allows proteolysis of PTH-rP.

Influence of Signalment
Species
None

Breed
None

Age
There is an increased incidence of PTH-rP–secreting neoplasms in older animals.

Gender
None

Pregnancy
None

LIMITATIONS OF THE TEST
Sensitivity, Specificity, and Positive and Negative Predictive Values
N/A

Valid If Run in a Human Lab?
Yes, if the assay has been validated for dogs.

Causes of Abnormal Results

High values	Low values
HHM	No clinical significance
Anal sac adenocarcinoma (dogs)	
Lymphoma (dogs and cats)	
Squamous cell carcinoma (cats)	
Other miscellaneous neoplasms	
Renal failure	

CLINICAL PERSPECTIVE
- PTH-rP levels are typically sought in animals with unexplained hypercalcemic.
- In hypercalcemic dogs with a diagnosis of lymphoma or anal sac adenocarcinoma, a PTH-rP assay is not necessary.

- It is important to consider other causes of hypercalcemia and to know that other tumors may cause hypercalcemia via mechanisms other than PTH-rP secretion.
- Patients with humoral hypercalcemia of malignancy may be intermittently hypercalcemic.
- Like PTH, PTH-rP promotes hypercalcemia. If the glomerular filtration rate is adequate, hypophosphatemia is promoted.
- PTH values are expected to be low in cases of PTH-rP–mediated hypercalcemia, but there are exceptions.

MISCELLANEOUS

ANCILLARY TESTS
- Concurrent iCa, phosphorus, and PTH are optimally evaluated along with PTH-rP.
- Vitamin D assay is recommended to rule out toxicosis if there is hypercalcemia, hyperphosphatemia, and low PTH and PTH-rP.
- Imaging, fine-needle aspiration, and/or biopsy can be used to detect and define a tumor in the body.
- BUN and/or creatinine concentration and urine specific gravity should be evaluated to rule out renal failure as a potential cause of elevated PTH-rP.

SYNONYMS
None

SEE ALSO
Blackwell's Five-Minute Veterinary Consult: Canine and Feline Topics
- Anal Sac Disorders
- Hypercalcemia
- Lymphoma—Cats
- Lymphoma—Dogs

Related Topics in This Book
- Calcitriol
- Calcium

- Parathyroid Hormone
- Phosphorus

ABBREVIATIONS
- HHM = humoral hypercalcemia of malignancy
- HPTH = hyperparathyroidism
- iCa = ionized calcium
- PTH = parathyroid hormone
- PTH-rP = parathyroid hormone–related protein

Suggested Reading
Blind E, Raue F, Meinel T, *et al.* Levels of parathyroid hormone–related protein in hypercalcemia of malignancy: Comparison of midregional radioimmunoassay and two-site immunoradiometric assay. *Clin Invest* 1993; 71: 31–36.
Feldman EC, Nelson RW. Hypercalcemia and primary hyperparathyroidism. In: *Canine and Feline Endocrinology and Reproduction*, 3rd ed. St Louis: Saunders Elsevier, 2004: 668–673.
Hutchesson AC, Hughes SC, Bowden SJ, Ratcliffe WA. In vitro stability of endogenous parathyroid hormone–related protein in blood and plasma. *Ann Clin Biochem* 1994; 31: 35–39.
Orloff JJ, Soifer NE, Fodero JP, *et al.* Accumulation of carboxy-terminal fragments of parathyroid hormone–related protein in renal failure. *Kidney Int* 1993; 43: 1371–1376.
Stockham SI, Scott MA. Calcium, phosphorus, magnesium, and their regulatory hormones. In: *Fundamentals of Veterinary Clinical Pathology*. Ames: Iowa State Press, 2002: 403–412.

INTERNET RESOURCES
Colorado State University, Hypertexts for Biomedical Sciences, Pathophysiology of the Endocrine System: Parathyroid hormone–related protein, http://www.vivo.colostate.edu/hbooks/pathphys/endocrine/thyroid/phrp.html.

AUTHOR NAME
Ryan M. Dickinson

PARTIAL THROMBOPLASTIN TIME, ACTIVATED

BASICS

TYPE OF SPECIMEN
Blood

TEST EXPLANATION AND RELATED PHYSIOLOGY
The activated partial thromboplastin time (aPTT) is a functional test of the intrinsic and common coagulation pathways. The aPTT *result* is the clotting time (in seconds) of an assay mixture containing a reagent that specifically initiates coagulation through activation of factor XII. The assay measures the enzyme or coenzyme activity of the intrinsic system factors (factors VIII, IX, XI, and XII), common system factors (factors II, V, and X) and is sensitive to a severe deficiency or inhibition of fibrinogen. Possible explanations for prolonged aPTT include intrinsic and common pathway factor deficiencies, coagulation inhibitors, and anticoagulant therapy. Coagulation inhibitors can be specific for 1 or more factors or nonspecific.

Specific coagulation inhibitors are primarily immunoglobulins directed against 1 or more antigenic sites on a specific coagulation factor. They usually develop in association with immune-mediated disease (e.g., systemic lupus erythematosus), with lymphoproliferative diseases, or after transfusion (i.e., alloimmunization). Nonspecific coagulation inhibitors include animal venoms, FDP, and plasma expanders that act via impairment or interference with factor activity and fibrin cross-linkage. The *lupus anticoagulant* refers to autoantibodies directed against phospholipid-binding proteins. In vitro, these antibodies prolong the aPTT; however, lupus anticoagulants are associated with the development of thrombosis in patients with immune disorders.

The aPTT assay end point of fibrin formation is detected as a change in light transmittance (by photoptical instruments) or viscoelasticity (by mechanical instruments).

INDICATIONS
- Screening test to detect coagulation factor deficiencies
- Assessing animals with acute or chronic hemorrhage, especially body-cavity bleeding, large hematoma, and/or hemorrhage into joints
- Screening test to detect coagulation inhibitors
- Monitoring unfractionated heparin (UFH) therapy

CONTRAINDICATIONS
None

POTENTIAL COMPLICATIONS
None

CLIENT EDUCATION
Blood coagulation is a complex process, and a combination of tests is often required for a comprehensive assessment of coagulation.

BODY SYSTEMS ASSESSED
Hemic, lymphatic, and immune

SAMPLE

COLLECTION
1.8 mL of venous blood

HANDLING
- Collect blood directly into sodium citrate (3.2% or 3.8%) anticoagulant.
- Combine exactly 1.8 mL of blood with exactly 0.2 mL of citrate; an exact ratio of blood to citrate (9 parts:1 part) is critical for valid results.
- Within 1 h of collection, perform point-of-care coagulation tests or centrifuge whole blood and transfer plasma into plastic or siliconized glass tube (without additives).

STORAGE
- Store in a refrigerator for assay within 4 h.
- Store in a freezer if assayed >4 h after collection.
- Ship overnight on cold packs.

STABILITY
- Room temperature: 1 h
- Refrigerated (2°–8°C): 4 h
- Frozen (−20°C): 2 weeks

PROTOCOL
None

INTERPRETATION

NORMAL FINDINGS OR RANGE
- Dogs: 10–17 s
- Cats: 14–18 s
- Reference values are from the Comparative Coagulation Section of the Cornell University Animal Health Diagnostic Center, but values significantly vary based on the choice of reagent and clot detection method.

ABNORMAL VALUES
- Shortening of the aPTT has little clinical relevance and often results from improper sampling technique that causes ex vivo factor activation.
- Prolongation of the aPTT beyond the reference range, or 1.5-fold greater than same-species control, is abnormal.

CRITICAL VALUES
The correlation between relative prolongation of aPTT and in vivo hemostatic failure varies for different disease syndromes and underlying causes of long aPTT. In general, combined mild to moderate deficiencies of several factors cause longer clotting times in the aPTT than does moderate deficiency of a single factor. Factor XII deficiency, and other contact group factor deficiencies, causes marked prolongation of aPTT, but does not cause a bleeding tendency.

INTERFERING FACTORS
Drugs That May Alter Results or Interpretation
Drugs That Interfere with Test Methodology
Oxyglobin [hemoglobin glutamer-200 (bovine); Biopure, Cambridge, MA] may interfere with end-point determination in photoptical, but not mechanical, clot-detection instruments.

Drugs That Alter Physiology
- Treatment with anticoagulant drugs may prolong aPTT.
- Therapeutic monitoring of UFH is based on attaining a target prolongation of aPTT. Prolongation of aPTT to 1.5–2.0 times the patient's baseline value is a generally accepted target for high-dose UFH therapy. Less commonly, the target aPTT is based on a heparin sensitivity curve supplied by the testing laboratory. The sensitivity curve relates clotting times in the aPTT throughout a range of heparin concentrations.
- Therapeutic levels of coumadin or low molecular weight heparins are monitored by measuring prothrombin time (PT) and factor Xa inhibition, respectively.

Disorders That May Alter Results
Severe hemolysis or lipemia may interfere with end-point determination in photoptical clot-detection instruments. These conditions do not interfere with fibrometer or mechanical end-point determinations.

Collection Techniques or Handling That May Alter Results
Appropriate sample collection techniques are critical for valid aPTT (and other clotting-time test) results. Sodium citrate must be used as an anticoagulant.

- Artifactual prolongation of aPTT results from blood collection into heparin (green top), EDTA (purple top), plain glass (red top) tubes, or into tubes containing a serum separator with clot activator.
- Inaccurate results are caused by excess or insufficient citrate anticoagulant due to high or low Hct (hemotocrit) or if insufficient blood is drawn.
- Poor venipuncture technique can alter results by causing ex vivo factor activation.
- Collection from an IV catheter can contaminate samples with heparin.

Influence of Signalment

Species
Factor XII deficiency (Hageman trait) is common in cats but rare in dogs.

Breed
- Factor XII deficiency (Hageman trait) is an autosomal recessive trait and has been reported in DSH, Siamese, and Himalayan cats, sharpeis, and miniature poodles.
- Factor XI deficiency has been reported in DSH cats, Kerry blue terriers, and springer spaniels.
- Inherited vitamin K–dependent factor deficiency has been reported as an autosomal recessive trait in Devon rex cats and as a congenital defect in a Labrador retrievers. All vitamin K–dependent factors (II, VII, IX, and X) are affected.

Age
None

Gender
Hemophilia A (factor VIII deficiency) and hemophilia B (factor IX deficiency) are both X-linked recessive traits and therefore much more common in male dogs and cats than in females.

Pregnancy
None

LIMITATIONS OF THE TEST
The sensitivity (and specificity) of aPTT varies in different assay/reagent systems. In general, aPTT prolongation is not observed unless factor activities fall below 30%–40%. Milder reductions in factor activity can be detected if multiple factors are deficient.

Sensitivity, Specificity, and Positive and Negative Predictive Values
N/A

Valid If Run in a Human Lab?
Yes—but interpretation of aPTT results requires same-species reference range. Human aPTT values are generally twice those of dogs and cats.

Causes of Abnormal Values

High values (prolonged aPTT)	Low values
Acquired factor deficiencies	Not clinically significant
Vitamin K deficiency (e.g., malabsorption, maldigestion, chronic oral antibiotics)	
Coumadin therapy (overdosage beyond target therapeutic range)	
Cholestatic disease	
Liver failure	
Anticoagulant rodenticide ingestion (e.g., vitamin K antagonism)	
Thromboembolic disease (local or disseminated; factor consumption)	
Heparin therapy	
Hereditary factor deficiencies (trait)	
Factor VIII deficiency (hemophilia A): most common hereditary coagulopathy; any breed and sporadic cases, X-linked recessive	
Factor IX deficiency (hemophilia B): any breed; sporadic cases, X-linked recessive	
Factor XI deficiency: DSH cats, Kerry blue terriers, and springer spaniels	
Factor XII deficiency (Hageman trait): DSH, Siamese, and Himalayan cats, sharpeis, and miniature poodles; not associated with a bleeding tendency	
Vitamin K–dependent factor deficiency: Devon rex cats, Labrador retrievers; combined prolongation of aPTT and PT	
Contact factor: prekallikrein and kininogen deficiencies cause long in vitro clotting time in the aPTT; not associated with a bleeding tendency	
Acquired inhibitors of coagulation	
Antibodies against coagulation factors	
Increased FDPs	
Snake venom	
Lupus anticoagulant (not associated with bleeding)	

PARTIAL THROMBOPLASTIN TIME, ACTIVATED

CLINICAL PERSPECTIVE
- Differentials for specific prolongation of aPTT include intrinsic factor deficiency, therapeutic UFH levels, and coagulation inhibitors such as the lupus anticoagulant and FDP.
- Disease conditions that prolong aPTT and additional coagulation screening tests (see the Ancillary Tests section) include liver disease, vitamin K deficiency, drug overdose or toxin, and disseminated intravascular coagulation.
- The clinical significance of long aPTT should be interpreted in the context of clinical presentation and the results of other tests of hemostasis. Inappropriate sampling techniques invalidate aPTT results.
- Mild to moderate deficiencies in factor VIII or IX (5%–15% of normal) are considered mild hemophilia, with clinical signs apparent primarily after surgery or injury. Severe and spontaneous hemorrhage is seen in hemophiliacs with severe (<1%) factor activity. In contrast to hemophilia, patients with factor XII deficiency (Hageman trait) do not express a bleeding tendency, regardless of their residual factor XII activity.

MISCELLANEOUS

ANCILLARY TESTS
- The workup of any patient with unexplained bleeding should include measurement of the PT and thrombin clotting time (TCT) (or fibrinogen) screening tests, in addition to aPTT.
- The pattern of abnormalities in coagulation screening tests varies for different disease conditions:
  - Specific prolongation of aPTT is an indication of an intrinsic system defect. A definitive diagnosis is made by specific factor assay.
  - Specific prolongation of PT indicates factor VII deficiency.
  - Combined prolongation of aPTT and PT indicates a common pathway or multifactor deficiency such as liver disease.
  - Prolongation of aPTT and PT (with normal TCT and fibrinogen) is often caused by vitamin K deficiency.
  - Prolongation of aPTT, PT, and TCT (with low fibrinogen) is most often caused by severe liver failure or hemorrhagic disseminated intravascular coagulation.

SYNONYMS
Activated partial thromboplastin time (aPPT)

SEE ALSO
Blackwell's Five-Minute Veterinary Consult: Canine and Feline Topics
- Chapters on hepatic diseases
- Anticoagulant Rodenticide Poisoning
- Disseminated Intravascular Coagulation

Related Topics in This Book
- Anticoagulant Screen
- Coagulation Factors
- Prothrombin Time

ABBREVIATIONS
- aPPT = partial thromboplastin time, activated
- DIC = disseminated intravascular coagulation
- DSH = domestic shorthair
- FDP = fibrin and fibrinogen degradation products
- PT = prothrombin time
- TCT = thrombin clotting time
- UFH = unfractionated heparin

Suggested Reading
Kitchen S, Jennings I, Woods TA, Preston FE. Wide variability in the sensitivity of APTT reagents for monitoring of heparin dosage. *J Clin Pathol* 1996; **49**: 10–14.
Mischke R, Nolte IJA. Hemostasis: Introduction, overview, laboratory techniques. In: Feldman BF, Zinkl JG, Jain NC, eds. *Schalm's Veterinary Hematology*, 5th ed. Baltimore: Lippincott Williams & Wilkins, 2000: 519–525.
Stokol TS, Brooks MB, Erb HN. Effect of citrate concentration on coagulation test results in dogs. *J Am Vet Med Assoc* 2000; **217**: 1672–1677.

INTERNET RESOURCES
Cornell University, College of Veterinary Medicine, Department of Population Medicine and Diagnostic Sciences: Comparative coagulation, http://www.diaglab.vet.cornell.edu/coag/clinical/diagnos.asp.
Massachusetts General Hospital, Pathology Service: Activated partial thromboplastin time, http://www.massgeneral.org/pathology/coagbook/CO003400.htm.

AUTHOR NAME
Marjory Brooks

BASICS

TYPE OF PROCEDURE
Diagnostic sample collection

PROCEDURE EXPLANATION AND RELATED PHYSIOLOGY
Pericardiocentesis (PC) is both a diagnostic and a therapeutic procedure undertaken to relieve cardiac compression caused by pericardial effusion (PE). PE may be neoplastic, idiopathic, traumatic, infectious, inflammatory, hemorrhagic, or metabolic in origin, or may result from late-stage CHF. Chronic PE typically produces gradual onset of clinical signs (weakness, right-sided CHF) and a classically globoid cardiac silhouette radiographically. Acute PE tends to cause rapid onset of clinical signs (collapse, cardiogenic shock, sudden death) and subtle radiographic changes.

Cardiac tamponade is hemodynamic instability (cardiogenic shock) resulting from PE and occurs when effusion is sufficient to substantially elevate the intrapericardial pressure; the latter may exceed diastolic intracardiac pressures. This may be observed echocardiographically as partial collapse of the right heart in diastole, particularly the right atrium. Cardiac tamponade is characterized clinically by signs of shock and generally necessitates emergency PC. Tamponade also enhances ventricular interdependence dramatically, whereby 1 ventricle fills at the expense of the other, and causes pulsus paradoxus, a palpable decrease in peripheral pulse pressure that occurs on inspiration. It is the intrapericardial pressure, not the effusion volume per se, that determines clinical and hemodynamic severity. Typically, medical therapies are relatively contraindicated (an exception is PE secondary to CHF), and PC may be necessary to stabilize the patient prior to surgery if the latter is contemplated.

INDICATIONS
- PE producing clinical signs due to cardiac compression
- Obtain a sample of PE for diagnostic analysis if a sufficient amount of PE is present such that the risk of PC is acceptable. Cytologic evaluation of PE is usually nondiagnostic.

CONTRAINDICATIONS
- An insufficient volume of PE such that the risk of PC outweighs a potential benefit (the less proficient the operator, the greater the risk)
- Relative contraindications may include hemorrhagic PE secondary to bleeding disorders or endocardial splitting where the concern is that relieving pericardial pressure may perpetuate hemorrhage.
- Not indicated for distention of the pericardium by solid tumors or abdominal contents (peritoneal-pericardial diaphragmatic hernia)

POTENTIAL COMPLICATIONS
- Puncture of cardiac chambers or great vessels; cardiac dysrhythmia, including life-threatening ventricular tachycardia; coronary laceration causing myocardial ischemia or infarction; exsanguination; death; pulmonary laceration or hemorrhage; pneumothorax; failure to relieve cardiac tamponade or obtain a diagnostic PE sample; or infection
- Complications are minimized by careful preparation and technique.
- Exsanguination is more likely to occur from failure to confirm the correct catheter position resulting in evacuation of blood from a ventricular chamber by the operator than from ventricular puncture.
- Subsequent constrictive or effusive-constrictive pericardial disease may be a late complication of PC.

CLIENT EDUCATION
- Clients should be informed of potential risks and complications of the procedure that relate not only to the skill of the operator, but also to the cause of the PE, which may not be known at the time of PC. Hemangiosarcoma is a common cause of PE with a poor average long-term prognosis regardless of the result of the procedure. PC also

may exacerbate hemorrhage of a large, friable tumor and may worsen tamponade or precipitate cardiopulmonary arrest.
- Effusions may recur in the near future or far future. Recurrences are cause dependent and difficult to predict.

BODY SYSTEMS ASSESSED
Cardiovascular

PROCEDURE

PATIENT PREPARATION
Preprocedure Medication or Preparation
- Medical treatment prior to emergency PC is relatively contraindicated (e.g., diuretics may be detrimental). The more debilitated the patient is, the greater is the need for the procedure.
- Specific therapies for underlying causes and conditions (e.g., rapid fluid administration for hemorrhage, antibiotics for sepsis) may be administered concurrently during rapid preparation for PC.
- An IV catheter facilitates sedation and treatment of emergent dysrhythmia.
- Echocardiographic diagnosis of small cardiac tumors may be facilitated by the presence of PE. Ultrasound examination of the heart should precede PC if the patient is stable.

Anesthesia or Sedation
- Recommendations are operator dependent and not universally endorsed among cardiovascular specialists.
- The author prefers combination IV sedation and analgesia with diazepam (0.2 mg/kg) and butorphanol (0.2 mg/kg) or with diazepam (0.2 mg/kg) and oxymorphone (0.1 mg/kg). Avoid agents promoting hypotension (e.g., acepromazine).

Patient Positioning
- The author prefers left lateral recumbency to facilitate directing the PC catheter toward the right ventral caudal aspect of the heart. This positioning applies to typical effusions, but the possibility exists of localized PE that is not accessible from this approach.
- Some specialists prefer ventral recumbency. In this position, a long catheter may necessitate positioning the patient near the edge of the operating table to enable proper angulation toward the ventral aspect of the heart from below the table surface.

Patient Monitoring
- ECG monitoring is essential.
- It may be valuable to determine the hematocrit of presumed PE during the procedure for comparison with peripheral blood because PE often appears similar and it is essential to confirm that the PC catheter is not in a cardiac chamber.

Equipment or Supplies (Figure 1)
- A large-bore, over-the-needle catheter is typically used: 18–14 gauge, 2–5$^1/_2$ inches (5.08–13.97 cm), depending on patient size.
- Small (3 mL) and large (10–50 mL) syringes, 3-way stopcock, extension tubing, collection tubes or apparatus for cytologic evaluation (EDTA) and culture submission, no. 10 and no. 11 surgical blades, and sterile surgical gloves
- 2% lidocaine for local anesthesia and for treatment of ventricular arrhythmias

TECHNIQUE
- The patient is sedated, positioned as already described, and gently restrained by an assistant. The default catheter entry location is at the intercostal space 5–7 of the right ventral thorax, at the level of the costal-chondral junction. The hair is clipped liberally here, and the suitability of the site is confirmed by using ultrasound. The transducer is twisted 90° to verify positioning in both perpendicular planes so that the greatest amount of PE is between the catheter and heart.

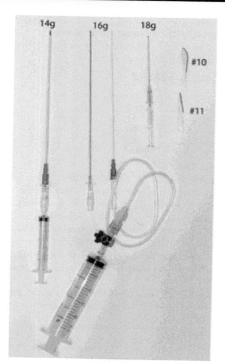

Figure 1

Instrumentation used for PC. A 14-gauge, $5^1/_2$-inch (13.97 cm) catheter and stylus are shown with a small syringe attached; i.e., configured to advance into the pericardial space. The sharp metal stylus is removed after the catheter is fully positioned, as demonstrated for the 16-gauge, $5^1/_2$-inch (13.97 cm) catheter, and an extension tube attached to the catheter for aspiration using a larger syringe and 3-way stopcock. An 18-gauge, 2-inch (5.08 cm) catheter is used for cats and similarly sized dogs. A no. 11 blade is ideal for creating a small stab incision at the entry site. The author uses a no. 10 blade to cut side holes in the distal end of the larger catheters (optional).

The operator plans for the catheter to intersect the pericardium at its ventral-lateral aspect, so the catheter is usually advanced dorsally and cranially; i.e., toward the opposite scapula (Figure 2). This technique leads to an oblique intersection of the catheter and pericardium, effectively increasing the "size" of the pericardial space; i.e., the distance in the direction of catheter advancement before reaching the heart. Avoidance of lung and dorsal cardiac structures (atria and great vessels) is confirmed (Figure 3).
• After a preliminary scrub, the site is infiltrated deeply with lidocaine (0.5–3.0 mL, depending on patient size), with a 24- to 22-gauge needle advancing all the way to the pleural space, with continuous injection while the syringe is being withdrawn. Needle entry should be near the center of the rib space, erring toward the caudal side of the space, so as to avoid the intercostal vessels situated at the caudal aspect of the rib. Proximity of the flexible catheter to a rib may result in kinking and obstruction as the patient breathes. A no. 11 blade is used to create a small stab incision at the site of needle entry and serves also to mark the site. The aseptic preparation of the skin is complete. At this point in the procedure, additional palpation of the skin is neither advantageous nor desirable.
• Using aseptic technique, the gloved operator attaches a sterile 3-mL syringe to the PC catheter, positions the point of the catheter at the predetermined location, stabilizing it near the distal end with 1 hand, and orients the direction of the catheter with the other hand, positioned at the syringe. As soon as the catheter tip is through the skin, a small amount of suction is applied with the syringe; this serves

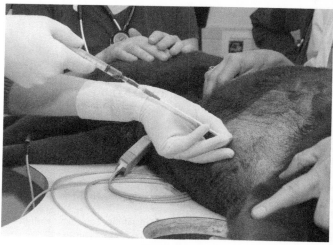

Figure 2

The photograph demonstrates catheter positioning and orientation for PC from the right ventral approach. While stabilizing the catheter near the entry point with 1 hand, the catheter is advanced cranially and dorsally with the other; i.e., toward the opposite scapula. A small degree of suction is maintained with the syringe so that pericardial fluid is aspirated at the moment of pericardial penetration. Subsequently, the syringe and stylet are held stationary while the flexible catheter is advanced well into the pericardium. The sharp metal stylet is withdrawn after the catheter is fully positioned.

a valuable sentinel function, ensuring that PE will be aspirated as soon as the catheter tip penetrates the pericardium. The entire apparatus is advanced linearly, in the predetermined direction only, with the proximal hand used both to advance the catheter and syringe and to apply mild suction. The ECG is monitored closely during this phase. A burst of ventricular premature complexes suggests that the catheter tip has contacted the epicardium and is cause to retract the catheter until the dysrhythmia abates. In contrast, contact of the catheter tip with the moving pericardium may impart a scratchy sensation to the catheter, which can alarm an inexperienced operator. There may be a sensation of popping through the pericardium with the catheter.
• When PE is aspirated, the catheter-stylus-syringe is advanced a short distance further (e.g., 2–4 mm), similar to catheterization of a peripheral vein. The hand closest to the animal stabilizes the syringe and stylus assembly while the other hand advances the flexible catheter off the stylus, well into the pericardial space. The distended pericardium may shrink substantially during the procedure, which will cause the catheter tip to exit the pericardial space if it is not advanced sufficiently. The metal catheter stylus is then fully withdrawn from the flexible over-the-needle portion. The operator stabilizes and repositions the latter for the rest of the procedure.
• Extension tubing is attached directly to the proximal catheter end, leading to a large syringe and interposed 3-way stopcock that is operated by an assistant. Typically, PE is grossly hemorrhagic in appearance, so it may be difficult to determine by inspection whether the fluid source is the pericardial space or blood from a cardiac chamber. If the cardiac rhythm is stable, there is adequate time to make this determination and it must be accurate. If the operator is reasonably certain of proper placement, then a small amount of presumptive PE (e.g., 5–20 mL) can be removed while the heart rate is observed on the ECG. With tamponade, even a small decompression of the pericardial space typically decreases heart rate demonstrably. A continual decrease in heart rate throughout the procedure is suggestive of correct catheter placement, whereas any trend toward increased heart rate should prompt the operator to suspend aspiration and reevaluate the

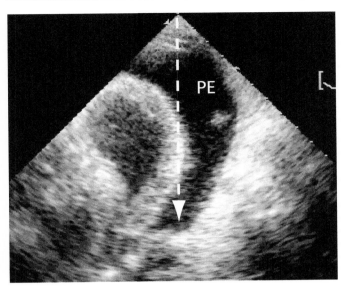

Figure 3

An echocardiograph acquired with the transducer at the same location and orientation (direction) as the catheter in Figure 2. The *dotted line* indicates structures encountered by the central ultrasound beam; i.e., in the path of the catheter. While this patient had a relatively small amount of pericardial effusion (PE), proper catheter positioning, orientation, and linear advancement minimize risk. Oblique orientation of the catheter, relative to the cardiac surface, increases the effective distance between the pericardium and heart.

catheter position. Other methods for confirming the source of hemorrhagic fluid include a hematocrit determination (PE should be clearly different from the peripheral blood, either increased or decreased, and supernatant is often xanthochromic) or clot determination (blood from a cardiac chamber clots quickly when placed in an appropriate collection tube; an activated clot-time collection tube containing diatomaceous material may be used). Once catheter tip positioning within the pericardial space is a certainty, PE can be evacuated rapidly by using the 3-way stopcock to alternately aspirate and expel PE into a collecting vessel.

• The author's preference is to evacuate the pericardial space as completely as possible (exceptions are atrial tear and bleeding disorder). Although this approach is not necessary for marked clinical improvement, in theory it maximizes the time interval before a subsequent PC and enables the clinician to best determine echocardiographically whether there has been additional effusion subsequent to the procedure. At some point during the procedure, it will become difficult to aspirate additional PE. This may be accompanied by a scratchy sensation transmitted to the catheter as it rubs against the pericardium and epicardium, ventricular dysrhythmias, or stuttering of the extension tubing caused by intermittent flow obstruction. As this occurs, the operator may slowly withdraw the catheter while the assistant maintains a small amount of suction with the syringe. Catheter withdrawal is paused at any location that results in additional aspiration of PE, and the process is repeated until the catheter is completely withdrawn. The catheter tip is inspected to assure that it is intact. The catheter may become obstructed during the procedure, so flushing with a small amount of heparinized saline may be beneficial, but excessive suction is not. The author routinely cuts 2 additional side holes near the catheter tip to help preclude catheter obstruction. At any time during the procedure, significant ventricular arrhythmias should prompt catheter repositioning, usually partial withdrawal, and consideration of treatment with an 2% lidocaine IV bolus (2–4 mg/kg = 1–2 mL/10 kg) if the dysrhythmia does not abate promptly.

• It is a common that the pericardial space is not evacuated entirely at the first attempt. If this occurs, subsequent attempts may be more difficult if the PE volume has been significantly reduced, and possibly unwarranted since marked clinical improvement may occur after removing a relatively small amount of PE. Furthermore, cardiac motion may continue to expel PE into the pleural space through a pericardial puncture, if present. The decision to attempt a subsequent PC is made on an individual basis.

• Prior to complete catheter withdrawal, chemotherapeutic or anti-inflammatory drugs are sometimes instilled into the pericardium after the majority of the contents have been aspirated. Drug choices depend on a definitive diagnosis prior to undertaking PC and are controversial. Water-soluble gas (e.g., carbon dioxide) may be instilled into the pericardial space for immediate radiographic examination (pneumopericardiography); the volume of gas should be less than the volume of PE removed.

SAMPLE HANDLING
Pericardial fluid of high cellularity is placed in EDTA for cytologic examination and then in suitable sterile transport media for microbiologic evaluation (bacterial and/or fungal).

APPROPRIATE AFTERCARE
Postprocedure Patient Monitoring
• In most cases, monitor patients for 12–24 h prior to their discharge. Monitoring should include heart rate, respiratory checks, and ECG, if available.
• Significant ventricular arrhythmias may develop.
• Iatrogenic pneumothorax is possible.
• Return of PE and clinical signs may be rapid if there is ongoing intrapericardial hemorrhage.

Nursing Care
None specific to PC. Other care may depend on the cause of PE.

Dietary Modification
N/A

Medication Requirements
• Ancillary medical treatments depend on the cause of the PE (e.g., neoplastic, infectious, idiopathic). Abdominal effusion stemming from tamponade-induced heart failure typically does not require the administration of diuretics or treatment other than PC.
• Fluid therapy if hemorrhagic PE causes hypovolemia

Restrictions on Activity
It is not known whether injudicious activity may hasten or precipitate the return of PE. Judicious exercise restriction may be warranted subsequent to PC.

Anticipated Recovery Time
PC typically produces dramatic and immediate improvement in hemodynamic parameters. However, dogs may remain somewhat subdued for 1–2 days.

 INTERPRETATION

NORMAL FINDINGS OR RANGE
N/A

ABNORMAL VALUES
• Cytologic evaluation of PE is notoriously nondiagnostic because the most common causes of PE—neoplasia and idiopathic ("benign") effusion—typically produce hemorrhagic effusions without identifiable cell types or features that differentiate the causative conditions. Unusual causes of PE that may be diagnosed cytologically include lymphoma, unusual tumors, and bacterial or fungal infections.

CRITICAL VALUES
• An increasing heart rate or clotting PE sample during PC. Check to ensure correct catheter placement.
• Ventricular tachycardia or more than occasional premature complexes. Reposition (partially withdraw) the catheter.

INTERFERING FACTORS
Drugs That May Alter Results of the Procedure
None

Conditions That May Interfere with Performing the Procedure
• A small (insufficient) volume of PE
• A bleeding disorder

Procedure Techniques or Handling That May Alter Results
None

Influence of Signalment on Performing and Interpreting the Procedure
Species
Cats and small dogs typically are more difficult subjects for PC because of the small size of their pericardial space.

Breed
N/A

Age
N/A

Gender
N/A

Pregnancy
N/A

CLINICAL PERSPECTIVE
• Significant clinical improvement can occur with removal of even a small volume of effusion.
• Hemodynamically significant PE requires PC.

MISCELLANEOUS

ANCILLARY TESTS
• Echocardiography may provide a definitive diagnosis at the time if an intrapericardial mass is clearly present.
• Cytologic and microbiologic examination of the PE
• Further evaluation may include CBC and biochemical analysis, evaluation for bleeding disorders, determination of toxoplasmosis titer (cats), thoracic radiographs and abdominal ultrasound in search of metastases, biopsy and histopathology, and thoracic exploration or thoroscopic surgery for partial pericardectomy.
• For dogs of typical signalment and without a visible mass on echocardiography, elevation in the level of serum cardiac troponin I suggests an increased probability of hemangiosarcoma.

SYNONYMS
None

SEE ALSO
Blackwell's Five-Minute Veterinary Consult: Canine and Feline Topics
• Anticoagulant Rodenticide Poisoning
• Atrial Wall Tear
• Chemodectoma
• Coccidioidomycosis
• Feline Infectious Peritonitis (FIP)
• Hemangiosarcoma, Spleen and Liver
• Myocardial Tumors
• Pericarditis

Related Topics in This Book
Troponins, Cardiac Specific

ABBREVIATIONS
• CHF = congestive heart failure
• PC = pericardiocentesis
• PE = pericardial effusion

Suggested Reading
Sisson D, Thomas WP. Pericardial disease and cardiac tumors. In: Fox PR, Sisson D, Moise NS, eds. *Textbook of Canine and Feline Cardiology,* 2nd ed. Philadelphia: WB Saunders, 1999: 400–425.
Smith FWK, Rush JE. Diagnosis and treatment of pericardial effusion. In: Bonagura J, ed. *Kirk's Current Veterinary Therapy XIII.* Philadelphia: WB Saunders, 2000: 772–777.
Tobias AH. Pericardial disorders. In: Ettinger SJ, Feldman EC, eds. *Textbook of Veterinary Internal Medicine,* 6th ed. St Louis: Saunders Elsevier, 2005: 1104–1118.

INTERNET RESOURCES
None

AUTHOR NAME
Donald J. Brown

BASICS

TYPE OF SPECIMEN
Blood

TEST EXPLANATION AND RELATED PHYSIOLOGY
Phosphorus, which is widely spread throughout the body, is a chief component of hydroxyapatite in bone and cellular membranes, found intracellularly and extracellularly, and is present in organic and inorganic forms. Within cells, significant amounts of phosphorus are in nucleic acids, phospholipids, phosphoproteins, and high-energy compounds (e.g., ATP). Phosphorus is an essential constituent of second messenger systems [e.g., cyclic adenosine monophosphate (cAMP)], is important for hemoglobin function through 2,3-diphosphoglycerate (2,3-DPG), and can act as a buffer for acid-base regulation.

Serum phosphorus is regulated through interactions with calcium, PTH, calcitonin, and vitamin D, and the kidneys, intestines, and bone. Phosphorus concentration is affected by dietary intake, renal excretion (which is enhanced by PTH), and calcium concentration, along with hormones that control calcium homeostasis. Calcitonin acts to increase renal excretion of phosphorus, and vitamin D promotes intestinal absorption. Rising phosphorus levels tend to decrease calcium concentrations directly through formation of calcium-phosphorus complexes that are deposited in soft tissues, and indirectly by inhibiting the renal enzyme responsible for the final step in vitamin D activation.

Phosphorus determination relies on a colorimetric method where phosphorus reacts with ammonium molybdate to form a complex. This complex reacts with an indicator substance to produce a colored product, the amount of which is proportional to the phosphorus concentration. Both organic and inorganic phosphorus compounds are present in blood, but common assays measure only inorganic phosphorus.

INDICATIONS
- Part of a routine biochemistry profile
- History and clinical signs associated with phosphorus imbalances generally reflect the underlying disease or condition rather than the serum abnormality.
- Animals with severe hypophosphatemia may exhibit the following:
  - Pallor and/or hemoglobinuria secondary to hemolytic anemia
  - Muscle weakness or pain associated with rhabdomyolysis
  - Depression; neurologic signs
  - Tachypnea, dyspenia, or shallow, rapid breathing because of hypoxia and/or compromised respiratory muscle function
  - Anorexia, vomiting, and nausea associated with intestinal ileus
- Animals with hyperphosphatemia may show signs of renal failure with or without uremia (e.g., polyuria-polydipsia, weight loss, anorexia, lethargy, vomiting, oral ulceration).
- Nonazotemic animals with hyperphosphatemia may show polyphagia, restlessness, and weight loss. If hyperphosphatemia is acute, the resulting hypocalcemia may cause tetany and/or animals may exhibit vascular collapse, or present with vomiting, bloody diarrhea, ataxia, and depression.

CONTRAINDICATIONS
None

POTENTIAL COMPLICATIONS
None

CLIENT EDUCATION
None

BODY SYSTEMS ASSESSED
- Endocrine and metabolic
- Hemic, lymphatic, and immune
- Gastrointestinal
- Musculoskeletal
- Neuromuscular
- Renal and urologic

SAMPLE

COLLECTION
1–2 mL of venous blood

HANDLING
- Collect the sample into red-top tube, serum-separator tube, or heparin (green top).
- Separate the serum (or plasma) from cells within 1 h of sample collection to avoid in vitro hemolysis.

STORAGE
- Separation from cells is recommended before the sample is stored.
- For short-term storage, refrigeration is recommended.
- For long-term storage, freezing is recommended.

STABILITY
- Refrigerated ($2°$–$8°$C): $\approx$1 week
- Frozen ($-20°$C): $\approx$6 months

PROTOCOL
None

INTERPRETATION

NORMAL FINDINGS OR RANGE
- Dogs: 2.9–5.3 mg/dL (0.94–1.71 mmol/L)
- Cats: 3.0–6.1 mg/dL (0.97–1.97 mmol/L)
- Reference intervals may vary depending on the laboratory and assay.

ABNORMAL VALUES
- Dogs: <2.9 or >5.3 mg/dL
- Cats: <3.0 or >6.1 mg/dL

CRITICAL VALUES
- Phosphorus concentration of <1.5 mg/dL (0.48 mmol/L): increased risk of hemolysis or neuromuscular dysfunction
- Phosphorus concentration of >10 mg/dL (3.23 mmol/L): increased risk of soft tissue mineralization when the [phosphorus] × [calcium] product exceeds 60–70

INTERFERING FACTORS
Drugs That May Alter Results or Interpretation
Drugs That Interfere with Test Methodology
- Drugs or substances that potentially cause artifactual decreases in serum phosphorus include phenothiazines, cefotaxime, citrates, mannitol, oxalate, and tartrates (which may decrease or inhibit color development of the indicator); and promethazine.
- Drugs or substances that potentially cause artifactual increases in serum phosphorus include aminosalicylic acid, bilirubin, detergents contaminating glassware, fat emulsions, hemoglobin, lipemia, methotrexate, naproxen, and rifampin.

Drugs That Alter Physiology
- Drugs that potentially cause decreases in serum phosphorus concentrations include acetazolamide, albuterol, aluminum-containing antacids, amino acids, anesthetic agents, anticonvulsants, corticosteroids, epinephrine, estrogens, fructose, glucose, hydrochlorothiazide (occasionally with prolonged treatment), insulin, isoniazid, magnesium hydroxide, and sucralfate.
- Drugs that potentially cause increases in serum phosphorus concentrations include alanine, aluminum hydroxide, anabolic steroids,

androgens, β-adrenergic blockers, ergocalciferol, furosemide, growth hormone, hydrochlorothiazide, medroxyprogesterone, minocycline, phosphates, vitamin D, and xylitol.

• Nephrotoxic drugs (e.g., aminoglycoside antibiotics, amphotericin B, tetracycline) that decrease GFR can also elevate phosphorus concentration.

Disorders That May Alter Results

• Hemolysis can potentially cause false increases in the phosphorus concentration because of the release of phosphates and phospholipids from erythrocytes.

• Depending on the assay methodology or the system, lipemia or hyperproteinemia may result in false increases. Hyperbilirubinemia may interfere with the assay, causing either false increases or decreases.

• Thrombocytosis and monoclonal gammopathies have been reported to cause false increases.

• In some dogs with immune-mediated hemolytic, anemia phosphorus may be spuriously low.

Collection Techniques or Handling That May Alter Results

• Poor sample collection technique may result in hemolysis, which can affect results.

• Failure to separate cells from serum or plasma within a short period may result in falsely increased phosphorus concentrations because intracellular phosphorus may leak from aging blood cells.

Influence of Signalment

Species
None

Breed
None

Age
• Young, growing dogs (up to ≈1 year of age) have higher serum phosphorus concentrations than adults (4–9 mg/dL) because of bone remodeling during growth.

• The effect of age is less pronounced in cats, although young cats tend to have slightly higher serum phosphorus concentrations than adults.

Gender
None

Pregnancy
None

LIMITATIONS OF THE TEST
Sensitivity, Specificity, and Positive and Negative Predictive Values
N/A

Valid If Run in a Human Lab?
Yes.

Causes of Abnormal Findings

High values	Low values
Young growing animals	Diabetes mellitus with ketosis (diabetic ketoacidosis)
Decreased GFR associated with prerenal, renal, or postrenal azotemia	Hyperinsulinism or insulin administration in diabetic patients
Administration of phosphate-containing fluids or phosphate-containing enema	Inadequate dietary intake of phosphorus or lack of dietary calcium
Tissue trauma or myopathies	Hypercalcemia of neoplasia (early stages before renal calcinosis)
Hemolysis	
Muscle necrosis	Primary hyperparathyroidism (early, before renal calcinosis)
Malignant hyperthermia	
Rhabdomyolysis	Administration of phosphate-binding antacids, diuretics, bicarbonate, hyperalimentation, prolonged diuresis, or glucose infusion
Tumor lysis syndrome	
Hypoparathyroidism	
Hypervitaminosis D	
Calciferol rodenticides	Eclampsia (dogs)
Excess dietary supplementation	Hypovitaminosis D (vitamin D deficiency)
Vitamin D–containing topical medications	
Hyperthyroidism (cats) (without renal insufficiency)	Malabsorption or starvation
	Respiratory alkalosis
Osteolytic bone lesions	Hyperadrenocorticism (uncommon)
Plant toxicity [e.g., jasmine (*Cestrum* sp.)]	
	Hypomagnesemia
Acromegaly	Canine Fanconi-like syndrome
Artifactual (e.g., delay in separating cells from serum; in vitro hemolysis)	Drugs (see Drugs That May Alter Results or Interpretation)
Drugs (see Drugs That May Alter Results or Interpretation)	

CLINICAL PERSPECTIVE

• Two common causes for hyperphosphatemia include young, growing animals or decreased GFR, which can be prerenal, renal, or postrenal.

• With severe hypophosphatemia (<1.0–1.5 mg/dL), there is an increased risk of hemolysis.

• When the [calcium] × [phosphorus] product exceeds 60–70, there is an increased risk of soft tissue mineralization.

MISCELLANEOUS

ANCILLARY TESTS
- CBC (especially PCV)
- Serum chemistry profile (especially BUN, creatinine, and calcium)
- Urinalysis (especially urine specific gravity)

SYNONYMS
- Inorganic phosphate
- Phosphate

SEE ALSO
Blackwell's Five-Minute Veterinary Consult: Canine and Feline Topics
- Hyperparathyroidism
- Hyperparathyroidism, Renal Secondary
- Hypoparathyroidism
- Oliguria and Anuria
- Hyperphosphatemia
- Phosphorus, Hypophosphatemia
- Polyuria and Polydipsia
- Renal Failure, Acute Uremia
- Renal Failure, Chronic
- Vitamin D Toxicity

Related Topics in This Book
- Calcitriol
- Calcium
- Creatinine
- Urea Nitrogen
- Urinalysis Overview

- Urine Fractional Excretion of Electrolytes
- Urine Specific Gravity

ABBREVIATIONS
- GFR = glomerular filtration rate
- PTH = parathyroid hormone

Suggested Reading

Ferguson DC, Hoenig M. Endocrine system. In: Latimer KS, Mahaffey EA, Prasse KW, eds. *Duncan and Prasse's Veterinary Laboratory Medicine Clinical Pathology,* 4th ed. Ames: Iowa State Press, 2003: 270–303.

Fettman MJ. Fluid and electrolyte metabolism. In: Thrall MA, ed. *Veterinary Hematology and Clinical Chemistry*. Philadelphia: Lippincott Williams & Wilkins 2004: 329–353.

Nelson RW, Turnwald GH, Willard MD. Endocrine, metabolic, and lipid disorders. In: Willard MD, Tvedten H, Turnwald GH, eds. *Small Animal Clinical Diagnosis by Laboratory Methods,* 4th ed. St Louis: Saunders Elsevier, 2004: 165–207.

Stockham SL, Scott MA. Calcium, phosphorus, magnesium, and their regulatory hormones. In: *Fundamentals of Veterinary Clinical Pathology*. Ames: Iowa State Press, 2002: 410–432.

Willard MD, DiBartola SP. Disorders of phosphorus. In: DiBartola SP, ed. *Fluid Therapy in Small Animal Practice,* 2nd ed. Philadelphia: WB Saunders, 2000: 163–174.

INTERNET RESOURCES
Cornell University, College of Veterinary Medicine, Clinical Pathology Modules: Phosphate, http://diaglab.vet.cornell.edu/clinpath/modules/chem/phos.htm.

AUTHOR NAME
Karen E. Russell

PIVKA TEST

BASICS

TYPE OF SPECIMEN
Blood

TEST EXPLANATION AND RELATED PHYSIOLOGY
Vit K is an essential cofactor for γ-glutamyl carboxylase, which catalyzes carboxylation of glutamic acid residues on coagulation factors II, VII, IX, and X, and coagulation inhibitors (proteins C and S), in the liver. This carboxylation enables coagulation factors to bind to calcium and phospholipid surfaces, which is essential for coagulation. With Vit K deficiency, inactive (noncarboxylated) Vit K–dependent factors, known as *proteins induced by vitamin K absence or antagonism* (PIVKA), accumulate and cannot participate in coagulation, resulting in hemorrhage. In essence, Vit K absence or antagonism causes a relative factor deficiency because of inactivity rather than lack of protein. Vit K is oxidized during carboxylation. It is reduced and regenerated by epoxide reductase. Inhibition of this enzyme (by anticoagulant rodenticides) prevents Vit K recycling, resulting in a relative Vit K deficiency. Vit K deficiency also results from dietary lack or malabsorption (Vit K is fat soluble).

In human medicine, immunoassays directly measure PIVKA. In animals, a modified PT assay is used instead. This assay differs from a routine PT by the use of bovine thromboplastin (which is particularly sensitive to factor X deficiency in human patients), adsorbed bovine plasma (which provides excess factor V and fibrinogen) and by dilution of patient plasma. The bovine thromboplastin is also inhibited by noncarboxylated or inactive factor X to a greater extent than the thromboplastin used in the traditional PT assay. Thus, the PIVKA test produces longer clotting times than the PT assay in human patients with elevated noncarboxylated coagulation factors. It is unclear whether this also occurs in animals.

INDICATIONS
- A diagnostic test for deficiencies of Vit K–dependent coagulation factors VII, II, IX, and X
- Diagnosis and monitoring of anticoagulant rodenticide toxicity
- A screening test for Vit K deficiency in animals with various illnesses (e.g., hepatic disease)

CONTRAINDICATIONS
None

POTENTIAL COMPLICATIONS
None

CLIENT EDUCATION
None

BODY SYSTEMS ASSESSED
Hemic, lymphatic, and immune

SAMPLE

COLLECTION
1–3 mL of venous blood

HANDLING
Citrate anticoagulant (blue-top tube) is required.

STORAGE
- Refrigerate the sample for short-term storage.
- Freeze the plasma for long-term storage.

STABILITY
- Room temperature: 6 h
- Frozen ($-20°C$): ≈2 weeks

PROTOCOL
None

INTERPRETATION

NORMAL FINDINGS OR RANGE
- Dogs: 16–19 s (Mount et al. 2003); 18–24 s (Rozanski et al. 1999)
- Cats: 16–25 s

ABNORMAL VALUES
- Values above the reference interval
- Values increased by >20% of a concurrently run control sample

CRITICAL VALUES
None

INTERFERING FACTORS
Drugs That May Alter Results or Interpretation
Drugs That Interfere with Test Methodology
Heparin prolongs the PIVKA clotting test in human patients.

Drugs That Alter Physiology
Vit K epoxide reductase antagonists (e.g., warfarin, sulfaquinoxaline)

Disorders That May Alter Results
- Defects in fat absorption or enterohepatic bile circulation (portosystemic shunts) can cause Vit K deficiency.
- Values may be prolonged in severe anemia.

Collection Techniques or Handling That May Alter Results
Activation of coagulation during collection may deplete coagulation factors in vitro and prolong the assay.

Influence of Signalment
Species
None

Breed
- An inherited defect in γ-glutamyl carboxylase in Devon rex cats
- Hereditary factor VII and X deficiencies have been reported in various purebred (and mixed breed) dogs and domestic shorthair (DSH) cats.

Age
None

Gender
None

Pregnancy
None

LIMITATIONS OF THE TEST
The PIVKA assay does not specifically detect inactive precursors and cannot discriminate between loss of activity (Vit K deficiency) and loss of protein (e.g., consumption in DIC, inherited factor deficiencies).
Sensitivity, Specificity, and Positive and Negative Predictive Values
N/A

Valid If Run in a Human Lab?
Yes.

Causes of Abnormal Findings

High values	Low values
Vit K deficiency	No clinical significance
Anticoagulant rodenticide toxicity	
Fat malabsorption	
Cholestatic liver disease	
Exocrine pancreatic insufficiency	
Inflammatory bowel disease	
Portosystemic shunt	
Dietary deprivation	
Inherited defect in γ-glutamyl carboxylase or Vit K epoxide reductase	
Deficiency of Vit K–dependent coagulation factors	
Inherited: factor VII, factor V, or factor X deficiency	
Acquired (e.g., DIC, hepatic necrosis, neoplasia)	

CLINICAL PERSPECTIVE

• The PIVKA test is markedly prolonged (>150 s) in dogs with anticoagulant rodenticide toxicity. However, the test is not specific for this toxicosis; values can be similarly prolonged in dogs with other disorders (e.g., DIC).

• In experimentally induced anticoagulant rodenticide toxicity in dogs, the PIVKA test was the first coagulation test to be prolonged and was more markedly increased than the PT or aPTT. However, the latter assays are usually prolonged in clinically affected patients, obviating the need for the PIVKA test.

• The PIVKA assay offers no clear diagnostic advantage over the PT assay and is not routinely performed by diagnostic laboratories.

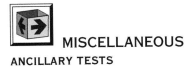

MISCELLANEOUS

ANCILLARY TESTS
• PT and aPTT

• Measurement of factor VII activity has replaced the PIVKA test for identification of Vit K–responsive coagulopathies.

SYNONYMS
None

SEE ALSO
Blackwell's Five-Minute Veterinary Consult: Canine and Feline Topics
Anticoagulant Rodenticide Poisoning
Related Topics in This Book
• Anticoagulant Screen
• Partial Thromboplastin Time, Activated
• Prothrombin Time

ABBREVIATIONS
• aPTT = activated partial thromboplastin time
• DIC = disseminated intravascular coagulation
• PIVKA = proteins induced by vitamin K absence or antagonism
• PT = prothrombin time
• Vit K = vitamin K

Suggested Reading
Center SA, Warner K, Corbett J, *et al.* Proteins invoked by vitamin K absence and clotting times in clinically ill cats. *J Vet Intern Med* 2000; 14: 292–297.
Giger U. Differing opinions on value of PIVKA test. *J Am Vet Med Assoc* 2003; 222: 1070–1071.
Mount ME, Kim BU, Kass PH. Use of a test for proteins induced by vitamin K absence or antagonism in diagnosis of anticoagulant poisoning in dogs: 325 cases (1987–1997). *J Am Vet Med Assoc* 2003; 222: 194–198.
Rozanski EA, Drobatz KJ, Hughes D, *et al.* Thrombotest (PIVKA) test results in 25 dogs with acquired and inherited coagulopathies. *J Vet Emerg Crit Care* 1999; 9: 73–78.

INTERNET RESOURCES
Cornell University, College of Veterinary Medicine, Clinical Pathology Modules: PIVKA, http://www.diaglab.vet.cornell.edu/clinpath/modules/coags/pivka.htm.

AUTHOR NAME
Tracy Stokol

PLATELET ANTIBODY DETECTION

BASICS

TYPE OF SPECIMEN
Blood

TEST EXPLANATION AND RELATED PHYSIOLOGY
The detection of antibodies directed against specific platelet surface glycoproteins may aid in the diagnosis of ITP. However, current assays cannot distinguish between true autoantibodies and those antibodies that adhere nonspecifically to platelet surface. Therefore, tests designed to detect platelet antibodies can only support the clinical diagnosis of ITP, and perhaps these tests are more appropriate for excluding rather than confirming the diagnosis. Some assays simply infer the presence of antibodies [e.g., the platelet factor 3 (PF3) immunoinjury test], whereas methods such as flow cytometry can actually quantify the presence of antibodies on the platelet surface (PSAIg). Performance of the PF3 immunoinjury test entails incubating serum from a thrombocytopenic patient with normal canine platelets. In the presence of autoantibodies directed against platelets, damaged platelets release PF3, which enhance clotting times compared with controls. Indirect measurements of anti–platelet antibodies can be performed via ELISA.

INDICATIONS
• Suspected primary or secondary ITP
• Severe thrombocytopenia

CONTRAINDICATIONS
None

POTENTIAL COMPLICATIONS
Depending on the assay selected, a prohibitively large amount of blood (e.g., 50 mL) may be required.

CLIENT EDUCATION
The present of antibodies directed against platelets does not confirm the diagnosis of ITP.

BODY SYSTEMS ASSESSED
Hemic, lymphatic, and immune

SAMPLE

COLLECTION
• Venous blood for anti–platelet antibody assays. The amount of blood required depends on the assay used and the patient platelet number. As much as 50 mL of blood may be required for patients with <10,000 platelet/μL. Flow cytometry may require as little as 7 mL of blood.
• Smears of aspirated bone marrow for detecting antibodies on megakaryocytes

HANDLING
• Flow cytometry: EDTA-anticoagulated or citrate/dextrose-anticoagulated blood, depending on the assay; check with the laboratory for the sample volume requirement and anticoagulant preference. Ship the sample on ice.
• ELISAs evaluating platelet-bindable antibodies require serum. Collect the blood into a plain red-top or serum-separator tube.
• Megakaryocyte immunofluorescence: Air-dry squash preparations of aspirated marrow.

STORAGE
• Serum: Freeze.
• Whole blood: Refrigerate for short-term storage, but process the sample as soon as possible.
• Bone marrow smears: Store at room temperature.

STABILITY
Not formally evaluated

PROTOCOL
None

INTERPRETATION

NORMAL FINDINGS OR RANGE
• A negative result (i.e., failure to detect platelet-bound antibodies) suggests that ITP is unlikely.
• The reference range depends on the assay employed.

ABNORMAL VALUES
A positive result (i.e., detection of PSAIg or anti–platelet antibodies) supports the diagnosis of ITP but cannot distinguish between primary and secondary forms of the disease.

CRITICAL VALUES
None

INTERFERING FACTORS
Drugs That May Alter Results or Interpretation
Drugs That Interfere with Test Methodology
None

Drugs That Alter Physiology
Immunosuppressive agents may decrease antibody production.

Disorders That May Alter Results
• Clotting of samples used to directly evaluate platelet-bound antibodies invalidates the test.
• Lipemia and hemolysis may interfere with some techniques.

Collection Techniques or Handling That May Alter Results
• Storing blood samples at room temperature or prolonged refrigeration may increase PSAIg as assayed by flow cytometry.
• False negatives if bone marrow aspirates have insufficient cellularity (absence of spicules)
• False positives if megakaryocytes are damaged during preparation of bone marrow smears

Influence of Signalment
Species
Evaluated in only dogs

Breed
None

Age
None

Gender
None

Pregnancy
None

LIMITATIONS OF THE TEST
• Indirect ELISA for platelet-bindable antibodies has the lowest sensitivity and specificity and is unreliable.
• Megakaryocyte immunofluorescence will be positive in ITP dogs only if antibodies are directed against an epitope shared by both the circulating platelets and the megakaryocytes.
• Flow cytometric tests are usually performed at research institutions.

Sensitivity, Specificity, and Positive and Negative Predictive Values
• Direct ELISA has a reported sensitivity of 94% and a reported specificity of 62%.
• Indirect ELISA has a reported sensitivity of 35% and a reported specificity of 80%.

- The PF3 immunoinjury test has a reported sensitivity ranging from 28% to 80%.
- Megakaryocyte immunofluorescence has a reported diagnostic sensitivity of ≈50%.

Valid If Run in a Human Lab?
No.

Causes of Abnormal Findings

High values	Low values
ITP	Not significant
Autoimmune disorder	
Drug reaction	

CLINICAL PERSPECTIVE
- Failure to detect PSAIg may exclude the diagnosis of ITP.
- The clinical diagnosis of ITP does not require the demonstration of PSAIg.

MISCELLANEOUS

ANCILLARY TESTS
- CBC and platelet count
- Bone marrow aspiration to rule out decreased production as a cause of thrombocytopenia
- Screen for tickborne diseases

SYNONYMS
- Direct megakaryocyte immunofluorescence assay
- Enzyme-linked immunosorbent assays (direct and indirect)
- Flow cytometric platelet immunofluorescence

- Platelet factor 3 immunoinjury test
- Platelet surface–associated immunoglobulin (PSAIg)

SEE ALSO
Blackwell's Five-Minute Veterinary Consult: Canine and Feline Topics
Thrombocytopenia, Primary Immune-Mediated
Related Topics in This Book
- Bone Marrow Aspirate and Biopsy
- Bone Marrow Aspirate Cytology: Microscopic Evaluation
- Platelet Count and Volume

ABBREVIATIONS
- ELISA = enzyme-linked immunosorbent assay
- ITP = immune-mediated thrombocytopenia
- PF3 = platelet factor 3
- PSAIg = platelet surface–associated immunoglobulin

Suggested Reading
Kristensen AT, Weiss DJ, Klausner JS, *et al.* Comparison of microscopic and flow cytometric detection of platelet antibody in dogs suspected of having immune-mediated thrombocytopenia. *Am J Vet Res* 1994; 55: 1111–1114.
Lewis DC, McVey DS, Shuman WS, Muller WB. Development and characterization of a flow cytometric assay for detection of platelet-bound immunoglobulin G in dogs. *Am J Vet Res* 1995; 56: 1555–1558.
Lewis DC, Meyers KM, Callan MB, *et al.* Detection of platelet-bound and serum platelet-bindable antibodies for diagnosis of idiopathic thrombocytopenic purpura in dogs. *J Am Vet Med Assoc* 1995; 206: 47–52.

INTERNET RESOURCES
None

AUTHOR NAME
Daniel L. Chan

BASICS

TYPE OF SPECIMEN
Blood

TEST EXPLANATION AND RELATED PHYSIOLOGY
Platelet numbers and volume are routinely assessed through hematologic samples. They provide important information regarding the adequacy of the bone marrow to produce platelets and indicate whether a consumptive or destructive process may be the source of thrombocytopenia and potentially compromised hemostasis. Platelet numbers are usually assessed by automated machines (e.g., aperture impedance flow automated hematology instruments, quantitative buffy coat analysis, flow cytometry), manually counted with a hemocytometer, or estimated on blood smears. The presence of platelet clumps may significantly underestimate platelet counts.

Mean platelet volume (MPV) reflects the average size of platelets in the circulation and is generally inversely related to platelet concentration. An increased MPV indicates larger-than-normal platelets and most often reflects release of immature platelets through increased thrombopoiesis in response to thrombocytopenia. A decreased MPV may be associated with excessive platelet destruction, insufficient megakaryocytes, or a lack of response by the bone marrow (e.g., toxic bone marrow injury).

INDICATIONS
- A minimal database in many diseases
- Physical findings indicating defects of primary hemostasis (e.g., petechiae, ecchymoses, mucosal bleeding, epistaxis)
- Patients requiring surgery or organ biopsies (e.g., liver, kidney)

CONTRAINDICATIONS
None

POTENTIAL COMPLICATIONS
Blood sampling in severely thrombocytopenic patients may cause hematoma formation.

CLIENT EDUCATION
None

BODY SYSTEMS ASSESSED
Hemic, lymphatic, and immune

SAMPLE

COLLECTION
1–3 mL of venous blood. To ensure a proper ratio of anticoagulant to blood, avoid underfilling or overfilling the blood-collection tube.

HANDLING
- Collect the sample into EDTA or sodium citrate anticoagulant.
- Invert the tube to mix the blood thoroughly with anticoagulant.
- Inspect the tube for blood clots that can invalidate the sample.

STORAGE
Refrigerate for short-term storage.

STABILITY
Platelet Numbers
- Room temperature: 5 h
- Refrigerated (4°C): 24 h

MPV
- Poor stability in EDTA with significant changes noted within 3 h even with refrigeration
- Better stability with citrate

PROTOCOL
None

INTERPRETATION

NORMAL FINDINGS OR RANGE
- Platelet count (varies with each laboratory):
  - Dogs: 170,000–575,000/μL
  - Cats: 200,000–680,000/μL
- MPV varies with the laboratory and the technique employed:
  - Technicon H-1 hematology analyzer (Bayer, Tarrytown, NY)
    - Dogs: 3.9–6.1 fL
    - Cats: 4.1–8.3 fL
  - Advia 120 (Bayer, Fernwald, Germany). New methodology is less likely to exclude larger platelets:
    - Dogs: 8.56–14.41 fL
    - Cats: 10.21–25.7 fL
  - Coulter S-Plus IV (Coulter Electronics, Hialeah, FL)
    - Dogs: 7.0–10.3 fL

ABNORMAL VALUES
Values above or below the reference interval

CRITICAL VALUES
- Platelet counts of <50,000 platelets/μL can be associated with spontaneous hemorrhage.
- Patients with significant thrombocytopenia (e.g., <50,000 platelets/μL) and evidence of bleeding into vital organs (e.g., CNS, eyes, pericardium) may require a fresh whole blood transfusion.

INTERFERING FACTORS
Drugs That May Alter Results or Interpretation
Drugs That Interfere with Test Methodology
None

Drugs That Alter Physiology
- Vincristine administration increases platelet numbers and may affect MPV.
- Drugs that cause thrombocytopenia through bone marrow suppression include chemotherapeutic agents, estrogens (in dogs), and occasionally phenylbutazone, sulfonamides, and griseofulvin.
- Drugs that can cause secondary immune-mediated thrombocytopenia (IMT) include gold salts and sulfonamides.

Disorders That May Alter Results
- Splenic disease and/or neoplasia may markedly decrease platelet numbers.
- Inflammatory disorders may increase platelet numbers.
- Severe hemorrhage may lead to secondary consumption of platelets rather than be the primary cause of bleeding.
- Severe lipemia may artifactually increase the platelet count if lipid droplets are included.

Collection Techniques or Handling That May Alter Results
- An improper ratio of blood to anticoagulant
- A traumatic and/or prolonged blood draw may trigger platelet clumping.
- EDTA-anticoagulated blood may interfere with the determination of MPV with some methodologies (e.g., electrical impedance methods).
- In rare dogs, EDTA will promote platelet clumping by unmasking antigenic sites on platelet membranes. In these dogs, the use of citrate anticoagulant will more reliably prevent platelet clumping.

Influence of Signalment
Species
Feline platelets are unreliably counted by electrical impedance methods. Manual counts are recommended.

Breed
• Greyhounds have lower platelet counts (80,000–148,000 platelets/μL).
• Cavalier King Charles spaniels tend to have lower counts and higher MPV. Automated counters often exclude giant platelets found in individuals of this breed.
• Otterhound thrombopathia is associated with enlarged platelets (increased MPV).

Age
None

Gender
None

Pregnancy
Expanded plasma volume associated with pregnancy may lower platelet counts.

LIMITATIONS OF THE TEST
• MPV is affected by sample age, temperature, and anticoagulant. These factors cause inaccuracies that make interpretation difficult.
• The presence of platelet clumps often invalidates platelet counts by any method. This is a particular problem in cats.
• Electronic impedance methods may exclude large platelets from evaluation, underestimating both the platelet count and MPV.

Sensitivity, Specificity, and Positive and Negative Predictive Values
An MPV of >12.0 fL in dogs has a reported 96% positive predictive value of normal to increased megakaryocytopoiesis in the bone marrow.

Valid If Run in a Human Lab?
Yes, for canine blood, but valid in cats only if the lab uses a hematology analyzer calibrated to run veterinary species and is willing to perform manual platelet counts.

Causes of Abnormal Findings

High values	Low values
Platelet count	Platelet count
Reactive thrombocytosis	Immune destruction
Inflammation	Consumption
Iron deficiency	Hemorrhage
Nonhemic neoplasia	Infection
Surgery/trauma	*Babesia* sp.
Rebound thrombocytosis	*Ehrlichia canis*
Hyperadrenocorticism	*Anaplasma phagocytophilum*
Splenectomy	*Histoplasma* sp.
Hemic neoplasia	Rocky Mountain spotted fever
Essential thrombocythemia	*Leishmania* sp.
Acute megakaryocytic leukemia	Thromboembolic disease (e.g.,
Other myeloproliferative	disseminated intravascular
disorders	coagulation)
	Hemodilution
	Impaired production (bone marrow
	disease)
MPV	MPV
Accelerated thrombopoiesis	Bone marrow failure
Congenital platelet disorder	Chemotherapeutic
(Cavalier King Charles	immunosuppression
spaniels or otterhounds)	Nonplatelet debris or lipid droplets
Mobilization of platelets from	(artifact)
spleen	IMT (occasionally)
FeLV infection	
Essential thrombocythemia	

CLINICAL PERSPECTIVE
• Platelet counts of <100,000 platelets/μL usually constitute significant thrombocytopenia, which merits evaluation of platelet production or consumption.
  • Moderate thrombocytopenia (e.g., 50,000–100,000/μL) suggests platelet consumption (e.g., hemorrhage, thrombosis, vasculitis, infection).
  • Severe thrombocytopenia (e.g., <20,000/μL) is more typical of IMT.
  • Thrombocytopenia due to bone marrow disease often occurs with other concurrent cytopenias.
• Platelet counts of >800,000 platelets/μL usually constitute significant thrombocytosis, which merits evaluation of platelet overproduction or bone marrow stimulation.
• A manual count is warranted if small platelet clumps or significant numbers of enlarged platelets are present. When large platelet clumps are present, an accurate count is not possible by any method.

MISCELLANEOUS
ANCILLARY TESTS
• The platelet count on a blood smear is estimated by determining the average number of platelets/100× oil-immersion field of view (minimum, 5 fields). In dogs and cats, each platelet seen corresponds to ≈15,000–20,000 platelets/μL. Conservative estimates can be made by using the following guidelines:
  • Normal dogs and cats have ≈10–25 platelets/100× hpf.
  • 8–10 platelets/100× hpf usually indicates >100,000 platelets/μL.
  • 6–7 platelets/100× hpf approximates 100,000 platelets/μL.
  • <3–4 platelets/100× hpf usually indicates <50,000 platelets/μL.
• CBC to look for other hematologic abnormalities
• Serologic evaluation or PCR to look for infectious agents

SYNONYMS
None

SEE ALSO
Blackwell's Five-Minute Veterinary Consult: Canine and Feline Topics
• Petechiae, Ecchymosis, Bruising
• Thrombocytopenia
• Thrombocytopenia, Primary Immune-Mediated

Related Topics in This Book
• Blood Smear Microscopic Examination
• Platelet Antibody Detection
• Platelet Function Tests

ABBREVIATIONS
• fL = femtoliter
• hpf = high-power field
• IMT = immune-mediated thrombocytopenia
• MPV = mean platelet volume

Suggested Reading
Prater R, Tvedten H. Hemostatic abnormalities. In: Willard MD, Tvedten H, eds. *Small Animal Clinical Diagnosis by Laboratory Methods,* 4th ed. St Louis: Saunders Elsevier, 2004: 92–112.
Stokol T. Disorders of haemostasis. In: Villiers E, Blackwood L, eds. *BSAVA Manual of Canine and Feline Clinical Pathology,* 2nd ed. Gloucester, UK: British Small Animal Veterinary Association, 2005: 83–98.

PLATELET COUNT AND VOLUME

Topper MJ, Welles EG. Hemostasis. In: Latimer KS, Mahaffey EA, Prasse K, Duncan JR, eds. *Duncan and Prasse's Veterinary Laboratory Medicine: Clinical Pathology,* 4th ed. Ames: Iowa State Press, 2003: 161–175.

Wilkerson MJ, Shuman W. Alterations in normal canine platelets during storage in EDTA anticoagulated blood. *Vet Clin Pathol* 2001; 30: 107–113.

INTERNET RESOURCES

AXIOM Veterinary Laboratories: Canine platelets and red blood cells, http://www.axiomvetlab.com/Canine%20platelets%20&%20red %20blood%20cells.html.

Cornell University, College of Veterinary Medicine, Clinical Pathology Modules: Hematology atlas, http://diaglab.vet.cornell.edu/clinpath/modules/heme1/intro.htm.

AUTHOR NAME

Daniel L. Chan

BASICS

TYPE OF SPECIMEN
Blood

TEST EXPLANATION AND RELATED PHYSIOLOGY
Practical assessment of hemostasis usually involves assessment of platelet numbers and secondary hemostasis (i.e., prothrombin time, activated partial thromboplastin time). However, an often overlooked aspect is platelet function, probably because precise platelet function cannot be routinely assessed. The only practical platelet function test that can be performed in routine practice is the buccal mucosal bleeding time (BMBT). However, this is a crude assessment of platelet function, with marked interobserver and intraobserver variability, and relies on subjective assessment rather than more objective measures afforded by more advance platelet function analyzers.

Platelet function analyzers (e.g., the PFA-100; Siemens, Deerfield, IL), which are being used increasingly in veterinary medicine, enable simulation of high-shear platelet function (adhesion and aggregation) within disposable test cartridges. With this technique, citrated blood is aspirated under constant negative pressure, and a microscopic aperture is cut into a membrane coated with specific platelet activators (e.g., collagen and epinephrine or ADP). These activators and high-shear forces cause platelet adhesion, activation, and aggregation that result in platelet plug formation and closure of the aperture. Platelet function is measured as a function of time (aperture-closure time). However, since this assay requires blood to be processed within 4 h of collection, platelet function analysis cannot be offered by diagnostic laboratories. Platelet aggregation is another facet of platelet function that can be measured, but this procedure is also limited by the need to perform analysis within 2 h of collection and therefore is not available for clinical cases seen in routine practice.

INDICATIONS
- Patients with defects of primary hemostasis but adequate platelet numbers
- Patients being administered platelet function–altering drugs and requiring surgery
- Patients at risk of having von Willebrand disease and requiring surgery or organ biopsies (e.g., liver, kidney)

CONTRAINDICATIONS
None

POTENTIAL COMPLICATIONS
Patients with severe thrombocytopathia may bleed profusely after BMBT is performed.

CLIENT EDUCATION
None

BODY SYSTEMS ASSESSED
Hemic, lymphatic, and immune

SAMPLE

COLLECTION
- PFA-100: 0.8 mL of venous blood is required for each cartridge.
- Platelet aggregation: Separation of platelet-rich plasma may require >10 mL of venous blood.

HANDLING
Citrate-anticoagulated blood for PFA-100 and for platelet-rich plasma is required for platelet aggregation.

STORAGE
Refrigerate the blood for aggregation and automated platelet function analyzers. Analyze the samples within 2–4 h of collection.

STABILITY
Poor

PROTOCOL
See the "Bleeding Time" chapter.

INTERPRETATION

NORMAL FINDINGS OR RANGE
- For BMBT, ranges of normal vary but generally should be <4.2 min in dogs and <3.3 min in sedated or anesthetized cats.
- For PFA-100, closure times of ≤98 or ≤300 s as measured with ADP or epinephrine as platelet agonists, respectively, may be considered normal.

ABNORMAL VALUES
- A BMBT of >5 min
- PFA-100 closure times of >98 or >300 s as measured with ADP or epinephrine as platelet agonists, respectively, may be considered abnormal.

CRITICAL VALUES
Unknown

INTERFERING FACTORS
Drugs That May Alter Results or Interpretation
Drugs That Interfere with Test Methodology
None

Drugs That Alter Physiology
- Aspirin
- Carbenicillin
- Cephalosporins
- Clopidogrel
- Dipyridamole
- Ibuprofen
- Indomethacin

PLATELET FUNCTION TESTS

- Levamisole
- Methylxanthines
- Nitrofurantoin
- Phenylbutazone
- Pimobendan
- Synthetic colloids
- Ticlopidine

Disorders That May Alter Results
- Congenital disorders of platelet function
- Disseminated intravascular coagulation
- Multiple myeloma
- Thrombocytopenia affects BMBT.
- Uremia
- Von Willebrand disease

Collection Techniques or Handling That May Alter Results
Atraumatic blood collection is necessary to minimize platelet activation.

Influence of Signalment
Species
- Cats reportedly have enhanced platelet aggregation compared with dogs.
- Feline platelets cannot be assessed via the PFA-100.

Breed
Abnormal platelet function reported in greyhounds, spitz (spitz thrombopathia), American cocker spaniels (subnormal ADP concentrations), basset hounds (basset hound thrombopathia), Great Pyrenees, and otterhounds (Glanzmann's thrombasthenia).

Age
None

Gender
None

Pregnancy
None

LIMITATIONS OF THE TEST
Sensitivity, Specificity, and Positive and Negative Predictive Values
PFA-100 (Couto et al. 2006)

ADP-Closure Time
- Sensitivity: 95.7%
- Specificity: 100%
- Positive predictive value: 100%
- Negative predictive value: 96.7%

Epinephrine-Closure Time
- Sensitivity: 95.7%
- Specificity: 82.8%
- Positive predictive value: 81.5%
- Negative predictive value: 96%

Valid If Run in a Human Lab?
No.

Causes of Abnormal Findings

Prolonged bleeding time/functional abnormalities	Shortened bleeding time
Von Willebrand disease	Not interpretable
Drug-induced thrombocytopathia	
Disseminated intravascular coagulation	
Congenital thrombocytopathia	
Thrombocytopenia (severe)	
Uremia	

CLINICAL PERSPECTIVE

For practical reasons, the BMBT will probably remain the only test routinely available in practice to assess platelet function. Increased availability of platelet function analyzers will likely increase our understanding of platelet physiology and the impact that different drugs and physiologic states have on platelet function.

MISCELLANEOUS

ANCILLARY TESTS

A von Willebrand factor assay is recommended if the results of the BMBT are abnormal.

SYNONYMS

- Platelet aggregometry
- Platelet function analyzer (e.g., the PFA-100)

SEE ALSO

Blackwell's Five-Minute Veterinary Consult: Canine and Feline Topics

- Petechiae, Ecchymosis, Bruising
- Thrombocytopathies

Related Topics in This Book

- Bleeding Time
- Platelet Count and Volume
- Von Willebrand Factor

ABBREVIATIONS

- ADP = adenosine diphosphate
- BMBT = buccal mucosal bleeding time

Suggested Reading

Callan MB, Giger U. Assessment of a point-of-care instrument for identification of primary hemostatic disorders in dogs. *Am J Vet Res* 2001; 62: 652–658.

Couto CG, Lara A, Iazbik MC, Brooks MB. Evaluation of platelet aggregation using a point-of-care instrument in retired racing greyhounds. *J Vet Intern Med* 2006; 20: 365–370.

Mischke R, Keidel A. Influence of platelet count, acetylsalicylic acid, von Willebrand's disease, coagulopathies, and haematocrit on results obtained using a platelet function analyser in dogs. *Vet J* 2003; 165: 43–52.

INTERNET RESOURCES

None

AUTHOR NAME

Daniel L. Chan

POTASSIUM

BASICS

TYPE OF SPECIMEN
Blood

TEST EXPLANATION AND RELATED PHYSIOLOGY
Potassium (K) is the principal cation of the intracellular fluid (ICF) compartment. Dietary K is nonselectively absorbed in the stomach and small intestine. The kidneys do not reabsorb K, so dietary absorption is essential to provide adequate amounts of K to the system.

Regulation of K homeostasis is controlled by renal excretion and by translocation of K from the extracellular space to the intracellular space. The latter is accomplished through hormonal influences and alterations of acid-base status. Initially, excess dietary K is redirected into the ICF by insulin and catecholamines. In metabolic acidosis, excess hydrogen ions are being buffered intracellularly, and, as a result, K leaves the cell. Metabolic alkalosis causes K to shift intracellularly.

Renal excretion of K is controlled by aldosterone, the amount of K intake, the degree of Na reabsorption, and rate of distal tubular flow. Aldosterone triggers reabsorption of Na (with passive absorption of chloride) in the distal nephron and the secretion of K. Aldosterone also increases the activity of the Na/K-ATPase pump in the distal convoluted tubule. Both of these actions increase secretion of K in the distal nephron.

The most important function of K is to create and maintain the normal resting-cell membrane potential. This is accomplished through preservation of the high intracellular to extracellular K ratio by means of the Na/K-ATPase pump. K also plays a critical role in neuromuscular transmission in cardiac and skeletal muscle. Of the 95%–98% of total body K located intracellularly, ≈60%–75% is located in muscle cells. Alterations of the resting-cell membrane potential can cause serious neuromuscular conduction abnormalities, so the K level must be maintained within a narrow range in the serum. Additionally, K is essential for normal function of enzyme systems that control synthesis of DNA, glycogen, and proteins.

K levels are measured in serum or plasma by dry-reagent methods, flame photometry, and direct or indirect potentiometry (ion selective). Because only 2%–5% of total body K is located extracellularly, measurement of serum K may not accurately reflect total body K. Point-of-care instruments that use direct ion-selective electrodes may have different ranges than indirect ion-selective electrodes and other traditional instruments that use dilution techniques.

INDICATIONS
- GI signs (e.g., vomiting, diarrhea, painful abdomen)
- Cardiac arrhythmias
- Skeletal muscle weakness or hyperexcitability
- Polyuria-polydipsia
- Renal disease
- Urethral blockage or uroabdomen
- Diabetic ketoacidosis (DKA)
- Monitoring therapy with insulin, angiotensin-converting enzyme (ACE) inhibitors, K-sparing diuretics, K supplementation (IV or oral), K penicillin G, or heparin

CONTRAINDICATIONS
None

POTENTIAL COMPLICATIONS
None

CLIENT EDUCATION
None

BODY SYSTEMS ASSESSED
- Cardiovascular
- Endocrine and metabolic
- Gastrointestinal
- Renal and urologic

SAMPLE

COLLECTION
0.5–1.0 mL of venous blood

HANDLING
Collect the sample into a red-top tube or serum-separator tube.

STORAGE
- Refrigeration is recommended for short-term storage.
- Freeze the serum or plasma for long-term storage.

STABILITY
- Room temperature: 1 day
- Refrigerated (2°–8°C): 1 week
- Frozen (−20°C): 1 year

PROTOCOL
None

INTERPRETATION

NORMAL FINDINGS OR RANGE
- Dogs and cats: 3.5–5.5 mEq/L
- Reference intervals may vary depending on the laboratory and assay.

ABNORMAL VALUES
Values above or below the reference range

CRITICAL VALUES
Immediate intervention is recommended if values are >7.5 or <2.5 mEq/L.

INTERFERING FACTORS
Drugs That May Alter Results or Interpretation
Drugs That Interfere with Test Methodology
None

Drugs That Alter Physiology
- Hypokalemia can be caused by loop and thiazide diuretics, acetazolamide, mineralocorticoids, insulin, glucose-containing fluids, K-free fluids, Na bicarbonate, amphotericin B, ammonium chloride, and K-free dialysate.
- Hyperkalemia can be caused by K chloride (IV or oral), digitalis overdose, trimethoprim, ACE inhibitors, K-sparing diuretics, nonspecific β blockers, and nephrotoxic NSAIDs.

Disorders That May Alter Results
- Thrombocytosis and leukocytosis may cause hyperkalemia (leak of K from cells).
- Hemolysis in dogs and cats with phosphofructokinase deficiency may cause hyperkalemia.
- Severe bilirubinemia may cause slightly increased levels of serum K if measured with ion-selective electrodes.
- Metabolic acidosis may cause hyperkalemia due to a normal physiologic response.

Collection Techniques or Handling That May Alter Results
- A poor venipuncture technique that causes hemolysis may increase levels of K in some dog breeds.
- K oxalate or EDTA anticoagulants cause an artificially high measured K value.
- Plasma K levels are higher than serum K levels.

Influence of Signalment
Species
None

Breed
- In vitro hemolysis of K-rich erythrocytes in the Akita and Shiba Inu breeds may cause pseudohyperkalemia (the use of lithium heparin collection tubes is recommended).
- In vivo hemolysis in phosphofructokinase deficiency in predisposed canine breeds (i.e., English springer spaniels, American cocker spaniels) may elevate serum K levels.

Age
In vitro hemolysis of K-rich erythrocytes in some neonates may cause pseudohyperkalemia.

Gender
See the Pregnancy section.

Pregnancy
Concurrent hyperkalemia and hyponatremia may occur in sick late-term pregnant dogs.

LIMITATIONS OF THE TEST
Sensitivity, Specificity, and Positive and Negative Predictive Values
N/A

Valid If Run in a Human Lab?
Yes.

CLINICAL PERSPECTIVE
- An Na/K ratio of <24 may be consistent with hypoadrenocorticism, but a similar ratio may occur with trichuriasis, repeated drainage of chylothorax, cavitary effusion, and illness during late-term pregnancy in dogs.
- If a pet is hyponatremic, hyperkalemic, and azotemic, consider renal failure or postrenal urinary obstruction or rupture. The use of radiography or ultrasonography may help to evaluate the kidneys and look for evidence of urinary tract blockage (e.g., urolithiasis) or may be used to diagnose uroperitoneum.
- If a pet is hypokalemic, hypochloremic, and alkalotic, consider imaging for upper GI obstruction.

MISCELLANEOUS

ANCILLARY TESTS
- Evaluation of Na, chloride, and magnesium levels to look for concurrent electrolyte derangements
- Blood-gas evaluation, anion gap to look for acid-base abnormalities
- An ACTH stimulation test to rule out hypoadrenocorticism
- Urinalysis to look for proteinuria, hematuria, pyuria, glucosuria, and ketonuria
- Determination of the urinary fractional excretion of K to rule out RTA
- Fecal flotation to rule out GI parasitism
- Electrocardiography to look for hyperkalemic arrhythmias
- Thoracic and abdominal radiography and ultrasonography to rule out cavitary effusion and look for enlargement or abnormal architecture of abdominal organs and evidence of an intact bladder

Causes of Abnormal Findings

High values	Low values
Pseudohyperkalemia	Pseudohypokalemia
Thrombocytosis (>1,000,000/μL)	Severe lipemia
Leukocytosis (>100,000/μL)	Decreased Intake
In vitro hemolysis of K-rich	Dietary deficiency
erythrocytes in certain canine	Administration of K-free IV fluids
breeds (e.g., Akita, Shiba Inu)	Increased loss: GI
and neonatal animals	Vomiting of K-rich stomach
Pregnancy (dogs)	contents
Phosphofructokinase deficiency	Diarrhea
(dogs)	Increased loss: renal/urinary
Increased intake	Chronic renal failure (cats)
Iatrogenic (IV or oral)	Diet-induced hypokalemic
Dietary	nephropathy (cats)
Diminished urinary excretion	Postobstructive diuresis
Postrenal obstruction	Diuresis caused by diabetes
Ruptured urinary tract	mellitus
Anuric/oliguric renal failure	Drugs (e.g., loop diuretics,
Hypoadrenocorticism	thiazide diuretics,
Certain GI disorders (e.g.,	amphotericin B, penicillin,
trichuriasis, salmonellosis,	albuterol overdose)
perforated duodenal ulcer)	Hyperadrenocorticism
Third-space losses	Dialysis
Repeated drainage of chylothorax	Hypomagnesemia
Medications (e.g., K-sparing	Hyperthyroidism (cats)
diuretics, ACE inhibitors,	Distal (type I) renal tubular
prostaglandin inhibitors, heparin)	acidosis (RTA)
Hyporeninemic hypoaldosteronism	Proximal RTA after bicarbonate
Translocation from ICF to ECF	therapy
DKA (i.e., insulin deficiency)	Primary hyperaldosteronism
Tissue necrosis (e.g., reperfusion	Translocation from ECF to ICF
following feline arterial	Insulin- or glucose-containing IV
thromboembolism, acute tumor	fluids
lysis, rhabdomyolysis, trauma)	Metabolic alkalosis
Medications (e.g., nonspecific β	Total parenteral nutrition
blockers)	Hypokalemic periodic paralysis in
Oleander toxicity	Burmese cats
Acute inorganic acidosis	Catecholamines

SYNONYMS
None

SEE ALSO
Blackwell's Five-Minute Veterinary Consult: Canine and Feline Topics
- Acidosis, Metabolic
- Diarrhea, Chronic—Cats
- Diarrhea, Chronic—Dogs
- Hyperkalemia
- Hypokalemia
- Hypoadrenocorticism (Addison's Disease)
- Renal Failure, Chronic
- Renal Tubular Acidosis
- Vomiting, Chronic

Related Topics in This Book
- ACTH Stimulation Test
- Anion Gap
- Bicarbonate
- Blood Gases
- Chloride
- Fecal Flotation
- Sodium
- Urine Fractional Excretion of Electrolytes

POTASSIUM

ABBREVIATIONS
- ACE = angiotensin-converting enzyme
- DKA = diabetic ketoacidosis
- ECF = extracellular fluid
- ICF = intracellular fluid
- K = potassium
- Na = sodium
- Na/K-ATPase = sodium-potassium-adenosine triphosphatase (Na/K pump)
- RTA = renal tubular acidosis

Suggested Reading

DiBartola SP, de Morais HA. Disorders of potassium: Hypokalemia and hyperkalemia. In: DiBartola SP, ed. *Fluid Therapy in Small Animal Practice*, 3rd ed. Philadelphia: WB Saunders, 1992: 91–121.

DiBartola SP, Green RA, de Morais HA, Willard MD. Electrolyte and acid-base disorders. In: Willard MD, Tvedten H, eds. *Small Animal Clinical Diagnosis by Laboratory Methods*, 4th ed. Philadelphia: WB Saunders, 2004: 117–122.

Manning AM. Electrolyte disorders. *Vet Clin North Am Small Anim Pract* 2001; 31: 1294–1300.

Schaer M, Halling KB, Collins KE, Grant DC. Combined hyponatremia and hyperkalemia mimicking acute hypoadrenocorticism in three pregnant dogs. *J Am Vet Med Assoc* 2001; 218: 897–899.

INTERNET RESOURCES
Cornell University, College of Veterinary Medicine, Clinical Pathology Modules, Routine Blood Chemistry: Electrolyes, Interpretation of Serum Potassium Results, http://diaglab.Vet.cornell.edu/clinpath/modules/chem/potass.htm.

AUTHOR NAME
Maria Vandis

BASICS

TYPE OF SPECIMEN
Blood

TEST EXPLANATION AND RELATED PHYSIOLOGY
As the time of ovulation approaches during estrus, ovarian follicular cells transform from estrogen-producing to progesterone-producing cells. LH causes ovulation and is responsible for this transformation. After ovulation, the follicles become corpora lutea, and progesterone is produced throughout pregnancy. The corpora lutea, which are the only significant source of progesterone in pregnant bitches and queens, are required to maintain pregnancy throughout gestation. Progesterone concentration must drop to basal levels for parturition to occur. The concentration remains at basal levels through anestrus, until ovulation during the next estrous cycle.

The LH surge and subsequent ovulation occur spontaneously in bitches, whereas, in queens, coital stimulation of the vagina is generally required to initiate the LH surge (induced ovulation). Noncoital ovulation also occurs fairly frequently in domestic shorthair cats. In bitches, progesterone concentrations begin to increase above basal levels as a preovulatory event. This initial rise occurs simultaneously with the LH surge. Therefore, progesterone can be used to approximate the LH surge and predict impending ovulation in bitches. In queens, the initial rise above basal progesterone concentration occurs after the LH surge. In bitches and queens, high progesterone concentrations are indicative that ovulation has occurred. The next cycle will not begin until sometime after progesterone has returned to basal levels.

The stage of the ovarian cycle during which progesterone concentrations are high is called *diestrus*. If conception has occurred, the length of diestrus will be the length of gestation. Gestation averages 65 days after breeding in queens and 63 days after breeding in bitches. If conception has not occurred in a queen that has ovulated, the corpus luteum (CL) will regress in ≈36–38 days. In other words, the duration of the CL depends on the presence of a viable pregnancy and vice versa. The bitch, on the other hand, is unique among common domestic animals in that the CL persists and produces progesterone for 2 months or longer, irrespective of pregnancy status.

A wide variety of laboratory methods are used to detect progesterone. These include RIA, which is considered to be the gold standard, and chemiluminescent immunoassay (CLIA). These are available from a variety of commercial laboratories. Lower values are obtained using CLIA techniques than using RIA. Therefore, it is important to use the reference ranges established by the laboratories for its methodology and validated for use in the particular species. The advantage of these methodologies is quantitative results. In-house tests based on ELISA and rapid immunomigration methods provide semiquantitative results that are below, between, or above the low-concentration standard control and the high-concentration standard control provided with the test kit.

INDICATIONS
- Assess aspects of ovarian function in bitches and queens.
- Determine the ovulation timing to determine breeding dates (bitches).
- Predict the whelping date (bitches).
- Confirm ovulation.
- Confirm an ovarian remnant.
- Assess CL function in cases of abortion:
  - Spontaneous pregnancy loss
  - Monitor the response to abortifacient drugs.
- Detect silent heat.
- Detect the presence of luteal cysts.
- 17-hydroxyprogesterone, a metabolite of progesterone, may occasionally be useful to assess adrenal gland function.

CONTRAINDICATIONS
None

POTENTIAL COMPLICATIONS
None

CLIENT EDUCATION
See the Clinical Perspective section.

BODY SYSTEMS ASSESSED
- Endocrine and metabolic
- Reproductive

SAMPLE

COLLECTION
1–3 mL of venous blood

HANDLING
- Collect the sample into a plain red-top tube. Do not use serum-separator tubes.
- Centrifuge and harvest the serum within 30–60 min.
- Because refrigeration of canine blood in serum tubes decreases progesterone significantly in freshly drawn samples, samples should be held at room temperature and serum separated as soon as possible. After 2 h at room temperature, refrigeration is no longer harmful.
- Some laboratories may accept heparinized plasma. Progesterone concentrations are higher in serum than in plasma. There was no decline in progesterone concentrations in canine blood drawn into heparinized tubes, regardless of storage temperature, for at least 5 h (Volkman 2006).
- Consult the laboratory for specific sample-handling recommendations.

STORAGE
Refrigerate or freeze the sample. Maintain the serum at room temperature for 2 h prior to refrigerating.

STABILITY
- Not stable after contact with serum-separator gel
- Decreased by prolonged contact with RBCs
- Refrigerated (2°–8°C): 1 week
- Immediate refrigeration of canine blood in serum tubes significantly decreases progesterone in freshly drawn samples (see the Storage section).
- Frozen (−20°C): 3 months

PROTOCOL
- See the Clinical Perspective section.
- To help detect ovarian remnant, progesterone can be evaluated anytime but might be particularly useful 7–10 days after clinical signs suggestive of estrus.

INTERPRETATION

NORMAL FINDINGS OR RANGE
- Units vary among laboratories. Conversion: ng/mL × 3.18 = nmol/L.
- Reference ranges through an estrous cycle vary among laboratories.
- Normal values vary among species and stage of estrous cycle.
- In general, values of ≤0.5 ng/mL (≈1.5 nmol/L) progesterone indicate no CL function, as during anestrus or in neutered animals.
- In general, the initial rise from anestrus progesterone concentrations to 1–2 ng/mL (≈3–6 nmol/L) is associated with the LH surge in bitches.

PROGESTERONE

- In general, progesterone reaches peak concentrations of 20–90 ng/mL ($\approx$60–180 nmol/L) within 30 days after ovulation and slowly decline thereafter throughout diestrus in bitches and pregnant queens.
- Progesterone concentration is similar in pregnant and pseudopregnant queens until about day 20, when it begins to decline in those pseudopregnant and remains high in those pregnant.
- In general, concentrations of >2 ng/mL ($\approx$6 nmol/L) are required to maintain pregnancy in bitches.

ABNORMAL VALUES
- Values above the basal reference levels for the laboratory should not be detected in ovariectomized females. This finding would be strongly suggestive of the presence of an ovarian remnant, even in the absence of overt signs of estrous behavior.
- Values above the basal reference levels for the laboratory should not be detected in males. This finding would be suggestive of a progesterone-producing testicular tumor.

CRITICAL VALUES
None

INTERFERING FACTORS
Drugs That May Alter Results or Interpretation
Drugs That Interfere with Test Methodology
Exogenous and endogenous steroid hormones, including 17-hydroxyprogesterone and other progestins, and deoxycorticosterone, may have some cross-reactivity with some progesterone assays.

Drugs That Alter Physiology
- Exogenous progestins, estrogen, and testosterone suppress gonadotropin-releasing hormone or LH and therefore progesterone secretion.
- Other drugs that affect gonadotropin–releasing hormone, LH, prolactin, or the CL directly can affect progesterone (examples are prostaglandin $F_{2\alpha}$; and dopamine agonists).

Disorders That May Alter Results
- Stage of the estrous cycle
- Pregnancy in cats
- Ovarian remnant
- Testicular tumor
- Luteal cysts
- Lipemia causes lower progesterone results.

Collection Techniques or Handling That May Alter Results
- Hemolysis does not interfere with RIA results but may interfere with ELISA.
- Storage time, temperature, contact with RBCs, contact with serum-separator gel, and anticoagulants affect the results. Species differences have also been noted.

Influence of Signalment
Species
- Queens: Coital stimulation induces the LH surge and ovulation. The progesterone concentration increases after the LH surge.
- Bitches: The progesterone concentration increases before ovulation and simultaneously with the LH surge. The CL persists for 60 days or longer, irrespective of pregnancy status.

Breed
None

Age
Adult

Gender
Used in females to detect presence of gonad and/or the stage of the estrous cycle

Pregnancy
- No effect in bitches. The CL persists (i.e., produces progesterone) for 60 days or longer after ovulation, irrespective of pregnancy status.
- Pregnancy does affect progesterone concentration in queens. In the absence of pregnancy in a queen that has ovulated, the CL will regress (i.e., stop producing progesterone) in $\approx$40 days rather than existing throughout the 65 days of gestation.

LIMITATIONS OF THE TEST
Quantitative results from RIA and CLIA; semiquantitative results from ELISA and rapid immunomigration
Sensitivity, Specificity, and Positive and Negative Predictive Values
N/A

Valid If Run in a Human Lab?
Yes, if the methodology used by lab has been validated for canine and feline specimens.

Causes of Abnormal Findings

High values	Low values
Functional CL	Normal anestrus
Ovarian remnant	Ovariohysterectomy
Luteal cyst(s)	Ovulation failure
	Premature luteolysis

CLINICAL PERSPECTIVE
- The initial rise above basal, anestrual concentrations coincides with the LH surge in bitches. Insemination should be done 4–6 days later. To detect the initial rise, samples should be taken every 2–3 days, beginning in proestrus. See Suggested Reading for details.
- Finding a high progesterone concentration indicates the presence of functional corpus luteum:
  - Ovulation has occurred within the past $\approx$60 days in bitches (pregnant or not) or within the past $\approx$30 days in nonpregnant queens.
  - A high progesterone concentration in a spayed female indicates the presence of an ovarian remnant, irrespective of previous signs of heat.
  - A high progesterone concentration in a female with prolonged anestrus or failure to cycle indicates either (a) a recent cycle was not observed (i.e., silent heat) or (b) luteal cysts.
  - A high progesterone concentration in breeding females found not to be pregnant indicates that ovulation failure is not the cause of infertility during that cycle. Furthermore, in queens, it indicates that coital stimulation was sufficient (i.e., multiple breedings probably occurred).
- A progesterone concentration lower than expected for the stage of gestation or $\leq$2 ng/mL ($\approx$6 nmol/L) indicates impending abortion or parturition.

MISCELLANEOUS
ANCILLARY TESTS
- Vaginal cytology for breeding management and identification of ovarian remnant
- LH for breeding management

SYNONYMS
None

SEE ALSO

Blackwell's Five-Minute Veterinary Consult: Canine and Feline Topics

- Abortion, Spontaneous, and Pregnancy Loss—Cats
- Abortion, Spontaneous, and Pregnancy Loss—Dogs
- Abortion, Termination of Pregnancy
- Breeding, Timing
- False Pregnancy
- Infertility, Female
- Ovarian Remnant Syndrome

Related Topics in This Book

- Luteinizing Hormone
- Relaxin
- Uterine Ultrasonography

ABBREVIATIONS

- CL = corpus luteum
- CLIA = chemiluminescent immunoassay
- LH = luteinizing hormone
- RIA = radioimmunoassay

Suggested Reading

Johnson CA. Disorders of the estrous cycle. In: Nelson RW, Couto CG, eds. *Small Animal Internal Medicine*, 3rd ed. St Louis: CV Mosby, 2003: 936–938.

Johnston SD, Root Kustritz MV, Olson PN. *Canine and Feline Theriogenology*. Philadelphia: WB Saunders, 2001.

Volkmann DH. The effects of storage time and temperature and anticoagulant on laboratory measurements of canine blood progesterone concentrations. *Theriogenology* 2006; 66: 1583–1586.

INTERNET RESOURCES

Root Kustritz MV. Use of commercial luteinizing hormone and progesterone assay kits in canine breeding management. In: Concannon PW, England G, Verstegen III J, Linde-Forsberg C, eds. Recent Advances in Small Animal Reproduction. Ithaca, NY: International Veterinary Information Service (IVIS), 2001; Document no. A1221.0501, http://www.ivis.org/advances/Concannon/root2/ivis.pdf.

AUTHOR NAME

Cheri A. Johnson

PROSTATIC WASH

BASICS

TYPE OF PROCEDURE
Diagnostic sample collection

PROCEDURE EXPLANATION AND RELATED PHYSIOLOGY
• Benign prostatic hyperplasia, prostatic neoplasia, and prostatitis are the most common diseases of the prostate in dogs. Differentiation of these 3 conditions requires initial evaluation of urinalysis, urine culture, and diagnostic imaging of the prostate.
• In many cases, although 1 of these differential diagnoses may be suspected after the initial evaluation, definitive diagnosis requires direct evaluation of cytologic or histopathologic prostatic samples. Prostatic wash is a minimally invasive method for obtaining prostatic fluid.
• Fluid obtained by prostatic wash may facilitate identification of neoplastic cells that have not exfoliated into urine sediment, may help in differentiating bacterial prostatitis from lower urinary tract infection without prostatic involvement, and is an alternative method for collection of prostatic fluid in stud dogs with reproductive failure.

INDICATIONS
• Suspected prostatic disease
• Collection of prostatic fluid from male dogs with reproductive failure
• Percutaneous aspiration of the prostate in dogs with suspected prostatic neoplasia may seed neoplastic cells to the abdomen along the needle track. Prostatic wash does not carry this risk.

CONTRAINDICATIONS
• None
• Severe balanophthitis is a relative contraindication for urethral catheterization.

POTENTIAL COMPLICATIONS
• Prostatic wash in animals with prostatitis (especially acute prostatitis) may cause or worsen bacteremia.
• Urethral trauma may occur during catheterization.
• Iatrogenic infectious cystitis may occur secondary to catheterization.

CLIENT EDUCATION
None

BODY SYSTEMS ASSESSED
• Renal and urologic
• Reproductive

PROCEDURE

PATIENT PREPARATION
Preprocedure Medication or Preparation
To maximize the likelihood of diagnostic sample collection in animals with suspected prostatitis, patients should have a prostatic wash performed prior to antibiotic therapy.

Anesthesia or Sedation
• The procedure can be performed in most animals without anesthesia or sedation.
• Aggressive animals or those with prostatic pain may require sedation or general anesthesia.

Patient Positioning
Lateral recumbency

Patient Monitoring
None

Equipment or Supplies
• Hair clippers
• Dilute povidone-iodine (Betadine) solution: 1 part povidone-iodine solution to ≈200 parts sterile saline. The color should be that of dilute tea.
• Two sets of 4 × 4-inch gauze sponges soaked in sterile saline and chlorhexidine or povidone-iodine solution
  • Povidone-iodine scrub should not be used on the genital mucous membranes.
• A sterile urinary catheter
  • A red rubber catheter of sufficient length to reach the urinary bladder should be used.
• Sterile lubricating jelly
• Sterile gloves for the person inserting the urinary catheter
• Gloves (nonsterile) for an assistant
• A syringe (6–20 mL)
• Sterile saline

TECHNIQUE
• Restrain the patient in lateral recumbency.
• Catheterize the patient by using sterile technique and remove all urine from the bladder (see the "Urethral Catheterization" chapter).
• Flush the urinary bladder 2–4 times with sterile saline. Remove and discard the saline and urine mixture after each flush.
• An assistant should palpate the prostate and prostatic urethra per rectum (see Figure 1).
  • The catheter is then withdrawn until the tip is approximately at the level of the prostate, as determined by the assistant's palpation.
• The prostate is vigorously massaged per rectum, including both downward massage and lateral movement.
• Inject 5–10 mL of sterile saline through the catheter into the urethra by using the syringe.
  • To minimize loss of fluid that occurs because of leakage around the catheter, manual occlusion of the urethral orifice should be maintained during saline injection and until the catheter is withdrawn.
• Aspirate the injected saline, which will contain any prostatic fluid and cellular debris.
  • Gentle negative pressure should be maintained while the catheter is advanced to the bladder, because most of the injected fluid will have flown cranially. Empty the bladder of all fluid. Aspiration then continues as the catheter is withdrawn from the urethra.
  • Aspiration while the catheter is in the urethra should be gentle to minimize trauma to the mucosa.

SAMPLE HANDLING
Prostatic fluid should be submitted for the following:
• *Cytologic analysis*: Cytopathologists should report the presence or absence of inflammatory cells, dysplastic or neoplastic cells, and infectious agents.
• *Culture*: Aerobic bacterial culture is usually sufficient for diagnosis of most cases of prostatitis. Mycoplasma and fungal cultures may be considered, depending on breed, concurrent physical examination findings, urinalysis and urine culture results, and cytopathologic findings of prostatic fluid.

APPROPRIATE AFTERCARE
Postprocedure Patient Monitoring
None

Nursing Care
None

Dietary Modification
None

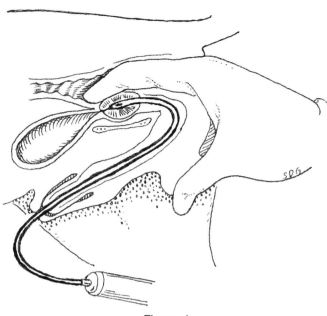

Figure 1

Sagittal section showing the recommended placement of the catheter tip and the assistant's finger for prostatic massage during prostatic wash.

Medication Requirements
- Administration of broad-spectrum antibiotics with an agent known to have good penetration into the prostate should be initiated following prostatic wash in those patients with suspected prostatitis, pending the results of bacterial culture.
- Antibiotics with good prostatic penetration include fluoroquinolones, sulfonamides, macrolides, and chloramphenicol.

Restrictions on Activity
None

Anticipated Recovery Time
Immediate

INTERPRETATION

NORMAL FINDINGS OR RANGE
- *Prostatic fluid appearance*: clear to white-tinged fluid that is usually not visible because of dilution in the saline used for sample collection
- *Prostatic fluid cytology*: low numbers of erythrocytes, leukocytes, and transitional epithelial cells that lack dysplastic or neoplastic criteria
- *Prostatic fluid culture*: There should be no bacterial growth.

ABNORMAL VALUES
- *Prostatic fluid cytology*: large numbers of inflammatory leukocytes (particularly neutrophils); transitional or prostatic epithelial cells with dysplastic or neoplastic changes
  - Dysplastic or neoplastic criteria may be seen in epithelial cells collected from animals with bacterial prostatitis, even in the absence of prostatic neoplasia. Differentiation of dogs with primary bacterial prostatitis from those with prostatic neoplasia and secondary bacterial prostatitis may require appropriate antibiotic therapy followed by repeat prostatic wash or, alternatively, percutaneous prostatic aspiration or biopsy. Patient signalment (neutered vs intact male dogs) and the appearance of the prostate on diagnostic images should also be used to prioritize differential diagnoses.

- *Prostatic fluid culture*: growth of bacterial or fungal agents
  - The most common agents of bacterial prostatitis are the same as those that cause bacterial urinary tract infections: *Escherichia coli*, *Staphylococcus* spp., *Proteus* spp., etc. Less commonly isolated bacteria from dogs with bacterial prostatitis include *Brucella canis* and *Mycoplasma* spp.
  - Low numbers of bacteria in animals with prostatitis (false negatives) may be due to antibiotic administration prior to sample collection. Low numbers of bacteria in animals without prostatitis (false positives) are most commonly due to contamination of the prostatic fluid sample by urethral flora.

CRITICAL VALUES
None

INTERFERING FACTORS
Drugs That May Alter Results of the Procedure
Antibiotic administration prior to sample collection may inhibit growth of bacteria in dogs with bacterial prostatitis.

Conditions That May Interfere with Performing the Procedure
- Functional or mechanical urethral obstruction
- Animals with acute prostatitis or metastasis of prostatic neoplasia to the lumbar vertebral bodies often have severe pain that precludes digital rectal examination and prostatic massage without heavy sedation or general anesthesia.

Procedure Techniques or Handling That May Alter Results
Poor technique during urethral catheterization can contaminate the sample with bacteria and result in a false-positive diagnosis of prostatitis.

Influence of Signalment on Performing and Interpreting the Procedure
Species
Prostatic disease is very rare in male cats, and thus the utility of prostatic wash for differentiation of types of prostatic disease has not been evaluated in this species. Regardless, the patient's size and the difficulty of catheterization will limit the ability to perform prostatic washes in cats; general anesthesia would be required.

Breed
None

Age
There are no significant age differences at presentation between dogs with bacterial prostatitis and dogs with prostatic neoplasia.

Gender
- The incidence of prostatic neoplasia is the same in neutered and castrated male dogs.
- Primary bacterial prostatitis is extremely rare in castrated male dogs. The most likely differential diagnosis in a castrated dog with suspected prostatic disease is neoplasia, even if urinalysis, urine culture, and prostatic fluid analysis indicate bacterial prostatitis.

Pregnancy
None

CLINICAL PERSPECTIVE
- Prostatic wash is a relatively easy method for obtaining diagnostic samples in patients with suspected prostatic disease.
- The correlation between cytologic and histopathologic diagnoses of samples obtained from dogs with prostatic disease is relatively high [80% in a recent study (Powe et al. 2004)]. The accuracy of the final diagnosis is likely improved by considering other factors, such as patient signalment, when interpreting results of prostatic wash fluid analysis.
- Thorough rectal palpation, abdominal radiographs, and ultrasonographic examination, urinalysis, and urine culture are the most useful adjunctive tests in patients with suspected or confirmed prostatic disease.

PROSTATIC WASH

MISCELLANEOUS

ANCILLARY TESTS
- *Brucella canis* rapid slide agglutination test (RSAT)
- Semen evaluation
- Urinalysis
- Urine culture

SYNONYMS
Prostatic massage

SEE ALSO
Blackwell's Five-Minute Veterinary Consult: Canine and Feline Topics
- Adenocarcinoma, Prostate
- Benign Prostatic Hyperplasia
- Brucellosis
- Prostate Disease in the Breeding Male Dog
- Prostatitis and Prostatic Abscess
- Prostatomegaly
- Transitional Cell Carcinoma, Renal, Bladder, Urethra
- Urinary Tract Infection, Bacterial

Related Topics in This Book
- Semen Analysis
- Semen Collection
- Urethral Catheterization

ABBREVIATIONS
None

Suggested Reading
Cornell KK, Bostwick DG, Cooley DM, *et al.* Clinical and pathologic aspects of spontaneous canine prostate carcinoma: A retrospective analysis of 76 cases. *Prostate* 2000; 45: 173–183.

Karwiec DR, Heflin D. Study of prostatic disease in dogs: 177 cases (1981–1986). *J Am Vet Med Assoc* 1992; 200: 1119–1122.

Powe JR, Canfield PJ, Martin PA. Evaluation of the cytologic diagnosis of canine prostatic disorders. *Vet Clin Pathol* 2004; 33: 150–154.

Read RA, Bryden S. Urethral bleeding as a presenting sign of benign prostatic hyperplasia in the dog: A retrospective study (1979–1993). *J Am Anim Hosp Assoc* 1995; 31: 261–267.

INTERNET RESOURCES
None

AUTHOR NAME
Barrak M. Pressler

PROTEIN ELECTROPHORESIS

BASICS

TYPE OF SPECIMEN
Blood

TEST EXPLANATION AND RELATED PHYSIOLOGY

Serum proteins are a heterogeneous category of molecules that can be separated into groups, or fractions, by electrophoresis. *Protein electrophoresis* is based on the principle that charged protein particles placed in an electric field will migrate within a support medium (cellulose acetate or agarose gel are most routinely used). The direction and speed of protein migration depend on several factors, including their net charge (+ or −), molecular size, and the type of gel used. In general, the sample is applied to the end closest to the cathode (negatively charged terminal), and the smaller and/or more negatively charged particles will migrate toward the anode (positively charged terminal) farther and faster than larger and/or less negatively charged particles. Protein bands form in the support medium at the end points of migration of the various proteins. The gel is stained, and the intensity of individual bands, corresponding to the protein concentration, is measured using a densitometer. This information is used to generate an *electrophoretogram*. The area under the curve of the electrophoretogram reflects the total quantity of stained protein, and the percentage of each protein fraction can be determined. Finally, to determine the approximate protein concentrations in each protein fraction, these percentages are multiplied by the total protein concentration obtained through chemical analysis (likely via biuret reaction).

The main fractions of proteins based on electrophoretic properties are albumin, and α-, β-, and γ-globulins, each of which may be further subdivided into zones (fast and slow) (Figure 1). Albumin migrates the farthest because of its small size and strong negative charge. The globulins are heterogeneous and are generally larger molecules with relatively weaker negative charge. The α-globulins migrate the farthest (of the globulins) and include some acute phase proteins (e.g., ceruloplasmin, haptoglobin, α_2-macroglobulin), lipoproteins (high-density lipoprotein), and pre-lipoproteins (very low-density lipoprotein). Acute inflammation is the most common reason for elevated α-globulins, although nephrotic syndrome can also increase this globulin fraction through increased lipoprotein production. Important

proteins of the β fraction include low-density lipoprotein and several other acute phase proteins, including fibrinogen, C-reactive protein, hemopexin, transferrin, and complement. Some immunoglobulins (IgM and IgA) will also migrate in this band. Increases in β-globulins can be seen with acute inflammation, conditions that cause antigenic stimulation, nephrotic syndrome, and active liver disease.

The γ fraction is composed primarily of immunoglobulins (IgG and IgE). Increases in γ-globulins, or *gammopathies*, are further classified as monoclonal or polyclonal, and these distinctions are made through examination of the electrophoretogram. Polyclonal gammopathies (Figure 1) are characterized by a wide γ-globulin fraction due to the presence of a variety of antibodies produced by a heterogeneous population of B lymphocytes and plasma cells. Sometimes, increased immunoglobulins will obscure the border between β and γ fractions. Polyclonal gammopathies can be seen with any process that causes chronic antigenic stimulation, including chronic infections (e.g., ehrlichiosis, FIP) or immune-mediated disease. Chronic liver disease can also lead to a polyclonal gammopathy, perhaps because of decreased liver clearance of antigens absorbed from the intestinal tract. Monoclonal gammopathies (Figure 1) consist of a single homogeneous protein and appear as a narrow peak with a base similar in width to the albumin band or a peak height at least 4 times the peak width. Monoclonal gammopathies are usually the result of a malignant clone of plasma cells (myeloma) or B lymphocytes (i.e., lymphoma, lymphoid leukemia).

INDICATIONS
• To screen for monoclonal gammopathy in animals with normoglobinulinemia or hyperglobulinemia
• To screen hypoglobulinemic patients for a γ-globulin deficiency suggestive of an immunodeficiency

CONTRAINDICATIONS
None

POTENTIAL COMPLICATIONS
None

CLIENT EDUCATION
None

BODY SYSTEMS ASSESSED
• Hemic, lymphatic, and immune
• Hepatobiliary

A. Normal

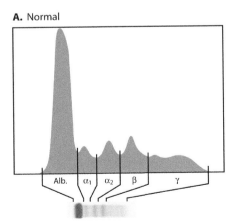

B. Polyclonal gammopathy

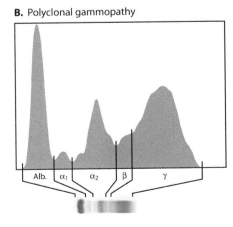

C. Monoclonal gammopathy

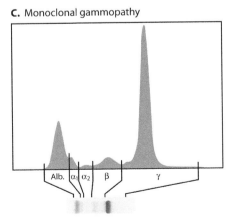

Figure 1

Examples of possible electrophoretograms: **(A)** normal, **(B)** a polyclonal gammopathy, and **(C)** a monoclonal gammopathy.

PROTEIN ELECTROPHORESIS

SAMPLE

COLLECTION
0.5–2.0 mL of venous blood

HANDLING
• Collect the sample into a plain red-top tube or serum-separator tube.
• Sodium heparin or lithium heparin anticoagulant also is acceptable.

STORAGE
Refrigeration is recommended for short-term storage. Freeze for long-term storage.

STABILITY
• Refrigerated (2°–8°C): 3 days
• Frozen (−20°C): 6 months

PROTOCOL
None

INTERPRETATION

NORMAL FINDINGS OR RANGE
Globulin concentrations; reference intervals may vary depending on the laboratory and assay:

Dogs
• α_1: 0.2–0.5 g/dL (2–5 g/L)
• α_2: 0.3–1.1 g/dL (3–11 g/L)
• β_1: 0.6–1.2 g/dL (6–12 g/L)
• β_2: N/A
• γ: 0.5–1.8 g/dL (5–18 g/L)

Cats
• α_1: 0.3–0.9 g/dL (3–9 g/L)
• α_2: 0.3–0.9 g/dL (3–9 g/L)
• β_1: 0.4–0.9 g/dL (4–9 g/L)
• β_2: 0.3–0.6 g/dL (3–6 g/L)
• γ: 1.7–2.7 g/dL (17–27 g/L)

ABNORMAL VALUES
Values above or below the reference range

CRITICAL VALUES
None

INTERFERING FACTORS
Drugs That May Alter Results or Interpretation
Drugs That Interfere with Test Methodology
None

Drugs That Alter Physiology
Corticosteroids may increase the α_2 fraction by elevating haptoglobin complexes.

Disorders That May Alter Results
Hemolysis may increase both the α_2 fraction, because of formation of haptoglobin-hemoglobin complexes, and the β-globulin peak, because of free hemoglobin.

Collection Techniques or Handling That May Alter Results
• Traumatic venipuncture causing in vitro hemolysis
• If plasma is used, fibrinogen, an acute phase protein, will run in the β_2-globulin peak. This protein is eliminated from serum through the process of clot formation.

Influence of Signalment
Species
Slight differences in migration exist for the same protein groups in different species.

Breed
None

Age
Minimal immunoglobulins are present at birth. The immunoglobulin concentration rises rapidly in newborns because of absorption of maternal immunoglobulins following ingestion of colostrum.

Gender
None

Pregnancy
Globulin concentrations may decrease during the third trimester of pregnancy and at whelping.

LIMITATIONS OF THE TEST
Calculated concentrations of the electrophoretic fractions are estimates of protein concentrations, and their accuracy can be affected by the substrate (cellulose vs agarose), type of stain, and how accurately individual protein bands are distinguished and marked for calculations. The latter can be a particular problem when proteins in different fractions begin to run together.

Sensitivity, Specificity, and Positive and Negative Predictive Values
N/A

Valid If Run in a Human Lab?
Yes.

CLINICAL PERSPECTIVE
• Most functional lymphoid neoplasms produce a monoclonal spike in the γ-globulin band. However, with IgM- or IgA-producing neoplasms, the monoclonal spike may appear in the β-globulin region.
• Occasionally, patients with myeloma or a lymphoid neoplasm will have 2 distinct malignant clones producing a biclonal gammopathy.
• Increased production of acute phase proteins can increase α and β fractions within 2 days after onset of inflammation, and this abnormality can persist as long as inflammation persists.
• Evaluation of the densitometer tracing is essential for identifying a monoclonal (vs polyclonal) gammopathy, and calculated concentrations of electrophoretic fractions are often not necessary.
• A marked polyclonal gammopathy is common in cats with FIP; α_2-globulins usually increase in early disease but switch to a γ-globulin response as clinical signs progress.
• Although some cases of *Ehrlichia canis* and FIP have been reportedly associated with monoclonal gammopathies, more likely multiple different IgG molecules are migrating into an extremely compact γ-globulin band (oligoclonal gammopathy).

MISCELLANEOUS

ANCILLARY TESTS
• Bone marrow aspiration is recommended in dogs and cats with monoclonal gammopathy to look for myeloma and lymphoid leukemia.
• Radiography can be used to look for lytic bone lesions recommended in animals with monoclonal gammopathy.

Causes of Abnormal Findings

High values	Low values
Albumin	Low albumin with decreased
Hemoconcentration	albumin/globulin ratio
α-Globulin	Decreased production
Inflammation (associated with a	Increased loss, selective (i.e.,
large variety of diseases; e.g.,	protein-losing nephropathy)
atopy, pyoderma, parvovirus	Sequestration (effusions)
enteritis, immune-mediated	Low albumin with normal
disease)	albumin/globulin ratio
Neoplasia (various)	Blood loss
Nephritic syndrome	Protein-losing enteropathy
Hepatic disease	Protein-losing dermatopathy
Spontaneous hyperadrenocorticism	Low γ-globulin
Diabetes mellitus	Failure of passive transfer
β-Globulin	Severe combined
Inflammation	immunodeficiency (dogs)
Nephrotic syndrome	Selective IgM, IgA, and IgG
Hepatic disease	deficiencies (dogs)
γ-Globulin, polyclonal	Transient
Infectious processes (e.g., bacterial,	hypogammaglobulinemia
rickettsial, viral, fungal, protozoal)	(dogs)
Immune-mediated diseases	
Liver disease (severe)	
γ-Globulin, monoclonal	
Lymphoid neoplasia (B cell)	
Plasma cell myeloma or	
plasmacytoma	
Lymphoma	
Lymphocytic leukemia	
Macroglobulinemia	
Nonneoplastic (infrequent)	
Canine ehrlichiosis*	
Canine amyloidosis	
Visceral leishmaniasis	
FIP*	
Immunoglobulin light chains	
(Bence-Jones proteins)	
Idiopathic	

*Usually polyclonal; possibly oligoclonal.

- In animals with a monoclonal gammopathy, immunoelectrophoresis can be used to identify the type of immunoglobulin present and is the ideal method for identification of light chains (Bence-Jones proteins).
- In hypoglobulinemic animals, radial immunodiffusion can quantify IgG, IgM, and IgA to better characterize an immunodeficiency.

SYNONYMS
None

SEE ALSO
Blackwell's Five-Minute Veterinary Consult: Canine and Feline Topics
- Immunodeficiency Disorders, Primary
- Multiple Myeloma

Related Topics in This Book
- Acute Phase Proteins
- Albumin
- Bence-Jones Proteins
- Globulins
- Immunoglobulin Assays
- Total Protein

ABBREVIATIONS
None

Suggested Reading

Evans EW, Duncan JR. Proteins, lipids, and carbohydrates. In: Latimer KS, Mahaffey EA, Prasse KW, eds. *Duncan and Prasse's Veterinary Laboratory Medicine Clinical Pathology*, 4th ed. Ames: Iowa State Press, 2003: 162–192.

Lassen ED. Laboratory evaluation of plasma and serum proteins. In: Thrall MA, ed. *Veterinary Hematology and Clinical Chemistry*. Philadelphia: Lippincott Williams & Wilkins, 2004: 401–412.

Stockham SL, Scott MA. Proteins. *In: Fundamentals of Veterinary Clinical Pathology*. Ames: Iowa State Press 2002: 251–276.

Thomas JS. Protein electrophoresis. In: Feldman BF, Zinkl JG, Jain NC, eds. *Schalm's Veterinary Hematology*, 5th ed. Ames, IA: Blackwell, 2006: 899–903.

INTERNET RESOURCES
None

AUTHOR NAMES
Rob Simoni and Joyce S. Knoll

PROTHROMBIN TIME

BASICS

TYPE OF SPECIMEN
Blood

TEST EXPLANATION AND RELATED PHYSIOLOGY
The prothrombin time (PT) is a functional test of the extrinsic and common coagulation pathways. The PT result is the clotting time (in seconds) of an assay mixture containing a tissue factor reagent that specifically initiates coagulation through activation of factor VII. The assay measures the enzyme or coenzyme activity of factor VII and the common system (factors X, V, and II) and is sensitive to severe deficiency or inhibition of fibrinogen. Prolongation of the PT therefore indicates extrinsic and/or common pathway factor deficiencies.

The PT assay end point of fibrin formation is detected as a change in light transmittance (by photoptical instruments) or viscoelasticity (by mechanical instruments).

INDICATIONS
- To screen for coagulation factor deficiencies
- To monitor coumadin therapy

CONTRAINDICATIONS
None

POTENTIAL COMPLICATIONS
None

CLIENT EDUCATION
A combination of tests is often required for a comprehensive assessment of coagulation.

BODY SYSTEMS ASSESSED
Hemic, lymphatic, and immune

SAMPLE

COLLECTION
1.8 mL of venous blood

HANDLING
- Collect blood directly into sodium citrate (3.2% or 3.8%) anticoagulant.
- Combine exactly 1.8 mL of blood with exactly 0.2 mL of citrate. An exact ratio of blood to citrate (9 parts:1 part) is critical for valid results.
- Within 1 h of collection, perform point-of-care coagulation tests or centrifuge whole blood and transfer plasma into plastic or siliconized glass tube (without additives).

STORAGE
- Store the sample in a refrigerator for assay within 4 h.
- Store the sample in a freezer if the sample is to be assayed in >4 h after collection.
- Ship the sample overnight on cold packs.

STABILITY
- Room temperature: 1 h
- Refrigerated (2°–8°C): 4 h
- Frozen (−20°C): 2 weeks

PROTOCOL
None

INTERPRETATION

NORMAL FINDINGS OR RANGE
- Dog PT: 13–18 s
- Cat PT: 14–22 s

Reference values are from the Comparative Coagulation Section of the Cornell University Animal Health Diagnostic Center. Values may vary based on reagents and instrumentation.

ABNORMAL VALUES
- Prolongation of the PT beyond the reference range, or 1.5 times greater than the same-species control
- Shortening of the PT has little diagnostic relevance and may reflect improper sampling.

CRITICAL VALUES
The correlation between relative prolongation of PT and in vivo hemostatic failure varies for different disease syndromes and underlying causes of long PT.

INTERFERING FACTORS
Drugs That May Alter Results or Interpretation
Drugs That Interfere with Test Methodology
Oxyglobin [hemoglobin glutamer-200 (bovine); Biopure, Cambridge, MA] may interfere with end-point determination in photoptical but not mechanical clot detection instruments.

Drugs That Alter Physiology
- Treatment with anticoagulant drugs may prolong the PT.
- Therapeutic monitoring of coumadin is based on attaining a target prolongation of PT of either 1.5 times the patient's baseline value or an international normalized ratio (INR) of 2–3. The *INR* is a transformation of the patient PT result that factors in variation between PT reagents and laboratory reference ranges and can be provided by the testing laboratory.
- Therapeutic levels of unfractionated heparin or low molecular weight heparins are monitored by measuring activated partial thromboplastin time (aPTT) and factor Xa inhibition, respectively.

Disorders That May Alter Results
Severe hemolysis or lipemia may interfere with photoptical, but not mechanical, clot-detection instruments.

Collection Techniques or Handling That May Alter Results
- Collection into heparin, EDTA, or plain glass tubes or into tubes containing serum-separator and clot activators
- Excessive or insufficient citrate anticoagulant because of high or low Hct, or incomplete blood draw
- Ex vivo factor activation because of poor venipuncture technique
- Heparin contamination of samples drawn via indwelling catheters

Influence of Signalment
Species
None

Breed
Hereditary factor VII deficiency reported as an autosomal trait in beagles, malamutes, Alaskan Klee Kais, deerhounds, and domestic shorthair cats

Age
None

Gender
None

Pregnancy
None

LIMITATIONS OF THE TEST
PT assays optimized for measuring human PT may be relatively insensitive to mild to moderate factor deficiencies in dogs and cats.

Sensitivity, Specificity, and Positive and Negative Predictive Values
N/A

Valid If Run in a Human Lab?
Yes—but same-species reference ranges are required.

Causes of Abnormal Values

High values (prolonged PT)	Low values
Hereditary factor VII deficiency	Not significant
Acquired factor VII deficiency	
Early or mild vitamin K deficiency	
Coumadin therapy	
Cholestatic disease	
Liver failure	
Anticoagulant rodenticide ingestion	
Consumptive coagulopathies	

CLINICAL PERSPECTIVE
• Coumadin and anticoagulant rodenticides impair hepatic production of functional vitamin K–dependent factors (factors II, VII, IX, and X). Factor VII has a short plasma half-life (<6 h), and so sensitive PT is prolonged before aPTT in early vitamin K–deficient states.
• Dogs and cats with active bleeding caused by vitamin K deficiency typically have prolonged aPTT and PT. Thrombin clotting time (TCT) and fibrinogen are insensitive to vitamin K deficiency.
• aPTT, PT, and TCT (with low fibrinogen) are most often prolonged by severe liver failure or hemorrhagic disseminated intravascular coagulation.
• Dogs and cats with hereditary factor VII deficiency have a prolonged PT but a normal aPTT.

MISCELLANEOUS

ANCILLARY TESTS
aPTT and TCT (or fibrinogen) screening tests

SYNONYMS
One-stage prothrombin time (OSPT)

SEE ALSO
Blackwell's Five-Minute Veterinary Consult: Canine and Feline Topics
• Chapters on hepatic diseases
• Anticoagulant Rodenticide Poisoning
• Disseminated Intravascular Coagulation

Related Topics in This Book
• Anticoagulant Screen
• Coagulation Factors
• Partial Thromboplastin Time, Activated
• PIVKA Test

ABBREVIATIONS
• aPTT = activated partial thromboplastin time
• INR = international normalized ratio
• PT = prothrombin time
• TCT = thrombin clotting time

Suggested Reading
Mischke R, Nolte IJA. Hemostasis: Introduction, overview, and laboratory techniques. In: Feldman BF, Zinkl JG, Jain NC, eds. *Schalm's Veterinary Hematology*, 5th ed. Baltimore: Lippincott Williams & Wilkins, 2000: 519–525.
Monnet E, Morgan MR. Effect of three loading doses of warfarin on the international normalized ratio for dogs. *Am J Vet Res* 2000; 61: 48–50.
Stokol TS, Brooks MB, Erb HN. Effect of citrate concentration on coagulation test results in dogs. *J Am Vet Med Assoc* 2000; 217: 1672–1677.

INTERNET RESOURCES
Cornell University, College of Veterinary Medicine, Department of Medicine and Diagnostic Sciences: Comparative diagnostics, http://www.diaglab.vet.cornell.edu/coag/clinical/diagnos.asp.

AUTHOR NAME
Marjory Brooks

PULMONARY FUNCTION TESTS

BASICS

TYPE OF PROCEDURE
Function tests

PROCEDURE EXPLANATION AND RELATED PHYSIOLOGY
The main function of the respiratory system is to transport air to and from (ventilate) the deep lung, thus delivering oxygen to the alveolar surface and, in return, removing carbon dioxide—all at a rate that matches the metabolic demand of the animal. If one considers the lung as 1 big ventilatory unit, the completeness of this gas exchange can be evaluated by using blood-gas analyses. On the other hand, PFTs assess the efficiency by which air is transported in and/or out of this ventilatory structure. When PFT data are combined with information on gas exchange, one can more objectively characterize respiratory dysfunction, allowing for more optimal management of the small-animal respiratory patient. This information would assist in assessing responses to specific drug treatment and in monitoring disease progression for prognostic purposes.

Although respiratory disease is common in companion animals, its development is often insidious, and, as a result, chronic disease processes can become well established prior to detection of significant abnormalities on routine physical examination or radiography. Fortunately, arterial blood-gas analysis, pulse oximetry, end-tidal carbon dioxide analysis, and related measurements are being used more routinely, enabling improved assessment of gas exchange and tissue oxygen delivery. However, comparable information on ventilation efficiency (i.e., changes in the mechanics of breathing) is still available only in select referral institutions. This latter topic will be expanded upon herein, with brief explanations of the approaches that are most applicable for use in companion animals.

Knowledge of basic respiratory physiology is fundamental to understanding how PFTs are used to characterize disease. Relationships exist between structural pathologic changes and resultant functional deficits. In general, increased oxygen demand (e.g., exercise) or conditions that impede the efficiency by which air can be transported in and/or out of the lung increase work for the respiratory muscles. Similarly, conditions that reduce efficiency of gas exchange at the alveolar surface, or reduce transport of oxygen-enriched blood throughout the body, also increase the work of breathing. To compensate, animals often minimize their activity levels, thus developing *exercise intolerance*. This relative lack of pulmonary reserve may be unmasked by increasing the animal's ventilatory efforts during testing. As airflow or gas exchange becomes more significantly compromised, resting or tidal breathing assessments may reveal an alternation in an animal's breathing strategy that is useful diagnostically.

PFT measurements are derived from key components of the ventilatory cycle. The inspiratory and expiratory phases of a breath are defined by changes in 3 interrelated variables: *volume*, *airflow*, and *pressure*. By simultaneously quantifying changes in these parameters, along with alterations in their temporal relationships, PFTs serve to localize disease and characterize changes into obstructive or restrictive patterns. Examples of PFTs include (in order of increasing complexity or invasiveness) spirometry, tidal breathing or augmented flow-volume (FV) loop analysis, plethysmography (including single-, double-, or head-out chamber variations on a theme), and measurements of upper airway resistance (Ruaw), lung resistance (R_L), total thoracic compliance, and static or dynamic lung compliance (C_{DYN}).

INDICATIONS
- Routine use of PFTs in veterinary medicine could enhance the earlier detection of respiratory disease, potentially enabling therapeutic intervention prior to the establishment of chronic, irreversible lung or upper airway remodeling.
- *Tidal breathing flow-volume loop (TBFVL) assessments.* Using TBFVL analysis, changes in airflow, volume, and the timing aspects of a breath can be assessed in conscious, nonsedated patients. The main disadvantage of this approach is its inherent insensitivity because measurements are not obtained during maximal ventilatory efforts. Nevertheless, TBFVL assessments have been used to characterize moderate airflow obstruction in both dogs and cats. Upper airway airflow obstruction can be differentiated into relatively fixed obstruction (e.g., pharyngeal mass) versus dynamic, largely inspiratory obstruction (e.g., laryngeal paralysis). Moderately severe lower airway obstruction can also be detected by using TBFVL analysis. For example, in cats with bronchopulmonary disease, prolonged expiratory-to-inspiratory time ratios and blunted midexpiratory and end-expiratory flow values can be observed, consistent with bronchoconstriction. Importantly, because of the ease with which this technique can be used in the same patient over time, one can monitor treatment response in individual cats following bronchodilator or anti-inflammatory therapy. Use of enhanced FV loop assessments may enable detection of changes (e.g., airflow decrements) in relatively incipient or mild disease.
- *Spirometry* and *dynamic lung volume* measurements can be used to assess the spontaneous ventilatory capability of patients recovering from ventilator support after thoracotomy or neuromuscular blockade.
- Similarly, related measurements (e.g., total thoracic compliance or static lung compliance) can be used in chronically ventilated patients to detect trends suggesting impending pulmonary edema or pneumonia.
- Ventilators used in small-animal critical care facilities may also provide information on peak flow rates, timing aspects of a breath, FV loops, and so forth. Although such data are usually obtained during mandatory (ventilator driven) breaths, these ventilators are also capable of displaying data from spontaneously triggered breaths. Since these machines are sufficiently sensitive to monitor neonates, infants, and adult humans, they are potentially capable of generating the range of breath volumes and flow rates needed to evaluate animals ranging in size from cats to large-breed dogs.
- *Whole-body plethysmography (WBP).* Because of its noninvasiveness, WBP has been used to assess cats with bronchopulmonary disease and dogs with chronic bronchitis or collapsing trachea. Importantly, WBP enables estimation of certain box flow signal-derived variables [e.g., enhanced pause (Penh)] that are purportedly related to the degree of bronchoconstriction present. Although experimental studies have shown that Penh does not always correlate with changes in airway resistance, a few studies using WBP in cats and dogs suggest that this parameter does have clinical utility. For example, one can nebulize aerosols directly into the chamber during testing. This approach has been used to evaluate acute bronchodilator response in asthmatic cats. In addition, one can deliver supplemental oxygen or carbon dioxide into the chamber to alter ventilatory effort during testing. Similarly, by nebulizing increasing concentrations of bronchoconstrictive agents (e.g., carbachol, methacholine) into the chamber, one can characterize a patient's degree of airway responsiveness.
- *Upper airway resistance (Ruaw) assessments.* Ruaw measurements can be obtained by using only local anesthesia and can be used in relatively large-breed dogs with suspect upper airway disease.

- *Lung mechanics.* For a more in-depth assessment of breathing mechanics, one must obtain information on the transpulmonary pressure changes occurring in conjunction with the flow and volume measurements. Accordingly, one can then calculate lung resistance (R_L), which is defined by the change in transpulmonary pressure occurring for a corresponding change in airflow. Increased R_L measurements are indicative of central with/or without peripheral *airway constriction* or *obstruction*. Alternatively, by measuring the volume of air transported in and/or out of the lung by a given change in pressure, one can assess C_{DYN}. Decreased C_{DYN} measurements reflect that the lung is *stiffer* than normal, possibly owing to extensive, small-airway constriction or, alternatively, development of diffuse infiltrative disease (e.g., pulmonary edema, pulmonary fibrosis). These measurements have been used to characterize cats with bronchopulmonary disease, specifically to establish (1) the degree of airway obstruction present; (2) the reversibility of the obstruction, if present; and (3) the degree of underlying nonspecific airway responsiveness present.

CONTRAINDICATIONS
Patients in overt respiratory distress should be considered extremely labile, and any additional stressors, including PFTs, should be delayed until better control over ventilation has been achieved. Of note, however, cats are seemingly quite tolerant of WBP. Hence, in a *hands-off*, minimally invasive manner, one may be able to place a dyspneic cat into a plethysmographic chamber, administer supplemental oxygen and various nebulized medications, and objectively monitor changes in relative airflow obstruction.

POTENTIAL COMPLICATIONS
Similar to those related to the use of anesthesia and endotracheal intubation in patients with respiratory disease

CLIENT EDUCATION
N/A

BODY SYSTEMS ASSESSED
Upper and/or lower respiratory tracts

PROCEDURE

PATIENT PREPARATION
Dependent on the type of test performed

Preprocedure Medication or Preparation
N/A

Anesthesia or Sedation
N/A

Patient Positioning
Standing, sitting, or sternal recumbency

Patient Monitoring
In patients undergoing assessments requiring general anesthesia, owing to the potentially labile nature of airway tone and patency, continuous monitoring of ECG and pulse oximetry are recommended during testing.

EQUIPMENT AND TECHNIQUE
- For acquisition of FV data, animals must be fitted with a tight-fitting face mask (see Figure 1) or be endotracheally intubated.
- *Spirometry* requires a spirometer that is connected to a face mask or endotracheal tube. To assess lung volume and airflow changes accurately, the spirometer must be calibrated and air leaks must be negligible.

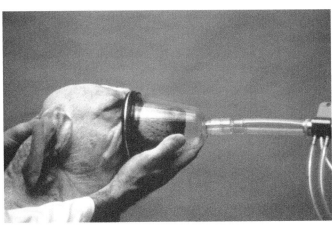

Figure 1

For tidal breathing flow-volume loop assessment, the animal's nose and mouth is enclosed in a snuggly fitting face mask. The mask must be connected to an appropriately sized, heated pneumotachograph and its associated pressure transducer.

- For *TBFVL analysis*, the animal's nose and mouth are enclosed in a snuggly fitting face mask. Some degree of patient cooperation (e.g., no excessive purring or growling) is needed in order to obtain breaths that are consistent and thus representative of the animal's resting airflow and breath-volume measurements. The mask must be connected to an appropriately sized, heated pneumotachograph and its associated pressure transducer (Figure 1). Electronic signals are processed by dedicated equipment.
- *Enhanced FV loop* assessments attempt to discern airflow decrements in relatively incipient or mild disease by inducing patients to breathe more maximally. Methods to increase respiratory drive have included drugs (e.g., doxapram), exercise, and increasing the percentage of inspired carbon dioxide (up to 10%).
- *Whole-body plethysmographs (WBPs)* are commercially available and include a variety of designs. To avoid excess dead space, plethysmography requires an appropriately sized body box for the patient under evaluation. WBPs can be sealed (pressure body boxes) or, more commonly, incorporate a known, biased flow (flow boxes). Pneumotachographs can be incorporated into the Plexiglas chamber itself. A double-chambered WBP (see Figure 1) enables discrimination of thoracic and nasal flow waveforms. Alternatively, for larger dogs, one can use a combination of face mask–derived (nasal) flow information with head-out plethysmography-derived (thoracic) flow data. Each type of plethysmograph has inherent advantages and disadvantages, the details of which are beyond the scope of this chapter.
- *Ruaw* measurements are obtained by inserting a catheter (connected to a pressure transducer) transtracheally into the lumen of the trachea, thus obtaining measurements of the pressure changes occurring across the upper airways during the breath. Simultaneous volume and airflow measurements are also needed and can be obtained noninvasively by using the aforementioned face-mask technique.
- To assess breathing mechanics, in addition to flow and volume measurements, one must obtain some estimate of the transpulmonary pressure changes occurring. In an anesthetized animal, a calibrated balloon-tipped catheter may be placed in the distal esophagus. The catheter is then connected to a pressure transducer. Alternatively, the

PULMONARY FUNCTION TESTS

animal may be placed in a head-out or closed (pressure) plethysmograph. Furthermore, to avoid the influence of the upper respiratory tract on these lung assessments, the animal is typically intubated. At isovolume conditions of the breath, R_L is calculated by dividing the change in transpulmonary pressure by the corresponding change in airflow. C_{DYN} is calculated at isoflow conditions by using the change in lung volume generated by a given change in pressure.

• Electronic signals obtained simultaneously from 2 or more pressure transducers must be calibrated and phase matched. Frequent recalibration of the system is needed to avoid erroneous information caused by signal drift.

• Preamplifiers, pulmonary mechanics analyzers, and specific software programs are needed to amplify, process, calculate, and store the vast amounts of data required to generate FV loops and other calculated indices (e.g., peak flow ratios, R_L, C_{DYN}, or Penh measurements).

• Owing to the specialized equipment and expertise necessary to perform these assessments, referral to veterinary pulmonary specialists will be necessary. Interested readers are referred to the references in the Suggested Reading section for more details on the use and interpretation of these testing procedures.

SAMPLE (DATA) HANDLING
One must establish and adhere to strict exclusion criteria for defining interpretable data. For example, excessively rapid respiratory rates (panting) or slow rates (breath holding) should not be used. For TBFVL assessments, breaths with inadequate loop closure or patient movement and/or vocalization should not be used. For enhanced FV loops, one should take care that the signals obtained do not go beyond the range or limit for the pneumotachograph and/or pressure transducer in use. For WBP, wide variations in box air temperature and humidification may influence the box flow signals. Likewise, disturbances in room pressure (e.g., doors opening and shutting) can affect the box flow signals.

APPROPRIATE AFTERCARE
Postprocedure Patient Monitoring
This is similar to general postanesthetic care provided for respiratory patients. Providing supplemental oxygen and having anticholinergic or bronchodilating medication available are recommended in order to ensure that patients recover fully from the testing procedure.

Nursing Care
N/A

Dietary Modification
N/A

Medication Requirements
N/A

Restrictions on Activity
N/A

Anticipated Recovery Time
N/A

INTERPRETATION

NORMAL FINDINGS OR RANGE
A general limitation in using PFTs to assess individual small-animal patients is the lack of specific reference values. Development of standardized, validated protocols will be necessary to generate such reference ranges. Further refinement will be needed to account for the wide differences in animal breeds and/or sizes. For upper airway assessments, refinement for differences in head and/or nasal shapes may also be necessary. Despite the current lack of reference values, PFTs are useful for monitoring an individual patient over time, with each test serving as a standard upon which to assess change.

ABNORMAL VALUES
N/A

CRITICAL VALUES
N/A

INTERFERING FACTORS
Drugs That May Alter Results of the Procedure
Essentially all clinically used premedicants, sedatives, or anesthetic agents potentially affect the upper and lower airway dilatory muscles, thus altering or minimizing the functional deficits that one is attempting to document.

Conditions That May Interfere with Performing the Procedure
N/A

Procedure Techniques or Handling That May Alter Results
N/A

Influence of Signalment on Performing and Interpreting the Procedure
Species
N/A

Breed
N/A

Age
N/A

Gender
N/A

Pregnancy
N/A

CLINICAL PERSPECTIVE
At present, clinical evaluation of small-animal respiratory patients is largely limited to (1) subjective assessment of the degree of respiratory compromise present, (2) localization of disease to the upper or lower air passageways versus the cardiovascular system, and (3) efforts to determine whether aberrant structural, infectious, or neoplastic processes exist. Increased availability of objective information on respiratory system dysfunction (i.e., PFTs) would enable improved assessment of disease severity, progression, and treatment response. Although specialized training and equipment are necessary to perform the tests discussed herein, such testing will improve our understanding of how specific diseases alter the basic physiologic processes of breathing, thus leading to better case management of small-animal respiratory patients.

MISCELLANEOUS

ANCILLARY TESTS
• Head, neck, or thoracic radiography with or without fluoroscopy
• Nasal, pharyngeal, laryngeal, tracheal, or bronchial endoscopic examination with or without biopsy
• Tracheal wash or bronchoalveolar lavage–derived cytology and/or evaluation for infectious agents
• Computed tomography or ultrasonographic imaging with or without lung aspiration

SYNONYMS
None

SEE ALSO
Blackwell's Five-Minute Veterinary Consult: Canine and Feline Topics
• Asthma, Bronchitis—Cats
• Bronchitis, Chronic (COPD)
• Hypoxemia

Related Topics in This Book
None

ABBREVIATIONS
- FV = flow-volume
- Penh = enhanced pause
- PFT = pulmonary function test
- R_L = lung resistance
- TBFVL = tidal breathing flow-volume loop
- WBP = whole-body plethysmography

Suggested Reading
Dye JA, Costa DL. Pulmonary mechanics. In: King LG, ed. *Textbook of Respiratory Disease in Dogs and Cats*. St Louis: Saunders Elsevier, 2005: 157–175.
Haskins SC. Interpretation of blood gas measurements. In: King LG, ed. *Textbook of Respiratory Disease in Dogs and Cats*. St Louis: Saunders Elsevier, 2005: 181–193.

Pilbeam SP. Ventilator graphics. In: Pilbeam SP, Cairo JM, eds. *Mechanical Ventilation,* 4th ed. St Louis: Mosby Elsevier, 2006: 177–228.
Rozanski EA, Hoffman AM. Lung mechanics using plethysmography and spirometry. In: King LG, ed. *Textbook of Respiratory Disease in Dogs and Cats*. St Louis: Saunders Elsevier, 2005: 175–181.
West JB, ed. *Pulmonary Pathophysiology: The Essentials,* 6th ed. Baltimore: Lippincott Williams & Wilkins, 2003.

INTERNET RESOURCES
None

AUTHOR NAME
Janice A. Dye

BASICS

TYPE OF PROCEDURE
Nuclear medicine

PROCEDURE EXPLANATION AND RELATED PHYSIOLOGY
The lungs function as a method to exchange both oxygen and carbon dioxide with the pulmonary circulatory system. This interaction occurs on the capillary level at the alveolus. Under optimum conditions, the ventilation of the alveoli is equal to the perfusion status to maximize gas exchange. When the lung is compressed or collapsed, as seen with atelectasis, the circulation will divert blood flow from these nonventilated areas to areas of better ventilation. When the arterial system is occluded by a pulmonary embolism, the ventilation to the lung remains normal, but the perfusion is clearly compromised. This study consists of the injection of a particulate form of albumin called *macroaggregated albumin* (MAA) into the venous system upstream from the capillary bed being investigated. (In this case, the pulmonary circulation is studied, so any peripheral venous injection site will work.) The MAA is bound to technetium 99m (^{99m}Tc) and is ≈10–90 μm in diameter. Because of this size, MAA will occlude the first capillary bed encountered. The ^{99m}Tc-MAA is injected IV, where the particles mix with the venous blood, travel into the pulmonary arteriole system, and then become lodged in the pulmonary capillary bed. As ^{99m}Tc-MAA accumulates, the gamma camera detects the radioactivity. Areas without radioactivity present (*photopenic* areas) are the result of vascular occlusion prior to the capillary bed. Differential diagnoses for photopenic areas include ventilation-induced perfusion abnormalities (e.g., recumbent atelectasis, pneumonia) or direct perfusion defects (e.g., pulmonary artery atresia or hypoplasia; pulmonary thrombosis or embolism). A complete thoracic radiographic study conducted immediately prior to the procedure is useful in helping to formulate an appropriate differential diagnoses.

INDICATIONS
• Acute onset of respiratory distress in a patient with thrombocytosis
• Acute onset of cyanosis
• Evaluation of pulmonary perfusion
• Evaluation of chronic obstructive lung disease
• Evaluation of the severity of pulmonary disease and its impact on the right heart and pulmonary arteries (cor pulmonale)
• Evaluation for the presence of right to left intracardiac or extracardiac shunts

CONTRAINDICATIONS
• Severe pulmonary hypertension. (Estimated peak systolic pulmonary artery pressure is >90 mmHg.)
• Animals in severe respiratory distress

POTENTIAL COMPLICATIONS
• The scan is generally considered safe.
• Though the typical dose of MAA occludes ≈0.1% of the pulmonary vasculature, in a severely compromised animal this may be enough to exacerbate the cyanosis and respiratory distress and could cause the patient's death.

CLIENT EDUCATION
Client education is based on the fact that specific state nuclear medicine regulations must be followed when animals are sent home. Over time, the MAA is broken down by the macrophage system, and a relatively small percentage of the radioactive sodium ^{99m}Tc-pertechnetate will be excreted into the kidney. Therefore, the urine will be radioactive for 60 h after injection. Since a minor amount of the ^{99m}Tc-MAA will be excreted, clients might not have to collect their animal's waste products, depending on what is required by state regulatory agency licensing.

BODY SYSTEMS ASSESSED
Respiratory

PROCEDURE

PATIENT PREPARATION
Preprocedure Medication or Preparation
• Care should be made to prevent recumbency-related atelectasis by maintaining patients in sternal recumbency before injecting the radiopharmaceutical.
• Thoracic radiographs should be obtained to identify any areas of increased pulmonary opacity (a reason for ventilation/perfusion abnormality) prior to the perfusion study.

Anesthesia or Sedation
• None is required.
• Sedation can be used if needed to control a patient.

Patient Positioning
The patient is maintained in sternal recumbency, and the gamma camera is rotated around the patient for collection of all images.

Patient Monitoring
Monitor respiration for signs of tachypnea or distress for 1 h after injection.

Equipment or Supplies
• A gamma camera with a general-purpose, low-energy collimator, with an acquisition computer workstation
• A 1- to 3-mL syringe containing 3–5 mCi (111–185 MBq) of ^{99m}Tc-MAA. This usually contains 300,000–500,000 particles of MAA. (The number of particles should be reduced to <100,000 if the patient's clinical signs are severe.)

TECHNIQUE
• The ^{99m}Tc-MAA should be administered via a cephalic catheter with the patient in sternal recumbency. Before radiopharmaceutical injection, the catheter should be flushed with saline to ensure that no clots have formed within the catheter system. (A clot containing a large number of radiopharmaceutical particles that dislodges can create an area of increased activity in the lungs.) The catheter is then flushed with saline. The syringe is discarded in the radioactive sharps container.
• At 5 min after injection, the patient is placed on the gamma camera in sternal recumbency.

- Static acquisitions are obtained by using a matrix size of 256 × 256 × 16 for a total image count of 250,000–500,000.
- Right lateral, right dorsal oblique, dorsal, left lateral, left dorsal oblique, and ventral images of the thorax are obtained.
- When imaging a right-to-left shunt, the head and abdomen should also be imaged (right lateral images only) to document the presence of radiopharmaceutical within the skull or abdomen (i.e., the renal bed).
- The radiopharmaceutical to be injected should be held in a specialized, lead syringe shield prior to injection.
- Rubber gloves and a laboratory coat should be worn to reduce the potential for personnel contamination.

SAMPLE HANDLING
None

APPROPRIATE AFTERCARE
Postprocedure Patient Monitoring
- After injection of the radiopharmaceutical, the needle is withdrawn and discarded in a radioactive materials sharps box.
- The patient should be monitored, and the exposure rates at the surface and at 1 m should be recorded and posted, with appropriate radioactive sign, on the animal's cage.
- Minimal interaction with the patient should be observed for 24 h to decrease personnel exposure.
- Urine may need to be collected and stored for 60 h (10 half-lives) before being discarded as general biologic waste.

Nursing Care
- After the procedure, minimal interaction with the patient is recommended to minimize the risk of contamination with radioactive material.
- Patients that are considered to be in severe respiratory distress prior to the study should be acutely monitored for any increased respiratory problems for 1 h after the study.

Dietary Modification
None

Medication Requirements
None

Restrictions on Activity
Patients should be isolated during hospitalization until the surface radioactive exposure is within an acceptable range.

Anticipated Recovery Time
Recovery of the patient is immediate although it will have surface radioactivity.

 INTERPRETATION

NORMAL FINDINGS OR RANGE
- A normal scintigraphic scan will have a uniform distribution of the ^{99m}Tc-MAA in all aspects of the lungs. This distribution is seen as uniform increased radioactivity with smooth margins and a central photopenic area indicating the location of the heart. The normal shape of the diaphragm is expected to be as seen on the thoracic radiographs.
- On the right lateral and ventral views, a photopenic area represents the cardiac notch associated with the lungs.

ABNORMAL VALUES
- An area of high-contrast photopenia (void of radioactivity) is seen distal to the vascular occlusion because the ^{99m}Tc-MAA is blocked from that area of the lung. This typically is lobar in location and has a wedge or triangular shape with the base of the wedge toward the periphery.
- Classically, a photopenic region appears as a wedge-shaped defect with a contour similar to that of the affected lung when a pulmonary embolus is present.
- The mottled appearance of the perfusion scan seen with chronic obstructive pulmonary disease is produced by hypoxic vasoconstriction of the pulmonary vasculature. This hypoxia is caused by decreased aeration of the lungs because of bronchoconstriction that causes secondary pulmonary vascular shunting to areas of more aerated lungs. Since the vasculature is not completely occluded, activity is still present, though not as much as in a normally aerated lung.
- A mottled peripheral photopenic appearance to the lungs may also occur because of multiple small emboli, disseminated intravascular coagulation (DIC), or in patients with heartworm disease.

CRITICAL VALUES
None

INTERFERING FACTORS
- Identification of thyroid tissue or the gastric mucosa indicates inadequate binding of the ^{99m}Tc-pertechnetate with the MAA. This study should be considered nondiagnostic for right-to-left shunt studies but may still be interpretable for the presence or absence of flow to all lung lobes.
- Photopenic regions can also be secondary to pulmonary masses (such as abscesses, tumors, or granulomas) or areas of ventilation abnormality (e.g., alveolar lung disease). These differential diagnoses can be excluded by obtaining radiographs prior to the pulmonary perfusion scan.

Drugs That May Alter Results of the Procedure
Administration of any respiratory depressants may decrease ventilation, thereby decreasing perfusion.

Conditions That May Interfere with Performing the Procedure
- Concurrent pneumonia would interfere with the results by decreasing aeration to the lung and thereby decreasing perfusion to that lung.
- Recumbency-related atelectasis interferes by similar mechanisms as those just mentioned.
- Right-to-left shunting of blood will cause the MAA to bypass the pulmonary capillary system and cause systemic emboli. Though this technique can be used to diagnose a right-to-left shunt, the number of MAA particles injected should be greatly reduced to avoid causing embolus-induced ischemia.

Procedure Techniques or Handling That May Alter Results
Excessive recumbency (right or left lateral) may produce atelectasis that will interfere with the results of the study.

Influence of Signalment on Performing and Interpreting the Procedure
Species
None identified

PULMONARY PERFUSION SCAN

Breed
None identified

Age
None identified

Gender
None identified

Pregnancy
None identified

CLINICAL PERSPECTIVE

Pulmonary perfusion scintigraphy is 1 of the few methods to evaluate the vascular status of the lungs. In human patients, the gold standard for the identification of pulmonary embolism is the use of contrast-enhanced helical computed tomography. This method has not gained the same acceptance in veterinary medicine, and the use of general anesthesia in a respiratory-compromised patient increases the risk of complication. Scintigraphy is generally safe and an effective, rapid method for assessing pulmonary perfusion in veterinary patients.

MISCELLANEOUS

ANCILLARY TESTS

- Thoracic radiography
- Echocardiography to assess for pulmonary hypertension

- Contrast-enhanced helical computed tomography to evaluate the pulmonary vessels

SYNONYMS

- Lung scan
- Pulmonary scan
- Pulmonary scintigraphy

SEE ALSO

Blackwell's Five-Minute Veterinary Consult: Canine and Feline Topics

- Atrial Septal Defect
- Atrial Tear
- Bronchitis, Chronic (COPD)
- Patent Ductus Arteriosus
- Pulmonary Thromboembolism
- Tetralogy of Fallot
- Ventricular Septal Defect

Related Topics in This Book

- Angiography and Angiocardiography
- Blood Gases
- Pulmonary Function Tests
- Thoracic Radiography

ABBREVIATIONS

- MAA = macroaggregated albumin
- MBq = megabecquerels (10^6 disintegrations per second)
- mCi = millicurie = 3.7×10^6 disintegrations per second or 1 Bq (becquerel)
- ^{99m}Tc = technetium 99m

Suggested Reading

Daniel GB, Koblik PD, Berry CR. Pulmonary and mucociliary scintigraphy. In: Daniel GB, Berry CR, eds. *The Textbook of Veterinary Nuclear Medicine*. Harrisburg, PA: American College of Veterinary Radiology, 2006: 303–328.

Hatabu H, Uematsu H, Nguyen B, *et al*. CT and MR in pulmonary embolism: A changing role for nuclear medicine in diagnostic strategy. *Semin Nucl Med* 2002; 32: 183–192.

Hood DM, Hightower D, Tatum ME. Lung perfusion imaging in the dog. *Vet Radiol* 1977; 18: 124–127.

Lamm WJ, Starr IR, Neradilek B, *et al*. Hypoxic pulmonary vasoconstriction is heterogeneously distributed in the prone dog. *Respir Physiol Neurobiol* 2004; 144: 281–294.

Thrall DE, Badertscher RR, Lewis RE, McCall JW. Scintigraphic evaluation of pulmonary perfusion in dogs with experimentally infected *Dirofilaria immitis*. *Am J Vet Res* 1979; 40: 1426–1432.

INTERNET RESOURCES

University of Tennessee, College of Veterinary Medicine: Nuclear radiology, http://www.vet.utk.edu/radiology/nuclear/index.php.

AUTHOR NAMES

Anthony Pease and Clifford Berry

BASICS

TYPE OF PROCEDURE
Electrodiagnostic

PROCEDURE EXPLANATION AND RELATED PHYSIOLOGY
A pulse oximeter is a noninvasive means of estimating arterial hemoglobin saturation (SpO_2). Hemoglobin changes its structural configuration when it participates in a chemical reaction, and each of the configurations has a different pattern of light reflection. At wavelengths of 660 nanometers (nm), which corresponds to the red region of the light spectrum, oxygenated hemoglobin (HbO_2) reflects light more effectively than does deoxygenated hemoglobin (Hb). This relationship is reversed at 940 nm (the infrared spectrum), where Hb reflects light more effectively than does HbO_2. Thus, when both wavelengths of light are passed through a sample of blood or a thin tissue bed with pulsatile flow, the intensity of light transmission at 660 nm is primarily a function of the concentration of HbO_2 in the sample, whereas the transmission at 940 nm is determined primarily by the concentration of Hb. The concentrations of HbO_2 and Hb are expressed in relative terms; that is, as the fraction of Hb that is in the oxygenated form. This is known as the percent oxyhemoglobin saturation (% saturation), and is derived as follows:

$$\text{\% saturation } (SpO_2) = (HbO_2/HbO_2 + Hb) \times 100$$

INDICATIONS
- Anesthesia monitoring and postoperative and/or recovery monitoring
- Cardiovascular monitoring
- Pulmonary function monitoring
- Patients on mechanical ventilation

CONTRAINDICATIONS
- Patient intolerance of the probe
- Mucosal or skin disease
- Pigmented skin

POTENTIAL COMPLICATIONS
Prolonged application of the probe can cause skin or mucosal pressure necrosis.

CLIENT EDUCATION
N/A

BODY SYSTEMS ASSESSED
- Cardiovascular
- Respiratory
- Hemic

PROCEDURE

PATIENT PREPARATION
Preprocedure Medication or Preparation
- Shave the area where medication has been applied to haired skin.
- Prepare a clean, moist mucosal surface.

Anesthesia or Sedation
Usually none is required, even in alert patients.

Patient Positioning
N/A

Patient Monitoring
If the patient is anesthetized or ventilated, standard monitoring should include heart rate, respiratory rate, ECG, and blood pressure, along with pulse oximetry.

Equipment or Supplies
Many pulse oximeters are commercially available.

TECHNIQUE
Commercially available veterinary pulse oximeters are quite simple in their designs and use. They come with an alligator-shaped probe (a transflectance probe) that can be easily placed at various sites on patients. Possible measurement sites include the tongue, lip, nasal septum, toe web, axilla, inguinal areas, prepuce, vagina, and tail base. A rectal (transflectance) probe may also be inserted. Pulse oximeters provide a pulse-rate signal-strength indicator. If the pulse rate reported by the pulse oximeter does not match the palpable pulse rate or if the signal strength indicator is low, then the reading is likely unreliable.

SAMPLE HANDLING
N/A

APPROPRIATE AFTERCARE
Postprocedure Patient Monitoring
N/A

Nursing Care
Probes placed in 1 location for prolonged periods may lead to pressure necrosis.

Dietary Modification
N/A

Medication Requirements
N/A

Restrictions on Activity
N/A

Anticipated Recovery Time
N/A

INTERPRETATION

NORMAL FINDINGS OR RANGE
95%–100% (with a good pulse signal)

ABNORMAL VALUES
Less than 95% can be considered abnormal.

CRITICAL VALUES
Less than 85%–90% in any patient

INTERFERING FACTORS
Drugs That May Alter Results of the Procedure
- Methylene blue (used to treat methemoglobinemia)
- Indigo carmine and indocyanine green (transiently)
- Lipid infusions

Conditions That May Interfere with Performing the Procedure
- Carboxyhemoglobinemia with carbon monoxide intoxication: falsely elevated
- Methemoglobinemia: falsely decreased
- Sulfhemoglobinemia and cyan methemoglobinemia (rare)
- Hypotension
- Intense vasoconstriction
- Lack of blood flow or poor blood flow to the area being measured
- Anemia
- Methylene blue administration
- Dark skin pigmentations
- Bilirubin and melanin do not interfere.
- Pulse oximetry becomes less accurate when arterial hemoglobin saturation (SaO_2) is <70%.
- Fingernail polish and/or onychomycosis
- Venous pulsations
- Edema

Procedure Techniques or Handling That May Alter Results
- Motion
- A poor signal or poor positioning of probe
- Ambient light (particularly fluorescent light)
- Poor sensor contact
- Infrared heating lamps

Influence of Signalment on Performing and Interpreting the Procedure

Species
N/A

Breed
The deeply pigmented skin of some breeds may falsely lower values.

Age
N/A

Gender
N/A

Pregnancy
N/A

CLINICAL PERSPECTIVE
The monitor, which is inexpensive and easy to use during anesthesia or for critical patients, lets clinicians know second by second whether immediate intervention may be required to improve oxygen saturation. It can be used to investigate problems associated with anesthesia and may eliminate catastrophic hypoxemia.

MISCELLANEOUS

ANCILLARY TESTS
Arterial blood-gas analysis

SYNONYMS
None

SEE ALSO
Blackwell's Five-Minute Veterinary Consult: Canine and Feline Topics
- Acetaminophen Toxicity
- Acute Respiratory Distress Syndrome
- Congestive Heart Failure, Left-Sided
- Cyanosis
- Drowning (Near Drowning)
- Pneumonia, Aspiration
- Pneumonia, Bacterial
- Pneumonia, Eosinophilic
- Pneumonia, Fungal
- Pneumonia, Interstitial
- Pulmonary Edema
- Pulmonary Edema, Noncardiogenic
- Pulmonary Thromboembolism
- Smoke Inhalation
- Tracheal Collapse

Related Topics in This Book
- Blood Gases
- Hematocrit
- Hemoglobin
- Methemoglobin
- Thoracic Radiography

ABBREVIATIONS
- HbO_2 = oxygenated hemoglobin
- SpO_2 = pulse oximetry–detected hemoglobin saturation

Suggested Reading
Darovic GO, ed. *Hemodynamic Monitoring: Invasive and Noninvasive Clinical Application,* 3rd ed. Philadelphia: WB Saunders, 2002: 263–281.
Marino PL, ed. *The ICU Book,* 2nd ed. Baltimore: Williams & Wilkins, 1998: 355–361.
Miller RD, ed. *Anesthesia,* 4th ed. New York: Churchill Livingstone, 1994: 1260–1265.

INTERNET RESOURCES
None

AUTHOR NAMES
Andrew Linklater and Marla Lichtenberger

RECTAL SCRAPING AND CYTOLOGY

 BASICS

TYPE OF PROCEDURE
Diagnostic sample collection

PROCEDURE EXPLANATION AND RELATED PHYSIOLOGY
This is a quick, relatively noninvasive, technique that sometimes can be used to diagnose certain colonic or rectal diseases. This is *different* from fecal cytologic evaluation, which looks for *Campylobacter* and clostridial spores (both findings are of questionable significance).

INDICATIONS
Chronic or very severe large-bowel disease (especially patients with hypoalbuminemia, weight loss, or both) in dogs that may have fungal disease (e.g., histoplasmosis) or algal disease (i.e., prototothecosis), and especially those with mucosal abnormalities on rectal palpation. The procedure is seldom indicated in cats.

CONTRAINDICATIONS
Severe coagulopathy

POTENTIAL COMPLICATIONS
- Excessive bleeding (rare)
- Perforation if an exceedingly improper technique is employed

CLIENT EDUCATION
- This test is specific for certain infections but is insensitive—if the results are negative, you have not eliminated any diseases.
- It is appropriate to evaluate rectal cytology before performing endoscopy in dogs with suspected fungal disease, especially if mucosal abnormalities are found on rectal examination.

BODY SYSTEMS ASSESSED
Gastrointestinal

 PROCEDURE

PATIENT PREPARATION
Preprocedure Medication or Preparation
None

Anesthesia or Sedation
Sedation with narcotics or even anesthesia with injectable propofol may be needed in animals that are in excessive pain during the rectal examination.

Patient Positioning
The procedure can be performed with the patient in any of several positions.

Patient Monitoring
None

Equipment or Supplies
- Examination gloves
- A small curette or similar instrument

TECHNIQUE
- A gloved finger is inserted into the rectum, and a complete rectal examination is performed.
- Next, a small curette is guided into the rectum with the finger, and the rectal mucosa is *gently* scrapped to obtain epithelial cells. The goal is to obtain mucosal epithelium, not feces. Blood should not be obvious after the procedure. The epithelial cells are spread on a glass slide, air-dried, and stained with new methylene blue, Diff-Quick, or a modified Giemsa.
- In larger dogs, one may tape the cap of a syringe casing to the tip of the index finger and use it to scrap the rectal mucosa.

SAMPLE HANDLING
The slide is handled routinely as any cytologic slide.

APPROPRIATE AFTERCARE
Postprocedure Patient Monitoring
None

Nursing Care
None

Dietary Modification
None

Medication Requirements
None

Restrictions on Activity
None

Anticipated Recovery Time
Immediate

 INTERPRETATION

NORMAL FINDINGS OR RANGE
No fungal organisms, no algae, and no appreciable inflammation

ABNORMAL VALUES
- Fungal organisms (e.g., histoplasmosis, typically found in macrophages)
- Algae (i.e., prototothecosis)
- Substantial numbers of neutrophils or eosinophils
- Malignant cells

CRITICAL VALUES
None

INTERFERING FACTORS
Drugs That May Alter Results of the Procedure
None known

Conditions That May Interfere with Performing the Procedure
Excessive rectal or anal pain makes sedation or anesthesia necessary.

Procedure Techniques or Handling That May Alter Results
None

Influence of Signalment on Performing and Interpreting the Procedure
Species
This procedure is almost never performed in cats.

Breed
None

Age
None

Gender
None

Pregnancy
None

CLINICAL PERSPECTIVE
- The test is specific but not necessarily sensitive for finding colonic histoplasmosis, a disease that is common in select geographic areas of the United States.
- The test may help detect severe colitis by finding substantial numbers of neutrophils, but this is a nonspecific finding that can occur in numerous disorders.
- Care must be taken before diagnosing a malignancy based solely on cytologic analysis because epithelial dysplastic changes are common in a variety of diseases.

MISCELLANEOUS

ANCILLARY TESTS

Colonoscopy and biopsy are required if rectal cytologic analysis is non-revealing in a dog that is suspected of having colonic histoplasmosis, prototothecosis, or rectal neoplasia.

SYNONYMS

Rectal scrape

SEE ALSO

Blackwell's Five-Minute Veterinary Consult: Canine and Feline Topics

Histoplasmosis

Related Topics in This Book

Colonoscopy

ABBREVIATIONS

None

Suggested Reading

Clinkenbeard KD, Cowell RL, Tyler RD. Disseminated histoplasmosis in dogs: 12 cases (1981–1986). *J Am Vet Med Assoc* 1988; 193: 1443–1447.

Jergens AE, Andreasen CB, Hagemoser WA, *et al.* Cytologic examination of exfoliative specimens obtained during endoscopy for diagnosis of gastrointestinal tract disease in dogs and cats. *J Am Vet Med Assoc* 1998; 213: 1755–1759.

INTERNET RESOURCES

None

AUTHOR NAME

Michael D. Willard

RED BLOOD CELL COUNT

BASICS

TYPE OF SPECIMEN
Blood

TEST EXPLANATION AND RELATED PHYSIOLOGY
RBCs are produced in bone marrow following stimulation by erythropoietin. Normally, they circulate for several months (dogs, 120 days; cats, 70 days) and are eventually removed by splenic macrophages.

Automatic cell counters provide the most accurate RBC counts. Manual hemocytometer counts are associated with a large degree of error. RBC count, hemoglobin concentration, and PCV are all measures of RBC mass and generally increase and decrease together, although changes may not be proportionate if RBC size and/or hemoglobin content are altered. Decreased RBC mass (anemia) can be caused by blood loss, increased RBC destruction (hemolysis), or decreased RBC production by bone marrow. An increased RBC count is frequently due to hemoconcentration (relative erythrocytosis). A true increase in RBC mass (absolute or relative erythrocytosis) is usually caused by increased erythropoietin secretion in response to hypoxia. Erythropoietin-secreting neoplasms and polycythemia vera, a neoplastic condition associated with uncontrolled production of RBCs, are rare.

INDICATIONS
To diagnose anemia or polycythemia

CONTRAINDICATIONS
None

POTENTIAL COMPLICATIONS
None

CLIENT EDUCATION
Consider a 12-h fast to prevent lipemia.

BODY SYSTEMS ASSESSED
Hemic, lymphatic, and immune

SAMPLE

COLLECTION
1–3 mL of venous blood

HANDLING
• EDTA is preferred, but heparin may be used.
• Transport the sample on ice.

STORAGE
Refrigerate the sample if it is not processed within 2–4 h.

STABILITY
• Room temperature: 2–4 h
• Refrigerated (2°–8°C): up to 2 days

PROTOCOL
None

INTERPRETATION

NORMAL FINDINGS OR RANGE
• Dogs: $5.4–7.8 \times 10^{6}/\mu L$ (SI units, $5.4–7.8 \times 10^{12}/L$)
• Cats: $5.8–10.7 \times 10^{6}/\mu L$ (SI units, $5.8–10.7 \times 10^{12}/L$)
• Reference intervals vary depending on the geographic location, laboratory performing the analysis, and age, gender, and breed of the patient.

ABNORMAL VALUES
Values above or below the reference interval

CRITICAL VALUES
An RBC count less than one-third of normal

INTERFERING FACTORS
Drugs That May Alter Results or Interpretation
Drugs That Interfere with Test Methodology
None

Drugs That Alter Physiology
• The RBC count may be lowered by drugs that damage bone marrow, including albendazole, sulfonamides, methimazole, estrogen, phenobarbital (in dogs), griseofulvin, and chloramphenicol (in cats).
• Chronic high levels of glucocorticoids may increase the RBC count.

Disorders That May Alter Results
• Decreased by overhydration
• Increased by dehydration
• Decreased by in vivo or in vitro hemolysis

Collection Techniques or Handling That May Alter Results
• Freezing blood will lyse RBCs.
• Difficult sample collection may activate platelets and cause clotting. An artifactually lowered RBC count may be obtained if the sample is processed (not recommended).

Influence of Signalment
Species
None

Breed
RBC counts are higher than average in some breeds (e.g., greyhounds, dachshunds).

Age
Young animals may have lower RBC counts.

Gender
Gender differences occur, but reference intervals are generated from both genders, masking the differences.

Pregnancy
Expanded plasma volume associated with pregnancy may lower the RBC concentration.

LIMITATIONS OF THE TEST
Sensitivity, Specificity, and Positive and Negative Predictive Values
N/A

Valid If Run in a Human Lab?
Yes—if a hematology analyzer is used that is calibrated to run veterinary species so that small feline RBCs are accurately counted.

Causes of Abnormal Findings

High values (polycythemia or erythrocytosis)	Low values (anemia)
Relative	Normal for age (i.e., neonates)
Hemoconcentration	Anemia of chronic disorders
Splenic contraction	Erythropoietin lack (chronic renal failure)
Absolute	Blood loss
Normal for breed	Trauma or surgery
(e.g., greyhounds)	GI ulceration or neoplasm
Hypoxia (heart or lung	Parasitism
disease)	Hemostasis defects
High altitude	Hemolysis
Erythropoietin-	Immune-mediated (primary or secondary)
producing tumors	RBC parasites
Primary erythrocytosis	Oxidants/Heinz body (e.g., acetaminophen,
(aka polycythemia	onions)
vera)	Zinc or copper toxicity
	Fragmentation (e.g., thrombosis, neoplasia,
	heartworm)
	Snake envenomation
	Endocrinopathies (e.g., hypothyroidism)
	Iron deficiency
	Bone marrow disease
	Infections (e.g., FeLV, FIV, panleukopenia,
	parvovirus, *Ehrlichia canis*)
	Myelophthisis
	Toxic bone marrow damage
	Pure red cell aplasia
	Erythroid myeloproliferative or
	myelodysplastic diseases
	Nutritional deficiencies (rare)

CLINICAL PERSPECTIVE
• Animals living in high altitudes have higher RBC counts than average because of physiologic response to decreased available oxygen.
• With bone marrow disease, leukopenia and thrombocytopenia are often seen before anemia, because of the long RBC life span.
• Decreases in both Hct and total protein suggest blood loss, although in stressed dogs, splenic contraction may temporarily mask decreased Hct.
• Increases in both Hct and total protein suggest hemoconcentration.

MISCELLANEOUS

ANCILLARY TESTS
• Evaluation of reticulocyte count and total protein
• Bone marrow aspiration and biopsy in animals with chronic nonregenerative anemia, if the underlying cause unknown
• A serum iron profile if iron-deficiency anemia is being considered
• A serum biochemical profile and urinalysis
• A coagulation profile if a coagulopathy is being considered
• Serologic evaluation or PCR for infectious organisms
• The Coombs' test as workup for immune-mediated hemolysis (not indicated if autoagglutination present)
• With polycythemia, thoracic radiography and evaluation of blood gases to look for evidence of hypoxia

SYNONYMS
None

SEE ALSO
Blackwell's Five-Minute Veterinary Consult: Canine and Feline Topics
• Anemia, Aplastic
• Anemia, Heinz Body
• Anemia, Iron-Deficiency
• Anemia, Metabolic (Anemias with Spiculated Red Cells)
• Anemia, Nonregenerative
• Anemia, Regenerative

Related Topics in This Book
• Blood Smear Microscopic Examination
• Red Blood Cell Indices
• Red Blood Cell Morphology
• Reticulocyte Count

ABBREVIATIONS
None

Suggested Reading
Stockham SL, Scott MA. Erythrocytes. In: *Fundamentals of Veterinary Clinical Pathology*. Ames: Iowa State Press, 2002: 85–154.
Thrall MA, ed. *Veterinary Hematology and Clinical Chemistry*. Philadelphia: Lippincott Williams & Wilkins, 2004.

INTERNET RESOURCES
Cornell University, College of Veterinary Medicine, Clinical Pathology Modules, Hemogram Basics: Hematology, http://www.diaglab.vet.cornell.edu/clinpath/modules/hemogram/cbc.htm.

AUTHOR NAME
Jennifer L. Brazzell

RED BLOOD CELL ENZYME ACTIVITY

BASICS

TYPE OF SPECIMEN
Blood

TEST EXPLANATION AND RELATED PHYSIOLOGY
Although RBC transport of oxygen and carbon dioxide does not require energy per se, energy in the form of ATP, NADH, and NADPH is required to keep RBCs circulating for months in a functional state. Mature RBCs depend solely on anaerobic glycolysis to generate ATP. Consequently, deficiencies in rate-controlling glycolytic enzymes, including PK and PFK, result in deficient ATP generation, shortened RBC life spans, and anemia. Methemoglobin, the oxidized form of hemoglobin, cannot bind oxygen. About 3% of hemoglobin within RBCs is oxidized to methemoglobin each day, but methemoglobin usually accounts for <1% of total hemoglobin because it is reduced back to hemoglobin by an NADH-dependent Cb5R enzyme. An inherited deficiency in this enzyme results in persistent methemoglobinemia with minimal or no clinical signs. Although not reported in small animals, a glucose-6-phosphate dehydrogenase deficiency in the pentose phosphate pathway that generates NADPH, or deficiencies in glutathione reductase and glutathione peroxidase, can increase susceptibility to oxidant injury, as suggested by the persistent observation of eccentrocytes and/or Heinz bodies.

INDICATIONS
• Unexplained persistent anemia with prominent reticulocytosis, especially in young animals, suggests PK or PFK deficiency.
• Unexplained episodes of intravascular hemolysis with hemoglobinuria, especially in English springer spaniels, suggests PFK deficiency.
• Persistent cyanotic-appearing skin and mucous membranes and methemoglobinemia (in the absence of other clinical signs) suggest cytochrome-b5 reductase (Cb5R) deficiency.

CONTRAINDICATIONS
None

POTENTIAL COMPLICATIONS
None

CLIENT EDUCATION
• Inherited RBC enzyme deficiencies cannot be cured, except by bone marrow transplantation.
• PK-deficient dogs generally do not live >3 years and die because of bone marrow and/or liver failure.
• Dogs with PFK deficiency may die during hemolytic crises, but many live to old age.
• Animals with Cb5R deficiency have normal life expectancies.

BODY SYSTEMS ASSESSED
Hemic, lymphatic, and immune

SAMPLE

COLLECTION
• 3–5 mL of venous blood
• Collect a sample from a healthy animal of the same species as the assay control.

HANDLING
• EDTA or heparin anticoagulant
• Refrigerate (do not freeze) until delivered to the laboratory.
• Ship samples by overnight express with ice packs to the appropriate laboratory. RBC enzyme assays are performed in a limited number of research laboratories.

STORAGE
Refrigerate.

STABILITY
1–2 days at 2°–8°C

PROTOCOL
None

INTERPRETATION

NORMAL FINDINGS OR RANGE
PK Activity
• Dogs: 4–14 U/g hemoglobin
• Cats: 11–49 U/g hemoglobin

PFK Activity
• Dogs: 8–14 U/g hemoglobin
• Cats: 1.0–3.6 U/g hemoglobin

Cb5R Activity
• Dogs: 8–15 U/g hemoglobin
• Cats: 6–16 U/g hemoglobin
• Reference values may vary depending on the laboratory and assay used.

ABNORMAL VALUES
• Values below the reference range indicate deficiency.
• The enzyme activities of heterozygous carriers are about half normal, but levels may fall within the reference range.
• Values above the reference range generally indicate reticulocytosis in animals without RBC enzyme deficiencies.
• PK-deficient dogs (but not cats) express another PK isoenzyme (M2) and can have normal or even high total PK activity. However, this enzyme is unstable when heated compared to the normal RBC isoenzyme. PK-deficient cats consistently have markedly reduced PK activity without heating.
• Dogs homozygous recessive for PFK typically have enzyme activities ≈20% of normal.
• Cb5R-deficient cats generally have enzyme activities of <20% of normal; in dogs, values range from 15% to 65% of normal, with an inverse relationship between methemoglobin concentration and enzyme activity.

CRITICAL VALUES
None

INTERFERING FACTORS
Drugs That May Alter Results or Interpretation
Drugs That Interfere with Test Methodology
None

Drugs That Alter Physiology
None

Disorders That May Alter Results
• Significant hemolysis can bias results toward reticulocytes, which do not readily hemolyze.
• Marked hemolysis (e.g., a sample frozen) renders results useless; enzymes are labile in hemolysates.

Collection Techniques or Handling That May Alter Results
• Rough sample handling that causes hemolysis
• Failure to refrigerate samples until assayed

Influence of Signalment
Species
PFK deficiency has been reported in only dogs.

RED BLOOD CELL ENZYME ACTIVITY

Breed
- PK deficiency: in many dog breeds and in Abyssinian, Somali, and domestic shorthair cats
- PFK deficiency: primarily in English springer spaniels; also reported in cocker spaniels and mixed-breed dogs
- Cb5R deficiency: in many dog breeds and in DSH cats

Age
PK deficiency is recognized primarily in young dogs. Other defects may not be recognized until middle age.

Gender
No gender predilection. These enzyme deficiencies are autosomal defects.

Pregnancy
None

LIMITATIONS OF THE TEST
Sensitivity, Specificity, and Positive and Negative Predictive Values
N/A

Valid If Run in a Human Lab?
Yes.

CLINICAL PERSPECTIVE
- Suspect hereditary PK and PFK enzyme deficiencies when other causes of anemia with prominent reticulocytosis are ruled out.
- PK-deficient dogs can have low, normal, or high enzyme levels, and any value below the reference interval in a dog with marked reticulocytosis is considered significant. Measurement of PK activity in hemolysates after heating or DNA-based assays may be needed to diagnose PK deficiency in some dogs.

MISCELLANEOUS

ANCILLARY TESTS
DNA-based assays have been developed for PFK and PK deficiency. Since several different mutations have been identified in canine PK deficiency, different assays must be developed and validated for each dog breed affected. When available, DNA-based assays can accurately identify heterozygous carriers that might be missed by enzyme assays.

SYNONYMS
- Inherited methemoglobinemia
- Phosphofructokinase
- Pyruvate kinase

SEE ALSO
Blackwell's Five-Minute Veterinary Consult: Canine and Feline Topics
- Methemoglobinemia
- Phosphofructokinase Deficiency
- Pyruvate Kinase Deficiency

Related Topics in This Book
- Heinz Bodies
- Methemoglobin

ABBREVIATIONS
- Cb5R = cytochrome-b$_5$ reductase
- DSH = domestic shorthair
- PFK = phosphofructokinase
- PK = pyruvate kinase

Suggested Reading
Harvey JW. Pathogenesis, laboratory diagnosis, and clinical implications of erythrocyte enzyme deficiencies in dogs, cats, and horses. *Vet Clin Pathol* 2006; 35: 144–156.

INTERNET RESOURCES
Penn Veterinary Medicine, University of Pennsylvania, PennGenn, Section of Medical Genetics, http://www.vet.upenn.edu/penngen.

AUTHOR NAME
John W. Harvey

RED BLOOD CELL INDICES

 BASICS

TYPE OF SPECIMEN
Blood

TEST EXPLANATION AND RELATED PHYSIOLOGY
Erythrocyte indices are generated to categorize anemias and narrow the list of differential diagnoses for anemia. The 4 commonly reported RBC indices are mean cell volume (MCV), mean cell (corpuscular) hemoglobin concentration (MCHC), mean cell (corpuscular) hemoglobin (MCH), and red cell distribution width (RDW).

MCV indicates the average size of RBCs in the sample. It is directly measured by most automated hematology analyzers, but it may be calculated if the PCV and absolute RBC count are known [PCV (%) × 10/RBC count = MCV fL (10^{-15} L)]. Automated hematology analyzers can sort RBCs based on their size and produce a histogram of cell size that is used to determine the mean cell volume. Increased MCV is termed *macrocytosis* and indicates the presence of RBCs that are larger than average. Decreased MCV is termed *microcytosis* and indicates the presence RBCs that are smaller than average.

MCHC is calculated from the hemoglobin (Hgb) concentration and the PCV [MCHC = Hgb (g/dL) × 100/PCV (%)]. It indicates the concentration of Hgb within an average RBC. Decreased MCHC is termed *hypochromasia* and indicates that, on average, the erythrocytes in the sample contain less Hgb per measure of volume. Increased MCHC is termed *hyperchromasia* and is almost always artifactual because Hgb synthesis stops when an optimal cytoplasmic Hgb concentration has been reached. However, true hyperchromasia can be seen rarely with pathologic conditions (e.g., spherocytes, eccentrocytes, pyknocytes) that cause loss of cell volume without a proportionate loss of hemoglobin.

MCH, which is calculated from the Hgb concentration and the RBC count [MCH = Hgb (g/dL) × 10/RBC count], does not generally provide any additional information over MCHC and is not typically interpreted. The MCHC calculation corrects for RBC volume and is considered a more accurate estimate of Hgb concentration per RBC.

RDW, which is the coefficient of variation of the RBC volume distribution, is calculated from the standard deviation (SD) of the RBC histogram and the MCV (RDW = MCV/SD). It is unitless and provides an index of the degree of size variation (anisocytosis) within the RBC population.

The most common categories of anemia based on classic RBC indices are (1) macrocytic, hypochromic, (2) normocytic, normochromic, and (3) microcytic with or without hypochromasia.

INDICATIONS
- To estimate RBC size and hemoglobin content to classify anemias
- To estimate the degree of anisocytosis

CONTRAINDICATIONS
None

POTENTIAL COMPLICATIONS
None

CLIENT EDUCATION
Consider a 12-h fast prior to sampling, since lipemia can interfere with results.

BODY SYSTEMS ASSESSED
Hemic, lymphatic, and immune

 SAMPLE

COLLECTION
1–3 mL of venous blood

HANDLING
- EDTA is preferred but heparin may also be used.
- Transport the sample on ice to the laboratory.

STORAGE
Anticoagulated blood samples should be refrigerated if not processed within 2–4 h.

STABILITY
- Room temperature: 2–4 h
- Refrigerated (2°–8°C): up to 48 h

PROTOCOL
None

 INTERPRETATION

NORMAL FINDINGS OR RANGE
Reference intervals vary depending on geographic location; the laboratory performing the analysis; and age, gender, and breed of the patient. The following intervals are only general guidelines:

Dogs
- MCV: 66–77 fL
- MCHC: 32–36 g/dL (SI units, 320–360 g/L)
- RDW: 12.5–16.5

Cats
- MCV: 39–55 fL
- MCHC: 30–36 g/dL (SI units, 300–360 g/L)
- RDW: 16–21

ABNORMAL VALUES
Values above and below the reference interval

CRITICAL VALUES
None

INTERFERING FACTORS
Drugs That May Alter Results or Interpretation
Drugs That Interfere with Test Methodology
The use of Oxyglobin [hemoglobin glutamer-200 (bovine); Biopure, Cambridge, MA] discolors the plasma and causes a falsely increased MCHC.

Drugs That Alter Physiology
None

Disorders That May Alter Results
- Iatrogenic or pathologic hemolysis of the sample can falsely increase MCHC, since calculation includes Hgb that is both within RBCs and free in the plasma.
- Increased sample turbidity caused by lipemia, large numbers of Heinz bodies, or WBC nuclei and/or cell stroma associated with severe leukocytosis can interfere with light transmission, falsely increasing MCHC. Lipemia may also cause in vitro hemolysis further falsely increasing MCHC.

• RBC agglutination may increase MCV as clusters of agglutinated RBCs may be measured as 1 large RBC.

• In cats, it may be difficult for automated analyzers to distinguish between the large platelets and small RBCs; enumeration of platelets as small erythrocytes may decrease MCV and increase MCHC and RDW.

• In vivo hyperosmolarity can lead to in vitro RBC swelling when placed in an iso-osmotic diluent. This results in an artifactually increased MCV and decreased MCHC.

• In vivo hypo-osmolarity can lead to in vitro RBC shrinkage when placed in an iso-osmotic diluent. This results in an artifactually decreased MCV and increased MCHC.

Collection Techniques or Handling That May Alter Results

• Traumatic venipuncture or inappropriate sample handling resulting in hemolysis may artifactually increase MCHC.

• RBC swelling or crenation because of inappropriate sample collection, handling, or storage may result in increased and decreased MCV, respectively.

• Excess EDTA in underfilled EDTA tubes draws fluid from RBCs and causes crenation resulting in artifactually decreased MCV.

Influence of Signalment

Species
Feline RBCs are smaller than canine RBCs, resulting in a lower MCV.

Breed
MCV: Healthy Shiba Inus, Akitas, Jindos, and possibly other dogs of Asian descent often have MCVs that are lower than average, whereas greyhounds normally have a higher MCV.

Age
Young animals (<3–4 months of age) have a low MCV.

Gender
None

Pregnancy
None

LIMITATIONS OF THE TEST
Sensitivity, Specificity, and Positive and Negative Predictive Values
N/A

Valid If Run in a Human Lab?
Yes—but only if the lab uses a hematology analyzer calibrated to run veterinary species. Human hematology analyzers may not correctly categorize small feline erythrocytes and large feline platelets, which could interfere with measurement of RBC count, MCV, and subsequently Hct (since it is calculated from measured RBC and MCV).

Causes of Abnormal Findings

	High values	Low values
MCV	Reticulocytosis	Iron deficiency
	FeLV infection	Portosystemic venous shunts
	Healthy greyhounds	Hepatic failure
	Congenital poodle	Healthy Asian breeds of dogs
	macrocytosis	(i.e., Shiba Inus, Akitas,
	Artifactual	Jindos)
	RBC agglutination	Young animals
	In vivo hyperosmolarity	Artifactual
		Excess EDTA
		In vivo hypo-osmolarity
MCHC	Artifactual	Reticulocytosis (it takes >20%
	Hemolysis, in vitro or	reticulocytosis for a detectable
	in vivo (intravascular)	decrease in MCHC)
	Lipemia	Iron deficiency
	Effect of excess EDTA	Hepatic failure (rare)
	Heinz bodies	In vivo hyperosmolarity (artifact)
	Severe leukocytosis	
	In vivo hypo-osmolarity	
	Marked spherocytosis	
RDW	Reticulocytosis	None
	Spurious due to artifacts	
	affecting MCV	

CLINICAL PERSPECTIVE

• Macrocytic, hypochromic anemias are most often caused by large numbers of immature, circulating reticulocytes that are larger and contain less hemoglobin.

• Macrocytic, hypochromic anemias are typically regenerative and secondary to recent hemorrhage or hemolysis. (Evaluation of erythrocyte shape changes on a peripheral blood smear may help to differentiate these differential diagnoses.)

• Normocytic, normochromic anemias are typically nonregenerative and may be secondary to anemia of chronic disease, lack of erythropoietin (chronic kidney disease), endocrinopathies (particularly hypothyroidism) or bone marrow disease/damage. The latter is often, but not always, accompanied by decreased WBC and/or platelet count(s).

• Regenerative anemia secondary to acute hemorrhage or hemolysis will often appear normocytic, and normochromic if they are of acute onset (<3 days) and the bone marrow has not had time to respond, or if anemia, and the associated response, is low grade. Because these

are mean values, reticulocytes must comprise a large percentage of the circulating RBCs before they will impact MCV and MCHC.
• Microcytic anemias with or without hypochromasia are typically secondary to iron deficiency that may develop as a result of chronic external hemorrhage (often into the GI tract).
• Macrocytosis in the absence of polychromasia on a feline blood smear is commonly associated with FeLV infection.
• In patients with an increased MCHC, plasma appearance should be checked for hemolysis or lipemia, which are the most common reasons for this finding.

MISCELLANEOUS

ANCILLARY TESTS
• A serum iron profile if iron-deficiency anemia is a consideration.
• Reticulocyte count: This test may identify a low-grade regenerative anemia associated with no changes in RBC indices.
• Bone marrow aspiration and biopsy may be warranted in animals with chronic, nonregenerative, normocytic, normochromic anemias if an underlying cause cannot be elucidated.
• Reticulocyte hemoglobin content: Classic RBC indices can be relatively insensitive in detecting changes associated with iron deficiency. Some of the more sophisticated hematology analyzers can specifically measure the hemoglobin content of reticulocytes, and this may prove to be more sensitive in detecting early iron deficiency or iron deficiency masked by concurrent disease.

SYNONYMS
• Mean cell (corpuscular) volume (MCV)
• Mean cell (corpuscular) hemoglobin (MCH)
• Mean cell (corpuscular) hemoglobin concentration (MCHC)
• Red cell distribution width (RDW)

SEE ALSO
Blackwell's Five-Minute Veterinary Consult: Canine and Feline Topics
• Anemia, Aplastic
• Anemia, Heinz Body
• Anemia, Iron-Deficiency
• Anemia, Nonregenerative
• Anemia, Regenerative

Related Topics in This Book
• Blood Smear Microscopic Examination
• Hematocrit
• Hemoglobin
• Red Blood Cell Count
• Red Blood Cell Morphology

ABBREVIATIONS
• Hgb = hemoglobin
• RDW = red cell distribution width

Suggested Reading
Steinberg JD, Oliver CS. Hematologic and biochemical abnormalities indicating iron deficiency are associated with decreased reticulocyte hemoglobin content (CHr) and reticulocyte volume (rMCV) in dogs. *Vet Clin Pathol* 2005; **34**: 23–27.
Stockham SL, Scott MA. Erythrocytes. In: *Fundamentals of Veterinary Clinical Pathology*. Ames: Iowa State Press, 2002: 85–154.
Lassen ED, Weiser G. Laboratory technology for veterinary medicine. In: Thrall MA, ed. *Veterinary Hematology and Clinical Chemistry*. Philadelphia: Lippincott Williams & Wilkins, 2004: 3–37.

INTERNET RESOURCES
Cornell University, College of Veterinary Medicine, Clinical Pathology Modules, Hemogram Basics: Hematology, http://www.diaglab.vet.cornell.edu/clinpath/modules/hemogram/cbc.htm.

AUTHOR NAME
Jennifer L. Brazzell

BASICS

TYPE OF SPECIMEN
Blood

TEST EXPLANATION AND RELATED PHYSIOLOGY
Changes in RBC morphology are determined through microscopic evaluation of a peripheral blood smear. It is imperative that RBC morphology be evaluated in the monolayer area, because RBCs will be distorted in the feathered edge and in thick areas of the smear. Evaluation at 1,000× magnification is needed to identify some RBC inclusions. Many RBC morphology changes are nonspecific and of little clinical significance unless found in marked numbers (e.g., anisocytosis, echinocytes, elliptocytes, codocytes, leptocytes). Other RBC morphology changes, however, are commonly associated with specific pathologic conditions or are indicative of a specific pathologic process (e.g., polychromasia, microcytic and hypochromic cells, spherocytes, autoagglutination, rouleaux, Heinz bodies, RBC parasites, viral inclusions). *Poikilocytosis* is a general term used to describe RBC morphologic changes when there is not a predominant shape change. When possible, more specific terms should be used to describe the poikilocytosis. The term *anisocytosis* refers to variation in RBC size and can refer to either RBCs that are larger (macrocytes) or smaller (microcytes) than normal.

INDICATIONS
• To aid in determination of a cause of anemia
• To aid in identification of toxicities (e.g., lead and zinc toxicity) or exposure to oxidants

CONTRAINDICATIONS
None

POTENTIAL COMPLICATIONS
None

CLIENT EDUCATION
None

BODY SYSTEMS ASSESSED
Hemic, lymphatic, and immune

SAMPLE

COLLECTION
• 1–3 mL of venous blood
• A drop of capillary blood can be used immediately to make a blood smear.

HANDLING
• EDTA is preferred.
• Heparin can be used but may change staining characteristics.
• Prepare direct smears immediately to prevent in vitro artifactual changes in RBC morphology.
• Transport blood on ice, but keep smears away from ice.

STORAGE
• Refrigerate the blood if the sample is not processed within 2–4 h.
• Store the blood smears at room temperature, protected from light.

STABILITY
• Room temperature: 2–4 h
• Refrigerated (2°–8°C): up to 48 h
• Unfixed (unstained) slides: ≈3 days
• Fixed slides (especially if permanently coverslipped): years

PROTOCOL
None

INTERPRETATION

NORMAL FINDINGS OR RANGE
• Dogs: Most RBCs have obvious central pallor; mild polychromasia (0–2/100× field).
• Cats: rouleaux, slight polychromasia (0–1/100× field), low numbers of Howell-Jolly bodies, and Heinz bodies in up to 10% of RBCs

ABNORMAL VALUES
• Any number of spherocytes is significant in dogs, and any number of schistocytes or keratocytes or autoagglutination is significant in dogs and cats.
• The presence of a marked (4+) morphology change is considered significant regardless of abnormality.

Guidelines for semiquantification of RBC abnormalities[a]

Morphology	1+	2+	3+	4+
Anisocytosis				
Dogs	7–15	16–20	21–29	>30
Cats	5–8	9–15	16–20	>20
Polychromasia				
Dogs	2–7	8–14	15–29	>30
Cats	1–2	3–8	9–15	>15
Hypochromasia	1–10	11–50	51–200	>200
Poikilocytosis	3–10	11–50	51–200	>200
Codocytes	3–5	6–15	16–30	>30
Spherocytes	5–10	11–50	51–150	>150
Echinocytes	5–10	11–100	101–250	>250
Schistocytes/keratocytes	1–2	3–8	9–20	>20

[a] Numbers are per 100× field. Assume that the monolayer contains 100–250 cells/100× field.
Modified from Weiss (1984).

CRITICAL VALUES
None

INTERFERING FACTORS
Drugs That May Alter Results or Interpretation
Drugs That Interfere with Test Methodology
None

Drugs That Alter Physiology
None

Disorders That May Alter Results
• Hemolysis can result in a thick pink background.
• Lipemia can cause RBCs to become smudged.
• Hyperglobulinemia can produce a thick blue background and rouleaux formation.
• Any thick background may distort RBCs or cause them to resemble spherocytes.

Collection Techniques or Handling That May Alter Results
• Use of blood >6–12 h old
  • Hematotropic mycoplasmas detach from RBCs.
  • RBCs may swell.
• Underfilling an EDTA tube may cause RBC shrinkage (crenation).
• Inappropriate drying of a smear may result in a refractile drying artifact.
• The use of an old stain or insufficient washing can result in stain precipitate easily mistaken for bacterial cocci or RBC parasites.

RED BLOOD CELL MORPHOLOGY

• Evaluation of RBCs in the feathered edge where they often resemble spherocytes

Influence of Signalment

Species

• Rouleaux, small numbers of Heinz bodies, and Howell-Jolly bodies are common in cats but not dogs.
• Spherocytes cannot be readily identified in cats because of their small RBCs without consistent central pallor.

Breed

Hereditary stomatocytosis has been reported in Alaskan malamutes, miniature schnauzers, and Drentse patrijshonds (Dutch partridge dogs).

Causes of Abnormal Findings

Age

Metarubricytes may be seen rarely in neonatal animals.

Gender

None

Pregnancy

None

LIMITATIONS OF THE TEST

Sensitivity, Specificity, and Positive and Negative Predictive Values

N/A

Valid If Run in a Human Lab?

Yes, if technologists are familiar with veterinary blood.

Shape change		Description	Associated with
Acanthocyte (spur cell)		Few asymmetrically distributed, irregular projections, often with blunt ends	RBC fragmentation (e.g., DIC, vasculitis hemangiosarcoma, glomerulonephritis Altered lipid metabolism (e.g., hepatic disease, hypercholesterolemia)
Agglutination		Clumping of erythrocytes together in clusters	Caused by immunoglobulins on RBC surfaces (e.g., IMHA, neonatal isoerythrolysis, transfusion reaction)
Basophilic stippling		Fine to coarse blue to purple dots (diffuse) that represent clumped ribosomes	Regenerative anemia Lead toxicity
Codocyte (target cell)		Central and peripheral distribution of Hgb	Regenerative anemia Iron-deficiency anemia Liver or kidney disease Lipid disorders
Dacrocyte		Resembles a teardrop	Artifactual Bone marrow disease (e.g., myelofibrosis, neoplasia)
Eccentrocyte (hemighost)		Hgb localized to part of cell, leaving an Hgb-poor area	Oxidative damage (e.g., onion, zinc, propofol, acetaminophen, benzocaine, vitamin K toxicosis)
Echinocyte (crenation; burr cell)		Spicules evenly spaced and symmetrical; may be sharp or blunt	Excess EDTA Old blood Glomerulonephritis Electrolyte disturbances Snake envenomation
Elliptocyte (ovalocyte)		Oval-shaped RBC	Bone marrow neoplasia Myelofibrosis Hepatic lipidosis Portosystemic shunts Glomerulonephritis Hereditary elliptocytosis
Ghost cell (hemolyzed cell)		Shell of RBC membrane without Hgb	Intravascular hemolysis
Heinz body		Irregularly round, inclusion, lighter pink than adjacent cytoplasm; along RBC margin or as small surface projections	Oxidized, denatured Hgb Cats: small numbers normal Increased with diabetes mellitus, lymphoma, or hyperthyroidism Increased with oxidative damage (e.g., onion, acetaminophen, vitamin K toxicosis)
Hgb crystal		RBC distorted by rectangular Hgb crystal	Common in cats (no clinical significance)

(Continued)

RED BLOOD CELL MORPHOLOGY

Shape change		Description	Associated with
Howell-Jolly body		Basophilic, dark purple spherical intracytoplasmic inclusion (nuclear remnant)	Common in cats Regenerative anemias Splenectomy
Hypochromasia		Central portion of cell is paler staining and has wider diameter than normal; thin rim of Hgb	Iron deficiency Must be differentiated from torocytes (artifact)
Macrocyte		Larger diameter than normal; may be polychromatophilic	Reticulocytosis FeLV infection In vitro cell swelling (e.g., prolonged storage, hypernatremic patients) Congenital poodle macrocytosis Myelodysplastic and myeloproliferative disorders
Microcyte		Smaller diameter than normal but not as dense as spherocyte; may be hypochromic	Iron deficiency Portosystemic venous shunts Healthy Asian breeds of dogs (e.g., Shiba Inus, Akitas)
Nucleated RBC		Usually polychromatophilic cells containing a condensed basophilic nucleus	Bone marrow damage (e.g., hypoxia, septicemia, endotoxemia, neoplasia) Lead toxicity Heart disease Endogenous or exogenous hypercortisolemia Splenectomy Dyserythropoiesis
Pincered cell		Knob joined to the cell by a pinched-off area	Intravascular trauma Pyruvate kinase deficiency
Polychromasia		Blue-gray cytoplasm (polychromasia); RBC is often larger than normal (macrocyte)	Regenerative anemias
RBC parasites or viral inclusion		Morphology depends on the organism	*Mycoplasma spp.*: epicellular organisms attached to external surface of RBC; small basophilic rods, cocci, or rings
			Babesia canis (large): piriform organisms in pairs or single with clear cytoplasm and red to purple nucleus
			Babesia gibsoni (small): signet ring–shaped intracytoplasmic inclusion
			Cytauxzoon felis: signet ring–shaped intracytoplasmic inclusion
			Distemper inclusions: basophilic to eosinophilic, variably sized round, oval, or irregular inclusions (may appear in WBC also)
Rouleaux		RBCs in a linear array (stacks of coins)	Normal in cats Hyperfibrinogenemia Hyperglobulinemia

(Continued)

RED BLOOD CELL MORPHOLOGY

Shape change		Description	Associated with
Schistocyte (includes RBC fragment, schizocyte, blister cell, keratocyte)		Small, triangular, comma-shaped, round, or irregularly shaped blister cells have intact or ruptured vesicle; keratocytes often have 2 membrane projections (horns)	RBC fragmentation (e.g., DIC, vasculitis hemangiosarcoma, glomerulonephritis)
Siderotic inclusions (Pappenheimer bodies)		Amorphous basophilic, cytoplasmic iron accumulations; often focal cluster near cell periphery (inclusions are Prussian blue positive)	Hemolytic anemia Lead toxicity Dyserythropoiesis Bone marrow neoplasia
Spherocyte		Decreased central pallor and diameter (MCV within normal limits); darker orange	IMHA; RBC transfusions RBC parasites Zinc toxicity Bee or snake envenomation
Stomatocyte		Cup-shaped with oval or elongated areas of central pallor	Artifact: thick blood film Immature erythrocytes Hereditary defect
Torocyte (donut cell)		Punched-out central clear space	Artifacts (do not confuse with codocytes)

CLINICAL PERSPECTIVE
- Polychromasia and anisocytosis represent reticulocytosis and a regenerative response to anemia.
- Any Heinz bodies in dogs indicate exposure to an oxidant and subsequent Heinz body hemolytic anemia.
- Increased Heinz bodies in cats are associated with several metabolic diseases, but oxidative toxicities should also be considered.
- Moderate to marked spherocytosis with or without autoagglutination is generally considered diagnostic for IMHA (primary or secondary).
- Increased numbers of schistocytes, keratocytes, and acanthocytes suggest RBC fragmentation.
- Microcytosis and hypochromasia, often with RBC fragmentation, are most frequently associated with iron deficiency.
- Uniformly macrocytic or microcytic RBCs are easily missed microscopically and more likely to be detected via RBC indices.

MISCELLANEOUS
ANCILLARY TESTS
- New methylene blue preparation to confirm Heinz bodies
- A serum iron profile
- A serum biochemical profile and urinalysis if organ dysfunction is a consideration
- A coagulation profile if a coagulopathy (e.g., DIC) is a consideration
- Coombs' testing may be considered (but not indicated if autoagglutination is present).

SYNONYMS
None

SEE ALSO

Blackwell's Five-Minute Veterinary Consult: Canine and Feline Topics
- Anemia, Heinz Body
- Anemia, Iron-Deficiency
- Anemia, Metabolic (Anemias with Spiculated Red Cells)
- Anemia, Regenerative

Related Topics in This Book
- *Babesia*
- Blood Smear Microscopic Examination
- Heinz Bodies
- Hemotrophic Mycoplasmas
- Red Blood Cell Count
- Reticulocyte Count

ABBREVIATIONS

- DIC = disseminated intravascular coagulation
- Hgb = hemoglobin
- IMHA = immune-mediated hemolytic anemia

Suggested Reading
Harvey JW. *Atlas of Veterinary Hematology.* Philadelphia: WB Saunders, 2001.
Weiss DJ. Uniform evaluation and semiquantitative reporting of hematologic data in veterinary laboratories. *Vet Clin Pathol* 1984; 13: 27–31.

INTERNET RESOURCES

Cornell University, College of Veterinary Medicine, Clinical Pathology Modules: Red blood cell morphology, http://www.diaglab.vet.cornell.edu/clinpath/modules/rbcmorph/rbcmorph.htm.

AUTHOR NAME

Jennifer L. Brazzell

RELAXIN

BASICS

TYPE OF SPECIMEN
Blood

TEST EXPLANATION AND RELATED PHYSIOLOGY
The principal site of relaxin production is the placenta. Therefore, it is considered to be a pregnancy-specific hormone in bitches and queens. Relaxin reaches detectable levels in serum or plasma as early as 20 days after the LH surge (or 20–35 days after a single breeding) (Steinetz et al. 2000). It reaches peak concentrations 30–35 days after the LH surge and remains high throughout pregnancy, until parturition or abortion, when it declines precipitously. Low levels may be detectable for 4 days postpartum in bitches. Although relaxin was detectable in the majority (80%) of bitches between days 20 and 28 after the LH surge, in 20% it was not detected until after day 30. Litter size may influence relaxin concentrations. Finding high concentrations of relaxin in serum or plasma confirms pregnancy. Declining or undetectable concentrations are found in cases of spontaneous abortion and following parturition. Relaxin is undetectable in pseudopregnant and nonpregnant bitches and queens.

There are 2 commercially available, in-house assays for relaxin. ReproCHEK is an ELISA microwell system in which 10 or more samples can be run simultaneously. Heparinized plasma or whole blood is required. Serum and EDTA samples *cannot* be used in this assay. ReproCHEK is for canine relaxin only. Witness Relaxin, which is a rapid immunomigration assay designed for single samples, can be used for canine and feline samples because it targets a different region of the relaxin hormone. Serum or plasma, *but not whole blood*, can be used in Witness Relaxin. Both assays are from Synbiotics (San Diego, CA).

INDICATIONS
- To detect pregnancy
- To monitor abortion

CONTRAINDICATIONS
None

POTENTIAL COMPLICATIONS
None

CLIENT EDUCATION
None

BODY SYSTEMS ASSESSED
Reproductive

SAMPLE

COLLECTION
0.5–1.0 mL of venous blood

HANDLING
ReproCHEK (Canine Only)
- Collect the sample into lithium heparin or sodium heparin (green-top tube).
- Either whole blood or heparinized plasma can be assayed.

Witness Relaxin (Canine or Feline)
- Collect the sample into a plain red-top tube, serum-separator tube, or lithium heparin or sodium heparin (green-top tube).
- Centrifuge the sample and use serum or plasma for the assay.

STORAGE
- It is recommended that the sample be tested immediately after collection.
- Refrigerate the sample for short-term storage.
- For use with the ReproCHEK, canine plasma samples may be frozen for longer storage.

STABILITY
- Room temperature: ≤4 h
- Refrigerated (2°–8°C): 2 days

PROTOCOL
Measure relaxin 20 or more days after the LH surge. Fewer false-negative results occur after day 30.

INTERPRETATION

NORMAL FINDINGS OR RANGE
Relaxin is reliably detected after days 30–35 of pregnancy and thereafter until parturition or abortion.

ABNORMAL VALUES
A drop in relaxin concentration during pregnancy indicates embryonic death and impending resorption or abortion.

CRITICAL VALUES
Undetectable relaxin in a previously pregnant animal indicates that the pregnancy has been lost.

INTERFERING FACTORS
Drugs That May Alter Results or Interpretation
Drugs That Interfere With Test Methodology
None

Drugs That Alter Physiology
Abortifacients

Disorders That May Alter Results
- Abortion
- Lipemia may color the background and obscure a positive result.

Collection Techniques or Handling That May Alter Results
Hemolysis may obscure a positive result.

Influence of Signalment
Species
- The ReproCHEK assay is specific for dogs.
- The Witness Relaxin assay can be used in dogs and cats.

Breed
None

Age
Sexually mature

Gender
Intact female

Pregnancy
Relaxin is detected only during pregnancy.

LIMITATIONS OF THE TEST
Sensitivity, Specificity, and Positive and Negative Predictive Values
- False-positive results have not been reported.
- False-negative results can (and do) occur early in pregnancy. To avoid this, test (or retest) after days 30–35.

Valid If Run in a Human Lab?
No.

High values (positive)	Low values (negative)
Pregnant	Not pregnant
	Pseudopregnant
	Abortion
	Early pregnancy (<35 days after breeding)

CLINICAL PERSPECTIVE
- Abdominal palpation, ultrasound, and relaxin can each be used to detect pregnancy in bitches and queens 20 or more days after breeding.
- Relaxin can be used to monitor spontaneous or induced abortion.
- Relaxin can be used to differentiate psuedopregnancy from pregnancy, although this is rarely necessary, especially in bitches in which the clinical signs of false pregnancy are seen at the end of diestrus, a time that is easily distinguishable from early pregnancy.

 MISCELLANEOUS

ANCILLARY TESTS
Abdominal palpation and ultrasonography to detect pregnancy

SYNONYMS
None

SEE ALSO
Blackwell's Five-Minute Veterinary Consult: Canine and Feline Topics
- Abortion, Spontaneous, and Pregnancy Loss—Cats
- Abortion, Spontaneous, and Pregnancy Loss—Dogs
- Abortion, Termination of Pregnancy

Related Topics in This Book
- Luteinizing Hormone
- Progesterone

ABBREVIATIONS
LH = luteinizing hormone

Suggested Reading
Buff S, Fontbonne A, Lopez P, *et al.* Circulating relaxin concentrations in pregnant and nonpregnant bitches: Evaluation of a new enzyme immunoassay for determination of pregnancy. *J Reprod Fertil Suppl* 2001; 57: 187–191.
Steinetz BG, Goldsmith LT, Brown MC, Lust G. Use of serum relaxin for pregnancy diagnosis in the bitch. In: Bonagura JD, ed. *Kirk's Current Veterinary Therapy XIII*. Philadelphia: WB Saunders, 2000: 924–925.
Verstegen JP. Physiology and endocrinology of reproduction in female cats. In: England G, Harvey M, eds. *Manual of Small Animal Reproduction and Neonatology*. Cheltenham, UK: British Small Animal Veterinary Association, 1998: 10–16.

INTERNET RESOURCES
None

AUTHOR NAME
Cheri A. Johnson

RENAL BIOPSY AND ASPIRATION

 BASICS

TYPE OF PROCEDURE
Biopsy

PROCEDURE EXPLANATION AND RELATED PHYSIOLOGY
Renal biopsy refers to the collection of renal tissue for histopathologic evaluation. *Renal aspiration* refers to needle aspiration of renal cortical or mass tissue for cytologic evaluation. Whereas renal aspiration is typically performed percutaneously (via ultrasound guidance or blindly), renal biopsies can be obtained percutaneously (via laparoscopy, the keyhole technique, ultrasound guidance, or blindly) or surgically. In all cases, care should be taken to collect only renal cortical tissue.

INDICATIONS
- When an accurate histologic diagnosis is likely to alter patient management or facilitate prognostication, as is most likely with acute renal failure (ARF) or protein-losing nephropathy (PLN)
- ARF that is either persistently severe or deteriorating despite appropriate medical management
- When PLN that is not associated with an identifiable underlying disease or proteinuria persists following effective treatment of a potential underlying disease
- Mass lesions or generalized lymphoma of the kidney may be diagnosed by renal aspiration; otherwise, a biopsy may be needed.

CONTRAINDICATIONS
- Uncorrectable coagulopathy
- Severe anemia
- Severe hydronephrosis
- Uncontrolled hypertension
- Large or multiple renal cysts
- Perirenal abscess
- Extensive pyelonephritis
- End-stage renal disease
- An inexperienced operator
- Incomplete patient immobilization
- See the "Laparoscopy" chapter for additional contraindications.

POTENTIAL COMPLICATIONS
- Hemorrhage (microscopic, macroscopic, perirenal, intrarenal, intra-abdominal)
- Death
- Thrombosis and infarction
- Biopsy of nonrenal tissue
- Hydronephrosis
- Renal scar formation and fibrosis
- Renal cyst formation
- Infection
- Arteriovenous fistula formation
- Renal aspiration is likely associated with a lower risk of these complications.
- See the "Laparoscopy" chapter for additional complications.

CLIENT EDUCATION
- General anesthesia is required for renal biopsy in most patients.
- Sedation is required for renal aspiration.
- Animals should not be fed on the day of the procedure.
- The most common complication of both procedures is hemorrhage. Gross hematuria may occur for up to 72 h after the biopsy procedure. Hemorrhage is severe enough to require a transfusion in up to 10% of dogs and 15% of cats undergoing renal biopsy.
- Death associated with renal biopsy is rare, reported in <3% of dogs and cats.

BODY SYSTEMS ASSESSED
Renal and urologic

 PROCEDURE

PATIENT PREPARATION
Preprocedure Medication or Preparation
- Withhold food the day of the procedure.
- Systemic hypertension and uremia should be controlled medically before biopsy.
- NSAIDs should be discontinued 5 days before the procedure.

Anesthesia or Sedation
Failure to properly immobilize the patient increases the likelihood of serious complications. Ideally, the patient should be immobilized by general anesthesia. Some patients who are very ill may be immobilized by sedatives alone; however, incomplete anesthesia of the peritoneum can result in sudden abdominal movement during the biopsy procedure.

Patient Positioning
- The right kidney is often preferred for renal biopsy in dogs. In cats, both kidneys are equally suitable for biopsy.
- The patient is placed in left lateral recumbency for biopsy of the right kidney or in right lateral recumbency for biopsy of the left kidney. Surgical biopsy samples are most often obtained with patients in dorsal recumbency.

Patient Monitoring
Appropriate anesthesia monitoring

Equipment or Supplies
Renal Biopsy
- Anesthetic agents and equipment
- Surgical skin-preparation supplies (e.g., clippers, povidone-iodine, alcohol)
- Needle biopsy: a disposable spring-loaded biopsy needle, or spring-loaded biopsy gun and disposable needle, 16 or 18 gauge, 9 cm long, with a cannula that does not move deeper into the tissue during activation
- Appropriate ultrasound, surgical, or laparoscopic equipment, dependent upon technique
- Tissue fixatives: formalin; 4% formalin plus 1% glutaraldehyde in sodium phosphate buffer for EM; Michel's solution or tissue-freezing material for IFA
- IV fluids

Renal Aspiration
- Sedatives
- Surgical skin-preparation supplies (e.g., clippers, povidone-iodine, alcohol)
- Ultrasound equipment
- A 6- or 12-mL needle and a 22-gauge needle
- Slides
- Romanovsky-type stain

TECHNIQUE
For All Percutaneous Methods
- The hair over the biopsy site is clipped and the skin aseptically prepared.
- A small stab incision is made through the skin at the site of needle entry.
- When possible, the tip of the needle should be placed just through the renal capsule prior to activation of the biopsy instrument to prevent sliding of the needle and tearing of the capsule.
- Penetration of the biopsy needle too deep beyond the renal capsule will limit the amount of renal cortex in the needle.
- The needle should be positioned at an angle that will ensure that only renal cortex is biopsied (Figure 1).

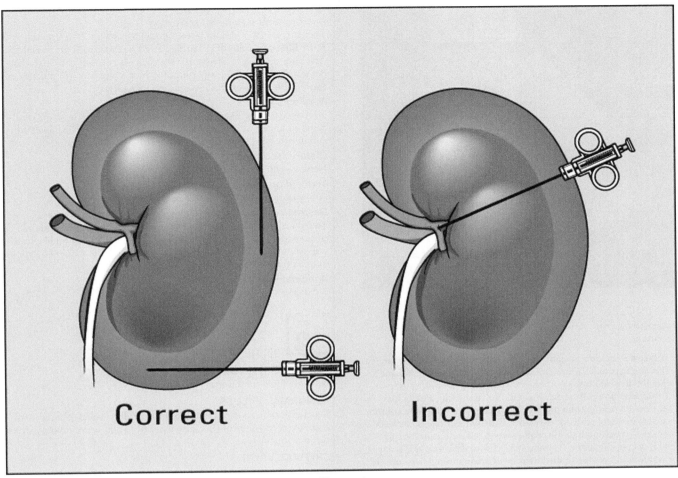

Figure 1

Schematic drawing showing the correct placement of the needle in the renal cortex. Note that the needle should not penetrate the medulla.

- At least 2 adequate samples should be taken by using the method required for the selected needle.
- Digital pressure should be applied to the kidney transabdominally for ≈5 min after biopsy to minimize hemorrhage.

Percutaneous Biopsy Using Ultrasound Guidance
Ultrasonography is used to examine the kidneys and guide correct placement of the needle. A sterile sleeve is placed over the ultrasound probe, and sterile coupling gel is applied. The kidneys are scanned for selection of the biopsy site. The tip of the biopsy needle is guided through the skin incision and the renal capsule with 1 hand while the probe is held with the other (Figure 2).

Percutaneous Biopsy Using the Keyhole Technique
With the dog in lateral recumbency, the dog's back should be facing the surgeon. An oblique, paralumbar 7.5- to 10-cm skin incision is made on a line that bisects the angle between the last rib and the edge of the lumbar musculature. Care should be taken not to make the incision too caudoventral, dorsal, or cranial because these errors may make it impossible to palpate the kidney; require the dissection of a large, vascular muscle mass; or lead to puncture of the intercostal artery, respectively. The muscle fibers are separated along muscle planes. A peritoneal incision is made that is large enough to enable easy insertion of the surgeon's index finger over the caudal pole of the kidney. The index finger holds the kidney against the edge of the lumbar musculature. The other hand inserts the biopsy needle through the separate stab incision in the lateral body wall and just through the renal capsule, while taking care to maintain the proper angle.

Blind or Palpation Technique
Either kidney is localized by palpation. The kidney is immobilized with 1 hand. The other hand advances the needle through the incision and directs it toward the cranial or caudal pole of the kidney. The tip of the needle is placed just through the capsule at an angle such that the needle will pass only through renal cortex.

Laparoscopic Biopsy
This rigid endoscopic procedure is performed under sterile conditions and enables direct visual inspection of the kidneys and visual control of the biopsy, leading to a higher likelihood that diagnostic tissue will be obtained. Laparoscopy requires appropriate equipment and operator expertise. A renal biopsy sample is obtained via an instrument that is introduced into the abdomen through a site that is separate from the trocar or Veress needle. Direct pressure can be applied with the laparoscope or laparoscopic tools if needed to control hemorrhage. (See the "Laparoscopy" chapter for a detailed description of the technique.)

Surgical Biopsy
A surgical wedge biopsy is preferred over a surgical needle biopsy. The surgical biopsy sample can be obtained through a paracostal incision if only 1 kidney is to be examined and biopsied or through a cranial midline abdominal incision if other intra-abdominal procedures are to be performed or both kidneys need to be examined prior to biopsy.

RENAL BIOPSY AND ASPIRATION

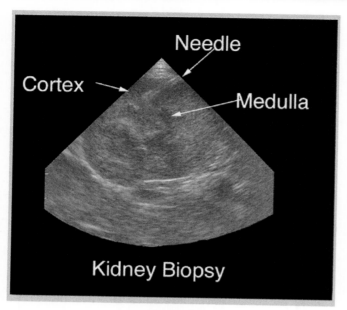

Figure 2

Ultrasonographic image of the kidney with the biopsy needle penetrating the renal cortex.

The paracostal incision is made with the patient in lateral recumbency. The incision is parallel and 2 cm caudal to the last rib. The oblique muscles are divided between fibers and retracted. The kidney is located after separating the transverse abdominal muscle. The kidney can be elevated through the incision by placing umbilical tape around both poles. In obese animals, exposure of the kidney may be difficult through the paracostal incision. Following exposure through either type of incision, the kidney is immobilized with thumb and forefinger prior to biopsy. A wedge-shaped incision is made through the capsule and into the cortex. Tissue forceps are used to lift the biopsy wedge gently while the scalpel blade is used to sever any remaining attachments. Monofilament, absorbable suture material (4-0) in a simple continuous pattern is used to close the renal capsule.

Renal Aspiration
Perform this procedure by using the method already described for ultrasound guidance or blind biopsy except that a syringe and 22-gauge needle are used instead of a biopsy needle.

SAMPLE HANDLING
• Microscopic examination of specimens using 10-fold magnification provides immediate verification that adequate biopsy samples, containing at least 5 glomeruli, have been obtained.
• For patients with PLN, 1 needle biopsy sample is put in formalin. One-half of the second piece is placed into a fixative for EM (e.g., 4% formalin plus 1% glutaraldehyde in sodium phosphate buffer) within 5 minutes of collection. The other half is frozen for IFA or put in ammonium sulfate-N-ethylmaleimide (i.e., Michel's solution). Wedge biopsies should be divided in a similar fashion; tissue for EM should be minced.
• For patients with ARF, formalin fixation may be all that is required for adequate histopathologic evaluation. Samples should also be collected for EM and IFA in the event that a glomerular disease is causing the ARF.
• Renal aspiration cytologic samples are processed for routine microscopic evaluation by spreading the cellular material across the slide, allowing the smear to air-dry, and staining the smear with some type of Romanovsky-type stain (e.g., Diff-Quick, Hema III, Giemsa, or Wright).

APPROPRIATE AFTERCARE
Postprocedure Patient Monitoring
The patient's PCV should be monitored for at least 24 h after the procedure. The color of the urine should be monitored for several days after the biopsy. Hematuria that persists beyond 72 h or severe hemorrhage developing any time after biopsy warrants reevaluation of the kidneys and biopsy site via ultrasonography.

Nursing Care
To reduce the likelihood that obstructing clots will form in the renal pelvis or ureter, isotonic fluids should be administered liberally IV in amounts needed to produce a diuresis for several hours after biopsy.

Dietary Modification
None specific to the procedure

Medication Requirements
Postoperative pain control may be needed.

Restrictions on Activity
To reduce the chances of dislodging a blood clot, the animal should be confined to a cage for 24 h after the procedure. Dogs should be leash walked only for 7–10 days after the procedure. Cats should be kept indoors for 7–10 days after the procedure.

Anticipated Recovery Time
7–10 days

INTERPRETATION
NORMAL FINDINGS OR RANGE
No pathologic conditions

ABNORMAL VALUES
Renal disease (e.g., membranoproliferative glomerulonephritis, membranous glomerulonephritis, hereditary nephritis, acute tubular necrosis); renal neoplasia

CRITICAL VALUES
None

INTERFERING FACTORS
Drugs That May Alter Results of the Procedure
None

Conditions That May Interfere with Performing the Procedure
• Coagulopathy, uncontrolled hypertension, and uremia are risk factors for complications, particularly serious hemorrhage, after biopsy.
• Operator inexperience or incomplete patient immobilization may increase the risk of complications.

Procedure Techniques or Handling That May Alter Results
• Take care not to crush the biopsy sample during or after its collection.
• Quickly place specimens into appropriate fixatives; drying of the specimen should be prevented.
• Use of only light-microscopic examination of the tissue to render a diagnosis is more subjective and may not be accurate, particularly in animals with PLN.

Influence of Signalment on Performing and Interpreting the Procedure
Species
Blind biopsy is more suitable for cats than for dogs. The keyhole technique has been described for dogs and is generally not used in cats. The right kidney is preferred for biopsy in dogs; either kidney is suitable for biopsy in cats.

Breed
Surgical biopsy of dogs that weigh <5 kg may be associated with fewer complications.

Age
None

Gender
None

Pregnancy
Avoid the use of percutaneous biopsy methods in pregnant animals.

CLINICAL PERSPECTIVE

- Percutaneous biopsy via ultrasound guidance is the method of choice for dogs weighing >5 kg and for all cats that do not have other contraindications for renal biopsy.
- The keyhole technique can be used in dogs when ultrasonography is not available.
- Blind biopsy can be used in cats when ultrasonography is not available.
- Compared with surgery, laparoscopy is less invasive, can be performed more quickly and has a lower rate of patient morbidity.
- Surgical biopsy may be the preferred method for small dogs (weighing <5 kg), animals with isolated areas (e.g., large cysts) in the kidney that need to be avoided, and animals that are undergoing laparotomy for another reason.
- Surgical biopsy may be safer in some animals that have other listed contraindications to biopsy (e.g., a large renal cyst).
- Disease-specific treatment may be indicated as determined by the histologic diagnosis.

MISCELLANEOUS

ANCILLARY TESTS
None

SYNONYMS
- Kidney aspirate
- Kidney biopsy

SEE ALSO

Blackwell's Five-Minute Veterinary Consult: Canine and Feline Topics
- Amyloidosis
- Glomerulonephritis
- Proteinuria
- Renal Failure, Acute Uremia

Related Topics in This Book
- Abdominal Ultrasonography
- Fine-Needle Aspiration
- Laparoscopy
- Renal Ultrasonography
- Tissue Biopsy: Needle and Punch
- Ultrasound-Guided Mass or Organ Aspiration

ABBREVIATIONS
- ARF = acute renal failure
- EM = electron microscopy
- PLN = protein-losing nephropathy

Suggested Reading
Vaden SL. Renal biopsy: Methods and interpretation. *Vet Clin North Am Small Anim Pract* 1004; 34: 887–908.

INTERNET RESOURCES
Jennette JC. Renal Pathology Tutorial. UNC Renal Nephropathology Laboratory, http://www.uncnephropathology.org/jennette/tutorial.htm.
Louisiana State University Health Sciences Center, Veterans Affairs Medical Center New Orleans: Handling the renal biopsy, http://www.medschool.lsuhsc.edu/pathology/pathist/DX_SERVICESh/andling_biopsy.htm.

AUTHOR NAME
Shelly L. Vaden

RENAL ULTRASONOGRAPHY

BASICS

TYPE OF PROCEDURE
Ultrasonographic

PROCEDURE EXPLANATION AND RELATED PHYSIOLOGY
The upper urinary tract is included in a complete abdominal ultrasonographic examination. The upper urinary tract examination includes each kidney and corresponding ureter. Ultrasonographic imaging of these organs does not rely on the function of the kidneys and is independent of radiography. Renal ultrasonography includes examining the entire kidney parenchyma and the collecting system. The ureter is examined at the renal pelvis and at the ureter's entrance into the bladder. Renal and ureteral diseases that affect the size, shape, contour, and echogenicity are often imaged and diagnosed with ultrasonography. Vascular flow within the kidneys can be assessed with Doppler interrogation.

INDICATIONS
- Azotemia
- Hematuria
- Pyuria
- A bladder mass
- A mass identified that, on abdominal radiographs or by palpation, is consistent with a renal or ureteral origin
- Suspected urinary tract calculi
- Suspected urinary tract obstruction
- Incontinence
- A trauma possibly involving the urinary tract
- Hypercalcemia
- Hypertension
- Abdominal or lumbar pain

CONTRAINDICATIONS
None

POTENTIAL COMPLICATIONS
- Bleeding may occur if kidney aspiration or biopsy is performed in conjunction with ultrasonography.
- Sedative drugs, the overall systemic condition of the patient, and the blood flow to the kidney may influence the appearance of the flow within the kidneys.

CLIENT EDUCATION
- The study requires clipping of the abdominal hair in most cases.
- The patient may need chemical restraint if unruly, in pain, or noncompliant.
- Aspirates may be needed if masses are detected.

BODY SYSTEMS ASSESSED
- Hemic, lymphatic, and immune
- Renal and urologic

PROCEDURE

PATIENT PREPARATION
Preprocedure Medication or Preparation
Enough hair is clipped over the abdomen so that the entire abdomen can be imaged.

Anesthesia or Sedation
- Sedation is administered only if the study may be compromised without it and if the patient is stable.
- Sedation may be required if aspirates are taken.
- Kidney biopsies require anesthesia.

Patient Positioning
Depending on the preference of the sonologist, the patient's conformation, and possible disease, the patient may be imaged in lateral or dorsal recumbency. An assistant holds the patient in position during the procedure.

Patient Monitoring
- Monitoring of respiration and heartbeat depends on the condition of the patient. If the patient is unstable or sedated, additional monitoring may be required.
- Laboratory results, including those for serum urea nitrogen and creatinine concentrations and a complete urinalysis, should be available prior to the examination.

Equipment or Supplies
- An ultrasound unit with transducers that have sufficient resolution and depth to image the kidneys in their entirety is required. This is usually 7 MHz or higher, depending on the size and conformation of the patient.
- Ultrasound gel for acoustic coupling
- Clippers
- Alcohol, often helpful for cleaning the skin
- Towels to remove the water-soluble gel when the study is completed
- Needles for aspiration (18–20 gauge) or for biopsy (16–18 gauge) and equipment for handling the samples (e.g., microscope slides, tissue fixatives)

TECHNIQUE
- The hair is clipped with a surgical blade from the level of the diaphragm to the pelvic limbs and from the epaxial muscles to the ventral midline.
- The animal is first placed in right lateral recumbency for imaging the left side.
- The skin is cleaned with alcohol.
- Ample ultrasound gel is applied.
- The transducer with the highest resolution (7–13 MHz) is chosen.
- The kidney is located in the dorsal midabdomen.
- The image is oriented such that the left side of the image on the screen should represent the cranial or dorsal aspect of the kidney.
- The kidney is imaged in both longitudinal (dorsal or sagittal) and transverse planes. Make sure to scan through the entire organ. The study should include the entire kidney from pole to pole and from side to side.
- Particular attention is made to the shape of the kidney, its margins, the corticomedullary distinction, and the size and echogenicity of the pelvis. The echogenicity within the kidney is evaluated as well as compared to the opposite kidney, the liver, the spleen, and the surrounding tissue. There is some variation in the relative echogenicity of the different organs with the degree of fat, the age, and even the transducer used (Figure 1).
- The length and width of the kidney, as well as the width of the proximal ureter, are measured.
- The patient is then placed in left lateral recumbency, and the right kidney and ureter are examined similarly to the left.
- Images and measurements are recorded as part of the medical record. Right or left indicator markers are recorded on the image.

SAMPLE HANDLING
None

APPROPRIATE AFTERCARE
Postprocedure Patient Monitoring
None is needed unless the kidney was aspirated or biopsied, in which case the patient should be monitored for potential postprocedural bleeding.

Nursing Care
None

Dietary Modification
None

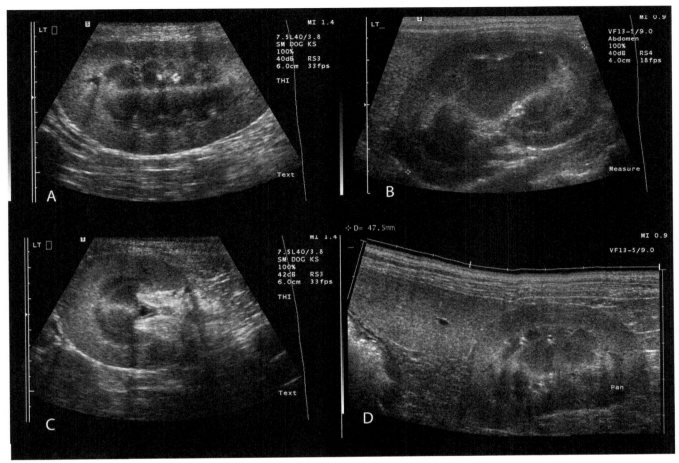

Figure 1

A: This is a dorsal plane through the kidney. This plane is a longitudinal one that divides the kidney into dorsal and ventral halves. **B:** This is a sagittal plane through the kidney. This plane is a longitudinal one that divides the kidney into right and left halves. **C:** This is a transverse plane through the kidney. Note the ureter and the renal pelvis. **D:** This image shows the echogenic relationship between the cortex of the kidney and the adjacent spleen. The spleen is typically more hyperechoic than the cortex, the cortex is more hyperechoic than the medulla, and the renal pelvis and diverticula are the most hyperechogenic.

Medication Requirements
None
Restrictions on Activity
None
Anticipated Recovery Time
Immediate

INTERPRETATION

NORMAL FINDINGS OR RANGE
The kidneys have a smooth contour. The cat kidney is more rounded whereas the dog kidney is more bean shaped. The size will vary depending on the species and the size of the patient. Cat kidneys are typically 3.6–4.2 cm long. The dog kidneys will increase with the weight and size of the dog. For a small dog of up to 15 lb (6.8 kg), they are typically up to 4.0 cm. There is a rough rule of thumb that the size of the kidney will increase by 1 cm for each 10 lb (4.5 kg) of weight. The renal pelvis wall and the fat in the peripelvic area and the diverticula are the most hyperechoic. The medulla is the most hypoe-

choic. The renal cortex should be equal or more hypoechoic compared to the liver and more hypoechoic than the spleen. It should be more hypoechoic than the perirenal fat. Each kidney should be compared to the opposite one and should be similar in appearance. The renal pelvis is typically collapsed or very mildly dilated if the urine volume has increased. The proximal ureter is usually 1–2 mm wide. The ureter throughout its course to the bladder is often not seen unless there is dilation and pathology. The ureteral papillae are normally seen in the dorsal trigone of the bladder as small projections into the lumen. Ureteral jets of urine can be seen entering the bladder especially with the aid of color Doppler. The identification of an ureteral jet is enhanced following the administration of furosemide. This diuretic will increase the flow rate, and volume, and decrease the specific gravity of the urine. This facilitates identification of the entrance of a ureter into the bladder.

ABNORMAL VALUES
- Irregular shape
- Small or enlarged kidneys
- A change in the overall echogenicity of the kidneys
- A focal increase in the echogenicity, such as can be seen from a calculus in the renal pelvis or within the parenchyma
- A dilated renal pelvis consistent with obstruction or infection

RENAL ULTRASONOGRAPHY

- Masses within the kidney
- Dilated ureters from obstruction or infection or congenital anomaly
- Mineralized concretions consistent with calculi with the ureters
- Ectopic ureters

CRITICAL VALUES
- Suspected ruptured ureter or kidney
- Excessive kidney bleeding associated with a mass or secondary to a biopsy, aspiration, or trauma
- Severe hydronephrosis with evidence for obstruction

INTERFERING FACTORS
Drugs That May Alter Results of the Procedure
- Diuretics may increase the size of the medulla and the collecting system, including the renal pelvis. This increase is usually mild.
- Sedative drugs may alter the blood flow within the kidneys, This can be monitored by pulsed-wave Doppler.

Conditions That May Interfere with Performing the Procedure
- A large mass may obscure a window to image the kidneys.
- An extraordinary amount of peritoneal gas may create enough artifact to obscure the kidneys. This is uncommon when imaging from a lateral approach.
- The ureters are not usually seen unless dilated. If the patient is moving during the examination, following the ureters is more difficult.
- A very critical patient
- Inability to apply any pressure to the abdominal cavity because of a very tense, painful abdomen, such as with pancreatitis, or because there is a mass such as a splenic hemangiosarcoma that may rupture if pressure is applied
- An intractable patient
- A patient's excessive panting

Procedure Techniques or Handling That May Alter Results
- Failure to scan the entire kidney and collecting system
- An oblique view through the kidney can foreshorten the size of the kidney and result in an erroneous measurement.

Influence of Signalment on Performing and Interpreting the Procedure
Species
- Feline kidneys may have more fat and may be more hyperechoic than canine kidneys.
- Feline kidneys are typically slightly rounder, whereas canine kidneys are more oblong.

Breed
Specific abnormalities are more commonly identified with a specific breed. These include congenital anomalies, as well as acquired diseases.

Age
- Older animals frequently have more degenerative changes in the kidneys.
- Congenital or developmental anomalies are detected more often in younger animals.

Gender
The kidneys may be slightly larger in males.

Pregnancy
With advancing pregnancy, mild pyelectasia may be present.

CLINICAL PERSPECTIVE
- Renal and ureteral ultrasonography has dramatically reduced the number of excretory urograms performed. Ultrasonography has the distinct advantage that it is easily conducted, usually requires no sedation, is noninvasive (unless an aspirate or biopsy sample is required), and the equipment can be relatively inexpensive. The internal architecture of the kidney is easily identified. Causes for renomegaly, renal masses, and suspected obstruction are easily discerned. Causes for hematuria or pyuria may be identified with renal sonography. Dilation of the ureters can be determined, as well as the cause and the site of obstruction.

- Ultrasonography can allow for the differentiation of chronic renal disease from acute renal disease as a cause for the clinical signs.
- Specific diseases such as ethylene glycol toxicity, leptospirosis, and renal dysplasia may be suspected based on their sonographic characteristics.
- If a mass is found, then the origin of the mass may be determined via ultrasonography-assisted aspiration, as well as regional metastasis.
- When a patient is azotemic, radiographic contrast procedures may not be indicated or productive. The sonographic appearance of the kidneys is not affected by kidney function.

MISCELLANEOUS

ANCILLARY TESTS
- Evaluation of serum urea nitrogen and creatinine concentrations
- Urinalysis
- Evaluation of serum calcium and phosphorus concentrations
- CBC
- Imaging of the parathyroid glands if hypercalcemia is present
- Abdominal radiography
- Thoracic radiography if neoplasia is suspected

SYNONYMS
- Renal sonography
- Upper urinary tract ultrasonography

SEE ALSO
Blackwell's Five-Minute Veterinary Consult: Canine and Feline Topics
- Adenocarcinoma, Renal
- Amyloidosis
- Congenital and Developmental Renal Diseases
- Glomerulonephritis
- Perirenal Pseudocysts
- Polycystic Kidney Disease
- Renal Failure, Acute Uremia
- Renal Failure, Chronic
- Transitional Cell Carcinoma, Renal, Bladder, Urethra

Related Topics in This Book
- General Principles of Ultrasonography
- Abdominal Ultrasonography
- Calcium
- Creatinine
- Lower Urinary Tract Ultrasonography
- Renal Biopsy and Aspiration
- Urea Nitrogen
- Urine Sediment

ABBREVIATIONS
None

Suggested Reading
Nyland TG, Mattoon JS, eds. *Small Animal Diagnostic Ultrasound.* Philadelphia: WB Saunders, 2002.

INTERNET RESOURCES
None

AUTHOR NAME
Kathy Spaulding

BASICS

TYPE OF SPECIMEN
Blood

TEST EXPLANATION AND RELATED PHYSIOLOGY
As RBC precursors mature in bone marrow, they extrude their nuclei and remove organelles (ribosomes and mitochondria) involved in synthesis of hemoglobin and cellular metabolism. Polychromatophils/reticulocytes are immature, anucleate RBCs containing cytoplasmic ribosomes and less than a full complement of hemoglobin. On a Wright-stained blood smear, these immature RBCs are larger and contain both eosinophilic hemoglobin and dispersed basophilic ribosomes and thus are described as *polychromatophilic*. The term *reticulocyte* refers to the appearance of aggregated, basophilic ribosomes within the cytoplasm of immature RBCs incubated with a vital stain such as new methylene blue (NMB) or brilliant cresyl blue. Incubation of whole blood with vital stain results in cytoplasmic precipitation of ribosomes in immature RBCs and enables visualization of reticulocytes. *Basophilic stippling* represents ex vivo aggregation of ribosomes that occurs during cell drying and before application of Wright's stain (without the addition of NMB). The terms polychromatophil and reticulocyte are considered synonymous and are used interchangeably. An increased number of reticulocytes is called *reticulocytosis*.

Reticulocytes mature in peripheral blood after their release from bone marrow. The youngest reticulocytes present in peripheral blood, which are called *aggregate reticulocytes*, contain large aggregates of precipitated ribosomes when stained with NMB. As aggregate reticulocytes mature, they become *punctate reticulocytes*, which contain small, punctate aggregates of ribosomes when stained with NMB. Canine reticulocytes mature quickly in peripheral blood and only aggregate reticulocytes are typically seen. Feline reticulocytes mature more slowly than canine reticulocytes and thus both aggregate and punctate reticulocytes are seen. Both aggregate and punctate reticulocytes can be enumerated when reticulocyte counts are performed in cats. Increased numbers of aggregate reticulocytes in a dog or cat support a current regenerative response to anemia. Increased numbers of punctate reticulocytes in cats indicate a bone marrow response to anemia that occurred up to 3–4 weeks previously. The number of aggregate reticulocytes seen with NMB-stained samples correlates with the number of polychromatophils seen on a Wright-stained blood smear. Feline punctate reticulocytes may not be visible as polychromatophils on Wright-stained blood smears.

Increased numbers of reticulocytes will be released from the bone marrow of cats and dogs with regenerative anemias. (These anemias may be macrocytic and hypochromic because of the release of larger, immature RBCs containing less hemoglobin.) The absence of reticulocytes supports the presence of a nonregenerative anemia and suggests that anemia is due to decreased RBC production. However, 3–4 days are required for bone marrow to respond to anemia, with maximum polychromasia and reticulocytosis achieved in ≈1 week, and thus increased aggregate reticulocytes may not initially be seen after acute hemorrhage or hemolysis.

Laboratories may report absolute reticulocyte count, reticulocyte percentage, corrected reticulocyte percentage, or reticulocyte production index (RPI = corrected reticulocyte percentage/reticulocyte maturation time). An absolute reticulocyte number per microliter of blood is considered the most consistent and diagnostically useful indicator of bone marrow reticulocyte production. Interpretation of reticulocyte percentage alone is not recommended because it does not take into consideration the patient's degree of anemia and will be elevated by the decrease in mature RBCs. A corrected reticulocyte percentage estimates the reticulocyte percentage if the patient was

not anemic. The RPI attempts to account for the longer life span of reticulocytes in peripheral blood. Unfortunately, the RPI requires that the reticulocyte maturation times (in health and during accelerated erythropoiesis) be known for all species. The reticulocyte maturation times for all species are not known, thus making the calculation of this index less than ideal and of questionable use in veterinary medicine.

We have traditionally relied on manual counting of reticulocytes, but newer automated hematology analyzers are capable of direct reticulocyte enumeration using fluorescent dyes with or without flow cytometry. The Advia 120 hematology analyzer (Siemens Medical Solutions Diagnostics, Tarrytown, NY) also can measure the hemoglobin content and volume of reticulocytes, which appear to be more sensitive indicators of iron-deficiency anemia.

INDICATIONS
• To determine whether the cause is decreased RBC production or increased RBC destruction or loss
• To evaluate the bone marrow erythroid response to anemia (i.e., to document the presence or absence of a regenerative response to anemia)

CONTRAINDICATIONS
None

POTENTIAL COMPLICATIONS
None

CLIENT EDUCATION
None

BODY SYSTEMS ASSESSED
Hemic, lymphatic, and immune

SAMPLE

COLLECTION
1–3 mL of venous blood

HANDLING
• EDTA is preferred. Heparin can be used but is not ideal.
• Transport the sample on ice to the laboratory.

STORAGE
Anticoagulated blood should be refrigerated if not processed within 2–4 h.

STABILITY
• Room temperature: 2–4 h
• Refrigerated (2°–8°C): stable for up to 48 h
• NMB-stained smears: stable for months to years if protected from light and humidity

PROTOCOL
• Mix equal volumes of blood and NMB or brilliant cresyl blue (which may be purchased or prepared in-house).
• Incubate the mixture at room temperature for 10–20 min.
• Prepare smears of stained blood and air-dry them.
• Examine 1000 RBCs and count the number of aggregate reticulocytes (in dogs and cats) and punctate reticulocytes (in cats).
• Calculate the reticulocyte percentage(s).
• Correct the count for the degree of anemia using 1 of the following methods:
  • Absolute reticulocytes count/μL = (% reticulocytes/100) × RBC count/μL
  • Corrected reticulocyte % = % reticulocytes × patient's PCV/average PCV for the species. A "normal" PCV is considered to be 45% in dogs and 37% in cats.

RETICULOCYTE COUNT

INTERPRETATION

NORMAL FINDINGS OR RANGE

Dogs

- Absolute reticulocyte count: <80,000/μL (SI units, <80 × 10^9/L)
- Corrected reticulocyte percentage: <1.5%

Cats

- Absolute aggregate reticulocyte count: <60,000/μL (SI units, <60 × 10^9/L)
- Absolute punctate reticulocyte count: <500,000/μL (SI units, <500 × 10^9/L)
- Corrected aggregate reticulocyte percentage: <0.4%
- Corrected punctate reticulocyte percentage: <10%

ABNORMAL VALUES

- Any increase above the reference interval suggests a regenerative response to anemia.
- The lack of an increase suggests the presence of a nonregenerative anemia.

CRITICAL VALUES

None

INTERFERING FACTORS

Drugs That May Alter Results or Interpretation

Drugs That Interfere with Test Methodology

None

Drugs That Alter Physiology

None

Disorders That May Alter Results

- Large numbers of mycoplasmal organisms may make differentiation of reticulocytes difficult.
- Large amounts of stain precipitate will make differentiation of reticulocytes difficult.

Collection Techniques or Handling That May Alter Results

None

Influence of Signalment

Species

- Cats normally have large numbers of circulating punctate reticulocytes.
- Dogs have a greater reticulocyte response than cats.

Breed

None

Age

None

Gender

None

Pregnancy

None

LIMITATIONS OF THE TEST

The degree of reticulocytosis must always be interpreted with knowledge of the severity and duration of the anemia.

Sensitivity, Specificity, and Positive and Negative Predictive Values

N/A

Valid If Run in a Human Lab?

Yes, but species-specific veterinary reference intervals should be used for interpretation.

Causes of Abnormal Findings

High values with anemia (regenerative anemia)	Low values with anemia (nonregenerative anemia)
Acute blood loss	Acute hemorrhage or hemolysis
Trauma	(<1–2 days duration) to which the
Neoplasia	bone marrow has not had time to
Surgery	respond
GI ulceration	Anemia of chronic disorders
Hemostasis defects	Erythropoietin lack (chronic kidney
Hemolysis	disease)
Immune mediated (primary	Endocrinopathies (e.g., hypothyroidism)
or secondary)	Iron deficiency (usually secondary to
RBC parasites	chronic external hemorrhage and
Oxidants (e.g.,	usually microcytic)
acetaminophen, onions)	Bone marrow disease (decreased
Zinc or copper toxicity	production)
Fragmentation (e.g.,	Infections (e.g., FeLV, FIV,
disseminated	panleukopenia, parvovirus,
intravascular coagulation,	*Ehrlichia canis*)
neoplasia, heartworm)	Myelophthisis
Snake envenomation	Toxic bone marrow damage
	Pure RBC aplasia
	Erythroid myeloproliferative or
	myelodysplastic diseases
	Nutritional deficiencies (rare)

CLINICAL PERSPECTIVE

- Anemia with appropriate reticulocytosis should prompt a search for blood loss or an underlying cause of hemolysis.
- Anemia without appropriate reticulocytosis should prompt a workup to rule out suppression of erythropoiesis by systemic disease. Evaluation of bone marrow may be necessary.
- Reticulocytosis may not be evident for 3–5 days after an acute hemolytic or hemorrhagic event.
- Reticulocytosis is typically more intense with hemolytic vs hemorrhagic diseases because the iron from hemolyzed RBCs is immediately available for reuse.
- Mild anemias (>30% in dogs; >20–25% in cats) may not provide enough stimulus for bone marrow to release reticulocytes into peripheral blood. Thus, reticulocytosis may not be appreciated even though marrow erythropoiesis may be increased.
- The duration of regenerative anemia in cats may be estimated by the pattern of reticulocyte response:
  - Marked aggregate reticulocytosis without punctate reticulocytosis suggests anemia of ≈3–5 days duration.
  - Marked punctate reticulocytosis without aggregate reticulocytosis suggests that a previous, resolved hemorrhagic or hemolytic event occurred up to 2–3 weeks earlier. (Punctate reticulocytes require ≈10–12 days to mature.)
  - The presence of both aggregate and punctate reticulocytosis suggests previous and ongoing hemorrhage or hemolysis.

MISCELLANEOUS

ANCILLARY TESTS
- Bone marrow aspiration and biopsy in animals with chronic nonregenerative, normocytic, normochromic anemias if the underlying cause cannot be elucidated
- A serum iron profile if iron-deficiency anemia is a consideration
- Evaluation of fecal occult blood to look for the source of blood loss
- A Coombs' test to identify immune-mediated hemolytic anemia

SYNONYMS
Retic count

SEE ALSO
Blackwell's Five-Minute Veterinary Consult: Canine and Feline Topics
- Anemia, Aplastic
- Anemia, Heinz Body
- Anemia, Iron-Deficiency
- Anemia, Nonregenerative
- Anemia, Regenerative
- Anemia of Chronic Renal Disease

Related Topics in This Book
- Blood Smear Microscopic Examination
- Coombs' Test
- Fecal Occult Blood
- Ferritin

- Hematocrit
- Hemoglobin
- Iron Level and Total Iron-Binding Capacity
- Red Blood Cell Count
- Red Blood Cell Morphology

ABBREVIATIONS
- RPI = reticulocyte production index

Suggested Reading
Steinberg JD, Olver CS. Hematologic and biochemical abnormalities indicating iron deficiency are associated with decreased reticulocyte hemoglobin content (CHr) and reticulocyte volume (rMCV) in dogs. *Vet Clin Pathol* 2005; 34: 23–27.
Thrall MA, ed. *Veterinary Hematology and Clinical Chemistry*. Philadelphia: Lippincott Williams & Wilkins, 2004.

INTERNET RESOURCES
Cornell University, College of Veterinary Medicine, Clinical Pathology Modules, Hemogram Basics: Hematology, http://www.diaglab.vet.cornell.edu/clinpath/modules/hemogram/retic.htm.
Cornell University, College of Veterinary Medicine, Clinical Pathology Modules: Red blood cell morphology, http://www.diaglab.vet.cornell.edu/clinpath/modules/rbcmorph/reticf.htm.

AUTHOR NAME
Jennifer L. Brazzell

RHEUMATOID FACTOR

BASICS

TYPE OF SPECIMEN
Blood

TEST EXPLANATION AND RELATED PHYSIOLOGY
The rheumatoid factor (RF) test detects the presence of RFs in canine serum. RFs are autoantibodies directed against the crystallizable fragments (Fc's) of the affected animal's own IgG. RFs may be IgG, IgM or IgA, or complexes of these immunoglobulins. A positive RF test and/or high titers for RFs are commonly associated with a diagnosis of erosive immune-mediated polyarthritis, which clinically and histologically resembles rheumatoid arthritis (RA) in people. Approximately 40%–75% of dogs with RA have positive RF test results. However, RFs are not specific for RA in dogs, and RFs may be found in patients whose serum contains circulating antibody-antigen complexes secondary to other disorders causing antigenic stimulation (e.g., SLE, Sjogren-like syndrome).

The most commonly used techniques to detect RFs are the Rose-Waaler agglutination test and the latex agglutination test. In the former, the patient's serum is mixed with rabbit IgG-sensitized sheep erythrocytes, and any RFs cause RBC agglutination. Agglutination test results are reported as positive or negative, and the titer may also be provided. The Rose-Waaler test best detects IgM because the test is more effective at agglutinating antigen-coated erythrocytes, so equivocal or negative results may occur if RFs are IgG or IgA. In the latex agglutination technique, latex beads coated with antigen bind to RF antibody. Drawbacks to the latex agglutination tests include poor specificity and poor correlation of the titers with results of the Rose-Waaler test. This low specificity limits its usefulness as a confirmatory test.

The RF agglutination tests are insensitive at diagnosing RA in dogs. Affected dogs tend to have naturally low titers, and, because RFs originate in the joints, serum levels may be below the detection limit. False-negative results may also occur if serum RFs, caught up in immune complexes, are pulled from serum. To complicate matters, certain dogs with RA may have fluctuating levels of measurable RFs.

Supplemental diagnostic tests such as joint radiography or other imaging, synovial fluid analysis, and synovial histopathologic evaluation may help to determine a definitive diagnosis.

INDICATIONS
- Shifting leg lameness
- Joint swelling affecting multiple sites
- Erosive arthropathy/polyarthritis
- Fever of unknown origin

CONTRAINDICATIONS
None

POTENTIAL COMPLICATIONS
None

CLIENT EDUCATION
None

BODY SYSTEMS ASSESSED
- Hemic, lymphatic, and immune
- Musculoskeletal

SAMPLE

COLLECTION
1–2 mL of venous blood

HANDLING
- Collect the blood sample in red-top tube or serum-separator tube.
- Sodium heparin or lithium heparin tubes may be accepted by some labs.

STORAGE
- Refrigeration is recommended for short-term storage.
- Do not freeze the serum.

STABILITY
- Room temperature: 1 day
- Refrigerated (2°–8°C): 1 week

PROTOCOL
None

INTERPRETATION

NORMAL FINDINGS OR RANGE
A negative test result

ABNORMAL VALUES
- A titer of >1:16 is considered positive for RFs.
- A titer of 1:8 is suspicious.

CRITICAL VALUES
None

INTERFERING FACTORS

Drugs That May Alter Results or Interpretation
Drugs That Interfere with Test Methodology
None

Drugs That Alter Physiology
None

Disorders That May Alter Results
None

Collection Techniques or Handling That May Alter Results
Freezing a sample may destroy RF activity and cause a false-negative result.

Influence of Signalment
Species
Dogs only

Breed
None

Age
None

Gender
None

Pregnancy
None

LIMITATIONS OF THE TEST
- Detection is difficult because of low levels of RF in dogs.
- The serum may not be of use in predicting the presence of RFs in synovial fluid.
- False negatives may be caused by immune-complex formation.
- There may be nonspecific agglutination with the latex agglutination test (false positive).

Sensitivity, Specificity, and Positive and Negative Predictive Values
The RF test is neither sensitive nor specific for the diagnosis of RA in dogs.

Valid If Run in a Human Lab?
Yes—if appropriate controls are used (e.g., unsensitized sheep erythrocytes).

Causes of Abnormal Findings

Positive result	Negative result
Canine RA (immune-mediated, erosive polyarthritis)	A normal dog
SLE	False-negative result
Sjogren-like syndrome	Serum RF levels too low for detection (sequestered in joint fluid and/or synovium)
Bacterial endocarditis	
Dirofilariasis	Frozen blood sample
Septic arthritis	Excessive immune complex formation
Miscellaneous arthropathies (e.g., osteoarthritis)	Fluctuation of titer levels may occur in normal and affected animals.
Chronic viral infections	Predominance of IgG or IgA

CLINICAL PERSPECTIVE

• Consider SLE if polyarthritis is accompanied by disease involving other tissues (e.g., skin lesions, hemolytic anemia, glomerular disease).
• A positive RF test should not be considered a definitive diagnosis of RA unless supported by other evidence of the disease. A definitive diagnosis depends on demonstrating at least 4 of 12 criteria established by the American Rheumatoid Arthritis Association, 1 of which is abnormal levels of serum RF (see the Internet Resources section).
• A negative result in a dog with clinicopathologic, radiographic, and/or histologic evidence compatible with RA may warrant repeat testing in case of a false-negative result.

MISCELLANEOUS

ANCILLARY TESTS
• Antinuclear antibody test
• Joint radiography

• Lupus erythematosus (LE) cell test
• Synovial fluid analysis

SYNONYMS
RF test

SEE ALSO
Blackwell's Five-Minute Veterinary Consult: Canine and Feline Topics
• Lupus Erythematosus, Systemic (SLE)
• Polyarthritis, Erosive, Immune-Mediated
• Polyarthritis, Nonerosive, Immune-Mediated
• Sjögren-like Syndrome

Related Topics in This Book
• Antinuclear Antibody
• Arthrocentesis with Synovial Fluid Analysis
• Lupus Erythematosus Cell Preparation

ABBREVIATIONS
• RA = rheumatoid arthritis
• RF = rheumatoid factor
• SLE = systemic lupus erythematosus

Suggested Reading
Bennett D. Immune-mediated and infective arthritis. In: Ettinger SJ, Feldman EC, eds. *Textbook of Veterinary Internal Medicine*, 6th ed. Philadelphia: WB Saunders, 2004: 1958–1965.
Werner LL, Turnwald GH, Willard MD. Immunologic and plasma protein disorders. In: Willard MD, Tvedten H, eds. *Small Animal Clinical Diagnosis by Laboratory Methods*, 4th ed. Philadelphia: WB Saunders, 2004: 301–303.

INTERNET RESOURCES
Arthritis Foundation, Disease Center: Rheumatoid arthritis, http://www.arthritis.org/conditions/DiseaseCenter/RA/default.asp.

AUTHOR NAME
Maria Vandis

RHINOSCOPY

BASICS

TYPE OF PROCEDURE
Endoscopic

PROCEDURE EXPLANATION AND RELATED PHYSIOLOGY
In this procedure, fiberoptics within rigid or flexible endoscopes or both are used to visualize structures of the nasal cavity, including the upper, middle, and ventral nasal meati. The nasopharynx is also viewed. Examination of the sinuses is generally not possible. Rhinoscopy is an important aid when collecting samples and performing certain therapeutic procedures within the nasal cavity.

INDICATIONS
- Rhinoscopy is indicated only when results of a systemic evaluation indicate that nasal disease is a primary problem. If the nasal disease appears to be secondary to an underlying disorder, rhinoscopy should be delayed until the primary problem is identified.
- Chronic nasal discharge (serous, serosanguinous, mucoid, or mucopurulent) that is unresponsive to conservative therapy and not diagnosed with preliminary diagnostics (CBC, chemistry panel, blood pressure, coagulation panel, CT or skull radiography, dental exam, with or without dental radiographs, and with or without submandibular lymph node aspirate)
- Epistaxsis
- Stertor
- Sneezing that is unresponsive to conservative therapy
- If nasal disease is suspected, these concurrent signs would also be indications for rhinoscopy:
  - Breathing difficulty
  - Facial swelling
  - Pawing or rubbing of the face and nose
  - Head shyness or pain when the nose is palpated
  - Depigmentation or ulceration of the nasal mucosa
  - Coughing or gagging

CONTRAINDICATIONS
- Most of the time, rhinoscopy is performed in patients with chronic problems; rarely are there acute indications. Hence, this procedure should be performed only in stable individuals that have had appropriate diagnostics performed previously.
- Caution must be used in patients that have had their cribiform plate destroyed.

POTENTIAL COMPLICATIONS
- Epistaxis is expected for 1–2 days after the procedure.
- Noisy breathing is frequent for 1–2 days after the procedure and may continue, depending on the disease process present.
- Occasionally, patients' nasal discharge may worsen.
- Aspiration of nasal discharge or irrigation fluid
- Disorientation and seizures if the cribiform plate is traversed

CLIENT EDUCATION
- Patients must be fasted a minimum of 12 h prior to the procedure.
- General anesthesia is required and has certain inherent risks.
- Patients typically are required to stay overnight to restrict activity and provide pain management, if necessary.
- Epistaxis is expected after the procedure. The client should be prepared to maintain the pet in an area that is easily cleaned.
- Rhinoscopy is a diagnostic tool and should not be expected to correct the underlying disorder.
- Given the anatomy of the nasal cavity, the entire cavity cannot be examined and, in some cases, a second rhinoscopy may be needed.

- Definitive diagnosis is not always possible with rhinoscopy, although a successful diagnosis has been reported in 90% of patients that have received a complete evaluation.
- Despite a definitive diagnosis, some conditions respond poorly to treatments, and some patients are no better or may even be worse after the diagnostics and treatments.

BODY SYSTEMS ASSESSED
Respiratory

PROCEDURE

PATIENT PREPARATION
Preprocedure Medication or Preparation
- Patients should be fasted for 12 h prior to this procedure.
- A preanesthetic serum biochemical panel and 3-view chest radiographs should be evaluated particularly in geriatric patients.
- A coagulation profile and evaluation of buccal mucosal bleeding time and blood pressure are recommended in animals with epistaxis.
- A full oral exam is required.
- The eyes should be examined to determine whether they can be retropulsed.
- Aural exams are recommended, particularly in young cats.
- Dental radiographs are recommended if unilateral disease is present.
- Ideally, a CT or magnetic resonance imaging of the nasal cavity is performed, although high-quality skull radiographs may be sufficient.
- Aspiration of the draining mandibular lymph nodes should be performed if neoplasia is a differential diagnosis or if the nodes are palpably enlarged.
- Opioids can be used during the premedication.
- The use of periprocedural antibiotics is not recommended.

Anesthesia or Sedation
General anesthesia is necessary for an adequate examination.

Patient Positioning
- Sternal recumbency
- The patient's head should be positioned with the tip of the nose angled slightly downward to allow for drainage of fluids and blood out of the nasal cavity through the nares rather than through the choana into the nasopharynx.

Patient Monitoring
Proper anesthetic monitoring should be used at all times.

Equipment or Supplies
- Equipment varies depending on the patient.
- A telescope, typically with 30° tip angle
- Sheaths are available with a port that enables the infusion of fluid into the nasal cavity. The use of a sheath will limit the length of scope that can be introduced into the nasal cavity. A sheath also increases the diameter that must be introduced into the nares, making it difficult to use in small dogs and cats.
- A light source
- A sterile fluid source (e.g., a 500-mL bag of 0.9% sodium chloride)
- A drainage bucket
- A flexible bronchoscope (5-mm outer diameter) to perform a retroflexion into the nasal cavity
- A sterile lubricant
- 4 × 4-inch gauze sponges
- Biopsy instrumentation
- A camera is optional but necessary for projection and recording of images.

- Foreign-object retrieval devices are optional.
- The use of phenylephrine (e.g., Neo-Synephrine) is optional but may help to control bleeding.
- Biopsy instrumentation

TECHNIQUE

- Consistent technique is important to ensure that an adequate endoscopic exam is performed in all patients. Techniques vary and are unique to each endoscopist.
- At the beginning of the procedure, the oral cavity should be examined thoroughly while the patient is under general anesthesia. All teeth and periodontal spaces should be inspected. The hard and soft palates should be visualized and palpated. The tonsils and the oropharynx should also be examined. In cats, virus-isolation swabs of the tonsillar crypts should be collected at this time.
- Deep nasal bacterial and fungal cultures can be obtained prior to rhinoscopy to help prevent sample contamination and dilution during the procedure. Sterile swabs can be passed into the nasal cavity after the external nares have been swabbed with povidone iodine. Although samples can be collected for cytologic analysis and culture via a saline nasal wash using 5 French sterile catheters, this technique is not recommended prior to examining the nasal cavity with the rhinoscope, because the fluid that remains can affect visualization.
- A flexible endoscope is introduced through the mouth and retroflexed over the soft palate so that the nasopharynx can be visualized. The exam of the nasopharynx is not complete until both choanae are visualized.
- If a flexible endoscope is not available, the nasopharynx can be examined with the aid of a light source, spay hook, and dental mirror, although visualization by this means is generally less than adequate.
- During this part of the procedure, red rubber latex urinary catheters (5 French for cats and small dogs; 8 French for breed dogs that are medium sized or large) can be introduced retrogradely through the nasal cavity and into the nasopharynx. Using the flexible endoscope as a guide, these catheters can be used to move mucus deposits and ensure that both nasal passageways are patent. However, this may alter the appearance of the nasal cavities when the rigid endoscope is introduced.
- After the nasopharyngeal exam is complete, the endoscope is removed from the mouth.
- The pharynx is then packed with 4 × 4-inch gauze sponges that have been moistened with saline to help prevent the aspiration of fluids that may enter the pharynx during the rhinoscopy. Gauze sponges must be counted to ensure that they are all removed at the end of the procedure.
- When examining the nasal cavities, the less affected side is typically examined first.
- Initially, the rigid telescope without a sheath is introduced into the nasal cavity. Care must be taken to avoid large movements because even normal nasal mucosa will bleed when traumatized. Diseased tissue will bleed even with light touch. To prevent inadvertent movements, your dominant hand holds the eyepiece end of the telescope and your nondominant hand, while resting on the animal's muzzle to ensure steadiness, guides the part of the telescope entering the nasal cavity.
- Each of the nasal meati is examined individually, starting with the ventral nasal meatus and then progressing to the middle and dorsal meati. Starting ventrally helps ensure visualization of the upper meati even if bleeding should occur.
- The exam is started in the rostral-most aspect of the nasal cavity and is finished when the caudal-most aspect of the cavity is reached or

when tissue occludes your view. After examining 1 meatus, the scope should then be completely removed from the nasal passages and then introduced into the next meatus.
- The scope can be passed the entire length of the ventral meatus, into the nasopharynx, provided there is not a large degree of inflammation or other obstruction.
- The endoscope should be advanced only if the operator is certain that the tip is within the lumen of the nasal cavity. Blind advancement is not advised.
- Examination can be nearly impossible if the nasal airways are occluded with nasal discharge or blood. Dry suction of material through a red rubber catheter or vigorous flushing with saline until the discharge appears clear followed by suction can be used to improve visualization.
- In most cases, the best visualization if bleeding and discharge obscure vision is with the use of a telescope sheath and constant saline irrigation. A fluid line can be used to run saline directly through the sheath during the exam. Pressure on the fluid bag is rarely necessary. By performing 2 exams, 1 in the dry nasal cavity and 1 during irrigation, an experienced operator can frequently obtain the most information within the shortest time.
- After the nasal cavity is examined, biopsy samples are obtained. If specific lesions are found, the endoscope can be used to guide the biopsy instrument to the abnormal area by sliding the forceps alongside the telescope. If the disease is diffuse, blind biopsy samples can be obtained. Blind biopsy samples should be taken from all representative areas of the nasal cavity. The medial cantus of the eye can be used as a guide to dictate the furthest distance the biopsy instrument can be passed safely. Minimally, biopsy samples should be obtained from the rostral, middle, and caudal aspects of the nose in all 3 meati on both sides of the nasal cavity. Adequate biopsies will cause bleeding.
- After obtaining all necessary samples, the gauze sponges should be removed from the caudal pharynx.
- The pharynx should be visually examined for fluid and discharge and suctioned, if necessary, before anesthesia is discontinued.

SAMPLE HANDLING

- Tissue for culture, if necessary, should be obtained at the beginning of the procedure.
- Impression smears can be made from biopsied tissue before it is placed in fixative.

APPROPRIATE AFTERCARE

Postprocedure Patient Monitoring

- Slowly waking or carrying the patient from anesthesia may be helpful to prevent the dislodging of clots from the nasal cavity. Bleeding is expected.
- To reduce the risk of aspiration, the patient should be swallowing at the time of extubation.

Nursing Care

Patients can be expected to sneeze blood clots and bleed for at least 12 h after the procedure. Most patients are hospitalized.

Dietary Modification

None

Medication Requirements

- If appropriate, anxious animals may be administered acepromazine to keep them calm in the first 12 h after the procedure.
- A second dose of pain medication is frequently administered prior to extubation and can be continued for the 12 h after the procedure, as necessary.

Restrictions on Activity
- Cage rest is recommended for the first 12 h after the procedure.
- Excessive activity is discouraged for an additional 24 h.

Anticipated Recovery Time
Most patients have recovered from the procedure within 2 days, although some will continue to have a small amount of epistaxis associated with sneezing.

INTERPRETATION

NORMAL FINDINGS OR RANGE
- The mucosa of the nasopharynx is homogeneously pink and should generally be smooth, with small changes in contour. In the caudal nasal cavity, along the midline, it is not unusual to note a slight roughened appearance to the mucosa. However, the mucosal integrity should be intact.
- No discharge should be visualized originating from the choanae.
- The nasal mucosa should be smooth and pink to red. Occasionally, the mucosa may appear pale, particularly if the rhinoscopy is performed with irrigation or if a topical vasoconstrictor is used.
- Blood vessels should be easily visualized traversing randomly beneath the mucosa.
- Turbinates appear organized, although their contours can be unpredictable, provided that the mucosa is intact, smooth, and gently curved. Normal turbinates can even have nodules or areas of thickening that distort their appearance.

ABNORMAL VALUES
- In an unexamined nasal cavity, the presence of blood or exudate is abnormal.
- Hyperemic, inflamed, friable mucosa is typical of any inflammatory process within the nasal cavity.
- Lack of turbinates, particularly if fungal mats are seen, may be consistent with an *Aspergillus* sp. infection. A large amount of mucopurulent discharge is typically present and not uncommonly can be found in a nasal cavity unaffected by the fungus. Early disease may be missed because the distortion of the turbinates may be overlooked. The ethmoid turbinates will appear to have more space surrounding them because they are degraded, and other turbinates will lose their rigidity as cartilage is lost. Depigmentation of the alar fold is occasionally seen, as well.
- Neoplasia typically appears as a space-occupying mass that distorts the turbinates. The neoplastic tissue is frequently obscured by exudates, hematomas, and necrotic or inflammatory tissue. The appearance of the tumor itself is highly variable.
- The nasal planum should be evaluated in both normal and abnormal nasal cavities for distortion, particularly if a tumor is suspected in the abnormal cavity.
- Polypoid masses may be consistent with *Rhinosporidium* sp. in dogs and nasopharyngeal polyps in cats.
- Foreign objects may be found within the nasal cavity or nasopharynx. Objects can be inhaled, or they can enter the nasal cavity through the nasopharynx when an animal vomits. These objects are frequently obscured from view by copious amounts of mucopurulent discharge. Organic debris, such as grass blades, can also degrade, making identification difficult
- Foreign objects may need to be removed with forceps rostrally through the nares, or they may need to be pushed caudally through the choana and into the nasopharynx for removal. Inspection for multiple foreign objects should be performed. Vigorous irrigation may be necessary to ensure that the nasal cavity is clear,

- Unilateral discharge that is identified ventrally in the nasal cavity is suspicious for dental disease. Frequently, the exudate associated with a tooth-root abscess is inspissated and can be removed in chunks. Occasionally, with dental disease, irrigation fluid from the nasal cavity can be noted running into the mouth along the affected tooth.
- In animals with rhinitis, the turbinates appear inflamed and thickened. Bacterial, allergic, and idiopathic rhinitis can all look similar. Histopathologic evaluation, as well as other ancillary diagnostics, are necessary in these cases to establish a diagnosis.
- Feline herpesvirus can cause turbinate erosion.

CRITICAL VALUES
None

INTERFERING FACTORS
Drugs That May Alter Results of the Procedure
Topical vasoconstrictors (e.g., phenylephrine or diluted epinephrine)

Conditions That May Interfere with Performing the Procedure
- Anatomic restrictions and the character of the nasal discharge are the 2 most common limiting factors.
- Iatrogenic hemorrhage

Procedure Techniques or Handling That May Alter Results
- Failure to obtain deep nasal bacterial and fungal cultures prior to rhinoscopy may cause sample contamination.
- Iatrogenic hemorrhage will obscure visualization.

Influence of Signalment on Performing and Interpreting the Procedure
Species
None

Breed
Patient size and anatomic differences can be limiting factors.

Age
None

Gender
None

Pregnancy
None

CLINICAL PERSPECTIVE
Insufficient biopsy samples can be a critical mistake when attempting to make a histologic diagnosis of a nasal problem. Many disease processes can be associated with an inflammatory process, and hence the appropriate diagnosis can be missed if biopsy samples are not appropriately representative.

MISCELLANEOUS

ANCILLARY TESTS
- Imaging of the nasal cavities should precede rhinoscopy in most cases.
- Depending on the lesion, prior to rhinoscopy, high-quality skull radiographs may provide sufficient information.
- CT and magnetic resonance imaging are superior imaging modalities of the nasal cavity. These images may be helpful in prioritizing a list of differential diagnoses, as well as in pinpointing areas of disease prior to rhinoscopy.
- Dental films provide excellent resolution when dental disease is a differential diagnosis for a unilateral nasal discharge.
- Cultures (bacterial and fungal) may be indicated in certain cases.
- Fungal serology may be warranted in certain cases.
- Virus isolation is recommended in cats with suspected viral rhinitis.

SYNONYMS
None

SEE ALSO
Blackwell's Five-Minute Veterinary Consult: Canine and Feline Topics
- Adenocarcinoma, Nasal
- Aspergillosis
- Epistaxis
- Nasal and Nasopharyngeal Polyps
- Nasal Discharge
- Sneezing, Reverse Sneezing, Gagging

Related Topics in This Book
General Principles of Endoscopy

ABBREVIATIONS
CT = computed tomography

Suggested Reading
Noone K. Rhinoscopy, pharyngoscopy, and laryngoscopy. *Vet Clin North Am Small Anim Pract* 2001; 31: 671–689.

INTERNET RESOURCES
None

AUTHOR NAME
Michael W. Wood

ROCKY MOUNTAIN SPOTTED FEVER

 BASICS

TYPE OF SPECIMEN
Blood
Tissue

TEST EXPLANATION AND RELATED PHYSIOLOGY
Rocky Mountain spotted fever (RMSF), a tickborne disease caused by the organism *Rickettsia rickettsii*, is an acute disease. Infected patients typically either succumb to the disease or recover within 2–4 weeks. Chronic RMSF has not been documented; therefore, testing patients with chronic signs of illness is not appropriate and can result in a misleading test interpretation.

• *IFA*: Detection of specific (hopefully) antibodies against the organism. Serum is the typical sample tested for antibodies, but they can also be detected in other biologic samples such as CSF. Many dogs with substantial exposure to ticks develop antibodies against avirulent spotted fever group rickettsiae that cross-react with *R. rickettsii*. Therefore, many dogs without RMSF will have detectable antibodies, and seroconversion between acute and convalescent samples is of utmost importance in achieving an accurate diagnosis.

• *PCR*: Amplification of a specific piece of organism DNA. *Rickettsia rickettsii* organisms live in vascular endothelial cells, and the testing of blood samples relies on infected endothelial cells entering the circulation. Alternatively, the organism detection can be attempted by using tissue samples. Obtain samples *before* treatment, because treatment may reduce the number of organisms and result in false-negative test results.

• *Direct IFA (dIFA)* antibody testing can be performed on biopsy samples of affected tissues (typically skin).

INDICATIONS
• Arthralgia
• Fever
• Hypoalbuminemia
• Lymphadenopathy
• Meningoencephalitis
• Myalgia
• Petechia
• Neurologic signs (Vestibular disease appears most common.)
• Thrombocytopenia
• Uveitis

CONTRAINDICATIONS
Patients with chronic illness

POTENTIAL COMPLICATIONS
None

CLIENT EDUCATION
• Infection occurs throughout the United States (except Maine), with the highest incidence in the eastern states.
• Owners of a dog with RMSF are at risk if exposed to the same infective tick population.
• Dogs with substantial tick exposure may have a positive serology test but not have RMSF.

BODY SYSTEMS ASSESSED
• Hemic, lymphatic, and immune
• Musculoskeletal
• Nervous
• Ophthalmic
• Renal and urologic

 SAMPLE

COLLECTION
• 2 mL of venous blood for PCR or IFA
• 0.5 mL of CSF for IFA or PCR
• Small (punch) biopsy of a lesion (petechia or necrosis) for dIFA or PCR

HANDLING
• IFA: Place in a red-top tube and ship overnight on ice.
• PCR: Collect blood into a purple-top tube and ship overnight on ice.
• Biopsy for PCR and dIFA: Place into a sterile container.
  • Ideally freeze the sample immediately, but methods are available that use formalin-fixed tissues.
  • Ship unfixed tissue overnight on dry ice.

STORAGE
• IFA: refrigerator or freezer
• PCR: refrigerator or freezer
• dIFA: freezer

STABILITY
• IFA
  • Refrigerated (2°–8°C): days
  • Frozen (−20° to −80°C): months to years
• PCR
  • Refrigerated (2°–8°C): days to weeks
  • Frozen (−20° to −80°C): months to years
• dIFA: Tissue is stable for several days at −20° to −80°C.

PROTOCOL
None

 INTERPRETATION

NORMAL FINDINGS OR RANGE
• IFA: either no detectable antibodies against *R. rickettsii* or no rising titer (≥4-fold increase) between acute and convalescent samples
• PCR: no detectable *R. rickettsii* DNA
• dIFA: no detection of *R. rickettsii* organisms

ABNORMAL VALUES
• IFA: A rising titer (≥4-fold increase) between the acute and convalescent samples indicates recent exposure and is consistent with infection. A single high titer (≥1:1,024) may be detected late in the disease course (i.e., >10 days after the onset of illness). A convalescent sample is still indicated as titers often continue to rise.
• PCR: The presence of *R. rickettsii* DNA indicates infection.
• dIFA: The presence of *R. rickettsii* organisms indicates infection.

CRITICAL VALUES
None

INTERFERING FACTORS
Drugs That May Alter Results or Interpretation
Drugs That Interfere with Test Methodology
None

Drugs That Alter Physiology
• PCR and dIFA: The administration of antirickettsial antibiotics (i.e., doxycycline) may result in false-negative results.
• IFA: The administration of antirickettsial antibiotics does not reduce antibody responses significantly, and seroconversion can still be detected.

Disorders That May Alter Results
None

Collection Techniques or Handling That May Alter Results
None

Influence of Signalment
Species
Dogs only

Breed
None

Age
IFA: Infected puppies may not have detectable antibodies.

Gender
None

Pregnancy
None

LIMITATIONS OF THE TEST
Negative tests do not rule out infection:
• Acute antibody titers may be negative because it may take a patient up to 3 weeks to develop antibodies.
• dIFA and PCR can be negative if the sample does not include infected vascular endothelial cells.

Sensitivity, Specificity, and Positive and Negative Predictive Values
• Sensitivity, specificity, and predictive values are unknown.
• Cross-reactive antibodies, to nonpathogenic spotted fever group rickettsiae, limit the specificity of antibody testing, but seroconversion is believed to be highly sensitive and specific for RMSF.
• In at least 1 experimental infection study (Breitschwerdt et al. 1999), PCR was superior to tissue culture for the detection of organisms after treatment, because of the persistence of nonviable DNA.

Valid If Run in a Human Lab?
Yes—but tests for antigen only (PCR or dIFA); canine antibody tests are invalid.

CLINICAL PERSPECTIVE
• IFA remains the method most commonly used to diagnose RMSF. Acute and convalescent titers and response to treatment are essential for confirmation.
• A similar constellation of clinical signs can be seen with Lyme disease, *Ehrlichia canis*, *Anaplasma phagocytophilum*, and systemic lupus erythematosus.

MISCELLANEOUS

ANCILLARY TESTS
• CBC including platelet count, serum biochemical profile, and urinalysis
• Arthrocentesis and/or collection of CSF, depending on the clinical signs

SYNONYMS
None

SEE ALSO
Blackwell's Five-Minute Veterinary Consult: Canine and Feline Topics
• Ehrlichiosis
• Lyme Disease
• Rocky Mountain Spotted Fever
Related Topics in This Book
• Antinuclear Antibody
• *Ehrlichial Anaplasma*
• Lyme Disease Serology

ABBREVIATIONS
• CSF = cerebrospinal fluid
• dIFA = direct immunofluorescence assay
• RMSF = Rocky Mountain spotted fever

Suggested Reading
Breitschwerdt EB, Papich MG, Hegarty BC, *et al.* Efficacy of doxycycline, azithromycin, or trovafloxacin for treatment of experimental Rocky Mountain spotted fever in dogs. *Antimicrob Agents Chemother* 1999; 43: 813–821.
Gasser AM, Birkenheuer AJ, Breitschwerdt EB. Canine Rocky Mountain spotted fever: A retrospective study of 30 cases. *J Am Anim Hosp Assoc* 2001; 37: 41–48.

INTERNET RESOURCES
None

AUTHOR NAME
Adam J. Birkenheuer

SCHIRMER TEAR TEST

BASICS

TYPE OF PROCEDURE
Function test

PROCEDURE EXPLANATION AND RELATED PHYSIOLOGY
The preocular tear film that bathes the surface of the cornea is essential in maintaining normal corneal health. The tear film serves many functions in addition to lubrication. It supplies oxygen to the cornea and contains many essential cytokines and growth factors important to the ocular surface. The tear film is essentially 3 layers. The aqueous middle layer of tears is the largest and is bordered by outer lipid and inner mucin layers. The aqueous layer is produced predominantly by the lacrimal gland in dogs and cats, with some contribution from the nictitans gland. Both quantitative and qualitative tear-film abnormalities occur. Qualitative tear-film abnormalities are more difficult to diagnose and are evaluated by the appearance of the corneal surface and tear-film break-up time. Quantitative tear-film abnormalities of the aqueous tear-film layer are the most common abnormality in small animals.

The Schirmer tear test (STT) measures the aqueous portion of the tear film. The standard STT measures tear-strip wetting over 1 min, which is composed of both the tears already present in the lacrimal lake together with those produced during the test period. The STT I, the most commonly used test in veterinary medicine, is performed in the absence of topical anesthesia and is a measure of both basal and reflex tearing. Reflex tearing occurs in response to any topical irritant, including the STT strip, and requires the ophthalmic branch of cranial nerve 5 (corneal sensation) as the afferent arm and the parasympathetic fibers in cranial nerve 7 as the efferent arm. The STT II, performed following the application of topical anesthesia, is a measure of basal tear secretion only, but is rarely used in veterinary medicine. The normal and abnormal ranges reported in this chapter are all in reference to the STT I.

The STT is essential in the diagnosis of dry eye or keratoconjunctivitis sicca (KCS) and should be performed on every dog with an ocular complaint. Clinical signs of KCS include mucoid to mucopurulent discharge, conjunctival hyperemia, superficial corneal vascularization, corneal pigmentation, and corneal ulceration. The corneal pigmentation is classically dorsal and central but progresses with severity and chronicity to involve the entire corneal surface and therefore interferes with vision. The STT is not routinely used in cats because quantitative abnormalities of the tear film in cats are much less common.

INDICATIONS
• Assessment of normal aqueous tear production
• Ocular discharge (especially mucoid)
• Ocular redness
• Ocular pain (e.g., squinting, blepharospasm)
• Corneal ulceration (especially nonhealing or recurrent corneal ulceration)
• Corneal pigmentation
• Corneal vascularization (superficial)
• Dull corneal appearance
• Epiphora

CONTRAINDICATIONS
Do not perform this test when a deep corneal ulcer is present because excessive manipulation of the eye could rupture the globe.

POTENTIAL COMPLICATIONS
• Corneal irritation
• Corneal trauma
• Corneal ulceration (unlikely)

CLIENT EDUCATION
None

BODY SYSTEMS ASSESSED
Ophthalmic

PROCEDURE

PATIENT PREPARATION
Preprocedure Medication or Preparation
• None
• This test should be performed before any drops, medications, or fluorescein stains are placed in the eye.
• The STT I specifically needs to precede the application of topical anesthesia.

Anesthesia or Sedation
Usually not required and can interfere with results

Patient Positioning
Sternal or sitting is easiest.

Patient Monitoring
None

Equipment or Supplies
• Commercial STT strips
• A watch or clock with a second hand

TECHNIQUE
• Use standardized sterile strips of filter paper.
• The round end of the test paper is bent at the notch while still in the envelope.
• Do not touch the notched end of the strip. Deposition of cutaneous oils and contaminants can interfere with strip absorbency.
• The notched end of the strip is then positioned in the lower conjunctival cul-de-sac at the junction of the lateral and middle thirds of the lower eyelid.
• Some animals will close their eyes or blink excessively. Restrain the animal from blinking by holding the eyelids closed to prevent dislodgement of the paper strip.
• Remove the paper strip at 60 s.
• The paper strip is measured on a millimeter scale on the envelope or on a scale embedded in the strip itself.
• Some strips are impregnated with blue dye, and either the leading edge of the dye or the leading edge of wetting is recorded.
• If convenient, both eyes may be tested at the same time.
• The results should be read immediately because the fluid or dye will continue to spread through the tear strip over time.

SAMPLE HANDLING
N/A

APPROPRIATE AFTERCARE
Postprocedure Patient Monitoring
None

Nursing Care
None

Dietary Modification
None

Medication Requirements
None

Restrictions on Activity
None

Anticipated Recovery Time
Immediate

INTERPRETATION

NORMAL FINDINGS OR RANGE
- For dogs, values of >15 mm/min are considered normal.
- The approximate average value reported for the STT I in dogs and cats is 18–22 mm of wetting/min.
- The approximate average value reported for the STT II in dogs and cats is 12 +/– 6 mm of wetting/min.

ABNORMAL VALUES
- For dogs, values of 10–15 mm/min are questionable. Values of <10 mm/min are abnormally low and suggest KCS.
- STT results in cats are more difficult to interpret because a value of zero may be normal in a stressed cat.
- In either species, a low STT result in combination with clinical signs in the abnormal eye is considered significant.

CRITICAL VALUES
N/A

INTERFERING FACTORS
Drugs That May Alter Results of the Procedure
- Any topical medication applied immediately prior to the test
- The administration of etodolac or sulfonamides can cause dry eye.
- If an animal is being treated concurrently with topical atropine or topical tropicamide, the STT results can be abnormally low as long as treatment continues.
- Drugs that can result in transient lower STT values when administered IM, SC, or IV include systemic atropine, general anesthetics, and sedatives (medetomidine, butorphanol, medetomidine-butorphanol, acepromazine-oxymorphone, diazepam-butorphanol, or xylazine-butorphanol).

Conditions That May Interfere with Performing the Procedure
- An aggressive animal that requires sedation prior to being handled
- Previous removal of the nictitans (third eyelid) gland

Procedure Techniques or Handling That May Alter Results
Excessive manipulation of the eyelids, administration of topical anesthesia, and exposure to other topical and systemic drugs (such as tranquilizers and atropine) should be avoided before the test.

Influence of Signalment on Performing and Interpreting the Procedure
Species
When a cat is stressed, its STT result can be zero.

Breed
Lower STT I values have been reported for Shetland sheepdogs.

Age
STT results may decrease slightly with age. These decreases are usually clinically insignificant.

Gender
None

Pregnancy
None

CLINICAL PERSPECTIVE
- The STT should be performed in every dog with ocular signs.
- A patient with a low STT result without concurrent clinical signs should have the test repeated and therapy initiated, if indicated.
- KCS is an extremely rare condition in cats, and the STT is not routinely performed. A low STT result in combination with clinical signs may be clinically important.

- The STT is not a linear test. A value of 5 mm in 30 s does not mean it will be 10 mm in 60 s. The test strip must be applied for the entire 60 s.
- Topical anesthesia blocks the reflex tearing elicited by the strips and can significantly affect the results for the STT I.
- Increased tear production because of corneal irritation during the test is of little significance in dogs and cats.
- An STT value of ≥15 mm in 60 s does not definitely rule out KCS. Animals can still have clinical dry eye because of other factors, which include increased evaporation of tears secondary to macropalpebral fissure or lagophthalmos. Clinical signs of dry eye in these cases may still improve with therapy.

MISCELLANEOUS

ANCILLARY TESTS
- STT II
- Phenol red thread test
- Tear-film break-up time

SYNONYMS
None

SEE ALSO
Blackwell's Five-Minute Veterinary Consult: Canine and Feline Topics
- Keratoconjunctivitis Sicca
- Conjunctivitis—Cats
- Conjunctivitis—Dogs
- Corneal Degeneration and Infiltrations
- Episcleritis
- Keratitis, Nonulcerative
- Keratitis, Ulcerative
- Ophthalmia Neonatorum
- Red Eye

Related Topics in This Book
Fluorescein dye test

ABBREVIATIONS
- KCS = keratoconjunctivitis sicca
- STT = Schirmer tear test
- STT I = Schirmer I tear test
- STT II = Schirmer II tear test

Suggested Reading
Gelatt KN. Ophthalmic examination and diagnostic procedures. In: Gelatt KN, ed. *Veterinary Ophthalmology*, 3rd ed. Philadelphia: Lippincott Williams & Wilkins, 1999: 427–466.
Hamor RE, Roberts SM, Severin GA, Chavkin MJ. Evaluation of results for Schirmer tear tests conducted with and without application of a topical anesthetic in clinically normal dogs of 5 breeds. *Am J Vet Res* 2000; 61: 1422–1425.
Hartley C, Williams DL, Adams VJ. Effect of age, gender, weight, and time of day on tear production in normal dogs. *Vet Ophthalmol* 2006; 9: 53–57.
Martin CL. Anamnesis and the ophthalmic examination. In: Martin CL, ed. *Ophthalmic Disease in Veterinary Medicine*. London: Manson, 2005: 11–38.
Saito A, Kotani T. Estimation of lacrimal level and testing methods on normal beagles. *Vet Ophthalmol* 2001; 4: 7–11.

INTERNET RESOURCES
None

AUTHOR NAME
Tammy Miller Michau

SEMEN ANALYSIS

BASICS

TYPE OF SPECIMEN
Tissue

TEST EXPLANATION AND RELATED PHYSIOLOGY
Semen analysis is an important part of a breeding soundness examination and can be an aid in documenting fertility problems. It can also help provide information regarding genital tract lesions.

The 4 essential components of canine semen evaluations are volume of the ejaculate (especially the second, sperm-rich fraction), percentage of progressive motile sperm, number of sperm per ejaculate, and percentage of morphologic normal sperm. In addition, semen pH, cytology (especially the presence of WBCs), and alkaline phosphatase (ALP) activity can be determined. Results are compared to values for normal ejaculates.

INDICATIONS
- To predict the fertility, based on semen characteristics, of a stud dog
- To diagnose inflammatory or neoplastic disease of the male reproductive tract

CONTRAINDICATIONS
None

POTENTIAL COMPLICATIONS
None

CLIENT EDUCATION
The ultimate proof of the true fertility of a stud dog is the number of pups sired.

BODY SYSTEMS ASSESSED
Reproductive

SAMPLE

COLLECTION
- Collect semen into a clean 50-mL urine cup or 50-mL vial or into a latex collection cone with an attached graduated centrifuge tube.
- For semen cultures, first wash prepuce and tip of the penis with sterile saline. The collection vials should be sterile.
- See the "Semen Collection" chapter for more details on procedure.

HANDLING
- Avoid contamination of genitalia or the collection vessel with disinfectant solution, glove power, or other foreign materials.
- Process the sample as soon as possible after collection.
- Avoid exposing the sample to fast temperature fluctuations and direct sunlight.

STORAGE
- Rapid cooling of dog semen can adversely affect spermatozoa viability (cold shock). See the "Semen Preservation" chapter for information on long-term semen storage.
- Air-dried smears: Store at room temperature, protected from light and humidity.

STABILITY
- Dog sperm seems to be more resistant to temperature fluctuation than is sperm of other domestics species.
- Dog semen does not undergo cold shock if temperatures are kept at >21°C (i.e., room temperature).
- The sample is not stable for long periods at ≥37°C.
- Unstained smears: 3 days
- Stained smears can be stored for years.

PROTOCOL
- Volume and color: Discard the first fraction and record the volume and color of the second and third fractions.
- Analyze the sperm motility immediately:
  - Place a drop of semen on a warmed microscopic slide covered with a warmed coverslip and observe with a 20× or 40× objective. The use of a phase contrast microscope with a stage warmer is optimal but not essential.
  - Highly cellular samples can be diluted with some prostatic fluid or with warm physiologic saline.
  - Visual estimation of sperm motility involves counting 10 sperm/field in 4–5 different fields of the slide. It should include the following:
    - Total sperm motility (percentage of sperm showing any kind of motility)
    - Progressive sperm motility (percentage of sperm moving rapidly and progressively forward in a straight line)
    - Sperm velocity (on a scale of 0–4)
    - For example, a motility value set of "85/80 (4)" would indicate that 85% of sperm were motile and 80% of sperm were progressively motile, exhibiting rapid and linear movement.
- Total sperm count is determined manually by using a hemocytometer and a microscope:
  - Dilute the sample 1:100 with saline or by using a WBC Unopette (20 μL of semen in 2 mL of diluent; Becton Dickinson, Sparks, MD) and charge the hemocytometer chamber with diluted sample.
  - Count all the sperm in the large central square on each side of the hemocytometer grid and calculate the average.
  - This count $\times 10^6$ = sperm/mL of semen (sperm concentration).
  - Total sperm count = sperm concentration × volume (mL) of semen.
- Sperm morphology
  - Make a smear of a sperm-rich fraction, air-dry, and stain with Diff-Quick, immersing the slide in each solution for 5 minutes.
  - Evaluate at least 100 sperm at 1,000× magnification (oil immersion).
- A pH test tape (0.5 increments) should be used to measure seminal plasma pH as soon as possible after collection.
- Cytologic evaluation: Process and evaluate the sperm-rich fraction and the prostatic fluid–rich fraction separately:
  - Prepare a smear of sediment obtained by centrifuging 0.5 mL of each fraction at 120 g for 7 min.
  - Alternatively, prepare the smears by using a cytocentrifuge technique.
  - Air-dry the smears and stain with Diff-Quick.
  - Examine the smears microscopically at 100× and 400× magnification.
- ALP can be measured by using a clinical chemistry assay.
- Semen culture (may be indicated by clinical signs, physical exam findings, and/or gross appearance of semen)
  - Culture is commonly used for aerobic bacteria because anaerobes are not usually found.
  - Submit the semen in a sterile container. Material on a Culturette is acceptable but not optimal.
  - For infertility workup, submit samples in special transport media for anaerobic culture (e.g., Port-A-Cul; Becton Dickinson), *Mycoplasma* culture (Aimes transport material) and *Ureaplasma* culture.

INTERPRETATION

NORMAL FINDINGS OR RANGE
- Volume varies from 2.5 to >80 mL, depending on the amount of prostatic fluid collected.

- The second fraction should be milky white.
- Total sperm per ejaculate varies with the size of the dog:
  - Small dogs: 400×10^6 sperm/ejaculate
  - Large dogs: $\approx 1.4 \times 10^9$ sperm/ejaculate
- Cytologic preparations contain spermatozoa, a few nondegenerate leukocytes, epithelial cells, and small numbers of bacteria.
- ALP is produced in the epididymis and is an excellent marker of ductal blockage. In normal semen samples, ALP is typically >5,000 IU/L.

Parameter	Normal values
First fraction	0.5–5.0 mL, clear
Second fraction (sperm rich)	1–4 mL, opalescent
Third fraction (prostatic)	1–80 mL, clear
Total ejaculate volume	2.5–80.0 mL
Sperm concentration	$4–400 \times 10^6$/mL
Total sperm per ejaculate	$300–2,000 \times 10^6$
Progressive forward motility (% total sperm)	>70%
Normal morphology (% total sperm)	>80%
pH	
Sperm-rich fraction	6.3–6.7
Prostatic fluid	5.5–7.1
Leukocytes/hpf in a centrifuged sample	0–3, first fraction
	0–3, second fraction
	0–6, total ejaculate
ALP	>5,000 IU/L

ABNORMAL VALUES

- Appearance
  - A yellow may represent urine in the ejaculate.
  - A red or brown indicates the presence of fresh or autolyzed RBCs due to either damage of blood vessels of the penis or prostatic disease.
  - A greenish or gray suggests inflammation, especially when tissue flecks are present.
- Sperm numbers
  - Oligozoospermia = decreased number of sperm in the ejaculate; $<200 \times 10^6$ sperm/ejaculate in dog weighing >4.5 kg.
  - Azoospermia = lack of sperm in the ejaculate.
- Sperm motility: <25% of sperm show progressive forward motility (asthenozoospermia). Some sperm may show side-to-side motion without forward progression or may move in small circles.
- Sperm morphology: <50% have normal morphology (teratozoospermia). Morphologic abnormalities include the following:
  - Detached or abnormally attached head
  - Double tail or coiled tail
  - Protoplasmic droplet
  - Abnormal midpiece
- Increased numbers of degenerating polymorphonuclear cells are an indication to culture.
- ALP of <5,000 IU/L suggests that either the epididymis is blocked or a complete ejaculate was not obtained. Male dogs with true

azoospermia, due to causes other than tubular blockage, usually have ALP concentrations of >5,000 IU/L.
- Semen cultures: >10,000 colony-forming units aerobic bacteria per milliliter of semen indicates infection. Lesser numbers of organisms likely reflect normal flora from the penile mucosa and distal urethra.

CRITICAL VALUES
None

INTERFERING FACTORS
Drugs That May Alter Results or Interpretation
Drugs That Interfere with Test Methodology
Disinfectant solution, glove power, or other foreign materials

Drugs That Alter Physiology
- Amphotericin
- Chemotherapeutic drugs
- Cimetidine
- Ketoconazole
- Steroids

Disorders That May Alter Results
- Congenital: fucosidosis or primary ciliary diskinesia
- Acquired: trauma, hematocele, hydrocele, fever, increased scrotal fat, heat stress, prostatitis, brucellosis, orchitis, epididymitis, testicular neoplasia, or testicular degeneration

Collection Techniques or Handling That May Alter Results
- The presence of a bitch in estrus may facilitate the collection of a representative sample.
- Rule out fear or discomfort problems interfering with collection.
- Contact with latex (an artificial vagina) or a lubricant may decrease spermatozoal motility.

Influence of Signalment
Species
Canine

Breed
None

Age
Sperm numbers rise after puberty and decrease with older age or with disease.

Gender
Male

Pregnancy
N/A

LIMITATIONS OF THE TEST
Individual sperm characteristics are poorly correlated with fertility. However, measuring multiple sperm attributes improves the ability to evaluate the fertilizing potential of dog sperm.

Sensitivity, Specificity, and Positive and Negative Predictive Values
N/A

Valid If Run in a Human Lab?
Not unless the lab is familiar with specifics about canine semen.

SEMEN ANALYSIS

Causes of Abnormal Results

Parameter	High values	Low values
Ejaculate volume	NS[a]	<1 mL Volume alone is not correlated with fertility.
Sperm count	NS	Fever Increased scrotal fat Heat stress Hydrocele Hematocele Transiently low with apprehension or prostatic pain
Sperm motility	NS	Primary ciliary diskinesia
Abnormal sperm morphology	Fever Infection Testicular trauma	NS
WBC	Brucellosis Epididymitis Orchitis Prostatitis	NS
ALP	NS	Blocked epididymis Collection of incomplete ejaculate

[a] NS, not significant.

CLINICAL PERSPECTIVE

• Considering the limited number of estrous cycles during a bitch's reproductive life, it is important to evaluate semen quality before using it to breed bitches artificially. Freezing semen of lower quality may result in very low postthaw sperm fertility.
• Evaluate findings in the light of medical history, clinical signs, and other laboratory data.
• The pH measured immediately after collection could be a useful parameter for antibiotic selection in a dog with infection.
• Morphologic abnormalities in the sperm midpiece or its attachment are most likely to be associated with infertility. With other abnormalities, semen can be used immediately, but cryopreservation may be unsuccessful.
• Sperm counts on ejaculates taken on different days under optimal conditions are necessary to confirm a low sperm count.
• *Mycoplasma* should be considered normal flora. However, a large number may cause problems, and mycoplasma has been suggested as a cause of canine infertility.

• Determine ALP concentrations if the sample is azoospermic to look for ductal blockage. Repeat the semen collection with the aid of a teaser bitch.

MISCELLANEOUS

ANCILLARY TESTS
• Semen culture for aerobic and anaerobic bacteria, mycoplasma, and ureaplasma
• Brucellosis

SYNONYMS
None

SEE ALSO
Blackwell's Five-Minute Veterinary Consult: Canine and Feline Topics
Infertility, Male—Dogs
Related Topics in This Book
• Bacterial Culture and Sensitivity
• Brucellosis Serology
• Semen Collection
• Semen Preservation

ABBREVIATIONS
ALP = alkaline phosphatase
HPF = high-powered field

Suggested Reading
Branam JE, Keen CL, Ling GV, Franti CE. Selected physical and chemical characteristics of prostatic fluid collected by ejaculation from healthy dogs and from dogs with bacterial prostatitis. *Am J Vet Res* 1984; 45: 825–829.
Johnston SD. Performing a complete canine semen evaluation in a small animal hospital. *Vet Clin North Am Small Anim Pract* 1991; 21: 545–551.
Johnston SD, Root Kustritz MV, Olson PNS. *Canine and Feline Theriogenology*. Philadelphia: WB Saunders 2001: 287–306.

INTERNET RESOURCES
Gradil CM, Yeager A, Concannon PW. Assessment of reproductive problems in the male dog. In: Concannon PW, England G, Verstegen III J, Linde-Forsberg C, eds. Recent Advances in Small Animal Reproduction. Ithaca, NY: International Veterinary Information Service (IVIS); last updated, April 19, 2006; Document no. A1234.0406, http://www.ivis.org/docarchive/A1234.0406.pdf.

AUTHOR NAME
Carlos M. Gradil

BASICS

TYPE OF PROCEDURE
Diagnostic sample collection

PROCEDURE EXPLANATION AND RELATED PHYSIOLOGY
Routine reproductive evaluations of male dogs are often requested by breeders to confirm fertility prior to purchase or sale, to check daily sperm output particularly in older stud dogs, to assess the potential of a stud dog as a provider of semen for chilled-semen or frozen-semen artificial insemination, or to address problems of apparent infertility or testicular abnormalities, or disorders of the prostate (e.g., prostatic infections). Such reproductive evaluations rely on appropriate and successful semen collection and accurate assessment of semen.

INDICATIONS
To predict the fertility of a stud dog by using laboratory and clinical evaluation

CONTRAINDICATIONS
- Edema or hematocele caused by trauma
- The breeding of males that have genetic abnormalities (e.g., cryptorchidism) should be avoided. This test may not be needed in such males.

POTENTIAL COMPLICATIONS
Hair may be drawn with the penis and irritate the penis and prepuce, especially in long-haired breeds. Therefore, the penis should be observed returning into the prepuce after semen collection and before the dog is released. Wait until the penis is flaccid and confirm that the prepuce is not retained behind the bulbus but has returned to the normal position.

CLIENT EDUCATION
- Provide the owner with genetic counseling stressing the importance of not using males that have genetic abnormalities (e.g., front-limb or rear-limb abnormalities, nondescended testicle or testicles) for breeding.

- If an ejaculate appears to be substandard, consider retaining the dog for several hours for a second collection, possibly under improved circumstances (e.g., without the owners present, in a quiet area, or in the presence of a submissive or estrous bitch).
- Consideration should be given to last time semen was collected from the dog, as well as possible recent pairings, breedings, and ejaculations, because these might affect the results of semen collection and evaluation.

BODY SYSTEMS ASSESSED
Reproductive

PROCEDURE

PATIENT PREPARATION
Preprocedure Medication or Preparation
- Allow a dog in a strange environment time to become accustomed to its surroundings.
- If a female is present, allow the dog to interact with her before semen collection.

Anesthesia or Sedation
None. A suitable quiet environment is recommended.

Patient Positioning
Semen from a stud dog, with or without a teaser bitch, should be collected while the dog is standing on a nonslippery surface.

Patient Monitoring
Monitor for signs of pain during pelvic thrusting.

Equipment or Supplies
A latex liner and a 15-mL graduated plastic tube or a 50-mL conical tube.

TECHNIQUE
- One can use clean hands or nonsterile or sterile gloves during semen collection. In either case, ensure that the genitalia and collection vessel are not contaminated with disinfectant solution, glove power, or other foreign materials.

SEMEN COLLECTION

- The presence of a bitch in estrus facilitates a good erection and collection.
- The prepuce should be gently pushed behind the bulbus glandis. The penis should be encircled with the fingers behind the bulbus glandis and slight pressure exerted; some dogs require some manipulation back and forth, but most do not. Failure to obtain an erection and pelvic thrusting should be countered by exertion of addition circumferential pressure by tightening the grip of the thumb and forefinger. Be prepared to allow the dog to step 1 leg over the collector's arm and hand at any time during the procedure.
- The semen is collected into a clean 50-mL urine collection cup or other type of paper cup, a 50-mL vial, or a latex collection cone with an attached graduated centrifuge tube. As an alternative, some people prefer to use a disposable baby-bottle liner. If the 50-mL vial is used, the rim of the vial should be encircled with the index finger and thumb to prevent the vial from cutting the penis. Using a set of stacked papers or Styrofoam cups allows easy switching from one to another to separate the second and third semen fractions. The first clear fraction flushes the urethra and should be discarded. The second cloudy sperm-rich fraction should be collected separately. The third fraction, which is clear, is a product of the prostate and should be evaluated in patients that are suspected to have prostatic disease.

SAMPLE HANDLING
The semen volume, color, and sperm motility and concentration, as well as the seminal plasma pH, cytology, and alkaline phosphatase, should be evaluated (see the "Semen Analysis" chapter).

APPROPRIATE AFTERCARE
Postprocedure Patient Monitoring
Observe the penis returning into the prepuce once collection is completed.

Nursing Care
Walking the dog or applying cold packs to its penis and prepuce will hasten the return of the penis to its normal position.

Dietary Modification
None

Medication Requirements
None

Restrictions on Activity
None

Anticipated Recovery Time
5–10 min

INTERPRETATION

NORMAL FINDINGS OR RANGE
Sperm concentrations: The total number of sperm for a small dog should be 400×10^6. Large dogs should yield an ejaculate with around 1.4×10^9 sperm.

ABNORMAL VALUES
- Less than 200 million sperm per ejaculate in dogs weighing >4.5 kg. *Note*: Sperm counts of ejaculates taken on different days under optimal conditions are necessary to confirm a low sperm count.
- WBCs per high-powered field should be ≤6.
- The pH of the third fraction (i.e., prostatic fluid) should be in the range of 6.3–6.7.
- An alkaline phosphatase activity of <5,000 IU/L in the seminal fluid from a normal intact male dog is indicative of an incomplete ejaculate.

CRITICAL VALUES
- No ejaculate = aspermia
- No sperm in the ejaculate = azoospermia

INTERFERING FACTORS
Drugs That May Alter Results of the Procedure
Steroids

Conditions That May Interfere with Performing the Procedure
- A noisy and busy environment
- Older dogs with age-related diseases or conditions; drugs, infectious diseases, or heat stress

Procedure Techniques or Handling That May Alter Results
The presence of a bitch in estrus. The use of prefrozen cotton sponges impregnated with vulvar secretion of bitches in estrus may facilitate the collection of a representative sample.

Influence of Signalment on Performing and Interpreting the Procedure

Species
Usually performed in dogs

Breed
None

Age
Dogs should be pubertal (i.e., ≥9 months of age).

Gender
Males should have testes that are of normal size and descended.

Pregnancy
N/A

CLINICAL PERSPECTIVE

Lack of breeding success is often multifactorial. Thus, a comprehensive reproductive exam or breeding soundness evaluation (BSE) will include examination of the genitalia, testis measurement, palpation of the testes and prostate, and semen evaluation, as well as ultrasonography of the testes and prostate in some cases. Testing for sexually transmitted disease, especially brucellosis, is a critical part of a BSE.

MISCELLANEOUS

ANCILLARY TESTS

- Measurement of testosterone and gonadotropins before and after gonadotropin-releasing hormone (GnRH) stimulation
- Ultrasonography of the reproductive tract
- Semen and/or urine cultures
- Serologic testing for canine brucellosis
- Measurement of thyroid hormones

SYNONYMS
Ejaculate

SEE ALSO
Blackwell's Five-Minute Veterinary Consult: Canine and Feline Topics
- Infertility, Male—Dogs
- Prostate Disease in the Breeding Male Dog

Related Topics in This Book
- Semen Analysis
- Semen Preservation

ABBREVIATIONS
BSE = breeding soundness evaluation

Suggested Reading
Johnston SD. Performing a complete canine semen evaluation in a small animal hospital. *Vet Clin North Am Small Anim Pract* 1991; 21: 545–551.
Olar TT, Amann RP, Pickett BW. Relationships among testicular size, daily production and output of spermatozoa, and extragonadal spermatozoal reserves of the dog. *Biol Reprod* 1983; 29: 1114–1120.

INTERNET RESOURCES
Gradil CM, Yeager A, Concannon PW. Assessment of reproductive problems in the male dog. In: Concannon PW, England G, Verstegen III J, Linde-Forsberg C, eds. Recent Advances in Small Animal Reproduction. Ithaca, NY: International Veterinary Information Service (IVIS); last updated, April 19, 2006; Document no. A1234.0406, http://www.ivis.org/advances/Concannon/toc.asp.

AUTHOR NAME
Carlos Gradil

SEMEN PRESERVATION

BASICS

TYPE OF PROCEDURE
Miscellaneous

PROCEDURE EXPLANATION AND RELATED PHYSIOLOGY
• Cryopreservation of dog semen has become a valuable tool to maintain and improve superior bloodlines. However, fertility after insemination with frozen-thawed semen varies because of the following:
  • The technique of semen collection
  • The extender and the final concentration of spermatozoa
  • Semen processing
  • The combination of extender and cooling rate during the freezing procedure
  • The thawing technique and the use of a thawing medium
  • Individual factors, individual ejaculates, or both
• Recent advances in dog semen–freezing techniques have evolved to improve postthaw longevity and motility of frozen-thawed spermatozoa and include the following:
  • Centrifugation
  • The use of membrane-stabilizing factors
  • Decreased glycerol concentrations
  • A high final concentration of spermatozoa
  • Two-step dilution
  • Moderate fast freezing combined with fast thawing
  • Computer-assisted freezing
  • The postthaw addition of a Tris buffer

INDICATIONS
Frozen semen is the best form of assurance that an outstanding dog's potential is preserved. Sperm can be stored in liquid nitrogen (LN_2) for many years without loss in viability.

CONTRAINDICATIONS
None

POTENTIAL COMPLICATIONS
N/A

CLIENT EDUCATION
• Semen is collected in routine fashion.
• Semen viability is reduced during freezing and subsequent thawing. An average dog can provide enough semen for 3 inseminations per ejaculate. Assuming a 50% chance of a litter resulting from 2 inseminations per cycle, then >1 ejaculate is required per litter. As a dog ages, the quality of the sperm cells gradually declines, and a decline in postthaw viability results; thus, the best time to freeze sperm is when he is young and highly fertile.
• Semen is frozen in either straws or pellets. Usually the final number of spermatozoa per straw or pellet is 100–200 million. Depending on the semen quality, typically 2–3 straws are used for each artificial insemination.

BODY SYSTEMS ASSESSED
Reproductive

PROCEDURE

PATIENT PREPARATION
Preprocedure Medication or Preparation
N/A

Anesthesia or Sedation
N/A

Patient Positioning
The semen should be collected while the dog is standing on a nonslippery floor. If a bitch in estrus is present, the dog should be allowed to mount her during the semen collection.

Patient Monitoring
N/A

Equipment or Supplies
• An LN_2 tank
• Uppsala Equex II extenders (which can be made as directed below or ordered from CaniRep HB, Fjällbo, Funbo, SE-755 97 Uppsala, Sweden; phone, +46 18 36 36 25; e-mail, Catharina.Lindeforsberg@gmail.com)
• Equex STM paste (Nova Chemical Sales, Scituate, MA)

Uppsala Equex-II extenders

	Extender 1	Extender 2	Thaw medium
Tris	3.025 g	3.025 g	3.025 g
Citric acid	1.7 g	1.7 g	1.7 g
Fructose	1.25 g	1.25 g	1.25 g
Streptomycin	0.1 g	0.1 g	0.1 g
Distilled water	to 77 mL	to 72 mL	to 100 mL
Benzylpenicillin	0.06 g (in 0.3 mL distilled water)	0.06 g (in 0.3 mL distilled water)	0.06 g (in 0.3 mL distilled water)
Glycerol	3 mL	7 mL	None
Equex	None	1 mL	None
Egg yolk	20 mL	20 mL	None
pH	6.72	6.74	6.76
Osmolarity	865 mOsm	1495 mOsm	324 mOsm

How to Make the Uppsala Equex II Extender
• Take the Equex from the refrigerator and leave it at 37°C for 30 min until it is of a liquid consistency.
• Weigh the amount of streptomycin, Tris, glucose, and citric acid.
• Take out 2 clean 100-mL measuring cylinders. Add distilled water up to 100 mL: for extender 1 = 100 − 23 mL (20 mL is egg yolk and 3 mL is glycerol); total, 77 mL of water. For extender 2 = 100 − 27 mL (20 mL is egg yolk and 7 mL is glycerol); total, 72 mL of water.
• Cover the cylinders carefully with Parafilm. Mix well and place it into solution by carefully tipping the cylinders back and forth, avoiding bubbles.
• Add glycerol: 3 mL in extender 1 and 7 mL in extender 2. A 5- or 10-mL syringe can be used for this. Avoid air bubbles in it and wipe off any glycerol sticking on the outside of the syringe.
• Add 1 mL of Equex to extender 2.
• Add the 20 mL of egg yolk to each extender. Avoid the remaining egg white by carefully rolling the yolk on filter paper.
• Cover the cylinders carefully with Parafilm again and mix well without creating bubbles.
• Check the pH and osmolarity.

TECHNIQUE
• The second sperm-rich fraction of the ejaculate is collected into a clean 50-mL urine-sample cup or other type paper cup, a 50-mL vial, or a latex collection cone with an attached graduated centrifuge tube. (See the "Semen Collection" chapter.)

• After assessing the motility and morphology and counting the total number of spermatozoa, the ejaculate is centrifuged at 700 g for 6 min. The supernatant is removed (and if it still contains spermatozoa it can be centrifuged again), and the pellet is diluted at room temperature in Uppsala Equex II/Extender 1 to a concentration of 400×10^6 spermatozoa/mL and allowed to equilibrate for 60–75 min to 4°C. An equal volume of Uppsala Equex II/Extender 2 is also cooled to 4°C and added slowly dropwise after the equilibration period. The sample is mixed carefully and 0.5-mL straws filled immediately, resulting in a final concentration of 200×10^6 spermatozoa/mL. In dogs of the smaller breeds, which produce fewer spermatozoa per ejaculate, it may be desirable to freeze the semen at a lower concentration to obtain more straws. The straws are frozen in LN_2 vapor in an LN_2 tank containing 15–18 mL of LN_2. The freezing is performed in 3 steps, with the goblets at the top of the canes and with the top of the canes 7, 13, and 20 cm (for 2 min, 2 min, and 1 min, respectively) below the opening of the tank, whereupon the canister is placed in the tank. Not more than 4 straws should be placed in each goblet, and not more than 4 goblets (i.e., a total of 16 straws) should be frozen in each batch.

• Alternatively, the straws can be frozen by using a Styrofoam box containing LN_2, with the straws lying horizontally on a rack placed 4 cm above the surface of the LN_2 for 10 min, whereupon the straws are immersed into the LN_2.

• The straws are best thawed in a water bath at 70°C for 8 s. (If this is impractical, they can be thawed at 37°C for 30–60 s.) Any water remaining on the outside of the straw should be carefully wiped off before the straw is opened. Each straw is emptied into 1 mL of the Uppsala Equex II/thaw medium at 37°C and left at this temperature for ≈5 min before the semen quality is assessed and artificial insemination is performed.

SAMPLE HANDLING
• Ensure there is no contamination of the collection vessel and materials that come into contact with sperm (e.g., disinfectant solution, glove power, or other contaminants).
• Avoid exposing the sample to fast temperature fluctuations and direct sunlight.

APPROPRIATE AFTERCARE
Postprocedure Patient Monitoring
N/A

Nursing Care
N/A

Dietary Modification
N/A

Medication Requirements
N/A

Restrictions on Activity
N/A

Anticipated Recovery Time
N/A

INTERPRETATION

NORMAL FINDINGS OR RANGE
General guidelines for adequate semen quality include >70% motility, at least 80% morphologically normal spermatozoa, few inflammatory cells, and ≈22 million spermatozoa per kilogram of body weight.

ABNORMAL VALUES
When in the presence of the following conditions, the specimen should not be frozen:

• Azoospermia: a lack of sperm in the ejaculate
• Oligozoospermia: a decreased number of sperm in the ejaculate (i.e., <200 million sperm per ejaculate)
• Teratozoospermia: <50% morphologically normal sperm
• Asthenozoospermia: <25% of sperm with progressive sperm motility

CRITICAL VALUES
If collected sperm numbers are marginal (<200 million sperm), wait 1 h and collect the semen a second time.

INTERFERING FACTORS
Drugs That May Alter Results of the Procedure
• Amphotericin
• Chemotherapeutic drugs
• Cimetidine
• Ketoconazole
• Steroids

Conditions That May Interfere with Performing the Procedure
An inadequate specimen: <200 million sperm, <70% motility, and/or <80% morphologically normal spermatozoa

Procedure Techniques or Handling That May Alter Results
• Use of substandard extenders (e.g., improper pH and osmolarity): Normal range values for pH are 6.72–6.76; osmolarity should be 324–1,495 mOsm, depending on the extender.
• Too fast or too slow an equilibration period between the extender and the sperm
• Inappropriate freezing and thawing rates
• Water contamination

Influence of Signalment on Performing and Interpreting the Procedure
Species
Canine

Breed
No breed predilection

Age
Semen numbers rise after puberty and decrease with older age or with disease.

Gender
Male

Pregnancy
N/A

CLINICAL PERSPECTIVE
Considering the limited number of estrous cycles during a bitch's reproductive life, it is important to freeze semen of good quality to assure high postthaw sperm fertility.

MISCELLANEOUS

ANCILLARY TESTS
Motility and viability can be assessed in a computer-assisted sperm analyzer and via fluorescence microscopy.

SYNONYMS
• Cold storage of semen
• Frozen semen

SEE ALSO
Blackwell's Five-Minute Veterinary Consult: Canine and Feline Topics
None

Related Topics in This Book
- Semen Analysis
- Semen Collection

ABBREVIATIONS

LN$_2$ = liquid nitrogen

Suggested Reading

Schafer-Somi S, Kluger S, Knapp E, *et al.* Effects of semen extender and semen processing on motility and viability of frozen-thawed dog spermatozoa. *Theriogenology* 2005; 66: 173–182.

INTERNET RESOURCES

Gradil CM, Yeager A, Concannon PW. Assessment of reproductive problems in the male dog. In: Concannon PW, England G, Verstegen III J, Linde-Forsberg C, eds. Recent Advances in Small Animal Reproduction. Ithaca, NY: International Veterinary Information Service (IVIS); last updated, April 19, 2006 Document no. A1234.0406, http://www.ivis.org/advances/Concannon/toc.asp.

Linde-Forsberg C. Regulations and recommendations for international shipment of chilled and frozen canine semen. In: Concannon PW, England G, Verstegen III J, Linde-Forsberg C, eds. Recent Advances in Small Animal Reproduction. Ithaca, NY: International Veterinary Information Service (IVIS); last updated, May 22, 2001; Document no. A1209.0501 (15 sid).

AUTHOR NAME

Carlos Gradil

BASICS

TYPE OF PROCEDURE
Radiographic

PROCEDURE EXPLANATION AND RELATED PHYSIOLOGY
Differential absorption of X-rays within the patient produce a negative image on radiographic film that is used to evaluate skeletal structures and, to a lesser extent, soft tissues. Because radiographs represent a 2-dimensional image of a 3-dimensional object, orthogonal (perpendicular) radiographs should be obtained at each location of interest. Collimation, positioning, and close object-to-film distance are important for obtaining diagnostic quality films. If possible, examinations should be performed with patients sedated or anesthetized to obtain highest-quality results and decrease radiation exposure to occupational personnel. Using a slow-film–screen combination will also produce higher-quality radiographs with better spatial resolution. Good positioning is extremely important and often requires the use of positioning aids such as tape, gauze, rope, sandbags, foam wedges, and troughs. Poor patient positioning severely compromises the diagnostic quality of the study and is a common cause of nondiagnostic studies and misdiagnosis.

INDICATIONS
- Lameness
- Musculoskeletal pain
- Musculoskeletal swelling or mass
- Conformation evaluation

CONTRAINDICATIONS
Care should be taken in performing examinations on animals suspected of vertebral fractures.

POTENTIAL COMPLICATIONS
Excessive movement of animals with vertebral fractures may cause further spinal cord trauma. Ideally, to minimize required patient movement, a horizontal beam radiograph (some X-ray machines can rotate the tube head horizontally) should be used for the ventrodorsal radiograph.

CLIENT EDUCATION
Because many animals require sedation or anesthesia for radiographic exams, it may be important to not feed the patient the morning of the visit.

BODY SYSTEMS ASSESSED
- Endocrine and metabolic
- Musculoskeletal
- Nervous
- Neuromuscular

PROCEDURE

PATIENT PREPARATION
Patient Preparation Preprocedure Medication or Preparation
Usually none. Ideally, splint or cast material should be removed before examination.

Anesthesia or Sedation
Exams are ideally performed with patients under sedation or anesthesia to aid in acquiring high-quality radiographs and to help decrease radiation exposure to occupational personnel. Some examinations, such as pelvic and spinal, should always be performed while patients are under anesthesia.

Patient Positioning
- At a minimum, orthogonal (perpendicular) radiographs should be made for each area of interest. This usually consists of a lateral and, depending on anatomic location, a craniocaudal, a dorsopalmar, a dorsoplantar, or a ventrodorsal radiograph.
- X-rays originate from a point source and diverge from the X-ray target to the size of the collimation field. X-ray beam divergence along with scatter are the primary reasons that studies should not cover large anatomic areas and should be tightly collimated and centered on the area of interest. This is particularly evident in spinal studies where the intervertebral disk spaces appear artifactually narrowed (because of beam divergence) at the periphery of the film, even though the patient is positioned appropriately. Increased scatter reduces contrast resolution and increases noise within the image, substantially affecting image quality.
- To ensure that the area being imaged is not oblique and is centered in the X-ray beam, care should be taken when positioning patients. Many times, this requires the use of positioning devices such as tape, gauze, sandbags, troughs, and foam wedges. Positioning devices also help decrease personnel exposure by enabling technicians to be further away from the patient.
- It is important that the area of interest be the side closest to the film. Minimizing object-to-film distance will help prevent geometric distortion and magnification, which result in a loss of spatial resolution.
- Most skeletal radiographs can be made on the tabletop. However, radiographs of anatomic areas thicker than ≈10 cm should be made within the X-ray table, where a grid helps remove scatter from the image. Do not forget to move the X-ray tube when transitioning to tabletop films to keep the same distance between the film and X-ray tube, at 40 inches (≈1 m).
- In some instances, additional specialty radiographs may need to be taken to further aid in diagnosis.

Patient Monitoring
Sedated or anesthetized patients should be monitored closely until fully recovered.

Equipment or Supplies
- An X-ray machine, preferably with horizontal beam capability
- A slow-screen–film combination
- A good technique chart
- Tape
- Gauze
- Rope
- Sandbags
- Troughs
- Foam padding or wedges
- A wooden spoon

TECHNIQUE
Standard Extremity Exams
- Extremity exams are typically centered on a long bone or joint.
- Examinations centered on long bones should include the complete joint proximal and distal to the long bone being examined. The X-ray beam should be centered on the middle of the long bone. This is the standard protocol for fracture cases. In cases where there is a large difference in anatomic thickness over an imaged region, 2 radiographs at different exposures may have to be made to obtain adequately exposed diagnostic quality radiographs.
- Exams centered on joints should be tightly collimated and centered under the X-ray beam. Small degrees of obliquity can significantly impact the appearance of joint spaces, making accurate interpretation difficult.

Pelvis
- The exam is best performed with patients under anesthesia.
- For extended leg (OFA view) and frogleg ventrodorsal radiographs, patients are placed in dorsal recumbency, with the thorax in a trough to aid with positioning.

- Straight positioning for extended leg (OFA view) ventrodorsal radiographs for evaluating for hip dysplasia is imperative for accurate interpretation. Ideal positioning will result in a symmetrical appearance to the obturator foramen, with parallel femurs and patellas centrally located. Any alteration from ideal positioning affects interpretation.
- Frogleg ventrodorsal pelvic radiographs are made similar to the extended leg (OFA) ventrodorsal radiographs, except the pelvic limbs are in a relaxed, abducted position. This view is excellent for evaluating the femoral head and neck.

SPINAL EXAMS
- The exam is best performed on anesthetized patients.
- The procedure is usually divided into cervical, thoracic, and lumbar exams. Tight collimation to the vertebral column and centering of it beneath the X-ray beam will produce the highest-quality radiographs and best visualization of intervertebral disk spaces.
- Straight radiographs are imperative. When evaluating radiographs for obliquity, look for superimposition of the transverse processes on the lateral radiograph and orientation of the spinous processes on the ventrodorsal radiograph.

SAMPLE HANDLING
N/A

APPROPRIATE AFTERCARE
Postprocedure Patient Monitoring
Sedated or anesthetized patients should be monitored closely until fully awake.

Nursing Care
None

Dietary Modification
None

Medication Requirements
None

Restrictions on Activity
None

Anticipated Recovery Time
None in cases without anesthesia or sedation. For sedated or anesthetized animals, the time depends on the patient's recovery from sedation or anesthesia.

INTERPRETATION

NORMAL FINDINGS OR RANGE
A wide variation of normal is seen. A large number of anatomic and radiographic atlases are available and should be consulted if there are questions. In addition, radiography of the opposite limb, for comparison, is often extremely useful with unilateral disease.

ABNORMAL VALUE
- Soft tissue abnormalities are usually classified as being intracapsular (within the joint capsule) or extracapsular (outside the joint capsule).
- Bony changes identified on radiographs are classified as being productive or lytic. Osteolysis (lysis of bone) requires approximately 30–60% bone mass loss before it is visualized radiographically. Periosteal reactions (new bone production) take ≈10–14 days before seen on radiographs, and most commonly occur after periosteal insult.
- Degenerative changes (osteophytes) result from periosteal new bone formed at the articular margin of a joint.
- Enthesophytes form when periosteal new bone forms at the origin or insertion of a tendon, ligament, or muscle.

CRITICAL VALUES
None

INTERFERING FACTORS
Drugs That May Alter Results of the Procedure
None

Conditions That May Interfere with Performing the Procedure
For pelvic exams, patients with severe canine hip dysplasia or lumbosacral transitional vertebra can be difficult to position adequately.

Procedure Techniques or Handling That May Alter Results
Patient obliquity and poor radiographic technique are the 2 most common reasons for nondiagnostic films and misdiagnosis.

Influence of Signalment on Performing and Interpreting the Procedure
Species
Skeletal differences between cats and dogs are relatively minor. Cats have long vertebral bodies, more prominent vertebral transverse processes, a more rectangularly shaped pelvis, completely mineralized clavicles, and a supratrochlear foramen of the humerus.

Breed
There is a wide variation in skeletal structures among breeds. If unilateral disease is present, the opposite leg may be invaluable for comparison.

Age
Immature patients can be challenging to interpret because of incomplete ossification of their bones. Anatomic and radiographic atlases can assist with interpretation. Again, radiography of the opposite limb may be useful with unilateral disease.

Gender
None

Pregnancy
None

CLINICAL PERSPECTIVE
- Skeletal radiography is most successful when used as a focused test, not as a large screening procedure.
- Orthogonal radiographs should be obtained at each location of concern.
- Focal exams, with tight collimation, appropriate X-ray beam centering, straight positioning, and proper technique will yield the best diagnostic results.
- The use of positioning devices with sedation or anesthesia will result in efficient radiographic studies of the highest quality, with limited exposure to occupational personnel.

MISCELLANEOUS

ANCILLARY TESTS
Computed tomography, nuclear medicine (bone scans), magnetic resonance imaging, and ultrasonography may be useful in some cases.

SYNONYMS
None

SEE ALSO
Blackwell's Five-Minute Veterinary Consult: Canine and Feline Topics
- Arthritis (Osteoarthritis)
- Arthritis, Septic
- Aspergillosis
- Ataxia
- Atlantoaxial Instability
- Anaerobic Infections
- Blastomycosis
- Chondrosarcoma, Bone
- Coccidioidomycosis

- Cruciate Ligament Disease, Cranial
- Fibrosarcoma, Bone
- Hemangiosarcoma, Bone
- Hip Dysplasia
- Histoplasmosis
- Hyperadrenocorticism (Cushing's Disease)—Cats
- Hyperadrenocorticism (Cushing's Disease)—Dogs
- Hyperparathyroidism
- Hypertrophic Osteodystrophy
- Hypertrophic Osteopathy
- Hypothyroidism
- Intervertebral Disc Disease, Cervical
- Intervertebral Disc Disease, Thoracolumbar
- Lameness
- Lead Poisoning
- Legg-Calvé-Perthes Disease
- Leishmaniasis
- Lumbosacral Stenosis and Cauda Equina Syndrome
- Malignant Fibrous Histiocytoma (Giant Cell Tumor)
- Mucopolysaccharidoses
- Multiple Myeloma
- Nail and Nailbed Disorders
- Neck and Back Pain
- Nocardiosis
- Osteochondrodysplasia
- Osteochondrosis
- Osteomyelitis
- Osteosarcoma
- Panosteitis

- Paralysis
- Patellar Luxation
- Peripheral Edema
- Pododermatitis
- Polyarthritis, Erosive, Immune-Mediated
- Polyarthritis, Nonerosive, Immune-Mediated
- Spondylosis Deformans

Related Topics in This Book
- General Principles of Radiography
- Bone Scan
- Computed Tomography
- Horizontal Beam Radiography
- Magnetic Resonance Imaging

ABBREVIATIONS

OFA = Orthopedic Foundation for Animals

Suggested Reading

Lavin LM. *Radiography in Veterinary Technology*, 3rd ed. Philadelphia: WB Saunders, 2003.

Morgan JP, ed. *Techniques in Veterinary Radiography*, 5th ed. Ames: Iowa State University Press, 1993.

Thrall DE, ed. *Textbook of Veterinary Diagnostic Radiology*, 4th ed. Philadelphia: WB Saunders, 2002.

INTERNET RESOURCES

Orthopedic Foundation for Animals (OFA), http://www.offa.org/.

AUTHOR NAME

Reid Tyson

SKIN BIOPSY

 BASICS

TYPE OF PROCEDURE
Diagnostic sample collection

PROCEDURE EXPLANATION AND RELATED PHYSIOLOGY
Full-thickness samples of lesional skin are collected for histopathologic examination. Sections are fixed in phosphate-buffered formalin solution and submitted to a diagnostic laboratory. The sections are then sectioned and stained with hematoxylin-eosin. Examination of appropriate samples under the microscope enables assessment of the tissue architecture and inflammatory or neoplastic processes.

Optimally, primary skin lesions are biopsied. Submission of samples to a veterinary pathologist with interest or expertise in dermatohistopathology is recommended. Veterinary dermatopathologists have adopted a system of pattern analysis. Specific histologic features are used to report a morphologic diagnosis that is associated with a particular set of diseases.

INDICATIONS
• The clinical presentation is unfamiliar.
• A lack of response to routine therapy has been observed.

CONTRAINDICATIONS
• Certain body areas, such as the footpad, nose, and pinnae, generally require deep sedation or full anesthesia. This may be contraindicated in compromised patients.
• Special care should be taken with patients who have bleeding disorders.
• Concurrent or recent treatment, particularly glucocorticoid therapy, will change the nature of lesions. Biopsy samples should be taken before treatment is started, or treatment should be discontinued before harvesting tissue.

POTENTIAL COMPLICATIONS
• Hemorrhage from the wound site
• Infection of the wound site
• Dehiscence of the wound
• Inappropriate healing may occur when infected or neoplastic areas of skin are biopsied or the patient is immunocompromised.

CLIENT EDUCATION
• The client should be educated in postoperative wound care.
• The client should be informed that general anesthesia may be required if the footpad, nose, or pinna is to be biopsied or if the lesions are painful.

BODY SYSTEMS ASSESSED
Dermatologic

 PROCEDURE

PATIENT PREPARATION
Preprocedure Medication or Preparation
• Usually none
• It is recommended, however, that secondary bacterial or *Malassezia* infections should be treated prior to biopsy, because the presence of these microorganisms and the associated inflammation can mask subtle underlying disease.

Anesthesia or Sedation
Light sedation is required for the majority of animals. The sedative should be chosen after the age and general health of the patient have been assessed. Full anesthesia is required when biopsying particularly sensitive areas, such as the footpad, nasal planum, pinna, and around mucous membranes. Painful dermatoses may also require anesthesia.

Patient Positioning
Patients should be positioned so that the affected areas of skin are well illuminated and easily accessible.

Patient Monitoring
Monitoring should be appropriate for the sedation or anesthesia used.

Equipment or Supplies
• Multiple 50- to 100-mL containers of 10% phosphate-buffered formalin. The biopsy sample should be placed in a minimum of 10-fold its volume of formalin.
• Biopsy punches (6–8 mm in diameter) or a scalpel handle and blade (for wedge biopsies)
• 1%–2% lidocaine solution
• A 3-mL syringe
• A 22-gauge (or smaller) needle
• A sterilized surgical pack containing gauze swabs, fine scissors, fine rat-toothed forceps, hemostats, and needle holders
• Nylon suture material for skin closure
• Clippers or scissors
• An indelible marker

TECHNIQUE
• Biopsy site selection is critical to the success of this technique. Optimally, primary skin lesions are selected and centered in the biopsy field. The tissue is usually sectioned through the center, which will ensure that the lesion is included in the tissue examined by the pathologist. For ulcerative skin disease, the sample should be harvested using a wedge technique across the margin of the ulcer. This will be cut along the longitudinal axis, allowing the junctional tissue between the normal and ulcerated skin to be examined. Deep lesions are poorly accessed with punch biopsies and, again, a wedge technique is indicated.
• For the majority of lesions, a 6- to 8-mm-diameter biopsy punch is optimal. Smaller-diameter punches are available but often provide insufficient diagnostic tissue. They can be used for small lesions on sensitive areas such as eyelid margins.
• In all cases, multiple biopsy samples (3–6) should be taken from the affected tissue.
• After being sedated or anesthetized, the patient should be positioned so the biopsy area is well illuminated and accessed easily. The areas should be lightly clipped (without touching the skin) or the hair is cut away with scissors. Do not scrub or surgically prepare the skin. The biopsy site is then outlined with a marker pen and 0.5–1.0 mL of lidocaine injected into the subcutaneous tissue below the site. Lidocaine is not required if the patient is fully anaesthetized.
• For the punch biopsy technique, the instrument is placed over the lesional skin, and unidirectional even pressure is applied. The circular blade should cut through the skin and hypodermis, leaving a cone of tissue attached at its base. The sample is then lifted gently with fine forceps by the base of the cone and, using curve scissors, detached below with forceps. Excessive manipulation of the sample at this stage can cause crush artifacts. Excess blood on the wound or biopsy sample can be removed by using a gauze swab lightly. The sample is then placed in formalin, and the jar is clearly labeled with the body site, lesion type, and patient identification. Additional samples should be placed in separate jars. Placing the biopsy sample on a card square prior to immersion in formalin limits tissue shrinkage. A line on the card indicating the direction of hair growth will facilitate orientation of the biopsy material for appropriate sectioning after submission.
• The wound is closed with a cruciate suture or an interrupted pattern.
• Wedge biopsy samples are harvested similarly, using a scalpel blade attached to a handle. Making impression smears from the cut margin of tissue is often a useful adjunctive technique.
• Clear information regarding the patient's signalment, duration of disease, previous or current treatment, and lesion description and body site should be provided to the pathologist. A list of clinical differential diagnoses is also very helpful.

APPROPRIATE AFTERCARE

The patient should be monitored for postsedation or postanesthetic recovery and hemorrhage from the biopsy site.

INTERPRETATION

NORMAL FINDINGS OR RANGE

The architecture of the skin varies with body site and species. An experienced pathologist should report on whether findings are within normal limits.

ABNORMAL VALUES

- The biopsy report should include a descriptive paragraph, morphologic diagnosis (pattern), and suggestions of differential diagnoses associated with that pattern. Results will reflect only the clinician's choice of lesion(s) to biopsy and should be interpreted in the context of all other abnormalities detected in that case. Many skin diseases look very similar histologically, so a definitive diagnosis requires clinical interpretation.
- In some cases, the pathologist may suggest additional staining techniques, which are usually used for 1 or 2 reasons: to view organisms which cannot be seen with routine hematoxylin-eosin staining or to further characterize an inflammatory or neoplastic infiltrate.

INTERFERING FACTORS

Drugs That May Alter Results of the Procedure

- Recent or concurrent glucocorticoid therapy can significantly alter both skin architecture and inflammatory processes.
- The administration of antimicrobials prior to biopsy may be recommended because secondary bacterial or *Malassezia* infections and the associated inflammation may mask underlying disease.

Conditions That May Interfere with Performing the Procedure

See the Contraindications section.

Procedure Techniques or Handling That May Alter Results

- Surgical scrubbing of the skin prior to biopsy will remove important architectural features on the epidermis or crust.
- The use of cautery will disrupt normal tissue architecture.
- Crush artifacts will result if the tissue is squeezed too hard.
- Failure to place the sample directly into formalin will result in tissue autolysis.
- The placement of large tissue samples in insufficient volumes of formalin will result in insufficient fixation of the tissue.

Influence of Signalment on Performing and Interpreting the Procedure

Species

The architecture of the skin varies with body site, age, and species. An experienced pathologist should report on whether findings are within normal limits.

Breed

None

Age

None

Gender

None

Pregnancy

None

CLINICAL PERSPECTIVE

Skin biopsy is an invaluable tool in veterinary dermatology; however, results reflect the lesions selected by the clinician. Lesion morphology changes considerably with the evolution of the disease, so select the newest lesions to biopsy and take multiple samples. Avoid treating first and biopsying later, with the exception of antimicrobial therapy. In some cases, skin biopsy is most useful in ruling out differential diagnoses. Never be afraid to call the pathologist and discuss the case or to request a second opinion from another pathologist.

MISCELLANEOUS

ANCILLARY TESTS

- Skin cytology
- Fine-needle aspiration cytology

SYNONYMS

None

SEE ALSO

Blackwell's Five-Minute Veterinary Consult: Canine and Feline Topics

Dermatoses

Related Topics in This Book

- Fine-Needle Aspiration
- Impression Smear
- Skin Surface and Otic Cytology

ABBREVIATIONS

None

Suggested Reading

Irhke PJ, Walder EJ, Affolter VK, Gross TL. *Skin Diseases of the Dog and Cat.* Ames, IA: Blackwell, 2005.

Yager JA, Wilcock BP. *Color Atlas and Text of Surgical Pathology of the Dog and Cat: Dermatopathology and Skin Tumors.* St Louis: Mosby-Year Book, 1994.

INTERNET RESOURCES

None

AUTHOR NAME

Hilary A. Jackson

SKIN SCRAPING AND TRICHOGRAM

BASICS

TYPE OF PROCEDURE
Diagnostic sample collection

PROCEDURE EXPLANATION AND RELATED PHYSIOLOGY
Samples are collected from the skin surface or hair follicles by scraping or plucking. These techniques are used to detect the presence of ectoparasites, to examine hair morphology, or both.

INDICATIONS
• When surface or follicular parasites are suspected
• To determine the growth phase of the hair
• To examine hair morphology in dysplastic or dystrophic follicular disease
• To detect dermatophyte arthrospores or hyphae on infected hair shafts

CONTRAINDICATIONS
None

POTENTIAL COMPLICATIONS
None

CLIENT EDUCATION
None

BODY SYSTEMS ASSESSED
Dermatologic

PROCEDURE

PATIENT PREPARATION
Preprocedure Medication or Preparation
Light manual restraint of patients

Anesthesia or Sedation
Not generally required

Patient Positioning
The patient should be positioned so that the affected areas of skin are well illuminated and easily accessible.

Patient Monitoring
None

Equipment or Supplies
• Microscope slides and coverslips
• A pencil or an indelible ink pen for labeling slides
• Mineral oil
• A size 10 blunted scalpel blade
• Curved hemostats

TECHNIQUE
• *Superficial skin scraping*: This technique is employed to identify surface parasites. Multiple scrapings (4–6) should be collected from diseased skin. Prior to collection, the hair should be gently clipped from the area by using scissors or clippers. A small quantity of mineral oil is dropped onto the center of a microscope slide. The blunted blade is dipped in this mineral oil and then scraped in wide arcs across the affected skin, taking care to collect as much surface scale as possible in the mineral oil on the blade. The sample is spread on the microscope slide, which is then labeled with the case identifier and body area from which the sample was collected.
• *Deep skin scraping*: This technique is employed to identify follicular parasites such as *Demodex* mites. Multiple scrapings (4–6) should be collected from diseased skin. The equipment and preparation are as described in the preceding paragraph. Thickened skin may be squeezed gently to encourage the extrusion of mites from hair follicles. Samples are harvested from a smaller area than for superficial skin scraping. The skin should be scraped until slight capillary ooze is observed, ensuring that the dermis has been reached. The sample is spread on the slide as described in the preceding paragraph.
• *Trichogram or hair plucking*: A technique employed to find follicular *Demodex* mites, dermatophyte arthrospores, or hyphae or to examine hair morphology. Curved hemostats are used to pull hairs gently from the affected skin. A rubber sleeve on the hemostat improves one's grip and minimizes damage to the hair shaft. For identification of *Demodex* mites or to examine hair morphology, hairs are then mounted in mineral oil on a microscope slide, taking care to lay them parallel for optimal examination. To examine for fungal elements, the preparation may be treated with an agent such as potassium hydroxide or chlorphenolic, although spores can be visualized on samples mounted in mineral oil alone.
• A coverslip is placed over the samples collected by the aforementioned methods, and slides are examined carefully under a microscope. Many surface ectoparasites can be easily detected under low-power magnification (10×). Visualization of *Demodex* mites and ectoparasite eggs is best done under higher power (40×). Examination of hairs for fungal elements requires oil immersion. To enhance contrast and improve visualization during examination of the slide, the microscope condenser should be lowered or the iris diaphragm aperture reduced.

APPROPRIATE AFTERCARE
None

INTERPRETATION

NORMAL FINDINGS OR RANGE
Skin Scrapings
No mites should be found in samples from normal dogs and cats. Although *Demodex* mites are present in very low numbers in normal animals, they are hard to detect. The finding of a single mite should therefore prompt additional scrapings and hair pluckings from the affected area. Occasional pollens, saprophytic fungal conidia, or strands of material such as carpet may be found in superficial samples.

Trichogram
The microscopic appearance of the distal end of the hair differs with the stage of growth of that hair. A growing hair (*anagen*) has a rounded or clublike morphology, whereas that of a resting hair (*telogen*) is pointed. In a sample from a normal hair coat, a mixture of anagen and telogen hairs is found, with the former population predominating. The precise ratio varies with breed, age, and season.

ABNORMAL VALUES
Superficial Skin Scrapings
The finding of any mites, lice, or their eggs is abnormal. In some cases, such as sarcoptic acariasis, mites or eggs can be difficult to find even after multiple skin scrapings. Thus, infestation cannot be definitely ruled out by using this technique. Surface-dwelling *Demodex* species, such as *Demodex gattoi* and *Demodex injae*, may also be detected with superficial skin scrapings.

Deep Skin Scrapings and Trichogram
The finding of any *Demodex* mites is considered diagnostic of demodicosis. Eggs may also be found by using these techniques.

Trichogram Examination for Hair Morphology
Telogen hairs will predominate in endocrine diseases such as hyperadrenocorticism. Uncommon diseases such as pili torti and trichorrhexis

nodosa will cause structural abnormalities of the hair shaft. Large aggregates of melanin associated with fractures of the shaft are seen in color-dilution alopecia. Fungal arthrospores and hyphae will be seen surrounding dermatophyte-infected hairs. A fractured hair shaft can be the result of trauma. This technique is often employed to demonstrate evidence of pruritus and self-trauma in cats with alopecia.

INTERFERING FACTORS
Drugs That May Alter Results of the Procedure
Recent glucocorticoid therapy may increase the chance of finding some ectoparasites.
Conditions That May Interfere with Performing the Procedure
None
Procedure Techniques or Handling That May Alter Results
• Failure to perform adequate depth or number of skin scrapings
• Nonsystematic examination of samples under the microscope
Influence of Signalment on Performing and Interpreting the Procedure
Species
In some cases of chronic canine pododemodicosis, *Demodex* mites can be very difficult to demonstrate. Hair plucking and deep scraping should be performed in these cases. However, sometimes mites may be demonstrable only in skin biopsy samples.

Breed
None

Age
None

Gender
None

Pregnancy
None

CLINICAL PERSPECTIVE
Skin scrapings and trichograms are invaluable and frequently used techniques in veterinary dermatology. The habitat of the suspected parasite should be considered when collecting specimens, and the samples should be examined carefully and completely under the microscope.

MISCELLANEOUS
ANCILLARY TESTS
• Skin biopsy may be required to demonstrate *Demodex* mites in cases of chronic canine pododemodicosis.
• A Wood's lamp examination and dermatophyte culture

SYNONYMS
Hair plucking

SEE ALSO
Blackwell's Five-Minute Veterinary Consult: Canine and Feline Topics
• Demodicosis
• Dermatophytosis
• Pododermatitis
• Sarcoptic Mange
Related Topics in This Book
None

ABBREVIATIONS
None

Suggested Reading
Curtis CF. Diagnostic techniques and sample collection. *Clin Tech Small Anim Pract* 2001; **16**: 199–206.
Moriello KA, Newbury S. Recommendations for the management and treatment of dermatophytosis in animal shelters. *Vet Clin North Am Small Anim Pract* 2006; **36**: 89–114.
Scott DW, Miller WH, Griffin CE. *Small Animal Dermatology*, 6th ed. Philadelphia: WB Saunders, 2001.

INTERNET RESOURCES
University of London, Royal Veterinary College, eMedia Review Site, Diagnosis in Dermatology: Skin scraping, http://www.rvc.ac.uk/review/Dermatology/Tests/Scraping.htm.

AUTHOR NAME
Hilary A. Jackson

SKIN SURFACE AND OTIC CYTOLOGY

BASICS

TYPE OF PROCEDURE
Diagnostic sample collection

PROCEDURE EXPLANATION AND RELATED PHYSIOLOGY
Samples are collected from the skin surface or ear canal by using a variety of techniques, mounted on a slide, and examined under high power with a microscope. These invaluable procedures enable the assessment of the type and number of organisms present on the skin and evaluation of the associated inflammatory response. Empirical treatment decisions are frequently made by using this information. Response to treatment can also be assessed.

INDICATIONS
• When exudate is visible in the ear canal or on the skin surface
• The contents of intact pustules can also be collected to determine their etiology.

CONTRAINDICATIONS
None

POTENTIAL COMPLICATIONS
None

CLIENT EDUCATION
None

BODY SYSTEMS ASSESSED
Dermatologic

PROCEDURE

PATIENT PREPARATION
Preprocedure Medication or Preparation
Light manual restraint of patients

Anesthesia or Sedation
Not generally required. Animals with painful otic disease may require sedation for collection of samples of diagnostic quality.

Patient Positioning
Patients should be positioned so that the affected areas of skin are well illuminated and easily accessible.

Patient Monitoring
None

Equipment or Supplies
• Microscope slides
• A pencil or an indelible ink pen for labeling slides
• Stain: Typically a modified Wright's stain such as Diff-Quick is employed.
• Cotton-tipped swabs
• Acetate tape: transparent, not frosted
• A sterile 22-gauge needle

TECHNIQUE
• A number of different techniques are described. The ideal technique varies with the sample site and quantity and quality of exudate present. For example, it is difficult to collect a direct impression smear from the interdigital skin; samples from this site are best collected by tape or swab. In all cases, the slide should be labeled with a case identifier and the body site from which it was harvested, particularly if immediate examination is not possible or if multiple samples from the same animal are being collected. For samples with a large lipid content, heat fixation is recommended prior to immersion in the alcohol fixative. In most other cases, air-drying is sufficient.
• Direct impression smear: The microscope slide is pressed directly onto the affected area of skin. This is best suited to relatively flat, accessible areas of the body. This technique may also be employed to collect samples directly from the exudates from draining tracts. In this case, prior to sample collection, the surface exudate should be wiped away and fresh exudate collected by squeezing the area gently. This avoids inadvertent assessment of surface colonization.
• Cotton-tipped swabs should be introduced into the affected ear canal or onto the affected area of skin, and a sample of the exudate is collected using moderate pressure. This is then rolled onto the microscope slide and dried and stained as directed by the manufacturer.
• Acetate tape: A 3- to 5-cm length of tape is cut, and the central portion is pressed repeatedly on the affected skin by using moderate pressure. This lifts organisms and cells off the immediate skin surface. After sample collection, affix the tape lightly to a microscope slide by each end, leaving the area on which the sample was harvested in a free loop in the center of the slide. This allows the sample area to be stained easily. When these samples are processed, the tape is stained directly. Do not dip it in the alcohol fixative because this will remove the gum and associated diagnostic sample from the tape. After staining, the tape is blotted and flattened onto the slide, gum-side down. The sample is viewed under the microscope through the tape. Microscope emersion oil can be applied directly to the tape for evaluation under high power.
• Cytology of intact pustules: The intact pustule is identified and ruptured gently by using a fine-gauge needle. The exposed pus is then collected onto a slide by pressing the slide gently onto the surface. Multiple samples from the same pustule can be collected by repeated application of the slide.

APPROPRIATE AFTERCARE
None

INTERPRETATION

NORMAL FINDINGS OR RANGE
Low numbers of coccoid bacteria and *Malassezia* may be found on normal skin. Numbers vary with the body area sampled and breed.

ABNORMAL VALUES
• There is much controversy over what constitutes "normal" flora and when numbers of organisms become clinically relevant. Publications vary in collection technique and the magnification under which samples were examined. This author recommends that samples are always examined under oil emersion at 100×. At this magnification, morphologic differences between organisms are clear. The finding of rod-shaped bacteria in skin or otic samples is generally abnormal.
• The finding of cocci supports a diagnosis of pyoderma, particularly if associated with the appropriate clinical signs (i.e., pustules, papules, collarettes). The presence of degenerate neutrophils and intracellular cocci is diagnostic.
• Most clinicians use a grading technique from 0 (normal) to 4+ (numerous).
• The clinical presentation should be taken into consideration when interpreting samples. Increasing evidence supports the idea that some animals develop a hypersensitivity response to *Staphylococcus* or *Malassezia* species, and, under these circumstances, even very few organisms can cause quite significant inflammation and pruritus.
• Finding nondegenerate neutrophils and numerous intact keratinocytes (acantholytic cells) in a sample from an intact pustule supports a diagnosis of pemphigus foliaceus, and a skin biopsy is warranted for definitive diagnosis.

INTERFERING FACTORS

Drugs That May Alter Results of the Procedure
Recent topical or systemic antimicrobial treatment can alter the numbers of organisms detected.

Conditions That May Interfere with Performing the Procedure
None

Procedure Techniques or Handling That May Alter Results
Failure to properly stain samples results in an underestimation of the number of organisms present. In this case, "ghost" outlines of the organisms may be apparent.

Influence of Signalment on Performing and Interpreting the Procedure

Species
Numerous *Malassezia* organisms may be found on certain dog breeds, such as basset hounds, with no apparent clinical signs.

Breed
None

Age
None

Gender
None

Pregnancy
None

CLINICAL PERSPECTIVE
These techniques are invaluable to the practice of veterinary dermatology, and, in most cases, empirical therapy based on skin surface or otic cytology is appropriate.

 MISCELLANEOUS

ANCILLARY TESTS
- Culture and sensitivity
- Fine-needle aspiration cytology
- Skin biopsy

SYNONYMS
None

SEE ALSO

Blackwell's Five-Minute Veterinary Consult: Canine and Feline Topics
- *Malassezia* Dermatitis
- Otitis Externa and Media
- Pemphigus
- Pyoderma

Related Topics in This Book
Skin Biopsy

ABBREVIATIONS
None

Suggested Reading
Bond R. *Malassezia* dermatitis. In: Greene CE, ed. *Infectious Diseases of the Dog and Cat*, 3rd ed. St Louis: Saunders Elsevier, 2006: 565–569.

INTERNET RESOURCES
None

AUTHOR NAME
Hilary A. Jackson

SKULL RADIOGRAPHY

BASICS

TYPE OF PROCEDURE
Radiographic

PROCEDURE EXPLANATION AND RELATED PHYSIOLOGY
Differential absorption of X-rays within the patient produces a negative image on radiographic film that is used to evaluate skeletal structures and soft tissues. Because radiographs represent a 2-dimensional image of a 3-dimensional object, multiple radiographic projections are required. The skull is anatomically very complex and often requires oblique or specialty radiographs that highlight certain anatomic regions, such as the tympanic bullae or temporomandibular joints. Collimation, positioning, and close object-to-film distance are important for obtaining diagnostic quality films. Occasionally, skull radiography may be performed with patients under sedation, but most examinations will require general anesthesia for best results. Using a slow-film–screen combination will produce higher-quality radiographs with better spatial resolution. Good positioning is extremely important and often requires the use of positioning aids such as tape, gauze, rope, sandbags, or foam wedges. Poor patient positioning severely compromises the quality of the study and is the most common reason for nondiagnostic studies and misdiagnosis.

INDICATIONS
- Head tilt
- Ophthalmic disease (e.g., exophthalmos)
- Oral disease
- Otitis
- Swelling or mass
- Trauma
- Upper airway disease

CONTRAINDICATIONS
None

POTENTIAL COMPLICATIONS
None

CLIENT EDUCATION
Do not feed patients the morning of the examination because skull radiography is typically performed with patients under general anesthesia. Skull radiography can be an extremely useful diagnostic tool for many diseases. However, because the skull is anatomically complex, more advanced imaging tools such as computed tomography (CT) or magnetic resonance imaging (MRI) may be needed.

BODY SYSTEMS ASSESSED
- Endocrine and metabolic
- Musculoskeletal
- Nervous
- Ophthalmic
- Respiratory

PROCEDURE

PATIENT PREPARATION
Preprocedure Medication or Preparation
None

Anesthesia or Sedation
Exams are typically performed with patients under general anesthesia to facilitate acquiring high-quality radiographs and patient positioning and to help decrease radiation exposure to occupational personnel.

Patient Positioning
- Use of an anatomic skull specimen can aid in visualization of patient positioning. It is particularly useful to understand the positioning differences between cats and brachycephalic dogs compared to dolichocephalic dogs.
- A baseline skull series consists of a minimum of 4 radiographic views; lateral, dorsoventral, and right and left lateral obliques.
- Depending on the area of clinical interest, additional specialty radiographs are often needed to highlight certain anatomic structures. Each skull series may be slightly modified to obtain optimum visualization of the anatomic structure of interest. The following are recommendations for typical studies with interest in a particular anatomic area:
  - *Dental series*: lateral, dorsoventral, and open-mouth right and left lateral obliques
  - *Mandible series*: lateral, dorsoventral, and open-mouth right and left lateral obliques. An intraoral ventrodorsal radiograph may be valuable for evaluating the rostral aspect of the mandible.
  - *Maxilla series*: lateral, dorsoventral, and open-mouth right and left lateral obliques. An intraoral dorsoventral radiograph may be valuable for evaluating the rostral aspect of the maxilla.
  - *Nasal and sinus series*: lateral, dorsoventral, right and left lateral obliques, intraoral dorsoventral, and a frontal sinus rostrocaudal radiograph
  - *Tympanic bulla series*: lateral, dorsoventral, right and left lateral obliques and open-mouth rostrocaudal radiographs
- Positioning for each of these projections depends on the anatomic shape of the patient's head. Cats and brachycephalic dogs have calvaria that are more round and are often more difficult to position appropriately, particularly for oblique radiographs.
- For the lateral view, the nose should be parallel to the cassette and the hemi-mandibles superimposed over each other. Foam wedges are often used under the nose and neck to help straighten the animal. In addition, tape is an invaluable resource in patients that are difficult to position. An empty syringe case or tape can be used to pry the mouth open for animals under general anesthesia. The open-mouth lateral radiograph can be useful in removing superimposition of the dental arcades and is more valuable than closed-mouth radiographs in some cases.
- For the dorsoventral view, the patient should be in sternal recumbency, and the body of the mandibles should be against the cassette. Again, tape may be needed to fix the patient in optimum position.
- Positioning for the left and right lateral oblique views depends on the anatomic area of interest and anatomic conformation of the skull. The degree of obliquity for ideal positioning and radiographic visualization of the mandible, maxilla, dental arcades, and tympanic bulla will be slightly different. The oblique view may be performed open-mouth to enable better visualization of some structures and to help remove superimposition.
- Intraoral views can be extremely useful for looking at the rostral nasal cavity, maxilla, and mandible. The radiographic cassette or non-screen film is placed into the anesthetized patient's mouth, corner first. For evaluating the nasal cavity and maxilla, the patient is placed in sternal recumbency, and intraoral dorsoventral radiography is performed. For evaluating the mandible, the patient is placed in dorsal recumbency, and intraoral ventrodorsal radiography is performed. The patient's thorax may be placed in a trough to help with positioning animals in dorsal recumbency. Because of the removal of superimposed structures, the diagnostic value of the intraoral radiograph is much better than the standard dorsoventral radiographs. However, the study is limited by how far caudally the radiographic cassette or nonscreen film can be inserted into the mouth. This is particularly difficult in brachycephalic dogs and cats.
- Rostrocaudal views are difficult to perform and require patients to be under general anesthesia and in dorsal recumbency. Placement of

the thorax into a trough aids positioning. For evaluation of the frontal sinuses, the nose should be pointing toward the tube head or approximately perpendicular to the table. Use of an anatomic model is extremely useful when trying to identify the optimum angle to orient the skull to obtain a "skyline" view of the frontal sinus. In some animals, particularly cats, it may be impossible to separate the frontal sinus from adjacent calvarial structures. For evaluation of the temporomandibular joints, open-mouth rostrocaudal radiography should be performed. Gauze or tape is tied around the maxilla and directed dorsally. Gauze or tape is also tied around the mandible and directed ventrally. Tension is applied to both the mandible and the maxilla, causing the mouth to widen. The X-ray beam is centered in the widened mouth.

Patient Monitoring
Patients should be closely monitored during anesthesia and recovery.

Equipment or Supplies
- An X-ray machine
- A slow-screen–film combination
- Nonscreen film
- A good technique chart
- Tape
- Gauze
- Rope
- Sandbags
- Troughs
- Foam padding and wedges

TECHNIQUE
- All skull radiographs are made tabletop and do not require the use of a grid.
- Remember to keep the tube-head to film distance static. Most systems require a 40-inch (1.016 m) tube-head to film distance. Intraoral radiography requires modification of the tube-head height because the radiographic cassette will be elevated off the table and within the patient's mouth.
- Ideally, the endotracheal tube should be removed from the area of interest. It is imperative to recognize that the endotracheal tube and tongue can artifactually cause opacity alterations that can mimic disease.
- Nonscreen film should be used for anatomic areas that require high detail, such as the dental arcade or nasal passages. The use of nonscreen film requires very long exposure times and produces extremely high-quality results. However, the radiation required for proper exposure necessitates that all personnel leave the room during the exposure and that the animal is under general anesthesia to prevent motion.
- X-rays originate from a point source and diverge from the X-ray target to the size of the collimation field. X-ray beam divergence along with scatter is the primary reason that studies should not cover large anatomic areas and should be tightly collimated and centered on the area of interest. Increased scatter reduces contrast resolution and increases noise within the image, substantially affecting image quality.
- It is important that the area of interest be the side closest to the film. Minimizing object-to-film distance will help prevent geometric distortion and magnification, which results in a loss of spatial resolution.

SAMPLE HANDLING
N/A

APPROPRIATE AFTERCARE
Postprocedure Patient Monitoring
Patients should be closely monitored until fully awake from anesthesia.

Nursing Care
None

Dietary Modification
None

Medication Requirements
None

Restrictions on Activity
None

Anticipated Recovery Time
This depends on the anesthesia protocol used on the patient.

INTERPRETATION
NORMAL FINDINGS OR RANGE
A wide variation of normal is seen. A large number of anatomic and radiographic atlases are available and should be consulted if there are questions.

ABNORMAL VALUES
- Soft tissue abnormalities can be difficult to detect because of the complex anatomy involved. Alterations in symmetry are often the earliest sign of soft tissue abnormalities. Soft tissue swelling or masses should be closely scrutinized for underlying bone involvement.
- Bone changes identified on radiographs are classified as being productive, lytic, or both. *Osteolysis* (lysis of bone) requires approximately 30–60% of bone mass loss before it is detectable on radiographs. *Periosteal reactions* (new bone production) take $\approx$10–14 days before being seen on radiographs, and most commonly occurs after periosteal insult. The type of periosteal reaction, bone lysis, and the zone of transition are all important in deciding the aggressiveness of a lesion.

CRITICAL VALUES
None

INTERFERING FACTORS
Drugs That May Alter Results of the Procedure
None

Conditions That May Interfere with Performing the Procedure
None

Procedure Techniques or Handling That May Alter Results
Poor patient positioning and radiographic technique are the 2 most common reasons for nondiagnostic films and misdiagnosis.

Influence of Signalment on Performing and Interpreting the Procedure
Species
Cats have small frontal sinuses that typically cannot be visualized on rostrocaudal radiographs. The anatomic shape of the feline and brachycephalic canine skulls is similar.

Breed
Large anatomic differences exist among brachycephalic, mesaticephalic, and dolichocephalic dogs. As such, each exam has to be somewhat tailored to the anatomic shape of the patient's skull. Anatomic models are a great resource for visualization of these anatomic differences.

Age
Immature animals will have open, flat bone physes (i.e., sutures). These sutures may mimic the appearance of calvarial fractures.

Gender
None

Pregnancy
None

SKULL RADIOGRAPHY

CLINICAL PERSPECTIVE
Performing skull radiography and interpreting the results can be challenging. However, skull radiography is extremely useful at identifying many common diseases seen regularly in clinical practice. Because of the complex anatomy of the skull, advanced imaging such as CT or MRI may have to be performed.

MISCELLANEOUS

ANCILLARY TESTS
In complex cases, CT or MRI may be required for further imaging.

SYNONYMS
None

SEE ALSO
Blackwell's Five-Minute Veterinary Consult: Canine and Feline Topics
- Adenocarcinoma, Salivary Gland
- Ameloblastoma
- Astrocytoma
- Brain Injury
- Ceruminous Gland Adenocarcinoma, Ear
- Chondrosarcoma, Nasal and Paranasal Sinus
- Chondrosarcoma, Oral
- Craniomandibular Osteopathy
- Epistaxis
- Epulis
- Fibrosarcoma, Nasal and Paranasal Sinus
- Gingival Hyperplasia
- Head Tilt
- Hyperparathyroidism
- Meningioma
- Nasal and Nasopharyngeal Polyps
- Nasal Discharge
- Nasopharyngeal Stenosis
- Oral Cavity Tumors, Undifferentiated Malignant Tumors
- Orbital Diseases (Exophthalmos, Enophthalmos, Strabismus)
- Osteosarcoma
- Otitis Externa and Media
- Otitis Media and Interna
- Ptyalism
- Rhinitis and Sinusitis
- Squamous Cell Carcinoma, Nasal and Paranasal Sinuses
- Squamous Cell Carcinoma, Nasal Planum
- Squamous Cell Carcinoma, Gingiva

Related Topics in This Book
- General Principles of Radiography
- Dental Radiography

ABBREVIATIONS
- CT = computed tomography
- MRI = magnetic resonance imaging

Suggested Reading
Lavin LM. *Radiography in Veterinary Technology*, 3rd ed. Philadelphia: WB Saunders, 2003.
Morgan JP, ed. *Techniques in Veterinary Radiography*, 5th ed. Ames: Iowa State University Press, 1993.
Thrall DE, ed. *Textbook of Veterinary Diagnostic Radiology*, 4th ed. Philadelphia: WB Saunders, 2002.

INTERNET RESOURCES
None

AUTHOR NAME
Reid Tyson

BASICS

TYPE OF SPECIMEN
Blood

TEST EXPLANATION AND RELATED PHYSIOLOGY
Sodium (Na) is the principal cation in the extracellular fluid (ECF) compartment. Na is primarily absorbed in the small intestine. Using ATP as an energy source, Na/K-ATPase pumps in the gut epithelial cells, actively pumps 3 Na ions out of the cells, and returns them to the ECF space in exchange for 2 K ions pumped into the enterocytes. In response to hypotension, Na may be almost completely reabsorbed by the colon. Na is freely filtered by the glomerulus, and almost 100% of filtered Na is reabsorbed by the kidneys. The bulk of the filtered Na load is transported in the early section of the proximal convoluted tubules, along with glucose, phosphate, amino acids, and bicarbonate, while Na is reabsorbed in the distal segment, along with chloride. Na is actively reabsorbed in the thick ascending limb of the loop of Henle.

Na is also the primary determinant of plasma osmolality. Na homeostasis is closely correlated with water homeostasis. Serum Na may not accurately reflect total body Na because serum Na represents the amount of Na relative to the total body water. If the total body water is very high (hypo-osmolality) or very low (hyperosmolality), the measured serum Na concentration may be within normal limits even though the total body Na is abnormal.

Water homeostasis is adjusted for changes in the plasma osmolality, serum Na level, and ECF volume. In cases of decreased ECF volume and hyperosmolality, thirst and ADH are stimulated, causing increased water retention. ADH decreases (by dilution) serum Na levels by increasing water reabsorption in the distal tubules. Decreased ECF volume also stimulates the release of aldosterone, which results in Na and water retention by the kidneys. Increased ECF volume causes release of atrial natriuretic factor. Atrial natriuretic factor increases the glomerular filtration rate, reduces aldosterone production, and decreases Na reabsorption in the collecting tubules, which decreases ECF volume through reduction in water and Na retention.

Hypernatremia is most commonly seen when water is lost (as pure water or as hypotonic fluid) in excess of Na or with increased intake of Na in excess of water. Hyponatremia is caused by loss of Na, increased water intake, or retention of excess body water. Renal excretion of Na and water is often compromised in patients who develop hyponatremia. Hypernatremia is associated with hyperosmolar states, whereas hyponatremia is usually associated with hypo-osmolar states but can be seen with high or normal osmolality.

Na is measured in serum or plasma by ion-specific potentiometry (direct or indirect), flame photometry, and dry-reagent methods. Point-of-care instruments using ion-selective electrodes may have different ranges than instruments that use dilutional techniques.

INDICATIONS
- Cavitary effusion
- Dehydration
- Edema
- GI signs (e.g., vomiting, diarrhea, weight loss, inappetence)
- Monitoring of diuretic therapy
- Monitoring of treatment for hypoadrenocorticism
- Muscle weakness
- Neurologic abnormalities (e.g., changes in mentation or behavior, seizures)
- Polyuria-polydipsia
- Renal disease

CONTRAINDICATIONS
None

POTENTIAL COMPLICATIONS
None

CLIENT EDUCATION
None

BODY SYSTEMS ASSESSED
- Endocrine and metabolic
- Gastrointestinal
- Hepatobiliary
- Renal and urologic

 SAMPLE

COLLECTION
0.5–1.0 mL of venous blood

HANDLING
Collect the sample into red-top tube, serum-separator tube, or lithium heparin.

STORAGE
- Refrigeration is recommended for short-term storage.
- Freeze the serum or plasma for long-term storage.
- Store in an airtight container to avoid evaporation.

STABILITY
- Room temperature: 1 day
- Refrigerated (2°–8°C): 1 week
- Frozen (−20°C): 1 year

PROTOCOL
None

 INTERPRETATION

NORMAL FINDINGS OR RANGE
- Dogs: 140–150 mEq/L
- Cats: 150–160 mEq/L
- Reference intervals may vary depending on the laboratory and assay.

ABNORMAL VALUES
Values above or below the reference intervals

CRITICAL VALUES
- In cats and dogs, neurologic abnormalities may occur when the Na level exceeds 170 mEq/L or falls below 125 mEq/L.
- The speed at which the Na level rises or falls (in <48 h) corresponds to the severity of clinical signs.

INTERFERING FACTORS
Drugs That May Alter Results or Interpretation
Drugs That Interfere with Test Methodology
None

Drugs That Alter Physiology
- Synthetic adrenocortical steroids (e.g., fludrocortisone, desoxycorticosterone acetate/pivalate), corticosteroids, lactulose, Na bicarbonate, Na phosphate enemas, hypertonic saline fluids, and amphotericin may cause hypernatremia.
- Loop and thiazide diuretics, K-sparing diuretics (i.e., spironolactone, triamterene), angiotensin-converting enzyme (ACE) inhibitors, Na-deficient fluids, trimethoprim combined with diuretics, NSAIDs, and sulfonylureas may cause hyponatremia.
- Mannitol therapy (hyperosmolar) may cause pseudohyponatremia.

Disorders That May Alter Results
- Dehydration may cause pseudohypernatremia.
- Hyperosmolar states (hyperglycemia) may cause pseudohyponatremia.
- Hyperproteinemia, hyperviscosity, and hyperlipemia/lipidemia may cause pseudohyponatremia.

Collection Techniques or Handling That May Alter Results
- Samples collected via IV catheters may cause spurious Na readings, depending on the fluid being administered.
- Samples combined with Na-containing anticoagulants may cause pseudohypernatremia.

Influence of Signalment
Species
None

Breed
None

Causes of Abnormal Findings

Age
None

Gender
See the Pregnancy section.

Pregnancy
Hyperkalemia and hyponatremia may be seen in ill, pregnant dogs.

LIMITATIONS OF THE TEST
Sensitivity, Specificity, and Positive and Negative Predictive Values
N/A

Valid If Run in a Human Lab?
Yes.

CLINICAL PERSPECTIVE
- Hypernatremia occurs when renal or GI loss of water exceeds loss of Na or in situations of decreased water intake.

High values	Low values
Pseudohypernatremia	Pseudohyponatremia (normal plasma osmolality)
Dehydration	Severe hyperproteinemia or hyperlipemia if ion-specific electrodes not used
Na-containing anticoagulants	
Pure water deficit (normovolemia)	Hyperosmolar hyponatremia (translational)
Primary hypodipsia	Hyperglycemia
Diabetes insipidus (central or nephrogenic)	Mannitol therapy (or any addition of exogenous solutes)
High environmental temperature (e.g., heatstroke, hyperthermia)	Hypo-osmolar hyponatremia due to:
Fever	Reduced renal excretion of free water
Restricted access to drinking water	Normovolemia
Hypotonic fluid loss (hypovolemia)	Decreased dietary Na intake
Renal	Na deficient (hypotonic) fluids
Osmotic diuresis (e.g., mannitol, hyperglycemia)	Thiazides (causing both Na and K depletion)
Diuretic therapy (loop diuretics)	SIADH (syndrome of inappropriate ADH secretion)
Chronic renal failure	Myxedema coma in hypothyroid canines
Nonoliguric acute renal failure	Hypervolemia
Postobstruction diuresis	Congestive heart failure
Extrarenal	Cirrhosis
GI (e.g., vomiting, diarrhea, small-intestinal obstruction)	Nephrotic syndrome with effusion
Third-space losses (e.g., pancreatitis, peritonitis)	Late-stage renal disease
Cutaneous (thermal burns)	Hypovolemia/dehydration
Increased Na gain (hypervolemia)	Renal losses
Hypertonic fluid administration (e.g., hypertonic saline,	Adrenal insufficiency
Na bicarbonate, parenteral nutrition, Na phosphate enema)	Osmotic diuresis
Hyperaldosteronism	Renal tubular acidosis
Salt toxicity	Loop diuretics and thiazides
Hyperadrenocorticism	Extrarenal Na losses
	GI losses (e.g., vomiting, diarrhea)
	Third-space losses (e.g., peritonitis, pancreatitis, uroabdomen, pleural or peritoneal effusion)
	Repeated drainage of chylothorax
	Cutaneous losses (burns)
	Blood loss
	Increased water intake in excess of normal renal excretory potential
	Primary polydipsia
	Accidental (e.g., near drowning)

- Hyponatremia is typically caused by excessive free water retention or by excessive loss of Na from the urinary or GI (especially large bowel) tracts.
- If the Na/K ratio is <19, strongly consider hypoaldosteronism if there are clinical signs that increase the index of suspicion.
- An Na/K ratio of <24 may be consistent with hypoadrenocorticism, but a similar ratio may occur with trichuriasis, repeated drainage of chylothorax, cavitary effusion, or uroabdomen.
  - In the abdominal fluid, a creatinine concentration >2 times that of serum level is consistent with uroabdomen in a patient with a suspect clinical presentation.
  - A similar abnormality of the Na/K ratio may occur with ill dogs in late-term pregnancy. The exact mechanism is unknown, but may be the electrolyte derangement caused by aldosterone inhibition secondary to increased concentrations of serum progesterone (Schaer et al. 2001).
- SIADH is infrequently reported in veterinary medicine. Possible causes found commonly in human medicine include neoplasia (e.g., a common paraneoplastic syndrome found with lung cancer) and selected drug therapies (e.g., cytotoxic chemotherapies, opioids, NSAIDS, thiazides) and in number of pulmonary and CNS disorders.

MISCELLANEOUS

ANCILLARY TESTS
- Evaluation of K and chloride concentrations to rule out concurrent electrolyte derangements
- Evaluation of blood gas, anion gap, and osmolality
- An ACTH stimulation test to rule out hypoadrenocorticism
- Fecal flotation to rule out GI parasitism (especially trichuriasis)
- Urinary fractional excretion of Na to rule out renal tubular acidosis
- A water-deprivation test (modified) to rule out diabetes insipidus
- Fluid analysis of any effusion

SYNONYMS
None

SEE ALSO
Blackwell's Five-Minute Veterinary Consult: Canine and Feline Topics
- Diarrhea, Chronic—Cats
- Diarrhea, Chronic—Dogs

- Gastrointestinal Obstruction
- Hypoadrenocorticism (Addison's Disease)
- Renal Failure, Chronic
- Renal Tubular Acidosis
- Vomiting, Chronic

Related Topics in This Book
- ACTH Stimulation Test
- Chloride
- Fecal Flotation
- Urine Fractional Excretion of Electrolytes

ABBREVIATIONS
- ACTH = adrenocorticotropic hormone
- ADH = antidiuretic hormone
- ADP = adenosine tri phosphate
- ECF = extracellular fluid
- K = potassium
- Na = sodium
- SIADH = syndrome of inappropriate ADH secretion

Suggested Reading

DiBartola SP. Disorders of sodium and water. In: DiBartola SP, ed. *Fluid Therapy in Small Animal Practice*, 2nd ed. Philadelphia: WB Saunders, 1992: 45–72.

DiBartola SP, Green RA, de Morais HSA, Willard MD. Electrolyte and acid-base disorders. In: Willard MD, Tvedten H, eds. *Small Animal Clinical Diagnosis by Laboratory Methods*, 4th ed. Philadelphia: WB Saunders, 2004: 117–135.

Manning AM. Electrolyte disorders. *Vet Clin North Am Small Anim Pract* 2001; 31: 1289–1294.

Schaer M, Halling KB, Collins KE, Grant DC. Combined hyponatremia and hyperkalemia mimicking acute hypoadrenocorticism in three pregnant dogs. *J Am Vet Med Assoc* 2001; 218: 897–899.

INTERNET RESOURCES
Cornell University, College of Veterinary Medicine, Clinical Pathology Modules, Routine Blood Chemistry: Electrolyes, http://diaglab.vet.cornell.edu/clinpath/modules/chem/lytes.htm.

AUTHOR NAME
Maria Vandis

SOMATOMEDIN C

BASICS

TYPE OF SPECIMEN
Blood

TEST EXPLANATION AND RELATED PHYSIOLOGY
The anabolic and growth-promoting effects of growth hormone (GH) are mediated by insulin-like growth factor I (IGF-I [somatomedin C]), which plays an essential role in proliferation and differentiation of cells, including cartilage and muscle.

IGF-I secretion depends on plasma GH and can be used for diagnosis of disorders related to acromegaly or GH deficiency and dwarfism. The stability of plasma concentrations allows interpretation of a single sample in contrast with GH, which is secreted in a pulsatile fashion. In GH deficiency, low plasma IGF-I concentrations are found. Decreased IGF-I concentrations are also found after prolonged fasting (because of malnutrition) and untreated diabetes mellitus. GH excess as seen in acromegaly is accompanied with increased plasma IGF-I concentrations. Acromegaly in dogs is almost exclusively found in intact females as a result of excessive GH secretion by mammary glands during the progesterone-dominated phase of the sexual cycle or due to progestin treatment for estrus prevention. In hypothyroidism also, elevated plasma GH is found with subsequently higher IGF-I concentrations. In cats, acromegaly is caused by a GH-producing pituitary tumor.

The IGFs are bound with high affinity to 6 different IGF-binding proteins. For adequate measurement of total plasma IGF-I concentrations, IGFs have to be separated from IGF-binding proteins. Currently no validated assays for free IGF-I concentrations are available for dogs and cats.

INDICATIONS
- Acromegaly
- Dwarfism

CONTRAINDICATIONS
Long-term fasting

POTENTIAL COMPLICATIONS
None

CLIENT EDUCATION
Food should be withheld from the patient for at least 8 h before testing.

BODY SYSTEMS ASSESSED
- Dermatologic
- Endocrine and metabolic
- Reproductive

SAMPLE

COLLECTION
2 mL of venous blood

HANDLING
- Choice of collection tube depends on the assay used. Check with the laboratory prior to collection.
  - A red-top tube or serum-separator tube, heparin, or EDTA can each be used for radioimmunoassays.
  - Avoid the use of EDTA for chemiluminescent assays.
- Centrifuge the sample for 10 min at 1500 *g* within a few hours after collection.

STORAGE
Freeze samples until analysis.

STABILITY
- Room temperature: 24 h
- Frozen (−25°C): 1 year

PROTOCOL
None

INTERPRETATION

NORMAL FINDINGS OR RANGE
Reference intervals may vary depending on the laboratory and assay.

Dogs
IGF-I concentrations are related to age and body size, with higher values seen in young dogs and larger breeds. Examples include the following:
- Toy poodles: 15 µg/L
- Cocker spaniels: 36 +/− 27 µg/L
- Beagles: 87 +/− 33 µg/L
- Keeshonds: 117 +/− 34 µg/L
- German shepherds: 280 +/− 23 µg/L
- Immature German shepherds and Great Danes may have plasma IGF-I concentrations of up to 345 and 300 µg/L, respectively.

Cats
Plasma IGF-I concentrations vary between 200 and 800 µg/L, with a significant relation found between total plasma IGF-I concentration and body weight.

ABNORMAL VALUES
Values above or below the age-specific and breed-specific reference intervals

CRITICAL VALUES
None

INTERFERING FACTORS
Drugs That May Alter Results or Interpretation
Drugs That Interfere with Test Methodology
Treatment with recombinant human IGF-I

Drugs That Alter Physiology
Drugs that stimulate or inhibit GH release will indirectly influence plasma IGF-I concentrations:
- Progestins stimulate mammary GH secretion: IGF-I may increase from 46 +/− 10 to 296 +/− 35 µg/L in progestin-treated beagles.
- Glucocorticoids may inhibit pituitary GH release.

Disorders That May Alter Results
- Prolonged fasting
- Liver disease
- In untreated diabetic cats, decreased values of 170 µg/L are found (range, 13–433 µg/L).

Collection Techniques or Handling That May Alter Results
None

Influence of Signalment
Species
None

Breed
Dogs
- Adult plasma IGF-I concentrations are breed (body weight) specific.
- Dwarfism in German shepherds is an autosomal recessive inherited abnormality. Six-month-old dwarfs have IGF-I concentrations of approximately 62 +/− 10 µg/L.

Cats
No breed-specific information is available.

Age
Shortly after birth, IGF-I concentrations rise with maximal concentrations around puberty. Adults have lower concentrations, which further decrease with age.

Gender
Male dogs and cats have slightly higher concentrations than (anestrous) females.

Pregnancy
During periods of elevated plasma progesterone concentrations such as metestrus and (pseudo)pregnancy, plasma IGF-I concentrations are elevated.

LIMITATIONS OF THE TEST
Sensitivity, Specificity, and Positive and Negative Predictive Values
N/A

Valid If Run in a Human Lab?
Yes.

Causes of Abnormal Findings

High values	Low values
Acromegaly	GH deficiency
Hypothyroidism	Severe, prolonged malnutrition
Progestin treatment	Untreated diabetes mellitus
Pregnancy and pseudopregnancy	Liver disease

CLINICAL PERSPECTIVE
• In cats, IGF-I concentrations of >1,000 μg/L are consistent with acromegaly caused by a pituitary somatotroph adenoma.
• German shepherds with congenital dwarfism should have a blunted GH stimulation test result.

MISCELLANEOUS
ANCILLARY TESTS
• Evaluation of fasting blood glucose and fructosamine concentrations to rule out diabetes mellitus
• A GH stimulation test to confirm GH deficiency:

• Collect blood before and 20 min after administration of either 1 μg human GH-releasing hormone or 10 μg/kg of clonidine (Catapresan; Boehringer, Ingelheim, DE).
• Healthy (anestrous) dogs have basal GH concentrations of 1.92 +/− 0.14 μg/L, which increase to 5–20 μg/L by 20 min after stimulation.
• Dogs with congenital pituitary dwarfism usually show no rise in plasma GH concentrations.
• In cats with suspected acromegaly, measure GH (basal concentration should be elevated). Visualize the pituitary by computed tomography.

SYNONYMS
Insulin-like growth factor I (IGF-I)

SEE ALSO
Blackwell's Five-Minute Veterinary Consult: Canine and Feline Topics
• Acromegaly—Cats
• Growth Hormone–Responsive Dermatoses

Related Topics in This Book
None

ABBREVIATIONS
• GH = growth hormone
• IGF-I = insulin-like growth factor I

Suggested Reading
Reusch CE, Kley S, Casella M, *et al*. Measurements of growth hormone and insulin-like growth factor 1 in cats with diabetes mellitus. *Vet Rec* 2006; 11: 195–200.
Rijnberk A, Kooistra HS, Mol JA. Endocrine diseases in dogs and cats: Similarities and differences with endocrine diseases in humans. *Growth Horm IGF Res* 2003; 13(Suppl A): S158–S164.

INTERNET RESOURCES
Cancer Genetics Web: IGF1, http://www.cancerindex.org/geneweb/IGF1.htm#contents.
Camacho-Hübner, C. The growth hormone-insulin-like growth factor axis. In: Grossman A, ed. Neuroendocrinology, hypothalamus, and pituitary. 2006; Endotext.org: Your endocrine source, http://www.endotext.org/neuroendo/neuroendo5a/neuroendoframe5a.htm.

AUTHOR NAME
Jan A. Mol

SPLENIC ULTRASONOGRAPHY

BASICS

TYPE OF PROCEDURE
Ultrasonographic

PROCEDURE EXPLANATION AND RELATED PHYSIOLOGY
Splenic ultrasonography is useful for determining the size and location of the spleen, as well as for evaluating it for focal or diffuse parenchymal abnormalities. The spleen is a dynamic organ, particularly in dogs, and thus ultrasonography may be helpful when splenomegaly is suspected. Splenic ultrasonography is also particularly helpful in identifying the origin of mass lesions, as well as in providing a means of obtaining cytologic samples for more definitive diagnosis.

INDICATIONS
- Abdominal mass(es)
- Hemoperitoneum
- Splenomegaly
- Trauma

CONTRAINDICATIONS
None

POTENTIAL COMPLICATIONS
None

CLIENT EDUCATION
- This is a noninvasive study and is tolerated well by most animals.
- Withholding food is helpful in improving the quality of the study results.
- To obtain satisfactory results, the hair must be clipped in the area to be imaged.

BODY SYSTEMS ASSESSED
Hemic, lymphatic, and immune

PROCEDURE

PATIENT PREPARATION
Preprocedure Medication or Preparation
- Withhold food 12 h prior to examination to improve the quality of the study results.
- The hair must be clipped using a no. 40 blade, and acoustic coupling gel applied to the skin.

Anesthesia or Sedation
Most examinations may be performed without sedation or general anesthesia. However, these may be required in anxious animals or those in pain. Sedate or place the animal under general anesthesia as needed to control its motion.

Patient Positioning
The examination may be performed with animals in dorsal or lateral recumbency.

Patient Monitoring
None

Equipment or Supplies
- Clippers with a no. 40 blade
- Acoustic coupling gel
- A high-frequency transducer (>7.5 MHz) for examination of the body and tail of the spleen because they are usually superficial
- A midfrequency to low-frequency transducer (2–5 MHz) for examination of the head of the spleen. A sector/vector format is often useful because the head is usually located within the costal arch, so a small footprint is necessary. Image depth should be adjusted because the head is located in the ventral abdomen, whereas the body and tail are often superficially located in the ventral abdomen.

TECHNIQUE
The entire spleen should be evaluated in 2 planes: parasagittal and transverse. To visualize the head of the spleen, the probe must be oriented craniolaterally beneath the left costal arch. (Point the probe toward the left elbow.) The spleen head will be visualized just lateral to the stomach fundus, with the head located in the dorsal abdomen. The head is held in place by the gastrosplenic ligament and will move with the stomach fundus provided this ligament remains in tact. The body and tail of the spleen may be visualized by moving the probe and keeping the splenic parenchyma on the ultrasound screen. The tail of the spleen may be located along the left body wall or may traverse the abdomen and be found on the right side. The splenic veins can be seen as hypoechoic tubular structures entering the hilus of the spleen. Often, fat can be seen originating and infiltrating around the entrance of the splenic veins and should not be confused with a focal mass.

SAMPLE HANDLING
N/A

APPROPRIATE AFTERCARE
Postprocedure Patient Monitoring
None

Nursing Care
None

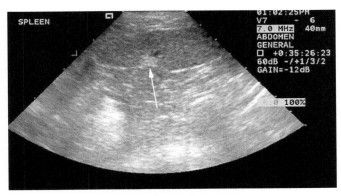

Figure 1

This is a parasagittal image of the body of the spleen. Notice the superficial location of the spleen and the fine, even echotexture. There is a small amount of fat adjacent to the splenic vein (*arrow*) that is not clinically significant.

Dietary Modification
Withhold food for 12 h prior to examination to improve the quality of the exam.

Medication Requirements
None

Restrictions on Activity
None

Anticipated Recovery Time
Immediate

 ## INTERPRETATION

NORMAL FINDINGS OR RANGE
The spleen is normally the most echogenic solid organ in the abdomen and has a fine echotexture. The margins should be smooth without evidence of masses. The splenic vasculature enters through the hilus, and the splenic veins are easily seen during gray-scale imaging. The splenic arteries may be identified by Doppler examination. Typically, the echogenicity of the spleen is compared to the cortex of the left kidney because they are often in close proximity: The spleen should be hyperechoic to the kidney cortex. Mild changes may be difficult to appreciate (Figure 1).

ABNORMAL VALUES
Diffuse Splenic Diseases
Most diffuse diseases cause overall enlargement and might alter the echogenicity. In general, ultrasonography may indicate enlargement or a change in echogenicity but is not specific for the exact cause of the infiltrate. A splenic aspirate is necessary to further define any potential changes.

Diseases to Consider for Diffuse Splenomegaly (Not Inclusive)
• *Splenic congestion*: This may cause normal hypoechoic or hyperechoic parenchyma. It may occur with changes in the systemic or portal circulation, hemolytic anemia, and administration of sedatives or anesthesia.
• *Splenic torsion*: This usually produces a diffusely hypoechoic spleen with multiple parallel echogenic lines. Splenic vein thrombosis may also cause a similar appearance (but can affect only a portion of the spleen). Doppler examination may be necessary to identify splenic vein thrombosis, although a thrombus may be visible on gray-scale images in some cases.
• *Infectious disease*: Systemic bacterial or fungal infection may cause splenomegaly but, in this author's experience, more often causes hypoechogenicity. However, a normal or hyperechoic spleen may also be seen.
• *Neoplasia*: Lymphoma, malignant histiocytosis, mastocytosis, or leukemia, and similar neoplasms may cause splenomegaly. Echogenic changes may be present (both hypoechogenicity and hyperechogenicity can be seen), but definitive diagnosis is not possible without cytologic examination of a splenic aspirate.

Diseases to Consider for Focal Splenomegaly (Masses)
• See Figures 2–5.
• *Hyperplastic nodules*: These are usually seen as isoechoic nodules or masses that may deform the splenic margin, and can also be hyper- or hypoechoic. If a nodule becomes large or if the vascular supply becomes compromised, a complex mass may be seen (cavitary). Differentiation of complex masses is not possible via ultrasonographic examination alone, so cytologic or histopathologic evaluation is necessary.
• *Neoplasia*: Hemangiosarcoma is one of the more common neoplasms of the spleen and is often seen as a large, complex cavitary mass of the splenic parenchyma. Other neoplasms, such as fibrosarcoma, osteosarcoma, and leiomyosarcoma, can also be seen. Peritoneal fluid may be seen in association with splenic neoplasia (often hemorrhage). Evaluation of other organs for metastasis should be attempted if neoplasia is suspected. In this author's experience, peritoneal or superficial metastasis may not be reliably noted during ultrasonography.
• *Abscesses*: These are usually difficult to differentiate from other focal lesions, although the presence of gas may shift abscess to the top differential diagnosis (hyperechoic foci with a discrete or "dirty" shadow).

SPLENIC ULTRASONOGRAPHY

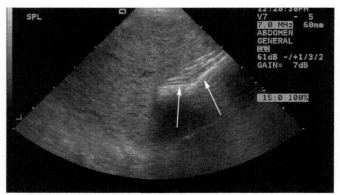

A

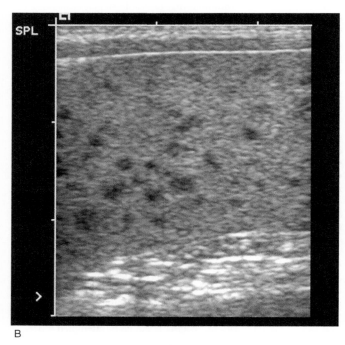

B

Figure 2

A: This is a parasagittal image of the head of the spleen of a dog. Notice the more dorsal location of this portion of the spleen and its location next to the stomach (*arrows*). There is a subtle change in the echotexture of the spleen, and it appears slightly coarser. **B:** This is a high-resolution image of the same spleen as in **A**. Notice the multiple hypoechoic areas scattered throughout the splenic parenchyma. Splenic aspiration was performed, and the cytologic diagnosis was lymphoma.

CRITICAL VALUES
A large splenic mass with hemoabdomen, splenic torsion, or extensive splenic vein thrombosis may warrant immediate surgery.

INTERFERING FACTORS
Drugs That May Alter Results of the Procedure
Opioids and some other sedatives, as well as general anesthesia, may cause splenic congestion and diffuse splenomegaly. Mild changes in echogenicity should be interpreted with caution when these drugs are administered.

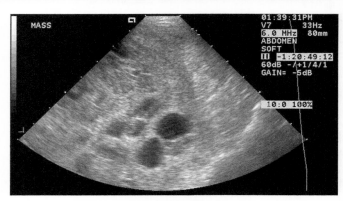

Figure 3

This is a parasagittal image of the tail of the spleen in a dog. Notice the multiple cavitations that are forming a mass in this portion of the spleen. The histopathologic diagnosis was hemangiosarcoma.

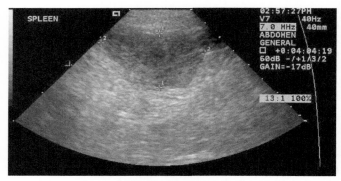

Figure 4

This is a parasagittal image of the body of the spleen in a dog. Notice the mass that is deforming the capsule and that the mass is similar in echogenicity to the rest of the spleen. This cytologic diagnosis after splenic aspirate was a hyperplastic nodule.

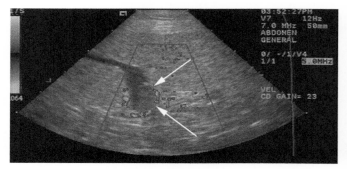

Figure 5

This is a parasagittal image of the body of the spleen in a dog. Notice the echogenic mass within the splenic vein (*arrows*), which is consistent with thrombosis.

Conditions That May Interfere with Performing the Procedure
None

Procedure Techniques or Handling That May Alter Results
None

Influence of Signalment on Performing and Interpreting the Procedure

Species
- Dogs: The spleen is more variable in size.
- Cats: The spleen is typically small and, in this author's experience, should not be more than 1 cm thick when imaged in a parasagittal plane.

Breed
None

Age
None

Gender
None

Pregnancy
None

CLINICAL PERSPECTIVE

Evaluation of the spleen should include assessment of the echogenicity of the splenic parenchyma, as well evaluation of the margins and focal enlargements. The spleen should be the most echogenic solid organ in the abdomen and have a fine echotexture. Ultrasonography is more sensitive than specific for disease etiology, so additional procedures such as splenic aspiration must be performed to define the cause of any changes that are observed.

 MISCELLANEOUS

ANCILLARY TESTS
Cytology of splenic aspirate

SYNONYMS
Splenic sonography

SEE ALSO

Blackwell's Five-Minute Veterinary Consult: Canine and Feline Topics
- Hemangiosarcoma, Spleen and Liver
- Splenic Torsion
- Splenomegaly

Related Topics in This Book
- General Principles of Ultrasonography
- Abdominal Ultrasonography
- Fine-Needle Aspiration
- Ultrasound-Guided Mass or Organ Aspiration

ABBREVIATIONS
None

Suggested Reading
Nyland TG, Mattoon JS, Herrgesell EJ, Wisner ER. Spleen. In: Nyland TG, Mattoon JS, eds. *Small Animal Diagnostic Ultrasound*, 2nd ed. Philadelphia: WB Saunders, 2002: 30–48.
O'Brien RT, Walker III KR, Osgood TL. Sonographic features of drug-induced splenic congestion. *Vet Radiol Ultrasound* 2004; 45: 225–227.
Sato MF, Solano M. Ultrasonographic findings in abdominal mast cell disease: A retrospective study of 19 patients. *Vet Radiol Ultrasound* 2004; 45: 51–57.
Saunders HM, Neath PJ, Brockman DJ. B-mode and Doppler ultrasound imaging of the spleen with canine splenic torsion: A retrospective evaluation. *Vet Radiol Ultrasound* 1998; 38: 349–353.

INTERNET RESOURCES
None

AUTHOR
Anne Bahr

T₃ SUPPRESSION TEST

BASICS

TYPE OF SPECIMEN
Blood

TEST EXPLANATION AND RELATED PHYSIOLOGY
During normal physiology, TRH released by the hypothalamus stimulates pituitary secretion of TSH, which, in turn, stimulates synthesis and secretion of T_4 from the thyroid gland. Active T_4 (and T_3) subsequently inhibits further TRH and TSH release, resulting in a decline in thyroid hormone levels (negative feedback inhibition). Feline hyperthyroidism is a disorder characterized by autonomous secretion of T_4 from a hyperplastic or adenomatous thyroid gland. Clinical signs are related to the thyrotoxic effects of excessive hormone and may include weight loss despite an excellent appetite, hyperexcitability, increased drinking and urination, and frequent vomiting. Diagnosis of feline hyperthyroidism is typically straightforward and consists of finding increased serum T_4 levels. However, some cats with signs suggestive of hyperthyroidism have T_4 levels within the reference interval or that are only slightly increased. This may occur in early disease or in the presence of a concurrent illness. Usually a second T_4 sample drawn days to weeks later is diagnostic, especially if a concurrent disease was successfully treated. Alternatively, a T_3 suppression test can be performed to aid in the definitive diagnosis of hyperthyroidism. In euthyroid cats, exogenously administered T_3 temporarily suppresses T_4 secretion, owing to intact feedback inhibition. In cats with hyperthyroidism, T_3 does not inhibit the autonomous secretion of T_4 from the hyperplastic or adenomatous gland.

INDICATIONS
Diagnosis of hyperthyroidism in cats with T_4 levels within the reference interval or only slightly increased

CONTRAINDICATIONS
Cats in which oral medications are contraindicated or not tolerated

POTENTIAL COMPLICATIONS
None

CLIENT EDUCATION
Oral medication must be successfully administered every 8 h for 7 doses. Failure to accomplish this renders the test invalid.

BODY SYSTEMS ASSESSED
Endocrine and metabolic

SAMPLE

COLLECTION
2.0 mL of venous blood at each time point

HANDLING
- Use a red-top tube. (Avoid the use of serum-separator tubes.)
- Spin and separate the serum.
- Refrigerate the serum sample and send it on ice packs to the laboratory.

STORAGE
Store the sample in a refrigerator or freezer.

STABILITY
- Room temperature: 5 days
- Refrigerated ($2°–8°C$): 2 weeks
- Frozen ($-20°C$): several months

PROTOCOL
- Draw blood for the baseline T_4 evaluation on day 1.

- Beginning the following morning, administer 25 μg of liothyronine (T_3) orally every 8 h for 7 doses (days 2–4). Liothyronine is available by prescription and is not licensed for use in cats.
- Draw blood for the T_4 evaluation 2–4 h after the final T_3 dose on day 4.
- Properly label the baseline and posttreatment samples and submit them to the laboratory.
- T_3 can be measured on both samples to confirm the successful administration of the tablets.

INTERPRETATION

NORMAL FINDINGS OR RANGE
Reference intervals may vary depending on the laboratory and assay.
Baseline
- T_4: 0.8–4.0 μg/dL (10.2–51.1 nmol/L)
- T_3: 32.5–130.0 ng/dL (0.5–2.0 nmol/L)

After Liothyronine Administration
- T_4: <1.5 μg/dL (<19.3 nmol/L) or <50% of the baseline
- T_3: increased over the baseline

ABNORMAL VALUES
- T_4 concentration after T_3 administration, >2.0 μg/dL (>25.7 nmol/L) or >65% of the baseline
- Failure of T_3 to increase over the baseline renders the test invalid.
- Inconclusive: T_4 concentration after T_3 administration, 1.5–2.0 μg/dL (19.3–25.7 nmol/L) or 50%–65% of the baseline

CRITICAL VALUES
None

INTERFERING FACTORS
Drugs That May Alter Results or Interpretation
Drugs That Interfere with Test Methodology
Levothyroxine (T_4)

Drugs That Alter Physiology
- Levothyroxine (T_4)
- Corticosteroids
- A number of medications can alter thyroid hormone levels in dogs. These drug effects have not been well characterized in cats.

Disorders That May Alter Results
Interference by hemolysis and lipemia is method dependent.

Collection Techniques or Handling That May Alter Results
- Prolonged storage at room temperature may falsely lower results.
- The use of serum-separator tubes is not recommended.

Influence of Signalment
Species
Primarily used in cats

Breed
None

Age
Hyperthyroidism is a disease of older cats.

Gender
None

Pregnancy
None

LIMITATIONS OF THE TEST
- The T_3 suppression test takes 4 days and depends on successful administration of oral medications.
- Its results may be inconclusive.

Sensitivity, Specificity, and Positive and Negative Predictive Values
N/A

Valid If Run in a Human Lab?
No—human assay lacks the necessary sensitivity to detect low T$_4$ levels.

Causes of Abnormal Results

Adequate suppression of T$_4$	Inadequate suppression of T$_4$
Normal thyroid function	Hyperthyroidism
	Failure to administer
	liothyronine properly

CLINICAL PERSPECTIVE
• The T$_3$ suppression test is used to diagnose hyperthyroidism in cats with consistent symptoms but in which T$_4$ levels are normal or only mildly increased, which may occur in cats with hyperthyroidism and concurrent disease.
• T$_3$ administration suppresses T$_4$ secretion in cats with normal thyroid function but will not suppress T$_4$ in cats with hyperthyroidism.
• An easier alternative is to retest T$_4$ in a few days or weeks or after concurrent disorders have been successfully treated.

MISCELLANEOUS

ANCILLARY TESTS
• Careful assessment of renal function is recommended prior to selecting treatment for hyperthyroidism. Resolution of the thyrotoxic state can worsen or unmask preexisting renal insufficiency.
• A TRH response test may be warranted in cats that are difficult to dose orally.

• The free T$_4$ test is more sensitive in detecting hyperthyroidism in mildly hyperthyroid cats than is a total T$_4$ measurement but occasionally has false-positive test results.
• Nuclear scintigraphy can be used to locate hyperplastic/adenomatous thyroid tissue prior to surgical treatment.

SYNONYMS
None

SEE ALSO
Blackwell's Five-Minute Veterinary Consult: Canine and Feline Topics
Hyperthyroidism
Related Topics in This Book
• Thyroid-Releasing Hormone Response Test
• Thyroxine (T$_4$), Free
• Thyroxine (T$_4$), Total

ABBREVIATIONS
• T$_3$ = triiodothyronine (hormone) or liothyronine (drug)
• T$_4$ = thyroxine, total (hormone) of levothyroxine (drug)
• TRH = thyroid-releasing hormone
• TSH = thyroid-stimulating hormone

Suggested Reading
Feldman EC, Nelson RW. Feline hyperthyroidism. In: Feldman EC, Nelson RW, eds. *Canine and Feline Endocrinology and Reproduction*, 3rd ed. St Louis: Saunders Elsevier, 2004: 86–151.

INTERNET RESOURCES
Bruyette D. Feline hyperthyroidism. In: Scherk M, ed. 26th Congress of the World Small Animal Veterinary Association (WSAVA), Vancouver, 2001, http://www.vin.com/VINDBPub/SearchPB/Proceedings/PR05000/PR00107.htm.
University of Georgia, College of Veterinary Medicine, Department of Pathology, Veterinary Clinical Pathology Clerkship Program: Stortz JS, Latimer KS, Tarpley HL, et al. 2004. Feline hyperthyroidism, http://www.vet.uga.edu/vpp/clerk/stortz.

AUTHOR NAME
Kristen R. Friedrichs

TAURINE

BASICS

TYPE OF SPECIMEN
Blood
Pet food
Tissue
Urine

TEST EXPLANATION AND RELATED PHYSIOLOGY
Taurine is a sulfur-containing amino acid. Unlike most other amino acids, it is not incorporated into proteins but rather remains as 1 of the most abundant free amino acids in the body. It is found in highest concentrations in cardiac muscle, skeletal muscle, central nervous system, WBCs, and platelets.

Taurine is involved with numerous metabolic processes, including retinal photoreceptor activity, development of the nervous system and stabilization of neural membranes, reduction in platelet aggregation, antioxidation, and reproduction. It plays a role in conjugation of bile acids and detoxification of xenobiotics via conjugation and excretion in bile. Taurine is also essential for normal myocardial function. Although the mechanisms underlying its effect on the heart remain unknown, evidence suggests that taurine plays a role in modulation of tissue calcium concentrations and availability, as well as inactivation of free radicals, membrane stabilization, and maintenance of osmolarity. Taurine deficiency can be associated with retinal degeneration, reproductive failure, growth retardation, and dilated cardiomyopathy.

Dietary taurine can be obtained primarily through animal-protein sources. Plant proteins are almost completely devoid of taurine. Taurine can also be synthesized from the precursor amino acids cysteine and methionine; however, the rate of synthesis varies within tissues and among species. For example, cats cannot synthesize adequate amounts of taurine, and therefore taurine is an essential amino acid in cats and must be provided in their diet. Taurine is a conditionally essential amino acid in dogs. Dogs generally can synthesize adequate quantities of taurine; in certain situations, however, synthesis is inadequate, and dietary taurine must be provided.

INDICATIONS
• Dilated cardiomyopathy
• Reproductive failure
• Retinal degeneration

CONTRAINDICATIONS
None

POTENTIAL COMPLICATIONS
None

CLIENT EDUCATION
• Collect the blood sample after the patient has fasted overnight.
• Assessment of both plasma and whole-blood taurine concentration provides the most accurate estimate of taurine status. If not possible, whole-blood taurine appears to be the best single measure.
• Taurine is inexpensive and safe to administer. If purchased through a health food store, the U.S. Pharmacopeia (USP) verification on the label ensures the purity of the ingredients.

BODY SYSTEMS ASSESSED
• Cardiovascular
• Ophthalmic
• Reproductive

SAMPLE

COLLECTION
• Venous blood: >1.5 mL is collected after the patient has fasted overnight. More is required when measuring both plasma and whole-blood taurine.
• Urine: >1 mL
• Pet foods: >10 g
• Skeletal and cardiac muscle: Contact the lab for a minimum sample size.

HANDLING
Plasma and Whole-Blood Taurine
• Heparin preferred (green top) or EDTA (purple top) tubes or a heparin-coated syringe
• When using a heparin-coated syringe
  • Remove the needle from patient's vein and draw an additional 1 mL of air into the syringe for mixing space in the syringe.
  • Remove the rubber stopper from green-top tube to reduce the risk of hemolyzing the sample.
• For plasma taurine determination
  • Immediately centrifuge the blood, separate the plasma from cells, and immediately freeze it (−70°C freezer, if available). Be careful to avoid contaminating the plasma with cells from the buffy coat. If the sample is hemolyzed, consider drawing a new sample.

- If centrifugation will be delayed, immediately place the glass blood tube on wet ice to decrease the chance of blood cells sticking to the glass and releasing taurine.

Urine
- 24-h urine collection
  - A sample from 24-h urine collection is required for measuring all 3 fractions of urine taurine (bound, unbound, total).
  - Pool the entire 24-h urine sample and then transfer a small aliquot (≥1 mL) into a plastic tube and freeze it until shipped.
- Fractional excretion of unbound and total taurine concentrations
  - Collect the sample after the patient has fasted overnight.
  - Transfer a small aliquot (≥1 mL) into a plastic tube and freeze it until shipped.
- Unbound and total taurine urine taurine/urine creatinine ratio
  - Collect the sample after the patient has fasted overnight.
  - Transfer a small aliquot (≥1 mL) into a plastic tube and freeze it until shipped.

Cardiac Muscle and Skeletal Muscle
Obtain a cardiac muscle sample by endomyocardial biopsy. Obtain a percutaneous skeletal muscle biopsy sample of cranial tibial muscle.

Ship Samples by Overnight Express Mail
- Plasma and whole blood can be shipped unfrozen on cold packs if shipped on the same day it is collected. Otherwise, ship samples frozen with cold packs on dry ice.
- Urine should be frozen immediately and shipped frozen.

STORAGE
- Store the plasma and/or whole blood in a refrigerator (2°–8°C) if the sample is being shipped on the day of collection.
- Freeze (−20°C) the plasma and/or whole blood in plastic tubes for storage overnight or longer.
- Freeze the urine immediately and keep it frozen during shipment.

STABILITY
- Samples are not stable at room temperature.
- Plasma and whole blood
  - Refrigerated (2°–8°C): 1 day
  - Frozen (−20°C): at least 3 months
- Store plasma, whole-blood, and urine taurine samples in an ultra-cold (−70°C) freezer for storage for >3 months.

PROTOCOL
24-h urine taurine collection
- Weigh dogs after emptying their urinary bladder. Collect their urine over the next 24 h.

- Record the total time for collection to the nearest minute.
- During the 24-h urine collection, freeze the samples collected. Briefly thaw and pool all samples at end of collection.
- Transfer >1 mL of pooled urine into a plastic tube and immediately freeze the sample until analyzed.

INTERPRETATION

NORMAL FINDINGS OR RANGE
- Dogs
  - Plasma, 60–120 nmol/mL
  - Whole blood, 200–350 nmol/mL
- Cats
  - Plasma, 60–120 nmol/mL
  - Whole blood, 300–600 nmol/mL
- Reference intervals may vary depending on the laboratory.

ABNORMAL VALUES
- Dogs
  - Plasma, <40 nmol/mL
  - Whole blood, <150 nmol/mL
- Cats
  - Plasma, <40 nmol/mL
  - Whole blood, <200 nmol/mL

CRITICAL VALUES
None

INTERFERING FACTORS
Drugs That May Alter Results or Interpretation
Drugs That Interfere with Test Methodology
None

Drugs That Alter Physiology
In cats (but not dogs), administration of antibiotics decreases fecal excretion of taurine and increases plasma and whole-blood taurine concentrations.

Disorders That May Alter Results
- Prolonged fasting in cats (>1 day) can produce plasma taurine levels below the reference range. Since cats cannot synthesize adequate quantities of taurine, plasma levels of taurine fall rapidly in fasting cats without a steady dietary source of taurine. Although whole-blood taurine levels also decrease during fasting, the decrease is not as severe.

TAURINE

• A significant postprandial increase in plasma, but not whole-blood, taurine concentration occurs in cats within 2 h of consuming a meal containing taurine.

• In dogs, plasma and whole-blood taurine concentrations are not affected by a recent meal or prolonged fasting. Dogs can synthesize taurine if dietary intake of taurine is inadequate.

• Cystinuria in dogs may decrease their plasma and whole-blood taurine concentrations.

• Cysteine is used to synthesize taurine endogenously, and it is theorized that excessive renal loss of cysteine may decrease endogenous taurine synthesis.

• In cats and dogs, taurine deficiency has been associated with diets that contain lamb or lamb meal and rice.

• In dogs, taurine deficiency has been associated with protein-restricted diets.

Collection Techniques or Handling That May Alter Results

• Type of anticoagulant used
  • Heparin is preferred and has been used to establish most reference ranges for cats and dogs.
  • Plasma taurine concentration is higher with heparin than with sodium citrate administration.

• Hemolysis falsely increases plasma, but not whole-blood, taurine concentration.

• Plasma taurine concentration increased by contamination with cells from the buffy coat or failure to immediately separate plasma from blood potentially leads to the spontaneous rupture of platelets.

• Hematuria may falsely increase urine taurine concentration.

• Refrigerating urine samples fails to prevent bacteria overgrowth, which could possibly alter results. Taurine is catabolized by a variety of microorganisms.

Influence of Signalment

Species

• Taurine is an essential amino acid in cats. Inadequate dietary intake of taurine can cause taurine deficiency.

• Cats are obligate carnivores. Therefore, their plasma and whole-blood taurine concentrations are usually higher than those of dogs.

• Taurine is not an essential amino acid in dogs, but taurine can become a conditionally essential amino acid.

Breed

• All breeds of cats can develop taurine deficiency from inadequate dietary taurine intake.

• Consider evaluating plasma and whole-blood taurine concentrations in any atypical breeds of dogs that develop dilated cardiomyopathy.

• Dog breeds with an association between taurine deficiency and dilated cardiomyopathy include American cocker spaniels, Newfoundlands, golden retrievers, Labrador retrievers, Dalmatians, English bulldogs, and Portuguese water dogs.

Age
None

Gender
Adult male cats may be at greater risk of developing taurine deficiency than adult female cats.

Pregnancy
Unknown

LIMITATIONS OF THE TEST
Unbound and total urine taurine fractional excretion and unbound and total urine taurine/creatinine ratios correlate well with 24-h urine taurine excretion in dogs. There is poor correlation for bound urine taurine. The same comparisons have not been evaluated in cats.

Sensitivity, Specificity, and Positive and Negative Predictive Values
N/A

Valid If Run in a Human Lab?
Yes—if appropriate methodology (e. g., an amino acid analyzer) is used.

Causes of Abnormal Findings

High plasma taurine values	Low plasma taurine values
Hemolysis	Prolonged (>1 day) fasting in cats
Contamination of sample with buffy coat	Dietary deficiency
Failure to centrifuge plasma sample immediately	
Cats receiving antibiotics	
Postprandial increase in cats within 2 h of consuming a taurine-content meal	

CLINICAL PERSPECTIVE
• Consider taurine deficiency in all cats with dilated cardiomyopathy.
• Consider dietary taurine deficiency as a potential cause of dilated cardiomyopathy in cats consuming improperly formulated homemade diets, boiled-meat diets, dog foods, or vegetarian diets.

- Consider taurine deficiency in atypical dog breeds with dilated cardiomyopathy.
- Consider taurine deficiency in any dog or cat breeds that develop dilated cardiomyopathy when consuming a diet of lamb meal and rice, a diet of lamb and rice, a vegetarian diet, or a protein-restricted diet not supplemented with taurine.
- Simultaneously evaluating plasma and whole-blood taurine concentrations appears to provide a better indicator of muscle taurine levels than evaluating either test alone.
- Analysis of skeletal or cardiac taurine samples is primarily limited to research situations and rarely would be indicated in clinical patients. Several studies in cats suggest that plasma or whole-blood taurine concentrations are correlated to muscle taurine concentrations.

MISCELLANEOUS

ANCILLARY TESTS
- Echocardiography: Diagnosis of dilated cardiomyopathy in all cats and certain breeds of dogs should increase the index of suspicion for taurine deficiency.
- Fundic exam: Evidence of degenerative retinopathy should increase the index of suspicion for taurine deficiency.

SYNONYMS
None

SEE ALSO
Blackwell's Five-Minute Veterinary Consult: Canine and Feline Topics
- Dilated Cardiomyopathy
- Retinal Degeneration
- Taurine Deficiency

Related Topics in This Book
- Carnitine
- Echocardiography

ABBREVIATIONS
None

Suggested Reading

Backus RC, Cohen GL, Pion PD, *et al.* Taurine deficiency in Newfoundlands fed commercially available complete and balanced diets. *J Am Vet Med Assoc* 2003; **223**: 1130–1136.

Fascetti AJ, Reed JR, Rogers QR, Backus RC. Taurine deficiency in dogs with dilated cardiomyopathy: 12 cases (1997–2001). *J Am Vet Med Assoc* 2003; **223**: 1137–1141.

Pion PD, Sanderson SL, Kittleson MD. The effectiveness of taurine and levocarnitine in dogs with heart disease. *Vet Clin North Am Small Anim Pract* 1998; **28**: 1495–1514.

INTERNET RESOURCES
None

AUTHOR NAME
Sherry Lynn Sanderson

TESTOSTERONE

BASICS

TYPE OF SPECIMEN
Blood

TEST EXPLANATION AND RELATED PHYSIOLOGY
Testosterone is produced by the interstitial (Leydig) cells of the testis under the control of hypothalamic gonadotropin-releasing hormone (GnRH) and pituitary luteinizing hormone (LH). In turn, testosterone feedback regulates GnRH and gonadotropin secretion. Testosterone is secreted in a pulsatile manner with pulses about every 80 min in male dogs. There is also a diurnal rhythm, with lowest concentrations in the morning. In cats, nadir concentrations may be below detectable levels. Testosterone has local effects and is also the major androgen in circulation. It also serves as a prohormone and may be converted by 5α-reductase to dihydrotestosterone or aromatized to estradiol-17β. These hormones also act locally at the tissue of origin, or they may enter circulation and act elsewhere. Testosterone causes differentiation of the Wolffian ducts, initiates and maintains spermatogenesis, and supports libido. Dihydrotestosterone causes virilization of external genitalia, prostate development, and development of masculine secondary sex characteristics at puberty.

Assays (RIA and chemiluminescent immunoassay) measure total testosterone, including both free and protein-bound hormone. There is little cross-reactivity (<5%) between the testosterone RIA and dihydrotestosterone. Because of its pulsatile secretion, stimulation tests are usually recommended over a single, random testosterone determination. An alternative would be to obtain serial samples through a pulse cycle; for example, every 20 min for 4 samples.

INDICATIONS
- To assess testicular function
- To differentiate bilateral cryptorchidism from previous castration
- To evaluate intersex animals

CONTRAINDICATIONS
None

POTENTIAL COMPLICATIONS
None

CLIENT EDUCATION
- Cryptorchid testes produce testosterone but not sperm. Affected males have typical masculine appearance and behavior despite the cryptorchid testicle(s) being sterile.
- Testosterone deficiency is rarely a cause of acquired infertility in dogs or cats.
- Congenital hypogonadism is associated with abnormally small testes, testicular dysfunction, and/or hypothalamic or gonadotropin dysfunction.

BODY SYSTEMS ASSESSED
Reproductive

SAMPLE

COLLECTION
1–2 mL of venous blood

HANDLING
- Use a plain red-top tube. (Avoid the use of serum-separator tubes.)
- Centrifuge and harvest the serum within 1 h.

STORAGE
Refrigerate or freeze the sample.

STABILITY
- Refrigerated (2°–8°C): ≈1 week
- Frozen (−20°C): ≈2 months

PROTOCOL
Variable. Consult the laboratory for the recommended protocol.
- Collect blood for a basal sample.
- Collect blood after administration of either human chorionic gonadotropin (hCG) or GnRH:
  - Protocol 1 (dogs and cats): 2–4 h after 40–50 IU/kg hCG IM
  - Protocol 2 (cats): 4 h after 250 IU/cat, hCG IM
  - Protocol 3 (dogs): 1 h after 0.22 μg/kg GnRH IV
  - Protocol 4 (dogs): 1 h after 1.0–2.2 μg/kg, GnRH IM
  - Protocol 5 (cats): 1 h after 25 μg/cat GnRH IM

INTERPRETATION

NORMAL FINDINGS OR RANGE
- Reference intervals vary tremendously among laboratories and protocols. Consultation is essential to proper interpretation.
- A high serum testosterone concentration indicates the presence of at least 1 testicle.
- At its nadir, the testosterone concentration in normal, and sexually intact male dogs and cats may overlap the reference range for castrated animals. However, testosterone significantly increases following administration of hCG or GnRH to intact males, including those that are cryptorchid or have had unilateral orchiectomy, whereas it does not increase in castrated animals. Reference ranges for castrated animals are generally 0 to <0.5 nmol.

ABNORMAL VALUES
Concentrations above the reference interval in a supposedly castrated animal

CRITICAL VALUES
None

INTERFERING FACTORS
Drugs That May Alter Results or Interpretation
Drugs That Interfere with Test Methodology
Testosterone RIA has high cross-reactivity (20%) with certain estrens and with nortestosterone.

Drugs That Alter Physiology
Progestins, estrogen, and testosterone suppress GnRH or LH and therefore testosterone.

Disorders That May Alter Results
- Castration causes an immediate drop in serum testosterone.
- Estrogen-producing testicular tumor
- Severe malnutrition
- Intersex conditions

Collection Techniques or Handling That May Alter Results
- Use of serum-separator tubes
- Failure to separate serum rapidly from RBCs

Influence of Signalment
Species
None

Breed
None

Age
Adult

Gender
Used to determine presence or absence of testicles

Pregnancy
Intersex animals are rarely fertile.

LIMITATIONS OF THE TEST
Sensitivity, Specificity, and Positive and Negative Predictive Values
A single, random, low value has no reliable diagnostic value.

Valid If Run in a Human Lab?
Yes, if the methodology has been validated for dogs and cats.

CLINICAL PERSPECTIVE
Low serum testosterone concentrations after hCG or GnRH administration to an otherwise healthy male indicate an absence of functional Leydig cells, which is consistent with castration.

MISCELLANEOUS

ANCILLARY TESTS
• Physical examination
  • Examine for testicle(s) in the scrotum or external inguinal area.
  • Examine the feline penis for presence of penile spines, which are androgen dependent and atrophy following castration.
  • The canine prostate is androgen dependent and involutes within weeks of castration. A normal-sized prostate gland in a supposedly castrated dog suggests either prostatic neoplasia or a retained testicle(s).

• Serum LH will be high in a castrated animal because negative feedback from testosterone is absent.
• Ultrasonography to locate cryptorchid testes

SYNONYMS
None

SEE ALSO
Blackwell's Five-Minute Veterinary Consult: Canine and Feline Topics
• Hyperandrogenism
• Infertility, Male—Dogs

Related Topics in This Book
• Abdominal Ultrasonography
• Luteinizing Hormone
• Semen Analysis

ABBREVIATIONS
• GnRH = gonadotropin-releasing hormone
• hCG = human chorionic gonadotropin
• LH = luteinizing hormone
• RIA = radioimmunoassay

Suggested Reading
Johnston SD, Root Kustritz MV, Olson PN. *Canine and Feline Theriogenology*. Philadelphia: WB Saunders, 2001.

INTERNET RESOURCES
None

AUTHOR NAME
Cheri A. Johnson

THORACIC RADIOGRAPHY

BASICS

TYPE OF PROCEDURE
Radiographic

PROCEDURE EXPLANATION AND RELATED PHYSIOLOGY
The differential absorption of X-ray photons by different tissue types within patients is what generates radiographic contrast. The thorax is well suited to imaging using ionizing radiation (radiography and CT), primarily because of the presence of air within the lungs. Other imaging technologies [diagnostic ultrasonography, magnetic resonance imaging (MRI), and nuclear medicine], though all very useful in specific intrathoracic diseases, do not provide as good an overview of thoracic pathology as do radiography and CT. Because radiographs are a 2-dimensional images of a 3-dimensional object, orthogonal (perpendicular) radiographs should be obtained. Atelectasis associated with recumbency necessitates that both lateral radiographs, in addition to an orthogonal VD or DV view, be obtained for an optimal exam. There are many situations in which both a DV view and a VD view should be considered. Collimation, adequate positioning, and selection of an optimum film/screen system or digital device are important in maximizing image quality. With respect to film/screen systems, standardization of processing parameters is important. If possible, thoracic radiographs should be acquired without patient sedation because sedation affects lung aeration and the conspicuity of pulmonary pathology. The thorax is a complex moving structure, so a radiograph taken at peak inspiration can look very different from a radiograph taken milliseconds later at peak expiration. One must realize that a single radiograph is only a "snapshot in time" and may not reflect intrathoracic physiology completely. The thorax also lends itself to digital imaging. The superior image latitude and ability to manipulate the images digitally during review are significant advantages of this technology.

INDICATIONS
- Assessment of cardiopulmonary anatomy and physiology
- Tumor staging
- Congenital or acquired heart disease
- Exercise intolerance
- Cough
- Evaluate for pulmonary metastases
- Esophageal disorders
- Mediastinal masses
- Chest wall mass or asymmetry
- Trauma

CONTRAINDICATIONS
There are no specific contraindications to thoracic radiography, though patients with severe cardiovascular compromise and spinal injuries should be handled with caution.

POTENTIAL COMPLICATIONS
- Cardiopulmonary decompensation of compromised patients because of physical or chemical restraint and forced positioning
- Exacerbation of spinal and severe orthopedic injuries by physical manipulation

CLIENT EDUCATION
- Veterinary patient radiation exposure from diagnostic radiography is clinically insignificant and highly unlikely to result in complications.
- Physical and chemical restraint of patients with severe cardiopulmonary function or spinal or severe orthopedic disease can exacerbate signs.
- In some situations, sedation may be required to enable optimal positioning and reduce patient stress.

BODY SYSTEMS ASSESSED
- Cardiovascular
- Hemic, lymphatic, and immune
- Respiratory

PROCEDURE

PATIENT PREPARATION
Preprocedure Medication or Preparation
- Assess patients for cardiopulmonary status and possible spinal instability.
- Unnecessary bandage material around the thorax should be removed.
- Collars and harnesses should be removed.
- Thoracic drainage tubes should be secured adequately to prevent accidental pullout during patient manipulation.
- Recumbent patients should be placed in sternal recumbency to enable optimal pulmonary aeration at least 10 min before radiography.
- Ideally, sedation should be avoided or minimized immediately before the procedure if it is not being used specifically for restraint during the procedure.

Anesthesia or Sedation
- Anesthesia and sedation can have a significant impact on the appearance of thoracic radiographs. All forms of chemical restraint potentially decrease lung aeration, and this can affect the conspicuity of pulmonary pathology. In addition, the apparent size of the heart alters relative to thoracic excursion, and drugs that cause bradycardia can make the heart appear larger than normal because of increased chamber filling.
- The decision to use anesthesia or sedation depends on many factors. Some state regulations in the United States prohibit radiographic personnel from physically restraining veterinary patients during radiography. Some practices make the decision not to directly engage personnel in patient restraint for radiation safety reasons. In these situations, physical restraint by ropes, tape, or sandbags is sometimes augmented by chemical restraint.
- When chemical restraint results in loss of the gag reflex, intubation is mandatory. When general anesthesia is used, positive pressure ventilation during the radiographic procedure should be employed to achieve optimal lung aeration. Anesthesia should be induced with the patient in sternal recumbency, and the patient should remain sternal where possible during the procedure. The time between induction and radiography should be minimized. The interpretation of screening thoracic radiographs made at the end of, or after another radiographic procedure may be complicated by variable degrees of pulmonary atelectasis and secondary mediastinal shift.

Patient Positioning
- The optimum radiographic study of the thorax comprises a minimum of 3 views: 2 lateral views and 1 orthogonal view. Ensuring the patient is straight is extremely important and often overlooked.
  - *Left lateral view*: The patient lies in left lateral recumbency. The radiographic beam enters the right side of the thorax (right to left, R-L lateral view—abbreviated to *left lateral view*).
  - *Right lateral view*: The patient lies in right lateral recumbency. The radiographic beam enters the left side of the thorax (left to right, L-R lateral view—abbreviated to *right lateral view*).
  - *VD view*: The patient is placed in dorsal recumbency. The radiographic beam enters the patient ventrally and exits dorsally.
  - *DV view*: The patient is placed in sternal recumbency. The radiographic beam enters the patient dorsally and exits ventrally.
- Patients are usually easier to position for a VD view as compared to a DV view, especially if the patient has hip osteoarthritis. However, the use of this view should be avoided in patients with severe

cardiopulmonary pathology, including large volumes of pleural fluid, because cardiopulmonary decompensation can result.
• The area imaged should extend from the level of the shoulder joints to at least the T12 vertebra. On the lateral views, the caudodorsal rib heads should be superimposed on each other. This is most easily effected by elevating the sternum to the same height as the spine with a small piece of nonradiopaque padding (e.g., foam pad). The sternum may need to be rolled toward the table rather than elevated in brachycephalic breeds or animals with a dorsoventrally compressed thorax. The forelimbs should be pulled cranially, and the head and neck slightly extended. The central beam (crosshairs) should be placed just caudal to the caudal aspect of the scapula in dogs and ≈1 inch (≈2.54 cm) caudal to that point in cats. Ventral flexion of the head and neck often results in dorsal displacement of the intrathoracic trachea, giving the false impression of a ventral cranial mediastinal mass.

Patient Monitoring
Sedated patients should be monitored. Patients should be returned to sternal recumbency between exposures to minimize recumbency-related atelectasis.

Equipment or Supplies
• All other factors being equal, with respect to thoracic radiographs, motion artifact and suboptimal patient positioning are the most common factors limiting the consistent production of good-quality images. Low-mA techniques (low-power machines) require a longer exposure time for a given mAs (mA × time in seconds = mAs). This increases the chances of motion artifact (radiographic blur), which is most critical in the thorax. Conveniently, the thorax has high inherent subject contrast and thus is well suited to a high-kVp technique, and this allows mAs to be kept at a minimum. Despite this, exposure time remains a significant limiting factor in thoracic radiography, and one should give preference to the purchase of equipment with a high-kVp output (125 or 150 kVp) and high mA output (300 mA or more). These machines often require more than single-phase power. High-frequency generators produce a more energetic beam than conventional generators and are preferred.
• As with all radiographic studies, a well-maintained automatic processor, appropriate film handling, and a modern film/screen system will eliminate many variables that adversely affect image quality.
• The selection of film type is important.
• Scatter (unwanted photons causing film exposure) is best controlled by the use of a grid. A grid should be used when patient thickness is >10 cm.
• There has been a dramatic upsurge in the adoption of digital imaging systems in the veterinary profession in recent years. This technology is extremely variable in price and image quality, so one should investigate a product and the vendor thoroughly before purchase is considered.

TECHNIQUE
• Thoracic radiographs should be made with a high kVp, at the maximal mA station available, and using as brief an exposure time as possible. The exposure should be made during peak inspiration to ensure optimal lung aeration. This affords the best opportunity to see most pulmonary pathology. Air within the lung provides the radiographic contrast needed to see most types of parenchymal pathology. The "down" lung in a lateral view is often minimally aerated, which often obscures pathology in that hemithorax. Acquiring both recumbent lateral views minimizes this problem.
• If pneumothorax or lung bullae are suspected but cannot be confirmed, repeat radiographs should be made at peak expiration. The reduced volume of air in the lung during peak expiration results in increased lung opacity increasing the conspicuity of any air trapped in the pleural space or in bullae.
• Positional radiographs made with a horizontal beam can be used to help gravitate fluid away from a region of interest to help in differentiating between mass or fluid.

• Repeat radiographs, made after removal of pleural fluid, will enable better assessment of an underlying cause for the fluid and the presence of concurrent pathology.
• A radiographic technique chart should be maintained and used to calculate the optimum machine settings. Variable kVp techniques are most commonly employed in veterinary medicine because they enable more exposure variation.
• If a radiograph is useful, but either too dark or too light, use the 10% rule: If too dark, decrease the kVp by 10%. If too light, increase the kVp by 10%.

SAMPLE HANDLING
• Radiographs are medicolegal documents and should be adequately permanently identified.
• Analog images should be permanently identified with the patient name, date of imaging, and clinic name.
• Digital radiographic images should be identified and stored using the medical image file format known as DICOM (Digital Imaging and COmmunications in Medicine).
• Radiographic images are part of the patient medical record and should be stored according to local regulations.

APPROPRIATE AFTERCARE
Postprocedure Patient Monitoring
Patients with severe cardiopulmonary compromise should be returned to the most comfortable position as soon as the exposure is made.

Nursing Care
None

Dietary Modification
None

Medication Requirements
None

Restrictions on Activity
None

Anticipated Recovery Time
Sedated patients will recover relative to the drugs and dose administered. As radiographic examinations are relatively quick, consideration should be given to the use of reversible agents.

INTERPRETATION
NORMAL FINDINGS OR RANGE
• Thoracic radiographs are probably more difficult to interpret than radiographs of any other region. Many texts include images of normal radiographic anatomy. An understanding of normal anatomy is essential before an effective radiographic interpretation is possible. Such resources should be readily available. Consideration should be given to maintaining a reference file of normal studies and of studies showing common pathology.
• The viewing environment is particularly important. Analog radiographs should be viewed on good-quality viewboxes in a quiet room with control of ambient lighting. Digital images should be viewed on well-calibrated monitors of adequate size, brightness, and pixel density.
• Radiographs should not be interpreted hastily. Sufficient time and attention should be dedicated to the exam. A systematic approach to radiographic evaluation is paramount to prevent important anomalies being overlooked.
• The radiographic exam should be assessed for radiographic quality before beginning interpretation. The initial radiographic evaluation should address such issues as the following:
  • Are there sufficient views? Is patient positioning adequate?
  • Are the images adequately identified? Are there any artifacts?
  • Is there sufficient contrast and detail? Is there sufficient film blackness?

- "Snapshot in time": Does the study accurately reflect the state of the thorax? Radiographs made at peak inspiration will not show dynamic principal bronchial or intrathoracic collapse. One must ensure that the clinical question has been answered. If the patient has a dry honking cough, exacerbated by excitement, radiographs made at peak expiration or during a coughing fit will probably be necessary to rule out bronchial or tracheal collapse.
- Recumbency has a profound effect on cardiopulmonary physiology, resulting in differences in the appearance of R and L lateral and DV and VD radiographs. Recumbency reduces aeration of the down lung. This reduces lesion conspicuity in the dependent hemithorax (silhouette sign). This is most pronounced when patients are in lateral recumbency but also occurs when in dorsal recumbency.
- Recumbent atelectasis is exacerbated by sedation, anesthesia, and patient size. To minimize this effect, take radiographs with the patient at full inspiration, minimize sedation, use positive pressure ventilation when the patient is anesthetized, make both lateral radiographs, and if necessary, a VD projection and a DV projection.
- *Right lateral recumbency*: The crura are parallel, the right crus cranial, there is more heart to sternal contact, the caudal vena cava inserts into the caudal aspect of heart, the cranial lobe vessels cross each other, the left lung is better visualized, and air is usually present in the gastric fundus.
- *Left lateral recumbency*: The crura diverge, the left crus is more cranial, and there is less heart to sternal contact compared to the right lateral view. The cranial lobe vessels are parallel, the right lung is better visualized, and air is usually in the pylorus. The cranial lobe-vessel-bronchus triad is more easily seen in the left lateral projection. In this projection, the right cranial lobe vessels are ventral, with the vein from the right cranial lung lobe always being the most ventral structure.
- The cranial lobe vessels are usually equal in size to the width of 4th rib at its most narrow point.
- *VD recumbency*: The crura have a convex appearance, and the descending aorta is more visible. One can usually detect smaller amounts of pleural fluid and see the heart better when large amounts of fluid are present. The cardiac silhouette is elongated and narrow, there is more space between the heart and diaphragm, and the caudal vena cava and accessory lung lobe appear larger.
- *DV recumbency*: The diaphragm has a dome appearance, the caudal lobar vessels are visualized better, the cardiac silhouette is readily obscured by fluid, and the cardiac silhouette is shorter, more oval, and more prone to cardiac apex shift.
- "Down" (recumbent) lung anatomy rises relative to "up" lung. This can be used to help differentiate the side of lesion and is the reason why the right cranial lobe vessels often cross the left cranial lobe vessels in the right lateral projection.

ABNORMAL VALUES
- A radiograph is a *summation shadowgram*. There is no depth of field. The orthogonal view, combined with an understanding of the basic principles of radiographic interpretation, enables clinicians to create a perception of the 3-dimensional structures being imaged. When 2 structures of the same opacity are in contact, the border between them cannot be defined. This, known as the *silhouette sign*, tells the clinician that these structures are in contact. Radiographic opacity is the result of summation of all structures in the plane parallel with the primary beam. For example, when vessels and ribs are superimposed, the radiographic opacity is a *summation* of these 2 structures (and all other structures in that plane). The resultant radiographic opacity can give the impression of a pulmonary mass and is a common cause of misdiagnosis, sometimes referred to as a *fakeout*.
- Radiographic interpretation is a skill that takes much time to master. Numerous texts are available that describe the radiographic manifestations of the common disorders of cats and dogs. These texts should be readily available to the interpreting clinician. Continuing education courses on all aspects of radiographic interpretation should be pursued.

- The advent of digital imaging has made second opinion by a boarded radiologist much easier than was possible previously, and this is considered a significant advantage of this technology. Many teleradiology interpretation services are available, some provided by vendors of imaging equipment and some independently by diplomates of the American College of Veterinary Radiology. It is expected that the use of such services will dramatically increase in the next decade as more veterinary clinics go online with digital imaging equipment and broadband Internet connections.

Pleural Cavity and Chest Wall
- The radiographic signs of pleural fluid include widened interlobar fissures (soft tissue opacity), retraction of lung from thoracic wall, soft tissue opacity in the space between lung and chest wall, increased opacity dorsal to sternum on lateral radiographs (i.e., scalloped margins), blunting of costophrenic sulci in the VD view, decreased visualization of the heart in the DV view, and obscured diaphragmatic outline in the DV and lateral views.
  - The VD is the best view for detecting small amounts of pleural fluid.
- *Pneumothorax*, defined as air within the pleural space, causes lung collapse and lack of the "heart cushion." There is a resulting mediastinal shift to the side of greatest lung collapse.
  - There is retraction of lung from chest wall, the space between lung and chest wall is radiolucent, and lung markings do not extend to thoracic wall. There is lung atelectasis with increased opacity and apparent dorsal displacement of the heart on lateral views. *Tension pneumothorax* occurs when the pleural pressure approaches or exceeds the atmospheric pressure. The large amounts of air in the pleural space displace the diaphragm caudally (i.e., *tenting*). The heart and mediastinum may be shifted away from the side of lung collapse (i.e., *paradoxical mediastinal shift*), especially if the mediastinum is intact as can sometimes occur normally or because of disease.
  - Conditions mimicking pneumothorax include hypovolemia, chondrodystrophic chest conformation, and skin folds on VD view.
- The ribs are commonly overlooked during radiographic evaluation. There may be congenital anomalies, fractures, primary tumors, or metastatic lesions. Metastatic rib carcinoma is a common cause of neoplastic pleural effusions.
- Diaphragmatic hernias may be congenital or acquired and result in abdominal contents in the thorax. There is often cranial displacement of abdominal structures, an absence of abdominal structures, displacement of thoracic structures, loss of the normal diaphragmatic outline, and sometimes pleural fluid. Peritoneal-pericardial diaphragmatic hernias may cause a large, round, misshapen cardiac silhouette, silhouetting of the diaphragm and caudal cardiac margin, and abdominal contents; especially gas-filled bowel or omentum may be apparent within the cardiac silhouette. A dorsal pericardial-peritoneal mesothelial remnant may be present.
- Sternal and costal cartilage anomalies are common. Young animals have incompletely calcified costal cartilage. Mature animals have varying calcification of costal cartilage and costochondral junctions. Chondrodystrophic breeds have enlarged costochondral junctions.
- Fractures and subluxations, and infrequently infections and tumors, can occur.

Mediastinum and Esophagus
- The *mediastinum* is defined as everything between right and left pleural sacs, bounded by mediastinal pleura. It extends from the thoracic inlet to diaphragm. It is fenestrated and may not contain unilateral disease. It is not a closed cavity and communicates with the neck and the retroperitoneal space.
- The *cranioventral mediastinal reflection* is the border between the right cranial lung lobe and the cranial part of the left cranial lobe. Cranially, the left lung extends to right, and, caudally, immediately cranial to the heart, the right lung extends to left of midline.

- The *caudoventral mediastinal reflection* is the border between the accessory lobe and the left caudal lobe. The left aspect of the accessory lobe crosses midline, pushing mediastinal pleura to the left.
- Mediastinal organs normally seen include the heart, trachea, caudal vena cava, aorta, thymus (in young animals), and esophagus (sometimes left lateral).
- Mediastinal abnormalities commonly identified radiographically include lymphomegaly, esophageal disorders, tracheal disorders, thymic masses, ectopic thyroid tissue, cysts and, less commonly, fluid. Mediastinal fluid, if present, is usually hemorrhage associated with a coagulopathy, exudate as with FIP, or esophageal rupture.
- Pneumomediastinum increases the conspicuity of mediastinal structures. Pneumomediastinum can progress to pneumothorax if distention is severe.
- Pneumothorax is very unlikely to progress to pneumomediastinum. Causes of pneumomediastinum include a tracheal laceration, neck wound, jugular vein puncture, transtracheal aspirate, endotracheal tube cuff overinflation, and retrograde flow along airways from intrapulmonary rupture. Mediastinal structures are readily visible as a result of the negative contrast afforded by the presence of gas, including the adventitial border of the trachea and esophagus, the ascending aorta, the left subclavian artery, and the brachiocephalic trunk.
- When a collapsing trachea and principal bronchi are suspected, radiographs should be made on peak expiration (cough) because these structures typically collapse on expiration.
- The esophagus, which is a conduit for ingesta, has a functional sphincter at both ends and is dorsal to the trachea. It is normally not completely visible on survey radiographs. Occasionally, it will contain a small amount of gas or fluid, especially in left lateral view.
  - The radiographic signs of generalized megaesophagus include the presence of a gas-filled or fluid-filled esophagus, ventral displacement of the trachea, and a converging funnel-shaped opacity in the caudal thorax on a VD view.
  - The radiographic signs of segmental megaesophagus include a focal mass effect or gas accumulation, trachea displaced ventrally if the abnormality is cranial to heart base, and a midline opacity on a VD view.
  - Vascular ring anomalies, which are more common in dogs, arise from aortic arch or subclavian abnormalities. The patient may also have generalized megaesophagus. One must assess the location of the compression relative to the heart base, and an attempt to assess esophageal motility caudal to the compression is important. Breeds predisposed to persistent right aortic arch include German shepherds, Great Danes, and Irish setters.
  - The most common consequence to esophageal dysfunction is *aspiration pneumonia*—an intense alveolar pattern, primarily in the ventral lung lobes, especially the right middle because this bronchus exits the principal bronchi ventrally. One must always assess the lungs for evidence of aspiration when signs of megaesophagus are present. In addition, assess the esophagus with a contrast study when there is evidence of aspiration because megaesophagus may not be evident on survey radiographs. A sliding hiatal hernia, not uncommon in the sharpeis, brachycephalic dog breeds, and Siamese cats, will result in a changing soft tissue opacity in the mid-caudodorsal thorax.

Heart

- The *cardiac silhouette* comprises the heart and pericardial fat. Patients with pericardial fluid have a rounded heart, and usually the border of the cardiac silhouette is sharp because the fluid dampens motion of the cardiac silhouette during exposure. Pericardial fat, masses, and peritoneal pericardial diaphragmatic hernias can alter the cardiac silhouette shape and opacity.
- Myocardial and valvular disorders usually cause cardiomegaly; specific chamber enlargement depends on the site of dysfunction.

Hypertrophic cardiomyopathy can be severe, but the external dimensions of the heart can be minimally altered, particularly in cats.

- Generally, there is a wide range of normal heart size and shape. Long, thin dogs have a long, thin heart, whereas short, squat, or muscular dogs have rounded, big hearts.
- There is greater sensitivity for seeing dilatory changes versus hypertrophy. Cardiomegaly may be artifact, false or real. Sedation, an expiratory radiograph, or obesity will give a false impression of cardiomegaly. Pericardial effusion and peritoneal-pericardial hernia will result in false cardiomegaly.
- Chamber dilation may be caused by a primary myocardial problem, volume overload, pressure overload, or turbulence. The radiographic changes caused by left atrial dilation include splitting of principal bronchi and elevation of the carina, seen on a lateral view and most commonly caused by mitral valve dysfunction resulting in volume overload.
- Changes caused by dilation in the VD or DV view include auricular enlargement (very common) manifesting as a bulge on VD images in the 2:00 to 3:00 o'clock position, and this is invariably associated with an enlarged left atrium.
- Main pulmonary artery dilation results in a bulge on VD images in the 1:00 to 2:00 o'clock position, and differentials include heartworm disease, pressure and flow disturbance as with pulmonic stenosis, and volume and pressure overload as with left-to-right shunts.
- Changes on VD images in the 11:30 to 12:30 o'clock position include enlargement of the aortic arch. Right atrial enlargement is much less common and manifests as a bulge at 09:30 to 11:30 o'clock position on a VD view.
- Left ventricular hypertrophy results in an elongated heart (most apparent on a VD view).
- Right ventricular hypertrophy results in the apex being elevated from the sternum, and the so-called reversed "D" on a VD view.
- Left heart failure increases hydrostatic pressure in the pulmonary venous and capillary bed and causes pulmonary edema.
- Right heart failure produces hepatomegaly, peritoneal effusion, and sometimes pleural effusion. The caudal vena cava size is not a sensitive indicator of right heart failure unless the CVC/Ao (caudal vena cava/descending aorta) ratio is >1.5.

Lung

- Radiographically, lung comprises connective tissue, the bronchial tree, afferent and efferent vessels and alveoli, and the terminal airspace. The ability to see vessels, bronchi, and some interstitial markings is normal.
- Lung pathology is classically categorized in 6 pulmonary patterns: normal, alveolar, interstitial (structured and unstructured), bronchial, vascular, and mixed. This classification is fraught with flaws, though, and many disease processes represent a transition through 2 or more classic patterns.
- Although technically not a pattern, determination of normal is obviously critical. There is a broad range of normal, depending on the age of the animal, its conformation, and the phase of respiration.

Alveolar Pattern

- The hallmark sign of alveolar lung disease is the *air bronchogram*: There is increased soft tissue opacity in the alveoli (due to blood, inflammation, or fluid), but bronchi feeding that region remain gas filled and readily visible. An air bronchogram does not have to be present for it to be classified as an alveolar pattern. There is loss of visualization of the vessels because the soft tissue infiltrate in the alveoli silhouettes with the vessels. The adventitial border of bronchial walls and other interstitial structures are not apparent.
  - The air bronchogram is not the only radiographic finding associated with an alveolar pattern. A *lobar sign*, which is the term used to describe the sharp demarcation between increased airspace opacity in the periphery of a lung lobe and adjacent normal lung, is invariably associated with an alveolar pattern.

- Two different mechanisms can produce an alveolar pattern: *consolidation* (fluid or cells in the alveoli) or *atelectasis* (collapse of the alveoli). Both increase soft tissue opacity in the alveolar space. Differential diagnoses, as well as diagnostic and treatment options, are different for these 2 findings.
- With consolidation, there is no mediastinal shift, the lung lobe is near normal size, and changes are not necessarily associated with pleural disease.
- With atelectasis, there is collapse of the alveoli (loss of air in the alveoli), a mediastinal shift, and the lung lobe is decreased in size. It is often associated with pleural disease, typically pneumothorax or pleural effusion.
- Causes of an alveolar lung pattern include atelectasis (e.g., recumbency), edema (e.g., left heart failure), hemorrhage (e.g., coagulopathy), inflammatory exudates (e.g., pneumonia), and infiltrate [e.g., pulmonary infiltrates with eosinophilia (PIE)].
- The most common cause of generalized alveolar lung disease is pulmonary edema, which can be due to increased hydrostatic pressure (e.g., left heart failure), reduced oncotic pressure (e.g., hypoalbuminemia), or increased capillary permeability (e.g., vasculitis).
- Focal alveolar lung disease has multiple causes. Prioritization of the differential is significantly influenced by the distribution and intensity of changes. An accurate medical history is important in ranking differentials.
- With a generalized alveolar pattern, consider permeability, hydrostatic, or oncotic causes. When a cranioventral pattern is present, consider pneumonia. With perihilar distributions, consider hydrostatic causes. When a caudodorsal distribution is present, consider permeability, hydrostatic, or oncotic causes.
- Usually, the intensity of opacification is most severe with inhalation pneumonia.

Interstitial Pattern

- This pattern is often divided into unstructured and structured. Patient factors and technical factors (e.g., underexposure, expiratory radiograph, obesity) can result in an apparent increase in unstructured lung opacity. For this reason, it is important that thoracic radiographs are made on *peak inspiration*. Expiratory films in particular may artifactually cause an unstructured interstitial pattern.
- When patient related, the hazy or amorphous increase in lung soft tissue opacity associated with an unstructured pattern can occur as a result of fluid, cells, or both in the interstitial space; fibrosis in the interstitial space; chronic inflammation; or as a normal aging change. When due to interstitial edema or infiltrate, vessels margins are fuzzy or indistinct, and there is peribronchial enhancement (i.e., the bronchi can be seen better) because of an increase in opacity of the interstitium. The adventitial border of bronchi is ill-defined, and the bronchus appears thick.
- A severe *unstructured* interstitial pattern may mimic a mild alveolar pattern. Sometimes one cannot distinguish between the 2 patterns. If in doubt, identify the pattern as alveolar because this is a more severe pattern.
- The second category—*structured*—can be divided into noncavitary and cavitary:
  - The common differentials for a structured noncavitary interstitial pattern include metastatic lung disease, primary lung mass, pulmonary osseous metaplasia, granulomas (e.g., fungal, eosinophilic, foreign body), abscess, and fluid-filled bullae. Miliary patterns are often associated with fungal infections.
  - Interstitial nodules must be differentiated from end-on vessels. An *end-on vessel* is usually located near other vessels, is the same size or smaller than associated longitudinal vessels, tends to follow a pattern, may be near a bronchus, typically is well defined with smooth margins, may have a tail, and is more opaque than expected for its size; whereas a pulmonary nodule does not have to be near vessels,

can be any size, is random in location, may not be near a bronchus, may be smooth or irregularly marginated, and has no tail.
  - Structured interstitial nodules must be differentiated from extrathoracic artifacts. Ectoparasites (e.g., ticks), skin masses, nipples, etc., can mimic a pulmonary nodule. Structures on the surface are often more opaque than expected because of the air–soft tissue interface. Paint barium paste on the cutaneous nodule to determine its location, if necessary.
  - Cavitated interstitial nodules include bullae, primary neoplasia, abscess, and parasitic nodules. Radiographically, these nodules appear as circumscribed lesions of various opacity (but by definition must contain gas), size, and number in the interstitial space. A horizontal beam may show a gas-fluid interface.

Bronchial Pattern

- Increased visualization of the bronchi may be due to an apparent increase in size of and number of bronchi. There is loss of the normal tapering, and bronchial walls become parallel and thickened. It can be difficult to distinguish primary bronchial disease from peribronchial enhancement, as is seen with diseases affecting the interstitium.
- The distinction between an end-on bronchus and a cavitary pulmonary nodule is important. Typically, an end-on bronchus is located near other bronchi, the same size or smaller than associated longitudinal bronchi, tends to follow a pattern, and may be near a vessel; whereas a cavitary nodule does not have to be near bronchi, can be any size, is random in location and does not have to be near a vessel.
- Bronchial wall mineralization is commonly associated with chronic inflammatory or allergic disease, metabolic diseases (e.g., hyperadrenocorticism) or can be a normal aging change.

Vascular Pattern

- In situations where there are enlarged arteries and normal veins, pulmonary hypertension, as with heartworm disease or chronic lung disease, should be considered. Enlarged arteries and enlarged veins are seen in pulmonary overcirculation, as in left-to-right shunts, in overhydration, and in concurrent heartworm disease and left heart dysfunction. Normal arteries and enlarged veins are seen with pulmonary venous hypertension as occurs with left heart dysfunction (e.g., mitral regurgitation, dilated cardiomyopathy, hypertrophic cardiomyopathy). Small arteries and small veins are associated with right-to-left shunts (tetralogy of Fallot), dehydration and circulatory collapse (e.g., hypoadrenocorticism), and severe pulmonic stenosis.
- Vessel mineralization is often associated with thromboembolism, lung trauma, and hypothyroidism.

CRITICAL VALUES
N/A

INTERFERING FACTORS
Drugs That May Alter Results of the Procedure
Many products used in the management of GI disorders are radiopaque and are apparent in survey radiographs. This may lead to confusion during radiographic interpretation.

Conditions That May Interfere with Performing the Procedure
Anesthesia and sedation of patients may cause transient pulmonary changes that are secondary to anesthesia and clinically insignificant. Anesthesia can cause pulmonary atelectasis and mediastinal shift, both of which are exacerbated by lateral recumbency for prolonged periods before radiography.

Procedure Techniques or Handling That May Alter Results
- A thorough understanding of the physics of radiography will enable clinicians to better troubleshoot problems that arise in the generation of radiographic images.
- The kVp primarily controls photon energy. The higher the kVp is, the more penetrating is the power of the beam. This results in a relative increase in the number of shades of gray and a radiograph with more latitude. This is preferred when imaging the thorax.

- The mAs primarily controls film blackness (essentially the number of photons hitting the film), although increasing the kVp does also increase film blackness. (More photons are generated at the anode and more photons penetrate the patient because of increased photon energy.)
- Small volumes of pleural fluid are more easily identified on a VD view because the fluid gravitates into the *dorsal gutters* (bilateral troughs created by the shape of the ribs), resulting in retraction of the dorsal borders as fluid tracks between lung lobes (so-called *interlobar fissures*).
- Large volumes of pleural fluid are more likely to obscure the heart on a DV view, because fluid gravitates to the sternum and silhouettes with the cardiac silhouette.
- Focal caudodorsal pulmonary pathology and the caudal lobar vessels are more easily seen on a DV view because the caudodorsal lung is better aerated in comparison to a VD view, the pathology is marginally magnified, and the normal vessels are more likely at right angles to the beam, increasing conspicuity.

Influence of Signalment on Performing and Interpreting the Procedure

Species

High-detail systems are needed to critically evaluate the fine trabecular detail in small bones and also the subtle pulmonary architecture in cats.

Breed

- Large-breed dogs are more difficult to image than are smaller breeds. The region of interest may not fit on a single cassette, and a higher exposure is required because the body part being imaged is often thicker (e.g., spine, thorax, abdomen, pelvis). This can result in motion artifact if a slow imaging system is used or the radiographic machine is low in mA output.
- Variation in thoracic conformation between dog breeds is considerable. The appearance of a normal thorax of a dolichocephalic breed is considerably different than that of a brachycephalic breed.

Age

There are changes in skeletal maturation with age.

Gender

None

Pregnancy

Unnecessary irradiation of pregnant bitches, particularly in the first trimester, should be avoided where possible. When necessary, well-collimated thoracic radiography is unlikely to result in clinically relevant fetal exposure.

CLINICAL PERSPECTIVE

Radiography is an extremely important tool in the diagnosis and management of a large number of small-animal disorders. A thorough understanding of the basic principles of diagnostic imaging will assist in ensuring consistently superior image quality. Many practices invest in physical resources, but fail to invest sufficient time and resources into technician training and clinician continuing education. A well-functioning radiography suite that produces good-quality images is a commonly undervalued resource in veterinary medicine.

 MISCELLANEOUS

ANCILLARY TESTS

- Diagnostic ultrasonography is extremely useful in evaluation of the heart and mediastinum and some pulmonary and pleural cavity disorders. Ultrasonography plays an important role in the acquisition of tissue samples for cytologic and histologic assessment, including mediastinal masses, pericardial and pleural effusions, and peripherally located pulmonary pathology.
- CT scanners, particularly those with helical and multislice functionality, can assist dramatically in the evaluation of thoracic pathology. Other modalities that complement diagnostic radiography include magnetic resonance imaging and, to a lesser extent, nuclear medicine.

SYNONYMS

Chest radiography

SEE ALSO

Blackwell's Five-Minute Veterinary Consult: Canine and Feline Topics

Many

Related Topics in This Book

- General Principles of Radiography
- Computed Tomography
- Magnetic Resonance Imaging

ABBREVIATIONS

- CT = computed tomography
- DV = dorsoventral
- kVp = kilovoltage peak
- mAs = milliampere seconds
- VD = ventrodorsal

Suggested Reading

Thrall D, ed. *Textbook of Veterinary Diagnostic Radiology*, 5th ed. St Louis: Saunders Elsevier, 2007.

INTERNET RESOURCES

None

AUTHOR NAME

Ian D. Robertson

THORACIC ULTRASONOGRAPHY

BASICS

TYPE OF PROCEDURE
Ultrasonographic

PROCEDURE EXPLANATION AND RELATED PHYSIOLOGY
Ultrasonography of the thorax for noncardiac abnormalities can be extremely informative but greatly limited in scope by the inflated lungs. Air impedes ultrasound-wave propagation, and acoustic windows needed to access thoracic pathology are provided when aerated lung is consolidated, collapsed, or displaced by a pleural effusion or mass. Thoracic radiographs must be obtained prior to the ultrasonographic study to first identify the abnormality prompting the need for ultrasonography. Because of aerated lung, the entire thorax cannot be imaged, so acoustic windows seen on the thoracic radiographs also guide the ultrasonographic exam.

INDICATIONS
- To determine the amount, character, and cause of a pleural effusion
- A possible cranial mediastinal mass
- Differentiating a pulmonary mass from a thoracic wall mass
- Differentiating a pulmonary consolidation from a mass
- A possible diaphragmatic hernia or rupture
- Ultrasound-guided diagnostic and therapeutic aspiration of pleural effusion
- Ultrasound-guided FNA and biopsy of masses

CONTRAINDICATIONS
- A normal thorax
- Nonconsolidating pulmonary disease (e.g., bronchitis, interstitial disease)
- Aerated lung between thoracic wall and targeted lesion
- A bilateral large-volume pneumothorax

POTENTIAL COMPLICATIONS
None

CLIENT EDUCATION
- Thoracic radiographs are needed prior to the ultrasonographic exam.
- Clipping of hair is required but often limited to small areas of the acoustic window.
- Pleural effusions in stable patients should not be removed prior to the ultrasonographic exam.
- Sedation is frequently required for ultrasound-guided FNA of pleural effusion and masses.
- General anesthesia is required for ultrasound-guided FNA or biopsy of pulmonary masses.

BODY SYSTEMS ASSESSED
- Hemic, lymphatic, and immune
- Respiratory

PROCEDURE

PATIENT PREPARATION
Preprocedure Medication or Preparation
- A pleural effusion in stable patients should not be removed prior to the ultrasonographic exam.
- A pneumothorax should be removed prior to the ultrasonographic exam.
- Patients should be fasted if there is the potential for ultrasound-guided FNA or biopsy, which might require sedation or general anesthesia.

Anesthesia or Sedation
- The patient's condition determines whether sedation is needed for aspiration of a pleural effusion.
- Sedation is generally needed for ultrasound-guided FNA of nonpulmonary masses (e.g., cranial mediastinal).
- Anesthesia is needed for pulmonary mass ultrasound-guided FNA or biopsy. Respiration must be suspended during the biopsy.
- Avoid the administration of sedatives or analgesics that cause hyperventilation.

Patient Positioning
- Patient positioning is determined by location of the lesion and acoustic windows: right or left lateral recumbency, sternal recumbency, or dorsal recumbency, as required.
- The chosen patient positioning and the ultrasound transducer location should take advantage of gravity's effect on a pleural effusion or on collapsed lung lobes.

Patient Monitoring
- Standard monitoring of pulse and respiration during the routine portion of the ultrasonographic exam
- Standard monitoring (e.g., oxygenation, blood pressure) during sedation or general anesthesia

Equipment or Supplies
- A diagnostic ultrasound machine, preferably with a higher-frequency (7.5–10.0 MHz) curvilinear, linear array, or phased array transducers
- Transducers with a small contact area (i.e., *footprint*) are preferred to mitigate intercostal access problems.
- Long [$1\frac{1}{2}$–$3\frac{1}{2}$ inches (3.81–8.89 cm)], 22- to 25-gauge needles for FNA techniques
- Larger-bore (14–18 gauge), fully or semiautomated needle biopsy devices for biopsy procedures
- A transducer needle guide if freehand needle techniques are too technically demanding for the operator

TECHNIQUE
- The transducer location and therefore skin-preparation site depend on the lesion and acoustic window location as determined from the thoracic radiographs.
- Intercostal, intercostal parasternal, substernal, and suprasternal are typical approaches.
- Stable patients with pleural effusion should not have the effusion removed prior to the ultrasonographic exam.
- Access to central pulmonary or hilar lesions or negating the limitations of a small pneumothorax may require scanning from the dependent aspect of the thorax (e.g., the left thoracic wall in left lateral recumbent patients). The technique is aided by anesthesia-induced dependent atelectasis. Dependent scanning is made easier by using a cardiac scanning table.

SAMPLE HANDLING
N/A

APPROPRIATE AFTERCARE
Postprocedure Patient Monitoring
Use ultrasonography or postprocedure thoracic radiography to monitor patients after lung or mass FNA or biopsy for pleural effusion or pneumothorax.

Nursing Care
None

Dietary Modification
None

Medication Requirements
None

Restrictions on Activity
To decrease the potential for hemothorax or pneumothorax, consider limiting patient activity after FNA or biopsy of a lung or mass.

Anticipated Recovery Time
Standard recovery from sedation or general anesthesia

 INTERPRETATION

NORMAL FINDINGS OR RANGE
• Information derived from ultrasonographic scanning of the normal thorax is limited to imaging the pleuropulmonary interface.
• The normal visceral or pulmonary pleural surface is characterized by a hyperechoic border sliding synchronously with respiration against the costal pleura lining the thoracic wall, has acoustic reverberation, and has no through sound transmission.

ABNORMAL VALUES
Pleural Effusion
The presence of pleural fluid reduces lung volume and is an excellent acoustic medium enabling ultrasonographic imaging of normally inaccessible deeper structures. Varying amounts of fluid separate the costal and pulmonary pleura. Fluid echogenicity varies with fluid type: anechoic (transudate) vs echogenic (cells, protein, fibrin). Chronic pleural effusions may be loculated with fibrin.

Mediastinal Masses
Ultrasonographic imaging of the mediastinum requires that aerated lung must be displaced by pleural effusion or the mediastinal mass contacts the thoracic wall. Mediastinal masses vary in appearance between and within diseases. Hypoechoic solid masses are most often due to lymphadenopathy. Cystic masses in cats may be idiopathic mediastinal cysts (large-volume anechoic fluid within a thin wall) or cystic thymoma (a thick, irregular wall with echogenic effusion).

Thoracic Wall vs Pulmonary Mass
Thoracic wall masses (i.e., neoplasia, abscess, granuloma, hematoma) are superficially located, may have a convex border bulging into the thoracic cavity, and move synchronously with the thoracic wall. The hyperechoic pleuropulmonary interface slides deep against the mass. Aggressive thoracic wall masses arising from or secondarily involving the ribs will create either an irregular or an absent rib interface. Pulmonary masses must be peripherally located and contact the thoracic wall or a pleural effusion in order to be imaged, whereas more centrally located masses require an acoustic window created by superficially collapsed or consolidated lung in order to be imaged. Pulmonary masses are differentiated from thoracic wall masses by synchronous movement with respiration and a sliding or gliding of the mass against the thoracic wall.

Pulmonary Mass vs Consolidation
The acoustic appearance of pulmonary masses varies depending on the mass structure. Most neoplastic masses are homogeneous and hypoechoic, with smooth borders between the mass and adjacent lung. Necrotic areas in masses appear as cavitated, complex echoic portions. Pulmonary consolidation often maintains the shape and angular-edge appearance of a normal lung lobe and involves the entire lung lobe or gradually blends with normal lung. The distinct delineation seen between pulmonary masses and aerated lung lobe is absent. Homogeneously consolidated lung parenchyma will resemble hepatic parenchyma. Air bronchograms, fluid bronchograms, and scattered echogenic foci caused by residual air also are seen in consolidated lung.

Diaphragmatic Hernia and Rupture
Ultrasonographic diagnosis relies on a high index of suspicion derived from thoracic radiographs but can still be a demanding study fraught with interpretation pitfalls. Diaphragmatic integrity and the presence of intrathoracic abdominal viscera must be assessed. With concurrent pleural or peritoneal effusions, gauging diaphragmatic integrity is easier by the transhepatic approach (with the transducer at the xiphoid). Do not incorrectly place the liver cranial to the diaphragm when a normal mirror-image artifact is seen. Traumatic diaphragmatic rupture is often accompanied by a pleural effusion; the liver is differentiated from consolidated lung lobes by following the portal vascular system and absence of fluid or air bronchograms. Congenital peritoneal-pericardial diaphragmatic hernias are characterized by abdominal viscera adjacent to the heart within the pericardial sac and loss of the midline diaphragmatic contour.

CRITICAL VALUES
A large-volume pleural effusion or pneumothorax causing respiratory distress requires immediate therapeutic intervention.

INTERFERING FACTORS
Drugs That May Alter Results of the Procedure
Sedatives or analgesics producing hyperventilation

Conditions That May Interfere with Performing the Procedure
• Panting or respiratory distress
• Unstable cardiovascular status

Procedure Techniques or Handling That May Alter Results
• An inappropriate transducer location that fails to take advantage of the acoustic windows
• The failure to use dependent transducer locations to take advantage of dependent atelectic lung or pleural effusion
• Draining of a pleural effusion prior to the ultrasonographic exam
• Basing the diagnosis of a diaphragmatic hernia or rupture on a normal mirror-image artifact in the liver

Influence of Signalment on Performing and Interpreting the Procedure
Species
None

Breed
None

Age
None

Gender
None

Pregnancy
None

CLINICAL PERSPECTIVE
• Noncardiac thoracic ultrasonography is a powerful imaging study that complements thoracic radiography.
• Thoracic radiography is required in order to identify a thoracic lesion prompting the ultrasonographic exam and to identify the lesion's location and ultrasonographic accessibility.
• Patients with intrathoracic structures that are obscured on radiographs by a pleural effusion are prime candidates for ultrasonography to determine whether underlying lesions are present (e.g., pulmonary, thoracic wall or mediastinal masses, diaphragmatic rupture).
• Patients with generalized pneumothorax or those with diffuse, nonconsolidating pulmonary infiltrative disease in which the lungs remain aerated are not good candidates for noncardiac thoracic ultrasonography.
• Ultrasound-guided FNA and biopsy of masses are additional relatively noninvasive diagnostic techniques.

 MISCELLANEOUS

ANCILLARY TESTS
• Positive contrast peritoneography can be used to detect suspected diaphragmatic rupture or hernia if the ultrasonographic exam results are inconclusive.

THORACIC ULTRASONOGRAPHY

- Thoracic radiography after removal of pleural fluid by thoracocentesis may indicate the present of lesions obscured on pre-tap radiographs or by partially aerated lung during ultrasonography.
- Pleural fluid analysis

SYNONYMS
None

SEE ALSO
Blackwell's Five-Minute Veterinary Consult: Canine and Feline Topics
- Lymphoma—Cats
- Lymphoma—Dogs
- Peritoneopericardial Diaphragmatic Hernia
- Pleural Effusion
- Squamous Cell Carcinoma, Lung
- Thymoma

Related Topics in This Book
- General Principles of Ultrasonography

- Thoracic Radiography
- Thoracocentesis and Fluid Analysis

ABBREVIATIONS
FNA = fine-needle aspiration

Suggested Reading

Reichle JK, Wisner ER. Noncardiac thoracic ultrasound in 75 feline and canine patients. *Vet Radiol Ultrasound* 2000; 41: 154–162.

Saunders HM, Keith D. Thoracic imaging. In: King LG, ed. *Textbook of Respiratory Disease in Dogs and Cats*. St Louis: Saunders Elsevier, 2004: 72–93.

Tidwell AS. Ultrasonography of the thorax (excluding the heart). *Vet Clin North Am Small Anim Pract* 1998; 28: 993–1015.

INTERNET RESOURCES
None

AUTHOR NAME
H. Mark Saunders

BASICS

TYPE OF PROCEDURE
Diagnostic sample collection

PROCEDURE EXPLANATION AND RELATED PHYSIOLOGY
Thoracocentesis or pleurocentesis can be performed for 1 of 2 purposes: diagnostic evaluation or therapeutic intervention. Diagnostic thoracocentesis can be essential for diagnosing the presence of pleural disease and evaluating the contents of the cavity, whether air or fluid. Pleural fluid can then be further evaluated grossly for color and consistency, and microscopically for cellularity and the presence of protein or organisms.

Therapeutic thoracocentesis is used to treat pleural effusion and pneumothorax resulting from a variety of causes. Typically, therapeutic thoracocentesis follows a positive diagnostic tap.

INDICATIONS
• When the presence of pleural air or fluid is suspected, especially in an animal with increased inspiratory effort and reduced breath sounds on thoracic auscultation
• Conditions leading to pleural space disease include trauma, hemorrhage, neoplasia, heart failure, chylothorax, spontaneous rupture of a pulmonary bulla, and infection.

CONTRAINDICATIONS
Thoracocentesis should not be performed on patients with abnormal hemostasis.

POTENTIAL COMPLICATIONS
• Lung puncture or laceration producing pneumothorax
• Hemorrhage, if the internal thoracic artery is lacerated
• If the fenestrated catheter technique is used, and the fenestrations are not small and smooth, the catheter can get caught on the skin and break, with pieces remaining in the patient.

CLIENT EDUCATION
Clients should be aware of the potential complications of the procedure and the potential severity of the underlying disease.

BODY SYSTEMS ASSESSED
• Cardiovascular
• Hemic, lymphatic, and immune
• Respiratory

PROCEDURE

PATIENT PREPARATION
Preprocedure Medication or Preparation
• Sedation may be necessary, especially in cats.
• Clip the hair over a large area of the lateral thorax. The point of needle insertion should be at the 7th or 8th intercostal space, dorsal to the costochondral arch.
• To remove fluid, the needle should enter at the level of the costochondral junction. To remove air, it should enter at the junction of the dorsal and middle thirds of the chest wall.
• Local anesthetic is generally not necessary for a diagnostic tap. However, local anesthesia is imperative for therapeutic thoracocentesis. Lidocaine should be injected SC and infused into the intercostal muscles.
• Dogs: Scrub the surface skin with povidone-iodine or chlorhexidine. Contact time should be at least 3 min and then wipe with alcohol.
• Cats: Scrub the surface skin with povidone-iodine because they can be sensitive to topical chlorhexidine. Allow a 3-min contact time and then wipe with alcohol.

• For diagnostic thoracocentesis, especially in an emergency setting, patient clipping and cleaning may need to be skipped.

Anesthesia or Sedation
• Selection should be based on the individual patient.
• Often, buprenorphine and acepromazine is sufficient in dogs and cats.

Patient Positioning
• The patient should be in a comfortable position that does not compromise its respiration. Typically, the patient is in sternal recumbency or standing.
• Sitting should be avoided because it interferes with accurate determination of landmarks.

Patient Monitoring
The patient's respiration, heart rate, and pulse should be monitored throughout the procedure.

Equipment or Supplies
Diagnostic Tap
A 3-mL syringe with a 22-gauge, 1-inch (2.54 cm) needle is needed for most dogs weighing >5 kg. A 25-gauge needle should be used in cats and dogs weighing <5 kg. A butterfly catheter can also be used in cats and small dogs.

Therapeutic Tap
• A 14- to 16-gauge, 3½- to 5¼-inch (8.89–13.34 cm) catheter for dogs
• A 16- to 20-gauge, 2- to 3½-inch (5.08–8.89 cm) catheter for cats and small dogs
• A no. 11 blade
• Sterile gloves
• A 3-mL syringe, non-Luerlocked
• A 60-mL syringe
• An IV fluid-extension set
• A 3-way stopcock
• A container for fluid

TECHNIQUE
Diagnostic Thoracocentesis
• Locate the desired point of insertion by counting to the 7th or 8th intercostal space. Position the needle in the junction of the dorsal and middle one-third of the thorax if air is suspected. The junction of the middle and ventral one-third of the thorax, above the costochondral arch, is the preferred site for aspiration of fluid.
• Stabilize both of your hands on the animal so that your hands and the needle move with the chest wall. Insert the needle through the skin; once in the subcutaneous space, apply 1–2 mL of vacuum. Slowly advance the needle perpendicular to the body wall while maintaining vacuum, all the while, along the cranial rib margin. Penetration of the pleura is indicated when the vacuum is suddenly lost (pneumothorax) or fluid enters the syringe (effusion).
• Do not advance the needle deeper than you have estimated the pleural space to be; use the rib as a landmark.
• Once the presence of pleural fluid or air is confirmed, withdraw the needle quickly to decrease the likelihood of lung laceration.

Butterfly Catheter Technique
• When using this technique, position the needle so that the bevel is facing cranially. Insert the catheter and, once in the subcutaneous space, apply 1–2 mL of vacuum with the attached extensions and a 60-mL syringe. Once the vacuum is lost, arch the needle caudally so that the point of the needle is furthest from the lung, and advance the needle. Hold the needle in place by pressing the wings of the catheter against the cranial rib so that the needle is less likely to lacerate the lung.
• To remove the needle, press down firmly on it and move it and skin cranially until the needle is no longer in the thoracic cavity. Then slide the needle out of the skin.

THORACOCENTESIS AND FLUID ANALYSIS

Therapeutic Thoracocentesis

- Locate the point of insertion by counting to the 7th or 8th intercostal space. Place the needle in the junction of the dorsal and middle one-third of the thorax if air is suspected. The junction of the middle and ventral one-third of the thorax, at or just above the costochondral arch, is the preferred site for fluid removal.
- Block with body wall and pleura with 0.5–1.0 mL of lidocaine and prepare the skin aseptically. If fluid is suspected, a few small fenestrations can be made in the catheter, starting 1 cm proximal to the tip to prevent clogging and increase yield. Use a no. 11 blade and, while wearing sterile gloves, make small V-shaped holes by joining cuts at a 45° angle. These holes should be no more that 20% of the circumference of the catheter. Rotate the catheter 90° at each fenestration to maintain the integrity of the catheter. Do not scoop holes out, and ensure that the edges are smooth to decrease the likelihood of the catheter getting caught on the skin and breaking.
- Lift the skin away from the body wall and make a stab skin incision that fully penetrates the dermis with the no. 11 blade.
- Attach the 3-mL syringe to the catheter-needle assembly.
- Stabilize your hands on the animal and your elbows or wrists on the table. If the animal is standing, you will be able to stabilize your hands only on the animal's thorax. Rest your dominant hand on the animal and use that hand to advance the catheter-needle assembly into the skin incision. The needle is advanced by the fingers of the dominant hand, which is in turn resting on the chest wall. Once the needle has entered the subcutaneous space, use your other hand to continuously apply 1–2 mL of vacuum. While maintaining the vacuum, advance the needle slowly along the cranial aspect of the rib until the vacuum is lost (or the fluid is observed), indicating that the pleural space has been entered.
- Once the needle has entered the pleural space, hold the needle hub stationary as you advance the catheter ≈1 cm over the needle. It is critical that the catheter is advanced and that the needle is not pulled backward out of the pleural space. Once the catheter has covered the tip of the needle, redirect the catheter-needle assembly to aim it cranially and as parallel to the body wall as practical. Holding the needle stationary, advance the catheter into the thorax, parallel to the spine (for air) or cranioventrally (for fluid).
- Remove the needle and have an assistant attach the extension that has been connected to the 3-way stopcock and syringe and begin aspiration. This catheter can potentially be left in place for a few hours if a waterproof tape butterfly is applied and sutured to the skin.

SAMPLE HANDLING

Samples may be placed in serum tubes and EDTA tubes for analysis. A slide should also be made for cytologic evaluation. If infection is suspected, a sample may also be saved for culture.

APPROPRIATE AFTERCARE

Postprocedure Patient Monitoring

- The patient's respiration rate and effort should be monitored after thoracocentesis. Deterioration suggests that either the condition is worsening or that an iatrogenic pneumothorax has developed.
- Monitor the heart rate, pulses, and capillary refill time.

Nursing Care

- No nursing care is necessary if the catheter is removed.
- If the catheter is kept in place because of continual production of air or fluid, the patient should be handled very carefully to ensure that the catheter stays in the pleural space. A butterfly of waterproof tape should be made and sutured to the patient to hold it securely. Administration of oxygen and analgesics to the patient may also be needed.

Dietary Modification

No dietary modifications are necessary for the procedure itself but may be needed based on underlying disease.

Medication Requirements

Based on underlying disease

Restrictions on Activity

The animal should remain quiet for a few hours after the thoracocentesis so that respiration rate and effort can be evaluated effectively. Further restrictions will be based on underlying disease.

Anticipated Recovery Time

The patient should recover as soon as the needle or catheter has been removed, and the sedation has worn off. Full recovery is based on the etiology of the underlying disease.

INTERPRETATION

NORMAL FINDINGS OR RANGE

A normal patient should not have any air or fluid in its pleural space.

ABNORMAL VALUES

- If air is found, this indicates a pneumothorax.
- If fluid is found, indicating pleural effusion, it can be due to a number of causes, which can often be distinguished from one another by fluid cytology.
- Transudates, modified transudates, and pseudochylous effusion can be found in patients with heart failure.
- The presence of bacteria or excessive numbers of neutrophils indicates a pyothorax.
- Chyle may be present and is defined by fluid analysis and comparison with serum. (Refer to the "Fluid Analysis" chapter for further details.)
- Cytologic evaluation will also provide an indication as to the likelihood of neoplasia.

CRITICAL VALUES

If air is continuously being produced and removed with the catheter apparatus, or if the fluid is indicative of a pyothorax, a chest tube should be placed to evacuate the pleural space more effectively.

INTERFERING FACTORS

Drugs That May Alter Results of the Procedure

None known

Conditions That May Interfere with Performing the Procedure

Inadequate sedation will prevent safe and adequate thoracocentesis.

Procedure Techniques or Handling That May Alter Results

- The fluid can be contaminated, invalidating the results of microbial culture, if the fluid is not handled aseptically.
- A fresh slide preparation should always be made, especially if there is delay in evaluating the EDTA sample.

Influence of Signalment on Performing and Interpreting the Procedure

Species
None

Breed
None

Age
None

Gender
None

Pregnancy
None

CLINICAL PERSPECTIVE

- If the clinician is unsure whether the patient has pleural space disease, a diagnostic thoracocentesis should first be performed, especially if the patient is not stable enough for radiography.

• If the results of the diagnostic thoracocentesis are positive, a therapeutic thoracocentesis is recommended if the animal has an increased inspiratory effort.

• The catheter technique is much safer than using a needle because it decreases the likelihood of lung laceration when properly performed, and it also enables repeated or continuous drainage, if required.

• Samples should be evaluated to guide the clinician on how to treat the patient properly.

MISCELLANEOUS

ANCILLARY TESTS

• Radiography following the procedure will assess the effectiveness of the thoracocentesis.

• Samples should be evaluated using appropriate fluid analysis, including cytologic evaluation. Based on these results, microbial culture of the fluid sample may be appropriate.

SYNONYMS
Chest tap

SEE ALSO
Blackwell's Five-Minute Veterinary Consult: Canine and Feline Topics
• Chylothorax
• Pleural Effusion
• Pyothorax

Related Topics in This Book
• Bacterial Culture and Sensitivity
• Fluid Analysis
• Thoracic Radiography
• Thoracic Ultrasonography

ABBREVIATIONS
None

Suggested Reading
Hawkins E. Clinical manifestations of the pleural cavity and mediastinal diseases. In: Nelson RW, Couto CG, eds. *Small Animal Internal Medicine*. St Louis: CV Mosby, 2003: 315–319.
Hawkins E. Diagnostic tests for the pleural cavity and mediastinum. In: Nelson RW, Couto CG, eds. *Small Animal Internal Medicine*. St Louis: CV Mosby, 2003: 320–326.
Mertens MM, Fossum TW, MacDonald KA. Pleural and extrapleural diseases. In: Ettinger SJ, Feldman EC, eds. *Textbook of Veterinary Internal Medicine*. Philadelphia: WB Saunders, 2005: 1272–1284.
Nelson OL. Pleural effusion. In: Ettinger SJ, Feldman EC, eds. *Textbook of Veterinary Internal Medicine*. Philadelphia: WB Saunders, 2005: 204–207.
Rozanski E, Chan DL. Approach to the patient with respiratory distress. *Vet Clin North Am Small Anim Pract* 2005: 315–316.

INTERNET RESOURCES
Washington State University, College of Veterinary Medicine, Small Animal Diagnostic & Therapeutic Techniques: Thoracocentesis, http://courses.vetmed.wsu.edu/samdx/thoracocentesis.asp.

AUTHOR NAME
Kielyn Scott

BASICS

TYPE OF PROCEDURE
Endoscopic

PROCEDURE EXPLANATION AND RELATED PHYSIOLOGY
This is a sterile procedure in which a rigid endoscope (telescope) is introduced into the thorax to view thoracic structures and obtain biopsy samples. Surgical procedures may also be performed. The technique enables exploration of, and surgery within, the thorax without the need for a full thoracic wall incision. The procedure is less painful and stressful than open surgery.

To view structures within the thorax, a pneumothorax must be created. The lung may need to be collapsed on the side being examined. Caution must be taken to assure that no respiratory compromise occurs. Negative pressure must be reestablished at the conclusion of the procedure.

INDICATIONS
- A need to evaluate the thoracic organs and their surfaces
- A need to biopsy lymph nodes, pleural surfaces, pericardium, or lung
- Lung, mediastinal, pleural, or other masses
- Spontaneous pneumothorax (to locate the bullae)
- Examination after trauma
- Chylothorax: thoracic duct evaluation and occlusion
- Pericardial fluid: pericardectomy
- Pleural foreign body removal

CONTRAINDICATIONS
An obvious need for open thoracic surgery

POTENTIAL COMPLICATIONS
- Cardiorespiratory compromise
- Internal organ damage
- Bleeding
- Need to convert to an open procedure
- Wound-healing complications
- Infection

CLIENT EDUCATION
- This procedure requires general anesthesia. The animal must not be fed for 12 h before surgery, unless this is an emergency examination for trauma.
- This is a sterile surgical procedure. The animal will be clipped for a full exploratory thoracotomy, and there may be a need to convert from a minimally invasive procedure to an open surgery.

BODY SYSTEMS ASSESSED
- Cardiovascular
- Hemic, lymphatic, and immune
- Respiratory

 PROCEDURE

PATIENT PREPARATION
Preprocedure Medication or Preparation
- The animal must not be fed for 12 h before the procedure.
- Routine preanesthetic drugs are administered.

Anesthesia or Sedation
General anesthesia

Patient Positioning
Depending on area being examined, lateral or dorsal recumbency

Patient Monitoring
Blood pressure measurement, pulse oximetry, ECG monitoring, and respiratory rate monitoring are used.

Equipment or Supplies
Basic
- Hair clippers
- Sterile preparation supplies
- 0° and 30° 2.7-, 5-, and 10-mm telescopes
- A video camera and monitor
- A light source and cable
- Thoracoscopic cannulae
- An endoscopic probe and retractors
- Endoscopic grasping forceps
- Endoscopic biopsy instruments
- A suction device
- Biopsy and aspiration needles
- Surgical instruments
- Suture material
- A scalpel blade

Additional
- A table that allows the animal to be easily tipped sideways, head down or head up
- Other telescopes: different viewing angles, smaller sizes, and operating telescope
- Specific instruments used to perform various thoracoscopic surgeries
- Devices to control hemorrhage (i.e., bipolar electrocautery, stainless-steel clips, stapling devices, harmonic scalpel)
- Special endotracheal tubes for 1-lung ventilation

TECHNIQUE

- Performing thoracoscopy requires special training. See the Internet Resources section for sources regarding basic equipment, videos, and training courses.
- The site of the telescope cannula placement is chosen according to the location of the suspected lesion. The paraxiphoid cannula is used for examining the pericardium, the ventral lungs, and the heart. The lateral telescope portals enable more extensive visualization of each hemithorax, especially the dorsal regions.
  - *Paraxiphoid telescope cannula*: The dog is anesthetized and placed in dorsal or dorsal oblique recumbency. Its hair is clipped over the entire ventral and lateral chest and cranial abdomen. Routine surgical preparation is performed. The patient is draped. A short skin incision is made lateral to the xiphoid. A hemostat is used to create a tunnel through the diaphragm and into the pleural space. The hemostat is directed lateral to midline to avoid the caudal mediastinal space. The cannula is placed using a blunt obturator. The obturator is removed, and air is allowed to enter the chest through the cannula, creating a pneumothorax. In many animals, the mediastinum is thin and easy penetrated by the telescope in order to visualize the opposite hemithorax. If the mediastinum is thick, it must be cut once instrument portals have been placed in the lateral thorax.
  - *Lateral telescope cannula*: The dog is anesthetized and placed in lateral recumbency. Its hair is clipped over the entire lateral chest. Routine surgical preparation is performed. The patient is draped. The portal is chosen to be close to, but not directly over, the lesion, unless an operating telescope is used. The obturator is removed, and air is allowed to enter the chest through the cannula, creating a pneumothorax.
- The telescope tip is placed in warm saline (to prevent fogging), and the light cable and camera are attached. The color balancing of the camera is performed, the orientation of the camera is selected, and the telescope is then introduced into the cannula. If an operating telescope (which has a channel for instruments) is used, this may be the only cannula placed.
- Once the camera is in place, exploration of the thorax may begin. It is critical that the operator know the orientation of the camera, and care must be taken to ensure that the orientation is not changed during exploration. Telescopes with angled lenses make visualizing thoracic structures easier because they enable the operator to "see around corners" but require some practice to maintain orientation. Camera fogging or obscured vision is controlled by keeping the telescope warm, by wiping the tip on the pleural surface, or by removing the telescope and wiping the tip with warm saline in a gauze sponge.

- Instrument portals, if needed, are placed through the lateral thoracic wall. The sites are chosen under visualization with the telescope so that the operating site is easily observed and the instruments will not interfere with each other or the telescope. A short skin incision is made over the chosen site, and a hemostat or a pair of dissecting scissors is used to dissect to the level of the pleura. The cannula is placed using a blunt obturator, but the cannula may be removed and the instrument placed directly through the defect if the cannula is hindering instrument manipulation. Instruments are always introduced into the thoracic cavity under direct visualization to ensure that no organ damage occurs.
- Thoracoscopic exploration enables clinicians to view the lesions within the thorax and to place biopsy or drainage needles under visualization. More substantial biopsy samples may be obtained using 5-mm oval cup (clamshell) biopsy forceps, guillotine sutures, or endoscopic stapling devices. Depending on the skill of the operator, correction or removal of a lesion may be performed by using a thoracoscopic or an open technique.
- Once the procedure is finished, the instruments are removed and the instrument portals are surgically closed. The muscle must be sutured if a 10-mm portal was created, but portals that are 5 mm or smaller may only need subcutaneous and skin sutures. A chest tube may be placed using the telescope for visualization of placement. Negative pressure is then reestablished using the chest tube. Alternatively, if the telescope cannula has a valve and a gasket, negative pressure can be reestablished using the cannula. Lung reexpansion is confirmed by observation, using the telescope, and then a suture is used to close the muscle defect rapidly while the cannula is removed. The subcutaneous tissues and the skin are then closed.

SAMPLE HANDLING

Biopsy samples are placed in formalin and submitted for histopathologic examination. Fluid samples are submitted for cytology and culture, as indicated.

APPROPRIATE AFTERCARE

Postprocedure Patient Monitoring

- Body temperature
- Heart and respiratory rate
- ECG
- Blood pressure, if indicated
- Sedation score
- Pain score
- Observation of incision sites

Nursing Care

- Provide a warm, quiet environment for anesthetic recovery.
- Monitor the chest tube and maintain a record of evacuations.

THORACOSCOPY

Dietary Modification
Feed the patient once it awakens from anesthesia.

Medication Requirements
Analgesics

Restrictions on Activity
Walk the patient on a leash until the incisions are healed and any sutures or staples are removed.

Anticipated Recovery Time
• Patients recover rapidly from minimally invasive surgery, usually within 12–24 h.
• The chest tube is removed once production of air has ceased and fluid production has ceased or decreased.
• Sutures or staples are removed 7–10 days after the procedure.

 INTERPRETATION

NORMAL FINDINGS OR RANGE
Normal size and shape of thoracic viscera and surfaces

ABNORMAL VALUES
• Abnormal size, shape, or color of thoracic viscera
• Presence of lung bullae
• Presence of mass or masses
• Diffuse neoplastic disease
• Pericardial or pleural effusion
• Presence of foreign bodies

CRITICAL VALUES
Any condition requiring immediate open surgery, such as severe thoracic trauma

INTERFERING FACTORS
Drugs That May Alter Results of the Procedure
None

Conditions That May Interfere with Performing the Procedure
• Hemorrhage
• Small patients
• Clinician inexperience

Procedure Techniques or Handling That May Alter Results
None

Influence of Signalment on Performing and Interpreting the Procedure
Species
Because of their small body size, thoracoscopy is more difficult to perform in cats than in dogs.

Breed
Thoracoscopy is more difficult to perform in small breeds than in larger breeds.

Age
None

Gender
None

Pregnancy
None

CLINICAL PERSPECTIVE
• This technique is used to explore the thorax and obtain biopsy samples, with minimal pain and stress for the animal. It is an ideal technique for use in medically compromised patients and provides a faster return to function in all patients.
• Results of the exploration and biopsies will enable development of a treatment plan or provide realistic expectations in the event of a terminal illness.

 MISCELLANEOUS

ANCILLARY TESTS
• Lung biopsy
• Thoracic radiography
• Thoracic ultrasonography

SYNONYMS
Minimally invasive surgery

SEE ALSO

Blackwell's Five-Minute Veterinary Consult: Canine and Feline Topics

- Adenocarcinoma, Lung
- Chylothorax
- Hemothorax
- Lung Lobe Torsion
- Mesothelioma
- Pericardial Effusion
- Pneumonia, Interstitial
- Pneumothorax
- Pulmonary Contusions
- Pulmonary Fibrosis
- Pyothorax
- Squamous Cell Carcinoma, Lung
- Thymoma

Related Topics in This Book

- General Principles of Endoscopy
- Laparoscopy

ABBREVIATIONS

None

Suggested Reading

Kovak JR, Ludwig LL, Bergman PJ, *et al.* Use of thoracoscopy to determine the etiology of pleural effusion in dogs and cats: 18 cases (1998–2001). *J Am Vet Med Assoc* 2002; 221: 990–994.

McCarthy TC, Monnet E. Diagnostic and operative thoracoscopy. In: McCarthy TC, ed. *Veterinary Endoscopy for the Small Animal Practitioner.* St Louis: Saunders Elsevier, 2005: 229–278.

Walton RS. Video-assisted thoracoscopy. *Vet Clin North Am Small Anim Pract* 2001; 31: 729–759.

INTERNET RESOURCES

BioVision Technologies: Veterinary endoscopy, http://www.biovisiontech.com/veterinary_products.html. Operating telescope equipment, videos, and training courses.

Storz: Laparoscopy/thoracoscopy, http://www.ksvea.com/small_laparoscopy.html. Equipment and videos.

University of Georgia, College of Veterinary Medicine: Minimally invasive surgery/endoscopic surgery, http://www.vet.uga.edu/mis/index.php. Examples of minimally invasive surgery and training courses.

AUTHOR NAME

Elizabeth M. Hardie

THYROGLOBULIN AUTOANTIBODY

BASICS

TYPE OF SPECIMEN
Blood

TEST EXPLANATION AND RELATED PHYSIOLOGY
Thyroglobulin (TG) is produced by thyroid follicular cells and stored in the follicular lumen. Thyroid cells concentrate and incorporate dietary iodine into TG and then further modify it to produce thyroid hormones. Approximately 50% of canine primary hypothyroid cases are the result of lymphocytic thyroiditis, which is thought to involve poor regulatory T-cell function and unabated helper and effector T-cell–mediated and plasma cell–mediated destruction of the thyroid gland. Thyroglobulin autoantibody (TGAA) is measured to detect lymphocytic thyroiditis in dogs.

There are 2 theories to explain TGAA in dogs with thyroiditis. The first is that TG is released into circulation following T-cell destruction of thyroid follicular cells, enabling subsequent (nonpathogenic) antibody production against the TG antigen. In contrast, the second theory is that TGAAs (as well as AAs to other antigens such as thyroidal microsomal antigen and colloid antigen 2) may be involved in the pathogenesis of thyroiditis. Presence of TGAA does not correlate with current thyroid gland function, and dogs with primary hypothyroidism caused by idiopathic thyroid atrophy may have no historic laboratory evidence of TGAA. Recent vaccination may increase TGAAs, but the values have been shown to decline to normal prior to the next scheduled vaccination. It is unknown whether these AAs affect thyroid function. Nonthyroidal illness (e.g., hyperadrenocorticism or hypoadrenocorticism, diabetes mellitus, dermatologic disorders) may be associated with equivocal results. Patients with equivocal results should be retested following alleviation/management of illness. In primary hypothyroidism, as thyroid tissue is progressively destroyed, TGAA levels may decline because less TG is produced in the gland.

Measurement of TGAAs
ELISAs are most commonly available. The ELISA compares specimen optical density to that of a negative control sample. Requiring that positive results be >200% negative of the negative control decreases the false-positive rate and improves specificity for thyroiditis. Equivocal results (increased TGAA levels that are <200% elevated above negative control) could be due to early disease or a false positive caused by nonthyroidal illness.

Radioimmunoprecipitation assays, complement fixation, fluorescent antibody, and passive hemagglutination are less commonly used.

INDICATIONS
Identification of dogs with lymphocytic thyroiditis

CONTRAINDICATIONS
None

POTENTIAL COMPLICATIONS
None

CLIENT EDUCATION
This is a screening test to identify dogs at risk of developing hypothyroidism. However, dogs with circulating TGAAs may not yet have clinical or laboratory evidence of the condition.

BODY SYSTEMS ASSESSED
Endocrine and metabolic

SAMPLE

COLLECTION
1–2 mL of venous blood

HANDLING
- Use a red-top tube. Avoid the use of serum-separator tubes.
- Centrifuge and separate the serum.
- Transfer the sample to plastic and freeze.
- Ship the frozen serum on ice packs to the laboratory.

STORAGE
Store the serum in a freezer.

STABILITY
N/A

PROTOCOL
None

INTERPRETATION

NORMAL FINDINGS OR RANGE
TGAAs: negative test result

ABNORMAL VALUES
- TGAA levels that are >200% of the control value
- TGAA levels that are increased but still <200% above the negative control are equivocal and warrant retesting.

CRITICAL VALUES
None

INTERFERING FACTORS
Drugs That May Alter Results or Interpretation
Drugs That Interfere with Test Methodology
None

Drugs That Alter Physiology
None

Disorders That May Alter Results
Lipemia or hemolysis

Collection Techniques or Handling That May Alter Results
Prolonged sample storage at room temperature promotes proteolysis.

Influence of Signalment
Species
Dogs only

Breed
- Several breeds reportedly have an increased risk for lymphocytic thyroiditis, including beagles, borzois, golden retrievers, English pointers, English setters, and boxers. Genetic links have been identified in beagles and borzois.
- Other studies dispute the influence of pedigree status.

Age
None

Gender
None

Pregnancy
None

LIMITATIONS OF THE TEST
Although sensitivity and specificity are reportedly high, some false-positive and false-negative results occur:
- Idiopathic thyroid atrophy may not be associated with TGAA.
- TGAA levels decline as thyroid tissue is progressively destroyed.

Sensitivity, Specificity, and Positive and Negative Predictive Values
- Sensitivity: 91%
- Specificity: 97%

Valid If Run in a Human Lab?
No—a canine-validated method is required.

Causes of Abnormal Results

Elevated TGAA level (>200% of negative control)	Negative or equivocal TGAA level (<200% of negative control)
Lymphocytic thyroiditis Postvaccination elevation of TGAA level (presumed transient)	Normal dogs may have low positive levels. Nonthyroidal illness Early or end-stage thyroiditis Thyroid atrophy

CLINICAL PERSPECTIVE

• TGAA-positive results correlate well with histologic evidence of thyroiditis, but this does not confirm hypothyroidism.
• A patient with thyroiditis is at increased risk of developing hypothyroidism; however, it is unknown when thyroid dysfunction will occur. Dogs with positive results should have thyroid panels (e.g., T_4, free T_4, cTSH) tested at future intervals and should be monitored for clinical signs of hypothyroidism.

 MISCELLANEOUS

ANCILLARY TESTS

• Mild normochromic, normocytic, nonregenerative anemia and hypercholesterolemia are typical findings in hypothyroid dogs.
• Free T_4 and cTSH
• T_4 AA

SYNONYMS

None

SEE ALSO

Blackwell's Five-Minute Veterinary Consult: Canine and Feline Topics
• Hypothyroidism
• Hyperthyroidism

Related Topics in This Book

• Thyroid-Stimulating Hormone
• Thyroxine (T_4), Free
• Thyroxine (T_4), Total

ABBREVIATIONS

• AA = autoantibody
• cTSH = canine thyroid-stimulating hormone
• T_4 = thyroxine
• TG = thyroglobulin
• TGAA = thyroglobulin autoantibody

Suggested Reading

Dixon RM, Mooney CT. Canine serum thyroglobulin autoantibodies in health, hypothyroidism and non-thyroidal illness. *Res Vet Sci* 1999; 66: 243–246.

Feldman EC, Nelson RW. Hypothyroidism. In: *Canine and Feline Endocrinology and Reproduction*, 3rd ed. St Louis: Saunders Elsevier, 2004: 90–93.

Nachreiner RF, Refsal KR, Graham PA, *et al.* Prevalence of autoantibodies to thyroglobulin in dogs with nonthyroidal illness. *Am J Vet Res* 1998; 59: 951–955.

Scott-Moncrieff JC, Azcona-Olivera J, Glickman NW, *et al.* Evaluation of antithyroglobulin antibodies after routine vaccination in pet and research dogs. *J Am Vet Med Assoc* 2002; 221: 515–521.

INTERNET RESOURCES

None

AUTHOR NAME

Ryan M. Dickinson

BASICS

TYPE OF PROCEDURE
Ultrasonographic

PROCEDURE EXPLANATION AND RELATED PHYSIOLOGY
Ultrasonography of the thyroid and parathyroid glands is an invaluable diagnostic tool for patients with cervical masses or nodules or for patients with abnormal calcium or thyroid hormone concentrations. Ultrasonography is a noninvasive, easy method to assess the origin of a mass, suspicion of metastasis, invasiveness of a mass, and relative blood supply. The changes seen with ultrasonography aid clinicians in deciding on further diagnostic tests that need to be performed or whether a patient is a candidate for surgery or radiation therapy. Fine-needle aspiration of abnormal tissue may be performed to further classify and determine a definitive diagnosis for a mass or nodule.

Hyperthyroid feline patients may undergo ultrasonography of the cervical region to better assess whether the disease is unilateral or bilateral. Nuclear scintigraphy is considered the gold standard for assessing feline patients with hyperthyroidism, because of its ability to determine the functional status of thyroid tissue. However, the equipment and radiation safety concerns limit the availability of this modality. If nuclear scintigraphy is unavailable, ultrasonography should be employed and can even be used with scintigraphy to provide surgeons with a noninvasive view of the tissues and surrounding structures. Deciding between various treatment protocols can be aided with the use of ultrasonography. Unilateral disease may be treated with unilateral thyroidectomy, whereas bilateral disease is best treated with iodine-131 therapy.

There are many causes of hypercalcemia, and patients that are exhibiting persistent hypercalcemia need to be further assessed for diseases such as primary hyperparathyroidism, secondary hyperparathyroidism due to renal disease or nutritional imbalances, and hypercalcemia of malignancy. By inspecting the size and architecture of the parathyroid glands, the clinician will be able to better diagnose the cause of the hypercalcemia and pursue treatment options.

INDICATIONS
• Cervical masses or nodules of unknown origin
• Abnormal blood calcium concentrations (increased or decreased) as seen with renal failure, hypercalcemia of malignancy, primary hyperparathyroidism, or secondary hyperparathyroidism
• Abnormal thyroid hormone profile, particularly cats with hyperthyroidism
• Reevaluation after thyroidectomy or parathyroidectomy

CONTRAINDICATIONS
None

POTENTIAL COMPLICATIONS
A compromised airway, or respiratory distress from other causes, may be exacerbated by a patient's positioning, stress of the procedure, or the pressure from the ultrasound probe in the region of the trachea (uncommon).

CLIENT EDUCATION
• Do not feed the patient on the morning of the exam in case sedation must be administered.
• Cervical masses of thyroid origin have a tendency to be very vascular, and hemorrhage secondary to aspiration may occur.

BODY SYSTEMS ASSESSED
Endocrine and metabolic

 PROCEDURE

PATIENT PREPARATION
Preprocedure Medication or Preparation
• The cervical region of the patient should be adequately clipped and cleaned from the larynx to the thoracic inlet.
• Alcohol should be applied to the skin for degreasing and cleaning purposes.
• An adequate amount of acoustic coupling gel should be applied to the cervical region.

Anesthesia or Sedation
• Most often, sedation or anesthesia is not required.
• Mild sedation or, infrequently, anesthesia will be required in uncooperative patients.
• Sedation or anesthesia is usually required for the aspiration of nodules or masses.

Patient Positioning
• There are 3 ways in which a patient may be positioned:
  1. Lateral recumbency (right and left) is used while the left and right thyroid and parathyroid glands are examined individually. This position may be more comfortable for the patient and require less restraint.
  2. Dorsal recumbency enables the examiner to see both the right and left sides without moving the patient.
  3. Sternal or sitting upright, with the patient facing the ultrasonographer, provides similar imaging as dorsal recumbency.
• In all positions, the neck should be extended to allow for better visualization of tissues.

Patient Monitoring
Mild patient restraint may be needed, and the patient should be monitored appropriately if sedation or anesthesia has been used. Patients with dyspnea due to an invasive cervical mass or other causes should be monitored closely for exacerbation of clinical signs during the exam.

Equipment or Supplies
• A 10- to 15-MHz linear array or microconvex curvilinear probe is ideal.
• A 7- to 10-MHz linear array or sector scanner transducer can be used.

THYROID AND PARATHYROID ULTRASONOGRAPHY

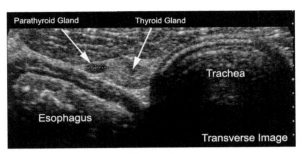

Figure 1

This transverse image of the cervical region in a normal dog depicts the normal anatomy and the left thyroid and parathyroid glands. This image was obtained using a 13.5-MHz linear probe.

- A standoff pad may be needed if a sector scanner is used.
- Ultrasound gel

TECHNIQUE

- The greatest challenge to ultrasonography of the cervical region in patients is the anatomy (Figure 1). It is very easy to mistake surrounding musculature, the mandibular salivary gland, or lymph nodes for the thyroid gland. The parathyroid glands may also be difficult to visualize because they can be very small or ectopic. Ectopic thyroid tissue may also be overlooked. Normal thyroid tissue is homogeneous and fusiform and is slightly hyperechoic to the surrounding musculature. The thyroid gland is located caudally and medially to the mandibular salivary glands and the submandibular and medial retropharyngeal lymph nodes. Several methods have been described that may aid the ultrasonographer in locating the thyroid glands (see the Suggested Reading section).
- One method is to first locate the carotid artery in a sagittal or long-axis plane immediately caudal to the larynx within the jugular groove (Figure 2). The probe is then positioned slightly ventrally and medially to image the thyroid gland in a long-axis or sagittal plane (oriented from cranial to caudal). If the probe is rotated too far, the tracheal wall is seen. The thyroid gland is very close to the trachea, and it may be difficult to image the thyroid gland in its entirety if it is located too dorsally, because the shadowing artifact created by the air in the trachea may hinder complete examination.
- Another method for locating the thyroid gland is to place the probe directly on the trachea, just caudal to the larynx in a cross-sectional or transverse plane (oriented from right to left). Then, slightly angle the probe to the right or left of the trachea, depending on which thyroid gland you wish to image. Slowly follow the length of the trachea from the larynx caudally toward the thoracic inlet. You will begin to see the thyroid gland immediately adjacent to the trachea, between the trachea medially and the common carotid artery laterally. The thyroid gland is triangular in this cross-sectional view and will have a distinct start and end. In contrast, the surrounding musculature can be followed along the length of the neck, with no definitive end point. The thyroid gland can then be viewed in the sagittal plane by simply rotating the probe 90°.

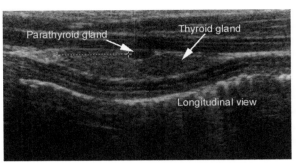

Figure 2

Longitudinal or sagittal image of the thyroid and parathyroid glands in a normal dog by using a 13.5-MHz linear probe. The *dotted line* indicates the distance from the cranial pole of the thyroid gland to the cranial pole of the parathyroid gland.

- Once the thyroid gland has been identified, parathyroid tissue can be located more easily. Most animals will have 4 parathyroid glands—2 on the left and 2 on the right—although oftentimes not all the parathyroid glands are seen with ultrasonography. The parathyroid glands may be embedded within the thyroid tissue, overlying the thyroid tissue, adjacent to the thyroid tissue, or not associated with the thyroid tissue at all. Normal parathyroid glands have been described as hypoechoic to anechoic compared to the thyroid tissue. They are usually oval to round. They may be located in any region of the thyroid gland or close to one another. Occasionally, an animal will have more than 4 parathyroid glands. Several structures may be confused with the parathyroid gland, which can make accurate interpretation difficult. Vessels, cysts (parathyroid or thyroid), thyroid lobules, and lymph tissue have all been described with a similar echogenicity and shape as the parathyroid glands and can be mistaken for parathyroid tissue. Oftentimes, not all of the parathyroid glands are seen with ultrasonography. Locating the parathyroid glands may be easier in larger patients.

SAMPLE HANDLING

If fine-needle aspiration is performed, the sample should immediately be placed on a slide and the sample spread similarly to a blood smear. These slides can then be stained to evaluate their contents.

APPROPRIATE AFTERCARE

Postprocedure Patient Monitoring

Watch the patient for hemorrhage only if aspirates have been taken from a vascular thyroid mass.

Nursing Care

None

Dietary Modification

None

Medication Requirements

None

Restrictions on Activity
None

Anticipated Recovery Time
Immediate

 INTERPRETATION

NORMAL FINDINGS OR RANGE
Thyroid Gland
- In dogs, the normal thyroid gland measures 2.5–5.0 cm long × 1.5 cm wide × 0.5 cm high. In cats, the normal thyroid is 2–3 cm long × 0.2–0.3 cm wide.
- A normal, well-demarcated, fusiform shape and homogeneous echotexture should be seen.

Parathyroid Gland
- It is hypoechoic to anechoic when compared to the thyroid tissue.
- Normal measurements have been reported to be 2.0–5.0 mm long and 0.5–1.0 mm wide.
- Length is likely the only reliable and reproducible measurement.
- No normal measurements have been reported in cats.
- The size of parathyroid gland appears to correlate with size of the patient, with larger dogs having glands that are slightly larger and easier to visualize.
- All parathyroid glands are not always seen.

ABNORMAL VALUES
Thyroid Gland
- Irregularly marginated, anechoic cystic structures may be seen within the parenchyma of the thyroid gland. Cysts should not be confused with thyroid vessels; color flow Doppler and orthogonal projections should be checked prior to diagnosis of a cystic structure. Cysts may also be confused with parathyroid glands, and cysts within the thyroid gland may occasionally have septations.
- Hypoechoic or heterogeneous and enlarged thyroid glands may be seen in cats because of hyperplastic transformation. Nodules and cystic structures may also be seen. These changes are bilateral 70% of the time.
- Thyroid gland enlargement with a nonuniform hypoechoic pattern (possible thyroiditis) is not commonly seen in animals.
- Heterogeneous, irregularly marginated nodules or masses (possible adenomas or carcinomas) are usually very vascular and may have mineralization within the mass.

Parathyroid Gland
- Enlarged or irregular single or multiple parathyroid glands may be secondary to parathyroid hyperplasia such as in nutritional hyperparathyroidism or renal secondary hyperparathyroidism, adenomas, or adenocarcinomas.

- One very enlarged parathyroid gland (>4 mm) with atrophy of other parathyroid glands is usually seen with a functional adenoma or adenocarcinoma.
- If a gland is small and difficult to visualize overall, it may be because hypercalcemia of malignancy is suppressing normal parathyroid tissue.

CRITICAL VALUES
None

INTERFERING FACTORS
Drugs That May Alter Results of the Procedure
None

Conditions That May Interfere with Performing the Procedure
- Ectopic thyroid or parathyroid tissue may be difficult to visualize or correctly identify.
- Prior surgery may disrupt normal anatomy. Hematomas or seromas in the region may further confuse the interpretation.
- Abnormal thyroid tissue may make interpretation of parathyroid gland images more difficult. Changes within the thyroid gland may cause the thyroid gland to be confused with the parathyroid glands or make visualization of parathyroid glands difficult.

Procedure Techniques or Handling That May Alter Results
- Inadequate clipping of hair
- Poor skin contact with probe
- Poor patient cooperation

Influence of Signalment on Performing and Interpreting the Procedure
Species
Cats may be more difficult to image because the small size of the thyroid and parathyroid glands and short neck prevent good probe contact.

Breed
Parathyroid glands may be more easily seen in larger dogs.

Age
None

Gender
None

Pregnancy
If any abnormalities in blood calcium concentrations exist, then concurrent changes with parathyroid glands may be seen.

CLINICAL PERSPECTIVE
- Ultrasonography of the thyroid and parathyroid glands is a non-invasive, easy method for assessing cervical masses, patients with hypercalcemia, or abnormal thyroid panels.
- Examination of the cervical region may be difficult for novice ultrasonographers because of the complex anatomy.

- Results of ultrasonography may help determine future treatments (i.e., surgery, medical management, radiation therapy or chemotherapy, or combination therapy).

MISCELLANEOUS

ANCILLARY TESTS
- Fine-needle aspiration of abnormal tissue can be performed.
- Nuclear scintigraphy of the thyroid gland may be performed if the origin of the tissue or mass is in question. However, very few neoplastic thyroid masses in dogs are functional.
- Nuclear scintigraphy should be used if ectopic thyroid tissue is suspected.
- Nuclear scintigraphy is the gold standard for assessing hyperthyroid feline patients.
- Computed tomography or magnetic resonance imaging with contrast medium can be used to further assess cervical region and invasiveness of mass.

SYNONYMS
None

SEE ALSO
Blackwell's Five-Minute Veterinary Consult: Canine and Feline Topics
- Adenocarcinoma, Thyroid—Dogs
- Hypercalcemia

- Hyperparathyroidism
- Hyperparathyroidism, Renal Secondary
- Hyperthyroidism
- Hypocalcemia
- Hypoparathyroidism
- Hypothyroidism

Related Topics in This Book
- General Principles of Ultrasonography
- Thyroid Scintigraphy
- Ultrasound-Guided Mass or Organ Aspiration

ABBREVIATIONS
None

Suggested Reading
Nyland TG, Mattoon JS, eds. *Small Animal Diagnostic Ultrasound.* Philadelphia: WB Saunders, 2002.
Wisner ER, Mattoon JS, Nyland TG, Baker TW. Normal ultrasonographic anatomy of the canine neck. *Vet Radiol* 1991; 32: 185–190
Wisner ER, Nyland TG. Ultrasonography of the thyroid and parathyroid glands. *Vet Clin North Am Small Anim Pract* 1998; 28: 973–991.

INTERNET RESOURCES
None

AUTHOR NAME
Sofija Rockov Liles

THYROID-RELEASING HORMONE RESPONSE TEST

BASICS

TYPE OF SPECIMEN
Blood

TEST EXPLANATION AND RELATED PHYSIOLOGY
During normal physiology, thyroid-releasing hormone (TRH) released by the hypothalamus stimulates pituitary secretion of TSH, which, in turn, stimulates synthesis and secretion of T_4 from the thyroid gland. Active T_4 (and T_3) subsequently inhibits further TRH and TSH release, resulting in a decline in thyroid hormone (negative feedback inhibition). Feline hyperthyroidism is a disorder characterized by autonomous secretion of T_4 from a hyperplastic or adenomatous thyroid gland. Clinical signs are related to the thyrotoxic effects of excessive hormone and may include weight loss despite an excellent appetite, hyperexcitability, increased drinking and urination, and frequent vomiting. Diagnosis of feline hyperthyroidism is typically straightforward and consists of finding increased serum T_4 levels. However, some cats with signs suggestive of hyperthyroidism have T_4 levels within the reference interval or that are only slightly increased. This may occur in early disease or in the presence of a concurrent illness. Usually a second T_4 sample drawn days to weeks later is diagnostic, especially if a concurrent disease was successfully treated. Alternatively, a TRH response test can be performed. TRH administered to a euthyroid cat significantly increases T_4 levels because of stimulation of TSH release. In cats with hyperthyroidism, autonomous secretion of T_4 results in persistent negative inhibition and atrophy of TSH-secreting cells. These cats have a blunted T_4 response to exogenous TRH.

The TRH response test may also be used to diagnosis primary and secondary hypothyroidism in dogs; however, owing to minor and inconsistent changes in T_4 and/or canine TSH in response to TRH, this test is not recommended.

INDICATIONS
Diagnosis of hyperthyroidism in cats with T_4 levels within the reference interval or only slightly increased

CONTRAINDICATIONS
None

POTENTIAL COMPLICATIONS
Administration of TRH can cause severe salivation, vomiting, tachypnea, and/or defecation that lasts for up to 4 h.

CLIENT EDUCATION
Administration of TRH may cause transient, but significant, salivation, tachypnea, vomiting, and defecation, but side effects should be resolved at the time of discharge.

BODY SYSTEMS ASSESSED
Endocrine and metabolic

SAMPLE

COLLECTION
2.0 mL of venous blood at each time point

HANDLING
- Use a red-top tube. (Avoid the use of serum-separator tubes.)
- Spin and separate the serum.
- Refrigerate the serum sample and send it on ice packs to the laboratory.

STORAGE
Store the sample in a refrigerator or freezer.

STABILITY
- Room temperature: 5 days
- Refrigerated (2°–8°C): 2 weeks
- Frozen (−20°C): several months

PROTOCOL
- Draw blood for baseline T_4.
- Administer 0.1 mg/kg TRH IV slowly over 1 min.
- Draw blood for T_4 4 h after TRH administration.
- TRH is available by prescription and is not licensed for use in cats.

INTERPRETATION

NORMAL FINDINGS OR RANGE
- A baseline T_4 concentration of 0.8–4.0 µg/dL (10.2–51.1 nmol/L)
- A T_4 level after TRH administration that is ≥2× the baseline T_4 concentration
- Reference intervals may vary depending on the laboratory and assay.

ABNORMAL VALUES
- A T_4 level after TRH administration that is <1.5× the baseline T_4 concentration
- Inconclusive: a T_4 level after TRH administration that is >1.5× but <2× the baseline T_4 concentration

CRITICAL VALUES
None

INTERFERING FACTORS
Drugs That May Alter Results or Interpretation
Drugs That Interfere with Test Methodology
Levothyroxine (T_4)

Drugs That Alter Physiology
- Levothyroxine (T_4)
- Corticosteroids
- A number of medications alter thyroid hormone levels in dogs. These drug effects have not been well characterized in cats.

Disorders That May Alter Results
Interference by hemolysis and lipemia is method dependent.

Collection Techniques or Handling That May Alter Results
- Prolonged storage at room temperature
- The use of serum-separator tubes

Influence of Signalment
Species
The test is used primarily in cats. The test is difficult to interpret in dogs, and not recommended.

Breed
None

Age
Hyperthyroidism is a disease of older cats.

Gender
None

Pregnancy
None

LIMITATIONS OF THE TEST
- The test may not accurately differentiate between hyperthyroid cats and euthyroid cats with severe systemic illness, because both may have a blunted T_4 response to TRH.
- In-office ELISAs may lack the necessary sensitivity to accurately detect the small changes in T_4 produced by TRH stimulation.

Sensitivity, Specificity, and Positive and Negative Predictive Values
N/A

Valid If Run in a Human Lab?
No—human assay lacks necessary sensitivity to detect low T_4 levels.

Causes of Abnormal Results

Adequate increase in T_4	Absent or blunted increase in T_4
Euthyroid state	Hyperthyroidism
	Euthyroid state with *severe*
	systemic illness

CLINICAL PERSPECTIVE
• The TRH response test is used to diagnose hyperthyroidism in cats with consistent symptoms but in which T_4 levels are normal or only mildly increased.
• An easier alternative is to retest the T_4 level in a few days or weeks or after concurrent disorders have been treated successfully.
• Cats with hyperthyroidism have a blunted T_4 response to TRH; however, this may also occur in cats with severe nonthyroidal illness.
• Intravascular administration of TRH may cause severe, but transient, autonomic symptoms.

MISCELLANEOUS

ANCILLARY TESTS
• Careful assessment of renal function is recommended prior to selecting treatment for hyperthyroidism. Resolution of the thyrotoxic state can worsen or unmask preexisting renal insufficiency.
• The free T_4 test is more sensitive in detecting hyperthyroidism in mildly hyperthyroid cats than is the total T_4 measurement, but has occasional false-positive test results.

• Nuclear scintigraphy can be used to locate hyperplastic/adenomatous thyroid tissue prior to surgical treatment.

SYNONYMS
TRH response test

SEE ALSO
Blackwell's Five-Minute Veterinary Consult: Canine and Feline Topics
Feline Hyperthyroidism

Related Topics in This Book
• T_3 Suppression Test
• Thyroxine (T_4), Free
• Thyroxine (T_4), Total

ABBREVIATIONS
• T_3 = triiodothyronine
• T_4 = thyroxine, total (hormone) or levothyroxine (drug)
• TRH = thyroid-releasing hormone
• TSH = thyroid-stimulating hormone (thyrotropin)

Suggested Reading
Feldman EC, Nelson RW. Feline hyperthyroidism. In: *Canine and Feline Endocrinology and Reproduction,* 3rd ed. St Louis: Saunders Elsevier, 2004: 86–151.

INTERNET RESOURCES
University of Georgia, College of Veterinary Medicine, Department of Pathology, Veterinary Clinical Pathology Clerkship Program: Stortz JS, Latimer KS, Tarpley HL, et al. Feline hyperthyroidism. 2004, http://www.vet.uga.edu/vpp/clerk/stortz.
Washington State University, College of Veterinary Medicine, Pet Health Topics: Hyperthyroidism in the cat. Last edited: May 29, 2008, http://www.vetmed.wsu.edu/clientED/hyperthyroidism.aspx.

AUTHOR NAME
Kristen R. Friedrichs

BASICS

TYPE OF PROCEDURE
Nuclear medicine

PROCEDURE EXPLANATION AND RELATED PHYSIOLOGY
The thyroid gland actively produces thyroxin and triiodothyronine from the amino acid tyrosine and the atomic ion, iodide (I^-). The iodide is then converted to iodine (I_2) within the thyroidal cell and bound to tyrosine. Of these molecules, 3 bound together form triiodothyronine (T_3) and 4 bound together form thyroxin (T_4). The T_3 and T_4 are then bound to proteins and secreted into a colloidal matrix as a central storage unit prior to release of the T_3 or T_4. To evaluate this process of iodide uptake by the thyroid and trapping of the thyroid hormone within the protein matrix of the colloid, 3 radiopharmaceuticals can be used: technetium 99m–pertechnetate ($^{99m}TcO_4^-$), the active transport mechanism at the level of the thyroid gland; and $^{123}I^-$ and $^{131}I^-$, which will be taken up by the active transport mechanism at the level of the external thyroid gland cell membrane and intracolloidal trapping or movement of the protein-bound radioactive I^- into the colloidal space, where it is stored for future use. A discrepancy (discordance) between the technetium and iodine radiopharmaceuticals has been seen in people but not in animals.

The thyroid tissues develop from the 4th pharyngeal arches and can migrate cranially to the base of the tongue or caudally to the cranioventral mediastinum (and can even be found in the heart-base area in the pericardial sac). In cats, enlarged thyroid glands may be palpable but are not necessarily present as a neck mass. In dogs, thyroid adenocarcinomas typically are nonfunctional (do not secrete excessive thyroid hormone) but will present as a large neck mass. Typically, on aspirates, these masses will be hemorrhagic, and the sample is nondiagnostic for an adenocarcinoma. In dogs, thyroid scintigraphy can be used to show the vascularity of the tumor (in the immediate dynamic vascular phase and in delayed static soft tissue imaging), as well as where the normal thyroid glands are located since they will not be suppressed from the lack of TSH in the euthyroid state. If the 2 thyroid glands can be clearly visualized and are normal in size, then the neck mass is originating from some other tissue. If only 1 normal-appearing gland is seen, and the contralateral side has a large amount of activity present, then the neck mass is an abnormal thyroid neoplasm. These 3 patterns of thyroid adenocarcinoma are seen with scintigraphy: a large, diffuse area of high radioactivity in the region of the thyroid gland, most common with follicular cell tumors; decreased activity in the region of the cervical mass with displacement of the normal-appearing contralateral thyroid gland, most common with stromal origin tumors; or irregular, variously sized, multifocal areas of radioactivity seen with mixed-cell tumor populations.

INDICATIONS
• Evaluation of cats with suspected hyperthyroidism
• Evaluation of cats with cranioventral thoracic masses or nodules for thyroidal origin
• Evaluation of neck masses in dogs for a relationship to the normal thyroid gland(s)
• Evaluation of dogs with functional thyroid carcinoma

CONTRAINDICATIONS
• There are no specific known contraindications to thyroid scintigraphy.

• The impact of methimazole on the uptake of sodium $^{99m}TcO_4^-$ has been studied in normal cats, but not in cats that are hyperthyroid. It is generally recommended that the cats be off of the methimazole for 2 weeks before the thyroid study.

POTENTIAL COMPLICATIONS
No immediate complications should be expected.

CLIENT EDUCATION
Client education is based on when the animal is sent home and based on state-specific nuclear medicine regulations. Both the radioactive iodide and the sodium pertechnetate will be excreted in the kidney, and therefore the urine will be radioactive for 60 h after injection (pertechnetate), 130 h for iodine 123, and 80 days for iodine 131. With minor amounts of the iodine 131 (a typical dose of 0.074–0.111 MBq or 200–300 μCi), clients will not have to collect waste products, but this depends on the individual's licensing requirements.

BODY SYSTEMS ASSESSED
Endocrine and metabolic

PROCEDURE

PATIENT PREPARATION
Preprocedure Medication or Preparation
• Removal of the patient from methimazole for 2 weeks prior to the scintigraphic study is recommended.
• In dogs, removal of thyroidal supplements that potentially block pertechnetate 99m or the iodide uptake at the cell receptor is recommended.
• Imaging procedures with iodinated contrast medium, such as excretory urography, should be avoided, if possible, since the contrast medium may cause iodine saturation in the hyperthyroid or hypothyroid animal and decrease the uptake of $^{99m}TcO_4^-$.
• The washout rate of competitive inhibition has not been determined for normal dogs and cats, but 2–3 weeks is currently recommended and appears to work well.
• The patient should have a catheter placed in a peripheral vessel for the radiopharmaceutical injection.

Anesthesia or Sedation
• None is necessary unless the dog or cat is fractious.
• Mild sedation can be used to ensure that the patient remains still during image acquisition.
• General anesthesia is typically needed if pinhole acquisitions (ventral images) of the thyroid are going to be acquired, because of the long acquisition times (5–8 min for 100,000-count images).

Patient Positioning
The patient is positioned in right lateral, left lateral, and sternal recumbency on the gamma camera for right lateral, left lateral, and ventral images, respectively. Centering is initially over the neck and then repeated over the thorax.

Patient Monitoring
None is required unless the patient is under general anesthesia.

Equipment or Supplies
• A gamma camera with a general-purpose, low-energy collimator with an acquisition computer workstation
• A 3-mL syringe with 300–600 μCi (11.1–22.0 MBq) of iodine 123 or iodine 131 for a dog or 200–400 μCi (7.4–14.8 MBq) of

iodine 123 or iodine 131 for a cat diluted to 1 mL. Typical dosing for pertechnetate 99m is 3–5 mCi (111–185 MBq) for a dog or a cat.

TECHNIQUE

- The $^{99m}TcO_4^-$ is injected into a cat via a peripheral catheter that is then flushed with saline and subsequently removed. The catheter and syringe are discarded into the radioactive sharps box. The patient is placed on the gamma camera after 20 min have passed. The cervical region is acquired as a static acquisition and at least 100,000 counts obtained. Left lateral, right lateral, and dorsal (or ventral) image planes are acquired. The camera is then centered over the thorax and left lateral, right lateral, and dorsal (or ventral) images are obtained. A static acquisition for the thorax is used, obtaining at least 250,000 counts. The matrix size for all acquisitions is 256 × 256 × 16 pixels.
- Radioactivity within the thyroid gland, which is seen as 2 focal areas of radioactivity in the midcervical region, is compared to that in the adjacent salivary tissue. In dogs, this tissue is the parotid salivary gland, and, in cats, the tissue is the zygomatic salivary glands. Regions of interest (ROIs) are drawn around the area of the thyroid gland and the salivary glands. A thyroid/salivary gland ratio is then created in which the number of counts in the thyroid gland divided by the total number of pixels in the ROI is in the numerator and the salivary gland counts divided by the total number of pixels in the ROI is in the denominator.
- The radiopharmaceutical for injection should be held in a specialized lead syringe shield prior to injection. Rubber gloves and a laboratory coat should be worn to reduce the potential for personnel contamination.

SAMPLE HANDLING

N/A

APPROPRIATE AFTERCARE

Postprocedure Patient Monitoring

- After injection of the radiopharmaceutical into the patient, the needle is withdrawn and discarded in a radioactive materials sharps box.
- The patient should be monitored and the exposure rates recorded at the surface and at 1 m and posted on the animal's cage with appropriate radioactive signage.
- There should be minimal interaction with the patient for 24 h.
- Feces and urine need to be collected and stored for 60 h (10 half-lives) before being discarded as general biologic waste.

Nursing Care

Minimal interaction with the patient after the procedure is recommended so as to minimize the risk of contamination with radioactive material.

Dietary Modification

None

Medication Requirements

None

Restrictions on Activity

None

Anticipated Recovery Time

If general anesthesia is used, recovery should take 15–30 min.

INTERPRETATION

NORMAL FINDINGS OR RANGE

- Sodium $^{99m}TcO_4^-$ has a chemical composition similar to the halogens, including iodide. The ionic charge (-1) and the atomic radius are similar, and therefore the $^{99m}TcO_4^-$ will be taken up by cell membrane receptors that concentrate the halogens. Specifically, these areas are the choroid plexus, the salivary glands, the gastric mucosa, and the thyroid glands.
- In normal dogs or cats, 2 focal regions of radioactivity are seen in the midcervical region that represent the thyroid glands.
- In cats, the normal thyroid/salivary gland ratio is 0.81:1 +/− 0.05 at 20 min. This ratio increases with a peak increase between 1 and 2 h (increased thyroidal gland uptake).
- In dogs, the thyroid/salivary gland ratio is 1.12:1 +/− 0.15 at 20 min. This ratio decreases over time in dogs because of increased salivary gland uptake and decreased thyroid gland uptake.

ABNORMAL VALUES

- Increased thyroid/salivary gland ratios are indicative of hyperfunctional tissue. If only 1 thyroid gland is identified, and it has an increased thyroid/salivary gland ratio, then the presumed functional adenoma is suppressing the contralateral gland. If 1 gland has an increased thyroid/salivary gland ratio while the other thyroid gland is barely detectable or has a similar activity as the ipsilateral thyroid gland, then both thyroid glands are abnormal. This is because the thyroid gland that has less activity is not complete suppressed as it should be if it were normal.

• The scintigraphic scan also provides anatomic information, and multifocal areas of increased activity is indicative of multinodular thyroid adenomas. These are primarily seen in cats.

• In dogs, thyroid adenocarcinomas are usually large at the time of presentation. The uptake may be more of a function of vascular capillary bed breakdown and size of the tumor than true active uptake of the radiopharmaceutical.

• Approximately 30% of cats have unilateral thyroid hyperplasia; 70% will be bilateral.

• Hypothyroidism is rare in cats and more common in dogs. This is characterized by decreased activity in the thyroid gland compared to the salivary glands. In cats, decreased activity can be seen if the patient has been previously treated with radioiodine or recent iodinated contrast medium administration associated with a specific contrast-imaging procedure.

• Mediastinal activity can be seen with metastatic disease or ectopic thyroid tissue. The cranial third of the thyroid gland is drained by the retropharyngeal lymph node, whereas the caudal two-thirds is drained by the cranial mediastinal lymph node.

• Activity can be seen in the esophagus due to swallowing of radioactive saliva. If mediastinal activity is seen, the mediastinum should be reevaluated in $\approx$1 h to verify that the activity is truly mediastinal and not esophageal.

• Pulmonary metastatic disease can be seen as focal areas of activity with metastatic thyroid adenocarcinoma.

CRITICAL VALUES
N/A

INTERFERING FACTORS
Drugs That May Alter Results of the Procedure
The administration of methimazole has been shown to increase thyroid uptake of $^{99m}TcO_4^-$ in normal cats, possibly because of increased circulating TSH. Increased thyroid uptake is seen for $\approx$15 days as part of a short-term rebound effect after withdrawal from the drug and may result in a false-positive result during thyroid scintigraphy.

Conditions That May Interfere with Performing the Procedure
None

Procedure Techniques or Handling That May Alter Results
• If a catheter is not used, an inadequate dose may be administered because of extravasation of radiopharmaceutical at the injection site.

• If an extension set is used, a portion of the radiopharmaceutical will bind to the plastic, also decreasing the dose that the patient receives.

Influence of Signalment on Performing and Interpreting the Procedure
Species
Cats may require a *pinhole* technique. This can be achieved with the zoom feature prior to image acquisition or can be done using a pinhole collimator. The advantage of this technique is increased image resolution; because of the small size of the image, the cat may need to be anesthetized to prevent its movement.

Breed
None

Age
Generally older animals suffer from hyperthyroidism.

Gender
None

Pregnancy
None for pregnancy; however, lactating cats have been shown to concentrate and excrete the sodium iodide and sodium pertechnetate in milk.

CLINICAL PERSPECTIVE
Thyroid scintigraphy is not only a functional imaging technique but also provides anatomic information. This procedure is the most effective for evaluating hyperthyroidism in cats and serves as a guide to determine thyroid gland uptake, as well as potential response to therapy. In addition, cats with bilateral increased activity identified during scintigraphy have a significantly higher risk of developing hypothyroidism compared to cats with a unilateral scintigraphic pattern.

MISCELLANEOUS

ANCILLARY TESTS

Determination of total T_4, T_3, and TSH concentrations

SYNONYMS

Thyroid scan

SEE ALSO

Blackwell's Five-Minute Veterinary Consult: Canine and Feline Topics
- Hyperthyroidism
- Hypothyroidism
- Adenocarcinoma, Thyroid—Dogs

Related Topics in This Book
- Thyroglobulin Autoantibody
- Thyroid and Parathyroid Ultrasonography
- Thyroid-Releasing Hormone Response Test
- Thyroid-Stimulating Hormone
- Thyroxine (T_4), Free
- Thyroxine (T_4), Total

ABBREVIATIONS
- MBq = megabecquerel = 1 disintegration per second
- μCi = microcurie = 3.7×10^4 disintegrations per second
- ROI = region of interest
- $^{99m}TcO_4^-$ = technetium 99m–pertechnetate
- TSH = thyroid-stimulating hormone

Suggested Reading

Adams WH, Daniel GB, Peterson MG, Young K. Quantitative ^{99m}Tc-pertechnetate thyroid scintigraphy in normal beagles. *Vet Radiol Ultrasound* 1997; 38: 323–328.

Beck KA, Hornof WJ, Feldman EC. The normal feline thyroid: Technetium pertechnetate imaging and determination of thyroid to salivary gland radioactivity ratios in 10 normal cats. *Vet Radiol* 1985; 26: 35–38.

Daniel GB, Nieckarz J, Sharp D, Adams WH. Quantitative thyroid scintigraphy as a predictor of serum thyroxin concentrations in normal and hyperthyroid cats. *Vet Radiol Ultrasound* 2002; 33: 313–320.

Nieckarz J, Daniel GB. The effect of methimazole on thyroid uptake of pertechnetate and radioiodine in normal cats. *Vet Radiol Ultrasound* 2001; 42: 374–382.

Nykamp SG, Dykes NL, Zarfoss MK, Scarlett JM. Association of the risk of development of hypothyroidism after iodine 131 treatment with the pretreatment pattern of sodium pertechnetate Tc 99m uptake in the thyroid gland in cats with hyperthyroidism: 165 cases (1990–2002). *J Am Vet Med Assoc* 2005; 226: 1671–1675.

INTERNET RESOURCES

University of Tennessee, College of Veterinary Medicine, Radiology: Nuclear medicine, http://www.vet.utk.edu/radiology/nuclear/index.php.

AUTHOR NAMES

Anthony Pease and Clifford R. Berry

THYROID-STIMULATING HORMONE

BASICS

TYPE OF SPECIMEN
Blood

TEST EXPLANATION AND RELATED PHYSIOLOGY
Thyroid hormone secretion is regulated through the hypothalamic-pituitary-thyroid axis. During normal physiology, thyroid-releasing hormone (TRH) from the hypothalamus stimulates thyroid-stimulating hormone (TSH) release from the pituitary, which in turn stimulates production and release of T_4 from the thyroid gland. Active T_4 subsequently inhibits further TRH and TSH release (negative feedback inhibition).

Canine primary hypothyroidism is a disorder caused by either destruction of thyroid tissue by immune-mediated thyroiditis or by idiopathic thyroid gland atrophy. This disorder is characterized by decreased thyroid hormone production by thyroid tissue and subsequent alleviation of negative feedback inhibition to the pituitary. In response to continued requirement for thyroid hormone production, the pituitary secretes larger amounts of TSH, which has a limited effect on the dysfunctional or atrophied thyroid tissue. Therefore, primary hypothyroidism is characterized by elevated TSH and low T_4 and/or free T_4 (fT_4) levels. Unfortunately, not all dogs with primary hypothyroidism have elevated TSH levels. This may be explained by pulsatile TSH secretion with episodic values within the reference interval (RI). There is also some thought that the current assay may miss some glycosylation forms of TSH, leading to false-negative results. Finally, chronic primary hypothyroidism might cause "exhaustion" of pituitary production of TSH. Sulfa drugs may inhibit thyroid gland production of thyroid hormone; therefore, sulfa-drug administration may mimic primary hypothyroidism in both clinical presentation and laboratory thyroid profile values.

Canine secondary hypothyroidism is caused by insufficient production of TSH from the pituitary. There is no direct damage to thyroid follicular cells in this disorder, but thyroid atrophy may be result from a lack of TSH stimulation. This disorder is characterized by low T_4, fT_4, and TSH values within the normal RI. Permanent causes of pituitary dysfunction (pituitary malformation or trauma) are uncommon. Glucocorticoids (naturally occurring or pharmaceuticals) and phenobarbital are 2 examples of drugs that may inhibit the production of TSH by an otherwise normal pituitary gland. Nonthyroidal illness can also inhibit pituitary release of TSH and possibly inhibit TRH release from the hypothalamus. Therefore, certain drugs and nonthyroidal illness may mimic laboratory thyroid profile values of secondary hypothyroidism. Laboratory testing for hypothyroidism should not be performed while a dog has a nonthyroidal illness or is receiving drugs that can alter thyroid hormone physiology.

Several types of canine TSH assays can be used by commercial laboratories, and all produce similar results. None of these assays are sufficiently sensitive to detect low TSH values, and therefore the low end of RI is designated as 0 mIU/L. Canine and feline TSH are similar, and the canine TSH assay can detect elevated feline TSH concentrations in the rare cases of feline hypothyroidism (typically secondary to surgical or radiation therapy for hyperthyroidism). However, the assay lacks the sensitivity necessary to detect the depression of feline TSH caused by hyperthyroidism.

INDICATIONS
• In conjunction with T_4 and/or fT_4 values, TSH levels can be used to either diagnosis or rule out primary hypothyroidism.
• To aid in differentiation between primary and secondary hypothyroidism

CONTRAINDICATIONS
• Avoid testing dogs with concurrent nonthyroidal illness.

• Avoid testing dogs on certain medications (see the Drugs That Alter Physiology section).

POTENTIAL COMPLICATIONS
None

CLIENT EDUCATION
A sample collected after withholding food for 8–12 h is preferred.

BODY SYSTEMS ASSESSED
Endocrine and metabolic

SAMPLE

COLLECTION
2 mL of venous blood

HANDLING
• Use a red-top tube. Do not use serum-separator tubes.
• Centrifuge the sample and then transfer the serum to a plastic tube and freeze it.
• Ship the frozen serum on ice packs to the laboratory.

STORAGE
Store the samples in a freezer.

STABILITY
Frozen ($-20°$C): 2 months

PROTOCOL
None

INTERPRETATION

NORMAL FINDINGS OR RANGE
• Dogs: 0–37 mIU/L (<0.5 ng/mL)
• Cats: 0–21 mIU/L
• RIs may vary depending on the laboratory and assay.

ABNORMAL VALUES
• Dogs: A TSH concentration of >37 mIU/L (>0.5 ng/mL) is consistent with primary hypothyroidism if there is concurrent decreased T_4 and/or fT_4 values.
• Cats: A TSH concentration of >21 mIU/L is consistent with primary hypothyroidism if there is concurrent decreased T_4 and/or fT_4 values.
• TSH values within the RI with concurrent decreased T_4 and/or fT_4 values may be due to secondary hypothyroidism, nonthyroidal illness, or certain drugs.

CRITICAL VALUES
None

INTERFERING FACTORS
Drugs That May Alter Results or Interpretation
Drugs That Interfere with Test Methodology
Administration of recombinant TSH will be detected by the assay.

DRUGS THAT ALTER PHYSIOLOGY
• Glucocorticoids, dopamine, cyproheptadine, and possibly phenobarbital and carprofen may inhibit release of TSH from the pituitary.
• Sulfonamides may interfere with T_4 production by thyroid follicular cells with indirect increase in TSH release from the pituitary.
• Prolonged administration of levothyroxine alters the hypothalamic-pituitary-thyroid axis. Thyroid supplements should be discontinued for 6–8 weeks before definitive thyroid function tests are performed.

Disorders That May Alter Results
Lipemia or hemolysis

Collection Techniques or Handling That May Alter Results
- Prolonged storage of serum at room temperature
- The use of gel-containing serum-separator tubes is not recommended.

Influence of Signalment
Species
This assay is used almost exclusively for dogs.

Breed
None

Age
Thyroid disease is more common in older animals.

Gender
None

Pregnancy
None

LIMITATIONS OF THE TEST
Sensitivity, Specificity, and Positive and Negative Predictive Values
- Specificity of the TSH test is higher when interpreted in context with concurrent T_4 and/or fT_4 values (specificity, 90%).
- Specificity of TSH alone: ≈82%
- Sensitivity: 76%–87%
- Diagnostic accuracy: 84%

Valid If Run in a Human Lab?
No—a species-validated assay is required.

Causes of Abnormal Findings

High values	Low values (within RI)
Primary hypothyroidism	Secondary hypothyroidism
Sulfa-drug effect	Chronic, nonthyroidal illness
Nonthyroidal illness	Glucocorticoid administration
	Hyperadrenocorticism
	Phenobarbital administration
	Chronic levothyroxine administration
	Primary hypothyroidism with false-negative result

CLINICAL PERSPECTIVE
- TSH alone is of limited diagnostic utility and should always be interpreted in context with physical examination findings and concurrent T_4 and/or fT_4 values.
  - An elevated TSH concentration with low T_4 and/or fT_4 values is consistent with primary hypothyroidism in a dog with a consistent medical history and physical examination findings.
  - Normal T_4, fT_4, and TSH values rule out hypothyroidism.
  - TSH levels are elevated in 7%–18% of dogs with normal T_4 and/or fT_4 values: This may be due to an early, compensated stage of primary hypothyroidism; retesting in 2–4 months may be warranted.
  - TSH levels are elevated in some dogs with nonthyroidal illness.
- Dogs with primary hypothyroidism may have normal TSH values because of fluctuation of pituitary TSH release, an inability of the assay to detect all TSH isoforms (uncommon), and pituitary exhaustion (uncommon).

- Secondary hypothyroidism, nonthyroidal illness, and certain drugs are associated with low T_4 and/or fT_4 values with a TSH within the normal RI.
- Although the canine TSH assay can be used to diagnose feline hypothyroidism, a feline-specific thyrotropin assay is needed to aid in diagnosis of feline hyperthyroidism.

MISCELLANEOUS
ANCILLARY TESTS
- Evaluation of T_4 and fT_4
- Consider canine TSH stimulation as warranted.
- Any required tests to rule out concurrent illness

SYNONYMS
- Canine TSH assay (cTSH assay)
- Thyrotropin assay

SEE ALSO
Blackwell's Five-Minute Veterinary Consult: Canine and Feline Topics
Hypothyroidism
Related Topics in This Book
- Thyroglobulin Autoantibody
- Thyroxine (T_4), Free
- Thyroxine (T_4), Total

ABBREVIATIONS
- fT_4 = free T_4
- RI = reference interval
- T_4 = thyroxine
- TRH = thyroid-releasing hormone
- TSH = thyroid-stimulating hormone (thyrotropin)

Suggested Reading
Daminet S, Ferguson DC. Influence of drugs on thyroid function in dogs. *J Vet Intern Med* 2003; 17: 463–472.
Feldman EC, Nelson RW. Hypothyroidism. In: *Canine and Feline Endocrinology and Reproduction,* 3rd ed. St Louis: Saunders Elsevier, 2004: 118–147.
Marca MC, Loste IO, González JM, *et al.* Evaluation of canine serum thyrotropin (TSH) concentration: Comparison of three analytical procedures. *J Vet Diagn Invest* 2001; 13: 106–110.
Peterson ME, Melian C, Nichols R. Measurement of serum total thyroxine, triiodothyronine, free thyroxine, and thyrotropin concentrations for diagnosis of hypothyroidism in dogs. *J Am Vet Med Assoc* 1997; 11: 1396–1402.
Scott-Moncrieff JC, Nelson RW, Bruner JM, Williams DA. Comparison of serum concentrations of thyroid-stimulating hormone in healthy dogs, hypothyroid dogs, and euthyroid dogs with concurrent disease. *J Am Vet Med Assoc* 1998; 212: 387–391.

INTERNET RESOURCES
Luechtefeld L. Thyroid diagnosis, treatment options evolve. Vet Pract News, http://www.veterinarypracticenews.com/vet-dept/canine-practice/thyroid-diagnosis-treatment-options-evolve.aspx.

AUTHOR NAME
Ryan M. Dickinson

THYROID-STIMULATING HORMONE STIMULATION TEST

BASICS

TYPE OF SPECIMEN
Blood

TEST EXPLANATION AND RELATED PHYSIOLOGY
During normal physiology, thyroid-releasing hormone (TRH) released by the hypothalamus stimulates pituitary secretion of TSH, which in turn, stimulates thyroid gland synthesis and secretion of T_4. Active T_4 [and triiodothyronine (T_3)] subsequently inhibits further TRH and TSH release, resulting in a decline in thyroid hormone (negative feedback inhibition). *Hypothyroidism*, a common endocrine disorder in dogs, is caused by idiopathic or immune-mediated destruction of thyroid tissue, leading to decreased production of thyroid hormones. Hypothyroidism is diagnosed by finding low T_4 levels in a dog with symptoms and clinical pathologic findings consistent with this disorder. However, there are numerous non-thyroid-related causes of low T_4. The TSH stimulation test is considered the gold standard for diagnosing hypothyroidism and will accurately differentiate hypothyroid dogs from euthyroid dogs with low T_4. In euthyroid dogs, administration of TSH will result in an appropriate increase in T_4. In contrast, dogs with hypothyroidism will fail to have an adequate increase in T_4 in response to TSH. Performance of the TSH stimulation test is limited by the availability and expense of TSH. The TSH stimulation test is rarely needed to diagnosis hypothyroidism in cats, an uncommon condition that is usually secondary to treatment of hyperthyroidism.

INDICATIONS
Definitive diagnosis of hypothyroidism, especially when T_4 may be spuriously decreased

CONTRAINDICATIONS
None

POTENTIAL COMPLICATIONS
An anaphylactic reaction to IV administration of TSH is rare.

CLIENT EDUCATION
An allergic reaction to TSH administration is rare.

BODY SYSTEMS ASSESSED
Endocrine and metabolic

SAMPLE

COLLECTION
2.0 mL of venous blood at each time point

HANDLING
- Use a red-top tube. Avoid the use of serum-separator tubes.
- Spin and separate the serum.
- Refrigerate the serum sample and send it on ice packs to the laboratory.

STORAGE
Store the serum in a freezer.

STABILITY
- Room temperature: 5 days
- Refrigerated (2°–8°C): 2 weeks
- Frozen (−20°C): several months

PROTOCOL
- Draw blood for a baseline T_4.
- Administer TSH IV.
  - Dogs: 0.1 IU/kg bovine TSH; maximum dose, 5 IU TSH or 50 μg recombinant human TSH (rh-TSH)
  - Cats: 0.5 IU/kg IV bovine TSH or 0.025–0.2 mg rh-TSH
- Draw blood for T_4 4–6 h (in dogs) or 6–8 h (in cats) after TSH administration.

INTERPRETATION

NORMAL FINDINGS OR RANGE
Reference intervals may vary depending on the laboratory and assay.

Dogs
- Baseline T_4 concentration: 1.0–3.5 μg/dL (12.8–45.0 nmol/L)
- T_4 concentration after administration of TSH: >3.0 μg/dL (>38.3 nmol/L) or >1.5× the baseline

Cats
- Baseline T_4 concentration: 0.8–4.0 μg/dL (10.2–51.1 nmol/L)
- T_4 concentration after administration of TSH: >3.0 μg/dL (>38.3 nmol/L) or >1.5× the baseline

ABNORMAL VALUES
- Canine T_4 concentration after administration of TSH: <1.5 μg/dL (19.3 nmol/L) or <1.5× the baseline
- Feline T_4 concentration after administration of TSH: <1.0 μg/dL (12.9 nmol/L) or <1.5× the baseline
- Nondiagnostic results
  - Canine T_4 concentration after administration of TSH: 1.5–3.0 μg/dL (19.3–38.6 nmol/L)
  - Feline T_4 concentration after administration of TSH: 1.0–3.0 μg/dL (12.9–38.6 nmol/L)

CRITICAL VALUES
None

INTERFERING FACTORS
Drugs That May Alter Results or Interpretation
Drugs That Interfere with Test Methodology
Levothyroxine (T_4)

Drugs That Alter Physiology
- Prolonged administration of levothyroxine alters the hypothalamic-pituitary-thyroid axis. Discontinue thyroid supplements 6–8 weeks prior to thyroid function testing
- Many commonly used drugs have the potential to decrease baseline T_4 values and variably affect free T_4 and TSH concentrations in dogs, including phenobarbital, glucocorticoids, sulfonamides, clomipramine, carprofen, etodolac, furosemide, methimazole, phenylbutazone, progestagens, and propylthiouracil. The effects these drugs have on response tests are less well characterized. Little is known about the effects of these drugs on the hypothalamic-pituitary-thyroid axis in cats.

Disorders That May Alter Results
Interference by hemolysis or lipemia is method dependent.

Collection Techniques or Handling That May Alter Results
- Prolonged storage at room temperature
- The use of serum-separator tubes is not recommended.

THYROID-STIMULATING HORMONE STIMULATION TEST

Influence of Signalment

Species
- Hypothyroidism is common in dogs.
- Hypothyroidism is uncommon in cats and typically secondary to treatment of hyperthyroidism.

Breed
Certain breeds, most notably greyhounds, have baseline T_4 levels that may fall outside accepted reference intervals; however, euthyroid greyhounds should increase T_4 by 1.5-fold in response to TSH administration.

Age
Older dogs may have a less vigorous response than younger dogs.

Gender
None

Pregnancy
None

LIMITATIONS OF THE TEST
- A lack of commercial bovine TSH and the expense of rh-TSH
- The presence of T_4 autoantibodies may interfere with RIA and chemiluminescent methods but not with ELISA.
- In-office ELISAs may lack the necessary sensitivity to accurately detect the changes in T_4 produced by TSH stimulation.
- Severe systemic illness may result in a subnormal response to TSH administration, mimicking true hypothyroidism.

Sensitivity, Specificity, and Positive and Negative Predictive Values:
N/A

Valid If Run in a Human Lab?
No—human assay lacks the sensitivity necessary to detect low T_4 levels.

Causes of Abnormal Results

Adequate stimulation of T_4	Inadequate stimulation of T_4
Euthyroid	Hypothyroidism
	Euthyroid with severe systemic illness

CLINICAL PERSPECTIVE
- The TSH stimulation test is the gold standard for diagnosis of hypothyroidism; however, owing to the unavailability of bovine TSH, this test is rarely performed. A recombinant form of human TSH is now available but is very expensive.

- The clinical diagnosis of canine hypothyroidism depends on finding signs and clinical pathologic changes suggestive of this disorder, combined with thyroid function tests, including T_4, free T_4, and TSH with or without thyroid hormone autoantibodies.

MISCELLANEOUS

ANCILLARY TESTS
Rule out nonthyroidal illness with appropriate diagnostic testing

SYNONYMS
TSH stimulation test (TSH stim)

SEE ALSO
Blackwell's Five-Minute Veterinary Consult: Canine and Feline Topics
Hypothyroidism
Related Topics in This Book
- Thyroid-Stimulating Hormone
- Thyroxine (T_4), Free
- Thyroxine (T_4), Total

ABBREVIATIONS
- rh-TSH = recombinant human TSH
- T_4 = thyroxine, total (hormone) or levothyroxine (drug)
- TRH = thyroid-releasing hormone
- TSH = thyroid-stimulating hormone

Suggested Reading
Feldman EC, Nelson RW. Hypothyroidism. *In: Canine and Feline Endocrinology and Reproduction*. St Louis: Saunders Elsevier, 2004: 86–151.

INTERNET RESOURCES
Bruyette D. Canine hypothyroidism. In: Scherk M, ed. 26th Congress of the World Small Animal Veterinary Association (WSAVA), Vancouver, 2001, http://www.vin.com/VINDBPub/SearchPB/Proceedings/PR05000/PR00158.htm.

AUTHOR NAME
Kristen R. Friedrichs

THYROXINE (T₄), FREE

BASICS

TYPE OF SPECIMEN
Blood

TEST EXPLANATION AND RELATED PHYSIOLOGY
Secretion of thyroid hormone is regulated through the hypothalamic-pituitary-thyroid axis (for a review, see the "Thyroxine (T₄), Total" chapter). T_4 constitutes most of the thyroid hormone secreted by the thyroid, and >99% of plasma T_4 is bound to proteins, with the remainder unbound [free T_4 (fT_4)]. Only fT_4 can enter peripheral tissue cells, and the plasma fT_4 concentration is strictly regulated. As with total T_4 (TT_4), nonthyroidal illness and certain drugs may decrease the fT_4 concentration. However, only severe illness or high/prolonged doses of drugs will alter the fT_4 concentration, making the fT_4 concentration more representative of thyroid hormone production than the TT_4 concentration.

A modified equilibrium dialysis followed by radioimmunoassay is the method of choice. Dialysis separates unbound T_4 (fT_4) from the protein-bound T_4 fraction and removes any T_4 autoantibodies that might interfere with the assay. Solid-phase radioimmunoassays (analog assays) and chemiluminescent assays are available (and often cheaper), but these tend to underestimate fT_4 concentrations in dogs and cats and are not recommended.

INDICATIONS
- Diagnosis of hypothyroidism in dogs with consistent clinical signs, physical exam findings, and clinical pathologic changes
- Confirmation of thyroid function in dogs with low TT_4 values but lacking classical signs of hypothyroidism
- Confirmation of thyroid function in cats with consistent clinical signs of hyperthyroidism (e.g., thyroid nodule, weight loss, tachycardia) but a TT_4 concentration in the upper 50% of the reference interval (RI) or only mildly increased

CONTRAINDICATIONS
Not recommended for patients without consistent clinical signs or exam findings, unless the TT_4 value is low

POTENTIAL COMPLICATIONS
None

CLIENT EDUCATION
None

BODY SYSTEMS ASSESSED
- Behavioral
- Cardiovascular
- Dermatologic
- Endocrine and metabolic
- Reproductive

SAMPLE

COLLECTION
0.5–2.0 mL of venous blood

HANDLING
- Use a red-top tube. Avoid the use of serum-separator tubes.
- Centrifuge and transfer the separated serum to a plastic tube and freeze it.
- Transport the sample on ice packs to the laboratory.

STORAGE
Store samples in a freezer.

STABILITY
- Room temperature: 5 days
- Refrigerated(2°–8°C): at least 2 weeks
- Frozen(−20°C): several months

PROTOCOL
None

INTERPRETATION

NORMAL FINDINGS OR RANGE
- Dogs: 8–26 pmol/L (0.8–2.5 ng/dL)
- Cats: 10–50 pmol/L (1–4 ng/dL)
- RIs may vary depending on the laboratory and assay.

ABNORMAL VALUES
Values above or below the RI

CRITICAL VALUES
None

INTERFERING FACTORS
Drugs That May Alter Results or Interpretation
Drugs That Interfere with Test Methodology
Levothyroxine

Drugs That Alter Physiology
- Decreased by administration of carprofen, etodolac, glucocorticoids, methimazole, phenobarbital, propylthiouracil, or sulfonamides in dogs. The effects of these drugs in cats are unknown but are assumed to be similar.
- Prolonged levothyroxine administration alters the hypothalamic-pituitary-thyroid axis and should be discontinued for 6–8 weeks before thyroid tests are performed.

Disorders That May Alter Results
- Lipemia or hemolysis
- T_4 autoantibody interferes with analog and chemiluminescent assays. The results of the modified equilibrium dialysis assay are not affected.

Collection Techniques or Handling That May Alter Results
- Prolonged storage of serum at room temperature
- Use of a serum-separator tube

Influence of Signalment
Species
- The most common thyroid disorder in dogs is hypothyroidism.
- The most common thyroid disorder in cats is hyperthyroidism.

Breed
- Golden retrievers, Doberman pinschers, dachshunds, cocker spaniels, Great Danes, boxers, poodles, German shepherds, Dalmatians, Irish setters, and miniature schnauzers have an increased risk of developing hypothyroidism.
- Sighthounds (e.g., greyhounds) have a lower fT_4 concentration than average dogs.
- Siamese and Himalayan cats have a decreased risk of hyperthyroidism.

Age
Thyroid disease is more common in older animals.

Gender
None

Pregnancy
Pregnancy may increase T$_4$ and fT$_4$ levels.

LIMITATIONS OF THE TEST
Sensitivity, Specificity, and Positive and Negative Predictive Values
Hypothyroid Dogs
- Sensitivity: 98%
- Specificity: 93%
- Diagnostic accuracy: 95%

Hyperthyroid Cats
- Sensitivity: 98%
- Specificity: 94%

Valid If Run in a Human Lab?
No—the test requires a method validated for use in dogs.

Causes of Abnormal Results

High values	Low values
Feline hyperthyroidism	Canine primary or secondary hypothyroidism
Overdose of thyroid supplementation	Certain drugs (fT$_4$ less affected than T$_4$)
Functional thyroid carcinoma in dogs (*rare*)	Nonthyroidal illness (fT$_4$ less affected than T$_4$)
	RI for some dog breeds is lower than in other dogs.

CLINICAL PERSPECTIVE
- Evaluation of the fT$_4$ concentration is the best single test to determine thyroid function but must be interpreted in context with patient's clinical signs, exam findings, chemistry, and hematology data.
- If possible, avoid using the test in patients with severe concurrent illness or those being administered certain drugs.
- In dogs, results of the fT$_4$ test are optimally interpreted in context with a concurrent endogenous TSH determination:
  - With a low fT$_4$ concentration accompanied by an elevated TSH concentration, suspect primary hypothyroidism.
  - With a low fT$_4$ concentration accompanied by a low normal TSH concentration, suspect secondary hypothyroidism (e.g., nonthyroidal disease).
- In cats, fT$_4$ is more sensitive than TT$_4$ for diagnosing hyperthyroidism that is early and/or mild or masked by concurrent nonthyroidal disease.

MISCELLANEOUS
ANCILLARY TESTS
- CBC, chemistry profile, and urinalysis
- Evaluation of canine TSH
- In cats, perform a triiodothyronine (T$_3$) suppression or thyroid-releasing hormone (TRH) response test if the fT$_4$ concentration fails to confirm suspected hyperthyroidism.

SYNONYMS
None

SEE ALSO
Blackwell's Five-Minute Veterinary Consult: Canine and Feline Topics
- Hyperthyroidism
- Hypothyroidism

Related Topics in This Books
- Thyroid-Stimulating Hormone
- Thyroxine (T$_4$), Total

ABBREVIATIONS
- fT$_4$ = free T$_4$
- RI = reference interval
- T$_4$ = thyroxine
- TSH = thyroid-stimulating hormone
- TT$_4$ = total thyroxine

Suggested Reading
Daminet S, Ferguson DC. Influence of drugs on thyroid function in dogs. *J Vet Intern Med* 2003; 17: 463–472.
Feldman EC, Nelson RW. Feline hyperthyroidism. In: *Canine and Feline Endocrinology and Reproduction*, 3rd ed. St Louis: Saunders Elsevier, 2004:152–218.
Feldman EC, Nelson RW. Hypothyroidism. In: *Canine and Feline Endocrinology and Reproduction*, 3rd ed. St Louis: Saunders Elsevier, 2004: 86–151.

INTERNET RESOURCES
None

AUTHOR NAME
Ryan M. Dickinson

THYROXINE (T$_4$), TOTAL

BASICS

TYPE OF SPECIMEN
Blood

TEST EXPLANATION AND RELATED PHYSIOLOGY
Requirements for thyroid hormone are regulated through the hypothalamic-pituitary-thyroid axis. During normal physiology, thyroid-releasing hormone (TRH) from the hypothalamus stimulates TSH release from the pituitary, which in turn stimulates production and release of T$_4$ from the thyroid gland. The majority of thyroid hormone released into plasma is in the form of T$_4$, with scant amounts of T$_3$ released. Active T$_4$ (and T$_3$) subsequently inhibits further TRH and TSH release, resulting in a negative feedback inhibition. Of plasma T$_4$, >99% is bound to proteins, with the remainder un-bound [free T$_4$ (fT$_4$)]. Only fT$_4$ can enter peripheral tissue cells. Protein-bound T$_4$ is a reserve supply for fT$_4$, and the levels of fT$_4$ are strictly maintained in healthy animals. T$_3$ is the active form of thyroid hormone, formed from deiodination of fT$_4$ after fT$_4$ enters a target cell.

Canine primary hypothyroidism is a disorder caused by either destruction of thyroid tissue by lymphocytes and plasma cells or by idiopathic thyroid gland atrophy. *Canine secondary hypothyroidism* is due to insufficient production of TSH from the pituitary, and permanent causes of pituitary dysfunction are uncommon. Clinical signs in hypothyroid dogs are the result of inefficient metabolism of several organ systems (a few examples include lethargy, weight gain, and symmetrical alopecia).

Feline hyperthyroidism is a disorder caused by autonomous secretion of T$_4$ from hyperplastic or adenomatous thyroid tissue. Excessive (toxic) levels of T$_4$ cause clinical signs such as hyperexcitability, weight loss despite good appetite, and polyuria-polydipsia. Nonthyroidal illness (neoplastic, inflammatory, metabolic, or hormonal etiologies) in either species can cause a net decrease in T$_4$ by altered protein binding of T$_4$ with increased T$_4$ clearance, by affecting TSH release by the pituitary, or T$_4$ production by thyroid follicular cells. Also, fT$_4$ deiodination to reverse T$_3$ (the inactive form of T$_3$) is promoted during nonthyroidal illness. Several drugs can alter thyroid physiology, as well. Therefore, euthyroid dogs with a nonthyroid illness or on certain medications may have T$_4$ values below the reference interval (RI). Likewise, a hyperthyroid cat with another illness or drug protocol may have T$_4$ values within the RI.

Measurement of T$_4$ Level
An RIA is considered the gold standard for measuring T$_4$. ELISA and chemiluminescent enzyme immunoassay (CEIA) have been validated in dogs and cats for T$_4$ measurement, and 1 study (Kemppaien 2006) demonstrated consistent results similar to T$_4$ results by RIA as long as assay-specific reference intervals are used for interpretation. Reference laboratories use RIA and/or CEIA, but most in-office T$_4$ assays rely on ELISA methodology.

INDICATIONS
Dogs
• To diagnose hypothyroidism in patients with consistent clinical signs, physical exam findings, and clinical pathologic changes
• To monitor T$_4$ levels in hypothyroid patients receiving thyroid hormone supplementation

Cats
• To diagnose hyperthyroidism in patients with consistent clinical signs, physical exam findings and clinical pathologic changes
• To perform follow-up monitoring for hyperthyroid cats that have received radioactive iodine or methimazole therapy

CONTRAINDICATIONS
Avoid testing animals that do not have clinical signs suggestive of thyroid disease.

POTENTIAL COMPLICATIONS
None

CLIENT EDUCATION
• Fasting of a new patient is recommended before collecting a sample.
• Adherence to a medication schedule is essential to proper therapeutic monitoring of T$_4$ levels.

BODY SYSTEMS ASSESSED
• Behavior
• Cardiovascular
• Dermatologic
• Endocrine and metabolic
• Reproductive

SAMPLE

COLLECTION
0.5–2.0 mL of venous blood

HANDLING
• Use a red-top tube. Avoid the use of serum-separator tubes.
  • Used for diagnostic laboratory assays and most in-office tests including Snap T$_4$ (IDEXX Laboratories, Westbrooke, ME) and Trilogy T$_4$ (Drew Scientific, Dallas, TX)
  • The use of heparinized whole blood or plasma is also acceptable for VetScan or VetScan VS2 T$_4$ (Abaxis, Union City, CA).
• Spin and separate the serum.
• Refrigerate the serum sample and transport it on ice packs to the laboratory.

STORAGE
Store the serum in a freezer.

STABILITY
• Room temperature: 5–8 days
• Refrigerated(2°–8°C): at least 2 weeks
• Frozen (−20°C): several months

PROTOCOL
None

INTERPRETATION

NORMAL FINDINGS OR RANGE
• Dogs: 1.2–5.2 μg/dL (15–67 nmol/L)
• Cats: 0.78–4.27 μg/dL (10–55 nmol/L)
• RIs may vary depending on the laboratory and assay.

ABNORMAL VALUES
• Canine hypothyroidism: T$_4$, <1.2 μg/dL (15 nmol/dL)
• Feline hypothyroidism: T$_4$, <0.78 μg/dL (10 nmol/dL)
• Feline hyperthyroidism: T$_4$, >4.27 μg/dL (55 nmol/L)

CRITICAL VALUES
None

INTERFERING FACTORS
Drugs That May Alter Results or Interpretation
Drugs That Interfere with Test Methodology
Levothyroxine (T$_4$)

Drugs That Alter Physiology
• Glucocorticoids (particularly immunosuppressive doses) can alter T$_4$ metabolism (net decrease in T$_4$) and can inhibit release of TSH from the pituitary.

• Phenobarbital (long term) can increase the rate of T_4 clearance perhaps with concurrent inhibition of TSH release.
• Sulfonamides can interfere with T_4 production by thyroid follicular cells.
• With acetylsalicylic acid, the T_4 turnover can increase within 24 h (with a net decrease in T_4) because of altered T_4 binding to proteins. Altered protein binding of T_4 can lead to a significant increase in fT_4 in short-term salicylate therapy.
• Prolonged levothyroxine administration alters the hypothalamic-pituitary-thyroid axis. Thyroid supplements should be discontinued for 6–8 weeks before definitive thyroid function tests are performed.
• Many other commonly used drugs can decrease baseline T_4 values and variably affect fT_4 and TSH in dogs, including carprofen, furosemide, methimazole, phenylbutazone, progestagens, and propylthiouracil. The effects these drugs have on response tests are unknown. The effects of these drugs in cats are less well characterized but should be assumed until proven otherwise.

Disorders That May Alter Results
• Lipemia or hemolysis
• T_4 autoantibodies (AAs) associated with lymphocytic thyroiditis may spuriously increase serum T_4 values by AAs interfering with the RIA or CEIA (the ELISA is not affected).

Collection Techniques or Handling That May Alter Results
• Prolonged storage of serum at room temperature
• The use of a gel-containing serum-separator tube is not recommended.

Influence of Signalment
Species
• Hypothyroidism is the most common thyroid disorder in dogs.
• Hyperthyroidism is the most common thyroid disorder in cats.

Breed
• Dog breeds at increased risk of developing hypothyroidism are golden retrievers, Doberman pinschers, dachshunds, cocker spaniels, Great Danes, boxers, poodles, German shepherds, Dalmatians, Irish setters, and miniature schnauzers. Other breeds may be overrepresented.
• The T_4 concentrations are higher in small breeds than in medium and large breeds of dogs but still fall within the RI.
• Sighthounds (e.g., greyhounds) have a naturally lower T_4 concentrations than other breeds, sometimes falling below the RI.
• Sprint racing increases the T_4 concentration of greyhounds. Racing long distances decreases the T_4 concentration of sled dogs.
• Siamese and Himalayan cats are at decreased risk for developing hyperthyroidism.

Age
• The serum T_4 concentration is lower, yet within the RI, in dogs >6 years old.
• Thyroid disease is more common in older animals.

Gender
None

Pregnancy
Pregnancy may increase T_4 and fT_4 levels.

LIMITATIONS OF THE TEST
In-office assays have a more limited dynamic testing range, and follow-up testing may be warranted for very high or very low values.

Sensitivity, Specificity, and Positive and Negative Predictive Values
Hypothyroid Dogs
• Sensitivity: 89%
• Specificity: 82%
• Diagnostic accuracy: 85%

Hyperthyroid Cats
• Sensitivity: 91%
• Specificity: 100%

Valid If Run in a Human Lab?
Yes—in cats, but not in dogs. The human T_4 assay lacks necessary sensitivity to detect accurately the low T_4 concentrations associated with canine hypothyroidism.

Causes of Abnormal Results

High values	Low values

Cats: hyperthyroidism caused by thyroid adenoma/adenomatous hyperplasia	Dogs
	  Primary hypothyroidism
	  Secondary hypothyroidism

Dogs
  False increase due to presence of anti-T_4 AAs (RIA)
  Overdose of levothyroxine supplementation
  Rare: functional thyroid carcinoma in dogs
	Nonthyroidal illness including hyperadrenocorticism
	    Pituitary failure
	    Certain drugs
	    May be normal for some breeds
	Cats: Following radioactive iodine or methimazole therapy for hyperthyroidism

CLINICAL PERSPECTIVE
• The serum T_4 concentration is not a definitive indicator of thyroid function. It must be interpreted in context with clinical signs, exam findings, chemistry, and hematology data.
• In dogs, the T_4 test is better for ruling out thyroid illness than confirming a diagnosis of thyroid illness.
• A full thyroid panel is optimal for evaluation of thyroid function.
  • If a low T_4 concentration is accompanied by an elevated TSH, this supports primary hypothyroidism.
  • If a low T_4 concentration is accompanied by a low normal TSH, consider a workup for secondary hypothyroidism, perhaps secondary to nonthyroidal disease.
• Cats with clinical signs of hyperthyroidism and a normal to mildly increased T_4 concentration should have the T_4 level rechecked in several weeks or, alternatively, measure fT_4 or perform a T_3 suppression test or a TRH response test.
• For monitoring of initiating levothyroxine supplementation in hypothyroid dogs, treat for 4–6 weeks and then measure the T_4 level 4–6 h after oral administration. Postpill total T_4 values are generally at the higher end of the RI or slightly above the RI.
• If an inappropriate diagnosis of hypothyroidism is suspected, discontinue thyroxine supplementation for 6 weeks before rechecking the T_4 level.
• Because of methodologic differences, it is difficult to compare in-office results to those obtained in a diagnostic laboratory. Results by different methods can differ significantly, and RIs and interpretive guidelines should reflect this difference.

MISCELLANEOUS
ANCILLARY TESTS
Dogs
• Chemistry profile and CBC looking for hypercholesterolemia and mild normochromic, normocytic, nonregenerative anemia
• Measure fT_4 and canine TSH levels to rule out secondary hypothyroidism.

Thyroxine (T$_4$), Total

Cats

- Chemistry profile looking for elevated ALT (toxic effects of excessive T$_4$ on hepatocytes) and alkaline phosphatase (bone isoform), with or without hyperglycemia
- Monitor BUN, creatinine, and urine specific gravity. Excessive T$_4$ levels may increase glomerular filtration rate sufficiently to mask underlying renal failure.
- fT$_4$, T$_3$ suppression, or TRH response test

SYNONYMS

None

SEE ALSO

Blackwell's Five-Minute Veterinary Consult: Canine and Feline Topics

- Hyperthyroidism
- Hypothyroidism

Related Topics in This Book

- Thyroglobulin Autoantibody
- Thyroid-Stimulating Hormone
- Thyroxine (T$_4$), Free

ABBREVIATIONS

- AA = autoantibody
- CEIA = chemiluminescent enzyme immunoassay
- fT$_4$ = free T$_4$
- RI = reference interval
- RIA = radioimmunoassay
- T$_3$ = triiodothyronine
- T$_4$ = thyroxine
- TRH = thyroid-releasing hormone
- TSH = thyroid-stimulating hormone

Suggested Reading

Daminet S, Ferguson DC. Influence of drugs on thyroid function in dogs. *J Vet Intern Med* 2003; 17: 463–472.

Feldman EC, Nelson RW. Feline hyperthyroidism. In: *Canine and Feline Endocrinology and Reproduction*, 3rd ed. St Louis: Saunders Elsevier, 2004: 152–218.

Feldman EC, Nelson RW. Hypothyroidism. In: *Canine and Feline Endocrinology and Reproduction*, 3rd ed. St Louis: Saunders Elsevier, 2004: 86–151.

Kemppainen RJ, Birchfield JR. Measurement of total thyroxine concentration in serum from dogs and cats by use of various methods. *Am J Vet Res* 2006; 67: 259–265.

INTERNET RESOURCES

Bell E, Latimer KS, LeRoy BE, Moore H. Canine Hypothyroidism, An overview; Veterinary Clinical Pathology Clerkship Program, 2005, http://www.vet.uga.edu/VPP/clerk/bell/index.php.

AUTHOR NAME

Ryan M. Dickinson

BASICS

TYPE OF PROCEDURE
Diagnostic sample collection

PROCEDURE EXPLANATION AND RELATED PHYSIOLOGY
Tissue biopsy, as collected by needle or punch, is an integral step in making a definitive diagnosis in tissues altered by disease. Histologic examination of biopsy samples by a trained pathologist provides a large amount of information regarding the nature of disease, enabling the diagnosis of inflammatory, hyperplastic, or neoplastic conditions. Collection of biopsy samples also enables application of immunohistochemical stains, an aid to diagnosis for cases not clearly categorized with routine histopathology, and frozen storage of tissues for molecular analysis.

INDICATIONS
- Evaluation of cutaneous and subcutaneous lesions or masses
- Evaluation of lymphadenopathy
- Evaluation of nodules, masses, or other identified changes within organs
- Evaluation of organs demonstrating altered function

CONTRAINDICATIONS
- Risk of hemorrhage when sampling cavitary masses
- Severe bleeding tendencies as with marked thrombocytopenia or other coagulopathies

POTENTIAL COMPLICATIONS
- Bleeding and bruising
- Pain and discomfort
- The release of bioactive substances (e.g., mast cell tumor)
- The potential spread of malignant neoplasia (rare)

CLIENT EDUCATION
Although risks are minimal, when tissue biopsy is performed, as collected by needle or punch, clients should be advised of the potential for hemorrhage, or other complications, relative to the site and nature of the tissue sampled.

BODY SYSTEMS ASSESSED
All

PROCEDURE

PATIENT PREPARATION
Preprocedure Medication or Preparation
The hair should be clipped and the skin aseptically prepared as indicated prior to tissue biopsy. (To maintain superficial tissue characteristics in some cases in which dermatologic disease is being assessed, such preparation might not be performed.)

Anesthesia or Sedation
- Local anesthesia (e.g., lidocaine) indicated for punch biopsy of superficial lesions, possibly in conjunction with sedation
- Heavy sedation or light anesthesia indicated for needle biopsy of very large or internal lesions sampled via ultrasound guidance

Patient Positioning
Any that enables optimal access to the tissue being biopsied

Patient Monitoring
- Monitoring for adequate analgesia and level of sedation
- Monitoring for bleeding at the biopsy site

Equipment or Supplies
- A sterile scrub
- Sterile gloves
- Sterile 4 × 4-inch gauze
- 1 mL of 2% lidocaine
- A jar containing 10% buffered formalin for the sample

Needle Biopsy
- An appropriately sized Tru-cut or other needle biopsy instrument
- A no. 11 scalpel blade
- A 25-gauge needle

Punch Biopsy
- An appropriately sized Keyes punch biopsy instrument
- Thumb forceps
- Metzenbaum scissors
- A needle holder
- 3–0 nonabsorbable suture

TECHNIQUE
Biopsies generally require 2 people: 1 to position the animal, monitor sedation or anesthesia, and assist with sample handling, and 1 to collect the sample. Clip an appropriately sized area and perform a surgical scrub. (Note that a surgical scrub might not be performed for evaluation of dermatologic lesions.)

Manual Needle Biopsy
Make a small skin incision with a no. 11 scalpel blade. While ensuring the bevel-containing Tru-cut needle is covered, insert the instrument into the tissue to be biopsied. Holding the instrument in place with the nondominant hand, use the dominant hand to advance and expose the bevel-containing needle inside the tissue. Gently press the instrument against the edge of the tissue and, holding the instrument stable with the dominant hand, with a single sharp motion advance the nondominant hand to close over the bevel-containing needle and thereby cut the tissue into the beveled groove. Remove the instrument, advance the dominant hand to expose the tissue caught within the bevel, and use a 25-gauge needle to peel the sample off the instrument. Place the sample in formalin (or liquid nitrogen for molecular analysis).

Automated Needle Biopsy
Make a small skin incision with a no. 11 scalpel blade. Pulling back the needle plunger until a click is heard charges the automated needle biopsy instrument. Insert the index and middle fingers through

TISSUE BIOPSY: NEEDLE AND PUNCH

the finger holes on the instrument and continuously hold back the needle plunger to ensure the bevel-containing needle remains covered as the instrument is inserted to the desired depth into the tissue to be sampled. Once inserted, gently advance the needle plunger part way to expose the bevel within the tissue. Press the instrument against the tissue, and while holding the instrument stable, press the needle plunger all the way in until a click is heard, which signifies the cutting of the tissue into the beveled groove. Remove the instrument, pull the plunger back until a click is again heard, advance the needle plunger part way to expose the tissue caught within the bevel, and use a 25-gauge needle to peel the sample off the instrument. Place the sample in formalin (or liquid nitrogen for molecular analysis).

Punch Biopsy
After infiltrating the area with 0.5–1.0 mL of local anesthetic (e.g., 2% lidocaine) and performing a final surgical scrub, place the Keyes biopsy instrument on the skin surface and rotate it *clockwise* to the level of the plastic hub. Then, remove the instrument and collect the sample from within the metal hub. If the biopsy core remains attached to the animal, gently lift the core tissue with thumb forceps and sever its attachment to underlying tissues by using Metzenbaum scissors. Place the sample in formalin (or liquid nitrogen for molecular analysis). Gently blot the area, as needed, with sterile gauze and close the skin wound with appropriately sized (generally, 3–0) nonabsorbable suture. Most commonly, a cruciate suture pattern is used.

SAMPLE HANDLING
Collected samples should be placed in 10% buffered formalin for submission (or in liquid nitrogen for potential molecular analysis).

APPROPRIATE AFTERCARE
Postprocedure Patient Monitoring
The patient may be monitored for evidence of hemorrhage (mucous membrane color and attitude, with or without PCV and total solids) in the hours after the procedure.

Nursing Care
This depends on the location biopsied.

Dietary Modification
None

Medication Requirements
None

Restrictions on Activity
Usually none, but restrictions vary with the location biopsied.

Anticipated Recovery Time
Usually immediate, but recovery time varies with the location biopsied.

INTERPRETATION

NORMAL FINDINGS OR RANGE
A portion of tissue for processing: a 0.5- to 2.0-cm-long core of tissue following Tru-cut needle biopsy, and a 4- to 8-mm-diameter core of tissue following punch biopsy

ABNORMAL VALUES
• Abnormal ratios, numbers, or types of cells present
• Infectious agents present
• Neoplastic cells present

CRITICAL VALUES
N/A

INTERFERING FACTORS
Drugs That May Alter Results of the Procedure
None

Conditions That May Interfere with Performing the Procedure
None

Procedure Techniques or Handling That May Alter Results
Failure to fix tissue adequately prior to processing for histologic evaluation may limit interpretation.

Influence of Signalment on Performing and Interpreting the Procedure
Species
None

Breed
None

Age
None

Gender
None

Pregnancy
None

CLINICAL PERSPECTIVE

Histologic (or molecular) analysis of biopsy samples collected by needle or punch is an integral step in evaluating microscopic tissue architecture and providing definitive diagnosis in tissues altered by disease. Histologic examination by a trained pathologist provides information regarding the nature of disease, enabling the diagnosis of inflammatory, hyperplastic, or neoplastic conditions. Collection of biopsy samples also enables application of immunohistochemical stains, an aid to diagnosis for cases not clearly categorized with routine histopathology.

 MISCELLANEOUS

ANCILLARY TESTS
Immunohistochemisty

SYNONYMS
None

SEE ALSO
Blackwell's Five-Minute Veterinary Consult: Canine and Feline Topics
Too many to list

Related Topics in This Book
- Bone Biopsy
- Fine-Needle Aspiration
- Impression Smear
- Liver Biopsy
- Muscle and Nerve Biopsy
- Renal Biopsy and Aspiration
- Skin Biopsy
- Ultrasound-Guided Mass or Organ Aspiration

ABBREVIATIONS
None

Suggested Reading
Gross TL, Ihrke PJ, Walder EJ, Affolter VK. *Skin Diseases of the Dog and Cat*, 2nd ed. Oxford: Blackwell Science, 2005.
Jubb KVF, Kennedy PC, Palmer N, eds. *Pathology of Domestic Animals*, vol 1, 4th ed. San Diego: Academic, 1993.
McGavin MD, Carlton WW, Zachary JF, eds. *Thomson's Special Veterinary Pathology*, 3rd ed. St Louis: CV Mosby, 2001.

INTERNET RESOURCES
None

AUTHOR NAME
Laurel E. Williams

TONOMETRY

BASICS

TYPE OF PROCEDURE
Pressure measurement

PROCEDURE EXPLANATION AND RELATED PHYSIOLOGY
The intraocular fluids that help maintain the shape of the eye consist of aqueous and vitreous humor. Aqueous humor is produced by the ciliary processes in the posterior chamber, travels through the pupil into the anterior chamber, and exits the eye primarily through the iridocorneal angle. The production of aqueous humor within the eye is balanced by the outflow resistance in the iridocorneal angle, resulting in a physiologic intraocular pressure (IOP).

Tonometry is the indirect measurement of IOP via indentation, applanation, or rebound techniques and is indicated in most ocular conditions. Tonometry is essential for the diagnosis of glaucoma, in which the IOP is usually high. Tonometry should always be performed prior to pharmacologic pupillary dilation during an ocular examination, because pupillary dilation is contraindicated if the IOP is elevated. All of the indirect tonometry techniques measure physical characteristics of the cornea and then estimate IOP, inherently introducing some degree of error.

Indentation tonometry is performed with a Shiötz tonometer. This method is archaic and has largely been replaced by applanation tonometry. In indentation tonometry, the cornea is indented by a weighted plunger within a footplate that has a curvature corresponding to the human cornea. The amount of corneal indentation is measured, and the tonometer scale reading is converted to an estimation of IOP by using the human calibration table. The result is inversely proportional to the IOP (i.e., the higher the scale reading, the lower the IOP). The Shiötz tonometer is more difficult to manipulate and can be less accurate than the applanation tonometers. This accuracy depends on the clinician, the patient, and the instrument. For example, the necessity of holding the instrument perfectly upright requires that the animal be placed in an uncomfortable position. Even more frustrating, the IOP obtained by this method is not always confirmed on referral to a specialist.

Applanation tonometry measures the amount of force or pressure needed to flatten a specific area of cornea. Handheld, battery-operated, applanation tonometers are very accurate and easy to use (i.e., Tonopen XL or Tono-Pen Vet; both from Reichert, Depew, NY). The Tonopen can be held horizontally, which enables the animal to be lightly restrained in a sitting or sternal position. The user should stand to the side of the patient when taking a reading, so that the corneal curvature can be visualized. Minimal to no pressure needs to be applied for the Tonopen to take a reading. If corneal indenting is visualized, the user is pressing too hard. Unlike the Shiötz tonometer, the Tonopen measures IOP in millimeters of mercury (mmHg) and does not require a conversion table. Tonopens average several readings and report a percent error to ensure accuracy. A reading with ≤5% error is the most accurate, and averages that are >5% error should be repeated. The tip of the Tonopen should be covered with a latex tip to prevent disease transmission and wicking of fluid. The small tip size, 1.0–1.5 mm in diameter, allows for measurement of IOP in pediatric patients, as well as a number of exotic animal species, such as ferrets.

Rebound tonometry, also called impact or dynamic tonometry, uses a probe that is electromagnetically propelled to come into contact with the cornea and then rebound from the corneal surface. The characteris-

tics of the rebound motion are used to estimate IOP. The inverse of the deceleration time is most closely correlated with IOP. It is commonly reported that a topical anesthetic is not required for this technique. Commercial handheld, battery-operated, rebound tonometers have become available for human patients (ICare; Tiolat Oy, Helsinki, Finland) and veterinary patients (TonoVet, Tiolat Oy, Helsinki), and studies are currently under way comparing their accuracy to that of the previous methods. The rebound tonometer is larger than the Tonopen and must be held parallel to the floor to function properly. However, it has been reported to provide accurate results and may be easier to use by inexperienced tonometrists. Although a choice of species-specific software is available, species-specific calibration curves are not published for this instrument. Measurements obtained with this tonometer compared to those with applanation tonometers can be extremely different, so tonometer-specific reference ranges must be established and consulted for each species.

INDICATIONS
- Red eye: conjunctival or episcleral hyperemia
- Blue eye: corneal edema
- Painful eye
- Decreased vision or loss of vision
- Anisocoria
- Fixed and midrange or dilated pupils
- Buphthalmos
- Conjunctivitis
- Anterior uveitis
- Hyphema
- Intraocular mass
- Breeds that are predisposed to glaucoma
- An animal of predisposed breed and with a history of glaucoma in the opposite eye
- Follow-up in animals with medically or surgically controlled glaucoma

CONTRAINDICATIONS
When the structural integrity of the globe is compromised, such as in deep corneal ulceration

POTENTIAL COMPLICATIONS
- Rupture of the globe if structural integrity is compromised (e.g., deep corneal ulcer)
- Corneal trauma and ulceration (more likely with the Shiötz than with applanation or rebound tonometers)

CLIENT EDUCATION
None

BODY SYSTEMS ASSESSED
Ophthalmic

PROCEDURE

PATIENT PREPARATION
Preprocedure Medication or Preparation
None

Anesthesia or Sedation
- Topical anesthesia (e.g., proparacaine hydrochloride) is required for indentation and applanation tonometry.
- Topical anesthesia may not be required with the rebound tonometer.

Patient Positioning
- Sternal recumbency or sitting is best for applanation and rebound tonometry.
- Indentation tonometry requires the patient to be either on its back or restrained with its nose pointed upward to allow for vertical positioning of the Shiötz tonometer.

Patient Monitoring
None

Equipment or Supplies
- Topical anesthesia (e.g., proparacaine hydrochloride)
- A tonometer
- A disposable cover if Tonopen is used

TECHNIQUE
Shiötz Technique
- Apply topical anesthetic to the cornea.
- Test the tonometer for accuracy by first calibrating it with the metal calibration standard supplied. When the instrument is placed on the standard, it should read zero on the scale. This means that the 5.5 g weight does not indent the metal standard.
- Add the 7.5 g weight because most dog and cat IOPs fall within this range.
- The animal should be placed on its back, or the animal's head should be elevated dorsally.
- Hold the eyelids open without putting pressure on the globe. This usually means positioning your fingers farther from the lid margins.
- The Schiötz tonometer must be held vertically and placed on the center of the cornea just long enough for the scale to be read.
- Take 2–3 readings.
- All readings should be relatively close to one another if they are accurate.
- The conversion table provided with the instrument (for human patients) appears to be reliable for IOP estimation in dogs and cats. It is not known how reliable it is in the face of an elevated IOP.
- Although there are conversion charts for dogs and cats, they should not be used because they result in higher readings and the misdiagnosis of glaucoma.

Applanation Tonometry
- Apply topical anesthetic to the cornea.
- Place a new disposable cover over the Tonopen tip.
- A handler should lightly restrain the animal and keep its nose pointing forward by holding under the muzzle. It is difficult to acquire a reading with the animal's nose pointed down.
- Stand to the side of the animal (the right side of the dog if you are right-handed and vice versa) so that you can visualize the corneal curvature.
- The Tonopen should be held in your dominant hand and the animal's eyelids opened with your nondominant hand.
- Turn on the Tonopen with firm pressure on the large black button on the handle. Press it only once. Pressing it twice initiates the calibration sequence.
- Once the Tonopen is ready to take measurements (acquires the double row of dashes), it will go into battery-saving mode after 15 s of nonuse and require that you press the button again.
- Minor movements away from the cornea and very gentle blotting of the cornea with the tip will enhance the reliability and reproducibility of the readings while reducing the number of readings necessary.
- You are pressing too firmly if the cornea indents when you contact it.

- It is best to take a reading from the center of the cornea, if possible.
- The *approach angle* of the Tonopen tip to the cornea is very important. The tip's flat surface should be exactly parallel to the corneal surface and the Tonopen itself perpendicular to the cornea. The approach angle of the Tonopen to the cornea must be changed, because of corneal curvature, if any area other than the central cornea is used.
- The approach angle is best achieved by viewing the interface between the cornea and the tip from the side as previously suggested.
- Whenever the cornea contacts the probe, an electronic tone will indicate whether a reading has been obtained.
- When the Tonopen is able to calculate an average value, a tone of a different pitch will sound, and no further readings can be obtained without restarting the Tonopen by using the large black button again.
- The number of readings required to achieve an average value varies depending on how dissimilar the readings are from one another and from the normal physiologic range.
- The digital screen at the end of the Tonopen opposite from the tip displays the IOP in mmHg.
- An estimate of the reliability (coefficient of variance) of the result also appears as a small bar above 1 of 4 percentage readings. This bar should be above the 5% mark, or tonometry should be repeated on that eye.

SAMPLE HANDLING
N/A

APPROPRIATE AFTERCARE
Postprocedure Patient Monitoring
None

Nursing Care
None

Dietary Modification
None

Medication Requirements
None

Restrictions on Activity
None

Anticipated Recovery Time
Immediate

 INTERPRETATION

NORMAL FINDINGS OR RANGE
- Across large populations, normal canine and feline IOP is reported as ≈10–25 mmHg. These values will change specifically with species and type of tonometer used.
- Significant variation is noted between individuals, technique, and time of day.
- Comparison of IOP between right and left eyes (if an option) is critical to interpretation of results.
- The IOP should not vary between eyes of the same patient by >5 mmHg.

ABNORMAL VALUES
- An IOP of <10 mmHg is suspicious for ocular inflammation but could be normal for some animals.
- An IOP of >25 mmHg is suspicious for glaucoma.

TONOMETRY

CRITICAL VALUES
An IOP of >25 mmHg

INTERFERING FACTORS

Drugs That May Alter Results of the Procedure
- Ketamine administration elevates the IOP in cats.
- Xylazine administration decreases the IOP in cats.
- It has been reported that topical 0.5% tropicamide, 1% cyclopentolate, and 1% atropine, in addition to causing mydriasis, raise the IOP in cats.
- It has been reported that lingual application of 0.5% tropicamide can also cause mydriasis and raise the IOP in cats.

Conditions That May Interfere with Performing the Procedure
- Curvature of the cornea must be constant with Shiötz tonometry. The tonometer underestimates IOP when megalocornea or buphthalmia are present and overestimates IOP when microphthalmos or microcornea is present.
- Severe corneal edema and corneal scarring may invalidate the result with Schiötz tonometry but is less important with applanation tonometry.
- Anterior lens luxation may result in the pressure of the lens being measured and not the IOP.
- It is often difficult to obtain a reading with the applanation tonometer when an IOP is significantly low (<5 mmHg).

Procedure Techniques or Handling That May Alter Results
- Artificial elevation of the IOP can be caused by excessive struggling by the patient, excessive pressure on the patient's eyelids (therefore indirectly on the globe), and pressure on the jugular veins during restraint.
- Nonvertical positioning of Shiötz tonometer will result in inaccurate readings.

Influence of Signalment on Performing and Interpreting the Procedure

Species
Normal cats may have slightly higher IOPs than normal dogs.

Breed
Breed differences are possible.

Age
IOP decreases with age in both dogs and cats by 2–4 mmHg.

Gender
Gender differences are possible.

Pregnancy
- Cats in estrus have been reported to have a higher IOP than those not in estrus.
- Pregnant cats with low progesterone levels have been reported to have a lower IOP than pregnant cats with high progesterone levels.

CLINICAL PERSPECTIVE
- An inherent variability of ≥2 mmHg exists with even the most accurate tonometer.
- A single tonometry reading is only a snapshot in a patient's IOP. A dog can have a normal IOP measurement and still develop acute congestive glaucoma 1 h later.

- The difference in IOP between 2 eyes in the same animal should be <5 mmHg.
- Diurnal variations occur in both dogs and cats. The IOP in normal dogs is 2–4 mmHg higher in the mornings and 6–10 mmHg higher in dogs with glaucoma. The IOP in cats is reported to be slightly higher in the evenings.
- It is important to remember that the ocular examination findings and a clinical assessment must also be used when interpreting the results of tonometry. For example, a patient with uveitis and secondary glaucoma may have an IOP that falls within the normal range.
- A low IOP is not a diagnosis in and of itself. A low IOP may be a normal aging change, and uveitis should not be diagnosed unless the clinical signs indicate it.
- The Tonopen appears to overestimate readings in the low range, is very accurate in the normal range, and underestimates IOP in the high range in people, dogs, and cats. The variations from real IOP are usually not clinically significant.
- The Tonopen XL designed for human use consistently underestimates the IOP in cats.
- The Tonopen requires gentle and repeated corneal touches that introduce variability that is operator dependent.
- With successive IOP measurements using applanation tonometry, the IOP will decrease slightly. Due to the minimal corneal contact, this may not occur with rebound tonometry. Progression of many of these diseases, especially glaucoma, can be monitored, and response to and adjustment of therapy should be based on repeated tonometry results. IOP can vary slightly with pulse rate, eyelid pressure, extraocular muscle tension, respiration, venous pressure, time of day, and blood osmotic changes.
- In dogs, the TonoVet underestimates IOP in the low normal range and overestimates IOP in the higher range.
- The Shiötz tonometer has a footplate that is designed to match the human corneal curvature. Larger eyes with a flatter cornea tend to give falsely low readings, whereas small eyes with greater corneal curvature (e.g., brachycephalic dogs) tend to give falsely elevated readings. Limbal readings may be also be higher than the central corneal readings.
- With Shiötz tonometry, the human conversion table gives the most accurate results for animal patients.

MISCELLANEOUS

ANCILLARY TESTS
- Gonioscopy
- Ocular ultrasound

SYNONYMS
None

SEE ALSO
Blackwell's Five-Minute Veterinary Consult: Canine and Feline Topics
- Anisocoria
- Anterior Uveitis—Cats

- Anterior Uveitis—Dogs
- Blind Quiet Eye
- Cataract
- Glaucoma
- Hyphema
- Hypopyon and Lipid Flare
- Lens Luxation
- Proptosis
- Red Eye
- Uveal Melanoma—Cats
- Uveal Melanoma—Dogs

Related Topics in This Book
None

ABBREVIATIONS
IOP = intraocular pressure

Suggested Reading
Gorig C, Coenen RTI, Stades FC, *et al.* Comparison of the use of new handheld tonometers and established applanation tonometers in dogs. *Am J Vet Res* 2006; 67: 134–144.

Knollinger AM, La Croix NC, Barrett PM, Miller PE. Evaluation of a rebound tonometer for measuring intraocular pressure in dogs and horses. *J Am Vet Med Assoc* 2005; 227: 244–248.

Martin CL. Anamnesis and the ophthalmic examination. In: Martin CL, ed. *Ophthalmic Disease in Veterinary Medicine*. London: Manson, 2005: 11–38.

Miller PE, Pickett JP, Majors LJ, Kurzman ID. Clinical comparison of the MacKay-Marg and Tono-Pen applanation tonometers in the dog. *Prog Vet Comp Ophthalmol* 1991; 1: 171–176.

Miller PE, Pickett JP, Majors LJ, Kurzman ID. Evaluation of two applanation tonometers in cats. *Am J Vet Res* 1991; 52: 1917–1921.

INTERNET RESOURCES
None

AUTHOR NAME
Tammy Miller Michau

TOTAL PROTEIN

BASICS

TYPE OF SPECIMEN
Blood

TEST EXPLANATION AND RELATED PHYSIOLOGY
The total protein (TP) concentration of the blood is composed of albumin and globulins. In serum, TP measurement includes albumin and all of the globulins except those consumed during clot formation (e.g., fibrinogen, factor V, factor VIII). In contrast, plasma proteins are measured in blood placed in an appropriate anticoagulant prior to clot formation. Differences between serum and plasma protein concentrations are generally clinically insignificant and largely reflect the presence of fibrinogen in plasma; fibrinogen accounts for ≈5% of plasma proteins.

The most common method for measuring serum TP using laboratory chemistry analyzers is by the *biuret reaction*, which is a colorimetric, spectrophotometric technique that measures the color change resulting from copper binding to peptide bonds. The TP concentration can also be estimated with a refractometer. The degree of light refraction (*refractive index*) of serum or plasma is proportional to the total solids present. Most of the total solids in serum or plasma are proteins, and the scale of the refractometer is calibrated to reflect this relationship.

INDICATIONS
- To assess hydration status
- To evaluate the cause of anemia, edema, or ascites
- To evaluate patients with unexplained weight loss, liver, renal, or GI disease

CONTRAINDICATIONS
None

POTENTIAL COMPLICATIONS
None

CLIENT EDUCATION
None

BODY SYSTEMS ASSESSED
- Cardiovascular
- Gastrointestinal
- Hemic, lymphatic, and immune
- Hepatobiliary

SAMPLE

COLLECTION
- Biuret reaction: 0.5–2.0 mL of venous blood
- Refractometer: 75 μL of venous blood (microhematocrit tube)

HANDLING
- Use a plain red-top tube or serum-separator tube (biuret reaction).
- The use of EDTA, sodium heparin, and lithium heparin is acceptable (biuret reaction).
- The use of a microhematocrit tube, heparinized or nonheparinized, is acceptable (refractometer).

STORAGE
Refrigerate or freeze the serum or plasma for long-term storage.

STABILITY
- Refrigerated (2°–8°C): 3 days
- Frozen (−20°C): 6 months

PROTOCOL
None

INTERPRETATION

NORMAL FINDINGS OR RANGE
Dogs
- Serum: 5.4–7.5 g/dL (54–75 g/L)
- Plasma: 6.0–7.5 g/dL (60–75 g/L)
Cats
- Serum: 6.0–7.9 g/dL (60–79 g/L)
- Plasma: 6.0–7.5 g/dL (60–75 g/L)
- Reference intervals may vary depending on the laboratory and assay.

ABNORMAL VALUES
Values above or below the reference range

CRITICAL VALUES
None

INTERFERING FACTORS
Drugs That May Alter Results or Interpretation
Drugs That Interfere with Test Methodology
Administration of dextran may cause increased levels in the biuret reaction.

Drugs That Alter Physiology
- The TP concentration is increased (mildly) by drugs that decrease protein catabolism (e.g., anabolic steroids such as estrogen or testosterone).
- The TP concentration is decreased (mildly) by drugs that increase protein catabolism (e.g., thyroxine, glucocorticoids).

Disorders That May Alter Results
- Hemolysis can cause false increases in the biuret reaction.
- Refractometer
  - Hemolysis may complicate the refractometer reading by obscuring the dividing line.
  - The TP value is increased by gross lipemia.
  - Hyperbilirubinemia may result in a spuriously high TP value.
  - The TP value is increased by high concentrations of glucose, urea, sodium, and chloride because of an increased refractive index (refractometer).

Collection Techniques or Handling That May Alter Results
- A slight difference between serum and plasma concentrations because of clot formation
- Traumatic venipuncture that causes hemolysis
- Collection of a sample from an animal that has not been fasted

Influence of Signalment
Species
None

Breed
None

Age
- Puppies and kittens may have lower TP concentrations than adult animals.
- TP generally increases with advancing age.

Gender
None

PREGNANCY
Serum TP progressively decreases during gestation.

LIMITATIONS OF THE TEST
Measurements are inaccurate for values of <1 g/dL.

Sensitivity, Specificity, and Positive and Negative Predictive Values
N/A

Valid If Run in a Human Lab?
Yes—but a refractometer calibrated for human samples may produce slightly different values than a veterinary refractometer with samples from dogs and cats.

Causes of Abnormal Findings

High values	Low values
Hemoconcentration (dehydration)	Hemodilution
Inflammation	Excess IV fluids (fluid overload)
Infectious	Congestive heart failure
Noninfectious (e.g., neoplasia, immune mediated, tissue damage)	Nephrotic syndrome
	Cirrhosis
	SIADH (syndrome of inappropriate ADH secretion)
Lymphoid neoplasia (e.g., B-cell lymphoma)	Loss of protein from vascular space
Multiple myeloma	Blood loss
	Protein-losing enteropathy
	Protein-losing nephropathy
	Exudative skin disease
	Deficient protein synthesis or increased protein catabolism
	Severe malnutrition or cachexia
	Maldigestion/malabsorption
	Hepatic insufficiency
	Failure of passive transfer
	Immunoglobulin deficiencies

CLINICAL PERSPECTIVE
• Concurrent evaluation of albumin and globulin concentrations can help determine the cause of an abnormal TP level.
• Increases in both TP and hematocrit suggest dehydration, whereas decreases in both suggest blood loss.
• Because of splenic contraction, a decreased TP may be the only sign of acute blood loss in stressed dogs.

MISCELLANEOUS

ANCILLARY TESTS
• Determination of the albumin and globulin concentrations
• Urinalysis and determination of the urine protein/creatinine ratio to look for proteinuria
• Evaluation of bile acids to assess liver function
• Serum protein electrophoresis

SYNONYMS
None

SEE ALSO
Blackwell's Five-Minute Veterinary Consult: Canine and Feline Topics
• Cirrhosis and Fibrosis of the Liver
• Multiple Myeloma
• Protein-Losing Enteropathy
• Proteinuria
Related Topics in This Book
• Albumin
• Globulins
• Protein Electrophoresis

ABBREVIATIONS
TP = total protein

Suggested Reading
Evans EW, Duncan JR. Proteins, lipids, and carbohydrates. In: Latimer KS, Mahaffey EA, Prasse KW, eds. *Duncan and Prasse's Veterinary Laboratory Medicine Clinical Pathology,* 4th ed. Ames: Iowa State Press, 2003: 162–192.
Kaneko JJ. Serum proteins and the dysproteinemias. In: Kaneko JJ, Harvey JW, Bruss ML, eds. *Clinical Biochemistry of Domestic Animals,* 5th ed. San Diego: Academic, 1997: 117–138.
Stockham SL, Scott MA. Proteins. In: *Fundamentals of Veterinary Clinical Pathology.* Ames: Iowa State Press, 2002: 251–276.

INTERNET RESOURCES
None

AUTHOR NAME
Rob Simoni

TOXOPLASMOSIS SEROLOGY

BASICS

TYPE OF SPECIMEN
Blood

TEST EXPLANATION AND RELATED PHYSIOLOGY
Domestic cats are the definitive host for *Toxoplasma gondii*, an intra-cellular coccidian. The major mode of transmission of *T. gondii* to cats and dogs is by ingestion of bradyzoite tissue cysts within intermediate vertebrate hosts. Infection occurs worldwide. Among cats and dogs in the United States, ≈30% are seropositive for *T. gondii*. Although exposure rates are high, latent infection is the norm and clinical disease (toxoplasmosis) is uncommon. Most cats and dogs mount an immune response that contains the infection, but the infection is not eliminated and organisms persist for life as tissue-encysted bradyzoites in latently infected dogs and cats. Immunosuppression may induce cyst rupture, multiplication of tachyzoites, and fulminating toxoplasmosis. The en-teroepithelial phase of primary infection in cats, during which oocysts are shed, is usually asymptomatic. Toxoplasmosis may result from replication of tachyzoites in tissues, during the extraintestinal phase of infection, in both primary and reactivated latent infections.

Definitive diagnosis of toxoplasmosis requires cytologic, histologic, or immunohistologic detection of *T. gondii* tachyzoites in body-cavity effusions, bronchoalveolar lavage fluid, or tissue biopsy samples. Serologic tests are a useful adjunct to the diagnosis of toxoplasmosis, although interpretation can be complicated. Measurement of both *T. gondii*–specific IgG and IgM antibody (Ab) titers simultaneously followed by a second IgG titer 2–4 weeks later is recommended as an aid to diagnosis of active infection. For paired IgG titers, both serum samples should be processed simultaneously at the same laboratory. Serologic tests that detect 1 or both classes of antibodies include the Sabin-Feldman dye test, IFA, ELISA, indirect hemagglutination test (IHA), latex agglutination test (LAT), and modified agglutination test. The Sabin-Feldman dye test is rarely used because of the requirement for live *T. gondii* tachyzoites as a substrate.

INDICATIONS
- To diagnose active infection in a dog or cat with disease of the res-piratory tract, CNS, liver, heart, eye (uveitis in cats), skeletal muscle (dogs), GI tract, or with multiorgan dysfunction
- To determine serostatus in queens with stillborn or fading kittens
- To determine serostatus before renal transplantation (recipient and donor) or before therapy with immunosuppressive drugs, especially cyclosporine

CONTRAINDICATIONS
None

POTENTIAL COMPLICATIONS
None

CLIENT EDUCATION
Although the Centers for Disease Control and the American Associa-tion of Feline Practitioners do not recommend testing healthy cats for *T. gondii* antibodies, serologic testing may be requested by cat owners because of a perceived risk of infection, particularly during pregnancy, from their own cats.
- Humans can be infected through ingestion of tissue cysts in un-dercooked meat directly, through contamination of food preparation areas, or through ingestion of oocysts from contact with unwashed vegetables, sandpits, gardening, or litter trays.
- Clients are at risk of infection from contact with pet cats during the period of oocyst shedding, which occurs during a primary in-fection. However, oocyst shedding lasts for only 1–2 weeks in most cats. Oocysts are not infective until sporulation, which usually occurs

1–5 days after excretion in feces. Infection from direct contact with cats is unlikely.
- Measures to minimize human infection risk include freezing or irradiation of meat to kill tissue cysts, avoiding undercooked or mi-crowaved meat and unpasteurized dairy products, washing vegetables and food preparation areas, and wearing gardening gloves. Litter trays should be cleaned daily with boiling water while gloves are worn, preferably by a nonpregnant household member.
- IgG-seropositive cats offer little risk of owner infection because the period of oocyst shedding has already passed and the risk of reshedding is low. IgM-seropositive cats are actively or recently infected and could be shedding oocysts.
- Measures to reduce the risk of seronegative pet cats acquiring in-fection include indoor housing, feeding of canned or pelleted pet foods only, and prevention of exposure to intermediate hosts (e.g., rodents, birds) and mechanical vectors (e.g., cockroaches). Raw-meat diets should be avoided, or only thawed, frozen meat should be fed, since freezing meat at −12°C for several days destroys most bradyzoite cysts. Although seropositive cats are generally immune to recurrent primary infection from ingestion of *T. gondii* oocysts, gut immunity to *T. gondii* can wane by 6 years after infection. Therefore, similar steps to prevent recurrent infection of seropositive cats are recommended.

BODY SYSTEMS ASSESSED
- Cardiovascular
- Dermatologic
- Gastrointestinal
- Hepatobiliary
- Musculoskeletal
- Nervous
- Ophthalmic
- Respiratory

SAMPLE

COLLECTION
0.5–1.0 mL of venous blood

HANDLING
Use a plain red-top tube or serum-separator tube. Centrifuge and separate the serum.

STORAGE
- Refrigerate or freeze the serum.
- For measurement of paired IgG titers, store the first sample frozen.

STABILITY
- Room temperature: several days
- Refrigerated (2°–8°C): days to weeks
- Frozen (−20°C): months to years

PROTOCOL
None

INTERPRETATION

NORMAL FINDINGS OR RANGE
Either no detectable antibodies against *T. gondii* or no rising titer (≥4-fold increase) between acute and convalescent samples

ABNORMAL VALUES
- IgM
  - Cats: IgM titers develop 1–2 weeks after infection and are usually negative by 12 weeks after acute infection.

- Dogs: IgM titers develop 1 week after infection and begin declining by 4 weeks after infection.
- IgG titers develop 2–4 weeks after infection. High IgG titers (e.g., >1:30,000) may persist for many years and merely reflect *T. gondii* antigen within tissues.
- A positive IgM titer greater than the least significant level of reactivity for that assay (usually >1:64) or a ≥4-fold increase in IgG in paired serum samples taken 2–4 weeks apart is considered diagnostic of recent or active infection.

CRITICAL VALUES
None

INTERFERING FACTORS
Drugs That May Alter Results or Interpretation
Drugs That Interfere with Test Methodology
None

Drugs That Alter Physiology
The administration of clindamycin to infected cats may blunt IgM responses, resulting in lower titers, but will not alter IgG responses.

Disorders That May Alter Results
- Concurrent FIV infection may cause persistent IgM titers for >12 weeks, perhaps because of a delayed Ab class shift from IgM to IgG.
- High doses of glucocorticoids administered to latently infected cats can alter *T. gondii*–specific Ab responses such that IgG titers may diminish and IgM titers may increase.

Collection Techniques or Handling That May Alter Results
- Failure to separate serum from cells, hemolysis, or anticoagulated blood samples
- Repeated freeze-thaw cycles

Influence of Signalment
Species
None

Breed
None

Age
- Maternally derived IgG antibodies in kittens wane by 8–12 weeks of age.
- Seroprevalence increases with age, reflecting an increased risk of exposure over time.
- Systemic toxoplasmosis is more common in kittens with transplacental or lactational infections.

Gender
None

Pregnancy
Infection is usually fatal in kittens born to queens undergoing primary infections during pregnancy.

LIMITATIONS OF THE TEST
- Because of the prevalence of latent infections, positive serology tests do not necessarily prove clinical toxoplasmosis.
- Up to 20% of cats may not develop positive IgM titers during active infection.
- IgM titers persist for >12 weeks after infection in some cats.

Sensitivity, Specificity, and Positive and Negative Predictive Values
Valid If Run in a Human Lab?
Yes—if using IHA (TMP-Test; Wampole Labs, Carter Wallace, Cranbury, NJ) or LAT (Toxo Test-MT; Eiken Chemical, Tokyo, Japan; and Synki, Chatsworth, CA). Other methods require species-specific reagents.

CLINICAL PERSPECTIVE
- In most cats with primary infections, clinical signs are absent or restricted to transient diarrhea. A small proportion of cats with primary infections and immunosuppressed cats with reactivated latent infections develop systemic signs, which may be acute or chronic. Infections may be focal (e.g., ocular) or widely disseminated, with clinical signs referable to organ involvement. Mortality rates among cats with acute, disseminated toxoplasmosis are high.
- Infections in dogs may be focal or disseminated and acute or chronic. Acute, disseminated infection is more common in young dogs. Neuromuscular infection is more common in older dogs.

ANCILLARY TESTS
- Ab coefficient values comparing *T. gondii* Ab titers in CSF or aqueous humor with Ab titers to another nonocular/non-CNS pathogen such as calicivirus can be used to differentiate local Ab production from passive diffusion of plasma Abs into the site. The coefficient is calculated as follows:

$$\frac{T.gondii \text{ Ab titer in CSF or aqueous humor}}{T.gondii \text{ Ab titer in serum}} \times$$

$$\frac{calicivirus \text{ serum Ab titer}}{calicivirus \text{ Ab titer in CSF or aqueous humor}}$$

- Ab coefficient values of >1, and particularly >8, are indicative of focal Ab production in CSF or aqueous humor and suggest focal CNS or ocular infection (uveitis).
- CBC and chemistry profile
  - Nonregenerative anemia, inflammatory leukogram, and eosinophilia are common. Leukopenia, with a degenerative left shift and lymphocytopenia, is often seen in cats with fulminating toxoplasmosis.
  - Serum biochemistry abnormalities depend on type and severity of organ involvement (e.g., pancreatitis, hepatitis and/or cholangitis, myositis).

Test	Class of Ab detected	Sensitivity	Specificity
IFA	IgG, IgM or IgA	High	Some false positives because of nonspecific binding of Ig Fc receptors (receptors against the Fc portion of immunoglobulin) on *T. gondii* tachyzoites
ELISA	IgG, IgM or IgA	High	Specificity at low serum dilutions may be lower than IFA, LAT or IHA.
IHA	IgG	Lowest sensitivity	
LAT	IgG	Lower sensitivity than IFA or ELISA	
Modified agglutination test (modified to destroy IgM Abs)	IgG	Highest sensitivity	High specificity
Uses acetone and formalin-fixed *T. gondii* tachyzoites		Increased Abs to formalin-fixed *T. gondii* are highly sensitive but not specific, as they may remain elevated for years.	Increased Abs to acetone-fixed *T. gondii* tachyzoites are diagnostic of acute infection of <12 weeks' duration.

TOXOPLASMOSIS SEROLOGY

- Imaging techniques for detection of effusion and specific organ involvement
- Cytologic examination of body-cavity effusions, or bronchoalveolar lavage fluid for tachyzoites
- Biopsy lesions to look for tachyzoites
- Immunohistochemical or immunofluorescence techniques increase the chance of detecting tachyzoites in cytologic or histologic samples.
- Oocyst shedding in cats can be detected by centrifugal fecal flotation using Sheather's sugar solution or zinc sulfate.
- PCR of CSF, skeletal muscle, or neural tissue can detect *T. gondii* DNA and distinguish it from *Neospora caninum*.

SYNONYMS
None

SEE ALSO
Blackwell's Five-Minute Veterinary Consult: Canine and Feline Topics
Toxoplasmosis
Related Topics in This Book
- Feline Coronavirus
- Feline Immunodeficiency Virus

ABBREVIATIONS
- Ab = antibody
- CNS = central nervous system
- CSF = cerebrospinal fluid
- FC = Fragment, crystallizable
- IHA = indirect hemagglutination test
- LAT = latex agglutination test

Suggested Reading
Dubey JP, Lappin MR. Toxoplasmosis and neosporosis. In: Greene CE, ed. *Infectious Diseases of the Dog and Cat,*. 3rd ed St Louis: Saunders Elsevier, 2006: 754–775.
Schatzberg SJ, Haley NJ, Barr SC, *et al*. Use of a multiplex polymerase chain reaction assay in the antemortem diagnosis of toxoplasmosis and neosporosis in the central nervous system of cats and dogs. *Am J Vet Res* 2003; 64: 1507–1513.

INTERNET RESOURCES
Feline Advisory Bureau (fab), Policy Statement 6: Cats and toxoplasmosis, http://www.fabcats.org/cat_group/policy_statements/toxo.html.

AUTHOR NAME
Vanessa R.D. Barrs

BASICS

TYPE OF PROCEDURE
Diagnostic sample collection

PROCEDURE EXPLANATION AND RELATED PHYSIOLOGY
Tracheal wash involves insertion of a catheter into the airway of a dog or cat, injection of sterile saline, and, for culture and cytologic evaluation, subsequent aspiration of the fluid that has contacted the airway lining. The catheter can be inserted through an oral approach using a sterile endotracheal tube or through a transtracheal approach by passing sterile tubing through a catheter that is inserted between tracheal rings.

INDICATIONS
Acute or chronic cough

CONTRAINDICATIONS
- Bleeding disorders
- Anesthetic contraindications
- Markedly fractious animals

POTENTIAL COMPLICATIONS
- Any anesthetic complication
- Subcutaneous emphysema
- Pneumomediastinum
- Hemorrhage
- Chondroma formation

CLIENT EDUCATION
- Cough may be transiently worsened after the procedure.
- Subcutaneous emphysema may be noted.

BODY SYSTEMS ASSESSED
Respiratory

PROCEDURE

PATIENT PREPARATION
Preprocedure Medication or Preparation
- Preoxygenate the patient for 5 min prior to the procedure.
- In cats with suspected bronchial disease, to counteract any tendency toward bronchoconstriction, consider the use of terbutaline (0.01 mg/kg SC q12h or 0.625 mg/cat PO q12h) in the 12–24 h prior to the procedure.
- Dogs with marked expiratory effort might also benefit from administration of terbutaline prior to the procedure.

Anesthesia or Sedation
- To perform a transoral tracheal wash, any sedation protocol can be used that enables easy intubation and 5–10 min of light anesthesia.
- Local anesthesia with lidocaine may be sufficient for a transtracheal wash in compliant patients. Alternately, mild sedation with valium and/or narcotics may be required.

Patient Positioning
Sternal recumbency

Patient Monitoring
- Pulse oximetry can be used throughout an endotracheal wash, along with any standard anesthetic monitoring.
- If SC emphysema or bleeding develops, the procedure should be aborted and stabilization procedures instituted with sedation and placement of the patient in an oxygen-enriched environment.

Equipment or Supplies
- Transoral tracheal wash: sedation protocol, sterile endotracheal tube, sterile catheter or tubing, syringes, and sterile saline
- Transtracheal wash: local anesthesia (lidocaine), jugular catheter or over-the-needle catheter and sterile tubing, syringes, and sterile saline

TECHNIQUE
- A transoral tracheal wash is appropriate for use in large and small dogs, pediatric patients, and in cats. A sterile endotracheal tube and a sterile polypropylene catheter (3.5–8.0 French) or red rubber catheter are needed. The animal is anesthetized with a short-acting anesthetic agent. The sterile endotracheal tube is passed into the trachea, taking care to avoid touching the oral mucosa or larynx with the end of the tube in order to limit contamination with oropharyngeal bacteria. An assistant holds the tube in place, and a sterile polypropylene catheter or red rubber tube is passed to the level of the carina. An aliquot of nonbacteriostatic saline (4–6 mL) is instilled into the airway, and gentle suction is used to retrieve the fluid and cells from the lower airway. Removal of fluid can be enhanced by having the assistant compress the chest or by stimulating a cough during suction. Fluid instillation and aspiration can be repeated 2–3 times until an adequate sample has been retrieved (0.5–1.0 mL is usually sufficient for culture and cytologic evaluation).
- A transtracheal approach is appropriate for use in dogs larger than 8–10 kg. This can be performed with a through-the-needle jugular catheter or with an over-the-needle catheter and sterile tubing. The ventral portion of the neck is clipped and lightly scrubbed with antiseptic solution followed by alcohol wipes, and a more complete surgical preparation is performed after local anesthesia is instilled. Lidocaine (0.25–0.5 mL) is used at the 2 sites that will be penetrated by the needle: in the skin and between the tracheal rings. The needle of the jugular catheter will penetrate the skin low on the neck, and the skin will then be drawn upward prior to the airway lumen being entered. This creates an SC seal that limits air leakage from the airway out through the skin. The catheter is inserted into

TRACHEAL WASH

the skin with the bevel of the needle facing downward. The skin is drawn upward to enter between 2 rings of the trachea at a site above the site where the skin was penetrated. The sterile tubing or catheter is passed down the neck. An aliquot of nonbacteriostatic saline (4–6 mL) is injected into the catheter and then withdrawn. Stimulation of a cough or a deep breath after instillation can facilitate retrieval of a cellular sample. As already described, fluid removal can be enhanced by having the assistant compress the chest or by stimulating a cough during suction. Fluid instillation and aspiration can be repeated 2–3 times until an adequate sample has been retrieved (0.5–1.0 mL is usually sufficient for culture and cytologic evaluation).

SAMPLE HANDLING
Airway samples are submitted for cytologic evaluation and for bacterial culture. Aerobic, anaerobic, and *Mycoplasma* cultures should be considered for individual cases, and the laboratory should be consulted for guidelines on sample submission. Aerobic culture can generally be submitted in a sterile red-top tube; however, some laboratories require Amies medium for *Mycoplasma* culture and an anaerobic culture tube to detect anaerobic bacteria.

APPROPRIATE AFTERCARE
Postprocedure Patient Monitoring
• Monitor respiratory rate and effort.
• Watch for respiratory distress or generation of SC emphysema.
• Monitor the transtracheal site for bleeding or swelling.

Nursing Care
• Keep the animal quiet during recovery.
• If distress develops, sedation and placement in an oxygen-enriched environment can be helpful.

Dietary Modification
Any animal undergoing a tracheal wash should be fasted for 12–24 h prior to the procedure, when possible.

Medication Requirements
None

Restrictions on Activity
• The use of leashes should be avoided for 1–3 days after a transtracheal wash.
• Normal activity levels can usually be resumed after 1 day.

Anticipated Recovery Time
1–2 h

INTERPRETATION

NORMAL FINDINGS OR RANGE
• Normal animals should have ciliated respiratory epithelial cells present on cytologic evaluation and rare inflammatory cells or macrophages.
• Culture of airway fluid in normal dogs and cats can reveal light growth of various types of bacteria, including *Pasteurella*, *Streptococcus*, *Staphylococcus*, *Acinetobacter*, *Moraxella*, *Enterobacter*, *Pseudomonas*, *Escherichia coli*, and *Klebsiella*.

ABNORMAL VALUES
• Large numbers of neutrophils or eosinophils are abnormal.
• Degenerate neutrophils and intracellular bacteria are typically found in infectious processes.
• Abnormal lymphocytes are suggestive of lymphoma.
• Airway parasites or protozoa may be evident on cytologic evaluation.
• Rarely, neoplastic cells may exfoliate into tracheal wash fluid.
• Infection can be documented by growth of a single species of pathogenic bacteria or by moderate growth of a mixed number of bacterial species.
• Detection of *Mycoplasma* in the lower airway of cats indicates infection.

CRITICAL VALUES
None

INTERFERING FACTORS
Drugs That May Alter Results of the Procedure
• Corticosteroids will reduce the flux of inflammatory cells into the airways.
• Antibiotics will suppress bacterial growth on culture.
• Cough suppressants may make it difficult to obtain fluid from the airways.

Conditions That May Interfere with Performing the Procedure
• Severe tracheal sensitivity and tracheal or airway collapse can be worsened by trauma associated with tracheal wash.
• Airway collapse can result in poor return of fluid.
• In obese animals, a transtracheal wash can be difficult to perform because of an inability to palpate and stabilize the trachea.

Procedure Techniques or Handling That May Alter Results

Upper airway contamination (indicated by the presence of squamous cells or *Simonsiella* bacteria on cytologic evaluation) influences culture results and increases the likelihood of growth of contaminating bacteria.

Influence of Signalment on Performing and Interpreting the Procedure

Species
- Dogs: Use a peroral or transtracheal approach, depending on size of the animal.
- Cats: Use a peroral approach.

Breed
- Caution should be employed when undertaking any respiratory procedure in brachycephalic animals.
- The size of animal will influence the decision to perform a peroral vs a transtracheal wash.

Age
Young dogs may be more likely to have *Bordetella* and/or *Mycoplasma* on culture than older dogs.

Gender
None

Pregnancy
None

CLINICAL PERSPECTIVE

Tracheal wash procedures are relatively safe and easy to perform. Results of culture and cytologic evaluation provide valuable information on appropriate treatment of respiratory patients.

MISCELLANEOUS

ANCILLARY TESTS

If results are nondiagnostic, bronchoscopy or lung biopsy could be indicated.

SYNONYMS

None

SEE ALSO

Blackwell's Five-Minute Veterinary Consult: Canine and Feline Topics
- Asthma, Bronchitis—Cats

- Bronchiectasis
- Bronchitis, Chronic (COPD)
- Cough
- Infectious Canine Tracheobronchitis (Kennel Cough)
- Pneumonia, Aspiration
- Pneumonia, Bacteria
- Pneumonia, Eosinophilic
- Pneumonia, Fungal
- Pneumonia, Interstitial
- Respiratory Parasites
- Tracheal Perforation

Related Topics in This Book

Bronchoscopy

ABBREVIATIONS

None

Suggested Reading

Dye JA, McKiernan BC, Rozanski EA, *et al.* Bronchopulmonary disease in the cat: Historical, physical, radiographic, clinicopathologic, and pulmonary functional evaluation of 24 affected and 15 healthy cats. *J Vet Intern Med* 1996; 10: 385–400.

Padrid PA, Hornof WJ, Kurpershoek CJ, Cross CE. Canine chronic bronchitis: A pathophysiological evaluation of 18 cases. *J Vet Intern Med* 1990; 4: 172–180.

Peeters DE, McKiernan BC, Weisiger RM, *et al.* Quantitative bacterial cultures and cytological examination of bronchoalveolar lavage specimens in dogs. *J Vet Intern Med* 2000; 14: 534–541.

Randolph JF, Moise NS, Scarlett JM, *et al.* Prevalence of mycoplasmal and ureaplasmal recovery from tracheobronchial lavages and of mycoplasma recovery from pharyngeal swabs in dogs with and without pulmonary disease. *Am J Vet Res* 1993; 54: 387–391.

Randolph JF, Moise NS, Scarlett JM, *et al.* Prevalence of mycoplasmal and ureaplasmal recovery from tracheobronchial lavages and of mycoplasma recovery from pharyngeal swabs in cats with and without pulmonary disease. *Am J Vet Res* 1993; 54: 897–900.

INTERNET RESOURCES

None

AUTHOR NAME

Lynelle R. Johnson

TRANSSPLENIC PORTAL SCINTIGRAPHY

BASICS

TYPE OF PROCEDURE
Nuclear medicine

PROCEDURE EXPLANATION AND RELATED PHYSIOLOGY
Transsplenic portal scintigraphy (TSPS) is a sensitive and specific imaging technique for diagnosis of macroscopic portosystemic shunts. TSPS has largely replaced per-rectal scintigraphy. With TSPS, one can inject a small volume of radiopharmaceutical with a relatively high count rate into the splenic parenchyma by using ultrasound guidance. This results in immediate transfer of the radiotracer from the splenic parenchyma into the portal circulation, resulting in a scintigraphic portogram during the first several seconds of acquisition. The radiopharmaceutical used is technetium 99m bound to a bilirubin analog (i.e., mebrofenin or disofenin) so that there is 95%–98% uptake by the hepatocytes on a first pass through the liver. The advantage of this procedure over the older, per-rectal procedure is much greater count rates and overall count density, making visualization of the radiotracer distribution easier. Furthermore, one is not count limited during acquisition. The images are much easier to interpret, and there is no dependency on the amount of radiopharmaceutical absorbed by the colon as with the per-rectal or transcolonic procedure. In addition, you do not have to block the large radioactive bolus that is left within the colon (because there is a <5% absorption rate) that will preclude evaluation of the first pass of the radiopharmaceutical through the liver.

INDICATIONS
• Evaluation of patients with suspected macroscopic intrahepatic or extrahepatic portosystemic shunts
• Follow-up evaluation for continued shunting or occlusion in dogs and cats after occlusion or ameroid constrictor placement
• Evaluation of hepatic function

CONTRAINDICATIONS
Bleeding disorders caused by the introduction of a needle into the splenic parenchyma for injection of the radiopharmaceutical

POTENTIAL COMPLICATIONS
• Splenic laceration and bleeding
• Peritoneal injection of the radiopharmaceutical, leading to a nondiagnostic study (no real patient complications) and study can be repeated immediately

CLIENT EDUCATION
• The patient will have to be held at the facility according to the state nuclear medicine license requirements. No follow-up for the patient is required once it is released to the owner.
• If there are specific at-home requirements for handling of the radioactive pet (assuming it is going home prior to the 60-h total decay period), these instructions should be presented to the client on paper and signed by the client with a copy being maintained in the medical record and the nuclear medicine license files.

BODY SYSTEMS ASSESSED
Hepatobiliary

PROCEDURE

PATIENT PREPARATION
Preprocedure Medication or Preparation
• The patient is fasted for 12 h.
• An IV catheter (cephalic) is placed.

• Enemas are not needed.
Anesthesia or Sedation
One-half to two-thirds of an induction dose of propofol is injected IV.

Patient Positioning
The patient is placed in right lateral recumbency on the gamma camera. The spleen is imaged using an ultrasound machine prior to anesthesia so that positioning of the patient is optimal for injection prior to induction. The image of the spleen of the patient should be optimized for the near field.

Patient Monitoring
ECG and pulse oximetry monitors are used as needed during the time the patient is under anesthesia.

Equipment or Supplies
• A gamma camera with general-purpose, low-energy collimator with acquisition computer workstation
• A 23-gauge, 1-inch (2.54 cm) needle
• A 1-mL (tuberculin) syringe with 0.2 mL containing ≈74 MBq (2 mCi) of ^{99m}Tc-mebrofenin (or ^{99m}Tc-disofenin)
• An ultrasound machine with a high-frequency transducer

TECHNIQUE
• The patient is placed in right lateral recumbency and the splenic images optimized using the ultrasound machine so that it is a near-field structure with the appropriate depth, gain, and focal zone settings. The spleen should be imaged in short axis (dorsal plane position of the probe on the dog or cat) so that it appears as a triangle on the screen. A splenic portal vessel should be present in the far-field side or mesenteric border of the image; however, the goal is to inject the radiopharmaceutical into the splenic parenchyma and not the splenic portal vessel.
• After injection of the radiopharmaceutical into the spleen, the needle is withdrawn and discarded in a radioactive materials sharps box. The needle should be withdrawn and moved away from the patient in such a way that there is no crosstalk of the radioactivity between the portal scintigraphic study and the residual radioactivity within the syringe. Typically, pulling the syringe ventrally will ensure this. The patient is still imaged by using ultrasound to evaluate for any potential splenic bleeding or complication.
• The nuclear medicine computer is set up for a dual-phase dynamic acquisition using a 256 (128) × 256 (128) × 16 matrix, and, if the patient is small (weighing <5 kg), a digital zoom factor of 1.5 or 2.0 is applied. The dual dynamic acquisition consists of an initial 1-min series of frames that are acquired at a rate of 4 frames/s and then a second dynamic data set where the frames are acquired at a rate of 2 s/frame for a total of 4 min after injection.
• If there is any question about hepatic function or biliary excretion, then a series of follow-up static images are obtained at 5, 10, 30, 60, and 120 min. The series consists of right and left lateral and ventral images that are acquired at 256 × 256 × 16, 1 min/frame for a count rate of 250,000 per image. Further imaging is used if the radioactivity is not seen to enter the gallbladder or empty from the gallbladder into the duodenum. These images can be made with the patient awake. A fatty meal can be fed to induce gallbladder contractions and help to define emptying into the duodenum.
• The radiopharmaceutical for injection should be held in a specialized lead syringe shield prior to injection.
• Rubber gloves and a laboratory coat should be worn to reduce the potential for personnel contamination.
• After injection, the ultrasound machine and probe should be monitored for any radioactive contamination by using a Geiger-Müller survey meter.

SAMPLE HANDLING
N/A

APPROPRIATE AFTERCARE
Postprocedure Patient Monitoring
• The patient should be monitored and the exposure rates recorded at the surface and at 1 m should be posted on the animal's cage with an appropriate radioactive sign. The ultrasound probe is monitored for potential contamination.
• The patient is monitored for normal recovery from the propofol anesthesia.

Nursing Care
• Not required for the procedure
• Specific care regarding recovery from anesthesia as is standard

Dietary Modification
No dietary restrictions are required afterward that are specific to the procedure.

Medication Requirements
None

Restrictions on Activity
None

Anticipated Recovery Time
Anesthetic recover should occur within 10–15 min after the dynamic acquisition has ended.

INTERPRETATION
NORMAL FINDINGS OR RANGE
• The transit of the radiopharmaceutical between the spleen, the liver, and then the heart occurs within seconds of injection. The needle (with syringe attached) is placed into the splenic parenchyma *adjacent* to a splenic portal vessel. It is easier to have the sonographer place the needle and have someone else make the actual injection. The dynamic acquisition is started, and several seconds are allowed to pass to make sure the study has started. The injection should be steady, but not administered as a rapid bolus. So that the air bubbles can be followed under ultrasound, it is best to draw a small amount of air into the end of the needle prior to placement in the spleen. The bubbles should be seen entering a splenic portal vessel and not the peritoneal space. The needle is withdrawn toward the bottom part of the camera and caudal aspect of the patient so that the needle (with leftover radioactivity) does not cross the cranial part of the patient and cause image degradation. The sonographer can then watch the radiopharmaceutical on the persistence oscilloscope above the gamma camera.
• The radiopharmaceutical should move from the spleen into the splenic portal system, portal vein, and hepatic portal capillary bed and be actively transported into the hepatocytes by the anion dye receptors (bilirubin receptors) found on the hepatocyte cell membrane. If the dog has highly increased bilirubin concentrations, the actual uptake of the radiopharmaceutical could be decreased by the competitive inhibition at the level of the cell membrane receptor. A small amount of radiopharmaceutical will not be taken up by the hepatocytes and will continue into the hepatic veins, caudal vena cava, and heart. This is because there is not 100% uptake of the radiopharmaceutical on a first pass. Portal streamlining can be seen where the radiopharmaceutical does not distribute itself equally within the portal circulation and follows the course of 1 of the 3 major divisional portal venous branches within the liver. Therefore, asymmetrical uptake of the radiopharmaceutical may occur.

ABNORMAL VALUES
• When macroscopic intrahepatic or extrahepatic portosystemic shunt(s) is present, the radiopharmaceutical will move from the portal vasculature across the shunt into the connecting returning venous route (azygos vein, caudal vena cava, or other venous structures) and enter the heart and then lungs. Thereby, the radiopharmaceutical will bypass the liver, and, even in the case of an intrahepatic shunt, there will be a lack of uptake by the liver (lack of visualization of the liver) and persistent radiopharmaceutical within the central circulation. Over time and recirculation, the radiopharmaceutical will be taken up by the liver. The overall liver size is typically small in animals with shunt vessels. Hepatic insufficiency will result in renal uptake and clearance of the radiopharmaceutical (its appearance in the kidneys and urinary bladder), which will be evident on the delayed static images.
• Calculation of a hepatic extraction fraction is a complex way to determine hepatic function, but is a relatively sensitive technique for determining changes in hepatic function over time, if applicable (see the references in the Suggested Reading section for further details).
• The shunt fraction can be calculated and should be <3% for the first 20 s of uptake of the radiopharmaceutical in the liver and within the blood pool of the heart in a normal dog or cat. The caveat is that dogs with microscopic portal vascular shunting or portal vascular dysplasia will have a normal TSPS (as with other imaging procedures, such as a portal angiogram).
• In the past (with transcolonic scintigraphy), a shunt fraction (percent radiopharmaceutical distribution in the liver as compared to the heart during the first 12–16 s of vascular transit) has been calculated and used to help evaluate patients for the presence or absence of a shunt. Some ambiguity in the drawing of the region of interest and experience of the interpreter has led to a falling out in the use of the shunt fraction calculation. With the current technique, a subjective review of the dynamic data set is all that is needed to determine the presence or absence of a macroscopic portosystemic shunt.

CRITICAL VALUES
None

INTERFERING FACTORS
Drugs That May Alter Results of the Procedure
None known

Conditions That May Interfere with Performing the Procedure
• Severe hyperbilirubinemia may inhibit hepatic uptake so that the functional aspects of the study may not be valid. However, the initial dynamic imaging sequence will still show whether there is a macroscopic portosystemic shunt.
• A large volume of ascites will probably preclude one from being able to perform the procedure.

Procedure Techniques or Handling That May Alter Results
If the splenic injection results in peritoneal accumulation of the radiopharmaceutical rather than uptake into the splenic portal system, then the study will be nondiagnostic and can be repeated immediately.

Influence of Signalment on Performing and Interpreting the Procedure
Species
• Smaller dogs and cats will require a digital zoom prior to study acquisition. Portosystemic shunts are more common in dogs than cats.
• Small-breed dogs tend to have single extrahepatic portosystemic shunts, whereas larger dogs tend to have intrahepatic portosystemic shunts.

Breed
The Yorkshire terrier breed is predisposed to single extrahepatic shunts and presumably has an unproven genetic defect that has a heritable character.

Age
Young animals (<2 years of age) typically present for imaging.

Gender
None known

Pregnancy
N/A

TRANSSPLENIC PORTAL SCINTIGRAPHY

CLINICAL PERSPECTIVE

TSPS can be used when ultrasound evaluation is equivocal or there is a reason to follow up a case in which a patient has had prior ameroid ring placement (banding). In addition, TSPS can provide information regarding hepatic function when mebrofenin or disofenin is used.

MISCELLANEOUS

ANCILLARY TESTS
- Abdominal ultrasonography
- Evaluation of bile acids
- Evaluation of BUN

SYNONYMS
- Portal scintigraphy
- Splenic portal scintigraphy

SEE ALSO

Blackwell's Five-Minute Veterinary Consult: Canine and Feline Topics
- Portosystemic Shunting, Acquired
- Portosystemic Vascular Anomaly, Congenital

Related Topics in This Book
- General Principles of Radiography
- Ammonia
- Bile Acids

ABBREVIATIONS

TSPS = transsplenic portal scintigraphy

Suggested Reading

Daniel GB, Bright R, Ollis P, Shull R. Per rectal portal scintigraphy using [99m]technetium pertechnetate to diagnose portosystemic shunts in dogs and cats. *J Vet Intern Med* 1991; 5: 23–27.

Daniel GB, DeNovo R, Bahr A, Smith GT. Evaluation of heart time-activity curves as a predictor of hepatic extraction of ^{99m}Tc-mebrofenin in dogs. *Vet Radiol Ultrasound* 2001; 42: 162–168.

Daniel GB, DeNovo RC, Sharp DS, *et al.* Portal streamlining as a cause of nonuniform hepatic distribution of sodium pertechnetate during per-rectal portal scintigraphy in the dog. *Vet Radiol Ultrasound* 2004; 45: 78–84.

Daniel GB, Koblik PD, Berry CR. Portal scintigraphy. In: Daniel GB, Berry CR, eds. *The Textbook of Veterinary Nuclear Medicine.* Harrisburg, PA: American College of Veterinary Radiology, 2006: 247–253.

Morandi F, Cole RC, Tobias KM, *et al.* Use of [99m]TcO$_4$(-) transsplenic portal scintigraphy for diagnosis of portosystemic shunts in 28 dogs. *Vet Radiol Ultrasound* 2005; 46: 153–161.

INTERNET RESOURCES

University of Tennessee, College of Veterinary Medicine, Radiology: Nuclear medicine, http://www.vet.utk.edu/radiology/nuclear/index.php.

AUTHOR NAMES

Anthony Pease and Clifford Berry

BASICS

TYPE OF SPECIMEN
Blood

TEST EXPLANATION AND RELATED PHYSIOLOGY
Triglycerides (TGs), which are among the major lipids in plasma, are synthesized in adipose tissue and the liver. Those produced in hepatocytes circulate as VLDLs. TGs are also the predominant form of dietary lipid. After ingestion, emulsified lipids in the jejunum are absorbed as micelles. Within enterocytes, micelles are broken down into fatty acids, monoglycerides, and cholesterol. TGs are assembled, and combined with apolipoproteins to form water-soluble chylomicra, which are secreted into intestinal lacteals. Chylomicra enter the general circulation through the thoracic duct and are carried to tissues, including muscle, adipose, and hepatocytes. Lipoprotein lipase on the surface of endothelial cells in these tissues hydrolyzes chylomicra TG, releasing fatty acids that are absorbed and used to synthesize TGs.

Hyperlipidemia, synonymous with hyperlipoproteinemia, refers to either hypertriglyceridemia or hypercholesterolemia, whereas *lipemia* refers to the cloudy or opaque appearance of serum or plasma as seen by the naked eye. Most TGs in a postprandial sample are in chylomicra, and postprandial hypertriglyceridemia peaks 2–6 h after eating. High-fat diets may cause lipemia because of high chylomicron content, but hypercholesterolemia does not produce cloudiness. Nearly all TGs in a fasting sample are in VLDLs synthesized by hepatocytes. Lipoproteins (chylomicra and VLDLs) are cleared from plasma by lipoprotein lipase; insulin, thyroid hormone, and heparin enhance clearance.

Hypertriglyceridemia is most commonly a physiologic phenomenon caused by inadequate fasting. Excess lipids present after at least a 12-h fast indicate a persistent, or pathologic, hyperlipidemia. Refrigeration may aid in evaluating plasma lipids: Specimen turbidity occurring after 4- to 8-h refrigeration indicates that VLDLs and/or chylomicra are present. A cream layer on top of a cleared zone suggests that chylomicra are likely present, but persistent turbidity generally implies presence of VLDLs. The presence of both conditions (i.e., a cream layer on top with turbidity below) suggests dual increases in chylomicra and VLDLs. Pathologic hypertriglyceridemia is generally secondary to underlying endocrine, pancreatic, hepatic, or renal disease. Primary hyperlipidemias, caused by genetic abnormalities, are rare.

INDICATIONS
- Screening for endocrinopathies, including diabetes mellitus, hypothyroidism, and hyperadrenocorticism
- Lipemia despite prolonged fasting

CONTRAINDICATIONS
None

POTENTIAL COMPLICATIONS
None

CLIENT EDUCATION
The patient should undergo a 12-h fast before testing.

BODY SYSTEMS ASSESSED
- Endocrine and metabolic
- Gastrointestinal
- Hepatobiliary
- Renal and urologic

SAMPLE

COLLECTION
1 mL of venous blood, preferably after a 12-h fast

HANDLING
Use a plain red-top tube, serum-separator tube, or heparin.

STORAGE
Refrigerate or freeze separated serum for long-term storage.

STABILITY
- Room temperature: 1 day
- Refrigerated (2°–8°C): 1 week
- Frozen (−20°C): 3 months; several years at −70°C

PROTOCOL
None

INTERPRETATION

NORMAL FINDINGS OR RANGE
- Dogs: 30–141 mg/dL (0.34–1.59 mmol/L)
- Cats: 19–146 mg/dL (0.21–1.65 mmol/L)
- Reference intervals may vary depending on the laboratory and assay.

TRIGLYCERIDES

ABNORMAL VALUES
Values above or below the reference interval

CRITICAL VALUES
None

INTERFERING FACTORS
Drugs That May Alter Results or Interpretation
Drugs That Interfere with Test Methodology
None

Drugs That Alter Physiology
• Decreased by heparin and L-asparaginase
• Increased by estrogen, glucocorticoids, progesterone acetate, and doxorubicin

Disorders That May Alter Results
• Hemolysis or bilirubinemia may falsely increase the TG value.
• TG concentration may increase with high-fat diets.
• Obese animals may have prolonged postprandial hyperlipidemia.

Collection Techniques or Handling That May Alter Results
• Contamination with glycerin (on vacuum-tube stoppers) and detergents may falsely elevate the TG concentration.
• Iatrogenic hemolysis

Influence of Signalment
Species
None

Breed
• Feline lipoprotein lipase deficiency has been reported as an autosomal recessive trait in Siamese, domestic shorthair, and Himalayan cats. Affected cats can have a TG concentration >10-fold normal, but normal cholesterol.
• Primary hyperlipidemia has been reported in miniature schnauzers, Brittany spaniels, beagles, and mixed-breed dogs.

Age
None

Gender
None

Pregnancy
None

LIMITATIONS OF THE TEST
Sensitivity, Specificity, and Positive and Negative Predictive Values
N/A

Valid If Run in a Human Lab?
Yes.

Causes of Abnormal Findings

High values	*Low values*
Physiologic/postprandial	Maldigestion/malabsorption
Primary hypertriglyceridemia	syndromes
Primary idiopathic	Exocrine pancreatic
hyperlipidemia of miniature	insufficiency
schnauzers (and other	Small-intestinal inflammation
breeds)	Portosystemic shunts
Feline lipoprotein lipase	Hyperthyroidism
deficiency	
Secondary hypertriglyceridemia	
Diabetes mellitus	
Acute pancreatitis	
Hypothyroidism*	
Nephrotic syndrome because of	
a protein-losing nephropathy*	
Hyperadrenocorticism or excess	
glucocorticoids*	

*Hypercholesterolemia with or without concurrent hypertriglyceridemia.

CLINICAL PERSPECTIVE
• If the TG concentration is increased, rule out a postprandial effect by collecting a second fasted sample. If persistent, rule out secondary causes.
• If the TG concentration is decreased, rule out liver, exocrine pancreatic, and intestinal disease.
• Chronic marked hypertriglyceridemia can cause secondary pancreatitis and seizures.

MISCELLANEOUS

ANCILLARY TESTS
• A full chemistry panel and urinalysis
• Evaluation of pancreatitis lipase immunoreactivity to rule out pancreatitis

- Thyroid and adrenal function tests
- Evaluation of bile acids to assess liver function or portal anomaly

SYNONYMS
None

SEE ALSO
Blackwell's Five-Minute Veterinary Consult: Canine and Feline Topics
- Cirrhosis and Fibrosis of the Liver
- Diabetes Mellitus with Hyperosmolar Coma
- Diabetes Mellitus with Ketoacidosis
- Diabetes Mellitus without Complication—Cats
- Diabetes Mellitus without Complication—Dogs
- Hyperadrenocorticism (Cushing's Disease)—Cats
- Hyperadrenocorticism (Cushing's Disease)—Dogs
- Hyperlipidemia
- Hypothyroidism
- Nephrotic Syndrome

Related Topics in This Book
- Albumin
- Bile Acids

- Glucose
- Pancreatic Lipase Immunoreactivity
- Urine Glucose
- Urine Protein

ABBREVIATIONS
- TG = triglyceride
- VLDL = very low density lipoprotein

Suggested Reading
Evans EW, Duncan JR. Proteins, lipids, and carbohydrates. In: Latimer KS, Mahaffey EA, Prasse KW, eds. *Duncan and Prasse's Veterinary Laboratory Medicine,* 4th ed. Ames: Iowa State Press, 2003: 162–192.

INTERNET RESOURCES
Cornell University, College of Veterinary Medicine, Clinical Pathology Modules, Specialized Chemistry Tests: Trigylerides, http://www.diaglab.vet.cornell.edu/clinpath/modules/chem/triglyc.htm.

AUTHOR NAMES
Rebekah Gray Gunn-Christie and J. Roger Easley

TROPONINS, CARDIAC SPECIFIC

BASICS

TYPE OF SPECIMEN
Blood

TEST EXPLANATION AND RELATED PHYSIOLOGY
Troponin is a protein that exists in skeletal and cardiac muscle and is involved in the calcium-dependent interaction of myosin with actin. Heart muscle cells contain 3 types of troponin (C, I, and T). Cardiac troponin C (cTnC) responds to calcium ions released from the sarcoplasmic reticulum, initiating the cross-bridge cycle with tropomyosin. Cardiac troponin I (cTnI) binds to the activated troponin C, restricting the interaction between actin and the myosin heads. Cardiac troponin T (cTnT) binds the whole troponin complex to tropomyosin.

Cardiac troponins I and T are specific markers of myocyte injury, ischemia, and necrosis. Cardiac troponin has a high specificity for cardiac muscle injury and therefore can help differentiate skeletal from cardiac muscle injury and is more specific for cardiac muscle injury than is creatine kinase MB isoenzyme. In human patients, cardiac troponin assays are used to help diagnose acute myocardial infarction. In dogs and cats with heart disease, modest elevations of cardiac troponin are common and tend to correlate with severity of disease. Cardiac troponin is also elevated in many animals with extracardiac diseases, such as gastric dilation and volvulus, and in this setting likely represents extension of hypoxic or toxic insult to the myocardium.

Cardiac troponin samples from veterinary patients are tested by using human medical immunoassays. A variety of cardiac troponin I assays are available but lack standardization, preventing direct comparison of results from different machines. In the author's experience, cardiac troponin I is more sensitive than troponin T. In animals with heart disease, circulating cardiac troponin is elevated but typically below values that are indicative of acute myocardial infarction. Thus, mild elevations in dogs and cats are thought to reflect low-level chronic damage to myocardial tissue rather than acute infarction. Serial cardiac troponin testing likely is more instructive than values obtained at a single point in time. The author stresses that, at the time of writing, cardiac troponin testing is relatively new in veterinary medicine, and concrete diagnostic, prognostic, and therapeutic recommendations based on assay results are not yet available.

INDICATIONS
- Suspected myocardial infarction
- Cardiomyopathy
- Gastric dilation and volvulus
- Arrhythmias (especially ventricular)
- Toxic myocardial disease (e.g., caused by doxorubicin)
- Infectious myocardial disease (e.g., *Babesia*, Chagas disease)
- Extracardiac diseases associated with hypoxia
- Differentiation of skeletal from cardiac muscle injury
- High creatine kinase value on routine blood screening

CONTRAINDICATIONS
Cardiac troponin concentrations are unlikely to assist in detection of asymptomatic (occult) cardiomyopathy (i.e., as a screening exam for mild heart disease) or in differentiating cardiac vs noncardiac causes of dyspnea and hypoxia (i.e., congestive heart failure vs primary respiratory disease).

POTENTIAL COMPLICATIONS
None

CLIENT EDUCATION
High test values do not pinpoint the cause of myocardial disease, and animals with cardiomyopathy can have normal troponin levels.

BODY SYSTEMS ASSESSED
Cardiovascular

SAMPLE

COLLECTION
1–3 mL of venous blood

HANDLING
- Most cardiac troponin assays accept either serum or heparinized or EDTA plasma.
- Some point-of-care tests use whole blood.

STORAGE
- Refrigerate the sample if the assay will be performed within 12 h after collection.
- Freezing (−20°C) the sample is recommended if analysis is delayed for >12 h after collection.

STABILITY
The stability of canine and feline troponin is largely unknown, and there are conflicting reports regarding the stability of canine cardiac troponin I at room temperature. Some of these differences are likely due to different rates of epitope degradation and differences in the antigen target(s) used by the various commercial tests. A single freeze-thaw cycle appears unlikely to affect test results significantly, and the author recommends freezing serum or plasma samples if the assay is not run the same day as sample collection. In general, handle veterinary samples according to the guidelines established for each specific test for collection, handling, and storage of human samples.

PROTOCOL
None

INTERPRETATION

NORMAL FINDINGS OR RANGE
In healthy animals, cardiac troponins I and T are typically undetectable (i.e., below the assay's lower limit of detection); however, the extreme sensitivity of newer assays indicates that mild increases of cardiac troponin (particularly troponin I) can occur in overtly healthy dogs. The author's experience using a variety of assays indicates that the normal troponin I concentration in dogs and cats is typically <0.08 ng/mL.

ABNORMAL VALUES
High cardiac troponin levels have been demonstrated over a wide range of cardiac and extracardiac diseases, including dilated cardiomyopathy, hypertrophic cardiomyopathy, congenital subaortic stenosis, mitral valve disease, pericardial effusion, hyperthyroidism, chest trauma, sepsis, gastric dilation and volvulus, babesiosis, and doxorubicin chemotherapy. In most cases, these elevations are relatively modest, and below the diagnostic threshold of acute myocardial infarction for human patients. In the author's experience, these elevations in troponin I are typically in the range of 0.1–0.8 ng/mL and likely reflect low-level myocardial hypoxia, ischemia, and myocardial cell damage.

CRITICAL VALUES
- Extremely high concentrations of cardiac troponin that are well above the diagnostic threshold of acute myocardial infarction in human patients are occasionally detected in dogs and cats. In the author's experience, these animals usually suffer from overt clinical disease in the form of congestive heart failure, arrhythmias, myocarditis, severe hypoxia, or significant trauma.
- In a small study of dogs with dilated cardiomyopathy, dogs with a cardiac troponin I level of >0.2 ng/mL had a worse prognosis than those with lower values.
- Serial tests that document increasing cardiac troponin concentrations over several days, weeks, or months are likely associated with poor outcome.

INTERFERING FACTORS
Drugs That May Alter Results or Interpretation
Drugs That Interfere with Test Methodology
None

Drugs That Alter Physiology
Doxorubicin cardiotoxicity can elevate troponin levels.

Disorders That May Alter Results
Chronic renal disease may falsely increase cardiac troponin concentrations.

Collection Techniques or Handling That May Alter Results
Excessive concentrations of heparin in plasma samples (because of underfilling of the collection tube) may interfere with some assays.

Influence of Signalment
Species
None

Breed
None established

Age
In overtly healthy Doberman pinschers, a significant increase in cardiac troponin I was associated with increasing age, but the magnitude of this change was so small as to be of negligible clinical importance.

Gender
None established

Pregnancy
None established

LIMITATIONS OF THE TEST
Sensitivity, Specificity, and Positive and Negative Predictive Values
- Although cardiac troponin assays are highly sensitive and specific for cardiac muscle injury, they are not specific with respect to etiology. Both cardiac and extracardiac diseases can elicit troponin elevations if the disease process injures cardiac tissue. In fact, in the author's experience, some of the most spectacular elevations occurred in dogs with primary respiratory disease and profound systemic hypoxia.
- Although most animals with moderate to advanced heart disease demonstrate elevated troponin concentrations, many do not, and, as such, cardiac troponin assays possess little value as a screening test for cardiac disease.
- Single measurements of cardiac troponin can help document cardiac injury and assess severity of disease. Serial measurements are more likely to provide prognostic information and indicate response to therapy.

Valid If Run in a Human Lab?
Yes.

Causes of Abnormal Findings

High values	Low values
Myocardial trauma	No pathologic causes
Feline hypertrophic cardiomyopathy	
Canine dilated cardiomyopathy	
Canine mitral valve disease	
Pericardial effusion	
Severe skeletal muscle injury	
Myocardial damage secondary to doxorubicin, babesiosis, gastric dilatation, and volvulus	
Systemic hypoxemia secondary to respiratory disease	

CLINICAL PERSPECTIVE
- Elevated cardiac troponin indicates myocardial tissue injury, often the result of hypoxia or ischemia.
- Most elevations in animals with cardiac disease are mild.
- Serial measurements likely are more useful than 1 measurement at a single point in time.
- Although specific for cardiac injury, cardiac troponin can be elevated in both cardiac and extracardiac disease and, as such, is not useful as a screening tool for cardiac disease.
- Magnitude of elevation correlates with severity of muscle injury but does not pinpoint the cause of the injury.
- High cTnI levels can be seen in cats with moderate to severe hypertrophic cardiomyopathy.
- Dogs with pericardial effusion caused by hemangiosarcoma (2.77 ng/dL; range, 0.09–47.18 ng/dL) are reported to have higher plasma levels of cTnI than dogs with idiopathic pericardial effusion (0.05 ng/dL; range, 0.03–0.09 ng/dL).
- The degree of elevation following gastric dilation and volvulus correlates with the severity of cardiac muscle injury and severity of arrhythmias.

 MISCELLANEOUS

ANCILLARY TESTS
Cardiac troponin assays are rarely performed in isolation, and ECG, echocardiographic, radiographic, arterial blood-gas measurement, blood pressure determination, and other cardiovascular diagnostic tests are often performed.

SYNONYMS
None

SEE ALSO
Blackwell's Five-Minute Veterinary Consult: Canine and Feline Topics
- Cardiomyopathy, Dilated—Dogs
- Cardiomyopathy, Hypertrophic—Cats
- Pericardial Effusion

TROPONINS, CARDIAC SPECIFIC

Related Topics in This Book
- Blood Gases
- Blood Pressure Determination: Noninvasive and Invasive
- Creatine Kinase
- Echocardiography

ABBREVIATIONS
- cTnC = cardiac troponin C
- cTnI = cardiac troponin I
- cTnT = cardiac troponin T

Suggested Reading

Herndon WE, Kittleson MD, Sanderson K, *et al.* Cardiac troponin I in feline hypertrophic cardiomyopathy. *J Vet Intern Med* 2002; 16: 558–564.

Oyama MA, Sisson DD. Cardiac troponin-I concentration in dogs with cardiac disease. *J Vet Intern Med* 2004; 18: 831–839.

Oyama MA, Solter PF. Validation of an immunoassay for measurement of canine cardiac troponin-I. *J Vet Cardiol* 2004; 6: 15–23.

Schober KA. Biochemical markers of cardiovascular disease. In: Ettinger SD, Feldman EC, eds. *Textbook of Veterinary Internal Medicine*, 6th ed. St Louis: Saunders Elsevier, 2005: 940–948.

Shaw SP, Rozanski EA, Rush JE. Cardiac troponins I and T in dogs with pericardial effusion. *J Vet Intern Med* 2004; 18: 322–324.

Sleeper MM, Clifford CA, Laster LL. Cardiac troponin I in normal dog and cat. *J Vet Intern Med* 2001; 15: 501–503.

Spratt DP, Mellanby RJ, Drury N, Archer J. Cardiac troponin I: Evaluation of a biomarker for diagnosis of heart disease in the dog. *J Small Anim Pract* 2005; 46: 139–145.

INTERNET RESOURCES
None

AUTHOR NAME
Mark A. Oyama

BASICS

TYPE OF SPECIMEN
Blood

TEST EXPLANATION AND RELATED PHYSIOLOGY
The assay for measurement of trypsin-like immunoreactivity (TLI) in serum is a species-specific immunoassay used to diagnose exocrine pancreatic insufficiency (EPI). The test primarily measures *trypsinogen*, the zymogen or inactive preform of trypsin in serum. Trypsinogen is synthesized and stored in pancreatic acinar cells, which, under physiologic conditions, release minute quantities of it into the vascular space. Trypsinogen and trypsin are not absorbed from the intestine. Therefore, the serum TLI concentration reflects the actual release of trypsinogen directly from the pancreas. As trypsin and trypsinogen are very similar, the TLI assay detects both trypsinogen and trypsin. The assay also detects a portion of trypsin that has been reversibly bound to α_1-proteinase inhibitor. Therefore, the assay is termed *trypsin-like* immunoreactivity.

The syndrome of EPI develops as a result of a lack of pancreatic acinar cells. This is most commonly caused by pancreatic acinar atrophy (an inherited trait in German shepherds) or chronic pancreatitis. The lack of acinar cells leads to a decrease in production and release of trypsinogen into the intestine and the blood. The resulting low serum concentrations of trypsinogen can then be observed when evaluating the serum TLI concentration. Clinical signs of EPI usually do not develop until the functional capacity of the pancreas is reduced to 10%–15% of normal.

High TLI concentrations are suggestive of pancreatitis, but the sensitivity of the TLI assay for pancreatitis is only 30%–60%. A normal TLI result does not exclude pancreatitis. Serum PLI concentration should be measured in patients with suspected pancreatitis.

INDICATIONS
Diagnostic test of choice for EPI in dogs and cats

CONTRAINDICATIONS
None

POTENTIAL COMPLICATIONS
None

CLIENT EDUCATION
To avoid lipemia, food should be withheld from the animal for 8–12 h before blood is drawn.

BODY SYSTEMS ASSESSED
Gastrointestinal

SAMPLE

COLLECTION
1–2 mL of venous blood

HANDLING
- Use a red-top or serum-separator tube.
- Separate the serum from the blood clot and transfer the serum into new tube with no additive.
- The serum can be shipped at ambient temperatures, although the addition of a cold pack is recommended to avoid high temperatures.

STORAGE
- Refrigeration is recommended for short-term storage (1–2 days), but room temperature is acceptable.
- Freezing is recommended for longer storage.

STABILITY
- Stable for several days at room temperature
- Refrigerated: (2°–8°C): up to 2 weeks
- Frozen (−20°C): up to several years

PROTOCOL
None

INTERPRETATION

NORMAL FINDINGS OR RANGE
- Dogs: 5.7–45.2 μg/L
- Cats: 12–82 μg/L
- Reference intervals may vary depending on the laboratory.

TRYPSIN-LIKE IMMUNOREACTIVITY

ABNORMAL VALUES
Values above or below the reference range

CRITICAL VALUES
None

INTERFERING FACTORS

Drugs That May Alter Results or Interpretation

Drugs That Interfere with Test Methodology
None

Drugs That Alter Physiology
None

Disorders That May Alter Results
Lipemia may affect the test results.

Collection Techniques or Handling That May Alter Results
Results may be affected by storage of sample at high temperatures.

Influence of Signalment

Species
The TLI assay is species specific. Indicate the species when submitting the sample.

Breed
None known

Age
None known

Gender
None known

Pregnancy
None known

LIMITATIONS OF THE TEST
Very rarely, EPI results from obstruction of the pancreatic duct, in which case the serum TLI concentration can be normal because the pancreas is functioning properly.

Sensitivity, Specificity, and Positive and Negative Predictive Values

Canine EPI
- Sensitivity: close to 100%
- Specificity: close to 100%

Feline EPI
- Sensitivity: unknown
- Specificity: 85%–100%

Canine and feline Pancreatitis
Sensitivity: 30%–60%

Valid If Run in a Human Lab?
No.

Causes of Abnormal Findings

High values	Low values
Pancreatitis Severe renal insufficiency may increase serum TLI concentrations because trypsinogen is eliminated through the kidney. This effect is usually minimal.	EPI

CLINICAL PERSPECTIVE
- In dogs, values <2.5 μg/L are diagnostic for EPI.
- In cats, values ≤8.0 μg/L are diagnostic for EPI.
- If the TLI concentration is in an equivocal range (dogs, 2.5–5.7 μg/L; cats, 8.1–12.0 μg/L), retest the patient after 3–4 weeks and perform other diagnostic tests to rule out other differential diagnoses.
- The most common causes of EPI are pancreatic acinar atrophy in German shepherd dogs and chronic pancreatitis in dogs of other breeds and in cats.
- If EPI due to obstruction of the pancreatic duct is suspected, which is associated with a normal serum TLI concentration, a fecal proteolytic activity assay may aid in the diagnosis.
- In dogs, values of >50 μg/L are consistent with pancreatitis; however, serum PLI concentration is more sensitive and specific for pancreatitis.
- In cats, values of >100 μg/L are consistent with pancreatitis; however, serum PLI concentration is more sensitive and specific for pancreatitis.

MISCELLANEOUS

ANCILLARY TESTS
- PLI assay, if the TLI concentration is above the cutoff for pancreatitis
- Evaluation of cobalamin and folate concentrations to assess small intestinal function
- Chemistry profile and urinalysis to rule out renal failure
- Fecal proteolytic activity assay

SYNONYMS
TLI

SEE ALSO
Blackwell's Five-Minute Veterinary Consult: Canine and Feline Topics
- Exocrine Pancreatic Insufficiency
- Pancreatitis
- Protein-Losing Enteropathy
- Small Intestinal Bacterial Overgrowth

Related Topics in This Book
- Cobalamin
- Folate
- Gastrointestinal Ultrasonography
- Pancreatic Lipase Immunoreactivity
- Pancreatic Ultrasonography

ABBREVIATIONS
- EPI = exocrine pancreatic insufficiency
- PLI = pancreatic lipase immunoreactivity
- TLI = trypsin-like immunoreactivity

Suggested Reading

Steiner JM, Williams DA. Serum feline trypsin-like immunoreactivity in cats with exocrine pancreatic insufficiency. *J Vet Intern Med* 2000; 14: 627–629.

Westermarck E, Wiberg M, Steiner JM, Williams DA. Exocrine pancreatic insufficiency in dogs and cats. In: Ettinger SJ, Feldman EC, eds. *Textbook of Veterinary Internal Medicine: Diseases of the Dog and Cat*, 6th ed. St Louis: Saunders Elsevier, 2005: 1492–1495.

Williams DA, Batt RM. Sensitivity and specificity of radioimmunoassay of serum trypsin-like immunoreactivity for the diagnosis of canine exocrine pancreatic insufficiency. *J Am Vet Med Assoc* 1988; 192: 195–201.

INTERNET RESOURCES

Texas A&M University, College of Veterinary Medicine, Gastrointestinal Laboratory, Assays: Serum trypsin-like immunoreactivity (TLI), http://www.cvm.tamu.edu/gilab/assays/TLI.shtml.

AUTHOR NAMES
Nora Berghoff and Jörg M. Steiner

ULTRASOUND-GUIDED MASS OR ORGAN ASPIRATION

BASICS

TYPE OF PROCEDURE
Ultrasonographic

PROCEDURE EXPLANATION AND RELATED PHYSIOLOGY
Percutaneous ultrasound-guided mass or organ aspiration is a technique that is commonly used to obtain material for cytologic examination as an aid in the definitive diagnosis of a disease process. Ultrasonography is typically sensitive but not specific for disease processes, and additional information such as that obtained from cytologic examination of cellular material is often helpful in determining a definitive diagnosis. In addition, because needle placement can be directly visualized in real time, precise placement in an area of interest is possible by using ultrasound guidance. This procedure is commonly used to obtain cellular material from the liver, spleen, and kidneys with diffuse, infiltrative disease, as well as masses anywhere within or on the body. A prerequisite is that the area to be aspirated must be visible during ultrasonography, and an unobstructed path for the needle trajectory must be identified. If there is gas or bone surrounding a lesion, then ultrasound guidance will likely not be possible.

INDICATIONS
Obtain a cellular or fluid sample for cytologic evaluation to further define or diagnose the etiology of an abnormality in an organ or mass.

CONTRAINDICATIONS
• Coagulopathy
• Superimposed structures in the path of the needle trajectory
• Patient noncompliance
• Inability to visualize the lesion definitively with ultrasonography

POTENTIAL COMPLICATIONS
• Sepsis or peritonitis if an abscess or infected lesion is sampled
• Hemorrhage, which is typically self-limiting unless a major vascular structure is damaged during the procedure or a severe coagulopathy is present
• Possible seeding of neoplasia along the needle tract (rare)

CLIENT EDUCATION
Typically, the client should be apprised of the possible complications, but no additional education is usually necessary. If general anesthesia is required (because of patient noncompliance or a difficult-to-reach lesion), then typical preparation instructions should be given (e.g., withhold food).

BODY SYSTEMS ASSESSED
• Cardiovascular
• Dermatologic
• Endocrine and metabolic
• Gastrointestinal
• Hemic, lymphatic, and immune
• Hepatobiliary
• Musculoskeletal
• Renal and urologic
• Reproductive
• Respiratory

PROCEDURE

PATIENT PREPARATION
Preprocedure Medication or Preparation
• Withhold food and water as needed if anesthesia is necessary to accomplish the procedure.
• The skin in the area to be aspirated should be removed of hair (typically using clippers with a no. 40 scalpel blade) and aseptically prepared.
• Alcohol may be used as an ultrasound-coupling agent to prevent any artifact that may occur in the cytologic preparation. (Ultrasound coupling gel can cause an artifact if it contaminates the slides during preparation.)
• To plan a safe needle trajectory, ultrasonography should be performed prior to the procedure.

Anesthesia or Sedation
• Many patients will tolerate this procedure without anesthesia, sedation, or the use of local anesthetics.
• If anesthesia or sedation is necessary, standard regimens may be used that are appropriate for the patient.
• It should be noted that protocols that cause panting or excessive splenic enlargement may make the procedure more difficult. For example, pure opioids may cause excessive panting and make it difficult to guide the needle into deep or small lesions.

Patient Positioning
Patients should be positioned to enable an unobstructed approach and placement of both the needle and the transducer. Typically, patients will be positioned in lateral or ventral recumbency, and they should be manually restrained if anesthesia is not used.

Patient Monitoring
None

Equipment or Supplies
Typically, a 22-gauge needle of appropriate length attached to a syringe (6 or 12 mL) is used. Small needles (23, 25, or 27 gauge) may be used particularly if hemorrhage is felt to be a significant risk. However, nondiagnostic samples may be obtained with these smaller-gauge needles. A more diagnostic sample for evaluation might be obtained by using 14- or 18-gauge needles.

TECHNIQUE
• There are 3 methods used to perform a percutaneous ultrasound-guided mass or organ aspiration. In any case, the shortest trajectory between the skin surface and the lesion should be chosen. Only 1 body cavity should be penetrated at a time. In addition, choice of transducer type can affect the ease of performing the procedure. Sector/vector-type transducers usually have a smaller footprint and thus are easier to manipulate when performing this procedure. A linear transducer may be difficult to use because it has a larger footprint.
   • *Indirect technique*: This technique involves using ultrasonography to identify the lesion to be sampled, and then the transducer is removed and the needle is passed blindly into the structure to be sampled. This technique may be used if the lesion is extremely large, and thus confirmation of needle placement is not necessary.

ULTRASOUND-GUIDED MASS OR ORGAN ASPIRATION

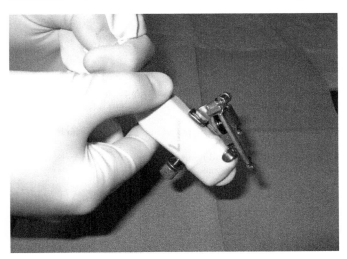

Figure 1

A transducer with a needle guide attachment in place. The guide will maintain the needle in the plane of the ultrasound beam and, combined with the software program on the machine, will enable specific placement of a needle or biopsy instrument in the area of interest.

• *Freehand technique*: The needle is held in 1 hand and the transducer is held in the other. The area of interest should be visualized, and the probe is manipulated such that the lesion is clearly visible. The needle should puncture the skin a few millimeters away from the transducer in order to facilitate needle visualization, as well as to protect against puncturing the transducer. The goal is to pass the needle within the plane (parallel) of the ultrasound beam. Do not pass the needle in a plane perpendicular to the ultrasound plane, because the length will not be visible. The more acute the needle angle is to the ultrasound beam, the more difficult it is to visualize the needle. Therefore, the needle should form at least a 45° angle with the transducer to facilitate its visualization. The needle is passed through the skin and then into the lesion of interest.

• *Guided technique*: The needle is held in place by using an attachable guide, which is coupled to the transducer (Figure 1). The ultrasound machine will have software that will show the projected trajectory of the needle. The area of interest is visualized, and the transducer is manipulated such that the projected path of the needle is superimposed over the area to be sampled. The needle is then passed through the needle guide attached to the transducer and into the patient.

• If using either the freehand or the guided technique, improved needle visualization may be obtained either by moving the needle slightly, by moving the needle in and out of the tissue, or by minimally adjusting the transducer to bring the needle more into the plane of the ultrasound beam.

• Using any of the aforementioned methods, the sample may be obtained either through direct aspiration with active suction applied to the syringe while the needle tip is in the lesion or through a nonaspiration technique whereby the needle is moved up and down in the area of interest several times before the needle is withdrawn from the patient.

• Any organ or mass can be aspirated by using any of these techniques. If a diffuse disease is suspected in the liver, it is usually best to aspirate the left side of the liver to help prevent possible laceration of the gallbladder. In addition, the spleen is typically sampled by using a nonaspiration technique to help prevent hemodilution of the sample. It may be advantageous to obtain at least 1 sample by using an active aspiration technique and 1 sample by using a nonaspiration technique (in organs other than the spleen) to maximize the chance of obtaining a diagnostic sample. Active aspiration may disrupt fragile cells such as seen in lymphoma.

• To practice aspiration or biopsy techniques, a biopsy phantom can be created. A biopsy phantom can enable one to improve the hand-to-eye coordination that is necessary to perform these techniques successfully, particularly the freehand technique, which requires more practice for proficiency (Figure 2).

• The simplest biopsy phantom uses a heavy plastic bag. (An empty IV saline bag works well.) Culinary gelatin is mixed at double the recommend concentration and poured into the bag. After 15–30 min of refrigeration, as the gelatin begins to set, targets are inserted into the middle of the gelatin. (Grapes, cherries, and chickpeas work well.) Care should be taken to not create any air bubbles. The gelatin is allowed to set completely, and then the bag is sealed. The outer surface can then be imaged and a needle passed easily through the bag to the target.

SAMPLE HANDLING
The cytologic sample should be placed onto a microscope slide. Disconnecting the needle from the syringe and filling it with air usually facilitates this. The needle is then reattached, and a rapid expulsion of the air in the syringe will force the cellular sample in the hub of the needle onto a microscope slide.

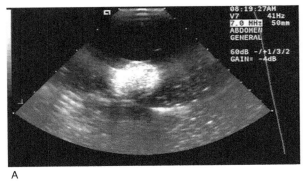

A

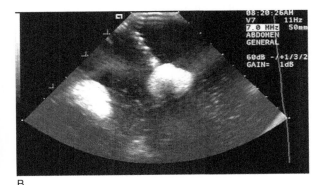

B

Figure 2

A: An ultrasound image of a biopsy phantom with a hyperechoic target lesion. **B:** An ultrasound image of the same biopsy phantom shown in **A**, with a needle placement into the target. Notice the entire length of the needle is visible as a hyperechoic line on the left side of the image, indicating that the needle is within the plane of the ultrasound beam.

ULTRASOUND-GUIDED MASS OR ORGAN ASPIRATION

APPROPRIATE AFTERCARE
Postprocedure Patient Monitoring
The patient should be monitored immediately after the procedure in order to verify that profuse hemorrhage is not occurring. The time line for duration of monitoring is variable depending on the individual patient and its specific problems.

Nursing Care
None

Dietary Modification
None

Medication Requirements
None

Restrictions on Activity
Excessive exercise should be avoided for a minimum of 12–24 h particularly if hemorrhage is likely.

Anticipated Recovery Time
Immediately

INTERPRETATION

NORMAL FINDINGS OR RANGE
N/A

ABNORMAL VALUES
N/A

CRITICAL VALUES
N/A

INTERFERING FACTORS
Drugs That May Alter Results of the Procedure
The use of opioids and other drugs that cause splenomegaly should be avoided because they may compromise the procedure.

Conditions That May Interfere with Performing the Procedure
• A lesion that is surrounded by air or bone and cannot be visualized by using ultrasound
• A patient's noncompliance

Procedure Techniques or Handling That May Alter Results
• Excessive hemodilution or rough handling of the material may result in a nondiagnostic sample.
• If appropriate orientation of the needle with the ultrasound plane is not maintained, then the needle might not be visualized in the ultrasound image and inappropriate sampling may occur.

Influence of Signalment on Performing and Interpreting the Procedure
Species
None

Breed
None

Age
None

Gender
None

Pregnancy
None

CLINICAL PERSPECTIVE
• Percutaneous ultrasound-guided mass or organ aspiration should be used to help further define the etiology of an infiltrative process or mass.
• This is a quick, safe, and easy procedure to perform as an initial diagnostic step.
• Both active aspiration and nonaspiration techniques may be necessary to obtain a diagnostic sample.

MISCELLANEOUS

ANCILLARY TESTS
If the cytologic sample is nondiagnostic, then a needle biopsy sample may be obtained by using the same principles as for obtaining a cytologic sample. Typically, sedation or general anesthesia is required for this procedure.

SYNONYMS
None

SEE ALSO
Blackwell's Five-Minute Veterinary Consult: Canine and Feline Topics
Many

Related Topics in This Book
• General Principles of Ultrasonography
• Fine-Needle Aspiration

ABBREVIATIONS
None

Suggested Reading
Nyland TG, Mattoon JS, Herrgesell EJ, Wisner ER. Ultrasound-guided biopsy. In: Nyland TG, Mattoon JS, eds. *Small Animal Diagnostic Ultrasound*, 2nd ed. Philadelphia: WB Saunders, 2002: 30–48.
Nyland TG, Wallack ST, Wisner ER. Needle-tract implantation following us-guided fine-needle aspiration biopsy of transitional cell carcinoma of the bladder, urethra, and prostate. *Vet Radiol Ultrasound* 2002; **43**: 50–53.
Pennick DG, Finn-Bodner ST. Updates in interventional ultrasonography. *Vet Clin North Am Small Anim Pract* 1998; **28**: 1017–1040.
Samii VF, Nyland TG, Werner LL, Baker TW. Ultrasound-guided fine-needle aspiration biopsy of bone lesions: A preliminary report. *Vet Radiol Ultrasound* 1999; **40**: 82–86.

INTERNET RESOURCES
None

AUTHOR NAME
Anne Bahr

BASICS

TYPE OF PROCEDURE
Radiographic

PROCEDURE EXPLANATION AND RELATED PHYSIOLOGY
An upper gastrointestinal (UGI) study is a radiographic study in which positive or negative contrast media, or both, are used to provide both morphologic and functional evaluation of the stomach and small intestine. The UGI study provides diagnostic information about the stomach and small intestine. A gastrogram or double-contrast gastrogram enables visualization of the stomach. A UGI study provides subjective physiologic information relative to gastric motility, pyloric outflow function, and small-bowel transit and assessment of animals with suspected partial or complete bowel obstruction. Sequential radiographs are obtained enabling visualization of the stomach, small intestine, cecum, and proximal large intestine.

INDICATIONS
- When a clinical diagnosis cannot be made from the combined clinical information derived from abdominal palpation, survey radiography, or ultrasonography
- In the assessment of animals with suspected partial or complete small-bowel obstruction

CONTRAINDICATIONS
If there is observable free peritoneal gas on survey films that is not due to recent celiotomy, a gastric or bowel perforation is likely and surgical intervention is advised rather than radiographic contrast procedures.

POTENTIAL COMPLICATIONS
- The most common complication is the aspiration of barium either during the swallowing process or as a sequel to emesis after the barium is deposited into the stomach. The clinical signs and adverse effects vary, depending on the volume of barium aspirated. With the administration of a large amount of aspirated barium, asphyxia and death may ensue. With the administration of a smaller volume of aspirated barium, either the barium will ultimately be removed by coughing or, if inhaled more deeply, become alveolarized and subsequently be identified in the terminal bronchioles, alveolar airspaces, or both. In animals that have alveolarized barium, radiographs obtained weeks or even years later may show barium in the alveoli or tracheobronchial lymph nodes. This has no known clinical significance.
- Barium may leak into the peritoneal cavity if there is a perforation of the stomach or small intestine. Leaked barium may cause a localized inflammatory reaction.

CLIENT EDUCATION
Clients should be informed about the value of the contrast study and that a definitive diagnosis may or may not be obtained. The potential complication of barium aspiration should also be discussed with the owners.

BODY SYSTEMS ASSESSED
Gastrointestinal

PROCEDURE

PATIENT PREPARATION
Preprocedure Medication or Preparation
If the UGI study is elective, withholding food and water for 12 h is optimum. Survey lateral and VD abdominal radiographs should be obtained just prior to any contrast study of the GI tract.

Anesthesia or Sedation
For single-contrast barium studies, anesthesia should not be used. Sedation can be used only when absolutely necessary to restrain an animal.

UGI Study
- Dogs: Acepromazine [1 mg/20 lb (9.07 kg) body weight IV] can be used, if needed, without causing any adverse effect on GI motility or small-bowel transit.
- Cats: Ketamine can be used [10 mg IV or 10 mg/lb (4.54 kg) body weight IM] with or without diazepam (1–3 mg IV or IM), if needed.

Pneumogastrogram
Sedation or general anesthesia is desired.

Double-Contrast Gastrogram
Sedation or general anesthesia is desired.

Patient Positioning
Recumbent lateral and VD projections are obtained. Opposite lateral and oblique projections may be helpful in assessing certain anatomic regions of the stomach, depending on the radiographic findings seen on the standard views.

Patient Monitoring
The only major potential problem is if an animal aspirates the barium mixture into its trachea or lung. If this is suspected, thoracic radiographs should be obtained. A small amount of barium aspirated is rarely of any clinical consequence. However, if a substantial amount of barium has been aspirated, suction should be used to remove as much barium as possible.

Equipment or Supplies
- Barium is available in concentrations of 30%–85% wt/vol and is prediluted with suspending agents to form a contrast medium that is homogeneous and provides adequate coating of the bowel and reliable transit time through the GI tract. A dilution of 30% wt/vol is advised for standard UGI studies.
- Recommended barium sulfate preparations: liquid barium sulfate [Barosperse (Lafayette Pharmaceuticals, Lafayette, IN), Novapaque (Picker International, Cleveland, OH), or E-Z-Paque (E-Z-EM, Westbury, NY)]

TECHNIQUE
UGI Study
- The preferred method is to instill the barium directly into the distal esophagus or stomach via an orogastric or nasogastric tube. With the animals sedated, with a mouth gag in place, most will tolerate a feeding tube placed within the esophagus. Palpation of the neck should document esophageal placement versus the misplacement of the tube in the trachea. The calculated volume of barium is infused (2.27–3.18 mL/kg body weight), and the tube is withdrawn. Alternatively, the animal can be given the barium by mouth, but this is time consuming and increases the possibility of the animal aspirating the barium, as well as not receiving the complete calculated dose.
- After the barium has been administered, lateral and VD radiographs of the abdomen should be immediately obtained. Additional radiographs are made, depending on the suspected diagnosis and the rapidity of gastric emptying and small-bowel transit as seen on the first radiographs. Radiographs are made periodically until either a diagnosis is made or the large bowel is visualized. Common times to obtain radiographs are 30 min and 1, 2, and 3 h. Oftentimes, in cats, the transit time is more rapid and the study is often completed in 45–60 min.

UPPER GASTROINTESTINAL RADIOGRAPHIC CONTRAST STUDIES

Pneumogastrogram

A pneumogastrogram consists of distending the stomach with room air, most often to outline a nonopaque gastric foreign body, such as a trichobezoar (hair ball), or to assess gastric wall thickness. An orogastric tube is placed, and air is infused to distend the stomach completely (2.27–3.18 mL/kg). Lateral and VD projections are then obtained. Following completion of the study, the gastric air is removed.

Double-Contrast Gastrogram

• A double-contrast gastrogram uses a small volume of positive contrast (barium) and a larger volume of negative contrast (air), enabling visualization of the mucosal folds and gastric wall.

• The use of sedation or general anesthesia is desired. Induction of gastric atony by using glucagon (0.10–0.35 mg IV prior to the procedure) will prevent spontaneous eructation. Glucagon administration is contraindicated in animals with diabetes mellitus.

• After the glucagon is administered, an orogastric tube is placed, and barium is infused into the gastric lumen at a dose of 0.45–0.91 mL/kg (85% wt/vol barium sulfate). Room air is then infused into the stomach at a dose adequate to fill the stomach completely (1.81–2.73 mL/kg). Right and left lateral, VD, and DV projections are then obtained. Additional oblique views may be helpful, depending on the results of the first radiographs and the location of the suspected gastric lesion. After completion of the study, the gastric air is removed.

SAMPLE HANDLING

As the radiographs are developed, they should be evaluated to determine whether additional views are needed (e.g., DV or oblique projections) and when subsequent radiographs should be made.

APPROPRIATE AFTERCARE
Postprocedure Patient Monitoring
None

Nursing Care
None

Dietary Modification
None

Medication Requirements
None

Restrictions on Activity
None

Anticipated Recovery Time
30 min to 1 h

INTERPRETATION

NORMAL FINDINGS OR RANGE

• The radiographic appearance of the stomach varies and depends on multiple factors, including species, body conformation, age, degree of gastric distention, type of gastric contents, and the position of the animal during radiography. Gastric motility can be observed directly with fluoroscopy and ultrasonography; static radiographic images provide a very limited assessment of motility. The rugal folds can usually be seen, but their appearance varies, depending on the degree of stomach distention. The folds appear larger in an empty stomach and flatter, smoother, and smaller in a distended stomach. The rate of pyloric emptying can be determined during a UGI study, but the rate of emptying may be delayed by various drugs, severe illness, and psychological factors (e.g., stress, fear, anxiety).

• During the UGI study, the small bowel from the pylorus to the ileocecal junction can be seen. Variance in diameter of the bowel because of peristalsis is expected. In the duodenum, pseudoulcers are commonly seen in dogs, and the "string of pearls" sign is common in cats due to strong circular muscle contractions. The normal mucosal border is highly variable in appearance but is usually smooth or finely irregular. There should not be any persistent filling defects. The transit time of barium from the stomach to the colon varies, ranging from 30 min to 2 h.

ABNORMAL VALUES

• Extra-gastric factors commonly due to localized or generalized hepatomegaly or splenic, pancreatic, and omental mass lesions, as well as gastric dilation and volvulus, affect the gastric position and shape. Gastric foreign bodies are usually easily identified if radiopaque, but soft tissue dense foreign bodies may require contrast evaluation to be identified. Gastric ulcers and tumors are usually not detectable on survey radiographs unless quite large and may be seen as masses projecting into the gastric lumen.

• Focal or generalized bowel ileus with delayed transit may indicate an obstructive process. Bowel transit can also be delayed in animals that are severely debilitated or by the effects of medication (e.g., anticholinergic drugs, narcotics, some tranquilizers). Mechanical ileus indicates obstruction due to foreign body, internal hernia, intussusception, or tumor, which may be identified as the barium reaches the site of obstruction. With functional ileus due to loss of peristalsis from viral disease (e.g., parvovirus), peritonitis, vascular compromise (e.g., ischemia, volvulus), spinal trauma, or dysautonomia, the bowel loops will be distended, and delayed transit should be expected. In infiltrative diseases, the mucosal appearance will often be altered and can be localized or diffuse. Examples of infiltrative disease include nonulcerative and ulcerative enteritis, inflammatory bowel disease (IBD), and neoplasia.

CRITICAL VALUES

• Obstruction, as evidenced by mechanical ileus, may require immediate surgical intervention.

• Leakage of contrast into the abdominal cavity, although rare, indicates a perforated bowel that requires immediate surgical intervention.

INTERFERING FACTORS
Drugs That May Alter Results of the Procedure
Gastric emptying and motility are delayed if narcotics, anticholinergic drugs, or tranquilizers have been used. Exceptions to this rule are acepromazine in dogs and ketamine combined with low-dose diazepam the cats.

Conditions That May Interfere with Performing the Procedure
Severe debilitation or clinical illness may alter gastric motility and small-bowel transit.

Procedure Techniques or Handling That May Alter Results
If insufficient barium has been administered, there will be incomplete gastric distention and poor visualization of the small intestine. A sufficient number of radiographs should be made so that the entire small intestine is visualized.

Influence of Signalment on Performing and Interpreting the Procedure
Species
None

Breed
None

Age
None

Gender
None

Pregnancy
None

CLINICAL PERSPECTIVE

Abdominal ultrasonography and endoscopy have replaced the need for barium GI studies in most clinical situations.

MISCELLANEOUS

ANCILLARY TESTS

• Barium-impregnated polyethylene spheres (BIPS) have been designed to study gastric and intestinal motility and to aid in confirming partial or complete bowel obstruction. They are inexpensive and easy to use, but provide no mucosal detail, and there is much controversy about their indications, applications, and usefulness.
• Nuclear scintigraphy has been determined to be the gold standard of gastric emptying and small-bowel transit.
• Computed tomography and magnetic resonance imaging are supplemental modalities that provide 3-dimensional view of the anatomy of the abdominal viscera.

SYNONYMS

Upper GI

SEE ALSO

Blackwell's Five-Minute Veterinary Consult: Canine and Feline Topics
• Gastric Motility Disorders
• Gastroesophageal Reflux
• Gastrointestinal Obstruction

Related Topics in This Book
• General Principles of Radiography
• Abdominal Radiography
• Abdominal Ultrasonography

• Barium-Impregnated Polyethylene Spheres (BIPS)
• Computed Tomography
• Esophagogastroduodenoscopy
• Gastrointestinal Ultrasonography
• Lower Gastrointestinal Radiographic Contrast Studies

ABBREVIATIONS

• DV = dorsoventral
• UGI = upper gastrointestinal
• VD = ventrodorsal
• wt/vol = weight/volume

Suggested Reading
Biery DN. The large bowel. In: Thrall DE, ed. *Veterinary Diagnostic Radiology*, 4th ed. Philadelphia: WB Saunders, 2002: 560–570.
Kealy JK, McAllister H. *Diagnostic Radiology and Ultrasonography of the Dog and Cat*, 4th ed. St Louis: Saunders Elsevier, 2005.
Mahaffey MB, Barber DL. The stomach. In: Thrall DE, ed. *Veterinary Diagnostic Radiology*, 4th ed. Philadelphia: WB Saunders, 2002: 615–638.
Owens JM, Biery DN. *Radiographic Interpretation for the Small Animal Clinician*, 2nd ed. Baltimore: Williams & Wilkins, 1999.
Riedesel EA. The small bowel. In: Thrall DE, ed. *Veterinary Diagnostic Radiology*, 4th ed. Philadelphia: WB Saunders, 2002: 639–659.

INTERNET RESOURCES

None

AUTHOR NAME

Jerry M. Owens

UREA NITROGEN

 BASICS

TYPE OF SPECIMEN
Blood

TEST EXPLANATION AND RELATED PHYSIOLOGY
Urea is a nitrogenous waste product used to assess glomerular filtration rate. Its synthesis depends on both liver function and protein balance (ammonia production). It is the principal end product of protein metabolism when ammonia, released during deamination of amino acids, is converted into urea in the liver through the urea cycle. Once formed, urea is carried from the liver via the vascular system and passively diffuses throughout total body water. A small amount of dietary urea is either absorbed directly or metabolized into ammonia by intestinal bacteria and absorbed.

Renal excretion is the most important factor in determining blood urea nitrogen (BUN) levels. Urea is freely filtered through the renal glomerulus, but then 50%–65% of the filtered urea is passively reabsorbed from the renal tubule. Some urea remains in the renal interstitium, contributing to medullary hypertonicity. The remaining urea is returned to the circulation. The amount of urea reabsorption is modulated by urine flow rate; rapid flow allows less reabsorption of urea and vice versa.

BUN can be measured by either wet spectrophotometric or dry-reagent reflectance methods [Vitros (Ortho-Clinical Diagnostics, Raritan, NJ), Reflotron Plus (Roche, Basel, Switzerland), and VetTest (IDEXX Laboratories, Westbrooke, ME)]. A crude estimate of BUN can be determined by placing a drop of fresh whole blood on a dipstick (e.g., Azostix reagent strips; Bayer, Miles Division, IN).

INDICATIONS
- Screen for renal function
- Marker of liver function/insufficiency

CONTRAINDICATIONS
None

POTENTIAL COMPLICATIONS
None

CLIENT EDUCATION
None

BODY SYSTEMS ASSESSED
- Hepatobiliary
- Renal and urologic

 SAMPLE

COLLECTION
0.5–2.0 mL of venous blood

HANDLING
- Use a plain red-top tube or serum-separator tube.
- The use of EDTA, sodium heparin, or lithium heparin anticoagulant is acceptable.

STORAGE
Refrigerate or freeze the separated serum or plasma for long-term storage.

STABILITY
- Room temperature: 1 day
- Refrigerated (2°–8°C): 1 week

PROTOCOL
None

 INTERPRETATION

NORMAL FINDINGS OR RANGE
- Dogs: 8–29 mg/dL (2.9–10.4 mmol/L)
- Cats: 15–33 mg/dL (5.3–11.8 mmol/L)
- Reference intervals may vary depending on the laboratory and assay.

ABNORMAL VALUES
Values above or below the reference interval

CRITICAL VALUES
None

INTERFERING FACTORS
Drugs That May Alter Results or Interpretation
Drugs That Interfere with Test Methodology
None

Drugs That Alter Physiology
- Increased (mildly) by drugs that increase protein catabolism (e.g., tetracycline)
- Decreased by drugs that decrease protein catabolism (e.g., anabolic steroids)
- Decreased by drugs that promote polyuria-polydipsia (e.g., glucocorticoids)
- Increased by nephrotoxic drugs, including amphotericin B, aminoglycoside antibiotics (e.g., amikacin, gentamicin, kanamycin, tobramycin), and high NSAID doses (e.g., aspirin, carprofen, phenylbutazone, ketoprofen)

Disorders That May Alter Results
Hemolysis can increase BUN results obtained by reflectance spectrophotometry through interference with light transmission.

Collection Techniques or Handling That May Alter Results
Contamination of the sample with quaternary ammonium disinfectants (e.g., benzalkonium chloride) can increase BUN results obtained by reflectance spectrophotometry.

Influence of Signalment
Species
None

Breed
None

Age
- Neonatal puppies ≤1 month of age have slightly increased urea levels; embryonic kidney development is not complete until at least week 3 of life.
- Puppies that are 2–3 months old have slightly decreased urea levels because of rapid growth and increased anabolic state.

Gender
None

Pregnancy
None

LIMITATIONS OF THE TEST
- The glomerular filtration rate must be reduced to ≤25% of normal before BUN levels rise above normal.
- Overhydration or dehydration can affect levels by altering tubular reabsorption.

Sensitivity, Specificity, and Positive and Negative Predictive Values
Ability of Azostix to identify abnormal BUN concentrations:
- Sensitivity: 86.4%
- Specificity: 90.3%
- Negative predictive value: 96.5%

• Positive predictive value: 65.5%. Test strips tend to underestimate BUN levels, missing a significant number of patients with elevated BUN.

Valid If Run in a Human Lab?
Yes.

Causes of Abnormal Findings

High values	Low values
Prerenal	Hepatic insufficiency
Dehydration, hypovolemia, or shock	Nonrenal causes of
Blood loss	polyuria-polydipsia
Burns	Significant protein loss into
Decreased cardiac output	urine or GI tract
Sepsis	Ascites
Renal	Low-protein diet or starvation
Causes of chronic renal failure	Overhydration
Acute tubular necrosis due to	
ischemia, nephrotoxins, severe	
intravascular hemolysis, or	
myoglobinuria	
Glomerulonephritis	
Pyelonephritis (e.g., leptospirosis)	
Postrenal	
Urinary tract obstruction	
Urinary tract rupture	
GI hemorrhage	
High-protein diet	
Increased protein catabolism due to	
fever or marked tissue necrosis	

CLINICAL PERSPECTIVE

• If urine is hypersthenuric [SG, >1.030 (dogs) or >1.035 (cats)], consider prerenal azotemia (decreased renal perfusion) or nonrenal factors.
• If urine in an azotemic animal is isosthenuric (SG, 1.008–1.012) or minimally concentrated (SG, 1.012–1.030), consider primary renal disease.
• BUN may be less accurate than creatinine as an indicator of renal disease.
• After a urinary tract rupture, BUN levels increase before serum creatinine.
• Abdominal fluid BUN that is ≥2-fold the simultaneous blood level is confirmatory for uroabdomen.

MISCELLANEOUS

ANCILLARY TESTS

• Urinalysis
• Ultrasonography to identify abdominal fluid in an animal with a ruptured bladder
• Fecal occult blood test
• Evaluation of serum or urine bile acid levels to assess liver function

SYNONYMS

Serum urea nitrogen (SUN)

SEE ALSO

Blackwell's Five-Minute Veterinary Consult: Canine and Feline Topics
• Cirrhosis and Fibrosis of the Liver
• Renal Failure, Acute Uremia
• Renal Failure, Chronic

Related Topics in This Book
• Bile Acids
• Creatinine
• Urinalysis

ABBREVIATIONS

• BUN = blood urea nitrogen
• SG = specific gravity

Suggested Reading
Hill D, Correa MT, Stevens JB. Sensitivity, specificity, and predictive values of reagent test strip estimations of blood urea nitrogen. *Vet Clin Pathol* 1994; 23:73–75.
Fettman MJ, Rebar A. Laboratory evaluation of renal function. In: Thrall MA, ed. *Veterinary Hematology and Clinical Chemistry*. Philadelphia: Lippincott Williams & Wilkins, 2004: 301–328.

INTERNET RESOURCES

University of Georgia, College of Veterinary Medicine, Veterinary Clinical Pathology Clerkship Program: McKee JA, Latimer KS, LeRoy BE. Blood urea nitrogen (BUN) concentration in dogs. 2004, http://www.vet.uga.edu/vpp/clerk/mckee/.

AUTHOR NAME

Joyce S. Knoll

BASICS

TYPE OF PROCEDURE
Diagnostic sample collection

PROCEDURE EXPLANATION AND RELATED PHYSIOLOGY
• Urinalysis is part of the minimum database for evaluation of ill dogs and cats and for routine health screening of all patients. Sterile sample collection is also required for culture and sensitivity testing of urine when infectious cystitis is suspected. In those cases where cystocentesis is contraindicated or unsuccessful at obtaining urine, urethral catheterization enables sterile urine samples to be collected with minimal risk to patients.
• Patients in need of exact calculation of urine output (e.g., those with anuric or oliguric renal failure), patients with functional or mechanical urethral obstruction, and many recumbent animals often require intermittent or indwelling urinary catheterization as part of their management plan.
• Urethral catheterization is required in order to perform other diagnostic procedures such as prostatic wash and voiding or catheter-assisted hydropropulsion of uroliths.

INDICATIONS
• Sterile urine collection when cystocentesis is contraindicated
• Temporary relief of urethral obstructions
• Collection of urine for fluid-output determination or metabolic testing (e.g., water-deprivation test; 24-h collection of urine for calculation of electrolyte excretion)
• Management of recumbent patients

CONTRAINDICATIONS
Severe vaginitis or balanophthitis

POTENTIAL COMPLICATIONS
• Iatrogenic bacterial or fungal cystitis
• Urethral trauma (perforations or tears)

CLIENT EDUCATION
None

BODY SYSTEMS ASSESSED
Renal and urologic

 PROCEDURE

PATIENT PREPARATION
Preprocedure Medication or Preparation
None

Anesthesia or Sedation
• Male dogs require minimal to no sedation.
• Female dogs and both male and female cats usually require heavy sedation or anesthesia.

Patient Positioning
• Male dogs: lateral recumbency
• Male cats: dorsal recumbency
• Female dogs and cats: sternal recumbency with their legs tucked underneath or extended over the edge of a table

Patient Monitoring
None

Equipment or Supplies
• Hair clippers
• Diluted povidone-iodine (Betadine) solution: 1 part povidone-iodine solution to ≈200 parts sterile saline (the color should be that of "dilute tea")
• A sterile 12-mL syringe
• Sterile gloves
• Sterile lubricating jelly
• Two sets of 4 × 4-inch gauze sponges soaked in sterile saline and chlorhexidine or povidone-iodine solution
    • Povidone-iodine scrub should not be used on the genital mucous membranes.
• A sterile urinary catheter (Foley catheter, red rubber catheter, or tomcat catheter of appropriate size)
• In female dogs, if the visualization method is being used (preferred):
    • A vaginal speculum
    • A light source
• If the urinary catheter will be indwelling:
    • A closed collection system
    • Materials for anchoring the catheter to the patient (e.g., bandage tape, suture material)

TECHNIQUE
Male Dogs
• For indwelling catheters, clip the hair on the distal one-third of the prepuce. Clipping the hair on the ventral abdomen around the preputial opening to a distance of 2–5 cm may also reduce the risk of iatrogenic infection.
• Flush the prepuce 3–5 times with 2–12 mL of dilute povidone-iodine solution (the volume depends on the size of dog) by using the sterile syringe.
• An assistant should exteriorize the penis. This is best done with the assistant standing at the dog's back (while the animal is in lateral recumbency), and the individual placing the catheter standing at the dog's ventrum.
• Clean the extruded penis with sterile 4 × 4-inch gauze sponges, alternating between chlorhexidine or povidone-iodine solution and sterile saline. A minimum of 3 scrubs should be performed with each solution.

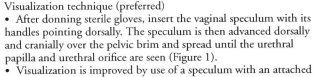
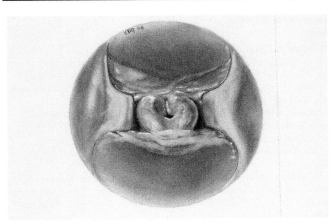

Figure 1

The vaginal vault of a female dog, as viewed during urethral catheterization. The urethral papilla with central orifice is located on the ventral midline.

- Flush the penis with 2–5 mL of dilute povidone-iodine solution.
- After donning sterile gloves, coat the distal catheter with the lubricating jelly. Using sterile technique, insert the urinary catheter. The catheter should be gently advanced until urine is seen in the distal end of the catheter. Some resistance may be encountered when the catheter passes around the ischial arch, but gentle pressure is usually sufficient to overcome this. Care should be taken not to advance the catheter too far into the bladder because in rare cases the catheter may knot inside the bladder, making removal difficult.
- Red rubber catheters can be used for indwelling or intermittent catheters in male dogs, but Foley catheters are preferred for indwelling catheters. Newer catheters (i.e., MilaCath; MILA International, Erlanger, KY) are made with nonlatex materials that may extend catheter life and are more pliable than red rubber.
    - If a Foley catheter is used, inflate the bulb with sterile saline after the catheter has been advanced to the bladder. Immediately connect a sterile, closed collection system to the indwelling catheter. Anchor the indwelling catheter as needed to prevent displacement. The most common method is to place bandage tape around the catheter ≈2–4 cm cranial to the preputial opening, with tabs on either side. Sutures are then passed through the tabs and attached to the body wall.

Female Dogs
- Clip the hair around the vulva, including the perineal area, to a distance of 2–5 cm from the vulva.
- Scrub the vulva and perivulvar area with sterile 4 × 4-inch gauze sponges, alternating between chlorhexidine or povidone-iodine solution and sterile saline. A minimum of 3 scrubs should be performed with each solution.

- Flush the vaginal vault 3–5 times with 2–12 mL of dilute povidone-iodine solution (the volume depends on the size of dog) by using the sterile syringe.
- Visualization technique (preferred)
    - After donning sterile gloves, insert the vaginal speculum with its handles pointing dorsally. The speculum is then advanced dorsally and cranially over the pelvic brim and spread until the urethral papilla and urethral orifice are seen (Figure 1).
    - Visualization is improved by use of a speculum with an attached light source or a headlamp or by an assistant who stands behind the individual placing the catheter and illuminates the vaginal vault with the light source.
    - The urethral papilla is on the ventral midline of the vaginal floor, distal to the cervix (Figure 1).
    - Coat the distal catheter with the lubricating jelly and then, using sterile technique, place the urinary catheter. Foley catheters are preferred for indwelling catheters. Red rubber catheters, though they can be used in female dogs, are easier to dislodge than in male dogs because a significantly shorter length of the catheter is inserted. Inflate the balloon if a Foley catheter is used.
- Digital palpation technique
    - After donning sterile gloves, insert the index finger of the nondominant hand into the vaginal vault, advancing cranially and dorsally over the pelvic brim until the urethral papilla is palpated at the fingertip.
    - Coat the distal catheter with the lubricating jelly and then, using sterile technique, place the urinary catheter. The catheter should be advanced along the ventral aspect of the inserted index finger and then guided into the urethral orifice by palpation.
- Anchor the urinary catheter to prevent displacement. Bandage tape can be used as described previously for male dogs, suturing the catheter to the body wall ventral to the vulva.

Male Cats
- Clip the hair around the prepuce, including the perineal area, to a distance of 1–2 cm from the preputial opening.
- An assistant should exteriorize the penis, which is best done with the assistant standing at the cat's head or side (while the animal is in dorsal recumbency).
    - Proper exteriorizing of the penis is critical for successful passage of urinary catheters in male cats. Gentle pressure at the base of the prepuce will cause the penis to extrude.
    - The penis should be completely exteriorized and pointed caudally, parallel to the spine. Attempting to pass the urinary catheter when the penis is not at the correct angle increases the risk of significant urethral trauma and will prevent the catheter from passing.
- Clean the extruded penis with sterile 4 × 4-inch gauze sponges, alternating between chlorhexidine or povidone-iodine solution and sterile saline. A minimum of 3 scrubs should be performed with each solution.
- After donning sterile gloves, coat the distal catheter with the lubricating jelly. Using sterile technique, place the urinary catheter. The

catheter should be gently advanced until urine is seen in the distal end of the catheter, taking care not to advance the catheter too far into the bladder.

- Tomcat catheters (close ended) can be used for intermittent catheterization; open-ended catheters are the preferred catheter for relieving urethral obstruction in male cats. Red rubber catheters or Foley catheters should be used for indwelling urinary catheters.
- Immediately connect a sterile, closed collection system for indwelling catheters.
- Anchor the catheter as needed to prevent displacement. The most common method for red rubber catheters is to tape the catheter to the cat's tail ≈2–4 cm caudal to the anus.

Female Cats
- Clip the hair around the vulva, including the perineal area, to a distance of 1–2 cm from the vulva.
- Scrub the vulva and perivulvar area with sterile 4 × 4-inch gauze sponges, alternating between chlorhexidine or povidone-iodine solution and sterile saline. A minimum of 3 scrubs should be performed with each solution.
- Flush the vaginal vault 3–5 times with 0.5–2.0 mL of dilute povidone-iodine solution (the volume depends on the size of cat) by using the sterile syringe.
- After donning sterile gloves, coat the distal catheter with the lubricating jelly. Using sterile technique, place the urinary catheter. The catheter should be gently advanced until urine is seen in the distal end of the catheter.
  - Urethral catheterization of female cats is performed blindly.
  - With the cat in sternal recumbency and its legs extended (which is most easily done with the legs allowed to dangle from the edge of a table), the catheter is inserted into the vulva and advanced slowly. The catheter usually enters the bladder without difficulty.
  - Tomcat catheters (open ended or close ended) can be used for intermittent catheterization. Red rubber catheters should be used for indwelling urinary catheters.
- Anchor the catheter as needed to prevent displacement. The most common method is to tape the catheter to the cat's tail ≈2–4 cm caudal to the anus.

SAMPLE HANDLING
- Samples collected for urinalysis should be analyzed immediately if possible; refrigeration for later analysis can alter some dipstick and sediment findings.
- Urine samples collected for culture should be refrigerated, ideally in a culture transport vial, until plated onto appropriate media.

APPROPRIATE AFTERCARE
Postprocedure Patient Monitoring
None
Nursing Care
Indwelling urinary catheters should be kept clean. The external portion of the catheter should be cleaned every 24 h with 4 × 4-inch gauze soaked in chlorhexidine or povidone-iodine solution and sterile saline.

Dietary Modification
None
Medication Requirements
- Prophylactic antibiotics for the prevention of urinary tract infection should not be administered to patients with indwelling urinary catheters. This practice increases the risk of hospital-acquired resistant infections and has not been shown to prevent infection.
- Animals with indwelling urinary catheters should have urine cultured at the time of catheter removal. Bacterial colonization of indwelling urinary catheters is possible, and therefore urine culture results drawn from indwelling catheters should be interpreted with caution.
- To treat any iatrogenically introduced bacteria, some clinicians advocate 3–5 days of antibiotic therapy with a first-line, broad-spectrum antibiotic (e.g., amoxicillin) after a single or intermittent catheterization.

Restrictions on Activity
Elizabethan collars should be placed on nonrecumbent patients with indwelling catheters.

Anticipated Recovery Time
Immediate

INTERPRETATION
NORMAL FINDINGS OR RANGE
N/A

ABNORMAL VALUES
N/A

CRITICAL VALUES
Urethral obstruction that cannot be relieved by urethral catheterization requires decompression by cystocentesis, followed by surgical intervention.

INTERFERING FACTORS
Drugs That May Alter Results of the Procedure
Drugs that increase urethral tone (e.g., phenylpropanolamine, diethylstilbestrol) may theoretically make catheterization more difficult. However, this is likely not clinically significant.

Conditions That May Interfere with Performing the Procedure
- Urethral obstruction by masses, inflammation, urethrospasm, uretholiths, matrix and mucous plugs, or extramural masses
- Pelvic trauma

Procedure Techniques or Handling That May Alter Results
Loss of sterility or contamination of the catheter during placement predisposes patients to development of iatrogenic urinary tract infection.

Influence of Signalment on Performing and Interpreting the Procedure
Species
See the Technique section.

Breed
None

Age
Placement of urinary catheters in neonatal or pediatric patients can be very difficult. Red rubber catheters are ideal because they are less likely to cause iatrogenic trauma during placement.

Gender
See the Technique section.

Pregnancy
None

CLINICAL PERSPECTIVE

• Urethral catheterization is underused as a method for obtaining sterile urine samples, particularly in those patients where repeated cystocentesis attempts are unsuccessful at obtaining a urine sample.
• If urine is being collected for culture, the first 3–10 mL of urine drawn from the catheter should be discarded, after which the sample for culture is collected. This is recommended because the distal urethra and vaginal vault are not sterile environments and often cause some contamination of the catheter tip during placement and because indwelling catheters may have bacterial colonization of the catheter lumen.

 MISCELLANEOUS

ANCILLARY TESTS
• Prostatic wash
• Urinalysis
• Urine culture

SYNONYMS
• Bladder catheterization
• Indwelling urinary catheter
• Urinary catheterization

SEE ALSO
Blackwell's Five-Minute Veterinary Consult: Canine and Feline Topics
• Renal Failure—Acute Uremia
• Urinary Tract Obstruction

Related Topics in This Book
• Bacterial Culture and Sensitivity
• Catheter-Assisted Stone Retrieval
• Prostatic Wash
• Urinalysis Overview
• Voiding Urohydropropulsion

ABBREVIATIONS
None

Suggested Reading
Smarick SD, Haskins SC, Aldrich J, *et al.* Incidence of catheter-associated urinary tract infection among dogs in a small animal intensive care unit. *J Am Vet Med Assoc* 2004; 224: 1936–1940.

INTERNET RESOURCES
None

AUTHOR NAME
Barrak M. Pressler

BASICS

TYPE OF SPECIMEN
Urine

TEST EXPLANATION AND RELATED PHYSIOLOGY
A urinalysis (UA) is a basic diagnostic screening test that is easy to perform, relatively inexpensive, and can be useful in evaluating renal/urologic and nonrenal conditions. A complete UA includes the following components:
• Physical characteristics: volume, color, transparency, odor, and solute concentration [e.g., urine specific gravity (USG)]
• Chemical characteristics: presence of bilirubin, blood, glucose, ketones, pH, and protein. Some tests available on dipsticks (e.g., urobilinogen, nitrite, leukocytes, esterase, USG) may be unreliable, of no value, or not validated for veterinary species.
• Microscopic evaluation of urine sediment: cells, crystals, casts, organisms, and other (e.g., sperm, lipid, mucus)
• Specifics about these components are discussed separately in the following chapters:
    • Urine Bilirubin
    • Urine Glucose
    • Urine Heme Protein
    • Urine Ketones
    • Urine pH
    • Urine Protein
    • Urine Sediment
    • Urine Specific Gravity

INDICATIONS
• Assessment of kidney function: concentrating ability of solutes (e.g., USG); filtering and resorptive handling of electrolytes, protein, glucose; and response to acid-base imbalance
• Detection of hemorrhage, inflammation, infection, or neoplasia in the urinary or genital tract
• Evaluation of systemic disorders or diseases

CONTRAINDICATIONS
None

POTENTIAL COMPLICATIONS
None

CLIENT EDUCATION
If an owner collects urine, it should be put into a clean container free of any type of contaminant.

BODY SYSTEMS ASSESSED
• Endocrine and metabolic
• Hemic, lymphatic, and immune
• Hepatobiliary
• Musculoskeletal
• Renal and urologic
• Reproductive

SAMPLE

COLLECTION
5–10 mL of urine collected by free catch of a voided sample, manual expression of the urinary bladder, catheterization, or cystocentesis

HANDLING
• Collect urine into a clean, dry container with a tight-fitting lid and free of potential contaminants (e.g., detergents, disinfectants). It should be labeled with appropriate information (e.g., patient and owner identification; date, time, and method of collection).
• Results are most accurate if urine is analyzed within 1–2 h after collection.
• The sample should be refrigerated if a delay in analysis is unavoidable.
• Refrigerated samples should be warmed to room temperature before analysis.

STORAGE
• Refrigeration can slow sample deterioration. The container should protect the sample from light and have a tight-fitting lid.
• Refrigeration may alter some results (e.g., increased crystal formation).
• Avoid freezing the urine because this will affect certain tests (e.g., urine sediment examination).
• Preservatives generally adversely affect chemical assays. No single preservative suits all testing requirements.

STABILITY
See specific chapters for information on individual components.

PROTOCOL
• Mix the sample and transfer it to a centrifuge tube.
• Evaluate the physical features of the urine (i.e., color, turbidity).
• Determine the USG by using a refractometer.
• Measure urine analytes by using a reagent strip.
    • Immerse a reagent strip into well-mixed, room-temperature urine and turn the strip on its side, tapping away excess urine.
    • Examine the color change of each analyte at the time indicated by the manufacturer and compare the color change to the reference chart.
    • Confirmatory tests are affected less by urine color and may be warranted to confirm specific dipstick analyte results. Such tests include the Ictotest (Bayer, Leverkusen, Germany) for bilirubin, the Acetest (Bayer, Leverkusen, Germany) for ketones, and sulfosalicylic acid test (SSA) for protein.
• Centrifuge the sample for 5–10 min at low RPM in a conical tube.
    • Ideally, the same volume of urine should be centrifuged each time, and reference values are based on 5 mL of urine. Analysis of smaller urine volume should be noted on the final report because that can result in less sediment.

• The recommended RPM is quite variable (500–3,000 RPM) because it is actually gravitation force (g-force) that is important. A g-force of ≈450 is recommended.

• The g-force generated depends on the length of the centrifuge arms (radius of rotation), determined by measuring the radius of the centrifuge arm from center to outermost portion (bottom) of a test-tube cup (in the horizontal position if the cup swings). See the Internet Resources section for a calculator that can be used to figure out the g-forces generated by your centrifuge at various RPM.

• Excessively high-speed centrifugation can distort cells or fragment fragile elements such as casts.

• Use urine supernatant to measure protein by the SSA method. If urine is bloody or extremely cloudy, double check the USG by using supernatant.

• Decant the supernatant, leaving ≈0.25 mL of urine sediment.

• Resuspend the sediment and transfer a drop to a microscope slide.

• Coverslip and examine the sample microscopically at 10× and 40×.

INTERPRETATION

NORMAL FINDINGS OR RANGE

• Fresh urine should be relatively clear, yellow, and have a slight odor. Intact male cats may have a strong urine odor.

• The USG should be evaluated based on the hydration status. In general, the urine concentration from a random urine sample is considered adequate if the USG is >1.030 and >1.035 in dogs and cats, respectively.

• Normal urine should have a pH between 6.0 and 7.5, and should be negative for protein, ketones, blood, bilirubin, and glucose. Some dogs with highly concentrated urine may show a trace to 1+ reaction for bilirubin and/or protein.

• Urine sediment should contain few cells and crystals and no casts. Lipid is seen occasionally in cat urine.

• See specific chapters for additional information on individual components of the UA.

INTERFERING FACTORS

Collection Techniques or Handling That May Alter Results

In general, strips should be stored at room temperature in the original container; protected from excessive light, moisture, and heat; not used past the expiration date; and discarded if any of the pads on the strips are discolored.

LIMITATIONS OF THE TEST

Valid If Run in a Human Lab?

Yes.

MISCELLANEOUS

SYNONYMS

None

ABBREVIATIONS

• SSA = sulfosalicylic acid
• UA = urinalysis
• USG = urine specific gravity

Suggested Reading

Chew DJ, DiBartola SP. Urinalysis interpretation. In: *Interpretation of Canine and Feline Urinalysis.* Wilmington, DE: Ralston Purina, 1998: 15–33.

Osborne CA, Stevens JB. Proteinuria. In: *Urinalysis: A Clinical Guide to Compassionate Patient Care.* Leverkusen, Germany: Bayer, 1999: 111–121.

INTERNET RESOURCES

Cornell University, College of Veterinary Medicine, Clinical Pathology Modules: Routine urinalysis, http://diaglab.vet.cornell.edu/clinpath/modules/ua-rout/ua-rout.htm.

Cornell University, College of Veterinary Medicine, Clinical Pathology Modules, Urine Sediment Atlas, http://diaglab.vet.cornell.edu/clinpath/modules/ua-sed/ua-intro.htm.

Kobuta, Laboratory Centrifuge: g-force calculation, http://www.centrifuge.jp/calculation/.

AUTHOR NAME

Karen E. Russell

URINE ALBUMIN

BASICS

TYPE OF SPECIMEN
Urine

TEST EXPLANATION AND RELATED PHYSIOLOGY
Microalbuminuria (MA) is a proven early predictor of nephropathy in people, particularly those with diabetes mellitus and essential hypertension. Likewise, MA has been shown to be an early indicator of disease in several models of progressive renal disease in dogs, with increasing magnitudes of urine albumin (UAlb) correlating with advanced disease. Similar models have not been available to study in cats. Albuminuria would be expected to increase whenever there is glomerular injury (from altered glomerular permeability, glomerular capillary hypertension, or both) that leads to albumin concentrations in the filtrate that are in excess of the tubular reabsorptive capacity. Glomerular injury can result from a variety of infectious, inflammatory, or neoplastic causes. Likewise, if there has been tubular injury and renal tubular cells can no longer resorb proteins, albuminuria will be present.

In addition to pathologic renal diseases, albuminuria can be caused by physiologic-renal or postrenal causes. Functional proteinuria is a poorly documented and unlikely physiologic cause of albuminuria in dogs and cats. Urinary tract inflammation and hemorrhage are postrenal causes of UAlb. Inflammation has a variable effect on UAlb concentrations. Hemorrhage does not increase the UAlb concentrations into the abnormal range until there is macroscopic hematuria or RBCs are too numerous to count (TNTC) via standard urinalysis.

The prevalence of MA in dogs and cats in the general population is ≈25%; however, this increases with advancing age. Of dogs and cats >12 years old, 50% or more have abnormally high UAlb concentrations. This age-associated increase in prevalence is most likely related to increases in the prevalence of kidneys diseases in older dogs and cats, as well as an increase in the prevalence of inflammatory, infectious, and metabolic conditions that are associated with glomerular injury.

By definition, *microalbuminuria* is the concentration of albumin in the urine that is greater than normal but below the limit of detection when conventional urine dipstick methodology is used. Therefore, the upper end of UAlb concentrations that are considered to be MA is typically 30 mg/dL (300 μg/mL). UAlb concentrations above this limit are often referred to as *overt albuminuria*. Proteinuria of this magnitude can often be detected by using the protein/creatinine ratio. The lower end of the MA range has been less easily defined because of the requirements that this concentration is greater than normal and reliably detectable but is generally considered to be >1 mg/dL. Thus, MA is the lowest detectable magnitude of abnormal urine protein.

Currently, the 2 commercially available methods for measuring UAlb are an *immunoturbidimetric test* (IT) and a *point-of-care immunoassay* (POC). The assays use the same species-specific antibody against either canine or feline albumin. The IT is quantitative, and the POC is semiquantitative. For the IT, samples must be sent to a reference laboratory, and results are not available immediately. The POC can be performed in house, and the results are available rapidly.

UAlb concentrations can be adjusted for differences in urine concentration by dividing by urine creatinine concentrations or dividing by (specific gravity − 1) × 100. Although UAlb excretion by dogs has been expressed as UAlb/creatinine ratio, the use of this ratio in dogs and cats has not been fully evaluated. Alternatively, urine can be diluted to a standard concentration (e.g., 1.010) prior to assay, which is the method being employed by the assays for UAlb in dogs and cats. This method of standardization appears to yield similar results to the UAlb/creatinine ratio in dogs.

INDICATIONS
- To assist in detection of early renal disease or occult systemic disease in middle-aged to older animals
- To screen dogs or cats of a breed known to have familial renal diseases, particularly those involving glomeruli. In such breeds, screening should generally start at an early age.
- To screen dogs or cats with systemic diseases that increase their risk of glomerular injury
- To monitor the progression of disease or response to treatment in animals with previously detected MA

CONTRAINDICATIONS
- Urinary tract infections can cause MA or overt albuminuria. As such, evaluation of UAlb concentrations is most meaningful in animals that are free of urinary tract infection.
- Macroscopic hematuria or RBCs that are too numerous to count via standard urinalysis

POTENTIAL COMPLICATIONS
None

CLIENT EDUCATION
This is a very sensitive test for urine protein. A positive result does not mean that the animal being tested has renal disease, particularly if it is a low positive. However, some animals with low positive test results will progress to a higher magnitude of albuminuria over time. There is greater concern that animals with increasing magnitudes of albuminuria or those with high or very high positive test results are experiencing ongoing glomerular injury. A complete systemic evaluation for those diseases known to be associated with glomerular injury and albuminuria is indicated in these animals. Repeat testing is indicated in any dog or cat that has a positive test result for UAlb.

BODY SYSTEMS ASSESSED
Renal and urologic

SAMPLE

COLLECTION
2 mL of urine collected by any method

HANDLING
- Quantitative IT: Samples can be sent on an ice pack to the laboratory but may be stable at room temperature, provided the sample does not have a large bacterial burden.
- POC: Use a fresh urine sample.

STORAGE
- Samples may be refrigerated (2°–7°C) for up to 24 h.
- Canine urine samples may be frozen (−20°C or lower) in vials with airtight seals. Feline urine samples should not be frozen.
- Warm the samples to room temperature before assaying.

STABILITY
- The stability of samples at room temperature has not been tested thoroughly. In theory, bacterial overgrowth, in samples left at room temperature or with prolonged refrigeration, could decrease UAlb.
- Refrigerated (2°–7°C): up to 24 h
- Frozen (−20°C): Canine UAlb is stable through multiple freeze-thaw cycles for up to 1 year. In ≈10% of feline samples, freeze-thawing will reduce UAlb. Because it is impossible to determine which samples will be affected, freezing of feline urine samples for UAlb determination is not recommended.

PROTOCOL
POC: Follow the manufacturer's guidelines.

INTERPRETATION

NORMAL FINDINGS OR RANGE
- POC: <1 mg/dL
- Quantitative IT: <2.5 mg/dL

ABNORMAL VALUES
- MA: POC, 1–30 mg/dL; quantitative IT, 2.5–30.0 mg/dL
- Overt albuminuria: >30 mg/dL

CRITICAL VALUES
None

INTERFERING FACTORS
Drugs That May Alter Results or Interpretation
Drugs That Interfere with Test Methodology
None known

Drugs That Alter Physiology
Administration of corticosteroids my increase the transglomerular movement of proteins, thereby transiently increasing the UAlb concentration in animals that previously had either normal UAlb or MA.

Disorders That May Alter Results
None known

Collection Techniques or Handling That May Alter Results
The UAlb results will be unreliable in the rare situation where the urine sample has macroscopic blood because of contamination during cystocentesis.

Influence of Signalment
Species
Assays are species specific.

Breed
Breeds known to have familial renal diseases, particularly those involving the glomeruli, may have a higher incidence of MA:
- Hereditary glomerulopathy: Bernese mountain dogs, bull terriers, Dalmatians, Doberman pinschers, English cocker spaniels, Newfoundlands, rottweilers, and soft-coated Wheaten terriers
- Familial amyloidosis: sharpeis, Abyssinians, beagles, and English foxhounds

Age
The prevalence of MA in dogs and cats increases with advancing age.

Gender
None

Pregnancy
None

LIMITATIONS OF THE TEST
Sensitivity, Specificity, and Positive and Negative Predictive Values
- The quantitative IT test is highly specific: The assay does not react with other proteins or albumins from other species.
- POC as compared to the quantitative IT in dogs and cats:
  - Specificity: >99%, with no false-positive results reported
  - Sensitivity: >95%

Valid If Run in a Human Lab?
No.

Causes of Abnormal Findings

High values	Low values
Renal	Not applicable
Physiologic	
Functional proteinuria (poorly documented)	
Glomerular injury	
Glomerular capillary hypertension	
Altered glomerular permeability	
Infectious diseases	
Inflammatory diseases	
Neoplastic diseases	
Diabetes mellitus	
Glucocorticoid excess	
Hyperadrenocorticism	
Exogenous glucocorticoid administration	
Hypertension	
Hyperthyroidism	
Tubulointerstitial renal disease	
Postrenal	
Urinary tract inflammation	
Urinary tract hemorrhage (macroscopic, or TNTC RBC/high-power field)	

CLINICAL PERSPECTIVE
- Standard urine dipsticks have relatively poor sensitivity and specificity. Thus, the POC for UAlb is a more accurate, reliable test for urine protein than is the standard urine dipstick.
- MA is the lowest detectable form of proteinuria. Proteinuria is a risk factor for renal morbidity, renal mortality, and all-cause mortality in dogs and cats.
- Proteinuric renal diseases are common in dogs. Dogs with a higher magnitude of proteinuria have a greater risk of development of a uremic crisis and death than do dogs with a lower magnitude. Furthermore, reduction of proteinuria, generally via administration of an angiotensin-converting enzyme (ACE) inhibitor, is believed to be renoprotective and therefore has the potential to slow the progression of renal disease.
- Cats with chronic renal failure and even mild proteinuria appear to have more slowly progressive disease when proteinuria is reduced via administration of an ACE inhibitor.
- Tests for UAlb can be used to detect proteinuria (POC or IT) and monitor proteinuria (IT) throughout treatment of renal diseases in dogs and cats.
- A positive test result for UAlb is not diagnostic for a specific condition. Rather, it alerts the clinician that the patient should be monitored. Some animals will have only transient albuminuria. Sequential positive tests over a period of weeks in the absence of postrenal causes of albuminuria should alert the clinician to ongoing renal damage. Greater concern should be given to patients with either persistently high positive test results or test results that are of increasing magnitude. Patients falling into this category should be systematically evaluated for disorders that may be causing renal injury. In 1 study, 56% of dogs with persistent MA were found to have a nonrenal systemic disease; an additional 31% were found to have renal disease (Whittemore et al. 2006).

URINE ALBUMIN

MISCELLANEOUS

ANCILLARY TESTS
- Urinalysis
- Urine protein/creatinine ratio
- Urine culture and susceptibility testing

SYNONYMS
Microalbuminuria

SEE ALSO
Blackwell's Five-Minute Veterinary Consult: Canine and Feline Topics
- Amyloidosis
- Glomerulonephritis
- Proteinuria
- Renal Failure, Acute Uremia
- Renal Failure, Chronic

Related Topics in This Book
- Bacterial Culture and Sensitivity Testing
- Urinalysis Overview
- Urine Protein
- Urine Sediment

ABBREVIATIONS
- ACE = angiotensin-converting enzyme
- IT = immunoturbidimetric test
- MA = microalbuminuria
- POC = point-of-care immunoassay
- TNTC = too numerous to count
- UAlb = urine albumin

Suggested Reading

Elliot J, Syme HM. Proteinuria in chronic kidney disease in cats: Prognostic marker or therapeutic target? [Editorial]. *J Vet Intern Med* 2006; 20: 1052–1053.

Lees GE, Brown SA, Elliot J, *et al.* Assessment and management of proteinuria in dogs and cats: 2004 ACVIM Forum Consensus Statement (small animal). *J Vet Intern Med* 2005; 19: 337–385.

Whittemore JC, Gill VL, Jensen WA, *et al.* Evaluation of the association between microalbuminuria and the urine albumin-creatinine ratio and systemic disease in dogs. *J Am Vet Med Assoc* 2006; 229: 958–963.

INTERNET RESOURCES
Heska, E.R.D.-Healthscreen, Urine Tests: Clinical data, http://www.heska.com/erd/clinical_data.asp.

AUTHOR NAME
Shelly L. Vaden

BASICS

TYPE OF SPECIMEN
Urine

TEST EXPLANATION AND RELATED PHYSIOLOGY
Conjugated bilirubin readily passes through the glomerulus and is not reabsorbed by renal tubules. Unconjugated bilirubin is bound to serum albumin and cannot pass through the glomerulus. The renal threshold for bilirubin is very low in dogs, and tubular epithelial cells contain glucuronyltransferase, which will conjugate bilirubin. Therefore, small, but detectable amounts of bilirubin may be present in the urine of healthy dogs even when serum bilirubin is normal.

Bilirubinuria can be seen following episodes of hemolysis that overwhelm the liver's ability to conjugate and excrete bilirubin, most frequently with immune-mediated hemolytic anemia or following internal hemorrhage. Excess conjugated bilirubin in hepatocytes leaks back into the circulation and is cleared by the kidney. Similarly, hepatobiliary disease can decrease the ability to excrete conjugated bilirubin into bile, with regurgitation of conjugated bilirubin into the bloodstream and clearance by the kidney.

Bilirubinuria is most often detected through the use of reagent strips [e.g., Multistix (Bayer, Leverkusen, Germany), Chemstrip (Roche, Basel, Switzerland)] and reported as negative or present in small (1+), moderate (2+), or large (3+) amounts. The level of bilirubinuria is affected by urine concentration. The Ictotest tablet test (Bayer) is also available as a screen for bilirubinuria. The Ictotest is more sensitive than dipsticks and should be used as a confirmatory test. Tests react with conjugated, but not unconjugated, bilirubin.

INDICATIONS
Bilirubinuria may precede clinical identification of jaundice or hyperbilirubinemia and therefore may serve as an early indicator of disease.

CONTRAINDICATIONS
None

POTENTIAL COMPLICATIONS
None

CLIENT EDUCATION
None

BODY SYSTEMS ASSESSED
- Hemic, lymphatic, and immune
- Hepatobiliary

SAMPLE

COLLECTION
Urine can be collected by any method.

HANDLING
- Collect the urine prior to medical therapy or contrast radiography.
- Use a clean sample container.
- Ideally assay within 30 min to 1 h. If analysis is delayed, refrigerate the sample.
- Rewarm the sample to room temperature before analysis.
- Avoid the use of centrifugation prior to examination for bilirubin. Precipitates of calcium carbonate and calcium phosphate may absorb bilirubin.

STORAGE
- Store in an opaque or amber container with a tight-fitting lid.
- Freezing is an acceptable method of urine preservation.

STABILITY
- Unstable at room temperature
  - Samples are degraded by exposure to light.
  - Samples may spontaneously hydrolyze to free bilirubin.
  - Samples may spontaneously oxidize to biliverdin, which is not detectable by routine methods.
- Refrigerated (2°–8°C): up to 12 h if protected from light
- Freeze for long-term storage.

PROTOCOL
See the "Urinalysis Overview" chapter.

INTERPRETATION

NORMAL FINDINGS OR RANGE
- Small amounts of bilirubin may be present in the concentrated urine of healthy dogs:
  - Concentrated urine (SG, 1.025–1.040) frequently contains small amounts (1+) of bilirubin.
  - Urine with an SG of >1.040 may contain moderate amounts (up to 2+) of bilirubin.
  - Dilute urine (SG, <1.025) should be bilirubin negative.
- Cat urine should be bilirubin negative.

URINE BILIRUBIN

ABNORMAL VALUES
- Any bilirubin in feline urine
- Any bilirubin in dilute canine urine
- 2+ to 3+ bilirubin can be abnormal in concentrated canine urine.

CRITICAL VALUES
None

INTERFERING FACTORS
Drugs That May Alter Results or Interpretation
Drugs That Interfere with Test Methodology
- False-positive results may be caused by administration of the following:
  - Indican or metabolites of etodolac
  - Phenazopyridine
  - Chlorpromazine metabolites
- False-negative results may be caused by ascorbic acid and nitrites.

Drugs That Alter Physiology
None

Disorders That May Alter Results
None

Collection Techniques or Handling That May Alter Results
- Prolonged exposure of the sample to light
- Urine at room temperature for >1 h before the test is performed
- Urine refrigerated for >12 h or tested before urine attains room temperature after refrigeration

Influence of Signalment
Species
Low levels of bilirubin can be seen in urine from healthy dogs.

Breed
None

Age
None

Gender
Incidental bilirubinuria is more common in healthy male dogs.

Pregnancy
None

LIMITATIONS OF THE TEST
Sensitivity, Specificity, and Positive and Negative Predictive Values
N/A

Valid If Run in a Human Lab?
Yes.

Causes of Abnormal Finding

High values	Low values
Prehepatic causes	Not significant
Hemolytic disorders that destroy erythrocytes	
Immune-mediated hemolysis (e.g., caused by infectious agents, drugs, autoantibodies, systemic lupus erythematosus)	
Infectious: *Mycoplasma* spp., FeLV, *Babesia*, *Ehrlichia*, *Cytauxzoon*, heartworm	
Prolonged fasting or starvation	
Fever	
Hepatic causes	
Adverse drug reactions	
Cholangiohepatitis	
Neoplasia	
Infectious canine hepatitis	
Hepatic lipidosis (in cats)	
Massive hepatic necrosis	
Systemic illness with hepatic involvement: leptospirosis (in dogs), histoplasmosis, or hyperthyroidism (in cats)	
Posthepatic causes	
Pancreatitis	
Neoplasia	
Cholangitis or cholangiohepatitis	
Ruptured gallbladder or bile duct	
Duct occlusion: cholelithiasis or liver flukes (in cats)	

CLINICAL PERSPECTIVE
- In animals with significant regenerative anemia, suspect that bilirubinuria is caused by hemolysis.
- In animals without anemia, especially if accompanied by elevated serum alkaline phosphatase and GGT, suspect that bilirubinuria is caused by hepatobiliary disease.
- Sepsis can decrease bilirubin uptake and cause bilirubinuria.
- Confirm weak positive dipstick reactions with the more sensitive Ictotest, especially if urine is discolored and color change is difficult to interpret.

MISCELLANEOUS

ANCILLARY TESTS
- Serum biochemistry including total serum bilirubin, ALT, AST, alkaline phosphatase, and gamma-glutamyltransferase
- CBC with blood smear evaluation
- Coombs' test
- PCR for RBC parasites

SYNONYMS
None

SEE ALSO
Blackwell's Five-Minute Veterinary Consult: Canine and Feline Topics
- Anemia, Immune-Mediated
- Anemia, Regenerative
- Anemia, Heinz Body
- Babesiosis
- Cholangitis/Cholangiohepatitis Syndrome
- Cholecystitis and Choledochitis
- Hemotrophic Mycoplasmosis (Haemobartonellosis)
- Hepatic Lipidosis

Related Topics in This Book
- Alkaline Phosphatase
- *Babesia*
- Bilirubin
- Gamma-Glutamyltransferase
- Hemotrophic Mycoplasmas

ABBREVIATIONS
SG = specific gravity

Suggested Reading
Gregory CR. Urinary system. In: Prasse KW, Latimer KS, Mahaffey EA, eds. *Duncan and Prasse's Veterinary Laboratory Medicine*, 4th ed. Ames: Iowa State Press, 2003: 239–240.
Osborne CA, Stevens JB. *Urinalysis: A Clinical Guide to Compassionate Patient Care*. Leverkusen, Germany: Bayer, 1999: 102–106.
Stockham SL, Scott MA. *Fundamentals of Veterinary Clinical Pathology*. Ames: Iowa State Press, 2002: 319–320.

INTERNET RESOURCES
None

AUTHOR NAMES
Angela Wilcox and Karen E. Russell

URINE FRACTIONAL EXCRETION OF ELECTROLYTES

BASICS

TYPE OF SPECIMEN
Blood
Urine

TEST EXPLANATION AND RELATED PHYSIOLOGY
This test compares the renal clearance of an electrolyte with the clearance of endogenous creatinine, an indicator of glomerular filtration rate. The most common electrolytes examined by this test are Na^+, K^+, Cl^-, and phosphorus (Pi), although renal handling of any solute can be assessed by this method. The concentrations of the electrolyte and of creatinine are determined in a urine sample and in a simultaneously drawn serum sample. The formula for the fractional excretion (FE) of an electrolyte is derived by dividing the clearance formula for the electrolyte by the clearance formula for creatinine and can be simplified and calculated as follows:

$$FE_{electrolyte} = \frac{[urine_{electrolyte}] \div [serum_{electrolyte}]}{[urine_{creatinine}] \div [serum_{creatinine}]}$$

$FE_{electrolyte}$ is often multiplied by 100% and expressed as a percentage.

The FE should reflect the manner in which the kidney handles the specific electrolyte. Normally, if an electrolyte is excreted by glomerular filtration alone, the FE = 1. If the electrolyte is filtered through the glomerulus and then reabsorbed by the renal tubules, the FE is <1. Conversely, if the electrolyte is filtered through the glomerulus and then undergoes net secretion by the renal tubules, the FE is >1.

Changes in FE may occur because of alterations in filtered load, tubular reabsorption or tubular secretion. FE should reflect an appropriate response to the load of the electrolyte. For example, increased Na^+ in the diet above the needs of the animal should increase FE_{Na} to eliminate excess Na^+ from the body. Conversely, an appropriate response to hyponatremia is a decrease in FE_{Na}, reflecting renal conservation.

INDICATIONS
• To evaluate renal tubular function
• To help to differentiate primary renal from extrarenal causes of azotemia

CONTRAINDICATIONS
• Diuretic therapy
• Fluid therapy
• Use of contrast media that is excreted by kidney

POTENTIAL COMPLICATIONS
None

CLIENT EDUCATION
The client should provide information on the type of diet and when the patient last ate. Fasting the patient overnight (for 15 h) may minimize the effect of diet.

BODY SYSTEMS ASSESSED
Renal and urologic

SAMPLE

COLLECTION
• 3–5 mL of urine collected by voiding, cystocentesis, or catheter. The urine may be collected either as a random spot sample or over a 24-h period.
• 3–5 mL of venous blood should be collected when the urine spot sample is obtained or midway during a 24-h urine collection.

HANDLING
• Centrifuge the urine to remove cells and debris.
• Separate the serum from the cells as soon as possible.

STORAGE
• Both the urine and the serum may be stored in a refrigerator or frozen. To avoid growth of bacteria, urine should not be stored at room temperature.
• For long-term storage (months), samples should be sealed to prevent evaporation of water and concentration of analytes, which can occur in frost-free freezers.

STABILITY
• Refrigerated (4°C): 1 week
• Frozen: prolonged stability

PROTOCOL
None

INTERPRETATION

NORMAL FINDINGS OR RANGE
Absolute normal ranges are not available because the FEs of electrolytes are affected by a variety of factors, including dietary intake, postprandial timing of sampling, circadian rhythm, and activity of neurohormonal systems such as the renin-angiotensin-aldosterone system. Below are approximate guidelines for dogs and cats expressed as percentages:

	Na^+	K^+	Cl^-	Pi
Dogs	<1%	<20%	<1%	<40%
Cats	<1%	5%–25%	<1%	<70%

ABNORMAL VALUES
Values above the reference intervals

CRITICAL VALUES
None

INTERFERING FACTORS
Drugs That May Alter Results or Interpretation
Drugs That Interfere with Test Methodology
Cephalosporins affect creatinine measurements.

Drugs That Alter Physiology
• Diuretics increase electrolyte excretion.
• Parenteral fluid therapy can affect electrolyte load.
• Glucocorticoids will affect renal excretion of electrolytes.
• Angiotensin-converting enzyme (ACE) inhibitors may decrease K^+ excretion.

Disorders That May Alter Results
• Measurement of creatinine concentration may be falsely decreased by bilirubin, hemolysis, or lipemia. The degree of interference depends on the specific methodology, and the laboratory performing the assay should be consulted.
• Measurement of creatinine may be falsely increased by the presence of noncreatinine chromagens in the serum, including such analytes as glucose, ketones, uric acid, and proteins. The degree of interference depends on the specific methodology, and the laboratory performing the assay should be consulted. Noncreatinine chromagens are not found in urine.

Collection Techniques or Handling That May Alter Results
Blood contamination of the urine (i.e., hematuria) can affect results.
Influence of Signalment
Species
None

Breed
A report in greyhounds (Bennett et al. 2006) proposed reference limits for this breed that were relatively similar to the aforementioned guidelines. However, a population of nongreyhound dogs was not evaluated under similar conditions to enable a true comparison.

Age
• The FEs of Na^+, K^+, Cl^-, and Pi tend to be lower in 4- to 6-week-old kittens compared to older kittens. However, all ages still fall within the aforementioned suggested guidelines.
• The FEs of Na^+, K^+, Cl^-, and Pi are slightly, but not significantly, higher in 9- to 21-week-old puppies compared to values reported for adult dogs.
• The FE of Ca^{+2} is reported to be higher in 6- to 9-week-old puppies compared to adult dogs.
• It is uncertain whether these age-related variations reflect real differences in renal tubular function or are influenced by composition of diets formulated for growth versus maintenance diets.

Gender
None

Pregnancy
Electrolyte imbalances may occur in some complicated pregnancies.

LIMITATIONS OF THE TEST
Sensitivity, Specificity, and Positive and Negative Predictive Values
N/A

Valid If Run in a Human Lab?
Yes.

Causes of Abnormal Findings

High values	Low values
$FE_{Na} > 1\%$	$FE_{Na} < 1\%$
Renal tubular disease	Dehydration
Chronic renal failure (some cases)	Prerenal azotemia
Acute on chronic renal failure	Nonrenal Na^+ loss, including
Fluid therapy	diarrhea, 3rd spacing
Diuretic therapy	Dietary Na^+ restriction
Hypoadrenocorticism	Hyperaldosteronism
Gentamicin toxicosis	Intratubular obstruction from
Ethylene glycol toxicosis	pigmenturia or contrast media
Fanconi's syndrome	
Dietary Na^+ excess	
FE_K	FE_K
Chronic renal failure	Extrarenal losses of K^+
Feline kaliopenic	Dietary K^+ restriction
polymyopathy-nephropathy	Hypoadrenocorticism
Renal tubular disease	
Gentamicin toxicosis	
Ethylene glycol toxicosis	
Fanconi's syndrome	
Dietary K^+ excess	
FE_{Pi}	FE_{Pi}
Chronic renal failure with renal	Decreased PTH
secondary hyperparathyroidism	
Primary hyperparathyroidism	
Nutritional secondary	
hyperparathyroidism	
Fanconi's syndrome	

CLINICAL PERSPECTIVE
• The FE must be interpreted in light of the serum concentrations of the electrolytes, the presence of azotemia, and dietary or therapeutic interventions. Changes in FE should be appropriate to the need of the patient to maintain homeostasis.
• In hyponatremic patients, FE_{Na} of $>1\%$ indicates that the kidney is the site of Na^+ loss, whereas FE_{Na} of $<1\%$ indicates renal conservation of Na^+ and an extrarenal route of Na^+ loss.
• The Cl^- fractional excretion usually follows a similar pattern to the FE_{Na}; however, there is a paucity of reports in the veterinary literature on the clinical utility of the Cl^- fractional excretion.
• In hypocalcemic patients, an increase in FE_{Pi} is usually mediated by an increase in PTH, whereas a decrease in FE_{Pi} suggests decreased PTH.
• Patients with severe glomerular disease but disproportionately less tubular damage may be azotemic but have concentrated urine and normal-appearing FE_{Na} because of glomerulotubular imbalance.
• Because of the variety of factors that can influence the FE of electrolytes, random spot urine samples show variable correlation with those obtained from 24-h urine collections. The influence of these factors may be minimized by collecting 24-h urine samples. However, because this procedure is cumbersome, 24-h collections are rarely done unless spot samples are equivocal.

MISCELLANEOUS
ANCILLARY TESTS
None

SYNONYMS
None

SEE ALSO
Blackwell's Five-Minute Veterinary Consult: Canine and Feline Topics
• Glomerulonephritis
• Polyuria and Polydipsia
• Renal Failure, Acute Uremia
• Renal Failure, Chronic

Related Topics in This Book
• Glomerular Filtration Rate
• Urine Gamma-Glutamyltransferase/Creatinine Ratio
• Urine Specific Gravity

ABBREVIATIONS
• Cl^- = chloride
• FE = fractional excretion
• FE_K = potassium fractional excretion
• FE_{Na} = sodium fractional excretion
• FE_{Pi} = phosphorus fractional excretion
• K^+ = potassium
• Na^+ = sodium
• Pi = phosphorus
• PTH = parathyroid hormone
• $[Serum_{creatinine}]$ = serum concentration of creatinine
• $[Serum_{electrolyte}]$ = serum concentration of the electrolyte
• $[Urine_{creatinine}]$ = urine concentration of creatinine
• $[Urine_{electrolyte}]$ = urine concentration of the electrolyte

Suggested Reading
Bennett SL, Abraham LA, Anderson GA, *et al*. Reference limits for urinary fractional excretion of electrolytes in adult non-racing Greyhound dogs. *Aust Vet J* 2006; 84: 393–397.
DiBartola SP, Chew DJ, Jacobs G. Quantitative urinalysis including 24-hour protein excretion in the dog. *J Am Anim Hosp Assoc* 1980; 16: 537–546.

Fettman MJ, Rebar A. Laboratory evaluation of renal function. In: Thrall MA, ed. *Veterinary Hematology and Clinical Chemistry.* Philadelphia: Lippincott Williams & Wilkins, 2004: 301–328.

Hoskins JD, Turnwald GH, Kearney MT, *et al.* Quantitative urinalysis in kittens from four to thirty weeks after birth. *Am J Vet Res* 1991; 52: 1295–1299.

Lane IF, Shaw DH, Burton SA, Donald AW. Quantitative urinalysis in healthy Beagle puppies from 9 to 27 weeks of age. *Am J Vet Res* 2000; 61: 577–581.

Laroute V, Chetboul V, Roche L, *et al.* Quantitative evaluation of renal function in healthy Beagle puppies and mature dogs. *Res Vet Sci* 2005; 79: 161–167.

Lefebvre HP, Dossin O, Trumel C, Braun J-P. Fractional exeretion tests: a cntical review of methods and applications in domestic animals. *Vet Clin Path* 2008; 37: 4–20.

Russo EA, Lees GE, Hightower D. Evaluation of renal function in cats using quantitative urinalysis. *Am J Vet Res* 1986; 47: 1308–1312.

INTERNET RESOURCES
None

AUTHOR NAME
M. Judith Radin

URINE GAMMA-GLUTAMYLTRANSFERASE/CREATININE RATIO

BASICS

TYPE OF SPECIMEN
Urine

TEST EXPLANATION AND RELATED PHYSIOLOGY
Gamma-glutamyltransferase (GGT) is most commonly assessed in relation to activity in hepatocytes and biliary epithelial cells. However, it is also present in renal tubular epithelial cells. Damage to renal tubular cells causes release of GGT into urine and increased urinary GGT activity. GGT activity in the urine is normalized to creatinine and reported as the urine GGT/creatinine ratio. Spot samples measuring urine GGT/creatinine ratio correlate with 24-h urine GGT measurements. The urine GGT/creatinine ratio can be increased by increased urinary GGT activity (renal tubular damage), and the urine GGT/creatinine ratio increases prior to detectable changes in serum creatinine, urine specific gravity, or urine protein/creatinine ratio in dogs with gentamicin-induced nephrotoxicosis. The urine GGT/creatinine ratio can also be increased by decreased urinary creatinine excretion (decreased GFR).

INDICATIONS
Evaluation for acute renal proximal tubular injury

CONTRAINDICATIONS
- Azotemia
- Severe glomerular damage

POTENTIAL COMPLICATIONS
None

CLIENT EDUCATION
None

BODY SYSTEMS ASSESSED
Renal and urologic

SAMPLE

COLLECTION
0.5 mL of urine (voided or by catheterization or cystocentesis)

HANDLING
Centrifuge the urine at 1,000–4,000 g for 5 min and transfer an aliquot of supernatant to a clean tube without additives.

STORAGE
Refrigeration is recommended.

STABILITY
Refrigerated (4°C): at least 4 days

PROTOCOL
None

INTERPRETATION

NORMAL FINDINGS OR RANGE
Reported in mixed units: GGT (IU/L)/creatinine (mg/dL). Reference intervals may vary depending on the laboratory and assay.
- Dogs: 0.39 +/− 0.18 (Grauer et al. 1995) or <0.42 (Gossett et al. 1987)
- Cats: 0.03–0.56 for 4-h urine collection (Bishop et al. 1991)

ABNORMAL VALUES
Values above the reference interval

CRITICAL VALUES
None

URINE GAMMA-GLUTAMYLTRANSFERASE/CREATININE RATIO

INTERFERING FACTORS
Drugs That May Alter Results or Interpretation
Drugs That Interfere with Test Methodology
None

Drugs That Alter Physiology
None

Disorders That May Alter Results
• Decreased GFR, with subsequent azotemia, increases the urine GGT/creatinine ratio. Urine creatinine excretion depends on GFR, such that, when GFR is decreased, urinary excretion of creatinine is decreased. This causes the urine GGT/creatinine ratio to increase independently of urinary GGT activity. The clinical utility of urine GGT/creatinine lies in detection of acute renal damage *before* the onset of azotemia.
• Severe glomerular damage allows passage of serum GGT into the urine and will cause the urine GGT/creatinine ratio to increase independently of renal tubular GGT excretion. This is a likely reason for the increased urine GGT/creatinine ratio reported in experimentally induced glomerulonephritis in cats.

Collection Techniques or Handling That May Alter Results
• Urine should be centrifuged to remove cells that may alter results.
• Freezing human and rat urine may inactivate urinary GGT, but this has not been reported in dogs and cats.

Influence of Signalment
Species
Inhibitors of GGT activity have been reported in the urine of some species, but this does not appear to be the case in dogs and cats.

Breed
None

Age
No correlation between age and urine GGT/creatinine was noted in dogs ranging in age from 6 months to 7 years.

Gender
None

Pregnancy
None

LIMITATIONS OF THE TEST
Sensitivity, Specificity, and Positive and Negative Predictive Values
N/A

Valid If Run in a Human Lab?
Yes.

Causes of Abnormal Findings

High values	Low values
Renal tubular damage	Not clinically significant
Decreased GFR	
Severe glomerular disease (e.g., glomerulonephritis in cats)	

CLINICAL PERSPECTIVE
• The urine GGT/creatinine ratio is useful in detecting *early* acute renal tubular damage from a variety of causes, including gentamicin-induced nephrotoxicity and other causes of renal tubular injury, such as pyometra.
• The magnitude of increase in the urine GGT/creatinine ratio correlates with the severity of renal tubular damage as assessed histopathologically.
• The urine GGT/creatinine ratio will increase independently of urinary GGT activity in conditions with decreased GFR or severe glomerular disease.

• Increased urine GGT/creatinine ratios have been reported in cats with experimentally induced glomerulonephritis and this finding may provide a sensitive indication of renal damage. The increased urinary enzyme activity is likely related to severe glomerular damage.

 MISCELLANEOUS

ANCILLARY TESTS

• Serum BUN and creatinine: If azotemia is present, an increased urine GGT/creatinine ratio may be due to decreased creatinine excretion (decreased GFR) rather than increased urinary GGT activity.
• Urine sediment evaluation, looking for casts or other abnormalities that might confirm renal tubular damage or suggest etiology

SYNONYMS

None

SEE ALSO

Blackwell's Five-Minute Veterinary Consult: Canine and Feline Topics
• Nephrotoxicity, Drug-Induced
• Renal Failure, Acute Uremia

Related Topics in This Book
• Creatinine
• Urea Nitrogen
• Urine Protein
• Urine Protein/Creatinine Ratio
• Urine Sediment

ABBREVIATIONS

GFR = glomerular filtration rate

Suggested Reading

Bain PJ. Liver. In: Latimer, KS, Mahaffey EA, Prasse KW, eds. *Duncan and Prasse's Veterinary Laboratory Medicine Clinical Pathology*. Ames: Iowa State Press, 2003: 193–214.

Bishop SA, Lucke VM, Stokes CR, Gruffydd-Jones TJ. Plasma and urine biochemical changes in cats with experimental immune complex glomerulonephritis. *J Comp Pathol* 1991; 104: 65–76.

Clemo FA. Urinary enzyme evaluation of nephrotoxicity in the dog. *Toxicol Pathol* 1998; 26: 29–32.

Gossett KA, Turnwald GH, Kearney MT, *et al.* Evaluation of gamma-glutamyl transpeptidase-to-creatinine ratio from spot samples of urine supernatant, as an indicator of urinary enzyme excretion in dogs. *Am J Vet Res* 1987; 48: 455–457.

Grauer GF, Greco DS, Behrend EN, *et al.* Estimation of quantitative enzymuria in dogs with gentamicin-induced nephrotoxicosis using enzyme/creatinine ratios from spot urine samples. *J Vet Intern Med* 1995; 9: 324–327.

Rivers BJ, Walter PA, O'Brien TD, *et al.* Evaluation of urine gamma-glutamyl transpeptidase-to-creatinine ratio as a diagnostic tool in an experimental model of aminoglycoside-induced acute renal failure in the dog. *J Am Anim Hosp Assoc* 1996; 32: 323–336.

Stockham SL, Scott MA. Enzymes. In: *Fundamentals of Veterinary Clinical Pathology*, 2nd ed. Ames: Iowa State Press, 2008: 639–674.

INTERNET RESOURCES

None

AUTHOR NAMES

Deanna M.W. Schaefer and M. Judith Radin

URINE GLUCOSE

 BASICS

TYPE OF SPECIMEN
Urine

TEST EXPLANATION AND RELATED PHYSIOLOGY
Glucose is freely filtered through the glomerular filtration barrier into the ultrafiltrate. Glucose reabsorption occurs at the proximal renal tubules via active transport in association with sodium reabsorption. A sodium-independent mechanism is responsible for transport of glucose into the interstitium, with subsequent uptake by renal peritubular capillaries. Although glucose is almost completely reabsorbed by this process, a small amount may be present in the urine of normal animals that is undetectable by commercial tests.

When urine glucose concentrations are at detectable levels by routine methods ($\geq$40 mg/dL, depending on test), the underlying cause for the glucosuria should be identified. Blood glucose levels should be measured to determine whether the patient is normoglycemic or hyperglycemic. When blood glucose levels surpass >280 mg/dL in cats and >180 mg/dL in dogs, the renal threshold for glucose transport is exceeded, resulting in glucosuria. Glucosuria can also occur with diseases that damage renal tubules or in genetic defects in excretion of glucose (e.g., Fanconi's syndrome). In these cases, renal epithelial cells are unable to reabsorb a normal, low-glucose load.

Methods for the semiquantitative measurement of urine glucose are colorimetric tests based on glucose oxidase/peroxidase activity or copper reduction. Reagent strips containing glucose oxidase react specifically with glucose, whereas tablets composed of cupric ions can be reduced by glucose, as well as other reducing substances in urine.

INDICATIONS
• A component of routine urinalysis
• Used to monitor response to insulin therapy in patients with diabetes mellitus
• Indicated in animals that are polyuric-polydypsic

CONTRAINDICATIONS
None

POTENTIAL COMPLICATIONS
None

CLIENT EDUCATION
• Collection cups must be free of cleaning solutions, such as hydrogen peroxide, baking soda, and bleach, which can cause false-positive urine glucose reactions.
• When monitoring diabetic pets:
   • It is essential to use nonexpired reagents that have been properly stored. Reagents may be adversely affected by exposure to heat, light, moisture, or chemical compounds and their fumes.
   • For diabetic dogs, reagent strips can be held directly in the urine stream. Evaluate the reagent pad within the time interval recommended by the manufacturer.
   • For diabetic cats, glucose indicator systems for the litterbox are available. The litterbox should first be cleaned with soap and water. Avoid the use of baking soda and bleach because these cause false-positive reactions.

BODY SYSTEMS ASSESSED
• Endocrine and metabolic
• Renal and urologic

 SAMPLE

COLLECTION
0.5–5.0 mL of urine collected by free catch of a voided sample, manual expression of the urinary bladder, catheterization, or cystocentesis

HANDLING
• Collect the urine into clean container free of additives, detergents, and chemicals.
• Ideally, perform the assay within $\leq$2 h.
• If analysis must be delayed, refrigerate the sample in a closed container.
• Allow refrigerated samples to warm to room temperature prior to analysis in order to avoid false-negative results for glucosuria from enzyme-dependent tests (glucose oxidase/peroxidase).

STORAGE
• Ideally, refrigerated samples should be analyzed within 6–8 h.
• Sodium fluoride can act as a preservative for glucose in the urine but will inhibit the enzymatic test found on many dipsticks so is not recommended for routine use.

STABILITY
• Glucose concentrations may decrease in unpreserved urine because of use by cells or bacteria.
• Refrigerated samples stored up to 12 h are probably adequate.

PROTOCOL
See the "Urinalysis Overview" chapter.

 INTERPRETATION

NORMAL FINDINGS OR RANGE
Negative reagent-strip assay

ABNORMAL VALUES
Detectable glucosuria is abnormal and should be interpreted in conjunction with blood glucose levels.

CRITICAL VALUES
None

INTERFERING FACTORS
Drugs That May Alter Results or Interpretation
Drugs That Interfere with Test Methodology
Glucose oxidase/peroxidase methods
• Drugs containing riboflavin, azo dyes, or nitrofurantoin may discolor the urine and interfere with interpretation of the reagent pad.
• False-positive results occur if chlorine, hydrogen peroxide, hypochlorite, or other oxidizing agents contaminate the sample or contact the reagent strip.
• Cephalexin administration has been associated with false-positive results in dogs.
• False-negative results for low levels of glucosuria (50–100 mg/dL) may occur with administration of tetracycline or salicylates or with urine ascorbic acid concentrations as low as 50 mg/dL. This level of ascorbic acid has been found in the urine of diabetic dogs and cats and in animals receiving vitamin C supplements.

• Formaldehyde exposure may also cause false-negative results because it inhibits enzymatic activity.

Copper reduction method
• This test method is not specific for glucose and will detect other reducing substances, such as fructose, galactose, lactose, maltose, and pentose.
• The administration of penicillin (high dosage), sulfonamides, chloral hydrate, salicylates, cephalexin, or enrofloxacin, and formaldehyde contamination have all been associated with false-positive reactions.
• Although ascorbic acid is a reducing substance, its concentration in urine is unlikely to be high enough to cause false-positive results.

Drugs That Alter Physiology
• Hyperglycemic glucosuria: parenteral solutions (e.g., dextrose, total parenteral nutrition), morphine, xylazine, phenothiazines, L-asparaginase, diazoxide, glucagon, epinephrine, adrenocorticotropic hormone (ACTH), progesterone, or glucocorticoids (less common)
• Normoglycemic glucosuria: associated with acquired Fanconi's syndrome secondary to toxicosis potentially caused by gentamicin, cephalosporins, streptozotocin, amoxicillin, lead, mercury, cadmium disinfectants containing *p*-chloro-*o*-benzylphenol, maleic acid, or cisplatin

Disorders That May Alter Results
• Substantial pigmenturia (e.g., bilirubinuria, hemoglobinuria) may interfere with the evaluation and interpretation of reagent pads.
• Elevated levels of glucuronic acid in the urine may cause false-positive results with the copper reduction method.

Collection Techniques or Handling That May Alter Results
• Sample contamination with cleaning solutions may cause false-positive reactions.
• The use of outdated or damaged reagent strips, excessive delay in testing, or improper storage may cause false-negative reactions.

Influence of Signalment
Species
None

Breed
• Congenital Fanconi's syndrome: basenjis, Shetland sheepdogs, miniature schnauzers, and Norwegian elkhounds
• Primary renal glucosuria: Scottish terriers
• Other congenital diseases associated with renal dysfunction: Norwegian elkhounds

Age
None

Gender
None

Pregnancy
Elevated progesterone levels in the diestrus phase of the estrous cycle may lead to the development of diabetes mellitus in bitches.

LIMITATIONS OF THE TEST
Sensitivity, Specificity, and Positive and Negative Predictive Values
Glucose Oxidase/Peroxidase Methods
• Although sensitivity may vary among brands, most tests will detect glucosuria at levels of <100 mg/dL. Some tests may be able to detect urine glucose levels as low as 40 mg/dL.
• These tests are specific for glucose and will not react with alternate reducing substances.

Copper Reduction Method
• This test has a sensitivity of ≈250 mg/dL for the detection of glucosuria.
• This test is not specific for glucose, as previously discussed.

Valid If Run in a Human Lab?
Yes.

Causes of Abnormal Findings

Hyperglycemic glucosuria	Transient glucosuria
	Stress (release of catecholamines and glucocorticoids)
	Pharmacologic agents (e.g., morphine, xylazine, phenothiazines, L-asparaginase, diazoxide)
	Persistent glucosuria
	Diabetes mellitus
	Hyperadrenocorticism
	Acute pancreatitis
	Acromegaly
	Pheochromocytoma
	Glucagonoma
	Chronic hepatic insufficiency (altered glucagon clearance)
Normoglycemic glucosuria	Congenital
	Fanconi's syndrome
	Primary renal glucosuria
	Congenital renal dysfunction
	Acquired
	Acute renal failure
	Fanconi's syndrome secondary to toxicosis (e.g., exposure to nephrotoxic drugs or heavy metals, such as cadmium, lead, or mercury)
	Chronic renal failure

CLINICAL PERSPECTIVE
Glucosuria should be interpreted in conjunction with blood glucose levels:
• Determination of whether glucosuria is transient or persistent can help identify underlying cause.
• Glucosuria with hyperglycemia suggests endocrine or metabolic disease.
• Glucosuria with normoglycemia suggests renal tubular disease.

 MISCELLANEOUS

ANCILLARY TESTS
• Blood or serum glucose
• Urine ketones
• Tests of urine fractional excretion may help document renal tubular defects.

SYNONYMS
None

SEE ALSO
Blackwell's Five-Minute Veterinary Consult: Canine and Feline Topics
• Diabetes Mellitus with Hyperosmolar Coma
• Diabetes Mellitus with Ketoacidosis
• Diabetes Mellitus without Complication—Cats
• Diabetes Mellitus without Complication—Dogs
• Fanconi's Syndrome
• Glucosuria
• Renal Failure, Acute Uremia
• Renal Failure, Chronic

URINE GLUCOSE

Related Topics in This Book
- General Principles for Performing Urine Tests
- Glucose
- Glucose Curve
- Glycosylated Hemoglobin
- Urinalysis Overview
- Urine Fractional Excretion of Electrolytes
- Urine Ketones

ABBREVIATIONS
None

Suggested Reading

Osborne CA, Stevens JB. Biochemical analysis of urine: Glucose. In: *Urinalysis: A Clinical Guide to Compassionate Patient Care.* Leverkusen, Germany: Bayer, 1999: 92–99.

Prasse KW, Mahaffey EA, Latimer KS, eds. *Duncan and Prasse's Veterinary Laboratory Medicine: Clinical Pathology,* 4th ed. Ames, IA: Blackwell, 2003: 238–239.

Rees CA, Boothe DM. Evaluation of the effect of cephalexin and enrofloxacin on clinical laboratory measurements of urine glucose in dogs. *J Am Vet Med Assoc* 2004; 224: 1455–1458.

Stockham SL, Scott MA. *Fundamentals of Veterinary Clinical Pathology,* 1st ed. Ames, IA: Blackwell, 2002: 315–317.

INTERNET RESOURCES
None

AUTHOR NAMES
Seth E. Chapman and Karen E. Russell

BASICS

TYPE OF SPECIMEN
Urine

TEST EXPLANATION AND RELATED PHYSIOLOGY
Macroscopic and microscopic detection of heme-containing substances (i.e., erythrocytes, hemoglobin, myoglobin) is part of the routine urinalysis. *Pigmenturia* (abnormal urine color) may suggest the presence of heme-containing substances. Red or reddish brown urine suggests the presence of erythrocytes, hemoglobin, or myoglobin, and brown-to-black urine suggests the presence of myoglobin or methemoglobin produced through oxidation of hemoglobin. In the absence of obvious pigmenturia, microscopic examination and chemical evaluation may reveal the presence of erythrocytes and/or heme-containing substances, respectively.

A positive dipstick reaction for urine heme protein indicates the presence of blood (hematuria), hemoglobin (hemoglobinuria), or myoglobin (myoglobinuria) in urine. Hematuria can result from hemorrhage or erythrocyte diapedesis occurring anywhere along the urogenital tract. General causes include trauma, inflammation, infection, neoplasia, infarction, and coagulopathy. Hemoglobinuria occurs with lysis of erythrocytes already present in urine or secondary to intravascular hemolysis with hemoglobinemia. With intravascular hemolysis, a reddish discoloration of the plasma occurs as hemoglobin is released and binds to plasma proteins (e.g., haptoglobin). It is transported to the liver, where it is further metabolized. With severe hemolysis, increased free hemoglobin accumulates and overwhelms haptoglobin binding. Free hemoglobin dissociates into dimers, which pass through the glomerulus and spill into urine. Myoglobin, a heme protein in skeletal muscle, is present in circulation in small concentrations and is cleared through the kidney. Myoglobinuria occurs secondary to marked muscle injury or necrosis.

Urine dipsticks have a reagent pad that tests for the presence of erythrocytes, hemoglobin, or myoglobin. A tablet is also available commercially. Both methods rely on the peroxidase-like activity of the heme moiety in hemoglobin and myoglobin, which interacts with a chromagen to produce a color change proportional to concentration of heme-containing compounds. The test is more sensitive for hemoglobin and myoglobin but will react with intact erythrocytes. If erythrocytes are present, they are first lysed, and the pad can appear speckled (suggesting small numbers of erythrocytes) or exhibit a solid color change (suggesting a large number of erythrocytes). Any positive reaction should be interpreted with the microscopic evaluation of urine sediment.

INDICATIONS
- Evaluation of urine for heme protein is part of a routine urinalysis.
- Documentation of intravascular hemolysis
- Aid in identifying the cause of pigmenturia
- Aid in identifying the cause of proteinuria

CONTRAINDICATIONS
None

POTENTIAL COMPLICATIONS
None

CLIENT EDUCATION
Blood or substances containing heme that come from blood (*hemoglobin*) or muscle (*myoglobin*) should not be present in urine from healthy cats and dogs. Determining whether blood or heme is present in urine is part of a routine urinalysis. A positive reaction is important to know but is not specific for a disease or condition. If detected, further tests may be needed.

BODY SYSTEMS ASSESSED
- Hemic, lymphatic, and immune
- Musculoskeletal
- Renal and urologic

SAMPLE

COLLECTION
- 0.5–5 mL of urine, collected by free catch of a voided sample, manual expression of the urinary bladder, catheterization, or cystocentesis
- Urine should be collected prior to diagnostic procedures or administration of therapeutic agents.

HANDLING
- Collect urine into clean container free of additives, detergents, and chemicals.
- The container should be labeled with appropriate information (e.g., patient and owner identification; date, time, and method of collection).
- Ideally, the assay should be performed within ≤2 h.
- The urine should be well mixed immediately prior to analysis to ensure that erythrocytes will not be allowed to settle out of the suspension and will be included in the analysis.

STORAGE
- Refrigerate the urine if the sample cannot be analyzed soon after collection.
- Refrigerated urine should be stored in a container that can protect it from light and has a tight-fitting lid.
- Refrigerated samples should be warmed to room temperature before analysis.

STABILITY
Refrigerated urine stored for up to 8 h is probably suitable for analysis.

PROTOCOL
See the "Urinalysis Overview" chapter.

INTERPRETATION

NORMAL FINDINGS OR RANGE
Urine should be free of heme protein.

ABNORMAL VALUES
- A positive test reaction indicates the presence of erythrocytes, hemoglobin, and/or myoglobin.
- A positive test reaction can occur with as few as 5–20 erythrocytes/μL urine.

CRITICAL VALUES
None

INTERFERING FACTORS
Drugs That May Alter Results or Interpretation
Drugs That Interfere with Test Methodology
- Metabolized methenamine releases formaldehyde, which can interfere with the test reaction and cause a negative test result.
- Large amounts of ascorbic acid (from urinary acidifiers, vitamin therapy, or drug preservatives) potentially interfere with color reaction on reagent pad, causing a false-negative test result.
- False-negative (or decreased) test results may be caused by captopril.

Drugs That Alter Physiology
None

URINE HEME PROTEIN

Disorders That May Alter Results
- Gross pigmenturia may interfere with interpretation of the color change on the reagent pad.
- False-negative results may occur with highly concentrated urine.
- Erythrocytes will lyse in alkaline urine. The reagent pad will be positive, but no or few erythrocytes may be found on sediment examination.
- False-positive results can occur in urine containing peroxidases from bacteria, leukocytes, epithelial cells, or spermatozoa (the latter being unlikely).
- False-negative results can occur in urine where large amounts of bacterial nitrites delay the reaction on the reagent pad.

Collection Techniques or Handling That May Alter Results
- Blood can be introduced into urine during collection by cystocentesis, by catheterization, or by applying pressure to the urinary bladder, resulting in a positive result.
- False-positive results can occur in urine containing or contaminated with any of the following:
  - Bleach (sodium hypochlorite)
  - Oxidizing agents in disinfectants or detergents
  - A large amount of iodide or bromide (unlikely)
- False-negative results can occur in urine where
  - Erythrocytes have settled and sample is poorly mixed before tested (common).
  - Formalin is used as a urine preservative.

Influence of Signalment
Species
None

Breed
- Episodes of intravascular hemolysis with hemoglobinuria, triggered by respiratory alkalosis, are seen in phosphofructokinase-deficient English springer spaniels and cocker spaniels.
- Myoglobinuria, triggered by exertional lactic acidosis, has been reported in Old English sheepdogs that have mitochondrial myopathy.
- Hemoglobinuria can be seen in Bedlington terriers that have copper-associated liver disease if stress triggers acute hepatic necrosis and acute hemolysis caused by release of copper.
- Porphyria is a rare cause of intravascular hemolysis and hemoglobinuria in Siamese cats.

Age
None

Gender
None

Pregnancy
None

LIMITATIONS OF THE TEST
Sensitivity, Specificity, and Positive and Negative Predictive Values
- The practical sensitivity for commonly available reagent strips is as few as 5–20 erythrocytes/μL, which corresponds to a free hemoglobin concentration of $\approx$0.015–0.062 mg/dL.
- The practical sensitivity for detection of myoglobin has not been established.

Valid If Run in a Human Lab?
Yes.

Causes of Abnormal Findings
Hematuria
Renal/urinary causes
- Cystitis and/or urethritis: urinary tract infection, idiopathic cystitis (cats), urolithiasis, cyclophosphamide, or parasites (*Capillaria plica*)
- Renal associated: nephrosis/nephritis, infarct, renal pelvic hematoma, or parasites (*Dioctophyma renale*)
- Neoplasia: transitional cell carcinoma

Nonurinary causes
- Hematuria due to a systemic coagulopathy: anticoagulant rodenticide or disseminated intravascular hemolysis
- Iatrogenic: catheterization or cystocentesis
- Genital tract contamination: estrus, vaginal disease, uterine disease, preputial disease, prostatic disease, or neoplasia

Hemoglobinuria
Renal/urinary causes
Lysis of erythrocytes in alkaline and/or dilute urine

Nonurinary causes
- Intravascular hemolysis with hemoglobinemia: immune-mediated hemolytic anemia, babesiosis, leptospirosis, zinc toxicosis, incompatible blood transfusion, snake envenomation, hypotonic fluid therapy, neonatal isoerythrolysis, hypophosphatemia, or hemolytic uremic syndrome
- Drugs or chemicals: acetaminophen, benzocaine, methylene blue, NSAIDs, or vitamin K
- Infectious: anthrax, aspergillosis, *Mycoplasma haemofelis* (in cats, rarely), or *M. haemocanis* (in dogs, rarely), babesiosis, or blastomycosis
- Physical insults: trauma, severe burns, electric shock, or heatstroke
- Toxic plants: onion or sago palm
- Hypophosphatemia
- Systemic lupus erythematosus
- Genetic/congenital: pyruvate kinase deficiency, phosphofructokinase deficiency (in dogs), copper-associated liver disease (in Bedlington terriers), or congenital porphyria (in cats)

Myoglobinuria
- Acute severe muscle injury or necrosis: trauma, toxic, or ischemic
- Excessive exertion
- Exertional lactic acidosis/myopathy in Old English sheepdogs

CLINICAL PERSPECTIVE
- A positive urine heme protein test indicates hematuria, hemoglobinuria, or myoglobinuria. Any positive reaction should be interpreted in conjunction with microscopic evaluation of the urine sediment.
  - Hematuria is indicated by the presence of erythrocytes in the urine sediment.
  - In the absence of RBCs, myoglobinuria is suggested by significantly elevated serum CK and AST activity and normal-looking plasma. The animal's hematocrit and erythrocyte count are often normal.
  - In the absence of erythrocytes, hemoglobinuria is suggested by a low hematocrit and low RBC count and red serum or plasma. Serum CK activity is often normal, but the AST concentration may be elevated because of release of RBC cytosolic enzyme.
  - In the absence of erythrocytes, if the urine specific gravity is <1.008 or the pH is >8, consider hematuria with artifactual erythrocyte lysis.
- Hematuria is more common than hemoglobinuria. Myoglobinuria is uncommon in dogs and cats.

MISCELLANEOUS
ANCILLARY TESTS
- Biochemistry profile including AST and CK
- CBC
- Urine protein
- Urine sediment examination

SYNONYMS
- Urine blood test
- Urine heme

- Urine occult blood test

SEE ALSO
Blackwell's Five-Minute Veterinary Consult: Canine and Feline Topics
- Hematuria
- Hemoglobinuria and Myoglobinuria

Related Topics in This Book
- Creatine Kinase
- Red Blood Cell Count
- Red Blood Cell Morphology
- Urine Protein
- Urine Sediment

ABBREVIATIONS
- CK = creatine kinase
- IMHA = immune-mediated hemolytic anemia

Suggested Reading
Chew DJ, DiBartola SP. Urinalysis interpretation. In: *Interpretation of Canine and Feline Urinalysis*. Wilmington, DE: Ralston Purina, 1998: 15–33.

Gregory CR. Urinary system. In: Latimer KS, Mahaffey EA, Prasse KW, eds. *Duncan and Prasse's Veterinary Laboratory Medicine Clinical Pathology*, 4th ed. Ames: Iowa State Press, 2003: 231–259.
Osborne CA, Stevens JB. Biochemical analysis of urine: Indications, methods, interpretation. In: *Urinalysis: A Clinical Guide to Compassionate Patient Care*. Leverkusen, Germany: Bayer, 1999: 86–124.
Stockham SL, Scott MA. Urinary system. In: *Fundamentals of Veterinary Clinical Pathology*, 2nd ed. Ames, IA: Blackwell, 2008: 415–494.

INTERNET RESOURCES
Cornell University, College of Veterinary Medicine, Clinical Pathology Modules, http://www.diaglab.vet.cornell.edu/clinpath/modules/index.htm.

AUTHOR NAME
Karen E. Russell

URINE KETONES

BASICS

TYPE OF SPECIMEN
Urine

TEST EXPLANATION AND RELATED PHYSIOLOGY
Ketones (i.e., acetoacetate, β-hydroxybutyrate, and acetone) are the end product of rapid or excessive fatty-acid breakdown and occur with a shift from carbohydrates to lipids for energy production. In dogs and cats, this is usually due to an absolute insulin deficiency or an increase in cortisol, growth hormone, or epinephrine. Increased ketogenesis can also be the result of a carbohydrate deficiency (e.g., starvation, late-stage pregnancy).

Ketones are freely filtered by the glomerulus and completely re-sorbed by the proximal tubules under normal circumstances. The renal threshold for ketones is low, and ketonuria is frequently detectable prior to the development of ketonemia. Only acetoacetate and acetone are detectable by reagent strips or tablet tests, which are based on the reaction of acetoacetate (more reactive) and acetone (less reactive) with nitroprusside.

Urine (and blood) can be screened for ketones by using either reagent strips or tablets. The test pads on reagent strips are impreg-nated with nitroprusside, and the intensity of the color (beige to purple) is proportional to the amount of ketones present. The Acetest (Bayer, Leverkusen, Germany) is a tablet test based on the same re-actions as reagent strips but contains lactose to improve the quality of the color changes. A positive reaction is indicated by a lavender to deep purple, depending on the concentration of ketones. The Acetest is more sensitive than reagent strips and will detect 5 mg/dL of ketones compared with 10 mg/dL for dipsticks.

INDICATIONS
- Evaluation of patients with diabetes mellitus for ketoacidosis
- Assessment of patients with diseases associated with increased gluco-neogenesis and/or excessive catabolism of lipids
- Detection of pregnancy toxemia (hypoglycemia)

CONTRAINDICATIONS
None

POTENTIAL COMPLICATIONS
None

CLIENT EDUCATION
None

BODY SYSTEMS ASSESSED
- Endocrine and metabolic
- Reproductive

SAMPLE

COLLECTION
1–5 mL of urine collected by any method

HANDLING
- Collect the urine prior to medical therapy or contrast radiography.
- Collect the urine into a clean, dry container with a tight-fitting lid and free of additives, detergents, and chemicals.
- Ideally, assay within ≤1 h. If analysis is delayed, refrigerate the sample in a closed container.
- Rewarm the sample to room temperature before analysis.

STORAGE
- Acetone is highly volatile, so it should be stored in containers with tight-fitting lids.
- Freezing is acceptable but will compromise components in sediment.

STABILITY
- Room temperature: 1 h
- Refrigerated (2°–8°C): 24 h

PROTOCOL
See the "Urinalysis Overview" chapter.

INTERPRETATION

NORMAL FINDINGS OR RANGE
Negative test result

ABNORMAL VALUES
Ketonuria in dogs and cats is abnormal.

CRITICAL VALUES
None

INTERFERING FACTORS
Drugs That May Alter Results or Interpretation
Drugs That Interfere with Test Methodology
- Substances containing free sulfhydryl groups such as captopril, D-penicillamine, 2-mercaptoproprionyl glycine, and cystine may cause false-positive results.
- Levodopa metabolites may cause false-positive reactions.
- Sulfobromophthalein or phenolsulfonphthalein dyes may lead to a reddish change in alkaline urine similar to a positive ketone reaction.

Drugs That Alter Physiology
None

Disorders That May Alter Results
Hemoglobinuria or myoglobinuria may interfere with interpretation of reagent strip color changes.

Collection Techniques or Handling That May Alter Results
- Delayed analysis, especially if the sample is left at room temperature
- Exposure of the reagent pad to heat, moisture, or light

Influence of Signalment
Species
None

Breed
None

Age
Young animals are more prone to developing ketonuria.

Gender
None

Pregnancy
Pregnancy toxemia (hypoglycemia and ketonemia) is a rare syndrome in the pregnant bitch.

LIMITATIONS OF THE TEST
Sensitivity, Specificity, and Positive and Negative Predictive Values
The lower limit of sensitivity is 5–10 mg/dL for acetoacetic acid and 70 mg/dL for acetone.

Valid If Run in a Human Lab?
Yes.

Causes of Abnormal Findings

High values	Low values
Impaired use of carbohydrates	Not significant
Diabetes mellitus	
Functional endocrine tumors (e.g., pituitary	
adenomas, adrenal tumors,	
glucagonomas)	
Glycogen storage disease	
Carbohydrate deficiency	
Starvation, anorexia, and/or persistent	
fever	
Persistent hypoglycemia (e.g., insulinoma)	
Strenuous exercise (dogs)	
Low-carbohydrate, high-fat diets	
Pregnancy toxemia	
Carbohydrate loss	
Renal tubular disorders	

CLINICAL PERSPECTIVE

- The Acetest should be performed as a confirmatory test when positive reagent strip test results are unexpected or occur in pigmented urine.
- Decreased tissue perfusion (e.g., shock) leads to increased production of β-hydroxybutyrate (β-OHB). Hence, severe ketosis may go undetected by routine laboratory tests.
- In diabetic animals, insulin treatment prompts metabolism of β-OHB to acetoacetate. Hence, the degree of ketonuria may appear to increase in some diabetic animals despite clinical improvement.
- β-OHB is best measured through a specific assay. Modification of the reagent-strip assay by premixing urine with 30% hydrogen peroxide to convert β-OHB to acetoacetate is not recommended because of the relative insensitivity of this method.
- In an animal with ketonurias, a decreased bicarbonate value and elevated anion gap suggest titration acidosis consistent with ketoacidosis.

MISCELLANEOUS

ANCILLARY TESTS

- Serum β-OHB, either using a handheld meter and a ketostrip (PrecisionXtra; Abbott, Alameda, CA) or enzymatically assayed by a diagnostic laboratory

- Serum biochemistry panel to evaluate glucose, anion gap, and total carbon dioxide

SYNONYMS
None

SEE ALSO
Blackwell's Five-Minute Veterinary Consult: Canine and Feline Topics
- Diabetes Mellitus with Hyperosmolar Coma
- Diabetes Mellitus with Ketoacidosis
- Diabetes Mellitus without Complication—Cats
- Diabetes Mellitus without Complication—Dogs
- Glucosuria

Related Topics in This Book
- General Principles for Performing Urine Tests
- Glucose
- Glucose Curve
- Glycosylated Hemoglobin
- Urinalysis Overview

ABBREVIATIONS
β-OHB = β-hydroxybutyrate

Suggested Reading
Gregory CR. Urinary system. In: Prasse KW, Latimer KS, Mahaffey EA, eds. *Duncan and Prasse's Veterinary Laboratory Medicine*, 4th ed. Ames: Iowa State Press, 2003: 231–259.
Hoenig M, Dorfman M, Koenig A. Use of a hand-held meter for the measurement of blood beta-hydroxybutyrate in dogs and cats. *J Vet Emerg Crit Care* 2008; 18: 86–87.
Osborne CA, Stevens JB. *Urinalysis: A Clinical Guide to Compassionate Patient Care*. Leverkusen, Germany: Bayer, 1999: 99–101.
Stockham SL, Scott MA. Urinary System. In: *Fundamentals of Veterinary Clinical Pathology*, 2nd ed Ames: Iowa State Press, 2008: 415–494.

INTERNET RESOURCES
None

AUTHOR NAMES
Angela Wilcox and Karen E. Russell

URINE PH

BASICS

TYPE OF SPECIMEN
Urine

TEST EXPLANATION AND RELATED PHYSIOLOGY
Acid-base homeostasis is regulated largely by the renal and respiratory systems. The kidneys excrete protons (usually in the form of phosphorus or ammonium) and/or retain bicarbonate. Urine pH can be used to estimate a patient's acid-base status, but should not be the only method used to evaluate that status. Abnormal plasma chloride and potassium levels can interfere with the kidney's ability to compensate for acid-base abnormalities.

Urine pH influences the types of crystals or uroliths that form in urine. Calcium oxalate, amorphous urate, uric acid crystals and cystine, and uric acid uroliths are typically found in acidic urine. Crystals found in alkaline urine include struvite (triple phosphate), amorphous phosphate, calcium carbonate, calcium phosphate, and ammonium biurate. Magnesium ammonium phosphate and calcium phosphate uroliths generally form in alkaline urine.

There are several possible methods for determining urine pH. Reagent strips designed for urinalysis are most commonly used. Reagent pads for pH determination on the dipstick contain 2 color indicators that enable pH detection in the broad range of 5–9. The reaction occurs fairly rapidly and needs to be read within the recommended time frame (generally 60 s). The urine pH is estimated to the nearest 0.5 pH unit. Pigmenturia or an abnormal urine color may interfere with reading the reaction and interpreting the results. Reagent strips should be stored according to the manufacturer's recommendations.

Although not commonly used in clinical practice because of their expense, pH meters are more accurate than reagent strips. Occasionally small, handheld pH meters are used to evaluate patients at risk of urolith formation or confirm results from a reagent pad if there is color interference. Certain types of pH paper, with a wide pH range (e.g., 5.5–9.0), can also be used to determine urine pH. Litmus paper or nitrazine paper is either too insensitive or has too narrow a detection range to be useful.

INDICATIONS
- Part of a routine urinalysis
- Estimation of the animal's acid-base status
- Helpful in predicting urolith formation and monitoring therapy for uroliths

CONTRAINDICATIONS
None

POTENTIAL COMPLICATIONS
None

CLIENT EDUCATION
- If urine is collected by the owner, an appropriate container should be provided to avoid possible contamination with detergents, disinfectants, or other substances, which can affect urine pH.
- Urine should be collected prior to a meal to avoid alkaline tide.

BODY SYSTEMS ASSESSED
- Endocrine and metabolic
- Renal and urologic

SAMPLE

COLLECTION
1–5 mL of urine collected by any method

HANDLING
Collect the urine into a clean, dry container with a tight-fitting lid and free of potential contaminants.

STORAGE
- Analyze the sample within 1–2 h after collection.
- If analysis will be delayed, the sample can be refrigerated in a container with a tight-fitting lid.
- Warm refrigerated samples to room temperature before analysis.

STABILITY
Refrigerated urine stored for up to 8 h is probably suitable for analysis.

PROTOCOL
None

INTERPRETATION

NORMAL FINDINGS OR RANGE
Typically, urine pH from normal dogs and cats falls between 6.0 and 7.5 but can range as widely as 5.5–8.0.

ABNORMAL VALUES
- <6.0
- >7.5

CRITICAL VALUES
None

INTERFERING FACTORS
Drugs That May Alter Results or Interpretation
Drugs That Interfere with Test Methodology
None

Drugs That Alter Physiology
- Acidifying agents: ammonium chloride, ascorbic acid, citric acid, furosemide, D,L-methionine, and phosphate salts
- Alkalinizing agents: acetazolamide, chlorothiazide, potassium citrate, sodium acetate, sodium bicarbonate, and sodium lactate

Disorders That May Alter Results
None

Collection Techniques or Handling That May Alter Results
- Urine becomes more alkaline with time; therefore, the pH should be determined on a fresh sample.
- Urine can become alkaline if contaminated with detergents or disinfectants.
- Collection of urine soon after a meal may show postprandial urine alkalinization (alkaline tide) in response to increased secretion of hydrogen chloride by the stomach.

Influence of Signalment
Species
None

Breed
None

Age
None

Gender
None

Pregnancy
None

LIMITATIONS OF THE TEST
Sensitivity, Specificity, and Positive and Negative Predictive Values
N/A

Valid If Run in a Human Lab?
Yes.

Causes of Abnormal Findings

High values (alkalinuria)	Low value (aciduria)
Vegetable or cereal-based diets	High-protein, meat, or milk-based diets
Postprandial alkaline tide	
Urine left exposed to air at room temperature or if there is a delay in urinalysis	Urinary tract infection with non–urease-producing organisms
Urinary tract infection with urease-producing organisms (e.g., *Proteus, Staphylococcus*)	Acidifying agents
	Metabolic or respiratory acidosis
	Catabolic states
Alkalinizing agents	Complete anorexia
Metabolic or respiratory alkalosis	Hypochloridemic, hypokalemic metabolic alkalosis from upper GI obstruction (i.e., paradoxical aciduria)
Distal renal tubular acidosis	
Proximal renal tubular acidosis (early)	
	Proximal renal tubular acidosis (if bicarbonate is depleted)
	Furosemide therapy

CLINICAL PERSPECTIVE
• Urine pH influences the types of crystals or uroliths that form in urine. It may be useful in predicting the type of urolith found prior to mineral analysis.
• If an acidotic patient has urine that is not acidic, consider renal tubular acidosis, a condition where the kidneys are not able to acidify urine.

 MISCELLANEOUS

ANCILLARY TESTS
• Blood-gas analysis
• Serum biochemistry profile (total carbon dioxide and anion gap)

SYNONYMS
None

SEE ALSO
Blackwell's Five-Minute Veterinary Consult: Canine and Feline Topics
• Chapters on specific types of urolithiasis
• Acidosis, Metabolic
• Alkalosis, Metabolic
• Crystalluria
• Renal Tubular Acidosis
Related Topics in This Book
• Urinalysis Overview
• Urolith Analysis

ABBREVIATIONS
None

Suggested Reading
Chew DJ, DiBartola SP. Urinalysis interpretation. In: *Interpretation of Canine and Feline Urinalysis*. Wilmington, DE: Ralston Purina, 1998: 15–33.
Osborne CA, Stevens JB. Biochemical analysis of urine: Indications, methods, interpretation. In: *Urinalysis: A Clinical Guide to Compassionate Patient Care*. Leverkusen, Germany: Bayer, 1999: 86–124.

INTERNET RESOURCES
Cornell University, College of Veterinary Medicine, Clinical Pathology Modules, http://www.diaglab.vet.cornell.edu/clinpath/modules/index.htm.

AUTHOR NAME
Karen E. Russell

URINE PROTEIN

BASICS

TYPE OF SPECIMEN
Urine

TEST EXPLANATION AND RELATED PHYSIOLOGY
Limited filtration of low molecular weight proteins (MW, <65 kD) occurs in the glomeruli. In health, most proteins are resorbed by the proximal tubules. There is minimal secretion of mucoproteins by the loop of Henle and distal tubules so that protein concentration in urine is negligible.

Proteinuria implies an abnormal amount of protein in the urine. This can be caused by prerenal factors that overload the renal tubules (e.g., hemoglobinuria, myoglobinuria, Bence-Jones proteinuria). Renal proteinuria can be caused by damage to either glomeruli or renal tubules, although moderate to marked protein is more typically associated with glomerular disease. Finally, mild proteinuria is commonly associated with inflammation or hemorrhage somewhere in the urogenital tract. Although these processes might be localized to the kidneys, they often involve the lower urinary tract (postrenal proteinuria). Evaluation of urine for protein is part of a routine urinalysis. Positive results should be interpreted with knowledge of the method of sample collection, urine specific gravity (USG), urine sediment, and other clinical findings. When detected, proteinuria should be confirmed with additional testing. The absence of proteinuria does not rule out renal disease.

Screening is usually done with urine dipsticks and is semiquantitative. Urine dipsticks have a reagent pad for detecting protein. The pad contains an acidic pH indicator that changes color when amino groups of negatively charged proteins bind and react with the indicator dye. The color change is proportional to the concentration of protein in urine. Reactions are graded as trace, 1+, 2+, 3+, or 4+ and detect protein concentrations in the approximate range of ≥30–2,000 mg/dL. The method is more sensitive for albumin; does not reliably detect globulins, Bence-Jones proteins, hemoglobin, or mucoproteins; and reacts poorly with cellular proteins (i.e., leukocytes, epithelial cells). A negative dipstick result does not rule out the presence of these proteins. Urine does not need to be centrifuged prior to performing this method.

Sulfasalicylic acid (SSA) is used as a confirmatory test for proteinuria and relies on acid precipitation of protein. A 5% stock solution of reagent-grade SSA is made, and equal parts of urine and the SSA solution are mixed. SSA denatures protein and causes increasing turbidity proportional to the protein concentration. It is also semiquantitative and is graded on a 1 to 4+ scale. SSA reacts better with albumin than globulins, can detect Bence-Jones proteins, and can be helpful in differentiating a false-positive reaction on the reagent pad because of alkaline urine. Urine should be centrifuged prior to performing this method so that any cloudiness in the urine sample does not interfere with interpretation of the results.

INDICATIONS
- Evaluation of urine for protein is part of a routine urinalysis.
- The potential loss of protein into the urine should be investigated in any hypoproteinemic animal.

CONTRAINDICATIONS
None

POTENTIAL COMPLICATIONS
None

CLIENT EDUCATION
- Detection of proteinuria is considered an abnormal finding that should be further investigated. Proteinuria can be due to renal or nonrenal causes.

- A negative urine dipstick protein result does not rule out renal disease.

BODY SYSTEMS ASSESSED
- Hemic, lymphatic, and immune
- Renal and urologic

SAMPLE

COLLECTION
- 0.5–5.0 mL of urine collected by free catch of a voided sample, manual expression of the urinary bladder, catheterization, or cystocentesis
- Urine should be collected prior to diagnostic procedures or the administration of therapeutic agents.

HANDLING
- Collect the urine into a clean, dry container that has a tight-fitting lid and is free of potential contaminants (e.g., detergents, disinfectants).
- The container should be labeled with appropriate information (e.g., patient and owner identification; date, time, and method of collection).

STORAGE
- Fresh or refrigerated urine samples can be used.
- Urine should not be frozen and thawed because this can precipitate or denature proteins and interfere with test results.

STABILITY
- Ideally, refrigerated samples should be analyzed within 48 h, although stability up to 4 weeks has been reported.
- Avoid the use of urine preservatives because these will interfere with protein determination.

PROTOCOL
See the "Urinalysis Overview" chapter.

INTERPRETATION

NORMAL FINDINGS OR RANGE
- Urine should be free of protein in normal dogs and cats.
- In moderately to highly concentrated urine samples (USG, >1.030), a trace or 1+ protein reaction on a urine dipstick may be seen as an artifact in healthy dogs and cats.

ABNORMAL VALUES
- Results should be interpreted in conjunction with the USG and urine sediment. The presence of proteinuria in poorly concentrated urine is clinically significant.
- Persistent proteinuria found on screening tests (i.e., urine dipsticks) should be confirmed with other tests such as SSA or urine protein/creatinine ratio.

CRITICAL VALUES
None

INTERFERING FACTORS
Drugs That May Alter Results or Interpretation
Drugs That Interfere with Test Methodology
- False-positive results on dipsticks can occur with either of the following:
  - Phenazopyridine
  - Acetazolamide (increases urine pH)
- False-positive results with SSA can occur with any of the following:
  - X-ray contrast media

- Tolbutamide
- Large doses of penicillin, cephaloridine, cephalothin, sulfisoxazole, or aminoglycosides
- Tolmetin sodium

Drugs That Alter Physiology
Prednisone can cause proteinuria. The mechanism is not known.

Disorders That May Alter Results
Reagent Pad
- Conditions leading to significant pigmenturia (e.g., hematuria, hemoglobinuria, myoglobinuria, bilirubinuria) may interfere with the interpretation of the color change on the reagent pad.
- False-positive results can occur with alkaline urine (pH, >8).
- Weak false-positive results (trace to 1+) can be seen as an artifact in moderately to markedly concentrated urine (SG, >1.030) if the buffering capacity of the test pad is overwhelmed.
- False-negative results can occur with Bence-Jones proteins.

SSA
- False-positive results with SSA can occur if urine is cloudy or if urine contains large numbers of crystals (coprecipitation of protein with crystals). Centrifugation and use of the supernatant will often resolve this problem.
- False-negative results with SSA can occur with either of the following:
  - Highly buffered alkaline urine
  - Cloudy urine that prevents reading changes in turbidity after the addition of SSA

Collection Techniques or Handling That May Alter Results
- The collection method (e.g., cystocentesis, catheterization) may introduce blood (and hence plasma protein) into a urine sample during collection.
- False-positive results on the reagent pads can occur with urine contamination with disinfectants (e.g., chlorhexidine, quaternary ammonium compounds such as benzalkonium chloride).
- False-positive results with SSA can occur if the sample is contaminated with the urine preservatives thymol and para-aminosalicylic acid.
- False-negative results on the reagent pads can occur if the urine sample has been acidified after collection.

Influence of Signalment
Species
None

Breed
- Hereditary glomerulopathy: Bernese mountain dogs, bull terriers, Dalmatians, Doberman pinschers, English cocker spaniels, Newfoundlands, rottweilers, and soft-coated Wheaten terriers
- Familial amyloidosis: sharpeis, Abyssinians, beagles, and English foxhounds
- Cutaneous and renal glomerular vasculopathy: greyhounds

Age
Neonatal puppies and kittens may have a mild, physiologic proteinuria that coincides with protein absorption from the gut. This proteinuria will peak at ≈20 h of life and can last for up to 10 days.

Gender
None

Pregnancy
None

LIMITATIONS OF THE TEST
Sensitivity, Specificity, and Positive and Negative Predictive Values

- Generally, reagent pads on a dipstick can detect protein in the range between 5–30 and 2,000 mg/dL or greater.
- The SSA test can detect protein in the range between 5 and 5,000 mg/dL or greater.
- The following approximate protein concentrations are needed to cause a trace to 1+ reaction on a reagent pad:
  - Albumin, 14–21 mg/dL
  - Hemoglobin, 5–50 mg/dL
  - α-Globulin, 20–30 mg/dL
  - β-Globulin, 40–50 mg/dL
  - γ-Globulin, >1,000 mg/dL
  - Light chains (κ and λ), 26–52 mg/dL

Valid If Run in a Human Lab?
Yes.

Causes of Abnormal Findings: Positive Results (Proteinuria)
Hematuria: Hemorrhage into the Urinary Tract
- Iatrogenic (i.e., artifact of catheterization, cystocentesis)
- Neoplasia
- Secondary to inflammation/infection
- Trauma

Inflammation within the Urinary Tract
- Bacterial infection
- Fungal infection (uncommon)
- Neoplasia
- Urolithiasis

Renal Disease
- Amyloidosis
- Glomerular: increased filtration of protein (acquired, congenital, or hereditary glomerulonephropathies)
- Parenchymal inflammation
- Tubular: increased secretion, failure of resorption, or leakage (toxicosis or hypoxia)

Nonrenal Proteinuria
- Bence-Jones proteinuria
- Cardiac disease with hypertension
- Fever
- Genital tract contamination: hemorrhage, infection, inflammation, or neoplasia
- Hemoglobinuria
- Muscular exertion (myoglobinuria)
- Shock

CLINICAL PERSPECTIVE
- Detection of proteinuria is considered an abnormal finding that should be further investigated.
- Proteinuria should be interpreted in conjunction with USG and microscopic examination of urine sediment.
  - The presence of increased numbers of RBCs suggests that proteinuria is caused by hemorrhage.
  - The presence of increased WBCs suggests that proteinuria is due to inflammation.
- Proteinuria can be due to renal or nonrenal causes.
- Persistent moderate to marked proteinuria (3 to 4+), in the absence of hemoglobinuria, myoglobinuria, hematuria, or pyuria, is generally caused by glomerular disease.
- Proteinuria caused by tubular disease is usually mild.
- A negative urine dipstick protein result does not rule out renal disease.
- If the urine is highly concentrated or alkaline, a weak positive (trace to 1+) dipstick protein result should be followed by other methods for documenting proteinuria, because it can be difficult to know whether the dipstick reaction is an artifact or a sign of a pathologic process.

URINE PROTEIN

MISCELLANEOUS

ANCILLARY TESTS
- Biochemistry panel (especially albumin)
- CBC
- Urine protein/creatinine ratio
- USG and sediment examination

SYNONYMS
None

SEE ALSO
Blackwell's Five-Minute Veterinary Consult: Canine and Feline Topics
- Amyloidosis
- Glomerulonephritis
- Hematuria
- Nephrotic Syndrome
- Paraproteinemia
- Proteinuria
- Pyuria

Related Topics in This Book
- Albumin
- Urine Albumin
- Urine Heme Protein
- Urine Protein/Creatinine Ratio
- Urine Sediment
- Urine Specific Gravity

ABBREVIATIONS
- SSA = sulfasalicylic acid
- USG = urine specific gravity

Suggested Reading

Chew DJ, DiBartola SP. Urinalysis interpretation. In: *Interpretation of Canine and Feline Urinalysis*. Wilmington, DE: Ralston Purina, 1998: 15–33.

Gregory CR. Urinary system. In: Latimer KS, Mahaffey EA, Prasse KW, eds. *Duncan and Prasse's Veterinary Laboratory Medicine Clinical Pathology*, 4th ed. Ames: Iowa State Press, 2003: 231–259.

Osborne CA, Stevens JB. Proteinuria. In: *Urinalysis: A Clinical Guide to Compassionate Patient Care*. Leverkusen, Germany: Bayer, 1999: 111–121.

Stockham SL, Scott MA. Urinary System. In: *Fundamentals of Veterinary Clinical Pathology*, 2nd ed. Ames, IA: Blackwell, 2008: 415–494.

INTERNET RESOURCES
Cornell University, College of Veterinary Medicine, Clinical Pathology Modules, http://www.diaglab.vet.cornell.edu/clinpath/modules/index.htm.
University of Iowa, Carver College of Medicine, Continuing Medical Education, Urinalysis: Part I, http://www.medicine.uiowa.edu/cme/clia/modules.asp?testID=19.

AUTHOR NAME
Karen E. Russell

BASICS

TYPE OF SPECIMEN
Urine

TEST EXPLANATION AND RELATED PHYSIOLOGY
The *urine protein/creatinine ratio* (UPC) is an index of magnitude of proteinuria used to assess patients with proteinuria caused by renal disease, and it has been shown to correlate well with 24-h protein excretion. Total daily creatinine excretion depends mostly on muscle mass and is therefore relatively constant in a single patient. Normal urine should contain little protein when compared with the creatinine level, because proteins (usually <60 kD) that are normally filtered through the glomerulus are almost completely reabsorbed by the proximal tubule. Thus, low UPC values are considered normal. Protein and creatinine levels are comparably affected by changes in urine volume; therefore, the UPC is not affected by urine concentration or volume. Causes of increased UPC can be divided into 3 categories:

- Prerenal proteinuria (tubular overload): increased filtered immunoglobulin fragments, free hemoglobin, or myoglobin
- Renal proteinuria: glomerular disease such as glomerulonephritis and amyloidosis, interstitial nephritis, tubular damage or defects, and *functional proteinuria* (altered renal physiology without renal lesions; e.g., due to exercise, extreme heat or cold, fever, seizures, venous congestion)
- Postrenal proteinuria: hemorrhage or exudative processes of the renal pelvis, ureter, bladder, urethra, and/or genital tract. This is the most common cause of a mild proteinuria, and it is typically associated with an active sediment.

UPCs tend to be highest in patients with glomerular lesions, and UPC monitoring is of greatest interest when proteinuria is caused by glomerular disease. Glomerular disease alters glomerular permeability and can be caused by glomerulonephritis (usually immune mediated), amyloidosis, glomerulosclerosis, or hereditary nephropathy. Measurement of the UPC is not recommended when active inflammation or macroscopic hemorrhage is observed; however, glomerular proteinuria may be present in addition to these conditions. Therefore, detection of a large amount of protein by dipstick and/or sulfasalicylic acid (SSA) turbidometric test warrants reevaluation of urine protein when postrenal diseases have resolved.

Urine protein and urine creatinine can be determined quantitatively and semiquantitatively. For quantitative determination using a chemistry analyzer, urine protein is measured with a colorimetric or turbidometric method. Creatinine is generally measured using either an enzymatic method (e.g., creatinine amidohydrolase) or Jaffe's reaction (picrate ion). The UPC is determined by dividing an individual's urine protein concentration (UP) by the urine creatinine concentration (UC): UP (mg/dL)/UC (mg/dL). When monitoring a patient's UPC, samples should be analyzed by a single laboratory to minimize analytical variation. Semiquantitative dipstick methods are available for UPC estimation, but little published information exists regarding their accuracy. A recent study (Welles et al. 2006) determined that the Multistix PRO (Bayer Corporation, Elkhart, IN) reported fairly reliable results in dogs but not cats.

The UPC in a single patient can vary substantially from day to day without a significant change in underlying renal disease. In general, values that differ by ≈50% or more are suggestive of an actual change in magnitude of proteinuria. Serial monitoring to determine trends is also recommended to determine whether the UPC is increasing or decreasing in a patient.

INDICATIONS
To assess magnitude of proteinuria when
- proteinuria is detected by urine dipstick or SSA test without concurrent inflammation, hemorrhage, and/or bacteria

- evaluating prognosis and progression of acute and chronic renal disease
- monitoring proteinuria-reducing therapy
- screening geriatric patients for renal disease
- a patient has chronic illnesses known to become complicated by glomerular disease (e.g., dirofilariasis, chronic bacterial infections, neoplasia, systemic lupus erythematosus)

CONTRAINDICATIONS
- Highly active urine sediment (WBCs with or without bacteria)
- Macroscopic hematuria
- Glucocorticoid therapy

POTENTIAL COMPLICATIONS
None

CLIENT EDUCATION
A normal result does not rule out renal disease, especially in cats.

BODY SYSTEMS ASSESSED
- Cardiovascular
- Endocrine and metabolic
- Renal and urologic

SAMPLE

COLLECTION
0.5–1.0 mL of urine collected by cystocentesis or midstream voided sample

HANDLING
- Centrifuge the urine (<2,000 RPM) for ≈5 min.
- Transfer a minimum of 0.5 mL of supernatant to a clean container.
- Transport the sample on ice to the laboratory.

STORAGE
Store in a refrigerator.

STABILITY
- Room temperature: at least 4 h (protein) and 3 days (creatinine)
- Refrigerated (2°–8°C): at least 3 days (protein) and 5 days (creatinine)
- Freezing is not recommended because proteins may precipitate out of solution.

PROTOCOL
None

INTERPRETATION

NORMAL FINDINGS OR RANGE
- Dogs: <0.5
- Cats: <0.4

ABNORMAL VALUES
- A single measurement where UPC is >2 (dogs) or >1 (cats)
- A UPC between 0.5–2 (dogs) or 0.4–1 (cats) on 3 or more consecutive measurements 2–4 weeks apart (persistent proteinuria)

CRITICAL VALUES
None

INTERFERING FACTORS
Drugs That May Alter Results or Interpretation
Drugs That Interfere with Test Methodology
Gentamicin may increase protein detected via the Ponceau S dye method (trichloroacetic acid solution).

Drugs That Alter Physiology
Drugs that may potentially increase proteinuria
- By glomerular mechanisms: D-penicillamine, methimazole, captopril, or pyrithioxine
- By tubular damage and/or interstitial nephritis: aminoglycosides, ampicillin, cephalosporins, rifampin, sulfonamides, allopurinol, or bisphosphonates
- By unknown mechanisms: prednisone

Drugs that may potentially decrease proteinuria
Angiotensin-converting enzyme (ACE) inhibitors may decrease proteinuria through their hemodynamic effects (i.e., decreased glomerular pressure), altering glomerular permselectivity, and/or preserving glomerular structure.

Disorders That May Alter Results
- Bilirubin, lipids, and acetoacetate may decrease measured creatinine, and acetone and glucose increase measured creatinine when determined by Jaffe's reaction.
- Severe IV hemolysis or rhabdomyolysis may increase protein.
- A high-protein diet can increase protein excretion in patients with glomerular disease.
- Active inflammation and macroscopic hematuria may increase protein, but microscopic hematuria alone appears to have little, if any, effect on the UPC.

Collection Techniques or Handling That May Alter Results
- Increased protein may be seen in voided samples because of urogenital contamination and with cystocentesis if collection is traumatic and causes gross hematuria.
- Failure to centrifuge the sample and separate the supernatant may increase protein measured by turbidometric methods.

Influence of Signalment
Species
Cats uncommonly have a UPC of >1.

Breed
- Hereditary glomerulopathy: Bernese mountain dogs, bull terriers, Dalmatians, Doberman pinschers, English cocker spaniels, Newfoundlands, rottweilers, and soft-coated Wheaten terriers
- Familial amyloidosis: sharpeis, Abyssinians, beagles, and English foxhounds
- Cutaneous and renal glomerular vasculopathy: greyhounds
- Fanconi's syndrome: basenjis

Age
Puppies may have mild transient increases in the UPC (usually a UPC of <2; higher if puppies are <3 days old). A similar phenomenon has not yet been reported in kittens.

Gender
None

Pregnancy
Unknown

LIMITATIONS OF THE TEST
- It cannot distinguish among the various causes of proteinuria. Screening for diseases that cause prerenal and postrenal proteinuria is necessary to determine the origin of the protein.
- The absence of proteinuria does not rule out renal disease, especially in cats.

Sensitivity, Specificity, and Positive and Negative Predictive Values
- An abnormal UPC can be more sensitive than serum creatinine evaluation in detecting renal disease.
- Specificity depends on appropriate screening for prerenal and postrenal causes of proteinuria. If proteinuria is determined to be persistent and renal in origin, a UPC of >2 is considered specific for pathologic renal disease.

Valid If Run in a Human Lab?
Yes.

Causes of Abnormal Findings: High Values
Postrenal
- Cystitis: bacterial, idiopathic cystitis (cats), mycotic (e.g., *Aspergillus*, *Candida*), or toxic (cyclophosphamide)
- Hemorrhage: trauma or coagulopathy
- Neoplasia: transitional cell carcinoma
- Pyelitis
- Ureteritis
- Urolithiasis
- If the sample is voided, consider a genital tract origin (e.g., normal secretions, inflammation, neoplasia) in addition to the aforementioned causes.

Renal
Glomerular
- Glomerulonephritis: membranous, mesangioproliferative, or membranoproliferative
  - Immune mediated: idiopathic, neoplasia (e.g., lymphoma, mastocytosis, leukemia, primary erythrocytosis), bacterial (e.g., chronic pyoderma, pyometra, septicemia, brucellosis, borreliosis), rickettsial (e.g., ehrlichiosis), parasitism (e.g., dirofilariasis, leishmaniasis, babesiosis, trypanosomiasis), pancreatitis, viral (e.g., FeLV, FIP, infectious canine hepatitis), or autoimmune disease (e.g., SLE)
  - Endocrine: hyperadrenocorticism
  - Infectious: infectious canine hepatitis virus
  - Cutaneous and renal glomerular vasculopathy of greyhounds
  - Drugs: sulfadiazine in Doberman pinschers
- Amyloidosis: reactive (secondary) to chronic systemic inflammatory diseases, plasma cell myeloma, or familial
- Glomerulosclerosis: diabetes mellitus, systemic hypertension, or idiopathic or end-stage glomerular disease
- Minimal change disease
- Hereditary glomerulopathy

Tubulointerstitial
- Acute or chronic tubulointerstitial nephritis: leptospirosis, infectious canine hepatitis, FIP, or fungal
- Tubular necrosis: hypoxia, drugs (aminoglycosides), or ethylene glycol
- Pyelonephritis
- Neoplasia: lymphoma or renal carcinoma
- Tubular defect: Fanconi's syndrome: acquired or hereditary
- *Dioctophyma renale*

Other
- Hyperthyroidism (cats)
- Hypertension

Functional (poorly documented in veterinary patients)
- Exercise
- Extreme heat or extreme cold
- Fever
- Seizures
- Venous congestion

Prerenal
- Intravascular hemolysis: immune-mediated hemolytic disease, zinc toxicity, babesiosis, or hypotonic fluid administration
- Neoplasia: plasma cell myeloma, or B-cell lymphoma or leukemia
- Rhabdomyolysis

CLINICAL PERSPECTIVE
- A persistently increased UPC with an inactive sediment and normal or decreased serum protein is supportive of renal disease.
- A UPC persistently of >2 may be an indication for treatment.
- The higher the UPC, the more likely glomerular disease is present.

• A single mildly elevated UPC (<2) may not be significant if it is due to transient proteinuria.

MISCELLANEOUS

ANCILLARY TESTS
• Abdominal ultrasound
• Antinuclear antibody test
• Blood pressure
• Chemistry panel (especially total protein and globulins)
• Radiography
• Renal biopsy
• Tests for infectious diseases (e.g., heartworm antigen test, FeLV/FIV, tick panel)
• Urine culture
• Urine sediment examination

SYNONYMS
None

SEE ALSO
Blackwell's Five-Minute Veterinary Consult: Canine and Feline Topics
• Amyloidosis
• Glomerulonephritis
• Hypoalbuminemia
• Nephrotic Syndrome
• Proteinuria

Related Topics in This Book
• Urine Heme Protein
• Urine Protein
• Urine Sediment

ABBREVIATIONS
• SLE = sytemic lupus erythematosus
• SSA = sulfasalicylic acid turbidometric [test]
• UPC = urine protein/creatinine ratio

Suggested Reading
Lees GE, Brown SA, Elliott J, *et al.* Assessment and management of proteinuria in dogs and cats: 2004 ACVIM Forum Consensus Statement (small animal). *J Vet Intern Med* 2005; 19: 377–385.
Nabity MB, Boggess MM, Kashtan CE, Lees GE. Day-to-Day Variation of the Urine Protein: Creatinine Ratio in Female Dogs with Stable Glomerular Proteinuria Caused by X-Linked Hereditary Nephropathy. *J Vet Intern Med* 2007; 21: 425–430.
Osborne CA, Stevens JB. Proteinuria. In: *Urinalysis: A Clinical Guide to Compassionate Patient Care.* Leverkusen, Germany: Bayer, 1999: 111–121.
Vaden SL, Pressler BM, Lappin MR, Jensen WA. Effects of urinary tract inflammation and sample blood contamination on urine albumin and total protein concentrations in canine urine samples. *Vet Clin Pathol* 2004; 33: 14–19.
Welles EG, Whatley EM, Hall AS, Wright JC. Comparison of Multistix PRO dipsticks with other biochemical assays for determining urine protein (UP), urine creatinine (UC) and UP:UC ratio in dogs and cats. *Vet Clin Pathol* 2006; 35: 31–36.

INTERNET RESOURCES
IDEXX Laboratories, IDEXX VetLab Suite: IDEXX VetTest chemistry analyzer, http://www.idexx.com/animalhealth/analyzers/vettest/chemistries/upc/faqs.jsp.

AUTHOR NAME
Mary B. Nabity

URINE SEDIMENT

BASICS

TYPE OF SPECIMEN
Urine

TEST EXPLANATION AND RELATED PHYSIOLOGY
Microscopic evaluation of urine is recommended on every urine sample, even when physical characteristics or the results from a urine dipstick are unremarkable. Components evaluated include cells, crystals, casts, organisms, and other elements (e.g., lipid, mucus). Erythrocytes can enter the urine anywhere in the urologic tract (i.e., kidneys, ureters, bladder, urethra) or genital tract. Neutrophils are the common leukocyte found in urine, but macrophages and lymphocytes can also be present. Epithelial cells include renal tubular cells, transitional cells, and squamous cells. Neoplastic cells are sometimes detected. Formation of crystals depends on urine pH and concentration [i.e., urine specific gravity (USG)] and the presence of oversaturated crystalogenic substances. Diet and some drugs may also influence crystal formation. The presence of crystals suggests an increased risk of urolithiasis, but it does not predict which animals may actually form uroliths or the type of urolith that may form. Casts originate in the tubular lumen and are composed of mucoprotein, cells, and cellular debris. The presence of casts may indicate renal proteinuria (hyaline) or tubular degeneration (cellular and/or granular).

INDICATIONS
• Microscopic examination of urine sediment is part of a routine urinalysis (UA).
• Many of the chemical results (e.g., urine heme protein, protein) should be interpreted in conjunction with the sediment findings.
• Part of the workup in an animal exposed to a nephrotoxic substance
• Stranguria or pollakiuria

CONTRAINDICATIONS
None

POTENTIAL COMPLICATIONS
None

CLIENT EDUCATION
Urine sediment is critical in diagnosing urinary tract infections.

BODY SYSTEMS ASSESSED
• Hemic, lymphatic, and immune
• Hepatobiliary
• Renal and urologic

SAMPLE

COLLECTION
• 0.5–5mL of urine collected by free catch of a voided sample, manual expression of the urinary bladder, catheterization, or cystocentesis. The method of collection may affect sediment makeup.
• As much a possible, it is important that a consistent volume of urine is used for sediment evaluation. This will enable findings to be semiquantitative and compared with reference values, and enable monitoring of the animal's response to treatment.

HANDLING
• Collect the urine into a clean container free of additives, detergents, and chemicals.
• Ideally, the assay should be performed in ≤2h.

STORAGE
• Refrigeration can aid in slowing cellular breakdown, but it enhances crystal formation.
• Do not freeze the urine.

STABILITY
Components analyzed in urine sediment (i.e., cells, casts, crystals, bacteria) do not hold up well in urine. Cells may lyse, and casts can break down. Crystals can dissolve or new crystals may form. Bacteria may die or multiply.
• Casts begin to deteriorate within 2 h.
• Cells can lyse or lose morphologic characteristics within 2–4 h, depending on urine osmolality.

PROTOCOL
• A standard volume of urine (usually 5mL) is centrifuged at a slow speed.
• The supernatant is removed and saved for biochemical or other tests.
• The pellet is gently resuspended in a small amount of urine (≤1mL), and a small drop is placed onto a glass slide with a coverslip.
• Microscopic examination is done at a low magnification [10× objective; low-power field (lpf)] and a high magnification [40× objective; high-power field (hpf)] with the condenser of the microscope lowered so that contrast is increased.
  • Several components (i.e., cells, casts) are quantified by the number per lpf or hpf.
  • Other components such as crystals, bacteria or other organisms, lipid, and mucus are either graded as present or absent or graded on a few (1+), moderate (2+), or many (3+) scale.
• Staining the urine sediment with a commercial, water-based stain or new methylene blue before examination may aid in identifying constituents and accentuate cellular detail.
• A cytologic preparation of urine sediment can be made by smearing a drop of sediment on a slide, allowing it to air-dry, and staining it with routine hematologic stains. This technique is useful in evaluating cells and identifying bacteria or other organisms.

INTERPRETATION

NORMAL FINDINGS OR RANGE
• Urine sediment is usually relatively inactive, containing few microscopically visible components, but it is not uncommon to find low numbers of cells or certain types of crystals, depending on method of collection.
• The following may be seen in urine from healthy dogs or cats:
  • WBCs: <2–5/hpf
  • RBCs: <2–5/hpf
  • Epithelial cells: <2/hpf
  • Casts: none or at most a few that are hyaline or granular
  • Crystals: Amorphous phosphate, bilirubin (in dogs), calcium oxalate dihydrate, calcium phosphate, and struvite are common in healthy animals. Ammonium biurate, sodium urates, and uric acid crystals are occasionally seen in urine from healthy animals.
  • Bacteria: usually none. Low numbers occasionally are seen in voided samples with genital tract contamination or samples taken from floors, tabletops, or litterboxes.

ABNORMAL VALUES
The following are considered abnormal in dogs or cats:
• WBCs: >5/hpf
• RBCs: >5/hpf

- Epithelial cells: >5/hpf
- Casts: the presence of >1–2/lpf (hyaline, granular) or any cellular (epithelial, RBC, WBC), waxy, fatty, and/or broad casts
- Crystals: the presence of calcium oxalate monohydrate, ammonium biurate, bilirubin, cholesterol, cystine, leucine, tyrosine, sodium urate, and/or uric acid (see this chapter's table)

CRITICAL VALUES
None

INTERFERING FACTORS
Drugs That May Alter Results or Interpretation
Drugs That Interfere with Test Methodology
Acidifiers or alkalinizers may modify crystal formation and composition.

Drugs That Alter Physiology
Sulfadiazine and metabolites, ampicillin, allopurinol, and radiopaque contrast agents (uncommon) have been associated with crystal formation in dogs and cats.

Disorders That May Alter Results
- Casts and cells, especially RBCs, may lyse in poorly concentrated (USG, <1.008) or alkaline urine, especially if a sample is several hours old.
- RBCs usually are crenated in highly concentrated urine. This may cause difficulties with identification.

Collection Techniques or Handling That May Alter Results
- Voided samples may contain more cells, have bacterial contamination, or contain material from the genital tract.
- Catheterized samples may contain more RBCs or epithelial cells (transitional or squamous cells).
- Samples obtained by cystocentesis generally have the least potential of contamination but may contain increased RBCs if blood vessels are damaged during urine collection.
- Refrigeration often enhances crystal formation.
- The use of certain urine preservatives may cause in vitro formation of tyrosine-like crystals.
- The use of stain can dilute sediment, lowering counts, and may introduce crystals and/or organisms (i.e., bacteria, yeast) that grow in stain.

Influence of Signalment
Species
- Lipid droplets are common in cats and are of no clinical significance.
- Low numbers of bilirubin crystals are sometimes seen in concentrated urine from healthy dogs.
- Cystinuria with cystine crystal formation is more common in dogs but occurs rarely in cats.

Breed
- Uric acid and ammonium biurate crystals are common in Dalmatians and English bulldogs.
- Cystinuria with cystine crystalluria has been reported in many breeds of dogs, including dachshunds, Newfoundlands, English bulldogs, Scottish deerhounds, mastiffs, and Scottish terriers.

Age
None

Gender
Sperm may be found only in the urine from intact males or recently bred intact females.

Pregnancy
None

LIMITATIONS OF THE TEST
- Crystals that form in vitro have no clinical significance.
- The number of casts is not an indication of the severity, duration, or potential reversibility of the underlying disease. The type of cast rarely denotes a specific diagnosis.

- A normal sediment does not rule out some type of urinary tract disease.

Sensitivity, Specificity, and Positive and Negative Predictive Values
N/A

Valid If Run in a Human Lab?
Yes.

CLINICAL PERSPECTIVE
- Urine sediment examination should always be part of a routine UA, even if physical and chemical characteristics are unremarkable.
- A standard volume of urine used for sediment examination should be established.
- Chemistry results (e.g., heme protein, protein) should be interpreted with knowledge of urine sediment.
- The urine pH can affect the type of crystals present, and the USG can affect urine sediment.
- The presence of crystals does not necessarily indicate the presence of a urolith, although high concentrations of crystals may predispose an animal to urolith formation. Clinical signs and hematuria may help identify those animals with uroliths.
- Cocci are difficult to identify unless in chains: Brownian movement of tiny particles of debris may resemble cocci. Suspected cocci should be verified by Gram staining an air-dried smear of sediment. Cocci will appear deep purple with a Gram stain, whereas debris/protein will be pink or perhaps colorless.
- Some sediment abnormalities (e.g., casts) can be an early sign of nephrotoxicity seen prior to the onset of serum chemistry abnormalities.
- The absence of pyuria or a failure to detect bacteria does not exclude an occult urinary tract infection. This is particularly common in conditions associated with dilute urine, such as diabetes mellitus and hyperadrenocorticism.

MISCELLANEOUS

ANCILLARY TESTS
- Biochemical profile
- CBC
- UA (including heme, protein, USG, pH)
- Urine culture to rule out occult infection
- Urolith analysis

SYNONYMS
None

SEE ALSO
Blackwell's Five-Minute Veterinary Consult: Canine and Feline Topics
- Crystalluria
- Cylindruria
- Dysuria and Pollakiuria
- Ethylene Glycol Poisoning
- Hematuria
- Pyuria
- Transitional Cell Carcinoma, Renal, Bladder, Urethra
- Urolithiasis, Calcium Oxalate
- Urolithiasis, Calcium Phosphate
- Urolithiasis, Cystine
- Urolithiasis, Struvite—Cats
- Urolithiasis, Struvite—Dogs
- Urolithiasis, Urate
- Urolithiasis, Xanthine

URINE SEDIMENT

Causes of Abnormal Findings

Element	Reference interval with lesion location	Etiology
Cells		
RBCs (hematuria)	<2–5/hpf	May be normal
	>5/hpf	
	Renal	Bleeding or vascular damage associated with glomeruli or tubules, calculi, renal vein thrombosis, vascular dysplasia, trauma, infarct, inflammation, or infection
	Lower urinary tract	Acute or chronic infection, calculi, neoplasia, or hemorrhagic cystitis
	Genital tract	Voided urine sample from animals in estrus
	Iatrogenic	Vessel damage from cystocentesis or catheterization
	Coagulopathy	Thrombocytopenia, thrombocytopathia, von Willebrand disease, or hereditary or acquired coagulopathies
WBCs (pyuria)	<2–5/hpf	May be normal
	>5/hpf	
	Renal	Inflammation from noninfectious causes: pyelonephritis/nephritis, urolithiasis (calculi), neoplasia, or necrosis
		Inflammation from infectious causes: pyelonephritis/nephritis, bacteria, fungal, or parasitic
	Lower urinary tract	Acute or chronic cystitis (infectious or noninfectious), calculi, neoplasia
	Genital tract inflammation	Voided urine sample with contamination from the prostate, prepuce, or vagina
Epithelial cells		
	Squamous epithelial cells	Insignificant finding in voided or catheterized samples
	Transitional cells	
	<2/hpf	May be normal or artifact of collection method
	>5/hpf	Hyperplasia secondary to inflammation, infection, or irritation, or due to cyclophosphamide administration
	Neoplastic cells	Transitional cell carcinoma cells occasionally found in urine; caution advised if cellular atypia noted in the presence of inflammation (may be difficult to differentiate hyperplasia from neoplasia)

Crystals (crystalluria)	**Type of crystal and typical conditions**	**Etiology**
	Urine pH acidic or neutral	
	Amorphous urate	Formed from yellow precipitates of sodium, potassium, magnesium, or calcium urate salts; normal in dalmatians and English bulldogs; also seen with liver disease or portal vascular anomalies
	Bilirubin	May be seen in healthy dogs, common in dogs with bilirubinemia or abnormal bilirubin metabolism, and uncommon in cats
	Calcium oxalate monohydrate	Common with ethylene glycol toxicosis
	Calcium oxalate dihydrate	Found in healthy dogs and cats, found in animals with uroliths composed mostly of calcium oxalate, and occasionally seen with ethylene glycol toxicosis
	Cystine	Rare; congenital renal tubular defect in reabsorption of cystine from the renal filtrate; cystinuria may result in cystine store for formation
	Sodium urate	May be seen concurrently with ammonium urate crystals
	Sulfa	Associated with sulfonamide administration
	Uric acid	Considered normal in dalmatians and English bulldogs, rarely seen in other healthy animals, and can be seen with liver disease or portal vascular anomalies

Element	Reference interval with lesion location	Etiology
	Urine pH alkaline and/or neutral	
	Ammonium urate (ammonium biurate)	Portosystemic shunts or hepatic diseases with hyperammonemia, can be seen rarely in healthy animals but are common in dalmatians and English bulldogs
	Amorphous phosphate	Amorphous form of calcium phosphate crystals that resemble amorphous urates; may be seen in healthy dogs and cats
	Calcium phosphate	Seen in healthy dogs and in dogs with persistently alkaline urine or with calcium phosphate uroliths
	Struvite (triple phosphate)	Common in cats and dogs with alkaline urine; composed of magnesium, ammonium, and phosphorus
	Other crystals	
	Ampicillin	Associated with ampicillin administration
	Cholesterol	Uncommon; associated with cellular membrane deterioration, occasionally seen with some renal diseases, and may be seen in healthy dogs
	Leucine	Rare; may suggest liver disease
	Tyrosine	Rare in dogs; can be associated with liver disease
	Xanthine	Rare; may be seen in animals treated with allopurinol

Casts (cylinduria)	**Type of cast**	**Etiology**
	Hyaline	A few can be normal with concentrated urine; >1–2/lpf associated with renal causes of proteinuria
	Cellular	
	WBC	Associated with tubular inflammation, infection (e.g., bacterial pyelonephritis, leptospirosis), or acute tubular necrosis
	Epithelial	Associated with degeneration/necrosis of tubules (e.g., ischemia, toxins, infarct)
	RBC	Rare; associated with hemorrhage into tubules
	Granular	A few can be normal with concentrated urine; >1–2/lpf associated with degeneration/necrosis of tubules (e.g., ischemia, toxins, infarct)
	Fatty	Common in cats with renal tubular degeneration
	Waxy	Associated with chronic degeneration/necrosis of tubules (e.g., ischemia, toxins, infarct)

URINE SEDIMENT

Element	Reference interval with lesion location	Etiology
Bacteria (bacteriuria)		Infection of the urinary tract, infection of the genital tract (voided sample), in vitro growth with delayed sample analysis, or contamination (voided and some catheterized samples)
Other organisms	Yeast	Often *Candida* spp.
	Fungi (hyphae or budding)	*Blastomyces* spp., *Cryptococcus* spp., or *Aspergillus* spp. (German shepherd dogs can have a disseminated infection)
	Nematode ova	*Dioctophyma renale* or *Capillaria plica*
	Microfilariae	Seen with significant hematuria
	Algae	*Prototheca* spp. (dogs can have disseminated infection)
Lipids		No clinical significance; may be normal; a common finding in cats
Mucus		Genital secretions, suggestive of urethral irritation; mucous strands may form linear structures resembling casts
Contaminants	Pollen grains	Occasionally found in urine sediment, not significant but may be potentially confused with other constituents
	Sperm	
	Glove powder	
	Fibers	

Related Topics in This Book
- Urinalysis Overview
- Urine Heme Protein
- Urine pH
- Urolith Analysis

ABBREVIATIONS
- hpf = high-power field (40×)
- lpf = low-power field (10×)
- UA = urinalysis
- USG = urine specific gravity

Suggested Reading
Chew DJ, DiBartola SP. *Interpretation of Canine and Feline Urinalysis*. Wilmington, DE: Ralston Purina, 1998.

Meyer DJ. Microscopic examination of the urinary sediment. In: Raskin RE, Meyer DJ, eds. *Atlas of Canine and Feline Cytology*. Philadelphia: WB Saunders, 2001: 261–276.

Osborne CA, Stevens JB. Urine sediment: Under the microscope. In: *Urinalysis: A Clinical Guide to Compassionate Patient Care*. Leverkusen, Germany: Bayer, 1999: 125–179.

INTERNET RESOURCES
Cornell University, College of Veterinary Medicine, Clinical Pathology Modules, http://www.diaglab.vet.cornell.edu/clinpath/modules/index.htm.

Hano J. Urine Sediment Atlas, http://www.meddean.luc.edu/lumen/MedEd/MEDICINE/PULMONAR/Renal/Atlas/urineatlas_f.htm.

AUTHOR NAME
Karen E. Russell

BASICS

TYPE OF SPECIMEN
Urine

TEST EXPLANATION AND RELATED PHYSIOLOGY
Urine solute concentration requires adequate renal function, which, in turn, depends on intake of fluid, glomerular filtration, renal tubular resorption and secretion, release and response to vasopressin, and the extent of extrarenal fluid losses. Renal tubular resorption and secretion of solutes and water regulate water balance and total solute concentration in urine. In health, urine solute concentration is expected to increase when the kidneys conserve water and decrease if the kidneys are diuresed. Urine solutes include electrolytes (e.g., sodium, potassium, chloride, calcium, magnesium, phosphorus, sulfate, NH_4^+) and metabolites [e.g., urea, creatinine (Cr), uric acid].

Urine solute concentration can be measured by *osmolality* or *refractometry*. Measurement of osmolality is the gold standard; refractometry closely correlates with osmolality. Urine specific gravity (USG), which is part of the complete urinalysis, is determined by refractometry and is the most common technique for assessing the ability of the kidneys to concentrate urine solutes.

The USG of plasma and glomerular filtrate ranges between 1.008 and 1.012. USG in this range is referred to as *isosthenuria* and implies that there is failure of the kidneys to concentrate urine. *Hypersthenuria* or *baruria* denotes concentrated urine with a USG that is increased and much greater than that of glomerular filtrate or plasma. Hypersthenuria (>1.035 in dogs and >1.040 in cats) is expected in dehydrated states. Hyposthenuria (USG, 1.001–1.007) signifies a dilute urine sample that is less than that of glomerular filtrate or plasma. It may be more clinically relevant to refer to the ability to concentrate or dilute urine as maximally concentrated, adequately concentrated, questionable, or inappropriate when interpreted in light of the hydration status and other findings in a patient.

Refractometry looks at the ratio of urine refractive index compared to that of water and depends on particle number, size, and weight. Measurement of refractive index is temperature dependent. Most refractometers made for clinical use are designed to be accurate between 16° and 38°C (60°–100°F). Refractometers that are made specifically for veterinary species are available. These have 2 scales for USG: 1 for dog and large-animal urine and a separate 1 for cat urine. Some reagent pads (dipsticks) provide a USG determination, but these are unreliable in veterinary species.

INDICATIONS
To screen renal function by assessing the ability of the kidneys to concentrate urine

CONTRAINDICATIONS
None

POTENTIAL COMPLICATIONS
None

CLIENT EDUCATION
- USG can be used to determine whether the kidneys can concentrate urine appropriately, which is an indication of renal function. The results must be interpreted with the knowledge of the hydration status of the animal and BUN and Cr concentrations.
- If urine is collected by the owner, then an appropriate container should be provided to avoid possible contamination with detergents, disinfectants, or other substances.

BODY SYSTEMS ASSESSED
- Endocrine and metabolic
- Hepatobiliary
- Renal and urologic

SAMPLE

COLLECTION
- Only a drop of urine is needed, collected by any method.
- The urine should be collected prior to diagnostic procedures or the administration of therapeutic agents.

HANDLING
- The urine should be collected into a clean, dry container that has a tight-fitting lid and is free of potential contaminants (e.g., detergents, disinfectants). It should be labeled with appropriate information (e.g., patient and owner identification; date, time, and method of collection).
- The urine should be analyzed within 1–2 h after collection.

STORAGE
- The sample should be refrigerated if it cannot be analyzed soon after collection.
- Store the sample in a container that can protect the sample from light and that has a tight-fitting lid.
- Refrigerated samples should be warmed to room temperature before analysis, because cold urine is denser and has a higher USG than warm urine.

STABILITY
Refrigerated urine stored for up to 8 h is probably suitable for analysis.

PROTOCOL
- The refractometer should be periodically calibrated using distilled water, which has a USG of 1.000.
- The urine sample need not centrifuged prior to determination of USG, because components of urine sediment (e.g., cells, casts, crystals) do not contribute significantly to osmolality.
- Clean the cover and surface of the refractometer with a small amount of distilled water and dry thoroughly. Close the cover and apply 1–2 drops of urine at the notched edge so that it flows over the surface by capillary action.
- Point the refractometer toward a light so that there is good contrast and the scale can be seen clearly. If needed, rotate the eyepiece to focus the scale. There should be a sharp dividing line between the light and dark contrast. The USG of the sample is that point of the scale where the dividing line lies.

INTERPRETATION

NORMAL FINDINGS OR RANGE
- USG is interpreted based on the hydration status of the patient and the serum BUN and Cr concentrations.
- Adequate renal concentrating ability is assumed if a random urine sample has a USG that is >1.030 in a dog and >1.035 in a cat.
- However, USG can range widely, from 1.015 to 1.045 and from 1.015 to 1.065 in an adequately hydrated dog and cat, respectively, and it is assumed that the animal does not have renal impairment if BUN and Cr concentrations are within the reference intervals.
- If dehydration exists, then the urine should be concentrated (hypersthenuria). USG should be >1.035 and >1.040 in dogs and cats, respectively.

ABNORMAL VALUES
- In the presence of increased serum BUN and Cr concentrations (azotemia), USG that is <1.030 and <1.035 in dogs and cats, respectively, is considered inadequate and implies impaired renal function.

URINE SPECIFIC GRAVITY

• USG that is persistently <1.030 (dogs) or <1.035 (cats) from successive urine samples in an animal that is not azotemic may be a sign of underlying renal or nonrenal disease.

CRITICAL VALUES
USG remains in the isosthenuric range (1.008–1.012) in animals with advanced or end-stage renal failure.

INTERFERING FACTORS
Drugs That May Alter Results or Interpretation
Drugs That Interfere with Test Methodology
In human patients, high doses of benzylpenicillin or carbenicillin are reported to increase USG.

Drugs That Alter Physiology
• Fluid therapy or administration of diuretics affects USG. These therapies increase urine production and volume, and urine is dilute as reflected by a low USG.
• Corticosteroids may interfere with renal concentrating mechanisms, resulting in lower USG.
• Administration of fluids containing glucose may cause a glucosuria and subsequent osmotic diuresis.
• USG may increase following IV administration of triiodinated radiopaque contrast agents because these agents are excreted into the urine.

Disorders That May Alter Results
Marked proteinuria or glucosuria may cause an artificial rise in USG.

Collection Techniques or Handling That May Alter Results
USG should be determined from a urine sample that has been collected prior to any treatments or diagnostic procedures.
Influence of Signalment
Species
None

Breed
None

Age
Neonatal puppies and kittens may not have the ability to concentrate urine as well as mature dogs and cats.

Gender
None

Pregnancy
None

LIMITATIONS OF THE TEST
Sensitivity, Specificity, and Positive and Negative Predictive Values
N/A

Valid If Run in a Human Lab?
Yes. However, refractometers specifically made to evaluate human samples may slightly underestimate the urine concentration in cats.

Causes of Abnormal Findings

USG	Interpretation of USG	Hydration status	BUN and Cr	Clinical condition
>1.035 (dogs) >1.040 (cats)	Maximal urine concentration (hypersthenuria)	Dehydrated states	Increased	Hypovolemia
>1.035 (dogs) >1.040 (cats)	Maximal urine concentration (hypersthenuria)	Normal hydration	Increased	Plasma hyperosmolality Decreased cardiac output
>1.030 (dogs) >1.035 (cats)	Adequate urine concentration	Normal hydration	Normal	Clinically normal
1.001–1.080	Variable urine concentration	Normal hydration	Normal	Random urine sample; may be clinically normal; recheck
1.015–1.030	Questionable urine concentration	Normal hydration	Normal	Random urine sample; may be clinically normal
				Diabetes mellitus (osmotic diuresis)
				Possible underlying renal disease, especially if USG remains in this range
1.015–1.030	Questionable urine concentration	Dehydrated states	Increased	Underlying renal disease and impaired concentrating ability
				Hypoadrenocorticism (impaired release and response to ADH)
				Diabetes mellitus (osmotic diuresis)
1.008–1.012	Inadequate urine concentration (isosthenuria)	Variable	Increased	Renal failure

1.001–1.007 (may actually range from 1.001 to 1.015)	Low urine concentration (hyposthenuria)	Variable	Normal or decreased	Diuretic therapy
				IV fluid therapy
				Medullary washout
				Central diabetes insipidus
				Hyperadrenocorticism
				Hyperthyroidism (cats)
				Hypoadrenocorticism
				Hypoparathyroidism
				Nephrogenic diabetes insipidus
				    Hypercalcemia
				    Liver disease
				    Pyometra
				    Hypokalemia
				    Psychogenic polydipsia
				Thyroiditis (dogs)

CLINICAL PERSPECTIVE
• USG should be interpreted in conjunction with knowledge of the hydration status and BUN and Cr concentrations.
• Approximately one-third of the nephrons from both kidneys must be functional to concentrate or dilute urine adequately. When the USG denotes an inadequate or inappropriate urine concentration, it is presumed that loss of function has occurred in at least two-thirds of the nephrons. At this point, the USG usually falls into the isosthenuric range of 1.008–1.012.
• In a polyuric animal, a USG of <1.008 suggests defective urine-concentrating ability secondary to an extrarenal disease (e.g., central diabetes insipidus or conditions that cause renal diabetes insipidus). Primary renal failure is unlikely since a USG of <1.008 demonstrates an ability to dilute the ultrafiltrate.
• Knowledge of USG is also needed for proper interpretation of several other tests (e.g., bilirubin, protein) that are part of the urinalysis.

 MISCELLANEOUS

ANCILLARY TESTS
• Biochemistry profile (especially BUN and Cr)
• CBC (especially PCV)

SYNONYMS
None

SEE ALSO
Blackwell's Five-Minute Veterinary Consult: Canine and Feline Topics
• Azotemia and Uremia

• Renal Failure, Acute Uremia
• Renal Failure, Chronic

Related Topics in This Book
• Creatinine
• Osmolality
• Urea Nitrogen

ABBREVIATIONS
• Cr = creatinine
• USG = urine specific gravity

Suggested Reading
Chew DJ, DiBartola SP. Urinalysis interpretation. In: *Interpretation of Canine and Feline Urinalysis*. Wilmington, DE: Ralston Purina, 1998: 15–33.
Gregory CR. Urinary system. In: Latimer KS, Mahaffey EA, Prasse KW, eds. *Duncan and Prasse's Veterinary Laboratory Medicine Clinical Pathology*, 4th ed. Ames: Iowa State Press, 2003: 231–259.
Osborne CA, Stevens JB. Urine specific gravity, refractive index, or osmolality: Which one would you choose? In: *Urinalysis: A Clinical Guide to Compassionate Patient Care*. Leverkusen, Germany: Bayer, 1999: 73–85.
Stockham SL, Scott MA. Urinary System. In: *Fundamentals of Veterinary Clinical Pathology*, 2nd ed. Ames, IA: Blackwell, 2002: 415–494.

INTERNET RESOURCES
Cornell University, College of Veterinary Medicine, Clinical Pathology Modules, http://www.diaglab.vet.cornell.edu/clinpath/modules/index.htm.

AUTHOR NAME
Karen E. Russell

UROLITH ANALYSIS

BASICS

TYPE OF SPECIMEN
Tissue

TEST EXPLANATION AND RELATED PHYSIOLOGY
The term *lith* is Greek and is translated as "stone." *Calculus* is a Latin term translated as "stone." *Uroliths* are aggregates of crystalline and matrix material that form in 1 or more locations within the urinary tract when urine becomes oversaturated with crystallogenic substances. Uroliths may be composed of 1 or more types of biogenic minerals that may be deposited in layers (laminations) or admixed throughout the stone. Each urolith may contain (1) a nidus, (2) a stone, (3) a shell, and (4) surface crystals. The *nidus* or nucleus of a urolith is an area of obvious initiation of urolith growth. The term *stone* refers to the major body of the urolith. The term *shell* designates a layer of precipitated material that completely surrounds the body of the stone, and the term *surface crystals* is used to describe an incomplete covering of the outermost surface of the urolith. It is useful to have these layers analyzed separately and their compositions reported.

Although 1 mineral type usually predominates, the composition of uroliths is frequently mixed. The center (nidus) may be composed of 1 mineral type, whereas outer layers may be composed of different mineral types. In addition to biogenic crystals, medications (e.g., sulfadiazine) may precipitate as crystals within the urinary tract and become incorporated into uroliths. A nidus is not visible in all uroliths. When a nidus is present, it does not invariably represent the geometric center of the urolith; however, a centrally located nucleus infers that the urolith was freely accessible from all sides and that growth proceeded at a similar rate on all sides. A nidus may be composed of minerals or structures such as suture material, hair, fleas, plant awns, metallic buck shot, or pieces of urinary catheter.

Layers of concentric rings (laminae or shells) surrounding the main portion of uroliths are common. They represent sequential periods of mineral-matrix deposition beginning at the core and moving outward. A visible difference in appearance between 2 consecutive layers of a stone should prompt suspicion of differences in their mineral composition; however, a difference in mineral composition between 2 layers may not exist. In addition to alternating bands of different mineral types, shells (laminations) may represent intermittent periods of growth during which a single type of mineral is deposited or alternating bands with different proportions of mineral and matrix. A urolith without a nidus or shell of different composition that contains ≥70% of 1 type of mineral is identified by that mineral. A urolith with <70% of 1 mineral is identified as a *mixed* urolith. A urolith with a nidus or stone and 1 or more surrounding layers of different mineral composition is called a *compound* urolith.

Two general methods of analysis are used: quantitative and qualitative. *Qualitative analysis* is performed using spot chemical test reagents to identify chemical radicals and ions. *Qualitative analysis* does not enable determination of approximate percentages of different minerals comprising the urolith. Also, crystalline components including silica and drugs cannot be identified. Quantitative analysis, which is the preferred method, includes optical crystallography, infrared spectroscopy, X-ray diffraction, energy-dispersive techniques, and other methods.

INDICATIONS
Complete knowledge of the entire urolith composition can help direct diagnosis, treatment, and prevention of further urolithiasis.

CONTRAINDICATIONS
None

POTENTIAL COMPLICATIONS
None

CLIENT EDUCATION
Although specific mineral types of uroliths often have characteristic shapes, colors, and surface features, the overlap in gross appearance between stones of different mineral types and the fact that some stones contain more than 1 mineral preclude a specific diagnosis of mineral type on the basis of gross morphologic characteristics of uroliths.

BODY SYSTEMS ASSESSED
Renal and urologic

SAMPLE

COLLECTION
- Do not submit just 1 urolith if many are collected. Uroliths of different mineral composition may form at different times in the same patient. Submit all of the uroliths or representative sizes and appearances of the uroliths.
- Do not fragment or crush uroliths because this will interfere with detection of layers composed of different mineral types.

HANDLING
- Package uroliths in noncrushable mailing containers. Samples in paper envelopes are often crushed as they pass through automated mail-sorting and postage-canceling devices.
- Avoid the use of formalin, which may alter the mineral composition of uroliths.

STORAGE
Store samples dry at room temperature.

STABILITY
Samples are stable indefinitely: The mineral composition of uroliths is unlikely to alter following collection from patients.

PROTOCOL
None

INTERPRETATION

NORMAL FINDINGS OR RANGE
None

ABNORMAL VALUES
The biogenic minerals identified in uroliths formed by cats and dogs include the following:
- Oxalates
  - Ca oxalate monohydrate (whewellite)
  - Ca oxalate dihydrate (wheddellite)
- Phosphates
  - Beta-tricalcium phosphate (whitlockite)
  - Ca phosphate carbonate (carbonate apatite)
  - Ca hydrogen phosphate dihydrate (brushite)
  - Ca phosphate (hydroxyapatite)
  - Magnesium ammonium phosphate hexahydrate (struvite)
  - Magnesium hydrogen phosphate trihydrate (newberyite)
- Purines
  - Uric acid
  - Ammonium urate
  - Other salts of urate (Ca and sodium urate)
  - Xanthine
- Cystine
- Silica

CRITICAL VALUES
None

INTERFERING FACTORS

Drugs That May Alter Results or Interpretation

Drugs That Interfere with Test Methodology

Drug metabolites may be incorporated into uroliths.

Drugs That Alter Physiology

Allopurinol may interfere with conversion of xanthine to uric acid and allantoin. As a consequence, xanthine uroliths may form.

Disorders That May Alter Results

• Urinary tract infections predispose patients to struvite uroliths.
• Primary hyperparathyroidism and other causes of hypercalcemia (and hypercalciuria) predispose patients to formation of Ca phosphate and Ca oxalate uroliths.
• A low-Ca diet can promote increased absorption of oxalates from the diet, predisposing patients to Ca oxalate uroliths.
• Conditions that cause hyperammonemia (and hyperammonuria), such as chronic hepatic insufficiency and portal vascular anomalies, can lead to urate uroliths.

Collection Techniques or Handling That May Alter Results

• Formalin may cause the transformation of struvite to newberyite.
• Submission of a sample of insufficient size for analysis

Influence of Signalment

Species

• Cats
  • 60% Ca oxalate
  • 30%–40% struvite
• Dogs
  • 40% Ca oxalate
  • 50% struvite
• In cats, sterile struvite uroliths are more common ($\approx$95%) than infection-induced struvite uroliths (<5%).
• In dogs, infection-induced struvite uroliths are more common (99%) than sterile struvite uroliths (<1%).

Breed

• Himalayan, Persian, Scottish fold, ragdoll, and Burmese cats appear to have increased risk for Ca oxalate uroliths.
• Six breeds represent 60% of Ca oxalate cases in dogs: miniature schnauzers, Lhasa apsos, Yorkshire terriers, bichon frises, shih tzus, and miniature poodles.
• Cystine uroliths may affect many breeds, especially dachshunds, English bulldogs, Newfoundlands, Staffordshire bull terriers, and Welsh corgis.

• Urate uroliths are more common in dalmatians, English bulldogs, and breeds at risk of portosystemic shunts (e.g., Yorkshire terriers).
• Naturally occurring xanthine uroliths have been reported in Cavalier King Charles spaniels and in cats.
• German shepherds, golden retrievers, and Labrador retrievers appear prone to silica uroliths.

Age

• Infection-induced struvite uroliths may occur at any age.
  • Of uroliths that affect dogs and cats that are <1 year of age, infection-induced struvite uroliths are most common.
  • Sterile struvite uroliths have not been reported in young cats.
• Ca oxalate uroliths occur more commonly in older (>7 years) dogs and cats.
• Canine cystine uroliths primarily affect adult dogs (mean age at diagnosis, 5 years; range, 3 months to 14 years).
• The mean age of detection of urate uroliths in dogs without portosystemic shunts is $3^{1}/_{2}$ years (range, 0.5 to >10 years). The mean age of detection of urate uroliths in dogs with portosystemic shunts is <1 year (range, 0.1 to >10 years).

Gender

• Struvite urethral plugs primarily affect male cats. These plugs are composed of $\geq$50% mucoid matrix, often with embedded struvite crystals, and are usually sterile.
• Struvite uroliths are more common in female dogs because of an increased incidence of urinary tract infections.
• In dogs, cystine uroliths are primarily detected in males but may affect females.
• No gender predisposition for cystine uroliths has been observed in cats.
• Ca oxalate uroliths are more common in males.

Pregnancy

None

LIMITATIONS OF THE TEST

Qualitative analysis is not recommended because of very poor sensitivity and specificity. Qualitative analysis does not enable determination of approximate percentages of different minerals comprising a urolith. Also, crystalline components, including silica and drugs, cannot be identified.

Sensitivity, Specificity, and Positive and Negative Predictive Values

N/A

Causes of Abnormal Findings

Uroliths in dogs and cats

Uroliths	% Uroliths		pH at which more soluble	Physical features	Predisposing causes
	Dogs	Cats			
Struvite	50	30–40	<6.5	Yellow to white, hard	Urinary tract infection
Ca oxalate	30–40	60	Not affected	White or cream, hard and brittle; jagged edges	Hypercalcemia Low Ca diet Chronic metabolic acidosis
Urate	8	2	>7	Green to yellow; concentric laminations	Chronic liver insufficiency Portal vascular anomalies Inherited defect in uric acid metabolism
Cystine	1	<1	>7	Yellowish, easily crushed	Cystinuria (inherited renal tubular transport defect)
Ca phosphate	<1	<1	<7	Hard, white to yellowish	Hypercalcemia
Silica	1	None	Not affected	Jackstone appearance (i.e., resemble toy jacks)	Diet high in silica (corn, soybean)

UROLITH ANALYSIS

Valid If Run in a Human Lab?
Yes, if quantitative methods of analysis are used.

CLINICAL PERSPECTIVE

• Hematuria is a common finding in the urinalysis from a dog or cat with urolithiasis. Other clinical signs include pollakiuria and stranguria.

• The presence of crystals in urine sediment does not indicate the presence of a urolith, although persistently large numbers of crystals can be a predisposing factor for urolith formation and growth.

• Uroliths may or may not be associated with urine crystals of the same type as present in the urolith.

• Approximately 10%–30% of cats with signs of feline lower urinary tract disease have urolithiasis. Most of the other cases are idiopathic, and this percentage has not been affected by changes in cat food composition.

• Urolith formation is a process that typically takes several weeks (e.g., infection-induced struvite) to months (e.g., Ca oxalate) rather than days. In fact, the most common cause of an apparent rapid recurrence of uroliths (within days) is incomplete removal at the time of surgery.

 MISCELLANEOUS

ANCILLARY TESTS

• Bacterial culture of urine and/or urolith
• Urinalysis

SYNONYMS

• Bladder stone
• Calculus stone analysis
• Urinary calculi
• Urinary stones

SEE ALSO

Blackwell's Five-Minute Veterinary Consult: Canine and Feline Topics

• Urolithiasis, Calcium Oxalate
• Urolithiasis, Calcium Phosphate
• Urolithiasis, Cystine
• Urolithiasis, Struvite—Cats
• Urolithiasis, Struvite—Dogs
• Urolithiasis, Urate
• Urolithiasis, Xanthine

Related Topics in This Book

• Urinalysis Overview
• Urine pH
• Urine Sediment

ABBREVIATIONS

Ca = calcium

Suggested Reading
Osborne CA, Lulich JP, Bartges JW, eds. The ROCKet science of canine urolithiasis. *Vet Clin North Am* 1999; **29**: 1–309.

INTERNET RESOURCES

University of Minnesota, College of Veterinary Medicine, Minnesota Urolith Center, http://www.cvm.umn.edu/depts/minnesotaurolithcenter/home.html.

AUTHOR NAMES

Carl A. Osborne, Jody P. Lulich, and Lisa K. Ulrich

BASICS

TYPE OF PROCEDURE
Ultrasonographic

PROCEDURE EXPLANATION AND RELATED PHYSIOLOGY
Ultrasonography is a safe, noninvasive method of examining morphology of the uterus. There is no known hazard to the operator or patient from ultrasonography. The exam consists of imaging through the ventral or lateral abdominal wall with ≥5-MHz ultrasound transducers. Real-time 2-dimensional (2-D) B-mode ultrasound scanners produce a tomographic (cross-sectional) gray-scale anatomic image of the soft tissues. Ultrasonography is an excellent method of identifying fluid versus soft tissue and easily identifies uterine abnormalities that produce luminal fluid. Fluids with low cellular or protein content (e.g., cystic uterine fluid) have no echoic interfaces within the fluid and appear black (anechoic) on the image. Fluids such as exudates (e.g., pyometra, mucometra) will show internal echoes and range from hypoechoic (dark gray) to hyperechoic (light gray). Ultrasonography cannot image through gas (e.g., GI tract) or mineral (e.g., bone, feces), which can prevent observation of early pregnancy or a uterine abnormality.

INDICATIONS
- Vaginal discharge
- Suspected uterine disease, such as pyometra
- Pregnancy evaluation
- Postpartum evaluation
- Female infertility
- Suspected mass in caudal abdomen in female dogs

CONTRAINDICATIONS
None

POTENTIAL COMPLICATIONS
None

CLIENT EDUCATION
- Patients should not be fed for 12 h before examination is possible. Water can be given up to the time of the examination.
- The hair covering the abdomen may need to be clipped for adequate imaging.
- This is an excellent method for evaluating the viability of fetuses.
- Estimation of fetal numbers with ultrasonography is inaccurate in litters of 6 or more.
- Early fetal death (in <25 days) and resorption may decrease birth number versus count determined via early ultrasonography of fetuses.

BODY SYSTEMS ASSESSED
Reproductive

PROCEDURE

PATIENT PREPARATION
Preprocedure Medication or Preparation
- Patient preparation consists of clipping the hair from the ventral abdomen along with cleaning the skin to enable proper acoustic coupling of the ultrasound transducer with the skin. Poor contact with the skin results in inferior-quality images.
- Avoid any procedure that will increase the amount of air within the GI tract, such as enemas or stress that causes aerophagia. Excessive GI gas will interfere with imaging of the uterus.
- Do not allow the patient to urinate immediately prior to procedure. The urine-filled bladder acts as a good landmark and acoustic window through which the uterine body can be imaged.

Anesthesia or Sedation
- Sedation is used depending on the temperament of the patient. The patient must lie still in dorsal or lateral recumbency while the procedure is performed. Excessive patient movement prevents adequate imaging of the uterus.
- Avoid sedation that produces panting. Motion produced by panting can severely degrade the quality of the examination.

Patient Positioning
Dorsal or lateral recumbency is used depending on the preference of the sonographer. The author uses dorsal recumbency.

Patient Monitoring
- No special monitoring is required.
- Monitoring of the patient is based on clinical signs.
- Dyspneic patients may not tolerate dorsal recumbency without oxygen supplementation.

Equipment or Supplies
- A diagnostic ultrasound scanner with high-resolution probes
- A ≥7-MHz transducer for best resolution of the uterus. A 5-MHz transducer may provide adequate resolution for moderate to severe uterine changes.
- Ultrasound acoustic coupling gel
- A clipper with no. 40 blade

TECHNIQUE
- Apply acoustic gel to the clipped area of the skin.
- Place the transducer on the ventral midline in transverse view (transverse to the long axis of the body) at the level of the urinary bladder.
- Move the probe cranially and caudally looking for a tubular hypoechoic structure immediately dorsal to the urinary bladder and ventral to the colon. The urine in the bladder is typically anechoic and provides a good acoustic window for viewing the uterine body and cervix. The colon usually contains hyperechoic gas and mineral content and shows as a crescent-shaped echogenic structure with acoustic shadowing.
- Follow the uterine body cranially to observe the bifurcation into the right and left uterine horns.
- If observable, follow each uterine horn cranially to the ovaries just caudal to the caudal pole of each kidney.
- Turn the probe 90° to obtain a long-axis view of the uterine body and cervix.
- Avoid confusing major vessels dorsal to the urinary bladder with a fluid-filled uterus by following the structure cranially and caudally with transverse scanning with 2-D gray-scale imaging or use Doppler imaging. The aorta and caudal vena cava branch as you progress caudally, whereas the uterus branches into left and right horns as you move cranially.

SAMPLE HANDLING
N/A

APPROPRIATE AFTERCARE
Postprocedure Patient Monitoring
Monitoring is only required for sedation or anesthesia if either has been used to immobilize the patient.

Nursing Care
Clean the acoustic gel from the skin following the procedure.

Dietary Modification
None following the procedure

Medication Requirements
None

Restrictions on Activity
None

Anticipated Recovery Time
None

INTERPRETATION

NORMAL FINDINGS OR RANGE
- The normal uterus may be too small to observe without higher-frequency transducers.
- The normal uterus in dogs is 3–8 mm in diameter in anestrus or late diestrus. Large dogs and multiparous dogs may have a slightly larger uterus.
- The normal uterus is a tubular hypoechoic structure immediately dorsal to the bladder.
- The cervix is slightly larger in diameter and is observed at, or slightly cranial to, the trigone of the bladder.
- The body of the uterus extends cranially to the middle to cranial one-third of the urinary bladder, where it bifurcates into the 2 uterine horns.
- The uterine horns are normally smaller in diameter than the uterine body and usually cannot be observed in an animal that is in anestrus.
- No definable layers are observed in the uterine wall.
- The uterus enlarges slightly during proestrus, estrus, and early pregnancy.
- Pregnancy evaluation at 21–31 days in dogs reveals 1 or more anechoic fluid-filled spherical to oblong blastocysts (embryonic vesicles) with echogenic embryos with observable heartbeats. The fetal heart rate is generally twice the maternal heart rate.
- Gestation age (GA) in dogs: +/−3 days
  - <40 days
    - $GA = (6 \times GSD) + 20$
    - $GA = (3 \times CRL) + 27$
  - >40 days
    - $GA = (15 \times HD) + 20$
    - $GA = (7 \times BD) + 29$
- GA in cats: +/−2 days
  - >40 days
    - $GA = (25 \times HD) + 3$
    - $GA = (11 \times BD) + 21$
- Normal involution of the canine uterus is complete in 3–4 weeks.
- Normal involution of the feline uterus is complete in 24 days.

ABNORMAL VALUES
- Observable fluid other than within an embryonic vesicle is abnormal. Fluid within the uterus may be observed with pyometra, mucometra, hematometra, or endometriosis. The fluid is usually easy to observe and is generally anechoic with endometriosis and echogenic to variable degrees with pyometra, mucometra, and hematometra.
- The presence of peritoneal effusion (especially echogenic fluid) along with a fluid-distended uterus could indicate rupture of a pyometra with resulting peritonitis.
- Focal uterine wall thickening and focal fluid accumulation may indicate a retained placenta or incomplete involution.
- Stump pyometras may present as pockets of echogenic fluid dorsal to the bladder or as complex masses.
- Masses within the uterus can indicate neoplasia such as adenoma, adenocarcinoma, leiomyoma, or leiomyosarcoma. Uterine neoplasia is rare.
- Bradycardia of the fetal heart rate indicates fetal distress.

CRITICAL VALUES
No luminal fluid or masses other than in embryonic vesicles should be seen in the normal uterus.

INTERFERING FACTORS
Drugs That May Alter Results of the Procedure
None

Conditions That May Interfere with Performing the Procedure
- Severe distention of the GI tract with gas and mineral content can hide underlying uterine changes because ultrasonography cannot image through these substances.
- An empty urinary bladder can be difficult to identify and make identification of the uterus difficult.

Procedure Techniques or Handling That May Alter Results
Lower-frequency transducers may not reveal mild uterine changes.

Influence of Signalment on Performing and Interpreting the Procedure
Species
The uterus of cats is slightly smaller than that of dogs, and pregnancy can be detected several days earlier in cats.

Breed
Larger-breed dogs will have slightly larger uterine bodies that may be easier to detect in both anestrus and estrus.

Age
Pyometra is more common in older, intact dogs.

Gender
Intact females only, except for uterine stump abscess or pyometra in neutered females

Pregnancy
Ultrasonography is more sensitive to fetal viability by evaluating heartbeat and movement.

CLINICAL PERSPECTIVE
- The normal uterus is not routinely observed in most dogs and cats without the use of higher-resolution transducers and skilled examination dorsal to the urinary bladder.
- Fluid within the lumen of the uterus is an abnormal finding and indicates abnormality. Anechoic luminal fluid is most compatible with a hydrometra or cystic endometriosis. Echogenic luminal fluid is most likely pyometra, mucometra, or hematometra.
- Ovariohysterectomy is the usual treatment when there are abnormal uterine findings.

MISCELLANEOUS

ANCILLARY TESTS
CBC and serum chemistries along with a medical history help differentiate pyometra, mucometra, and endometriosis.

SYNONYMS
Transabdominal uterine sonography

SEE ALSO
Blackwell's Five-Minute Veterinary Consult: Canine and Feline Topics
- Infertility, Female
- Metritis
- Pyometra and Cystic Endometrial Hyperplasia
- Retained Placenta
- Subinvolution of Placental Sites

Related Topics in This Book
General Principles of Ultrasonography

ABBREVIATIONS
- BD = body diameter
- CRL = crown-rump length
- GA = gestational age
- GSD = gestational sac diameter
- HD = head diameter

Suggested Reading

Beck KA, Baldwin CJ, Bosu WTK. Ultrasound prediction of parturition in queens. *Vet Radiol* 1990; **31**: 32–35.

England GCW. Ultrasonographic assessment of abnormal pregnancy. *Vet Clin North Am Small Anim Pract* 1998; **28**: 849–868.

England GCW, Allen WE. Studies on canine pregnancy using B-mode ultrasound: Diagnosis of early pregnancy and the number of conceptuses. *J Small Anim Pract* 1990; **31**: 321–323.

England GCW, Allen WE, Porter DJ. Studies on canine pregnancy using B-mode ultrasound: Development of the conceptus and determination of gestational age. *J Small Anim Pract* 1990; **31**: 324–329.

Nyland TG, Mattoon JS, eds. *Small Animal Diagnostic Ultrasound*, 2nd ed. Philadelphia: WB Saunders, 2002.

Toal RL, Walker MA, Henry GA. A comparison of real-time ultrasound, palpation and radiography in pregnancy detection and litter size determination in the bitch. *Vet Radiol* 1986; **27**: 102–108.

INTERNET RESOURCES

None

AUTHOR NAME

George A. Henry

BASICS

TYPE OF PROCEDURE
Radiographic

PROCEDURE EXPLANATION AND RELATED PHYSIOLOGY
Vaginography is the process of retrograde distention of the vestibule and vagina (with secondary reflux commonly noted into the urethra) by use of sterile, iodinated (ionic or nonionic) contrast medium, room air (see the Contraindications section), or soluble gas (CO_2 or N_2O) to define the lumen and the walls. An alternative procedure is vaginoscopy. In general, vaginourethrography is only a morphologic study and provides little physiologic information except for what can be garnered from an assessment of acquired or congenital abnormalities and their expected effects on coitus, insemination, continence, fertility, and vaginal birth.

INDICATIONS
- Locate, assess, and, as necessary, determine the continuity of the vestibule and vagina in selected patients with lower urogenital tract clinical signs but particularly in patients with acute trauma.
- Define the contents of the vestibule or vagina for anything that is clinically suspicious (e.g., uroliths, polyps, masses, foreign bodies).
- Assess the relevance of the lower genital tract in hematuria, pyuria, stranguria, and pollakiuria.
- Assess the relationship between the vestibule, the constrictor vestibule muscle, or the vagina with the external urethral orifice, the urinary bladder, the urethra, and their surrounding structures (e.g., compressed or distorted vagina or vestibule; vaginourethral or rectovaginal fistula).
- Assess the vagina for leaks in unusual cases of peritoneal or retroperitoneal fluid or both.
- Assess the vagina and vestibule for abnormalities that might contribute to recurrent urinary tract infections.

CONTRAINDICATIONS
- Do not use room air in any patient with visible hematuria because this can result in a systemic fatal air embolism.
- Avoid aggressive distention in patients with recent bladder, urethral, uterine, or vaginal surgery.

POTENTIAL COMPLICATIONS
- Introduction or spread of resistant lower urogenital tract organisms into the bladder, the peritoneal or retroperitoneal cavities, or the uterus
- Although unlikely, fatal air embolism when room air is used in the face of gross hematuria, particularly after urethral or bladder trauma or extensive vaginal bleeding

CLIENT EDUCATION
- The animal should not have any food for at least 18 h prior to the procedure unless it is an emergency.
- The animal will need a cleansing, tepid water enema at least 2 h before the procedure unless it is an emergency.
- There is limited, although not insignificant, risk of an iatrogenic complication (e.g., vestibular or vaginal tear or excoriation) as a result of the catheterization and filling aspects of the procedure.

BODY SYSTEMS ASSESSED
- Renal and urologic
- Reproductive

PROCEDURE

PATIENT PREPARATION

Preprocedure Medication or Preparation
- Withhold food for at least 18 h prior to the procedure unless it is an emergency.
- Administer a cleansing, tepid water enema at least 2 h before the procedure unless it is an emergency.
- Be sure there are no physiologic contraindications to the necessary sedation or anesthesia.

Anesthesia or Sedation
In general, the contrast vaginourethrography is best performed with heavy sedation or anesthesia to assure adequate positioning and limit the likelihood of the patient's reaction compromising the study (e.g., balloon catheter blown out) or causing patient injury (e.g., catheter ripped out).

Patient Positioning
Right recumbent and dorsally recumbent (VD) views are indicated before contrast-medium administration and thereafter. Where applicable, the opposite recumbent [e.g., left or sternally (DV) recumbent] or oblique views may facilitate wall or lumen assessment.

Patient Monitoring
General observation of the patient's well-being as would be expected for any patient under sedation or anesthesia

Equipment or Supplies
- Sodium-based, ionic (diatrizoate or iothalamate) or nonionic (iopamidol or iohexol) iodinated contrast media
- An appropriately sized balloon catheter (Foley or Swan-Ganz) that can be placed and sufficiently distended to prevent leakage of the injected materials from the vestibule and vaginal opening. The appropriate size of the catheter will depend on the patient size.

• An otoscope or vaginoscope with a 1- to $1\frac{1}{2}$-inch (2.54–3.81 cm) small-bore cone is quite helpful in both examining the vestibule and locating the external urethral orifice, particularly in small, fat, female dogs and in most female cats.

• Radiographic facilities capable of creating adequate abdominal views

• Materials used in harvesting samples (e.g., culture equipment, microscope slides, coverslips)

• Syringes (appropriate size depending on the volume of contrast media to be used)

• A 3-way stopcock

• A source of CO_2 or N_2O for the pneumovaginogram or double-contrast vaginogram if the patient has gross hematuria or active bleeding from the vagina. *Note*: Never directly distend the vagina from the compressed gas source, always use a syringe filled with the gas via the 3-way stopcock, and then inject the gas manually.

• Appropriate, noninjurious antiseptic cleansing materials and disposable gauze or swabs to cleanse the urogenital area prior to any attempts to catheterize (e.g., topical chlorhexidine or dilute iodine solutions suitable for surgical preparation)

TECHNIQUE
Expose the survey radiographs to ensure that the patient has been adequately prepared and that the radiographic techniques are adequate.

Vaginography
• This generally is performed *only* as a positive-contrast study, but negative-contrast (gas based) or double-contrast studies can be used where deemed needed.

• After cleansing the vaginal orifice and surrounding structures, distend the vestibule and vagina by placing a balloon catheter just inside the labia and optimally inflating it. Minimally traumatic forceps (sponge, placental, or Pennington) can facilitate keeping the balloon in the vagina when adequate distention alone fails. The balloon catheter should be prefilled with the material of choice, and retrograde filling should continue until mild resistance to injection is noted (preferably before pressure-induced leakage occurs around the balloon). This applies to either the preferred positive-contrast (a solution containing ≈150 mg/mL of iodine as sterile diatrizoate or iothalamate) or negative-contrast [usually room air is used (see the Contraindications section)] studies.

Radiographic Views and Filming Sequence
Expose a lateral and VD view centered on the pelvis immediately after administration of contrast material. Expose oblique or DV and opposite lateral views to clarify intramural or attached versus free intraluminal filling defects.

SAMPLE HANDLING
None

APPROPRIATE AFTERCARE
Postprocedure Patient Monitoring
• Be sure that the patient recovers promptly and completely from the sedation or anesthesia.

• Monitor any procedure-induced vaginal bleeding or hematuria. Repeat vaginoscopy to verify that there is no laceration and treat as though bleeding is caused by vaginitis or cystitis with antibiotics if bloody discharge or bloody urine persists for more than 1 or 2 voidings after the catheter is removed.

• Be sure the patient can urinate voluntarily once recovered from the sedation or anesthesia.

• Monitor for any evidence of procedure-induced urinary tract infection and treat as necessary.

Nursing Care
None

Dietary Modification
None

Medication Requirements
Antibiotics as necessary to treat procedure-induced urinary tract infection

Restrictions on Activity
None

Anticipated Recovery Time
Only as long as it takes to recover from the sedation or anesthesia

 INTERPRETATION

NORMAL FINDINGS OR RANGE
The normal canine vagina and vestibule, when distended, approach the diameter of the normally distended colorectal structures (Figure 1). There is a mild narrowing at the level of the constrictor vestibuli muscle. This narrowing is ≈50% of the vaginal or vestibular diameter, although more dramatic narrowing to no less than 0.35 times the DV vaginal diameter has been suggested to be normal and usually in a transverse plane at or just proximal to the tuber ischii. The narrowing is also referred to as a vestibulovaginal junction. The external urethral orifice is usually just distal to the narrowed region and is centered on the floor of the proximal vestibule. The mucosal surfaces of the vestibule and vagina are smooth, with no sharp crevices or irregularities. There are no clefts, bands, or duplicate tubes in the normally distended female lower genital tract. It is normal (and often preferable) to have reflux from the vestibule into the external urethral orifice, filling the urethra and demonstrating its continuity to the level of the

VAGINOGRAPHY

urinary bladder. Unless the bitch or queen is in or very near estrus or has been primed with estrogen, the cervix is usually sufficiently tight to limit reflux of contrast medium into the uterus. The vagina should be approximately centered in the pelvis, and the cervix should be visualized as a beanlike filling defect at the proximal tip of the vagina, just anterior to the pelvic inlet, at about the transverse plane of the urinary bladder trigone.

ABNORMAL VALUES

In general, the abnormalities found include atresia or stricture (particularly at the interface between the vagina and vestibule), duplicate vaginal tubes or a central cleft, persistent or imperforate hymen, a malpositioned external urethral orifice (at or proximal to the constrictor vestibuli plane), masses originating in the wall that project into and distort the lumen (usually tumors but occasionally blood clots, polyps, or granulomas), and foreign bodies. On occasion, abnormal connections can be identified, including an ectopic ureter connected to the vagina or a fistula between the vagina and the colon, the urinary bladder, or the peritoneal cavity. A uterine stump granuloma can distort the otherwise bean-shaped appearance of the cervix. Keep in mind that a contrast vaginourethrogram and a good vaginoscopic examination are generally complementary. Although the urethra can be at least partially distended using retrograde vaginourethrography, it is not a substitute for (and is often more difficult than) a retrograde urethrocystogram.

CRITICAL VALUES

None

INTERFERING FACTORS

Drugs That May Alter Results of the Procedure

None

Conditions That May Interfere with Performing the Procedure

- Stricture of the external labia, limiting access to the vestibule
- Contraindication for sedation or anesthesia in all but the most depressed patients

Procedure Techniques or Handling That May Alter Results

- None, unless there is iatrogenic overdistention or rupture of the vagina or vestibule or if there is iatrogenic catheter trauma or perforation
- *Beware* of contrast-medium effects on urinalysis results probably for at least 24 h, including specifically false increases in urine specific gravity and some interference with the successful growth of some organisms in samples submitted for bacterial culture.

Influence of Signalment on Performing and Interpreting the Procedure

Species

Catheter size and availability may be more limited for cats.

Breed

None

Age

None, provided the patient can endure the physiologic effects of sedation or anesthesia

Gender

Only females

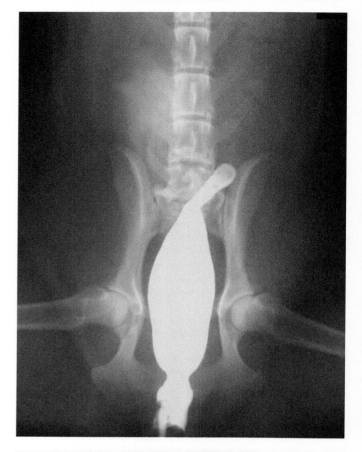

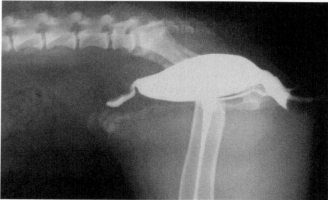

Figure 1

Ventrodorsal (above) and right lateral (below) views of a normal female canine contrast vaginourethrogram. Courtesy of Dr. Gary R. Johnston.

Pregnancy
Radiation effects on first-trimester fetuses can be problematic, so this procedure is, therefore, a risk-benefit judgment for pregnant patients.

CLINICAL PERSPECTIVE

Contrast vaginography provides morphologic (i.e., size, shape, location, surface characteristics) information on the vestibule, vagina, and the urethra. Similar information cannot be garnered from transrectal or intrapelvic ultrasonography (which requires specialized transducers) unless the vagina and vestibule are distended. In addition, contrast vaginourethrography requires a commitment to heavy sedation or even general anesthesia and appropriate distention to limit equivocation and interpretive error. Contrast vaginourethrography provides little information on sphincter function unless apparent morphologic distortion is directly associated with sphincter region.

MISCELLANEOUS

ANCILLARY TESTS
None

SYNONYMS
* Contrast vaginography
* Retrograde vaginourethrography

SEE ALSO
Blackwell's Five-Minute Veterinary Consult: Canine and Feline Topics
* Urolithiasis, Calcium Oxalate
* Urolithiasis, Calcium Phosphate
* Urolithiasis, Cystine
* Urolithiasis, Struvite—Cats
* Urolithiasis, Struvite—Dogs
* Urolithiasis, Urate
* Urolithiasis, Xanthine
* Uterine Tumors
* Vaginal Malformations and Acquired Lesions
* Vaginal Tumors

Related Topics in This Book
* General Principles of Radiography
* Cystourethrography
* Excretory Urography
* Lower Urinary Tract Ultrasonography
* Uterine Ultrasonography

ABBREVIATIONS
* DV = dorsoventral
* VD = ventrodorsal

Suggested Reading
Allen WE, France C. A contrast radiographic study of the vagina and uterus of the normal bitch. *J Small Anim Pract* 1985; **26**: 153–156.
Burk RL, Feeney DA. The abdomen. In: *Small Animal Radiology and Ultrasonography: A Diagnostic Text and Atlas*, 3rd ed. Philadelphia: WB Saunders, 2003: 427–428.
Crawford JT, Adams WM. Influence of vestibulovaginal stenosis, pelvic bladder, and recessed vulva on response to treatment for clinical signs of lower urinary tract disease: 38 cases (1990–1999). *J Am Vet Med Assoc* 2002; **221**: 995–999.
Feeney DA, Johnston GR. Uterus, ovaries and testes. In: Thrall DE, ed. *Textbook of Veterinary Diagnostic Radiology*, 4th ed. Philadelphia: WB Saunders, 2002: 603–614.
Gibbs PEC, Latham J. An evaluation of positive contrast vaginourethrography as a diagnostic aid in the bitch. *J Small Anim Pract* 1984; **24**: 531–549.
Kyles AE, Vaden S, Hardie EM, Stone EA. Vestibulovaginal stenosis in dogs: 18 cases (1987–1995). *J Am Vet Med Assoc* 1996; **209**: 1889–1893.
Root MV, Johnston SD, Johnston GR. Vaginal septa in dogs: 15 cases (1983–1992). *J Am Vet Med Assoc* 1995; **206**: 56–58.

INTERNET RESOURCES
University of Minnesota, Veterinary Radiology, http://www.cvm.umn.edu/vetrad/.

AUTHOR NAME
Daniel A. Feeney

VOIDING UROHYDROPROPULSION

BASICS

TYPE OF PROCEDURE
Miscellaneous

PROCEDURE EXPLANATION AND RELATED PHYSIOLOGY
Voiding urohydropropulsion (VU) enables safe and rapid removal of small urocystoliths of any mineral composition. This technique is designed to take advantage of the effects of gravity on urolith position in the urinary bladder and of dilation of the urethral lumen that occurs during the voiding phase of micturition. Special equipment is not required.

INDICATIONS
• Removal of urocystoliths from asymptomatic and symptomatic dogs or cats
• This procedure is ideal for expulsion of recurrent uroliths in patients that are regularly monitored.
• Other material (e.g., crystalline debris, blood clots) in the urinary bladder can also be removed.

CONTRAINDICATIONS
• Uroliths larger than the most narrow portions of the urethra (e.g., greater than ≈5 mm in diameter in a 20-kg male dog) are unlikely to pass.
• Urethroliths are usually too large to pass further distally through the urethra.
• Urinary tract infection may result in vesicoureteral reflux of bacteria to the kidney.
• Uroliths, once detected radiographically, are usually too large to pass through the normal urethra of male cats.
• The urinary bladder may be too fragile to manually express following recent surgery (within 1–3 months).

POTENTIAL COMPLICATIONS
• Bladder rupture
• Incomplete urolith removal
• Transient hematuria
• Transient pollakiuria
• Urethral obstruction
• Urinary tract infection

CLIENT EDUCATION
• To minimize anesthetic complications, withhold food 12 h prior to VU.
• If complete urolith removal is unsuccessful, surgery or other forms of urolith removal should be considered.
• Uroliths that become lodged in the urethra during VU are easily flushed back into the urinary bladder. These uroliths that are too large to pass through the urethra will require other methods of correction.

BODY SYSTEMS ASSESSED
Renal and urologic

PROCEDURE

PATIENT PREPARATION
Preprocedure Medication or Preparation
To minimize retrograde reflux of bacteria into the kidney, ensure that there is no urinary tract infection prior to VU.

Anesthesia or Sedation
• General anesthesia is the standard of care to minimize pain and ensure urethral relaxation.
• Additional urethral anesthesia can be achieved with epidural anesthesia or intraurethral instillation of local anesthetic agents (e.g., carbocaine, lidocaine).

Patient Positioning
Just prior to bladder evacuation, position the patient such that the spine is approximately vertical.

Patient Monitoring
None

Equipment or Supplies
• Flexible urinary catheters: typically, flexible 8 French, 21 inches (53.3 cm) or longer
• Sterile physiologic solution (e.g., normal saline, lactated Ringer's solution)
• A large-volume syringe (20–60 mL): A drip set can be used to administer larger volumes of fluid.
• A 3-way stopcock
• Sterile water-soluble lubricant
• Supplies to facilitate transurethral catheterization of the female (e.g., vaginoscope, otoscope)

TECHNIQUE
• Anesthetize the patient.
• Attach a 3-way stopcock to the end of the urinary catheter.
• Use the urinary catheter to fill the urinary bladder.
• Position the patient such that the spine is approximately vertical.
• Agitate the bladder from side to side to facilitate movement of stones into neck of the urinary bladder.
• Manually express the urinary bladder to evacuate its contents (i.e., fluids and uroliths).
• This procedure should be repeated until no uroliths are detected in the expelled fluid.

SAMPLE HANDLING
Submit the uroliths for quantitative mineral analysis.

APPROPRIATE AFTERCARE
Postprocedure Patient Monitoring
Perform medical imaging (e.g., radiography) or endouroscopy to verify that all uroliths have been evacuated.

Nursing Care
None

Dietary Modification
None needed for the procedure

Medication Requirements
• Administer a prophylactic antimicrobial agent for 3–5 days.
• Short-term (24 h) medication to minimize pain can also be considered but should not be necessary in every patient.

Restrictions on Activity
None

Anticipated Recovery Time
Postprocedural hematuria and dysuria should resolve in 12 h to 2 days.

 INTERPRETATION

NORMAL FINDINGS OR RANGE
• Most uroliths are expelled during the first voiding.
• A forceful urine stream indicates proper bladder filling, adequate forceful bladder expression, and passage of uroliths without obstruction.

ABNORMAL VALUES
If no stones are expelled, consider that the diagnosis was incorrect or spontaneous urolith passage prior to VU.

CRITICAL VALUES
Bladder rupture during manual expression requires diagnostic radiography to assess the extent of the lesion and the need for surgical correction.

INTERFERING FACTORS
Drugs That May Alter Results of the Procedure
Phenlypropanolamine administration increases urethral pressure. The clinical implications of these physiologic changes in anesthetized patients are not known.

Conditions That May Interfere with Performing the Procedure
Urethral tumors and urethral strictures may impede urolith passage.

Procedure Techniques or Handling That May Alter Results
None

Influence of Signalment on Performing and Interpreting the Procedure
Species
The urethra of cats is usually smaller than that of dogs of equal size, limiting the size of cystoliths that can be removed by VU.

Breed
The urethral diameter in large breeds is larger and should accommodate removal of larger uroliths.

Age
None

Gender
The urethra of male dogs is smaller than that of females, thereby limiting the size of cystolith that can be removed by VU and increasing the risk of urethral obstruction. We do not perform VU routinely in male cats to remove uroliths without surgical backup.

Pregnancy
None

CLINICAL PERSPECTIVE
• When the likelihood of success is uncertain (e.g., male patients, larger uroliths, uroliths with a spiked contour, a novice veterinarian), plan surgical backup or other alternative methods of urolith removal.
• When monitoring patients with recurrent uroliths, waiting until they develop clinical signs often results in uroliths that are too large to remove by VU.
• Previous urethrostomies may heal with deposition of fibrous tissue and subsequent stricture formation narrowing the urethral lumen, which may impede urolith passage.

 MISCELLANEOUS

ANCILLARY TESTS
If all uroliths have not been removed, consider medical dissolution, basket retrieval, lithotripsy, or surgery as alternatives.

SYNONYMS
None

SEE ALSO
Blackwell's Five-Minute Veterinary Consult: Canine and Feline Topics
• Urolithiasis, Calcium Oxalate
• Urolithiasis, Calcium Phosphate
• Urolithiasis, Cystine
• Urolithiasis, Struvite—Cats
• Urolithiasis, Struvite—Dogs
• Urolithiasis, Urate
• Urolithiasis, Xanthine

Related Topics in This Book
• Catheter-Assisted Stone Retrieval
• Urolith Analysis

ABBREVIATIONS
VU = voiding urohydropropulsion

Suggested Reading
Lulich JP, Osborne CA, Carlson M, *et al*. Nonsurgical removal of urocystoliths in dogs and cats by voiding urohydropropulsion. *Am J Vet Med Assoc* 1993; **203**: 660–663.
Lulich JP, Osborne CA, Sanderson SL, *et al*. Voiding urohydropropulsion: Lessons from 5 years of experience. *Vet Clin North Am Small Anim Pract* 1999; **29**: 283–291, xiv.

INTERNET RESOURCES
None

AUTHOR NAMES
Jody Lulich and Carl Osborne

VON WILLEBRAND FACTOR

 BASICS

TYPE OF SPECIMEN
Blood

TEST EXPLANATION AND RELATED PHYSIOLOGY
Von Willebrand factor (vWF) is an adhesive plasma glycoprotein required for platelet plug formation and control of small-vessel hemorrhage. vWF is synthesized in endothelial cells and megakaryocytes and undergoes extensive posttranslational processing resulting in formation and release of large subunit complexes (multimers). Large vWF multimers support platelet adhesion through interactions with subendothelial collagen and platelet membrane receptors. In addition, plasma vWF acts as a carrier protein for coagulation factor VIII, thereby enhancing thrombin generation at sites of platelet activation and vessel injury.

Hereditary vWF deficiency (vWD) is a common bleeding disorder of dogs. Subcategories of vWD (types 1, 2, and 3 vWD) are defined by the amount of residual protein and its multimeric structure. *Type 1* vWD refers to a partial quantitative vWF deficiency, with normal vWF multimer structure. *Type 2* vWD is a quantitative defect, and affected dogs also lack the most active, high molecular weight vWF multimers. *Type 3* vWD is the most clinically severe form, defined by the complete absence of vWF protein.

Von Willebrand factor concentration (vWF:Ag) is routinely measured in quantitative assays, with ELISA the most accurate method. Functional analyses of vWF can be performed based on vWF-dependent platelet agglutination, however these tests are difficult to standardize. Assays to measure vWF-collagen binding have been developed to screen for vWF functional defects. Evaluation of vWF multimeric structure is performed using Western blot analyses.

INDICATIONS
- To diagnose and classify vWD
- To monitor the efficacy of treatment with desmopressin and/or transfusion support to increase vWF to hemostatic levels and control hemorrhage in vWF-deficient patients
- To predict the carrier status for the vWD trait

CONTRAINDICATIONS
None

POTENTIAL COMPLICATIONS
None

CLIENT EDUCATION
Screening for trait before surgery or breeding is useful, especially in breeds with a high prevalence (i.e., Doberman pinschers) or severe forms (i.e., Scottish terriers and German shorthair pointers) of vWD.

BODY SYSTEMS ASSESSED
Hemic, lymphatic, and immune

 SAMPLE

COLLECTION
Venous blood: 1.8 mL (2-mL draw tube) or 2.7 mL (3-mL draw tube)

HANDLING
- Sodium citrate anticoagulant or EDTA anticoagulant
- Tube method: Collect blood directly into the tube by using a Vacutainer or butterfly needle. Allow the vacuum to fill the tube to the appropriate level.

- Syringe method: Draw exactly 1.8 mL of blood into a syringe containing exactly 0.2 mL of citrate.
- Centrifuge within 1 h of collection and transfer the plasma to plastic or siliconized glass tubes (no additives).

STORAGE
Store the plasma in a freezer.

STABILITY
Frozen (−20°C): 2 weeks

PROTOCOL
None

 INTERPRETATION

NORMAL FINDINGS OR RANGE
- The normal canine and feline vWF:Ag range is 70%–180% of the control.
- The normal canine vWF:CB is ≥50%. The normal ratio of vWF:Ag to vWF:CB is 1:1.
- Reference intervals are from the Comparative Coagulation Section of the Cornell University Animal Health Diagnostic Center. The values may vary depending on the laboratory.

ABNORMAL VALUES
- Values of vWF:Ag that are <50% indicate vWF deficiency.
- A ratio of vWF:Ag to vWF:CB that is >2 is evidence of type 2 vWD.

CRITICAL VALUES
- A vWF:Ag of <1% is diagnostic for severe, type 3 vWD.
- A vWF:Ag of <25% is associated with greatest risk of clinical expression of type 1 and 2 vWD.

INTERFERING FACTORS
Drugs That May Alter Results or Interpretation
Drugs That Interfere with Test Methodology
None

Drugs That Alter Physiology
Desmopressin (DDAVP) may induce a transient increase in vWF:Ag.

Disorders That May Alter Results
- Low vWF:Ag: endocrinopathy (especially hypothyroidism), immune-mediated disorders, and cardiac valvular defects associated with decreased synthesis or increased clearance of vWF
- High vWF:Ag: systemic inflammatory syndromes (vWF is an acute phase protein) and pregnancy

Collection Techniques or Handling That May Alter Results
- Poor venipuncture technique and failure to draw blood directly into the anticoagulant
- Clot formation depletes vWF, causing false depression of the vWF:Ag and vWF:CB.

Influence of Signalment
Species
- Most common hereditary bleeding disorder in dogs
- Rare in cats

Breed
See this chapter's table.

Age
None

Gender
None

Pregnancy
vWF:Ag increases during pregnancy.

LIMITATIONS OF THE TEST
Sensitivity, Specificity, and Positive and Negative Predictive Values
N/A

Valid If Run in a Human Lab?
No—species-specific assays are required.

Classification of Von Willebrand Disease

Type	Clinical and laboratory features	Reported breeds
Type 1 vWD	Mild to moderate bleeding tendency Low vWF:Ag and vWF:CB (ratio, 1:1) Normal vWF multimers	Airedale, Bernese mountain dog, Doberman pinscher, dachshund, corgi, miniature pinscher, and schnauzer, among others
Type 2 vWD	Moderate to severe bleeding tendency Low vWF:Ag and vWF:CB (ratio, >2) Lack of high molecular weight multimers	German wirehaired pointer, German shorthaired pointer, and Cavalier King Charles spaniel
Type 3 vWD	Severe bleeding tendency No detectable vWF:Ag or vWF:CB	Scottish terrier, Shetland sheepdog, Dutch kooiker, and sporadic cases

CLINICAL PERSPECTIVE
• Typical signs of vWD include mucosal hemorrhage (e. g., epistaxis, gingival hemorrhage, GI bleeding) and prolonged posttraumatic or surgical hemorrhage.
• The clinical severity of type 1 vWD correlates with severity of vWF deficiency. The risk of abnormal bleeding is greatest for dogs with an vWF:Ag of <25%.

MISCELLANEOUS

ANCILLARY TESTS
• Buccal bleeding time and/or PFA-100 (platelet function analyzer) closure time (nonspecific tests of platelet function)

• Coagulation assays and platelet function studies to rule out coagulation factor deficiency or platelet dysfunction

SYNONYMS
None

SEE ALSO
Blackwell's Five-Minute Veterinary Consult: Canine and Feline Topics
Von Willebrand Disease
Related Topics in This Book
• Bleeding Time
• Partial Thromboplastin Time, Activated
• Platelet Count and Volume
• Platelet Function Tests
• Prothrombin Time

ABBREVIATIONS
• vWD = von Willebrand Disease
• vWF:Ag = von Willebrand factor antigen
• vWF:CB = von Willebrand factor collagen-binding assay

Suggested Reading
Brooks MB, Catalfamo JL. Platelet disorders and von Willebrand disease. In: Ettinger S, Feldman E, eds. *Textbook of Veterinary Internal Medicine*, 6th ed. St Louis: Saunders Elsevier, 2004: 1918–1929.
Meyers KM, Wardrop KJ, Meinkoth J. Canine von Willebrand disease: Pathobiology, diagnosis, and short term treatment. *Compend Contin Educ Pract Vet* 1992; **14**: 13–22.

INTERNET RESOURCES
Cornell University, College of Veterinary Medicine, Department of Population Medicine and Diagnostic Sciences, Comparative coagulation: Canine von Willebrand disease, http://www.diaglab.vet.cornell.edu/coag/clinical/vonwill/.
Massachusetts General Hospital, Pathology Service, Coagulation Test Handbook: Von Willebrand Factor, http://www.massgeneral.org/pathology/coagbook/co006200.htm.

AUTHOR NAME
Marjory Brooks

WATER-DEPRIVATION TEST, MODIFIED

 BASICS

TYPE OF PROCEDURE
Functional test

PROCEDURE EXPLANATION AND RELATED PHYSIOLOGY
Polydipsia and polyuria are routinely characterized as high water consumption >100 mL/kg/day and urine production >50 mL/kg/day, respectively. Many of the diagnostic tests used to determine the common causes of polydipsia and polyuria are available through point-of-care machines or major commercial laboratories. Because direct determination of antidiuretic hormone (ADH) concentration, also known as arginine vasopressin, in small animal patients is not widely available, indirect testing is used to assess the presence of ADH and its activity on the kidneys in a clinical setting. The modified water-deprivation test enables the assessment of this hormonal pathway.

In normal animals, ADH is produced in the hypothalamus and then stored and released from the posterior pituitary in response to increasing osmolality and decreasing blood volume. ADH then travels in the vasculature to the kidneys and, at the level of the nephron, binds to receptors on cells of the collecting ducts to promote water reabsorption. The result is total body water retention and increasing urine concentration.

INDICATIONS
To distinguish psychogenic polydipsia from central diabetes insipidus (CDI) and primary nephrogenic diabetes insipidus (NDI), generally in animals with hyposthenuria

CONTRAINDICATIONS
• Dehydration, azotemia, or systemic illness
• Patients that have not been evaluated for other common causes of polyuria and polydipsia by means of routine testing such as a CBC, biochemical profile, urinalysis with culture, or appropriate endocrine testing to evaluate for hyperadrenocorticism (especially dogs) or hyperthyroidism (especially cats) should not undergo a modified water-deprivation test.
• Patients with repeated fixed isosthenuria (urine specific gravity, 1.008–1.015) and high normal kidney values should be suspected to have renal insufficiency and not be evaluated with a modified water-deprivation test without further renal evaluation.
• Patients with recent history of receiving medication that may contribute to polyuria and polydipsia, such as corticosteroids, diuretics, and anticonvulsants, should not undergo the modified water-deprivation test until after a sufficient washout period.

POTENTIAL COMPLICATIONS
• Central nervous system injury caused by hypernatremic hypertonic dehydration
• Unrecognized renal insufficiency worsened by generalized dehydration
• Water intoxication, if the animal has an uncontrolled urge to consume water rapidly after the test

CLIENT EDUCATION
• Hospitalization is required.
• The testing process is time consuming and may require >1 day.
• The patient may require referral to a 24-h-care hospital for evaluation during continuation of the test.
• The administration of additional diagnostics may be necessary to obtain a definitive diagnosis and prognosis.

BODY SYSTEMS ASSESSED
• Endocrine
• Renal and urologic

 PROCEDURE

PATIENT PREPARATION
Preprocedure Medication or Preparation
• Complete evaluation for other causes of polyuria and polydipsia prior to the modified water-deprivation test.
• Repeated urinalyses or at least 3 repeated measurements of urine specific gravity should be part of the diagnostic evaluation prior to a modified water-deprivation test.
• To lessen the impact of medullary washout, the owner should measure and record the pet's 24-h water consumption (in mL/kg/day) several days prior to the test. Water intake should be gradually reduced from that value recorded at >3–4 days to the value recorded at ≈80–100 mL/kg/day just before the test.
• Withhold food for 12 h before the start of the test.

Anesthesia or Sedation
None

Patient Positioning
N/A

Patient Monitoring
Monitor for any signs of dehydration, altered mentation, or systemic illness such as weakness or vomiting during the testing.

Equipment or Supplies
• An accurate body-weight scale with appropriate subunits of measurement (i.e., ounces or one-tenth of a kilogram)
• A urinary catheter for either intermittent or indwelling catheterization (e.g., polypropylene catheter or Foley catheter)
• A calibrated refractometer
• Point-of-care biochemical testing for BUN, serum creatinine, and serum electrolyte concentrations.
• ADH (i.e., vasopressin) or an analog. Because no veterinary products are available, products approved for human patients are used in an extralabel fashion. Vasopressin is available as Pitressin (Monarch Pharmaceuticals, Bristol, TN) or as a generic with a concentration of 20 units/mL in variously sized vials. Desmopressin, a synthetic vasopressin analog, is available as DDAVP (Rhone-Poulenc Rorer, Collegeville, PA) or as a generic and can be obtained as an intranasal spray or injection. The intranasal preparation is available in 2.5- and 5-mL bottles at a concentration of 100 µg/mL. Although this can be administered effectively intranasally in dogs and cats, it is far easier to administer this form into the conjunctival sac; the expected response is similar. The injectable desmopressin is available in 4 or 15 µg/mL but may be cost prohibitive. The oral formulation is not recommended for use during the modified water-deprivation test.

TECHNIQUE
Part 1
• The test should be performed at the start of the day, although this is less critical if the hospital has veterinarians and staff on site 24 h a day.
• Perform a physical examination, including assessment of hydration and neurologic status.
• Empty the urinary bladder via catheterization or, though much less desirable, by manual expression, cystocentesis, or voluntarily patient voiding.
• Determine the animal's body weight by using the same scale that will be used for the remainder of the test.
• Determine the immediate preprocedure BUN, serum creatinine, serum electrolyte concentrations, and the urine specific gravity.
• Serum and urine are collected and saved for osmolality at the start of test, as well.
• The patient is hospitalized and confined, without food or water, to a run or cage.

• The body weight is determined, and hydration and neurologic status are examined every hour and recorded.
• The bladder is emptied by catheterization, and urine specific gravity is checked and recorded every 2 h, as well as at the end of part 1.
• Repeat the testing of BUN, serum creatinine, and serum electrolytes every 4 h, as well as at the end of the part 1.
• Part 1 is completed when the patient has either demonstrated a urine specific gravity of ≥1.030, lost 5% of its body weight, appears clinically dehydrated, becomes azotemic (BUN, >30 mg/dL; or creatinine, >1.6 mg/dL) or hypernatremic, or appears neurologically inappropriate or systemically ill.
• Serum and urine are collected and saved for osmolality at the completion of part 1.
• Upon completion of part 1, blood can be obtained to determine the vasopressin concentration, although handling and storage should be discussed with the recipient laboratory prior to the water-deprivation test.
• Animals found to have a urine specific gravity of ≥1.030 do not need to proceed to part 2 of the modified water-deprivation test.

Part 2
• Animals that did not develop azotemia, hypernatremia, neurologic abnormalities, or signs of systemic illness may be tested further for response to exogenous ADH stimulation. Those that have developed these abnormalities should be given medical attention, and part 2 is not initiated.
• Food and water are withheld until the end of the test.
• Either vasopressin or desmopressin is administered to the patient parenterally.
• If vasopressin is selected, 0.5 units/kg with a maximum dose of 5 units is administered IM. If desmopressin is selected, 20 µg (4 drops) of the intranasal preparation is administered into a conjunctival sac, or 5 µg of injectable preparation is administered IV. Neither IV nor SC administration of the intranasal product is advised due to the lack of sterility of the product and variable absorption in a dehydrated state, respectively.
• If vasopressin has been administered, the bladder is emptied completely at 30, 60, and 90 min, and the urine specific gravity and osmolality are measured at each sampling.
• The time to peak effect of desmopressin is variable. Therefore, the bladder is emptied every 2 h for at least 8 h after desmopressin administration or until urine specific gravity is ≥1.010.

Other Considerations
• If the patient has not met any of the criteria for completion of part 1 by the regular closing time of the initiating hospital, a couple of options exist: (1) the veterinarian performing the test and appropriate staff stay until completion of the test, (2) the patient is referred with complete and detailed records, including weight at the time of referral, to an overnight hospital that can continue (weighing the patient upon admission) and complete the test, or (3) the test is aborted and appropriate postprocedure aftercare is followed to minimize health risks.
• If part 1 is aborted because of time constraints, and referral to a 24-h hospital is not possible for future testing, further modification of the test can be considered. This adjustment should never be made during the first attempt at water-deprivation testing. This adjustment entails starting a new test at 10 p.m. to midnight on a new day, following the similar starting protocol of emptying the bladder, checking urine specific gravity and body weight, and confining the patient without food and water until early the following morning. The patient is looked after by nighttime hospital staff making rounds or by the owner with the pet at home. Then, early the next morning (e.g., 6 a.m.) the body weight is checked along with urine specific gravity and bladder emptying, and the test is continued until completion, as previously described.

SAMPLE HANDLING
• Store samples for serum and urine osmolality in a refrigerator in properly labeled airtight containers.
• Samples for endogenous vasopressin assay should be stored according to the receiving laboratory's specifications.

APPROPRIATE AFTERCARE
Postprocedure Patient Monitoring
Monitor the reintroduction of water, watching for signs of vomiting or changes in mentation.

Nursing Care
After the modified water-deprivation test, gradually reintroduce small amounts of water (10 mL/kg) every 20–30 min for 2–4 h so as to not allow large quantities to be consumed rapidly.

Dietary Modification
None

Medication Requirements
None

Restrictions on Activity
None

Anticipated Recovery Time
A recovery time of 2–4 h, provided the reintroduction of water proceeds without incident

INTERPRETATION
NORMAL FINDINGS OR RANGE
• A urine concentration of ≥1.030 or a urine osmolality of >1,200 mOsm/kg is considered normal following part 1 of the modified water-deprivation test.
• Normal results also are identified commonly in dogs with psychogenic polydipsia and rarely in dogs with hyperadrenocorticism after part 1 of the modified water-deprivation test.
• Endogenous vasopressin concentrations of >6 pg/mL following water deprivation and a subsequent loss of 5% of body weight are normal but may also be seen with NDI and, rarely, psychogenic polydipsia.

ABNORMAL VALUES
• A urine specific gravity of >1.007 to ≤1.030 or a urine osmolality of >310 to ≤1,000 mOsm/kg following part 1 is consistent with partial CDI, hyperadrenocorticism, or psychogenic polydipsia with substantial medullary washout. A further increase in urine specific gravity or urine osmolality by >10% after vasopressin or desmopressin administration suggests partial CDI or hyperadrenocorticism.
• A urine specific gravity of ≤1.007 or a urine osmolality of ≤300 mOsm/kg following part 1 is typical for either complete CDI or primary NDI. These dogs cannot eliminate urine with a higher osmolality than their serum. Following administration of vasopressin or desmopressin, a change in urine specific gravity to ≥1.010 or a change in urine osmolality by >10% of the value obtained at the end of part 1 is consistent with complete CDI.
• Following water deprivation and a subsequent loss of 5% of body weight, an endogenous vasopressin concentration of ≤6 pg/mL is suggestive of CDI or psychogenic polydipsia.
• Many other diseases causing polyuria and polydipsia can have abnormal water-deprivation test results (e.g., chronic renal failure with fixed isosthenuria), which underscore the need for the previously mentioned diagnostics prior to a water-deprivation test.

CRITICAL VALUES
None

WATER-DEPRIVATION TEST, MODIFIED

INTERFERING FACTORS
Drugs That May Alter Results of the Procedure
- Corticosteroids
- Anticonvulsants
- Diuretics
- A severely protein-restricted diet may lead to medullary washout in normal animals and should be identified prior to commencement of the modified water-deprivation test.

Conditions That May Interfere with Performing the Procedure
Conditions known to causes polyuria and polydipsia—including renal failure, hypercalcemia, hypokalemia, pyelonephritis, liver insufficiency, diabetes mellitus, pyometra (and prostatitis), primary renal glycosuria, hyperthyroidism, hyperadrenocorticism, hypoadrenocorticism, and polycythemia—can potentially cause abnormal results and should be treated and controlled prior to considering a water-deprivation test.

Procedure Techniques or Handling That May Alter Results
Vasopressin is stored at room temperature, whereas desmopressin is stored by refrigeration. Always check the package insert for additional handling information.

Influence of Signalment on Performing and Interpreting the Procedure
Species
- Since passing a urinary catheter repeatedly in cats is typically more difficult, the use of an indwelling urinary catheter should be considered. Alternatively, though less preferable, a combination of voluntary voiding, manual expression, or cystocentesis is used to collect urine samples and empty the bladder during testing.
- Normal cats typically can concentrate urine to a specific gravity of ≥1.035 when they are dehydrated.

Breed
None

Age
Renal development in both puppies and kittens continues after birth for several weeks. Although their urine-concentrating ability approaches that of adults by 2 months of age, caution should used in diagnosing partial CDI in immature animals with a urine specific gravity of >1.015 to ≤1.030 following a modified water-deprivation test because maximal concentrating ability may not be reached until 3–4 months of age.

Gender
Urinary catheters may be difficult to place in female dogs and female cats.

Pregnancy
To the author's knowledge, the safety of this test has not been evaluated in pregnant animals and therefore its use in pregnant animals should be avoided.

CLINICAL PERSPECTIVE
- Many of the causes of polyuria and polydipsia can and should be ruled in or out by safe and widely available laboratory tests prior to a modified water-deprivation test.

- A modified water-deprivation test is a valuable functional diagnostic test for differentiating psychogenic polydipsia from CDI and primary NDI.
- Because hyperadrenocorticism is relatively common in dogs and because of the potential for its misdiagnosis as partial CDI based on modified water-deprivation test results, a thorough evaluation for typical and atypical hyperadrenocorticism should be considered either prior to a modified water-deprivation test or if results suggest partial CDI.

MISCELLANEOUS

ANCILLARY TESTS
- Pituitary imaging (magnetic resonance imaging or computed tomography)
- Hickey-Hare test (saline-infusion test)

SYNONYMS
None

SEE ALSO
Blackwell's Five-Minute Veterinary Consult: Canine and Feline Topics
- Diabetes Insipidus
- Hyposthenuria
- Polyuria and Polydipsia

Related Topics in This Book
Desmopressin Response Test

ABBREVIATIONS
- ADH = antidiuretic hormone
- CDI = central diabetes insipidus
- NDI = nephrogenic diabetes insipidus

Suggested Reading
Barsanti JA, DiBartola SP, Finco DR. Diagnostic approach to polyuria and polydipsia. In: Bonagura JD, ed. *Kirk's Current Veterinary Therapy XIII: Small Animal Practice.* Philadelphia: WB Saunders, 2000: 831–835.
Feldman EC, Nelson RW. Water metabolism and diabetes insipidus. In: Feldman EC, Nelson RW, eds. *Canine and Feline Endocrinology and Reproduction*, 3rd ed. Philadelphia: WB Saunders, 2004:2–44.

INTERNET RESOURCES
None

AUTHOR NAME
Nathan L. Bailiff

WHITE BLOOD CELL COUNT AND DIFFERENTIAL

BASICS

TYPE OF SPECIMEN
Blood

TEST EXPLANATION AND RELATED PHYSIOLOGY
The two components to the WBC count are a total leukocyte count and a differential cell count. The total number of WBCs measured in the peripheral circulation is expressed as the number of leukocytes per unit volume of blood. The WBC count is related to the balance of marrow production and tissue consumption, although numbers of circulating lymphocytes are relatively independent of marrow activity in the adult because most lymphocyte production occurs in the peripheral lymphoid tissue. The distribution of leukocytes between circulating and marginal pools in response to glucocorticoids or endotoxin may impact the measured individual leukocyte numbers and total WBC count without changing the actual numbers of cells in the blood (see the "White Blood Cells: Neutrophils" chapter for further details). Numbers of cells measured in the peripheral circulation reflect cells that are in transit at a single time point and do not always represent tissue concentrations accurately, particularly for eosinophils.

A variety of methods are used to measure the total WBC count. Automated analyzers can use impedance, optical, or quantitative buffy coat analysis. Some instruments report a total nucleated cell count, which may include nucleated erythroid precursors, in which case the WBC count must be corrected mathematically. Other analyzers perform the correction automatically and report a true WBC count. Manual methods include hemocytometer counts or estimation of WBC counts by blood smear microscopic examination. One suggested formula for estimating the WBC count is the average number of WBCs at 10× magnification × 100. It is important that at least 10 microscopic fields be examined from all portions of the smear, including the feathered edge and the butt end.

Five types of WBCs can be found in a routine blood sample: neutrophils, lymphocytes, monocytes, eosinophils, and basophils. All of these cell types (as well as erythrocytes and platelets) arise from a pluripotential stem cell in the bone marrow. Through the effects of cytokines and growth factors, increased leukocyte production can be triggered by a variety of conditions, including infections, tissue damage, allergic reactions, and immune-mediated disease. In addition, DNA damage can lead to uncontrolled proliferation of hematopoietic cells, resulting in either lymphoma or leukemia. Acute leukemia (lymphoblastic or myeloid) occurs when proliferating precursors fail to differentiate and remain as blasts. With chronic leukemia, precursors fully differentiate, resulting in increased numbers of morphologically normal cells (e.g., erythrocytes, neutrophils, small lymphocytes).

WBCs can be divided into granulocytes and agranulocytes. Granulocytes, including neutrophils, eosinophils, and basophils, have cytoplasmic granules and multilobed nuclei. Agranulocytes include monocytes and lymphocytes. These cells lack cytoplasmic granules and generally have an irregularly round to bean-shaped nucleus.

In the differential cell count, the relative proportion of each type of leukocyte is determined and expressed as a percentage. An increase in the percentage of 1 type of leukocyte results in a decreased percentage of other types of leukocytes. Because of this, percentages can be difficult to interpret. Absolute leukocyte numbers are determined by multiplying the total leukocyte count by the percentage of each cell type in the differential cell count (e.g., absolute lymphocyte count = total WBC count ×% lymphocytes). Absolute counts are the most reliable values for clinical interpretation.

Many automated analyzers report partial or complete differential cell counts; however, manual differential cell counts based on microscopic classification of a minimum of 100 leukocytes remains the gold standard because of the limitations of automated differential cell counts, frequent flagging of suspect automated differential cell counts by the analyzers, and the inability of automated analyzers to identify important morphologic abnormalities. At a minimum, scanning of a blood smear is recommended to verify the accuracy of automated WBC and differential cell counts.

INDICATIONS
- Marker of inflammation or allergic reactions
- Marker of hematopoietic neoplasia/leukemia
- Assessment of the animal for evidence of immunosuppression
- Assessment of marrow function

CONTRAINDICATIONS
None

POTENTIAL COMPLICATIONS
None

CLIENT EDUCATION
None

BODY SYSTEMS ASSESSED
Hemic, lymphatic, and immune

SAMPLE

COLLECTION
1–3 mL of venous blood

HANDLING
EDTA is the anticoagulant of choice.

STORAGE
- Refrigeration is recommended for short-term storage of blood.
- Stained smears should be protected from light.

STABILITY
- Whole blood
  - Several hours at room temperature
  - 1–2 days at 2°–8°C
- Stained smears are stable for many years if protected from light.

PROTOCOL
- A manual differential count is performed at 50–100× magnification by zigzagging back and forth across the monolayer of the smear just behind the feathered edge (see the "Blood Smear Microscopic Evaluation" chapter).
  - As one moves toward the back of the smear, extensive RBC overlap should trigger a change in direction.
  - The feathered edge, where RBCs are organized into clusters separated by large areas of white space, should be avoided.
- All leukocytes should be identified and counted. These counts are used to determine the percentage of each cell type. Typically, 100 WBCs are identified.
- Nucleated RBCs (nRBCs) are tallied separately.

INTERPRETATION

NORMAL FINDINGS OR RANGE
- Dogs: 6,000–17,000/μL (6.0–17.0 × 10^3/μL; 6.0–17.0 × 10^9/L)
- Cats: 5,500–19,500/μL (5.5–19.5 × 10^3/μL; 5.5–19.5 × 10^9/L)
- Reference intervals may vary depending on the laboratory and assay.

WHITE BLOOD CELL COUNT AND DIFFERENTIAL

ABNORMAL VALUES
- Values above or below the reference range
- If the absolute numbers of each type of leukocyte are within the reference intervals, a slight deviation of the total WBC count from the reference interval is of questionable clinical significance.

CRITICAL VALUES
Dogs and cats with WBC counts of ≥50,000/μL and neutrophil counts of ≥25,000/μL may be associated with a high mortality rate.

INTERFERING FACTORS
Drugs That May Alter Results or Interpretation
Drugs That Interfere with Test Methodology
None

Drugs That Alter Physiology
- Numerous and by a variety of mechanisms. Always consider idiosyncratic reactions to any drug.
- Glucocorticoids can cause leukocytosis.
- Drugs associated with leukopenia/pancytopenia include albendazole, captopril, cephalosporins, chloramphenicol, cimetidine, diazoxide, estrogen, griseofulvin, hydralazine, metamizole, methimazole, penicillium, phenobarbital, phenylbutazone, primidone, propranolol, propylthiouracil, sulfonamides, and numerous chemotherapy drugs.

Disorders That May Alter Results
- The WBC count may be artificially increased by hyperlipidemia or clumped platelets.
- The WBC count may need to be corrected in conditions that cause increased circulating nRBCs (e.g., regenerative anemia, lead toxicity, bone marrow damage or disease). The corrected WBC count = WBC count × 100/100 + the number of nRBCs observed per 100 WBCs identified in the differential count.

Collection Techniques or Handling That May Alter Results
- The use of poorly mixed or clotted blood may lower the WBC count.
- Aging artifacts associated with prolonged or inappropriate storage may interfere with accurate microscopic classification of leukocytes.

Influence of Signalment
Species
Reference intervals are species specific.

Breed
Low WBC counts may be normal in Belgian Tervurens and in greyhounds.

Age
The WBC count may be slightly higher in individuals that are <2 months of age. Young animals sometimes show a marked mature lymphocytosis, possibly related to response to antigenic stimulation such as vaccination. This abnormality should not be associated with clinical signs and resolves over time.

Gender
None

Pregnancy
The WBC count may be slightly increased during pregnancy, generally deviating only slightly from the reference intervals.

LIMITATIONS OF THE TEST
Abnormalities indicate a pathologic process but do not provide a specific diagnosis without additional workup.

Sensitivity, Specificity, and Positive and Negative Predictive Values
N/A

Valid If Run in a Human Lab?
Yes—if validated instrumentation is used and trained personnel perform the testing.

Causes of Abnormal Findings

High values	Low values
Inflammation	Excessive peripheral demand (e.g.,
Tissue necrosis	overwhelming inflammation and/or
Corticosteroid effects	endotoxemia)
Hyperadrenocorticism	Decreased production
Glucocorticoid therapy	Aplastic anemia
Endogenous cortisol release	Immune-mediated precursor
due to stress of disease	destruction
Epinephrine effects	Aleukemic acute leukemia
Acute lymphoblastic leukemia	Infectious disease
Chronic lymphocytic leukemia	*Parvovirus*
Acute myeloid leukemia	FeLV
Lymphoma	FIV
Chronic myeloid leukemia	Early canine hepatitis
Leukocyte adhesion molecule	Canine distemper
deficiency	*Histoplasma capsulatum*
	Cryptococcus neoformans
	Rickettsial disease
	Drug effects (see the section Drugs
	That Alter Physiology)
	Myelodysplastic syndrome
	Belgian Tervurens and greyhounds
	Cyclic hematopoiesis

CLINICAL PERSPECTIVE
- Small deviations from the reference interval may be age or breed related or normal for that individual.
- Infectious, inflammatory, and drug-related changes are more common than inherited or neoplastic conditions.
- A drastic decrease in WBC count may indicate bone marrow failure.
- Serial WBC counts and differential counts may have diagnostic and prognostic value.
- In the absence of infectious or inflammatory disease, obtain a thorough drug history. Some drugs are more likely than others to cause leukopenia/neutropenia; however, idiosyncratic reactions to any drug are possible in individual animals.
- Chronic myeloid leukemia can be difficult to distinguish from inflammation and is diagnosed by ruling out other causes.

MISCELLANEOUS

ANCILLARY TESTS
- Aerobic and anaerobic cultures to work up infectious disease
- Bone marrow biopsy indicated with unexplained leukopenia, bicytopenia, or pancytopenia
- Immunophenotyping by flow cytometry, immunohistochemistry, or immunocytochemistry may be needed to identify atypical cells.

SYNONYMS
- Diff
- Leukocyte count

SEE ALSO

Blackwell's Five-Minute Veterinary Consult: Canine and Feline Topics

- Canine Parvovirus Infection
- Cyclic Hematopoiesis
- Feline Immunodeficiency Virus Infection (FIV)
- Feline Leukemia Virus Infection (FeLV)
- Feline Panleukopenia
- Immunodeficiency Disorders, Primary
- Leukemia, Acute Lymphoblastic
- Leukemia, Chronic Lymphocytic
- Lymphoma—Cats
- Lymphoma—Dogs
- Myelodysplastic Syndromes
- Myeloproliferative Disorders
- Pencytopenia

Related Topics in This Book

- Blood Smear Microscopic Examination
- Bone Marrow Aspiration and Biopsy
- Complete Blood Count
- White Blood Cells: Eosinophils

- White Blood Cells: Lymphocytes
- White Blood Cells: Neutrophils

ABBREVIATIONS

nRBC = nucleated red blood cell

Suggested Reading

Lucroy MD, Madewell BR. Clinical outcome and associated diseases in dogs with leukocytosis and neutrophilia: 118 cases (1996–1998) *J Am Vet Med Assoc* 1999; **214**: 805–807.

Lucroy MD, Madewell BR. Clinical outcome and diseases associated with extreme neutrophilic leukocytosis in cats: 104 cases (1991–1999) *J Am Vet Med Assoc* 2001; **218**: 736–739.

Mitzner BT. Why automated differentials fall short. *J Am Anim Hosp Assoc* 2001; **37**: 117–118.

Weiser G, Thrall MA. Introduction to leukocytes and the leukogram. In: Thrall MA, ed. *Veterinary Hematology and Clinical Chemistry.* Philadelphia: Lippincott Williams & Wilkins, 2004: 125–130.

INTERNET RESOURCES

None

AUTHOR NAME

Leslie Sharkey

BASICS

TYPE OF SPECIMEN
Blood

TEST EXPLANATION AND RELATED PHYSIOLOGY
Basophils, which are produced in the marrow, circulate and enter tissues, where they may persist for up to 2 weeks under appropriate conditions. The specifics of basophil function are still being investigated; however, they are likely to participate in the regulation of immune responses, especially those with a hypersensitivity component. Like eosinophils, basophils are larger than neutrophils, have segmented nuclei, and contain cytoplasmic granules with shape and staining characteristics that vary by species. Feline basophils have numerous rather indistinct, pale lavender granules that often result in the cytoplasm having a cobblestone appearance. When these granules overlay the nucleus, they cause chromatin to appear moth-eaten. Canine basophils have lavender cytoplasm containing small numbers of dark purple (metachromatic) granules. Both types of basophils are easily mistaken for monocytes.

INDICATIONS
- Screening for hypersensitivity disorders or parasitism
- Paraneoplastic reaction associated with a variety of malignancies

CONTRAINDICATIONS
None

POTENTIAL COMPLICATIONS
None

CLIENT EDUCATION
None

BODY SYSTEMS ASSESSED
Hemic, lymphatic, and immune

SAMPLE

COLLECTION
1–3 mL of venous blood

HANDLING
EDTA is the preferred anticoagulant although lithium heparin can also be used.

STORAGE
- Refrigeration is recommended for short-term storage of blood.
- Stained smears should be protected from light.

STABILITY
- Whole blood is stable for several hours at 25°C or up to 2 days at 4°C.
- Stained smears are stable for many years if protected from light.

PROTOCOL
None

INTERPRETATION

NORMAL FINDINGS OR RANGE
Basophils are not usually found in a routine differential count.
- Dogs: 0–100/μL (0–0.1 × 10^3/μL; 0–0.1 × 10^9/L)
- Cats: 0–100/μL (0–0.1 × 10^3/μL; 0–0.1 × 10^9/L)
- Reference intervals may vary depending on the laboratory and assay.

ABNORMAL VALUES
Values above the reference range

CRITICAL VALUES
None

INTERFERING FACTORS
Drugs That May Alter Results or Interpretation
Drugs That Interfere with Test Methodology
None

Drugs That Alter Physiology
None

Disorders That May Alter Results
None

Collection Techniques or Handling That May Alter Results
Aging artifacts may interfere with accurate microscopic classification of leukocytes.

Influence of Signalment
Species
Reference intervals are species specific.

Breed
None

Age
None

Gender
None

Pregnancy
None

LIMITATIONS OF THE TEST
Because of their indistinct granules, these cells tend to be overlooked by automated hematology analyzers and are identified only through microscopic examination of a blood smear.

Sensitivity, Specificity, and Positive and Negative Predictive Values

N/A

Valid If Run in a Human Lab?

Yes—if the blood smears are examined by personnel familiar with the unique appearance of canine and feline basophils.

Causes of Abnormal Findings

High values	Low values
Hypersensitivity disorders	Because basophil reference intervals
Parasitism	extend to zero, basopenia is difficult
Mast cell tumor	to document and is not considered
Thymoma	clinically significant.
Basophilic leukemia	
Associated with other	
myeloproliferative diseases	

CLINICAL PERSPECTIVE

- Basophilia is most often accompanied by eosinophilia.
- Because of the imprecision of leukocyte differential counts, only substantial basophilia or persistent mild basophilia ($>300/\mu L$) should be considered clinically significant.
- Substantial basophilia without eosinophilia might suggest a myeloproliferative disorder.

MISCELLANEOUS

ANCILLARY TESTS

- Bone marrow aspiration if a myeloproliferative disorder is present.
- Fecal float
- Heartworm antigen test
- Radiographs or ultrasound to rule out neoplasia

SYNONYMS

Basos

SEE ALSO

Blackwell's Five-Minute Veterinary Consult: Canine and Feline Topics

- Baylisascariasis
- Heartworm Disease—Cats
- Heartworm Disease—Dogs
- Hookworms (Ancylostomiasis)
- Liver Fluke Infestation
- Myelodysplastic Syndromes
- Myeloproliferative Disorders
- Roundworms (Ascariasis)
- Whipworms (Tricuriasis)

Related Topics in This Book

- Blood Smear Microscopic Examination
- Bone Marrow Aspirate and Biopsy
- White Blood Cell Count and Differential

ABBREVIATIONS

None

Suggested Reading

Stockham SL, Scott MA eds. Leukocytes. In: *Fundamentals of Veterinary Clinical Pathology*, 2nd ed. Ames: Iowa State Press, 2008:55–106.

Scott MA, Stockham SL. Basophils and mast cells. In: Feldman BF, Zinkl JG, Jain NC, eds. *Schalm's Veterinary Hematology*, 5th ed. Ames, IA: Blackwell, 2001: 308–317.

Weiser G, Thrall MA. Introduction to Leukocytes and the Leukogram. In: Thrall MA, ed. *Veterinary Hematology and Clinical Chemistry*. Philadelphia: Lippincott Williams & Wilkins, 2004: 125–130.

INTERNET RESOURCES

Cornell University, College of Veterinary Medicine, Clinical Pathology Modules, Leukocytes: Basophils, http://www.diaglab.vet.cornell.edu/clinpath/modules/heme1/baso.htm.

Merck Veterinary Manual: White blood cells, http://www.merckvetmanual.com/mvm/index.jsp?cfile = htm/bc/10103.htm.

Rebar AH, MacWilliams PS, Feldman BF, et al. Basophils: Overview, quantity, morphology. In: Rebar AH, MacWilliams PS, Feldman BF, et al., eds. A Guide to Hematology in Dogs and Cats. Jackson, WY: Teton NewMedia, http://www.ivis.org/docarchive/A3307.0505.pdf.

AUTHOR NAME

Leslie Sharkey

WHITE BLOOD CELLS: EOSINOPHILS

 BASICS

TYPE OF SPECIMEN
Blood

TEST EXPLANATION AND RELATED PHYSIOLOGY
Eosinophils are produced in the bone marrow and are present in the blood circulating pool and the blood marginated pool for minutes to hours. Eosinophils migrate into tissues in response to chemical signals and can persist in tissues for an extended period. Hence, eosinophil numbers in the circulation do not always parallel tissue concentrations. Eosinophils generally reside in the skin and along mucosal surfaces. The exact function of eosinophils is still under investigation, although increased numbers in the circulation may be associated with hypersensitivity disorders, with immune response to parasites, and with neoplasms such as mast cell tumor and lymphoma. Eosinophils may also have an immunomodulatory function. Interleukin 5 produced by lymphocytes and mast cells appears to be an important regulator of eosinophil numbers and function.

Eosinophils are slightly larger than neutrophils and have segmented nuclei and characteristic red-to-orange granules that have species-specific morphology and staining. Canine eosinophils have round granules that can vary significantly in size. Feline eosinophil granules are small and slightly rod shaped. In tissue cytologic samples and peripheral blood smears, eosinophil granules may consolidate into 1 or more very large granules. The major effector proteins in the granules include major basic protein, eosinophil peroxidase, eosinophil cationic protein, and eosinophil-derived neurotoxin. Selective degranulation can occur, resulting in the release of specific granule proteins.

INDICATIONS
• Marker for hypersensitivity disorders or parasitism
• Paraneoplastic reaction associated with mast cell tumor or lymphoma

CONTRAINDICATIONS
None

POTENTIAL COMPLICATIONS
None

CLIENT EDUCATION
None

BODY SYSTEMS ASSESSED
Hemic, lymphatic, and immune

 SAMPLE

COLLECTION
1–3 mL of venous blood

HANDLING
EDTA is the preferred anticoagulant although lithium heparin can also be used.

STORAGE
• Refrigeration is recommended for the short-term storage of blood.
• Stained smears should be protected from light.

STABILITY
• EDTA blood is stable for several hours at 25°C or up to 24 h at 4°C.
• Stained smears are stable for many years if protected from light.

PROTOCOL
None

 INTERPRETATION

NORMAL FINDINGS OR RANGE
• Dogs: 100–1,200/μL (0.1–1.2 × 10^3/μL; 0.1–1.2 × 10^9/L)
• Cats: 0–1,500/μL (0–1.5 × 10^3/μL; 0–1.5 × 10^9/L)
• Reference intervals may vary depending on the laboratory and assay.

ABNORMAL VALUES
Values above or below the reference range

CRITICAL VALUES
None

INTERFERING FACTORS
Drugs That May Alter Results or Interpretation
Drugs That Interfere with Test Methodology
None

Drugs That Alter Physiology
Glucocorticoids can cause eosinopenia.

Disorders That May Alter Results
None

Collection Techniques or Handling That May Alter Results
Artifacts caused by aging may interfere with the accurate microscopic classification of leukocytes.

Influence of Signalment
Species
Reference intervals are species specific.

Breed
Many greyhounds and some golden retrievers have abnormal eosinophil granules that resist staining with Romanovsky stains, especially quick stains [e.g., Diff-Quick (Andwin Scientific, Woodland Hills, CA) or Hema III (Protocol, Fisher Diagnostics, Middletown, VA)]. Granule contents appear to have dropped out, giving their eosinophils a vacuolated appearance similar to toxic neutrophils or monocytes.

Age
None

Gender
None

Pregnancy
None

LIMITATIONS OF THE TEST
None

Sensitivity, Specificity, and Positive and Negative Predictive Values
N/A

Valid If Run in a Human Lab?
Yes—if validated instrumentation is used by trained personnel.

Causes of Abnormal Findings

High values	Low values
Hypersensitivity disorders	Because some eosinophil reference
Parasitism	intervals extend to zero,
Ectoparasites	eosinopenia is not a recognized
Heartworms	abnormality in cats.
Tissue nematodes,	In dogs, eosinopenia is of
trematodes, and protozoa	questionable clinical significance
Lymphoma	with the exception of
Hypoadrenocorticism	characterizing corticosteroid
Mast cell tumor	effects or when associated with
Idiopathic eosinophilic	bone marrow hypoplasia or
syndromes	aplasia.
Eosinophilic leukemia	

CLINICAL PERSPECTIVE

- Small deviations from the reference interval may be age or breed related or normal for that individual. A change in percentage of eosinophils, with a normal absolute eosinophil count, is clinically insignificant.
- Eosinophil numbers in the circulation may be within reference intervals despite elevations in tissue concentrations. Therefore, a normal CBC cannot be used to rule out disorders associated with increased eosinophils.
- Eosinophil granule contents can damage normal cells, as well as the parasites they may be responding to, resulting in secondary lesions in affected tissues.

MISCELLANEOUS

ANCILLARY TESTS

- Fecal float
- Heartworm antigen test
- Radiography or ultrasonography to rule out neoplasia
- Bone marrow aspiration if a myeloproliferative disorder is suspected

SYNONYMS

None

SEE ALSO

Blackwell's Five-Minute Veterinary Consult: Canine and Feline Topics

- Atopy
- Baylisascariasis
- Eosinophilic Granuloma Complex
- Flea bite hypersensitivity and Flea Control
- Heartworm Disease—Cats
- Heartworm Disease—Dogs
- Hookworms (Ancylostomiasis)
- Liver Fluke Infestation
- Mast Cell Tumors
- Myeloproliferative Disorders
- Neosporosis
- Roundworms (Ascariasis)
- Tapeworms (Cestodiasis)
- Toxoplasmosis
- Whipworms (Tricuriasis)

Related Topics in This Book

- • Blood Smear Microscopic Examination
- Complete Blood Count
- White Blood Cell Count and Differential

ABBREVIATIONS

None

Suggested Reading

Iazbik MC, Couto CG. Morphologic characterization of specific granules in Greyhound eosinophils. *Vet Clin Pathol* 2005; **34**: 140–143.

Stockham SL, Scott MA, eds. Leukocytes. In: *Fundamentals of Veterinary Clinical Pathology*, 2nd ed. Ames: Iowa State Press, 2008: 55–106.

Weiser G, Thrall MA. Introduction to leukocytes and the leukogram. In: Thrall MA, ed. *Veterinary Hematology and Clinical Chemistry*. Philadelphia: Lippincott Williams & Wilkins, 2004: 125–130.

INTERNET RESOURCES

Cornell University, College of Veterinary Medicine, Clinical Pathology Modules, Leukocytes: Eosinophils, http://www.diaglab.vet.cornell.edu/clinpath/modules/heme1/eos.htm.

Rebar AH, MacWilliams PS, Feldman BF, et al. Eosinophils: Overview, quantity, morphology. In: Rebar AH, MacWilliams PS, Feldman BF, et al., eds. A Guide to Hematology in Dogs and Cats. Jackson, WY: Teton NewMedia, 2005, http://www.ivis.org/docarchive/A3306.0405.pdf.

AUTHOR NAME

Leslie Sharkey

BASICS

TYPE OF SPECIMEN
Blood

TEST EXPLANATION AND RELATED PHYSIOLOGY
Unlike other leukocytes, lymphoid precursors disperse to peripheral tissues such as the thymus, spleen, lymph nodes, and mucosa, where they continue to develop and proliferate. Lymphocyte life span varies from hours to years. A variety of lymphocyte subsets (B cells, natural killer cells, T cells, and their subtypes) have distinct immunologic functions and are identifiable by special methods that characterize surface protein expression. These subtypes are not, however, distinguishable at the light-microscopic level, so only a total peripheral lymphocyte count in cells per microliter is reported as part of the CBC. The absolute lymphocyte count reflects only the numbers of lymphocytes that are in transit between lymphoid tissues. Like neutrophils, lymphocytes in the blood are distributed between circulating and marginated pools, and shifts between these pools can be reflected in peripheral cell counts. Lymphocytosis can be caused by excitement (epinephrine secretion), persistent antigenic stimulation causing lymphoid hyperplasia, or lymphocytic neoplasm (i.e., lymphoma or leukemia). Lymphopenia can be caused by redistribution of lymphocytes to body compartments (e.g., effect of cortisol secretion or antigenic recruitment), loss of lymph, or lympholysis (e.g., viral infection, cortisol).

Changes in lymphocyte morphology can be as diagnostically significant as changes in lymphocyte numbers. Typical mature lymphocytes are smaller than neutrophils, with scant pale blue cytoplasm and a round nucleus. Atypical lymphocytes that either are reacting to antigenic stimulation (i.e., reactive lymphocytes) or are neoplastic (i.e., lymphoma, acute lymphoblastic leukemia) generally have 1 or more features typical of cells undergoing proliferation. These include an increased size (as large or larger than neutrophils), increased nuclear size (nuclear diameter greater than a canine RBC), increased cytoplasm volume, and deeply basophilic cytoplasm, sometimes with a prominent pale, perinuclear Golgi zone. Nuclei often appear to stain lighter because of a dispersed chromatin pattern, sometimes with prominent nucleoli. Some atypical lymphocytes have nuclei that are cleaved or slightly lobular. Reactive lymphocytes are usually small to medium sized, although large lymphocytes can be seen with severe antigenic stimulation. Morphologic features cannot reliably distinguish reactive from neoplastic lymphocytes and must be interpreted along with other findings such as animal age, evidence of inflammation, or immune-mediated disease.

Granular lymphocytes, which can sometimes also be seen in the circulation, contain variable numbers of eosinophilic granules that cluster to 1 side of the nucleus. These cells are likely natural killer cells or T cells. Rarely, cytoplasmic inclusions or vacuoles may indicate congenital disease (i.e., storage diseases).

INDICATIONS
- A marker of antigenic stimulation
- A screen for leukemia/lymphoma

CONTRAINDICATIONS
None

POTENTIAL COMPLICATIONS
None

CLIENT EDUCATION
None

BODY SYSTEMS ASSESSED
Hemic, lymphatic, and immune

SAMPLE

COLLECTION
1–3 mL of venous blood

HANDLING
EDTA is the preferred anticoagulant although lithium heparin can also be used.

STORAGE
- Refrigeration is recommended for the short-term storage of blood.
- Stained smears should be protected from light.

STABILITY
- Whole blood is stable for several hours at 25°C or up to 48 h at 4°C.
- Stained smears are stable for many years.

PROTOCOL
None

INTERPRETATION

NORMAL FINDINGS OR RANGE
- Dogs: 1,000–5,000/μL (1.0–5.0 × 10^3/μL; 1.0–5.0 × 10^9/L)
- Cats: 1,500–7,000/μL (1.5–7.0 × 10^3/μL; 1.5–7.0 × 10^9/L)
- Reference intervals may vary depending on the laboratory and assay.

ABNORMAL VALUES
Values above or below the reference range

CRITICAL VALUES
None

INTERFERING FACTORS
Drugs That May Alter Results or Interpretation
Drugs That Interfere with Test Methodology
None

Drugs That Alter Physiology
- Corticosteroids can cause lymphopenia.
- Epinephrine can cause lymphocytosis.
- Immunosuppressive drugs can cause lymphopenia.

Disorders That May Alter Results
None

Collection Techniques or Handling That May Alter Results
Artifacts caused by aging may interfere with the accurate microscopic classification of leukocytes.

Influence of Signalment
Species
Reference intervals are species specific.

Breed
Some bassett hounds have a combined immunodeficiency associated with lymphopenia.

Age
- Puppies and kittens may have higher lymphocyte counts than mature animals.
- Increased reactive lymphocytes are common in puppies and kittens with antigenic stimulation, particularly after vaccination.

Gender
None

Pregnancy
None

LIMITATIONS OF THE TEST
• Antigenic stimulation causes tissue lymphocyte changes that are not consistently reflected in the peripheral blood. Lymphocyte counts are often within reference intervals.
• Morphologic features cannot consistently distinguish reactive from neoplastic lymphocytes.

Sensitivity, Specificity, and Positive and Negative Predictive Values
N/A

Valid If Run in a Human Lab?
Yes—if validated instrumentation is used by trained personnel.

Causes of Abnormal Findings

High values	Low values
Chronic antigenic stimulation	Glucocorticoids
Infectious agents	Exogenous
Chronic canine ehrlichiosis	Endogenous (e.g., Cushing's
Rocky Mountain spotted fever	disease, stress of chronic
Leishmaniasis	disease)
Brucellosis	Viral infections
Chronic fungal infection	Canine distemper
Encephalitozoonosis	Parvovirus (canine and feline)
Noninfectious agents	FeLV
Nonlymphoid neoplasm	FIV
Immune-mediated disease	Canine hepatitis
Physiologic shift	Coronavirus enteritis
(epinephrine/norepinephrine)	Acute inflammation
Excitement (esp. young cats)	(redistribution of
Pain	lymphocytes)
Exercise effect	Immunosuppression
Hypoadrenocorticism	Chemotherapeutic drugs
Neoplasia	Radiation
Lymphoma	Loss of lymph
Chronic lymphocytic leukemia	Chylous effusion
Acute lymphoblastic leukemia	Protein losing enteropathies
	Congenital immunodeficiency

CLINICAL PERSPECTIVE
• Physiologic response to epinephrine can produce a lymphocytosis as high as 20,000 lymphocytes/μL.
• In dogs and cats with >20,000 lymphocytes/μL, consider chronic lymphocytic leukemia.
• In dogs, chronic ehrlichiosis (*Ehrlichia canis*) can cause severe lymphocytosis of up to >40,000 lymphocytes/μL.
• Consider lymphoma or acute leukemia if atypical lymphocytes or blasts are found in the CBC.
• Lymphopenia should not be interpreted as evidence of bone marrow suppression, because lymphoid proliferation occurs largely in peripheral lymphoid tissues and is relatively independent of marrow activity in adults.
• The absence of lymphopenia in an obviously stressed or sick animal should indicate that hypoadrenocorticism should be considered.
• Antigenic stimulation or excitement is much more likely than chronic lymphocytic leukemia in puppies and kittens.
• Lymphopenia is more common than lymphocytosis in animals with lymphoma—recirculating lymphocytes are unable to migrate through effaced nodes.
• In patients with lymphoma, atypical neoplastic lymphocytes are an uncommon finding in their CBC.

MISCELLANEOUS
ANCILLARY TESTS
• Bone marrow aspiration or biopsy to look for leukemia or stage V lymphoma
• Radiography or ultrasonography
• Fine-needle aspiration or biopsy of lymphoid tissue to evaluate unexplained lymphocytosis or morphologically abnormal lymphocytes
• An *Ehrlichia canis* antibody titer or PCR test
• Specific tests for other infectious agents
• An adrenocorticotropic hormone (ACTH) stimulation test
• Immunophenotyping to identify specific cell surface markers can help characterize abnormal circulating cells and distinguish lymphocyte subsets.
• An antigen receptor gene rearrangement PCR test to look for evidence of lymphoma

SYNONYMS
Lymphs

SEE ALSO
Blackwell's Five-Minute Veterinary Consult: Canine and Feline Topics
• Chapters on specific infectious agents
• Immunodeficiency Disorders, Primary
• Leukemia, Acute Lymphoblastic
• Leukemia, Chronic Lymphocytic
• Lymphadenopathy
• Lymphoma—Cats
• Lymphoma—Dogs
• Mucopolysaccharidoses

Related Topics in This Book
• Blood Smear Microscopic Examination
• Complete Blood Count
• White Blood Cell Count and Differential
• White Blood Cells: Neutrophils

ABBREVIATIONS
None

Suggested Reading
Avery PR, Avery AC. Molecular methods to distinguish reactive and neoplastic lymphocyte expansions and their importance in transitional neoplastic states. *Vet Clin Pathol* 2004; **33**: 196–207.
Heeb HL, Wilkerson MJ, Chun R, Ganta RR. Large granular lymphocytosis, lymphocyte subset inversion, thrombocytopenia, dysproteinemia, and positive *Ehrlichia* serology in a dog. *J Am Anim Hosp Assoc* 2003; **39**: 379–384.
Schultze AE. Interpretation of canine leukocyte responses. In: Feldman BF, Zinkl JG, Jain NC, eds. *Schalm's Veterinary Hematology*, 5th ed. Ames, IA: Blackwell, 2001:366–378.
Weiser G. Interpretation of leukocyte responses in disease. In: Thrall MA, ed. *Veterinary Hematology and Clinical Chemistry*. Philadelphia: Lippincott Williams & Wilkins, 2004: 135–148.

INTERNET RESOURCES
Rebar AH, MacWilliams PS, Feldman BF, et al. Lymphocytes: Overview, quantity, morphology. In: Rebar AH, MacWilliams PS, Feldman BF, et al., eds. A Guide to Hematology in Dogs and Cats. Jackson, WY: Teton NewMedia, 2005, http://www.ivis.org/docarchive/A3309.0705.pdf.
Wikipedia: Reactive lymphocyte, http://en.wikipedia.org/wiki/Reactive_lymphocyte.

AUTHOR NAME
Leslie Sharkey

WHITE BLOOD CELLS: MONOCYTES

BASICS

TYPE OF SPECIMEN
Blood

TEST EXPLANATION AND RELATED PHYSIOLOGY
Monocytes are produced primarily in the bone marrow and circulate in the blood before migrating into tissues to become macrophages. Monocytes/macrophages are phagocytic cells capable of clearing infectious organisms and debris but also play an important role in regulation of hematopoiesis, inflammation, tissue remodeling, immune recognition, and immune surveillance. Like neutrophils and lymphocytes, blood monocytes are found in circulating and marginated pools, and shifts may alter the monocyte count (in cells per microliter) in the CBC (see the "White Blood Cells: Neutrophils" chapter). As a result, monocytosis can occur in response to increased levels of cortisol or as a result of glucocorticoid therapy in dogs. Monocytosis can also be seen in association with acute and chronic inflammation (both suppurative and pyogranulomatous), tissue necrosis, internal hemorrhage, hemolysis, trauma, or immune-mediated disease.

On peripheral blood smears, monocytes appear to be the largest cells and often contain relatively abundant grainy, blue-gray cytoplasm that may have variable numbers of small, clear vacuoles. In some monocytes, fine pink lysosomal granules are visible in the cytoplasm. Nuclei are pleomorphic and can be round, oval, bean shaped, bilobed, or somewhat segmented, with a fine, lacy chromatin pattern. Monocytes with segmented nuclei may be confused with large toxic neutrophils, although monocytes will not contain Döhle bodies. Monocytes with oval nuclei may resemble reactive or atypical lymphocytes.

INDICATIONS
A marker of inflammation and/or tissue degeneration and necrosis

CONTRAINDICATIONS
None

POTENTIAL COMPLICATIONS
None

CLIENT EDUCATION
None

BODY SYSTEMS ASSESSED
Hemic, lymphatic, and immune

SAMPLE

COLLECTION
1–3 mL of venous blood

HANDLING
EDTA is the anticoagulant of choice.

STORAGE
- Refrigeration is recommended for the short-term storage of blood.
- Stained smears should be protected from light.

STABILITY
- EDTA blood is stable for several hours at 25°C or up to 24 h at 4°C.
- Stained smears are stable for many years if protected from light.

PROTOCOL
None

INTERPRETATION

NORMAL FINDINGS OR RANGE
- Dogs: 0–1,200/μL (0–1.2 × 10^3/μL; 0–1.2 × 10^9/L)
- Cats: 0–800/μL (0–0.8 × 10^3/μL; 0–0.8 × 10^9/L)
- Reference intervals may vary depending on the laboratory and assay.

ABNORMAL VALUES
Values above the reference range

CRITICAL VALUES
None

INTERFERING FACTORS
Drugs That May Alter Results or Interpretation
Drugs That Interfere with Test Methodology
None

Drugs That Alter Physiology
Glucocorticoids may cause monocytosis in dogs.

Disorders That May Alter Results
None

Collection Techniques or Handling That May Alter Results
Artifacts caused by aging may interfere with the accurate microscopic classification of leukocytes.

Influence of Signalment
Species
Reference intervals are species specific.

Breed
None

Age
None

Gender
None

Pregnancy
None

LIMITATIONS OF THE TEST
None

Sensitivity, Specificity, and Positive and Negative Predictive Values
N/A

Valid If Run in a Human Lab?
Yes—if validated instrumentation is used by trained personnel.

Causes of Abnormal Findings

High values	Low values
Inflammation	Because monocyte reference intervals extend to zero, monocytopenia is not a recognized abnormality.
Septicemia	
Bacterial endocarditis	
Hemolysis	
Immune-mediated disease	
Pyogranulomatous disease	
Trauma or tissue necrosis	
Glucocorticoid response	
Stress of chronic disease	
Hyperadrenocorticism	
Corticosteroid therapy	
Neoplasia	
Nonhematopoietic neoplasms	
Monocytic leukemia	
Malignant histiocytosis	
Administration of G-CSF	
Recovery from marrow damage	
Rebound from cyclic hematopoiesis	

CLINICAL PERSPECTIVE

Small deviations from the reference interval may be age or breed related or normal for that individual. A change in the percentage of monocytes with a normal absolute monocyte count is clinically insignificant.

MISCELLANEOUS

ANCILLARY TESTS
- Bone marrow aspiration if a myeloproliferative disorder is suspected
- Heartworm antigen test
- Radiography or ultrasonography to rule out neoplasia

SYNONYMS
Monos

SEE ALSO
Blackwell's Five-Minute Veterinary Consult: Canine and Feline Topics
- Endocarditis, Inefective
- Histoplasmosis
- Leishmaniasis
- Myeloproliferative Disorders

Related Topics in This Book
- Blood Smear Microscopic Examination
- Complete Blood Count
- White Blood Cell Count and Differential

ABBREVIATIONS
G-CSF = granulocyte–colony-stimulating factor

Suggested Reading
Schultze AE. Interpretation of canine leukocyte responses. In: Feldman BF, Zinkl JG, Jain NC, eds. *Schalm's Veterinary Hematology,* 5th ed. Ames, IA: Blackwell, 2001: 366–378.
Weiser G. Interpretation of leukocyte responses in disease. In: Thrall MA, ed. *Veterinary Hematology and Clinical Chemistry.* Philadelphia: Lippincott Williams & Wilkins, 2004: 135–148.

INTERNET RESOURCES
Cornell University, College of Veterinary Medicine, Clinical Pathology Modules, Leukocytes: Monocytes, http://www.diaglab.vet.cornell.edu/clinpath/modules/heme1/monocyte.htm.
Rebar AH, MacWilliams PS, Feldman BF, *et al*. Monocytes: Overview, quantity, morphology. In: Rebar AH, MacWilliams PS, Feldman BF, *et al*., eds. A Guide to Hematology in Dogs and Cats, Jackson, WY: Teton, 2005, NewMedia, http://www.ivis.org/docarchive/A3308.0605.pdf.

AUTHOR NAME
Leslie Sharkey

WHITE BLOOD CELLS: NEUTROPHILS

BASICS

TYPE OF SPECIMEN
Blood

TEST EXPLANATION AND RELATED PHYSIOLOGY
Neutrophils are the predominant circulating leukocyte in dogs and cats. Increased neutrophil production can be stimulated by infections (especially bacterial) and tissue damage. The *absolute neutrophil count* reflects a balance between bone marrow production and tissue consumption, as well as shifts between circulatory pools. Neutrophils in blood are either free flowing (the *circulating pool*) or loosely adherent to endothelium (the *marginated pool*). Only neutrophils in the circulating pool are included in the neutrophil count. Glucocorticoids and epinephrine cause a shift from the marginated pool to the circulating pool, causing an apparent increase in circulating neutrophils, whereas endotoxin has the opposite effect. Marginated neutrophils may reenter the circulating pool or migrate into tissues. Neutrophils circulate for ≈6 h.

Neutrophil morphology is diagnostically significant. If tissue demand for circulating neutrophils exceeds supply, immature neutrophils with incompletely segmented nuclei (*band neutrophils*) will be released in increased numbers (*left shift*). Toxic change, another indicator of significant inflammation, occurs secondary to the effects of inflammatory cytokines or bacterial toxins on cell development in the marrow. Toxic change is characterized by cytoplasmic basophilia and vacuolization, and the presence of amorphous blue-gray aggregates of endoplasmic reticulum (*Döhle bodies*). Small Döhle bodies can be normal in cat neutrophils. Hypersegmentation indicates an in vivo or in vitro aging change. Rare neutrophil morphologic abnormalities include inherited disorders (e.g., Pelger-Huët anomaly, mucopolysaccharidosis, Chediak-Higashi syndrome) and the presence of infectious agents (e.g., distemper virus, *Ehrlichia* sp., *Anaplasma* sp.).

INDICATIONS
- A marker of inflammation or hematopoietic neoplasia/leukemia
- A screen for congenital or infectious diseases affecting neutrophils

CONTRAINDICATIONS
None

POTENTIAL COMPLICATIONS
None

CLIENT EDUCATION
None

BODY SYSTEMS ASSESSED
Hemic, lymphatic, and immune

SAMPLE

COLLECTION
1–3 mL of venous blood

HANDLING
EDTA is the preferred anticoagulant although lithium heparin can also be used.

STORAGE
- Refrigeration is recommended for the short-term storage of blood.
- Stained smears should be protected from light.

STABILITY
- Whole blood is stable for several hours at 25°C or up to 48 h at 4°C.
- Stained smears are stable for many years.

PROTOCOL
None

INTERPRETATION

NORMAL FINDINGS OR RANGE
Reference intervals may vary depending on the laboratory and assay.
Dogs
- Segmented neutrophils: 3,000–11,500/μL (3.0–11.5 × 10^3/μL; 3.0–11.5 × 10^9/L)
- Band neutrophils: 0–300/μL (0–0.3 × 10^3/μL; 0–0.3 × 10^9/L)
Cats
- Segmented neutrophils: 2,500–12,500/μL (2.5–12.5 × 10^3/μL; 2.5–12.5 × 10^9/L)
- Band neutrophils: 0–300/μL (0–0.3 × 10^3/μL; 0–0.3 × 10^9/L)

ABNORMAL VALUES
Values above or below the reference range

CRITICAL VALUES
- A value of < 1,000 segmented neutrophils/μ indicates increased risk of infection, especially with disruption of barriers such as skin and mucosa.
- Neutrophil counts of ≥25,000/μL may be associated with a high mortality rate.

INTERFERING FACTORS
Drugs That May Alter Results or Interpretation
Drugs That Interfere with Test Methodology
None

Drugs That Alter Physiology
- Increased segmented neutrophils caused by glucocorticoids
- Drugs associated with neutropenia or pancytopenia include albendazole, captopril, cephalosporins, chloramphenicol, cimetidine, diazoxide, dipyrone, estrogen, griseofulvin, hydralazine, methimazole, penicillium, phenobarbital, anticonvulsants, propranolol, propylthiouracil, sulfonamides, and numerous chemotherapy drugs.

Disorders That May Alter Results
None

Collection Techniques or Handling That May Alter Results
Aging may alter leukocyte morphologic features.

Influence of Signalment
Species
None

Breed
Low neutrophil counts may be normal in Belgian Tervurens or in greyhounds.

Age
Slightly higher values are seen in individuals that are <2 months of age.

Gender
None

Pregnancy
Slightly higher values may be seen.

LIMITATIONS OF THE TEST
Sensitivity, Specificity, and Positive and Negative Predictive Values
N/A

Valid If Run in a Human Lab?
Yes—if validated instrumentation is used by trained personnel.
Causes of Abnormal Findings

High values	Low values
Inflammation	Excessive peripheral demand
Corticosteroid effects	(e.g., overwhelming
Hyperadrenocorticism	inflammation and/or
Glucocorticoid therapy	endotoxemia)
Endogenous cortisol release due	Decreased production
to stress of disease	Aplastic anemia
Epinephrine effects	Immune-mediated precursor
Chronic myeloid leukemia	destruction
Leukocyte adhesion molecule	Myelodysplastic syndrome
deficiency	Aleukemic acute leukemia
	Infectious disease
	Parvovirus
	FeLV
	FIV
	Early canine hepatitis
	Canine distemper
	Histoplasma capsulatum
	Cryptococcus neoformans
	Rickettsial disease
	Drug effects (see the section
	Drugs That Alter
	Physiology)
	Cyclic hematopoiesis

CLINICAL PERSPECTIVE
- Small deviations from the reference interval may be age or breed related or normal for that individual. A change in the percentage of neutrophils with a normal absolute neutrophil count is clinically insignificant.
- Chronic myeloid leukemia, presenting with a neutrophilia, is diagnosed by ruling out causes of inflammation.

MISCELLANEOUS
ANCILLARY TESTS
- Aerobic and anaerobic cultures to work up infectious disease
- Bone marrow biopsy indicated with unexplained neutropenia

SYNONYMS
- Band neutrophils
- Bands
- Polymorphonuclear cells (PMNs)
- Polys
- Segmented neutrophils (Segs)

SEE ALSO
Blackwell's Five-Minute Veterinary Consult: Canine and Feline Topics
- Cyclic Hematopoiesis
- Feline Immunodeficiency Virus Infection (FIV)
- Feline Panleukopenia
- Histoplasmosis
- Immunodeficiency Disorders, Primary
- Myelodysplastic Syndromes
- Myeloproliferative Disorders
- Pelger-Huet Anomaly

Related Topics in This Book
- Blood Smear Microscopic Examination
- White Blood Cell Count and Differential

ABBREVIATIONS
None

Suggested Reading
Brown RM, Rogers KS. Neutropenia in dogs and cats. *Comp Contin Educ Pract Vet* 2001; **23**: 534–542.
Lucroy MD, Madewell BR. Clinical outcome and associated diseases in dogs with leukocytosis and neutrophilia: 118 cases (1996–1998) *J Am Vet Med Assoc* 1999; **214**: 805–807.
Lucroy MD, Madewell BR. Clinical outcome and diseases associated with extreme neutrophilic leukocytosis in cats: 104 cases (1991–1999) *J Am Vet Med Assoc* 2001; **218**: 736–739.

INTERNET RESOURCES
None

AUTHOR NAME
Leslie Sharkey

WOOD'S LAMP EXAMINATION

 BASICS

TYPE OF PROCEDURE
Diagnostic sample collection

PROCEDURE EXPLANATION AND RELATED PHYSIOLOGY
A Wood's lamp is an ultraviolet light source filtered through a cobalt or nickel filter. When hair infected with certain species of dermatophyte are illuminated with the lamp, metabolites produced by the dermatophyte fluoresce an apple green.

INDICATIONS
As an initial screening test for the presence of dermatophytosis. Hairs that fluoresce with illumination under a Wood's lamp should be plucked and submitted for dermatophyte culture to confirm infection.

CONTRAINDICATIONS
None

POTENTIAL COMPLICATIONS
None

CLIENT EDUCATION
None

BODY SYSTEMS ASSESSED
Dermatologic

 PROCEDURE

PATIENT PREPARATION
Preprocedure Medication or Preparation
Light manual restraint of the patient

Anesthesia or Sedation
Not generally required

Patient Positioning
The patient should be positioned so that skin lesions can be easily examined under Wood's lamp illumination.

Patient Monitoring
None

Equipment or Supplies
• A darkened room
• A Wood's lamp

TECHNIQUE
The Wood's lamp should be switched on a minimum of 5 min prior to use because the wavelength emitted is temperature dependent. Examination should take place in a darkened room. Optimally, the patient should be allowed time to adjust to the darkened environment before the lamp is used. The Wood's lamp should be held directly over lesional skin at a distance of 5–10 cm and illumination of the area continued for 3–5 min because fluorescence may not occur immediately.

APPROPRIATE AFTERCARE
None

 INTERPRETATION

NORMAL FINDINGS OR RANGE
Sebum, dust, and scale on the skin or hair coat may fluoresce under Wood's lamp illumination. These commonly take on a bluish hue and should not be interpreted as positive.

ABNORMAL VALUES
Positive fluorescence, indicated by an apple green or blue-green coloration of the hair, is suggestive of a dermatophyte infection. The only pathogen of veterinary importance that fluoresces is *Microsporum canis*, and not all strains of this dermatophyte will fluoresce.

INTERFERING FACTORS
Drugs That May Alter Results of the Procedure
• Shampoos, topical creams, or ointments can change or mask the fluorescence of affected hairs.
• Recently administered systemic tetracycline or doxycycline can cause hairs to fluoresce.

Conditions That May Interfere with Performing the Procedure
None

Procedure Techniques or Handling That May Alter Results
Failure to warm the Wood's lamp prior to use or illuminate the hair coat for a sufficient period may lead to false-negative results.

Influence of Signalment on Performing and Interpreting the Procedure
Species
Microsporum canis is a pathogen more commonly found on cats than dogs. The Wood's lamp is therefore a more reliable screening procedure in cats.

Breed
None

Age
None

Gender
None

Pregnancy
None

CLINICAL PERSPECTIVE

The Wood's lamp examination should be used as a screening tool only. When positive fluorescence is seen, the fluorescing hairs should be plucked for dermatophyte culture and trichogram examination. In cases where dermatophytosis is suspected but the Wood's lamp examination results are negative, a sample for culture should always be submitted.

 MISCELLANEOUS

ANCILLARY TESTS

- Dermatophyte culture
- Trichogram

SYNONYMS
None

SEE ALSO
Blackwell's Five-Minute Veterinary Consult: Canine and Feline Topics
Dermatophytosis
Related Topics in This Book
Skin Scraping and Trichogram

ABBREVIATIONS
None

Suggested Reading
Moriello KA. Diagnostic techniques for dermatophytosis. *Clin Tech Small Anim Pract* 2001; **16**: 219–224.
Moriello KA, Newbury S. Recommendations for the management and treatment of dermatophytosis in animal shelters. *Vet Clin North Am Small Anim Pract* 2006; **36**: 89–114.

INTERNET RESOURCES
None

AUTHOR NAME
Hilary A. Jackson

ZINC

 BASICS

TYPE OF SPECIMEN
Blood

TEST EXPLANATION AND RELATED PHYSIOLOGY
Zinc (Zn) is an essential dietary micromineral required for the function of numerous enzyme systems. Zn imbalances include deficiency, which may present in zinc-responsive dermatosis (ZRD), and toxicosis. Both forms of ZRD reported in dogs are treated by supplementation. Syndrome I occurs in Siberian huskies and related breeds fed diets containing adequate zinc. Syndrome II may occur in any breed because of a Zn-deficient diet and has been associated with generic dog food. Serum Zn concentrations may not be diagnostic for Zn-responsive dermatosis; thus, response to treatment and skin biopsy and histopathology may be necessary to rule out this disease.

Zinc is toxic in large doses, and toxicosis is usually caused by foreign body ingestion. U.S. pennies minted since 1982 and Canadian pennies minted between 1997 and 2002 are significant sources of Zn exposure. Other sources of exposure include galvanized metal knobs, screws, nails, nuts, washers, and other hardware; small toys like Monopoly pieces; topical Zn oxide ointments; Zn dust from industrial sites; and Zn supplements. Zn poisoning causes multiple organ system failure.

Zn is measured using graphite furnace atomic absorption spectrometry.

INDICATIONS
- Appropriate clinical signs of Zn-responsive dermatosis
  - Crusting and scaling of the muzzle, footpads, mucocutaneous junctions, and pressure points
- Suspect ingestion of a Zn-containing foreign body in these cases:
  - If the patient has a history of exposure
  - If coins or hardware are observed in the GI tract on radiographs
- Clinical signs
  - GI distress: anorexia, vomiting, diarrhea
  - Intravascular hemolysis and secondary icterus
  - Pancreatitis
  - Renal failure

CONTRAINDICATIONS
None

POTENTIAL COMPLICATIONS
None

CLIENT EDUCATION
- Serum Zn concentrations may be low or normal in dogs with ZRD.
  - Diagnosis of ZRD may be based on histopathology or response to treatment.
- Serum and plasma Zn concentrations are elevated in Zn toxicosis.

BODY SYSTEMS ASSESSED
- Dermatologic
- Gastrointestinal
- Hemic, lymphatic, and immune
- Hepatobiliary
- Renal and urologic

 SAMPLE

COLLECTION
- Use 1 mL of whole blood in a trace mineral collection tube.
- Avoid sample contact with rubber in a syringe since it may be contaminated with zinc.
- Avoid the use of hemolysed serum or plasma.

HANDLING
- Collection into trace-element collection tube (royal blue–capped tube) or zinc-free heparinized tube is preferred.
- If using a red-top tube, avoid sample contact with rubber stoppers, which may be contaminated with zinc.
- Centrifuge the sample promptly.
- Transfer the plasma or serum into a plastic vial or another trace-mineral tube.
- Ship the sample on ice to the laboratory.

STORAGE
Keep the sample refrigerated.

STABILITY
Zn is stable in serum or plasma.

PROTOCOL
None

 INTERPRETATION

NORMAL FINDINGS OR RANGE
- Dogs: 0.70–2.00 ppm
- Cats: 0.50–1.10 ppm
- Values may vary depending on the laboratory and assay.

ABNORMAL VALUES
- The serum Zn range in a study of dogs with ZRD was ≈0.23–0.66 ppm.
- Dogs may show clinical Zn toxicosis with serum Zn concentrations of ≥10.00 ppm.

CRITICAL VALUES
Animals with serum Zn concentrations of >10.00 ppm and clinical signs consistent with Zn toxicosis require therapy.

INTERFERING FACTORS
Drugs That May Alter Results or Interpretation
Drugs That Interfere with Test Methodology
None

Drugs That Alter Physiology
Chelation therapy may decrease serum Zn concentrations.

Disorders That May Alter Results
- Zn concentration may be increased by the following:
  - Hemolysis
  - Dehydration

Collection Techniques or Handling That May Alter Results
- Rubber test tube caps may be contaminated with Zn.
- Hemolysis may increase Zn.

Influence of Signalment
Species
- ZRD is reported more frequently in dogs.
- Zinc toxicosis is reported more frequently in dogs.

Breed
Dog breeds predisposed to ZRD syndrome II include Siberian huskies, Alaskan malamutes, and Samoyeds.

Age
- Serum Zn concentrations may be higher in neonates than adults.
- Dogs that are >7½ years of age may have decreased serum Zn.
- ZRD syndrome II usually occurs in dogs that are >1 year of age.

Gender
- Female dogs tend to have higher serum Zn concentrations than males.
- Signs of ZRD in females may resolve after ovariohysterectomy.

Pregnancy
Decreased serum Zn levels are reported in pregnant women.

LIMITATIONS OF THE TEST
- False positives may occur due to improper sample handling.
- Normal serum Zn levels do not rule out Zn-responsive dermatosis.

Sensitivity, Specificity, and Positive and Negative Predictive Values
N/A

Valid If Run in a Human Lab?
Yes.

Causes of Abnormal Findings

High values	Low values
New pennies	Dietary deficiency
Galvanized metal	Hepatopathies
Topical Zn oxide ointments	Hypothyroidism
Zn dust from industrial sites	Inflammation
Zn supplements	Stress

CLINICAL PERSPECTIVE
- ZRD is caused by dietary deficiency or breed predisposition.
- Adequate Zn levels do not rule out ZRD.
- Ingested Zn foreign bodies may be visible on radiographs.
- Oxidative damage to RBCs can result in Heinz body formation. Some dogs will have spherocytosis and be Coombs positive; this can be mistaken for immune-mediated hemolytic anemia.
- Clinical Zn toxicosis may affect multiple organs, including the GI tract, liver, kidneys, and pancreas.

MISCELLANEOUS

ANCILLARY TESTS
- Zn-responsive dermatosis
  - Hepatic and renal Zn analysis
  - Skin biopsy
- Zn toxicosis
  - Abdominal radiography
  - Evaluation of urea, creatinine, and urine specific gravity to look for acute renal failure
  - Hepatic and pancreatic enzymes
  - CBC and evaluation of RBC morphologic features
  - Coagulation panel
  - Hepatic and renal Zn analysis

SYNONYMS
None

SEE ALSO
Blackwell's Five-Minute Veterinary Consult: Canine and Feline Topics
- Anemia, Heinz Body
- Zinc Toxicity

Related Topics in This Book
Heinz Bodies

ABBREVIATIONS
- Zn = zinc
- ZRD = zinc-responsive dermatosis

Suggested Reading
Dziwenka MM, Coppock R. Zinc. In: Plumlee KH, ed. *Clinical Veterinary Toxicology*. St Louis: CV Mosby, 2003: 221–226.
Van Den Broek AHM. Diagnostic value of Zn concentrations in serum, leucocytes, and hair of dogs with zinc-responsive dermatosis. *Res Vet Sci* 1988; **44**: 41–44.
White SD, Bourdeau P, Rosychuk RA, *et al.* Zinc-responsive dermatosis in dogs: 41 cases and literature review. *Veterinary Dermatology* 2001; **12**: 101–109.

INTERNET RESOURCES
Beasley V. Nephrotoxic metals and inorganics. In: Beasley V, ed. Veterinary Toxicology, 1999, http://www.ivis.org/advances/Beasley/Cpt6B/ivis.pdf.

AUTHOR NAME
Karyn Bischoff

APPENDIX 1. TABLES OF LABORATORY NORMAL VALUES

The following reference intervals are used by the Cummings School of Veterinary Medicine (Tufts University, North Grafton, MA) and are provided as a general guideline. However, since results can significantly vary depending on methodology, type of instrumentation, and reagents used, it is strongly recommended that one use reference intervals specifically developed by the laboratory analyzing your patient samples.

Hematology reference intervals

Test	Units	Dogs	Cats
RBC count	$\times 10^6/\mu L$	5.8–8.5	6.8–10.0
Hemoglobin	g/dL	14.0–19.1	10.5–14.9
Packed cell volume (PCV)	%	39–55	31–46
Hematocrit (Hct)	%	40.0–56.0	31.0–49.0
MCV	fL	60.0–75.0	39.0–56.0
MCH	Pg	19.1–26.2	13.8–17.1
MCHC	g/dL	33.0–36.0	30.5–36.2
Red cell distribution width (RDW)		14.5–19.9	17.9–24.8
WBC count	$\times 10^3/\mu L$	4.9–16.9	4.5–15.7
Neutrophils	$\times 10^3/\mu L$	2.8–11.5	2.1–10.1
Bands	$\times 10^3/\mu L$	0.0–0.3	0.0–0.3
Lymphocytes	$\times 10^3/\mu L$	1.0–4.8	1.1–6.0
Monocytes	$\times 10^3/\mu L$	0.1–1.5	0.0–1.6
Eosinophils	$\times 10^3/\mu L$	0.1–1.25	0.0–1.9
Basophils	$\times 10^3/\mu L$	0.0–0.3	0.0–0.3
Platelets	$\times 10^3/\mu L$	181–525	183–643

Cell counts were determined by using a CellDyn 3700 (Abbott Laboratories, Abbott Park, IL), using Abbott reagents. Differential leukocyte counts were determined manually. Automated differential counts may vary, with a higher proportion of monocytes and few basophils.

Clinical chemistry reference intervals

Test	Canine	Feline	Common units	$\times$ Conversion factor = international units
Albumin	2.8–4.0	2.4–4.0	g/dL	$\times 10 = g/L$
Alkaline phosphatase	12–121	10–72	IU/L	
Alanine aminotransferase (ALT)	18–86	29–145	IU/L	
Ammonia	1–55	30–65	*mu*g/dL	$\times 0.587 = \mu mol/L$
Amylase	409–1203	496–1874	IU/L	
Aspartate aminotransferase (AST)	16–54	12–42	IU/L	
Bilirubin, total	0.1–0.3	0.1–0.3	mg/dL	$\times 17.1 = \mu mol/L$
Calcium, total	9.4–11.6	8.9–11.5	mg/dL	$\times 0.25 = mmol/L$
Chloride	106–116	110–125	mEq/L	$\times 1 = mmol/L$
Cholesterol	82–355	77–258	mg/dL	$\times 0.026 = mmol/L$
Creatine kinase	48–400	14–528	IU/L	
Creatinine	0.6–2.0	0.9–2.1	mg/dL	$\times 88.4 = \mu mol/L$
Gamma-glutamyltransferase (GGT)	2–10	0–5	IU/L	
Globulin, calculated	2.3–4.2	2.5–5.8	g/dL	$\times 10 = g/L$
Glucose	67–135	70–120	mg/dL	$\times 0.0555 = mmol/L$
Lipase[a]	53–770	17–179	IU/L	
Magnesium, total	1.8–2.6	2.0–2.7	mg/dL	$\times 0.411 = mmol/L$
Sodium/potassium (Na/K) ratio	29–40	28–43		
Phosphorus	2.6–7.2	3.0–6.3	mg/dL	$\times 0.323 = mmol/L$
Potassium	3.9–5.6	3.6–5.4	mEq/L	$\times 1 = mmol/l$
Sodium	143–154	149–162	mEq/L	$\times 1 = mmol/l$
Total CO_2 (bicarbonate)	15–28	13–22	mEq/L	$\times 1 = mmol/l$
Total protein	5.5–7.8	6.0–8.4	g/dL	$\times 10 = g/L$
Triglycerides	30–321	25–191	mg/dL	$\times 0.0113 = mmol/L$
Urea (BUN)	8–30	15–32	mg/dL	$\times 0.357 = mmol/L$
Venous blood gas[b]				
pH	7.36–7.44	7.36–7.44		
PCO_2	36–40	36–40	mmHg	
HCO_3^-	20–24	20–24	mEq/L	$\times 1 = mmol/L$
BE (base excess) = +/−4	−4 to +4	−4 to +4		
PO_2 (at sea level)	90–100	90–100	mmHg	

Unless indicated, values were obtained on a Hitachi 911 chemistry analyzer (Roche Diagnostics, Indianapolis, IN), using Roche reagents.
[a] Obtained using lipase reagent from Equal Diagnostics (Exton, PA).
[b] Values obtained using a Nova Critical Care Xpress (Nova Biomedical, Waltham, MA).

AUTHOR NAME
Joyce S. Knoll

Guidelines for drug monitoring are listed in the accompanying table. Veterinarians can use local hospitals and diagnostic laboratories that have the capability of performing drug analysis. Because of large individual variations in pharmacokinetics for the drugs listed, monitoring is advised for the following conditions: (1) in treating animals refractory to medication despite an adequate dose, (2) in treating animals showing toxicity despite an adequate dose, (3) in assessing owner compliance, (4) when switching medications (e.g., from a brand name to a generic) and the need to establish a baseline, (5) when checking for drug interactions (e.g., checking to determine whether interactions are occurring with cyclosporine administration), and (6) in examining individual patients for pharmacokinetic differences such as altered absorption or elimination.

THERAPEUTIC DRUG MONITORING: CONSIDERATIONS

TIMING OF SAMPLE

For drugs with a short half-life, more than 1 sample (3 samples are ideal) is the most useful for determining individual pharmacokinetic parameters. Alternatively, a peak (C_{MAX}) and a trough (C_{MIN}) can be collected to determine the bounds of high and low concentrations at steady state. For drugs with a long half-life (e.g., digoxin, bromide, phenobarbital), a single sample during the dosing interval is sufficient. If one suspects altered clearance rates, more samples can be collected to assess half-life, however. For cyclosporine, a single trough sample has been used for many years, but now recommendations are changing to a single 2-h sample (C_2). For cyclosporine a "trough" usually refers to a 12-h sample, even though this drug is used once a day, or once every other day in some patients.

ASSAY

The assay will vary by laboratory. Many automated chemistry machines used for biochemical analysis have drug-detection kits that can be added to their menus. Some laboratories use radioimmunoassay (RIA) methods, whereas others use other immunoassay methods (e.g., chemiluminescence). One of the popular benchtop assay machines is the fluorescence polarization immunoassay by Abbott Laboratories (Abbott Park, IL), known commonly as the TDx method. Rarely is high-performance liquid chromatography (HPLC) used because of the expense and slow turnaround time, but it is still considered the gold standard for specificity. This assay reports a true value, except for cyclosporine. For cyclosporine, the TDx assay overestimates the true value in dogs and cats. Therefore, in cats the TDx value should be multiplied by a factor of 0.5 to obtain the true value. For dogs, multiply the TDx value by 0.65 to obtain the true value.

TYPE OF SAMPLE

The type of sample will vary according to the specific assay. Most assays allow the use of serum, some require plasma, and for some assays either is acceptable. Samples should be collected and centrifuged as soon as possible. Avoid the use of serum-separator tubes because they may lower drug concentrations by adsorbing drug into the matrix. Some assays are specific about storage of samples. The use of plastic cryovial-type tubes are acceptable for most assays. For cyclosporine, the assay specifically calls for whole blood, not plasma, collected in an EDTA tube.

Examples of drugs that can be measured in most routine clinical or diagnostic laboratories are listed in the accompanying table.

Test	Specimen	Timing of sample	Tube	Storage	Effect of interference	Reference range
Amikacin	Serum or plasma, 0.5 mL	1, 2, and 4 h after the dose, preferably. Other strategies for collecting 2 or 3 samples also have been used to assess clearance.	Red top or lavender top	30 days at −20°C	Hemolysis: no effect Icterus: no effect Lipemia: no effect Cross reactivity: <1% interference with other drugs and antibiotics, except tobramycin, with which there is high cross-reactivity.	Peak. 40 µg/mL Trough, <0.8 mcg/ml Other methods to assess clearance are possible if >2 samples are collected.
Bromide (potassium or sodium bromide)	Serum, 0.5 mL	Anytime during the dosing interval	Red top	60 days at −20°C	No interference with other drugs Bromide and phenobarbital can be analyzed in same sample. Hemolysis: no effect Icterus: no effect Lipemia: no effect	100–200 mg/dL (with phenobarbital) 200–300 mg/dL (monotherapy)
Cyclosporine	Whole blood, 1.0 ml	Trough (12 h after the last dose). Alternatively, peak concentrations at 2 h have been used.	Lavender top	30 days at −20°C	Because of metabolites, the assay overestimates true cyclosporine concentrations by 1.5- to 2-fold. For a true level, correct the result by × 0.7 in dogs and ×0.5 in cats.	300–600 ng/mL at 12 h (may vary with disease)

Test	Specimen	Timing of sample	Tube	Storage	Effect of interference	Reference range
Digoxin	Serum, 0.5 mL	Anytime during dosing interval; generally 4–6 h after dosing.	Red top	7 days at 2°–8°C 2 months at −20°C	Hemolysis: no effect Bilirubin: No effect Lipemia: No effect Heparin tube: decrease by 5% EDTA tube: decrease by 7% Do not use serum-separator tubes.	0.8–2.5 ng/mL
Gentamicin	Serum or plasma, 0.5 mL	1, 2, and 4 h after the dose, preferably. Other strategies for collecting 2 or 3 samples also have been used to assess clearance.	Red top or lavender top	30 days at −20°C	Hemolysis, icterus, and lipemia produce a <5% error in the assay. Cross-reactivity: <1% interference with other drugs and antibiotics.	Peak, 20 µg/mL Trough, <0.27 µg/mL Other methods to assess clearance are possible if >2 samples are collected.
Phenobarbital	Serum or plasma, 0.5 mL	Anytime during the dosing interval	Red top or lavender top	2 days at 2°–8°C 1 month at −20°C	Bilirubin: no effect Hemolysis: no effect EDTA or heparin tube: no significant effect. Do not use serum-separator tubes.	15–40 µg/mL
Theophylline	Serum, 0.5 mL	Ideally, a peak and trough should be collected. If that is not possible, collect a trough immediately before the next dose.	Red top	30 days at −20°C	Hemolysis and icterus produce a < 5% error in the assay. Lipemia produces a <10% error. Cross-reactivity: <1% interference with other drugs, and 1.5% cross-reactivity with theobromine	10–20 µg/mL In some patients, trough concentrations of 5 µg/mL have been effective.
Vancomycin	Serum, 0.5 mL	Ideally, collect peak and trough sample. If it is not possible, collect a single trough sample prior to the next dose.	Red top	30 days at −20°C	Hemolysis, icterus, and lipemia produce a <5% error in the assay. Cross-reactivity: <1% interference with other drugs, and 1.5% cross-reactivity with theobromine	Peak, 30–40 µg/mL Trough, above 5 µg/mL

AUTHOR NAME

Mark Papich

APPENDIX 3. REFERRAL LABORATORIES

This appendix is divided into 2 sections. The first section includes a partial list of referral laboratories that offer a wide range of test options, along with contact information. The second section is divided into test categories and lists laboratories that offer certain types of specialized tests. The laboratories mentioned may offer tests in addition to those listed.

Laboratory name and address	*Laboratory name and address*

Full Service Laboratories

Antech Diagnostics
Suite 200
17672-A Cowarn Avenue
Irvine, CA 92714
Telephone: 800–745-4725
http://www.antechdiagnostics.com

Athens Diagnostic Laboratory College of Veterinary Medicine
University of Georgia
Athens, GA 30602
Telephone: 706–542–5568
Fax: 706–542-5977

Colorado State University
Veterinary Diagnostic Laboratory
300 West Drake
Fort Collins, CO 80523
Telephone: 970–297-1281
Fax: 970–297-0320
http://www.dlab.colostate.edu

IDEXX Laboratories, Inc.
One IDEXX Drive
Westbrook, Maine 04092
Telephone: 1–800-548–6733
Fax: 1–207-556–4346
http://www.idexx.com

Kansas State University College of Veterinary Medicine
Veterinary Diagnostic Laboratory
1800 Denison Avenue
Mosier Hall
Manhattan, KS 66506
Telephone: 785–532-5650
Fax: 785–532-4481
www.vet.ksu.edu

Michigan State University
Animal Health Diagnostics Laboratory
4125 Beaumont Road
Lansing, MI 48910–8104
Telephone: 517–353-1683
http://www.animalhealth.msu.edu

Oregon State University College of Veterinary Medicine
Veterinary Diagnostic Laboratory
30th & Washington Way
Magruder Hall, Room134
PO Box 429
Corvallis, OR 97339–0429
Telephone: 541–737-3261
Fax: 541–737-6817
http://oreganstate.edu/vetmed/vdl/vdl.htm

Arizona Veterinary Diagnostic Laboratory
2831 North Freeway
Tucson, AZ 85705
Telephone: 520–621-2356
http://www.microvet.arizona.edu

Auburn University College of Veterinary Medicine
Clinical Pathology
252-A Greene Hall
Auburn University, AL 36849
Telephone: 334–844-2653
http://www.vetmed.auburn.edu/index.pl/clinical_pathology

Cornell University College of Veterinary Medicine
Upper Tower Road
Ithaca, NY 14853
Telephone: 607–253-3900
Fax: 607–253-3943
http://diaglab.vet.cornell.edu/service/

Iowa State University College of Veterinary Medicine
Veterinary Diagnostic Laboratory
Ames, IA 50011
Telephone: 515–294-1950
http://www.vetmed.iastate.edu/departments/VDPAM/vdl.aspx

Louisiana Animal Disease Diagnostic Laboratory
1909 Skip Bertman Drive
Room 1519
Baton Rouge, LA 70803
Telephone: 225–578-9777
Fax: 225–578-9784
http://laddl.lsu.edu

Murray State University Veterinary Diagnostic & Research Center
PO Box 2000 North Drive
Hopkinsville, KY 42240
Telephone: 270–886-3959
http://breathitt.murraystate.edu/bvc

Texas Veterinary Medical Diagnostic Laboratory (TVMDL)
1 Sippel Road
College Station, TX 77843
Telephone: 979–845-3414 or 1–888-646–5623
Fax: 979–845-1794
http://tvmdl.tamu.edu

Laboratory name and address

Laboratory name and address

University of Illinois College of Veterinary Medicine
Veterinary Diagnostic Laboratory
1231 VMBSB
2001 South Lincoln
Urbana, IL 61802–6199
Telephone: 217–333-1620
http://vetmed.illinois.edu/vdl/

University of Tennessee
2407 River Drive
Room A105
VTH
Knoxville, TN 37996–4543
Telephone: 865–974-5638
Fax: 865–974-7147
http://www.vet.utk.edu/diagnostic/

University of Minnesota
Veterinary Diagnostic Laboratory
1333 Gortner Avenue
St. Paul, MN 55108
Telephone: 800–605-8787
Fax: 612–624-8707
http://www.vdl.umn.edu/vdl/ourservices/home.html

Washington State University
Washington Animal Disease Diagnostic Laboratory
7613 Pioneer Way East
Puyallup, WA 98371–4919
Telephone: 253–445-4537
Fax: 253–445-4544
http://www.vetmed.wsu.edu/depts–waddl

Specific Laboratory Testing

Allergy testing

Greer Veterinary
PO Box 800
639 Nuway Circle
Lenoir, NC 28645
Telephone: 877–777-1080
Fax: 877–777-1090
http://www.greerlabs.com/vet/vet.index.php

Heska Veterinary Diagnostic Laboratories
1613 Prospect Parkway
Fort Collins, CO 80525
Telephone: 888–437-5237
Fax: 970–484-8210
http://www.heska.com

Amino acid and taurine analysis

University of California–Davis
Amino Acid Analysis Laboratory
Department of Molecular Biosciences
School of Veterinary Medicine
1091 Haring Hall
Davis, CA 95616–8741
Telephone: 530–752-7578
Fax: 530–752-6253
http://www.vetmed.ucdavis.edu/vmb/aal/aal.html

Blood typing

Midwest Animal Blood Services
4983 Bird Drive
Stockbridge, MI 49285
Telephone: 877–517-6227
Fax: 517–851-7762
http://www.midwestabs.com

University of Pennsylvania
Section of Medical Genetics–PennGen
Transfusion Medicine Laboratory
Matthew J. Ryan Veterinary Hospital
Philadelphia, PA 19104–6010
Telephone: 215–898-3375 or 215–898-8894
Fax: 215–573-2162
http://www.vet.upenn.edu/penngen

APPENDIX 3. REFERRAL LABORATORIES

Laboratory name and address	*Laboratory name and address*

Endocrinology tests

Bet Labs
Suite 102
1501 Bull Lee Road
Lexington, KY 40511
Telephone: 859–273-3036
Fax: 859–273-0178
http://www.betlabs.com

University of Tennessee
Clinical Endocrinology Service
2407 River Drive
Room A105
VTH
Knoxville, TN 37996–4543
Telephone: 865–974-5638
Fax: 865–974-7147
http://www.vet.utk.edu/diagnostic/endocrinology

Michigan State University
Animal Health Diagnostics
Endocrine Diagnostic Laboratory DCPAH
Telephone: 517–353-0621
(See the related entry under full service laboratories for
additional contact information.)

Genetic testing

HealthGene
2175 Keele Street
Toronto, Ontario
M6M 3Z4 Canada
Telephone: 877–371–1551
http://www.healthgene.com

University of Pennsylvania
Section of Medical Genetics
Matthew J. Ryan Veterinary Hospital
Philadelphia, PA 19104–6010
Telephone: 215–898-3375 or 215–898-8894
Fax: 215–573-2162
http://www.vet.upenn.edu/penngen

Veterinary Genetics Laboratory University of California
Old Davis Road
Davis, CA 95616–8744
Telephone: 530–752-2211
Fax: 530–852-3556
http://www.vgl.ucdavis.edu

Wisdom Panel
(Mixed Breed Analysis)
Telephone: 1–888-K9.Pet.Test
http://www.Wisdompanel.com/vet

GI and pancreatic tests (TLI, PLI, B12, folate)

IDEXX Laboratories
(See the related entry under full service laboratories for contact
  information.)

Texas A&M University College of Veterinary Medicine
Gastrointestinal Laboratory
4474 TAMU–GI Lab
College Station, TX 77843–4474
Telephone: 979–862-2861
Fax: 979–862-2864
http://www.cvm.tamu.edu/gilab

Glycated hemoglobin

Louisiana Animal Disease Diagnostic Laboratory
(See the related entry under full service laboratories for contact
  information.)

Hemostasis tests

Cornell University
Comparative Hematology Section
Diagnostic Laboratory
College of Veterinary Medicine
(See the related entry under full service laboratories for contact
  information.)

Laboratory name and address | *Laboratory name and address*

Immunoassays (quantitative immunoglobulins, Coombs', etc.)

Kansas State University College of Veterinary Medicine
Clinical Immunology/Flow Cytometry Laboratory
Telephone: 785–532-4617
(See the related entry under full service laboratories for additional contact
    information.)

VMRD
Veterinary Medical Research & Development
PO Box 502
Pullman, WA 99163
Telephone: 509–334-5815 or 800–222-8673
Fax: 509–332-5356
http://www.vmrd.com/products/services/

Veterinary Animal Disease Diagnostic Laboratory
Clinical Immunology Laboratory
1243 Veterinary Pathobiology Building
Purdue University
West Lafayette, IN 47907
Telephone: 765–494-9676

Immunophenotyping

Colorado State University
Clinical Immunopathology
Veterinary Diagnostic Laboratory
(See the related entry under full service laboratories for contact information.)

IHC Services
1344 Highway 71
West Smithville, TX 78957
Telephone: 512–237–3730
Fax: 512–237-2133

Kansas State University
College of Veterinary Medicine
Clinical Immunology/Flow Cytometry Laboratory
Telephone: 785–532-4617
(See the related entry under full service laboratories for contact information.)

University of California–Davis
VMTH Pathology
Room 1025
Davis, CA 95616
Telephone: 530–752-3901

Molecular diagnostics (infectious disease PCR assays)

Athens Diagnostic Laboratory College of Veterinary Medicine
University of Georgia
(See the related entry under full service laboratories for contact information.)

Auburn University College of Veterinary Medicine
Molecular Diagnostics Laboratory
(See the related entry under full service laboratories for contact
    information.)

DyNAgenics Veterinary Diagnostics
PO Box 39079
12445 East 39th Avenue, Suite 201
Denver, CO 80239
Telephone: 303–576-6800
Fax: 303–307-8333
http://www.dynagenics.com

Lucy Whittier Molecular and Diagnostic Core Facility
University of California
Department of Medicine & Epidemiology
School of Veterinary Medicine
2108 Tupper Hall
Davis, CA 95616
Telephone: 530–742–7991
Fax: 530–754-6862
http://www.vetmed.ucdavis.edu/taqmanservice/diagnosics.html

Vector Borne Disease Diagnostic Laboratory
North Carolina State University
College of Veterinary Medicine
Room 462 A
4700 Hillsborough Street
Raleigh, NC 27606
Telephone: 919–513-6500
http://www.cvm.ncsu.edu/vth/ticklab.html

APPENDIX 3. REFERRAL LABORATORIES

| *Laboratory name and address* | *Laboratory name and address* |

Neuromuscular tests (2MM antibody, acetylcholine receptor antibody, etc.)

Comparative Neuromuscular Laboratory
9500 Gilman Drive
Basic Science Building, Room 2095
University of California, San Diego
La Jolla, CA 92093–0709
Telephone: 858–534-1537
Fax: 858–534-7319
http://vetneuromuscular.ucsd.edu/

California Animal Health & Food Safety Laboratory System
University of California–Davis
Thurman Laboratory
West Health Sciences Drive
Davis, CA 95616
Telephone: 530–752–8700
Fax: 530–752-6253

Michigan State University
Animal Health Diagnostics Laboratory
Toxicology Section
B619 W. Fee Hall
East Lansing, MI 48824–1316
Telephone: 517–355-0281

Washington State University
Washington Animal Disease Diagnostic Laboratory
(See the related entry under full service laboratories for contact information.)

Minnesota Urolith Center College of Veterinary Medicine
Department of Small Animal Clinical Sciences
University of Minnesota
St. Paul, MN 551108
Telephone: 612–625-4221
Fax: 612–624-0751
http://www.cvm.umn.edu/depts/minnesotaurolithcenter/home.html

Urolithiasis Laboratory
PO Box 25375
Houston, TX 77265–5375
Telephone: 800–235-4846
http://www.urolithiasis-lab.com

Toxicology

Cornell University College of Veterinary Medicine
Diagnostic Laboratory
(See the related entry under full service laboratories for contact information.)

Texas Veterinary Medical Diagnostic
1 Sippel Road
College Station, TX 77843
(See the related entry under full service laboratories for contact information.)

Urolith analysis

Urinary Stone Analysis Laboratory
Department of Medicine
School of Veterinary Medicine
University of California–Davis
Davis, CA 95616
http://www.vetmed.ucdavis.edu/vmth/small_animal/laboratory/default.

AUTHOR NAME
Joyce S. Knoll

INDEX

Text in **boldface** denotes chapter discussions.